Biochemistry and Molecular Biology Compendium

Biochemistry and Molecular Biology Compendium

Second Edition

Roger L. Lundblad

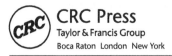

CRC Press
Taylor & Francis Group
Boca Raton London New York

CRC Press is an imprint of the
Taylor & Francis Group, an **informa** business

CRC Press
Taylor & Francis Group
6000 Broken Sound Parkway NW, Suite 300
Boca Raton, FL 33487-2742

First issued in paperback 2022

© 2020 by Taylor & Francis Group, LLC
CRC Press is an imprint of Taylor & Francis Group, an Informa business

No claim to original U.S. Government works

ISBN 13: 978-1-03-240105-8 (pbk)
ISBN 13: 978-1-138-05458-5 (hbk)
ISBN 13: 978-1-315-16662-9 (ebk)

DOI: 10.1201/b22194

Publisher's Note
The publisher has gone to great lengths to ensure the quality of this reprint but points out that some imperfections in the original copies may be apparent.

Visit the Taylor & Francis Web site at
http://www.taylorandfrancis.com

and the CRC Press Web site at
http://www.crcpress.com

This edition is dedicated to my daughters, Christy Smith and Cindy Maciariello, who will forever regret asking me how a firefly makes light.

Contents

Preface

As with first edition of the *Biochemistry and Molecular Biology Compendium,* this current work has been a learning process for me. Unlike other encyclopedic works where individual sections are written by experts, the current work has been written by a single individual best known as classical protein chemist (aka dinosaur) as opposed to someone skilled in proteomics. This has the advantage that the writer has no specific bias and needs to understand the various abbreviations and acronyms that have invaded article titles and abstracts with no explanation. The meaning of such abbreviations and acronyms is known, but frequently disputed, by the members of a specific group (Houck, J.C., Hinman, J.W., Glenn, E.M., Rebuck, J.W., and Forscher, B.K. Introduction, *Biochem. Pharmacol.* 17(Suppl. 1), v–vi, 1968; Chies, J.A.B. and Veit, T.D., Lost in a tsunami of references: the Babel tower strikes again, *Tissue Antigens,*75, 657, 2010); however, an individual outside of this group struggles to find an approved interpretation. Notwithstanding this issue, it is my hope that the information is useful. I feel a bit like the great Samuel Johnson in his compilation of "A dictionary of the English language in which the words are deduced from their originals and illustrated in their different significations by examples from the best writers" (8th edition, London, 1799). The preface describes a situation similar to mine in assembling content and ends with "The orthography and etymology, though imperfect, are not imperfect for lack of care, but care will not always be successful, and recollection or information come too late for use."

I wrote in the preface for the first edition about the importance of visiting libraries and not just relying on electronic access. There is much to be learned by consulting earlier works, such as those by John Edsall on the physical chemistry of amino acids and proteins.

Acknowledgements

The author acknowledges the support of the University of North Carolina at Chapel Hill Libraries and the advice of Professor Bryce Plapp at the University of Iowa in the preparation of this material. The author also acknowledges the support of Chuck Crumly of CRC Press for his support and guidance in this project and Jessica Vega of CRC Press for her endurance in the processing of text to book.

Author

Roger Lauren Lundblad is a native of San Francisco, California. He received his B.S. degree from Pacific Lutheran University and his Ph.D. degree in Biochemistry from the University of Washington. He spent two years as a research associate at the Rockefeller University in New York before joining the faculty of the University of North Carolina at Chapel Hill, rising to the rank of Professor of Pathology, Biochemistry, and Periodontics. He spent a decade at the Hyland Division of Baxter Healthcare before returning to Chapel Hill where he is a writer and consultant. He continues his relationship with the University of North Carolina at Chapel Hill as an Adjunct Professor of Pathology.

1 Abbreviations and Acronyms

2D-DIGE	two-dimensional difference gel electrophoresis
2DE	two-dimensional electrophoresis
A	absorbance
A1GP	α-1-glycoprotein
A23187	a calcium ionophore, Calcimycin
AAAA	Association Against Acronym Abuse
AAG box	an upstream *cis*-element
AAS	aminoalkylsilane; atomic absorption spectroscopy
AAT	amino acid transporter; alpha-1-antitrypsin
AAV	adenoassociated virus
ABA	abscisic acid, a plant hormone
ABC	ATP-binding cassette; antigen-binding cell
ABC-A1	ABC transporter A1
ABC-Transporter Proteins	ATP-binding cassette transporter proteins
ABE	acetone butanol ethanol
Abl	retroviral oncogene derived from Abelson murine leukemia
ABRC	ABA response complex
ABRE	ABA response element
7-ACA	7-aminocephalosporanic acid
ACES	2-[(2-amino-2-oxyethyl)amino]-ethanesulfonic acid
ACSF	artificial cerebrospinal fluid
ACS	active sequence collection; acute coronary syndrome
Ach (AcCho)	acetylcholine
AChR (AcChoR)	acetylcholine receptor
ACME	arginine catabolic mobile element
ACTH	adrenocorticotropin
ACN	acetonitrile
Acrylodan	6-acryloyl-2-(dimethylamino)-napthalene
AD	adverse event
ADA	adenosine deaminase; antidrug antibody
ADAM	a disintegrin and metalloproteinase
ADAMTS	a subfamily of disintegrin and metalloproteinase with thrombospondin motifs
ADCC	antibody-dependent cell-mediated cytotoxicity as in NK cells attacking antibody-coated cells
ADH	alcohol dehydrogenase; antidiuretic hormone
ADME	adsorption, distribution, metabolism, excretion
ADME/T	adsorption, distribution, metabolism, excretion/toxicology
AdoMet	*S*-adenosyl-l-methionine
ADR	adverse drug reaction
AE	adverse event
AEC	alveolar epithelial cell
AFLP	amplified fragment length polymorphism
AFM	atomic force microscopy
AGE	advanced glycation end products
AGO	argonaute protein family
AGP	acid glycoprotein
AID	activation-induced cytodine deaminase
AKAP	A-kinase anchoring proteins
Akt	a protein kinase
Akt	a retroviral oncogene derived from AKT8 murine T cell lymphoma
Alk	anaplastic lymphoma kinase; receptor member of insulin superfamily
ALL	acute lymphocytic leukemia
ALP	alkaline phosphatase
ALS	anti-lymphocyte serum
ALT	alanine aminotransferase
altORF	alternative open reading frame
ALV	avian leukosis virus
AML	acute myeloid leukemia
AMPK	AMP-activated protein kinase
AMS	accelerator mass spectrometry
AMT	accurate mass tag
AAA	abdominal aortic aneurysm; AAA+. ATPases associated with various cellular activities

ANDA	Abbreviated New Drug Application
ANOVA	analysis of variables (factorial analysis of variables)
ANS	1-anilino-8-napthlenesulfonate; autonomic nervous system
ANTH	AP180 N-terminal homology as in ANTH domain
2-AP	2-aminopyridine
6-APA	6-aminopenicillanic acid
APAF1	apoptotic protease activating factor 1
Apg1	a serine/threonine protein kinase required for vesicle formation which is essential for autophagy
API	active pharmaceutical ingredient
APL	acute promyelocytic leukemia
ApoB	apolipoprotein B
APPs	acute phase proteins
AQP	adenosine tetraphosphate
ARAP3	a dual Arf and Rho GTPase activating protein
ARD	acute respiratory disease; acireductone dioxygenase; automatic relevance determination; acid rock drainage
ARE	AU-rich elements
ARF	ADP-ribosylation factor
ARL	Arf-like
ARM	arginine-rich motif
ARS	automatic replicating sequence or autonomously replicating sequence
ART	mono-ADP-ribosyltransferase; family of proteins, large group of A-B toxins
AS	antisense
ASD	alternative splicing database; http://www.ebi.ac.uk/asd
ASPP	ankyrin-repeat, SH3-domain and proline-rich-region-containing proteins
AST	aspartate aminotransferase
ATAC	assay for transposable accessible chromatin
ATAC-seq	assay for transposable accessible chromatin with NGS
ATC	aspartate transcarbamylase domain
ATCase	aspartate transcarbamylase
ATP	adenosine-5′-triphosphate
ATD	arrival time distribution
ATPγ S	adenosine-5′-3-O-(thiotriphosphate)
ATR-FTIR	attenuated total reflectance-Fourier transform infrared

ATR-IR	attenuated total reflection infrared
ATS	automatic transfer switch
AVT	arginine vasotocin
Axl	anexceleko; used in reference to a receptor kinase related to the Tyro 3 family
BA	betaine aldehyde
BAC	bacterial artificial chromosome; also blood alcohol concentration
BAD	a member of the Bcl02 protein family considered to be a proapoptotic factor
BADH	betaine aldehyde dehydrogenase
BAEC	bovine aortic endothelial cells
BAEE	benzoyl-arginine ethyl ester
BALT	bronchial associated lymph tissue
BBB	blood–brain barrier
B-CAM	basal cell adhesion molecule
BCG	bacille-Calmette-Guérin
BCR	breakpoint cluster region; B-cell receptor
BCR-ABL	BCR-ABL is the fused gene that results from the *Philadelphia chromosome*; the BCR-ABL gene produces the *Bcr-Abl* tyrosine kinase
Bcl-2	protein family regulating apoptosis
BCIP	5-bromo, 4-chloro, 3-indoyl phosphate
BCS	biopharmaceutical classification system for describing the gastrointestinal absorption of drugs; also Budd-Chiari syndrome
BDH	d-β-butyrate dehydrogenase
BDNF	brain-derived growth factor
BEBO	an unsymmetrical cyanine dye for binding to the minor grove of DNA; 4-[(3-methyl-6-(6-methyl-benzothiazol-2-yl)-2,3,-dihydro(benzo-1,3-thiazole)-2-methylidene)]-1-methyl-pyridinium iodide
BET	refers to an isotherm for adsorption phenomena in chromatography; acronym derived from Stephen Brunauer, Paul Emmet, and Edward Teller
BEVS	Bacillus expression vector system
B/F	bound/free
bFGF	basic fibroblast growth factor
BFP	blue fluorescent protein
BFS	blow-finish-seal
BGE	background electrolyte

Bicine	*N, N*-bis(2-hydroxyethyl)glycine
BiFC	bimolecular fluorescence complementation
BIND	biomolecular interaction network database
BiP	immunoglobulin heavy chain-binding protein
***Bis*-TRIS**	2,2-bis-(hydroxymethyl)-2,2′,2″ nitriloethanol
BHK	baby hamster kidney
BLA	Biologic License Application
BLAST	basic local alignment search tool
BME	2-mercaptoethanol; β-mercaptoethanol
BMP	bone morphogenic protein
BopA	a secreted protein required for bio-film formation
BPTI	bovine pancreatic trypsin inhibitor
BCRA-1	breast cancer 1; a tumor suppressor gene associated with breast cancer
BRE-luc	a mouse embryonic stem cell line used to study bone morphogenetic protein
BRET	bioluminescence resonance energy transfer
BrdU	bromodeoxyuridine
Brig	polyoxyethylene lauryl ether
BSA	bovine serum albumin
BsAB	bispecific antibody
BTEX	benzene, toluene, ethylbenzene, and *o-/p*-xylene
BUN	blood urea nitrogen
bZIP	basic leucine zipper transcription factor
C1INH	C1 inhibitor; inhibitor of activated complement component 1, missing in hereditary angioneurotic edema
CA125	cancer antigen 125; a glycoprotein marker used for prognosis in ovarian cancer; also referred to as MUC16
CAD	multifunctional protein which is responsible for the *de novo* pyrimi-dine biosynthesis; caspases-activated DNAse; charged aerosol detection
CAK	Cdk-activating kinase
CALM	clathrin assembly lymphoid myeloid leukemia as in CALM gene
CAM (CaM)	calmodulin; cell adhesion molecule
CAMK	calmodulin kinase, isoforms I, II, III
CaMK	Ca^{2+}/calmodulin-dependent protein kinase

CAPA	corrective and protective action
CAPS	cleavable amplified polymorphic sequences; also cationic antimicrobial peptide
CAR	chimeric antigen receptor
CAR-T	chimeric antigen receptor T cell
CArG	a promoter element $[CC(A/T)_6G]$ gene for smooth muscle α-actin
CASP	critical assessment of structural prediction
CASPASE	cysteine-dependent aspartate-specific protease
CAT	catalase; chloramphenicol acetyl transferase
CATH	class, architecture, topology, homologous superfamily; hierarchical classification of protein domain structure; informal for catheter
CATP	chloramphenicol acetyltransferase
CBE	changes being effected
CBER	Center for Biologics Evaluation and Research
Cbl	a signal transducing protein downstream of a number of receptor-couple tyrosine kinases; a product of the *c-cbl* proto-oncogene
Cbs	chromosomal breakage sequence
CBz	carbobenzoxy
CCC	concordance correlation coefficient
CCD	charge-coupled device
CCK	choleocystokinin
CCS	rotationally average collision cross section
CCV	clathrin-coated vesicles
CD	clusters of differentiation; circular dichroism; cyclodextrin
CDC	complement-dependent cytotoxicity; complement-mediated cell death
CDK (cDK)	cyclin-dependent kinase
cDNA	complementary DNA
CDR	complementary determining region
CDTA	1,2-cyclohexylenedinitriloacetic acid
CE	capillary electrophoresis
CDS	coding sequence
CEC	capillary electrochromatography
CE-SDS	capillary electrophoresis in the presence of sodium dodecyl sulfate
CELISA	cellular enzyme-linked immunosorbent assay; enzyme-linked immunosorbent assay on live cells

CERT	ceramide transport protein	**CMC**	chemistry, manufacturing and controls; critical micelle concentration
CEPH	Centre d'Etude du Polymorphisme Humain	**CMCA**	competitive metal capture analysis
CEX	cation exchange	**CML**	chronic myelogenous leukemia
CFA	complete Freund's adjuvant	**CML**	carboxymethyl lysine
CFD	computational fluid dynamics	**CMO**	contract manufacturing organization
CFP	cyan fluorescent protein	**CNA**	bacterial cell wall collagen-binding
CFR	Code of Federal Regulations		protein
CFTR	cystic fibrosis transmembrane conductance region	**Cn**	calcineurin
Cfuc	colony forming unit	**CNC**	Cap'n'Collar family of basic leucine zipper proteins
CGE	capillary gel electrophoresis	**CNE**	conserved noncoding elements
CGH	comparative genome hybridization	**dCNE**	duplicated CNE
CGN	*cis*-Golgi network	**COACH**	comparison of alignments by constructing hidden Markov models
CH	calponin homology		
CHAPS	3-[(3-cholamidopropyl) dimethylammonio]-1-propane-sulfonic acid	**CoA**	coenzyme A
		COA(CofA)	Certificate of Analysis
		COFFEE	consistency based objective function for alignment evaluation
CHCA	α-cyano-4-hydroxycinnamic acid		
CHEF	chelation-enhanced fluorescence	**COFRADIC**	combined fractional diagonal chromatography
CHES	2-(*N*-cyclohexylamino)ethanesulfonic acid		
		COG	conserved oligomeric Golgi; cluster of orthologous groups
ChiP	chromatin immunoprecipitation		
ChiP-seq	ChiP followed by NGS DNA sequencing	**COPD**	chronic obstructive pulmonary disease
CHMP	Committee for Medicinal Products for Human Use	**COS**	cell line derived from African green monkeys
CHO	Chinese hamster ovary; carbohydrate	**Cot ½ DNA**	a method for measuring genome complexity by determining the time required for one-half of DNA in a sample to renature compared a standard sample (not currently in use as determined by literature search)
CIC	circulating immune complex		
CIC	Capicua transcriptional repressor gene		
CID	collision-induced dissociation; collision-induced dimerization		
CIDEP	chemically induced dynamic electron polarization	**COX**	cytochrome C oxidase
		Cp	ceruloplasmin
CIDNP	chemically induced dynamic nuclear polarization	**Cp and Cpk**	measures of process capability
		CPA	carboxypeptidase A
CIEEL	chemically initiated electron exchange luminescence	**CPB**	carboxypeptidase B
		CPD	cyclobutane pyrimidine dimer
CIP	clean in place	**CPDK**	calcium-dependent protein kinase
CLIP	class-II-associated invariant chain (Ii) peptide	**CpG**	cytosine-phosphate-guanine
		CpG-C	cytosine-phosphate-guanine class C
CLT	clotvinazole [1-(α2-chlorotrityl) imidazole]	**COG**	cluster of orthologous genes
		CPP	cell penetrating peptide; combinatorial protein pattern; critical process parameter
CLU	clusterin		
CLUSTALW	a general purpose program for structural alignment of proteins and nucleic acids; http://www.ebi.ac.uk/clustalw/		
		CPSase	carbamoyl-phosphate synthetase
		CPY	carboxypeptidase Y
		CQA	critical process attribute
cM	centimorgan	**CRAC**	calcium-release activated calcium (channels)
CM	carboxymethyl		

CRE	cyclic AMP response element	**DALI**	distance matrix alignment; http://www2.ebi.ac.uk/dali/
Cre1	cytokine response 1; a membrane kinase	**DANSYL**	5-dimethylaminonapthalene-1-sulfonyl; usually as the chloride (DANSYL chloride)
CREA	creatinine		
CREB	cAMP-response element binding protein	**DAP**	DNAX-activation protein; also diaminopimelic acid
CRISPR	clustered regularly interspaced single palindromic repeats	**DAP12**	DNAX activating protein of 12 kDa mass
CRM	certified reference material	**DAS**	distributed annotated system; downstream activation site
CRO	contract research organization		
CRP	C-reactive protein; cAMP receptor protein	**DAVID**	database for annotation, visualization and integrated discovery
CRY	chaperone	**DBMB**	Dulbecco's modified Eagle medium
CS	chondroitin sulfate		
CSF	colony stimulating factor; cerebral spinal fluid	**DBD-PyNCS**	4-(3-isocyanatopyrrolidin-1-yl)-7-(N,N-dimethylaminosulfonyl)-2-benzoxadiazole
CSP	cold-shock protein		
CSR	cluster-situated regulator; class-switch recombination	**DBS**	dried blood spot
		DBTC	"Stains All"; 4,5,4',5'-dibenzo-3,3'-diethyl-9-methylthiacarbocyanine bromide
CSSL	chromosome segment substitution lines		
Ct	chloroplast		
CT	charge transfer	**DC**	dendritic cell
CTB	cholera toxin B subunit	**DCC**	dicyclohexylcarbodiimide
CTD	C-terminal domain	**DCCD**	N,N'-dicyclohexylcarbodimide
CTL	cytotoxic T lymphocyte	**DD**	differential display
CTLA	cytotoxic T lymphocyte-associated antigen	**DDA**	data directed analysis
		DDBJ	DNA Databank of Japan; http://www.ddbj.nig.ac.jp
CTLL	cytotoxic T-cell lines		
CTPSase	CTP synthetase	**DDRs**	discoidin domain receptors (DDR1, DDR2)
CtrA	a master regulator of cell cycle progression		
		DDR1	discoidin domain receptor 1, CAK, CD167a, PTK3, Mck10
CV	coefficient of variation		
CV-1	cell line derived from African green monkey	**DDR2**	discoidin domain receptor 2, NTRK3, TKT, Tyro10
Cvt	cytosome to vacuole targeting	**DEAE**	diethylaminoethyl
CW	continuous wave (nonpulsed source of electromagnetic radiation)	**DEG**	differentially expressed gene(s)
		DEP	diethylpyrocarbonate (ethoxyformic anhydride)
CYP	cytochrome P450 enzyme		
Cst3	cystatin 3	**DEX**	dendritic-cell-derived exosomes
CZE	capillary zone electrophoresis	**DFF**	DNA fragmentation factor
D	diffusion	**DFP**	diisopropylphosphorylfluoridate (diisopropylfluorophosphate, isofluorophate)
D_{ax}	axial dispersion coefficient		
DAB(p-dab)	p-dimethyl amino azobenzene		
dABs	domain antibodies		
DABSYL	N,N-dimethylaminoazobenzene-4'-sulfonyl-usually as the chloride, DABSYL chloride	**DHFR**	dihydrofolate reductase
		DHO	dihydroorotase domain
		DHOase	dihydroorotase
		DHPLC (dHPLC)	denaturing HPLC
DAD	diaphanous-autoregulatory domain		
DAF	decay accelerating factor	**DHS**	DNAse I hypersensitivity site
DAG	diacyl glycerol	**DI**	deionized as in DI water (DIW)

DIP   database of interacting proteins—http://dip.doe-mbi.ucla. edu; also dictionary of interfaces in proteins—http://drug-redesign.de/superposition.html; also used to designate an enzyme inactivated by diisopropylphosphoryl fluoridate (DFP) such as DIP-trypsin

Dipso   3-[*N*,*N*-bis(2-hydroxyethyl)amino]-2-hydroxypropane sulfonic acid

DLS   dynamic light scattering

DM   an accessory protein located in the lysosome associated with MHC-class-II antigen presentation. It is located in the endosomal/lysosomal system of APC

DMBA   7,12-dimethylbenzo[α]anthracene

DMD   Duchenne muscular dystrophy; also Doctor of Dental Medicine

DMF   dimethylformamide; decayed, missing, filled (dentistry); drug master file

DMS   dimethyl sulfate; dried media spot

DMSO   dimethyl sulfoxide

DMT1   divalent metal transporter 1

ssDNA   single-stranded DNA

DNAa   a bacterial replication initiation factor

DNAX   DNAase III, tau and gamma subunits

dNPT   deoxynucleoside triphosphate

DNAse I deoxyribonuclease I

DO   an accessory protein located in the lysosome associated with MHC-class-II antigen presentation. DO has an accessory role to DM

DOAC   direct oral anticoagulants; also known as NOAC (new/novel oral anticoagulants)

DOE   design of experiments

DOI   digital object identifier

DOTA   tetraazacyclodedecanetetraacetic acid

DPE   downstream promoter element

DPI   dual polarization interferometry

DPM   disintegrations per minute

DPN   diphosphopyridine dinucleotide (currently NAD)

DPPC   dipalmitoylphosphatidylcholine

DPPE   1,2-dipalmitoyl-*sn*-glycerol-3-phosphoethanolamine

DPTA   diethylenetriaminepentaacetic acid

DQ   design qualification

dsDNA   double-stranded DNA

dsRNA   double-stranded RNA

dsRBD   double-stranded RNA binding domain

DRE   dehydration response element; dioxin response element

DRT   dimensionless retention time (a value for chromatography)

DSA   donor-specific anti-HLA antibodies

DSB   DNA double-strand break

DSC   differential scanning calorimetry

DSP   downstream processing

DTAF   dichlorotriazinyl aminofluorescein

DTE   dithioerythritol

DTNB   5,5′-dithio-bis(2-nitrobenzoic acid) Ellman's reagent

DTT   dithiothreitol

DUP   a duplicated yeast gene family

DVDF   polyvinyl difluoride

E1   ubiquitin-activating enzyme

E2   ubiquitin carrier protein

E3   ubiquitin-protein isopeptide ligase

E-64   *trans*-epoxysuccinyl-L-leucylamino-(4-guanidino)-butane, proteolytic enzyme inhibitor

EAA   excitatory amino acid

EBA   expanded bead adsorption

EBV   Epstein–Barr virus

EBPR   enhanced biological phosphate removal

EDC(EADC) 1-ethyl-3-(3-dimethylaminopropyl) carbodiimide *N*-ethyl-*N*′-(3-dimethyl-aminopropyl) carbodiimide

ECD   electron-capture detection

ECF   extracytoplasmic factor; extracellular fluid

ECM   extracellular matrix

EDC   1-ethyl-(3-dimethylaminopropyl)-carbodiimide

EDI   electrodeionization

EDTA   ethylenediaminetetraacetic acid, Versene, (ethylenedinitrilo) tetraacetic acid

EEO   electroendoosmosis

EEOF   electroendoosmotic flow

EF   electrofiltration

EFPIA   European Federation of Pharmaceutical Industries and Associations

EGF   epidermal growth factor

EGFR	epidermal growth factor receptor; Erb-1; HER1	**Ero1p**	a thiol oxidase which generates disulfide bonds inside in the endoplasmic reticulum
EGTA	ethyleneglycol-bis(β-aminoethylether)-N,N,N',N'-tetraacetic acid	**ERSE**	endoplasmic reticulum (ER) stress response element
eIF	eukaryotic initiation factor	**ES**	embryonic stem as in embryonic stem cell
EK	electrokinetic	**ESC**	embryonic stem cell
EKLF	erythroid Krüppel-like factor	**ESI**	electrospray ionization
ELSD	evaporative light scattering detection	**ESR**	electron spin resonance; erthyrocyte sedimentation rate
ELISA	enzyme-linked immunosorbent assay (enzyme-linked immunoassay)	**ESS**	exonic splicing silencer
EM	electron microscopy	**EST**	expressed sequence tag
EMA	European Medicines Agency (formerly EMEA)	**ETAAS**	electrothermal atomic absorption
		5,6-ETE	5,6-epoxyeicosatrienoic acid
EMBL	European Molecular Biology Laboratory	**ETD**	electron transfer dissociation
EMCV	encephalomyocarditis virus	**ETS**	family of transcription factors
EMF	electromotive force	**EUROFAN**	European functional analysis network—http:// mips.gsf.de/proj/ eurofan/; also European Programme for the Study and Prevention of Violence in Sport
EMMA	enhanced mismatch mutation analysis		
EMSA	electrophoretic mobility shift assay		
ENaC	epithelial Na channel		
EndoG	endonuclease G	**Exo1**	exonuclease 1
ENTH	epsin N-terminal homology as ENTH-domain	**EXP1**	expansion gene
		FAAH	fatty acid amide hydrolase
ENU	N-ethyl-N-nitrosourea	**Fab**	an antigen binding fragment from immunoglobulin; consists of a light chain and segment of the heavy chain amino-terminal to the hinge region linked by a disulfide bond; obtained from the papain digestion of IgG
EO	ethylene oxide		
EOF	electroosmotic flow		
EPC	endothelial progenitor cell		
Eph	a family of receptor tyrosine kinases; function as receptors/ligands for ephrins		
EPL	expressed protein ligation	**Fab'**	an antigen binding fragment from immunoglobulin; consists of a light chain and segment of the heavy chain containing the hinge region; linked by a disulfide bond and obtained by reduction of an $F(ab')_2$ obtained from the pepsin digestion of IgG. A dimeric derivative as compared to Fab or Fab'. contains two antigen binding sites
EPO	erythropoietin		
Epps	4-(2-hydroxyethyl)-1-piperazinepropanesulfonic acid		
EPR	electron paramagnetic resonance		
EPS	emergency power supply		
EPSS	emergency power supply system		
ER	endoplasmic reticulum		
ERAD	endoplasmic reticulum-associated protein degradation		
ErbB2	epidermal growth factor receptor, HER2	**FAB**	fast atom bombardment
		FAB-MS/MS	fast atom bombardment-mass spectrometry/mass spectrometry
ErbB3	epidermal growth factor receptor, HER3	**FACE**	fluorophore-assisted carbohydrate electrophoresis
ErbB4	epidermal growth factor receptor, HER4		
		FACS	fluorescence-activated cell sorting
ERK	extracellular-regulated kinase	**FADD**	Fas association death domain
Erk ∫	P 42/44 extracellular signal-regulated kinase	**FAD**	flavin adenine dinucleotide
		FAK	focal adhesion kinase

FAME	fatty acid methyl ester	**FTIR-ATR**	Fourier-transformed infrared
FAR	failure analysis report		reflection-attenuated total reflection
FBS	fetal bovine serum	**FLAG™**	an epitope "tag," which can be used
Fc	region of an immunoglobulin repre-		as a fusion partner for recombinant
	senting the C-terminal and contains		protein expression and purification
	various effector functions such as	**FlhB**	a component of the flagellum-
	activation of cells		specific export apparatus in bacteria
FcR	cell surface receptor for the Fc	**FLIP**	fluorescence loss in photobleaching
	domain of IgG; separate types are	**FLK-1**	receptor for vascular endothelial
	FcαR and FcγR		growth factor (VEGF)
FcRn	neonatal Fc receptor	**FLT-1**	receptor for vascular endothelial
FDA	fluorescein diacetate; Food and Drug		growth factor receptor
	Administration	**FMEA**	failure mode evaluation and analysis
FDA483	A form prepared at the end of an	**fMLP(FMLP)**	*N*-formyl methionine leucine
	FDA inspection, which contains		phenylalanine
	a list of observations that may	**fMOC**	9-fluorenzylmethyloxycarbonyl
	be violations of law. Since this	*Fms*	retroviral oncogene derived from SM
	information is accessible under the		feline sarcoma
	FOA act, it may also be used to	**FB**	fibronectin
	obtain competitive intelligence	**Fok1**	a type IIS restriction endonucle-
FDC	follicular dendritic cells		ase derived from *Flavobacterium*
FDP	fibrin/fibrinogen degradation		*okeanokoites*
	products	*Fos*	retroviral oncogene derived from
FCCP	carbonyl cyanide		FBJ murine osteosarcoma
	p-trifluoromethoxyphenyl-hydrazine	**FOX**	forkhead box
FD&C	Food Drug and Cosmetic Act	**FpA**	fibrinopeptide A
FEAU	2'-fluoro-2'-deoxy-β-D-	**FPC**	fingerprinted contigs
	arabinofuranosyl-5-ethyluracil	**FPLC**	fast protein liquid chromatography
FEN	flap endonuclease	**Fps**	retroviral oncogene from Fujiami
FERM	as in FERM-domain (four-point-one;		avian sarcoma
	ezrin, radixin, moesin)	**FRAP**	fluorescence recovery after
FFAT	two phenylalanyl residues in an		photobleaching
	acidic tract	**FRET**	fluorescence resonance energy trans-
FIAU	2'-fluoro-2'-deoxy-β-D-		fer; Förster resonance energy transfer
	arabinofuranosyl-5-iodouracil	**FSSP**	fold classification based on structure
FecA	ferric citrate transporter		alignment of proteins; http://www2.
FEN	flap endonuclease		ebi.ac.uk/dali/fssp/fssp.html
Fes	retroviral oncogene derived from ST	**FT**	Fourier transform
	and GA feline sarcoma	**FTE**	full-time equivalent
FFAP	free fatty acid phase	**FT-IR**	Fourier transform–infrared
FFPE	formalin-fixed, paraffin-embedded	**FU**	fluorescence unit
FGF	fibroblast growth factor	**5-Fu**	5-fluorouracil
FGFR	fibroblast growth factor receptor	**Fur**	ferric uptake receptor
Fgr	retroviral oncogene derived from GR	*Fur*	gene for Fur
	feline sarcoma	**FYVE**	a zinc-binding motif; acronym
FIBC	flexible intermediate bulk container		derived from four proteins
FIGE	field-inversion gel electrophoresis		containing this domain
FITC	fluoroscein isothiocyanate	**G**	guanine
FTIR	Fourier-transformed infrared	**Gα**	heterotrimeric G protein, α-subunit
	reflection	**Gβ**	heterotrimeric G protein, β-subunit

Gγ	heterotrimeric G protein, γ-subunit	GLC	gas–liquid chromatography
G-6-PD	glucose-6-phosphate dehydrogenase	GlcNac	N-acetylglucosamine
GABA	gamma (g)-aminobutyric acid	GLD	gelsolin-like domain
GAG	glycosaminoglycan	GLP	good laboratory practice(s)
Gal-3	galactan-3 as in galactin-3 protein	GLPC	gas–liquid phase chromatography
GalNac	N-acetylgalactosamine	GlpD	glyceraldehyde-3-phosphate dehydrogenase
GALT	gut-associated lymphoid tissues		
GALV	gibbon ape leukemia virus	GLUT	a protein family involves in the transport of hexoses into mammalian tissues
GAMP	good automated manufacturing product		
		Glut4	facilitative glucose transporter which is insulin-sensitive
GAPDH	glyceraldehyde 3-phosphate dehydrogenase		
		Glut5	a fructose transporter, catalyzes the uptake of fructose
GAPS	GTPase activating proteins		
GAS6	a protein, member of the vitamin K-dependent protein family	GM	genetically modified
		GM-CSF	granulocyte-macrophage colony stimulating factor
GASP	Genome Annotation Assessment Project; http://www. fruitfly.org/ GASP1/; also growth advantage in stationary phase		
		GMP	current good manufacturing practice
		cGMP	current good manufacturing practice
GBD	GTPase binding domain	GMP-PDE (cyclic GMP-PDE)	cyclic GMP-phosphodiesterase
GC	gas chromatography; granular compartment		
		GNSO	5-nitrosoglutathione
GC-MS	gas chromatography-mass spectroscopy	GPC	gel permeation chromatography
		GPCR	G-protein coupled receptor
GC-MSD	gas chromatography-mass selective detector	GPI	glycosyl phosphatidylinositol
		GPx	glutathione peroxidase
GcrA	a master regulator of cell cycle progression	GRAS	generally regarded as safe
		GRIP	a Golgi-targeting protein domain
G-CSF	granulocyte colony stimulating factor	GRP	glucose-regulated protein
		Grp78	a glucose regulated protein; identical with BiP
GCP	good clinical practice		
GDH	glutamate dehydrogenase	GSC	gas–solid chromatography; glioma stem cell; glioblastoma stem-like cell
GDNF	glial-derived neurotrophic factor		
GdnHCl	guanidine hydrochloride	GSH	glutathione
GDUFE	generic drug user fee amendments	GST	glutathione-S-transferase; gene trap sequencing tag
GEFs	guanine nucleotide exchange factors		
GF-AAS	graphite furnace atomic absorption spectroscopy	GTF	general transcription factor
		GTST(GST)	gene trap sequence tags
GFC	gel filtration chromatography	GTP (cGTP)	good tissue practice (current good tissue practice)
GFP	green fluorescent protein		
GGDEF	a protein family	GUS	beta-glucuronidase
GGT	gamma-glutamyl transferase	GVDH	graft-versus-host disease
GGTC	German Gene Trap Consortium; a reference library of gene trap sequence tags (GTST); http://www. genetrap.de/	GXP(s)	A generic acronym for good practices including but not limited to good clinical practice, good laboratory practice, good manufacturing processes
GHG	greenhouse gas		
GI	gastrointestinal; genomic islands	HA	hemagglutinin-A; hyaluronic acid; hydroxyapatite, $Ca_{10}(PO_4)_6(OH)_2$
cGK	cyclic GMP (cGMP)-dependent protein kinase		

HABA	[2-(4′-hydroxyazobenzene)] benzoic acid	**HMGR**	3-hydroxy-3-methylglutamyl-coenzyme A reductase
HACCP	hazard analysis, critical control point	**HMP**	herbal medicinal product(s)
HAPT	haptoglobin	**HMT**	histone
HAS	hyaluronan synthase	**hnRNA**	heterologous nuclear RNA
HAT	histone acetyltransferase; hypoxanthine, aminopterin and thymidine	**hpRNAi**	hairpin RNA interference
		HOG	high-osmolarity glycerol
HBSS	Hanks balanced salt solution	**HOPE**	Hepes-glutamic acid-buffer mediated organic solvent protein effect
H/D	hydrogen/deuterium exchange		
HAD	heteroduplex analysis	**HOX(_HOX, hox_)**	describing a family of transcription factors
HCP	host cell protein, refers to protein derived from the cell line used to expressed recombinant proteins	**HPAED-PAD**	high-performance anion-exchange chromatography-pulsed amperometric detection
HCIC	hydrophobic charge induction chromatography	**5-HPETE**	5-hydroperoxyeicosatetranenoic acid
HDAC	histone deacetylase	**HPRD**	human protein reference database
HDL	high-density lipoprotein	**HPRT**	hypoxanthine phosphoribosyl transferase
HDLA	human leukocyte differentiation antigen		
		HRP	horse radish peroxidase
HD-ZIP	homeodomain-leucine zipper proteins	**HRR**	homologous recombination repair
		HPLC	high-performance liquid chromatography (high-pressure liquid chromatography)
HEPT	height equivalent to plate number		
HeLa cells	a immortal cell line derived from human cervical cancer cells, acronym is from the patient's name, Henrietta Lacks	**uHPLC**	ultra-high-performance liquid chromatography
		HS	heparan sulfate
		HSA	human serum albumin
HEPA	high-efficiency particulate air as in HEPA-filtration	**HSB**	homologous synteny blocks
		HSC	hematopoietic stem cell
ERV	human endogenous retrovirus	**HSCQ**	heteronuclear single quantum correlation
HDPE	high-density polyethylene		
20-HETE	20-hydroxyeicosatetranenoic acid	**HSCT**	hematopoietic stem cell transplantation
HETP	plate height (chromatography)		
HexNac	_N_-acetylhexosamine	**HSE**	heat shock element
HP-LPME	hollow-fiber liquid-phase microextraction	**Hsp**	heat-shock protein
		Hsp70	heat shock protein 70
HGH	human growth hormone	**HS-SDME**	head space single-drop microextraction
HGP	human genome project		
HH	hereditary hemochromatosis	**HS-SPME**	head space solid-phase microextraction
HHM	hidden Markov models		
HIC	hydrophobic interaction chromatography	**5-HT**	5-hydroxytryptamine
		HTF	_Hpa_II tiny fragments; distinct fragments from the _Hpa_II digestion of DNA; _Hpa_II is a restriction endonuclease
HILIC	hydrophilic interaction liquid chromatography		
His-Tag (**His₆**; **H₆**)	histidine tag—a hexahistidine sequence		
		HTH	helix-turn-helix
HLA	human leukocyte associated antigen	**HTS**	high-throughput screening
		htSNP	haplotype single nucleotide polymorphism
HLA-DM	enzyme responsible for loading peptides onto MHC class II molecules		
		HUGO	human genome organization
HLA-DO	protein factor which modulates the action of HLA-DM	**HUVEC**	human umbilical vein endothelial cells

IAA	iodoacetic acid
IAEDANS	*N*-iodoacetyl-*N'*-(5-sulfo-1-napthyl) ethylenediamine
IBD	identical-by-descent; also inflammatory bowel disease
IC	ion chromatography
ICAM	intercellular adhesion molecule
ICAT	isotope-coded affinity tag
ICH	intracerebral hemorrhage; a gene related to *Ice* involved in programmed cell death; historically, international chick unit; International Conference for Harmonisation
ICPMS	inductively coupled plasma mass spectrometry
ID	internal diameter
IDA	interaction defective allele
IdeS	a protease from *Streptococcus pyogenes* which specifically cleaves IgG on the carboxyl side of the hinge region in a manner similar to pepsin
IDMS	isotope dilution mass spectrometry
IEC	ion-exchange chromatography
IEF	isoelectric focusing
IES	internal eliminated sequences
IFE	immunofixation electrophoresis
IFN	interferon
IEX	ion-exchange chromatography
Ig	immunoglobulin
IGF	insulin-like growth factor
IGFR	insulin-like growth factor receptor
Ihh	Indian hedgehog
I*k*B	NF-*k*B inhibitor
IIoT	industrial internet of things
I*k*K	I*k*B kinase
IL	interleukin, e.g. IL-2, interleukin-2; IL-6, interleukin-6
iLAP	integrated lysis and purification
ILGF	insulin-like growth factor
ILGFR	insulin-like growth factor receptor
ILK	integrin-linked kinase
IMAC	immobilized metal-affinity chromatography
IMINO	Na$^+$-dependent alanine-insensitive proline uptake system (SLC6A20)
IMMS	ion mobility mass spectrometry
IMP	integrin-mobilferrin pathway membrane protein system involves in the transport of ferric iron; also inosine-5′-monophosphate
IMS	ion mobility separation
IND	investigation new drug application
IoT	internet of things
IP$_3$	inositol 1,4,5-triphosphate
IPG	immobilized pH gradient
IPTG	isopropylthio-β-D-galactopyranoside
IQ	installation qualification
IR	inverted repeat; insulin receptor
IRB	institutional review board
IRES	internal ribosome entry site
IRS	insulin receptor substrate
ISE	ion-specific electrode
ISO	International Organization for Standardization
ISS	immunostimulatory sequence; also intronic splicing silencer
ISS-ODN	immunostimulatory sequence-oligodeoxynucleotide
ISSR	inter-simple sequence repeats
IT	isotocin
ITAF	IRES trans-acting factor
ITAM	immunoreceptor tyrosine-based activation motif
ITC	isothermal titration calorimetry
iTRAQ	isobaric tags for relative and absolute quantitation of proteins in proteomic research
JAK	Janus kinase
JNK	*c*-Jun *N*-terminal kinase
KARAP	killer cell activating receptor-associated protein
Kb, kb	kilobase
KDR	kinase insert domain-containing receptor; KDR is the human homolog of the mouse FLK-1 receptor. The KDR and FLK-1 receptors are also known as VEGFR2. See VEGFR
KEGG	Kyoto encyclopedia of genes and genomes
Kit	mast/stem cell growth factor receptor, CD 117
Kit	retroviral oncogene derived from HZ4 feline sarcoma
KLF5	Kruppel-like factor 5, a transcription factor
KRED	aldo/keto reductases
LAD	ladder logic; left anterior descending (artery)
LAK	lymphokine-activated killer cells
LAL	limulus amebocyte lysate (assay)

LATE-PCR	linear-after-the-exponential-PCR	**LOT**	the entire content of a production
LB	Luria–Bertani		batch of a therapeutic product
Lck	member of the Src family of protein		(drug or biologic)
	kinases	**LOQ**	limit of quantitation
LC$_{50}$	median lethal concentration in air	**LP**	lysophospholipid
LC/MS	liquid chromatography/mass	**LPA**	lysophosphatidic acid
	spectrometry	**LPH**	lipotropic hormone
LC/MS/MS	liquid chromatography/mass	**LPME**	liquid-phase microextraction
	spectrometry/mass spectrometry	**LPS**	lipopolysaccharide
LCR	low-copy repeat; locus control	**LR**	linear range
	region; low-complexity region	**LTB$_4$**	leukotriene B$_4$
LCST	lower critical solution temperature	**LTH**	luteotropic hormone
LD	as in LD motif, a leucine/aspartic	**Ltk**	leukocyte tyrosine kinase
	acid-rich protein-binding domain;	**LRP**	low-density lipoprotein receptor-
	also used to refer to peptidases		related protein
	without stereospecificity; also longin	**LSC**	liquid-solid chromatography
	domain; linkage disequilibrium;	**LSPR**	localized surface plasmon resonance
	lactate dehydrogenase	**LTR**	long terminal repeat
LD$_{50}$	median lethal dose	**LUCA**	last universal cellular ancestor
LDL	low-density lipoprotein	**Lys-C**	a protease with specificity for
LEAC	linear elution adsorption		cleavage at lysine carboxyl group
	chromatography	**LZ**	leucine/isoleucine zipper
LECE	ligand exchange capillary	**M13**	a bacteriophage used in phage
	electrophoresis		display
LED	light emitting diode	**MΦ**	macrophage
LLDPE	linear low-density polyethylene	**Mab**	monoclonal antibody
LDPE	low-density polyethylene	**MAC**	membrane attack complex
Lek	lymphocyte-specific protein tyrosine	**MAD** .	multiwavelength anomalous
	kinase		diffraction
LFA	lymphocyte function-associated	*Maf*	retroviral oncogene derived from
	antigen		AS42 avian sarcoma
LGIC	ligand-gated ion channel	**MAGE**	microarray and gene expression
LH	luteinizing hormone	**MALDI-TOF**	matrix-assisted laser desorption
LIF	laser-induced fluorescence		ionization time of flight mass
LIM	a domain involved in protein-protein		spectrometry
	interaction, originally described in	**MALLS**	multiangle laser light scattering
	transcription factors LIN1, ISL1, and	**MAP**	mitogen-activated protein; usually
	MED3		referring to a protein kinase such as
LIMS	laboratory information management		MAP-kinase
	systems	**MAPK**	MAP-kinase
LINE	long interspersed nuclear element	**MAPKK**	MAP-kinase kinase
LLC	liquid-liquid chromatography	**MAPKKK**	MAP-kinase kinase kinase
LLE	liquid-liquid extraction	**MAR**	matrix attachment region
LLOD	lower limit of detection	**MASE**	matrix-solid phase extraction
LLOQ	lower limit of quantification	**Mb, mb**	megabase (10^6)
LNA	locked nucleic acid	**MB**	molecular beacon
Lnr	initiator element	**MBL**	mannose-binding lectin
lncRNA	long, noncoding RNA	**MBP**	myelin basic protein; maltose-
lnRNP	large nuclear ribonucleoprotein		binding protein
LOD	limit of detection; log^{10} of odds	**MCA**	4-methylcoumaryl-7-acetyl
LOLA	list of lists—annotated	**MCAT**	mass coded abundance tag

MCD	magnetic circular dichroism
MCM	mini-chromosome maintenance
MCS	multiple cloning site
M-CSF	M-colony stimulating factor (macrophage-colony stimulating factor)
MDA	malondialdehyde
MDMA	3,4-methylenedioxymethamphetamine
MDCK	Madin-Darby canine kidney
MEF	mouse embryonic fibroblasts
MEF-2	myocyte enhancer factor 2
MEGA-8	octanoyl-*N*-methylglucamide
MEGA-10	decanoyl-*N*-methylglucamide
MEK	mitogen-activated protein kinase/ extracellular signal regulated kinase; also methylethyl ketone
MELC	microemulsion liquid chromatography
MELK	multi-epitope-ligand-kartographie
MEM	minimal essential medium
Mer	a receptor protein kinase; also Mertk, Mer tyrosine kinase
MES	2-(*N*-morpholinoethanesulfonic acid)
Met	receptor for hepatocyte growth factor
MFB	membrane fusion protein
MGO	methylglyoxal
MGUS	monoclonal gammopathy of undetermined significance
MHC	major histocompatibility complex
MIAME	minimum information about a microarray experiment
Mil	retroviral oncogene derived from Mill Hill-2 chicken carcinoma
MIP	molecularly imprinted polymer; macrophage inflammatory protein; methylation induced premeiotically
MIPS	Munich Information Center for Protein Sequences
miRNA	microRNA
MIS	Mullerian inhibiting substance
MLCK	myosin light chain kinase
MLCP	myosin light chain phosphatase
MMP	matrix metalloproteinase
MMR	mismatch repair
MMTV	mouse mammary tumor virus
MODR	method operable design region
MOPS	3-(*N*-morpholino)propanesulfonic acid; 4-morpholinopropanesulfonic acid
MOPSo	3-(*N*-morpholino)-2-hydroxypropanesulfonic acid

Mos	retroviral oncogene derived from Moloney murine sarcoma
MPD	2-methyl-2,4-pentanediol
MPSS	massively parallel signature sequencing
MQTT	message queuing telemetry transport
MR	magnetic resonance
MRI	magnetic resonance imaging
MRM	multiple reaction monitoring
mRNA	messenger RNA
miRNA	microRNA
MRP	migratory inhibitory factor-related protein
MRTF	myocardin-related transcription factor
MS	mass spectrometry, also mechanosensitive (receptors), multiple sclerosis
MS/MS	mass spectrometry/mass spectrometry
MS³	tandem mass spectrometry/mass spectrometry/mass spectrometry
MSDS	material safety data sheet(s)
MSP	macrophage stimulating protein
Mt	mitochondrial
mt-DNA	mitochondrial DNA
MTBE	methyl-*t*-butyl ether
MTOC	microtubule organizing center
mTOR	a eukaryotic regulatory of cell growth and proliferation; mechanistic target of rapamycin
MTSP	membrane type serine proteases
mTRAQ	MRM tags for relative and absolute quantitation
MTT	methylthiazoletetrazolium
MTX	methotrexate
MU	Miller units
Mu	mutator
MuRF (MURF)	muscle-specific RING finger proteins
MUSK	muscle skeletal receptor tyrosine kinase
MuDPiT	multidimensional protein identification technology
MuLV	Muloney leukemia virus
MWCO	molecular weight cut-off
My	million years
Myb	retroviral oncogene derived from avian myeloblastosis
Myc	retroviral oncogene derived from MC29 avian myelocytomatosis
MYPT	myosin phosphatase-targeting

Mys	myristoylation site	**NIRF**	near infrared fluorescence
NAA	neutron activation analysis	**NIST**	National Institute of Standards and
Nabs	neutralizing antibodies		Technology
nAChR	nicotinic acetylcholine receptor	**NK**	natural killer (as in cytotoxic T cell)
(nAcChoR)		**NKCF**	natural killer cytotoxic factor
NAD	nicotinamide adenine dinucleotide	**NKF**	*N*-formylkynurenine
	(DPN)	**NMDA**	*N*-methyl-D-aspartate
NADP	nicotinamide adenine dinucleotide	**NME**	new molecular entity
	phosphate (TPN)	**NMM**	nicotinamide mononucleotide
NAO	nonanimal origin	**NMR**	nuclear magnetic resonance
NASH	nonalcoholic steatohepatitis	**NO**	nitric oxide
NAT	nucleic acid amplification testing;	**NOE**	nuclear Overhauser effect
	nucleic acid testing	**NOESY**	nuclear Overhauser effect
Nbs$_2$	Ellman's reagent; 5,5′-dithiobis		spectroscopy
	(2-nitrobenzene acid)	**NOHA**	*N*^{w}-hydroxy-L-arginine
NBD	nucleotide-binding domain	**NORs**	specific chromosomal sites of
NBD-PyNCS	4-(3-isothiocyanato pyrrolidin-1-yl)-		nuclear reformulation
	7-nitro-2,1,3-benzoxadiazole	**NOS**	nitric oxide synthetase
NBE	new biological entity	**iNOS**	inducible oxide synthetase
NBS	*N*-bromosuccinimide	**NPC**	nuclear pore complex
NBT	nitroblue tetrazolium	*p***NPP**	*p*-nitrophenyl phosphate
NCBI	National Center for Biotechnology	**NSAID**	nonsteroid anti-inflammatory drug(s)
	Information	**NSF**	*N*-ethylmaleimide sensitive factor;
NCE	new chemical entity		National Science Foundation;
NCED	9-*cis*-epoxycarotenoid dioxygenase		*N*-ethylmaleimide-sensitive fusion
ncRNA	noncoding RNA	**Nt, nt**	nucleotide
NDA	New Drug Application	**NTA**	nitriloacetic acid
n-DAMO	nitrite-dependent anaerobic methane	**NTPDases**	nucleoside triphosphate diphospho-
	oxidation		hydrolases; also known as apyrases,
NDB	nucleic acid databank		E-ATPases
NDMA	*N*-methyl-D-aspartate	**NuSAP**	nucleolar spindle-associated protein
NDSB	3-(1-pyridinio)-1-propanesulfonate	**OCED**	Organization for Economic
	(nondetergent sulfobetaine)		Cooperation and Development
NEM	*N*-ethylmaleimide	**OCT**	optical coherence tomography
NEO	neopterin	**ODMR**	optically detected magnetic
NEP	nucleus-encoded polymerase		resonance
	(RNA polymerase)	**ODN**	oligodeoxynucleotide
NeuAc	*N*-acetylneuraminic acid	**OEM**	original equipment manufacturer
NeuGc	*N*-glycolylneuraminic acid	**OFAGE**	orthogonal-field-alternation gel
NF	National Formulary		electrophoresis
NFAT	nuclear factor of activated T cells, a	**OHQ**	8-hydroxyquinoline
	transcription factor	**OLED**	organic light emitting diode
NF-κB	nuclear factor kappa B, a nuclear	**OMG**	Object Management Group
	transcription factor	**OMIM**	Online Mendelian Inheritance in
NGF	nerve growth factor		Man (database) OMIM220100; avail-
NGFR	nerve growth factor receptor		able at http://www.ncbi.nlm.nih.gov
NGS	next generation sequencing	**OMP**	outer membrane protein; a protein
NHEJ	nonhomologous end-joining		family associated with membranes
NHS	*N*-hydroxysuccinimide	**OMT**	outer membrane transport
Ni-NTA	nickel-nitrilotriacetic acid	**OOS**	out of specification
NIR	near infrared	**OOT**	out-of-tolerance; out-of-trend

OPG	osteoprotegerin
OPV	organic photovoltaic as in organic photovoltaic cells
ORC	origin recognition complex
ORD	optical rotatory dispersion
ORF	open reading frame
ORFan	orphan open-reading frame
ORFeome	the protein-coding ORFs of an organism
uORF	upstream open reading frame
OSBP	oxysterol-binding proteins
OTCE	optically transparent carbon electrodes
OTFT	organic thin-film transistor
OTU	operation taxonomic unit
OVA	ovalbumin
OQ	operational qualification
OXPHOS	oxidative phosphorylation
OYE	old yellow enzyme
p53	a nuclear phosphoprotein which functions as a tumor suppressor
PA	peptide amphiphile
PAC	P1-derived artificial chromosome
PACAP	pituitary adenyl cyclase-activating polypeptide
PAD	peptidylarginine deiminase; protein arginine deiminase (EC 3.5.5.15)
PADGEM	platelet activator-dependent granule external membrane protein; GMP-140
PAGE	polyacrylamide gel electrophoresis
PAH	polycyclic aromatic hydrocarbon
PAK	P21-activated kinase
PAO	a redundant gene family (seri*pao*parin)
PAR	protease-activated receptor; proven acceptable range
PARP	poly(ADP-ribose) polymerase
PAS	preautophagosomal structure; periodic acid Schiff; preapproval supplement (prior approval supplement)
PAT	process analytical technology/process analytical technologies
PAT1	H$^+$-coupled amino acid transporter (slc36a1)
PAZ	a protein interaction domain; PIWI-argonaute-zwille
PBP	periplasmic binding protein
PBM	PDZ-binding protein
PBS	phosphate-buffered saline

PBST	phosphate-buffered saline with Tween-20
PC	polycystin; phosphatidyl choline
PCA	principal component analysis
PCAF	p300/CBP-associated factor, a histone acetyltransferase
PCB	polychlorinated biphenyl
PCNA	proliferating cell nuclear antigen; processing factor
PCOOH	phosphatidyl choline hydroperoxide
PCR	polymerase chain reaction
PDB	Protein Data Bank
PDE	phosphodiesterase
PDGF	platelet-derived growth factor
PDGFR	platelet-derived growth factor receptor
pDNA	plasmid DNA
PDI	protein disulfide isomerase
PDMA	polydimethylacrylamide
PDMS	polydimethylsiloxane
PDZ	as in PDZ domains; acronym derived from the first three proteins: postsynaptic density protein 95 (PSD-95), disks large (Dlg), and zona occludens 1 (ZO-1) proteins
PE	phycoerythrin; polyethylene
PEC	photoelectrochemistry
PECAM-1	platelet/endothelial cell adhesion molecule-1
PEEK	polyether ether ketone
PEF	polyethylene furanoate
PEG	poly(ethylene) glycol
PEI	polyethyleneimine
PEL	permissible exposure limit
PEND protein	a DNA-binding protein in the inner envelope membrane of the developing chloroplast
PEP	phosphoenol pyruvate
PEPCK-C	phosphoenolpyruvate carboxykinase, cytosolic form
PERK	double-stranded RNA-activated protein kinase-like ER kinase
PES	photoelectron spectroscopy
PET	positron emission tomography; polyethylene terephthalate
PEP	plastid-encoded polymerase (RNA polymerase)
Pfam	a protein family database; protein families database of alignments
PFE	pressure-fluid extraction
PFGE	pulsed-field gel electrophoresis

PFK	phosphofructokinase		**PNP**	p-nitrophenol (4-nitrophenol)
PFU	plaque forming unit		**POD**	peroxidase
PG	phosphatidyl glycerol; prostaglandin		**POET**	pooled ORF expression technology
3-PGA	3-phospho-D-glycerate		**POINT**	prediction of interactome database
PGO	phenylglyoxal		**Pol II**	RNA polymerase II
PGP-Me	archaetidylglycerol methyl phosphate		**POTRA**	polypeptide translocation associated
PGT box	an upstream *cis*-element		**PP**	polypropylene
PGx(PGX)	pharmacogenetics (PGx) is the use of genetic information to guide drug choice; prostaglandins (PGX) include thromboxanes and prostacyclins		**PPAR**	peroxisome proliferator activated receptor
			PPase	phosphoprotein phosphatase
			PQ	performance qualification
PH	pleckstrin homology		**PQL**	protein quantity loci
PHA	polyhydroxyalkanoates		**PS**	position shift polymorphism
PHD	plant homeodomain		**PS-DVB**	polystyrene-divinylbenzene
pHB(p-HB)	4-hydroxybenzoic acid (p-hydroxybenzoate)		**PSG**	pregnancy-specific glycoprotein(s)
			PS-1	presenilin-1
PhRMA	Pharmaceutical Research and Manufacturers Association		**PSI**	photosystem I
			psi	pounds per square inch
PI	propidium iodide		**PSI-BLAST**	position specific interactive BLAST; position-shift iterated BLAST (software program)
Pi	isoelectric point			
PIC	pre-initiation complex—complex of GTFs			
			PSII	photosystem II
PINCH	PINCH-protein; particularly interesting *cis*-his-rich protein		**PTB**	polypyrimidine-tract-binding protein; a repressive regulator of protein splicing; also pulmonary tuberculosis
PIP$_3$	phosphatidylinositol-3,4,5-triphosphate			
PIP$_n$	polyinositol polyphosphate		**PTC**	point to consider, plasma thromboplastin component (alternative name for blood coagulation factor IX, Christmas factor)
PIP$_n$S	polyinositol polyphosphates			
Pipes	1,4-piperzainediethanesulfonic acid			
PIRL*b*	paired immunoglobulin-like type 2 receptor *b*			
			PTD	protein transduction domain
PIWI	P-element induced wimpy testis		**PTEN**	phosphatase and tensin homolog deleted on chromosome 10
PKA	protein kinase A; cAMP-dependent kinase			
			PTFE	polytetrafluoroethylene
pKa	acid dissociation constant		**PTH**	phenylthiohydantoin
PKC	protein kinase C		**PTGS**	post-transcriptional gene silencing
PKG	cGMP-dependent protein kinase		**PTK**	protein-tyrosine kinase
Pkl	paxillin kinase linker		**PTM**	post-translational modification
PLA	polylactide		**PTPase**	protein tyrosine phosphatase
PLL	poly-L-lysine		**PUFAs**	polyunsaturated fatty acids
PLC	programmable logic controller		**PVA**	polyvinyl alcohol
PLOT	porous-layer open-tubular		**PVDF**	polyvinylidine difluoride
PLP	pyridoxal-5-phosphate		**QA**	quality assurance
PMA	phenyl mercuric acetate; phorbol-12-myristate-13 acetate		**QbD**	quality by design
			QC	quality control
PMCA	plasma membrane Ca^{2+} as PMCA-ATPase, a PMCA pump		**QMA**	quaternary methyl amine
			QP	qualified person (also responsible protein)
PMSF	phenylmethylsulfonyl fluoride			
PNA	peptide nucleic acid; p-nitroanilide		**QSAR**	quantitative structure–activity relationship(s)
PNGase	endoglycosidase			
PNGase-F	peptide N-glcyanase-F		**Q-TOF**	quadrupole time of flight

QTL	quantitative trait loci	**RGS**	regulator of G-protein signaling
QTPP	quality target product profile	**RHD**	Rel homology domain
R$_f$	retardation factor	**Rheb**	Ras homologue enriched in brain
RA	rheumatoid arthritis	**RhoA**	Ras homologous; signaling pathway
RAB-GAP	Rab-GTPase-activating protein	**RLD**	reference listed drug
RACE	rapid amplification of cDNA ends	**RI**	random integration
raf	retroviral oncogene derived from 3611 murine sarcoma	**RING**	really interesting new protein
		RIP	repeat-induced point mutation
RAGE	receptors for advanced glycation end products; receptors for AGE; recombinase-activated gene expression	**RIS**	radioimmunoscintigraphy
		RISC	RNA-induced silencing complex
		RIT	radioimmunotherapy
		RM	reference material
RAMP	receptor activity modifying protein	**RNA**	ribonucleic acid
RANK	receptor activator of NF-*k*B	**RNA-Seq**	RNA sequencing by NGS technology for analysis of transcriptome
RANK-L	receptor activator of NF-*k*B ligand		
Rap	a family of GTPase-coupled signal transduction factors which are part of the RAS superfamily	**RNAi**	RNA interference
		RNAse/RNAase	ribonuclease
		RNAse III	a family of ribonucleases (RNAses)
Rap1	a small GTPase involved in integrin activation and cell adhesion	**RNC**	ribosome-nascent chain complex
		snRNP	small nuclear ribonucleoprotein particle
RAPD	randomly amplified polymorphic DNA		
		RNS	reactive nitrogen species
RARE	RecA-assisted restriction endonuclease	**RO**	reverse osmosis
		ROCK (ROK)	Rho kinase
RAS	GTP-binding signal transducers	**ROESY**	rotating frame Overhauser effect spectroscopy
H-*ras*	retroviral oncogene derived from Harvey murine sarcoma		
		RON	receptor for macrophage stimulating protein
K-*ras*	retroviral oncogene derived from Kirsten murine sarcoma		
		ROS	reactive oxygen species
RC	recombinant cogenic	**RP**	reverse-phase; a nuclear serine/threonine protein kinase; responsible person (RP)
RCA	rolling circle amplification		
RCCX	RP-C4-CYP21-TNX module		
RCFP	reef coral fluorescent protein	**RP-CEC**	reverse-phase capillary electrochromatography
RCR	rolling circle replication		
RDP	receptor component protein	**RP-HPLC**	reverse-phase high-performance liquid chromatography
rDNA	ribosomal DNA		
REA	restriction enzyme analysis	**RPA**	replication protein A
Rel	avian reticuloendotheliosis	**RPEL**	a protein motif involved in the cytoskeleton
REMI	restriction enzyme-mediated integration		
		RPC	reverse-phase chromatography
REMS	risk evaluation and mitigation strategy	**RPMC**	reverse phase microcapillary liquid chromatography
RET	receptor for the GDNF family		
RF	a transcription factor, RFX family	**RPMI 1640**	growth media for eukaryotic cells
Rfactor	final crystallographic residual	**RPTP**	receptor protein-tyrosine kinase
RFID	radio frequency identification device	**RRM**	RNA-recognition motif
RFLP	restriction fragment length polymorphism	**rRNA**	ribosomal RNA
		RRS	Ras recruitment system; resonance Raleigh scattering
RFP	request for proposal(s)		
RGD	a signature peptide sequence-arginine-glycine-aspartic acid found in protein that bind integrins	**R, S**	designating optical activity of chiral compounds, where R is rectus (right) and S is sinester (left)

RSD	root square deviation; relative standard deviation
RT	reverse transcriptase; also room temperature
RTD	residence time distribution
RTK	receptor tyrosine kinase
RT-PCR	reverse transcriptase-polymerase chain reaction
RTX	repeat in toxins; pore-forming toxin of *E. coli* type (RTX toxin); also rituximab, resiniteratoxin, renal transplantation
Rub1	a ubiquitin-like protein, Nedd8
S1P	sphingosine-1-phosphate
S100	S100 protein family
SA	salicylic acid
SAGE	serial analysis of gene expression
SALIP	saposin-like proteins
SAM	self-assembling monolayers
SAMK	a plant MAP kinase
SAMPL	selective amplification of microsatellite polymorphic loci
Sap	saposin
SAP	sphingolipid activator protein; also serum amyloid P, shrimp alkaline phosphatase
SAR	scaffold associated region; structure-activity relationship
SATP	heterobifunctional crosslinker; *N*-succinimidyl-*S*-acetylthiopropionate
SAXS	small angle X-ray scattering
SCADA	supervisory control and data acquisition
scFv	single chain Fv fragment of an antibody
SCF	supercritical fluid
SCID	severe combined immunodeficiency
SCOP	structural classification of proteins; http://scop.mrc-lmb.cam.ac.uk/scop
SCOPE	structure-based combinatorial protein engineering
SDS	sodium dodecyl sulfate
SDS-PAGE	sodium dodecyl sulfate-polyacrylamide gel electrophoresis
SEC	secondary emission chamber for pulse radiolysis; size exclusion chromatography
Sec	secretory—usually related to protein translocation
SELDI	surface-enhanced laser desorption/ionization
SELEX	systematic evolution of ligands by exponential enrichment
SEM	scanning electron microscopy
SERCA	sarco/endoplasmic reticulum Ca^{2+} as in SERCA ATPase, a calcium pump
SEREX	serological identification of antigens by recombinant expression cloning
SERS	surface-enhanced Raman spectroscopy
SFC	supercritical fluid chromatography
SHAP	serum-derived hyaluron-associated protein
SH2	*Src* homology domain 2
SH3	*Src* homology domain 3
Shh	sonic hedgehog
shRNA	small hairpin RNA
SHO	yeast osmosensor
SIFT	selected ion flow tube mass spectrometry
SILAC	stable-isotope labeling with amino acids in cell culture
(p)SILAC	pulsed stable isotope labeling with amino acid in cell culture
SIMK	a plant MAP kinase
SINE	short interspersed nuclear element
SINS	sequenced insertion sites
SIP	steam-in-place
SIPK	salicylic-acid-induced protein kinase
siRNA	small, interfering RNA
SIRS	systemic inflammatory response syndrome
Sis	retroviral oncogene derived from simian sarcoma
SISDC	sequence-independent site-directed chimeragenesis
Ski	retroviral oncogene derived from avian SK77
Skp	a chaperone protein
S+/L-	an indicator cell line containing murine sarcoma virus (S+) but does not contain murine leukemia virus (L−) used to detect replication competent retroviruses such as murine leukemia retroviruses
SLAC	serial lectin affinity chromatography
SLE	systemic lupus erythematosus; supported liquid extraction
SLICE	seamless ligation cloning extract
SLN1	yeast osmosensor

S/MAR	scaffold and matrix attachment region	**SRCD**	synchrotron radiation circular dichroism
Smad	small mothers against decapentaplegic (proteins)	**SRP**	signal recognition particle
		SRF	serum response factor, a ubiquitous transcription factor
SMC	smooth muscle cell		
SNAP-tag	a modified form of the DNA repair enzyme, O^6-alkylguanine-DNA-alkyltransferase, which can execute a self-labeling reaction with O^6-benzylguanine derivatives	**SRM**	selected reaction monitoring
		SRPK	SR protein kinase
		SPR	structure-property relationship
		SRS	sequence retrieval system; SOS recruitment system
SNAREs	soluble N-ethylmaleimide-sensitive factor (NSF, N-ethylmaleimide-sensitive factor) protein attachment protein receptors; can be either R-SNAREs or Q-SNARES depending on sequence homologies	**SRWC**	short rotation woody crop
		SSA	serum amyloid protein
		SSC	saline sodium citrate
		ssDNA	single-stranded DNA
		SSLP	simple sequence length polymorphism
SNDA	supplemental new drug application	**SSR**	simple sequence repeats
SNM	SNARE motif	**ST**	structured text
SNP	single nucleotide polymorphism	**STAT**	signal transducers and activators of transcription
snRNA	small nuclear RNA		
snoRNA	small nucleolar RNA	**STC**	sequence-tagged connector
snRNP	small nuclear ribonucleoprotein particle	**STL**	stereolithography
		STM	sequence-tagged mutagenesis
SNV	single nucleotide variant	**STORM**	systematic tailored ORF-data retrieval and management; stochastic optical reconstruction microscopy
SOC	soil organic carbon; store-operated channel		
SOCS	suppressors of cytokine signaling	**STR**	short tandem repeats
SOD	superoxide dismutase	**STREX**	stress-axis related exon
SOD1s	CuZn-SOD enzyme (intracellular)	**STRING**	search tool for the retrieval of interacting genes/proteins
SOP	standard operating procedure		
sORF	short open reading frame	**stRNA**	small temporal RNA
SOS	response of a cell to DNA damage; salt overly sensitive (usually plants); son of Sevenless (signaling cascade protein)	**SUB**	single use bioreactor
		SUMO	small ubiquitin-like (UBL) modifier; small ubiquitin-related modifier; sentrin
SPA	scintillation proximity assay	**SUPAC**	scale-up and postapproval changes
SPC	statistical process control	**SurA**	a chaperone protein
SPE	solid-phase extraction	**SUS**	single use system
SPECT	sporozite mineneme protein essential for transversal; also single-photon emission computed tomography	**SV40**	simian virus 40
		SVS	seminal vesicle secretion
		$S_{w,20}$	sedimentation coefficient corrected to water at 20°C
SPIN	surface properties of protein–protein interfaces (database)		
		SWI/SNF	switch/sucrose-nonfermenting (a nucleosome remodeling complex)
SPP	signal peptide peptidase; superficial porous particles		
		TAC	transcription-competent artificial chromosome
SPR	surface plasmon resonance		
SQL	structured query language	**TACE**	tumor necrosis factor α-converting enzyme; also trans-catheter arterial chemoembolization
SR	as in the SR protein family (serine- and arginine-rich proteins); also sarcoplasmic reticulum; also scavenger receptor		
		TAFs	TBP-associated factors

TAFE	transversely alternating-field electrophoresis	**TI-VAMP**	tetanus neurotoxin-insensitive VAMP
TAFI	thrombin-activatable fibrinolysis inhibitor	**TLCK**	tosyl-lysyl chloromethyl ketone
TAG	triacyl glycerol	**TLR**	toll-like receptor
TAME	tosyl-arginine methyl ester	T_m	tubular membrane
TAP	tandem affinity purification; also transporter associated with antigen processing	**TM**	transmembrane
		TMAO	trimethylamine oxide
		TMD	*trans*-membrane domain
TAR	transformation-associated recombination; *trans*-activation response region	**TMS**	trimethylsilyl; thimersol
		TMV	tobacco mosaic virus
		TNA	treose nucleic acid
TAT	*trans*-activator of transcription	**TNB**	5-thio-2-nitrobenzoate
TATA	as in the TATA box, which is a TATA-rich region located upstream from the initiation RNA-synthesis initiation site in eukaryotes and within the promoter region for the gene in question. Analogous to the Pribnow box in prokaryotes	**TNBS**	trinitrobenzenesulfonic acid
		TnC	troponin C
		TNF	tumor necrosis factor
		TnI	troponin I
		TnT	troponin T
		TNF-α (TNFα)	tumor necrosis factor-α
		TNR	transferrin receptor
		TNX	tenascin-X
TBA-Cl	tetrabutylammonium chloride	**TPD**	temperature programmed desorption
TBP	TATA-binding protein; telomere-binding protein	**TOC**	total organic carbon
		TOCSY	total correlated spectroscopy
TCA	trichloroacetic acid; tricarboxylic acid	**TOF**	time of flight (in mass spectrometry)
		TOP	5′ tandem oligopyrimidine (terminal oligopyrimidine) tract
TCEP	tris (2-carboxyethyl)phosphine hydrochloride		
		TOPRIN	Topoisomerase and Primase in reference to a domain
TCR	T-cell receptor		
TE	therapeutic equivalence; transposable elements	**OR**	target of rapamycin; mTOR, mammalian target of rapamycin; dTOR, *Drosophila* target of rapamycin
TEA	triethylamine		
TEAA	triethylammonium acetate	**TORCOID**	TORC1 organized in inhibited domains
TEF	toxic equivalency factor		
TEM	transmission electron microscopy	**TOX**	toxicology
TEMED (TMPD)	*N,N,N′,N′*-tetramethylethylenediamine	**TPCK**	tosylphenylalanylchloromethyl ketone
		TPEN	*N′,N′*-tetrakis-(2-pyridyl-methyl) ethylenediamine
TEV	tobacco etch protease		
TF	tissue factor; transcription factor	**TPN**	triphosphopyridine dinucleotide (now NADP)
TFA	trifluoroacetic acid		
TFIIIA	transcription factor IIIA	**TRADD**	a scaffold protein
TGN	*trans*-Golgi network	**TRAIL**	tumor necrosis factor (TNF)-related apoptosis-inducing ligand
TGS	transcriptional gene silencing		
TH	thyroid hormone	**TRAP**	tagging and recovery of associated proteins as in RNA TRAP; also thrombin receptor activation peptide
THF	tetrahydrofuran		
TIGR	The Institute for Genomic Research		
TIM	translocase of inner mitochondrial membrane		
TIP	tonoplast intrinsic protein(s)	**TRE**	thyroid hormone response elements
TIR	toll/IL-1 receptor	**TRH**	thyrotropin-releasing hormone

TRI	as in TRI reagents such as TRIZOL™ reagents used for RNA purification from cells and tissues
TRIC	trimeric intracellular cation (channel)
Tricine	N-(2-hydroxy-1,1-bis(hydroxymethyl) ethyl) glycine
TRIF	TIR domain-containing adaptor-inducing interferon-β
Tris	tris-(hydroxymethyl)aminomethyl methane; 2-amino-2-hydroxymethyl-1,3-propanediol
bis-Tris	2-[bis(2-hydroxyethyl)amino]-2-(hydroxymethyl) propane-1,3-diol
Trk	neurotrophic tyrosine kinase receptor
TRL	time-resolved luminescence
TRP	transient receptor potential as in TRP-protein
TRs	thyroid receptors
Trx	thioredoxin
TSE	transmissible spongiform encephalopathy
TSP	thrombospondin; traveling salesman problem
TTSP	transmembrane type serine proteases
TUSC	Trait Utility System for Corn
Tween	polyoxyethylsorbitan monolaurate
TWIG	traveling wave ion guide
TX	thromboxane, also treatment
TyroBP	tyro protein tyrosine kinase binding protein, DNAX activation protein 12, DAP12, KARAP
UAS	upstream activation site
UBL	ubiquitin-like modifiers
UCDS	universal conditions direct sequencing
UDP	ubiquitin-domain proteins; uridine diphosphate
UDP-GlcNAc	uidine-5′-diphospho-N-acetylglucosamine
UNG	uracil DNA glycosylase
UPA	universal protein array; urokinase-like plasminogen activator
UPR	unfolded protein response
URL	uniform resource locator
URS	upstream repression site
USP	United States Pharmacopeia

USP-NF	United States Pharmacopeia–National Formulary
USPS	ubiquitin-based split protein sensor
UTR	untranslated region
VAMP	vesicle-associated membrane protein
VAP	VAMP-associated protein
VASP	vasodilator-stimulate phosphoprotein
VDAC	voltage-dependent anion-selective channel
VCAM	vascular cellular adhesion molecule
VDJ	variable diversity joining; regions of DNA joined in recombination during lymphocyte development; see VDJ recombination
VDR	vitamin D receptor
VEGF	vascular endothelial growth factor
VEGFR	vascular endothelial growth factor receptor
VGH	nonacronymial use; a neuronal peptide
V_H	variable heavy chain domain
VICKZ	a family of RNA-binding proteins recognizing specific *cis*-acting elements
VIGS	virus-induced gene silencing
VIP	vasoactive intestinal peptide
VLP	virus-like particle
VLDL	very-low-density lipoprotein
VNC (VNBC)	viable, but noncultivatable (bacteria)
VNTR	variable number tandem repeat; variable number of tandem repeats
VOC	volatile organic carbon
VPAC	VIP PACAP receptors
VSG	variable surface glycoproteins
VSP	vesicular sorting pathway
Vsp10	a type I transmembrane receptor responsible for delivery of protein to lysozyme/vacuole
vsp10	gene for Vsp10
WBOT	wide-bore open-tubular
WGA	whole-genome amplification
WFI	water for injection
WT, Wt	wild type
XBP	x-box binding protein
XO	xanthine oxidase
XPS	x-ray photoelectron spectroscopy
Y2H	yeast two-hybrid
YAC	yeast artificial chromosome
YCp	yeast centromere plasmid

YEp	yeast episomal plasmid
YFP	yellow fluorescent protein
Z	benzyloxycarbonyl
ZDF	Zucker diabetic factor
Zif	zinc finger domain peptides (i.e., Zif-1, Zif-3)
ZIP	leucine zipper
b-ZIP	basic leucine zipper
ZPA	zone of polarizing activity
ZZ Domain	a tandem repeat dimer of the immu-noglobulin-binding protein A from *Staphylococcus aureus*

It is recognized that there are likely some omissions in this list. Many journals (e.g. *Journal of Biological Chemistry*) have a list of abbreviations/acronyms that show which ones can be used in title and which are restricted to text. The works cited below discuss some of the issues with the use of acronyms.

Ali, H., and Ali-Mulla, F., Defining umbilical cord blood stem cells, *Stem Cell Discov.* 2, 15–23, 2012.

Anon., NUAP (No unnecessary acronyms please), *Nat. Methods* 8, 521, 2011.

Bettuzzi, S., Introduction: Clusterin, *Adv. Cancer Res.* 104, 1–8, 2009.

Charde, M., Shukla, A., Bukhariya, V., Mehta, J., and Chakole, R., A review on the significance of microwave-assisted techniques in green chemistry, *Int. J. Phytopharm.* 2, 39–50, 2012.

Dobson, G.P., Letson, H.L., Sharma, R., Sheppard, F.R., and Cap, A.P., Mechanisms of early trauma-induced coagulopathy: The clot thickens or not? *J. Trauma Acute Care Surg.* 79, 301–309, 2015.

Freire, C., Fernandes, D.M., Nunes, M., and Araujo, M., Poly-oxometalate-based modified electrodes for electrocataly-sis: From molecular sensing to renewable energy-related applications, in *Advanced Electrode Materials,* ed. A. Tiwani, F. Kuralay, and L. Uzun, pp. 147–212, John Wiley & Sons, Hoboken, NJ, 2017.

Jones, D.S.J., Pujado, P.R., and Treese, S.A., Dictionary of abbreviations, acronyms, expressions, and terms used in petroleum processing and refining, in *Handbook of Petroleum Processing*, ed. S.A. Tresse, P.R. Pujado, and D.S.J. Jones, Springer AG, Switzerland, 2015.

Linecker, M., Kron, P., Lang, H., de Santibañes, E., and Clavien, P.A. Too many languages in the ALPPS: Preventing another tower of Babel? *Ann. Surg.* 263, 837–838, 2016.

Murray, K.K., Boyd, R.K., Eberlin, M.N., et al., Definition of terms relating to mass spectrometry (IUPAC recom-mendations 2013), *Pure Appd. Chem.* 85, 1515–1609, 2013.

O'Conner, P.B., Dreiseward, K., Strupat, K., and Hillenkamp, F., MALDI mass spectrometry interpreted, in *MALDI MS*, ed. F. Hillenkamp and P. Katalinic, Wiley/Blackwell, Weinheim, Germany, 2014.

Pinh, N., and Kunej, T., Toward a taxonomy for multi-Omics science? Terminology development for whole genome study approaches by Omics technology and hierarchy, *OMICS* 21, 1–16, 2017.

Seah, M.P., Summary of ISO/TC 201 standard: ISO 18115-2:2013-surface chemical analysis—vocabulary—terms used in scanning probe microscopy, *Surf. Interface Anal.* 46, 361–364, 2013.

Seah, M.P., Summary of ISO/TC 201 standard—ISO 18115-1:2013-surface chemical analysis—vocabulary—general terms and terms used in spectroscopy, *Surf. Interface Anal.* 46, 357–360, 2013.

Stohner, J., and Quack, M., Conventions, symbols, quantities, units and constants for high-resolution molecular spectroscopy, in *Handbook of High-Resolution Spectroscopy*, ed. M. Quack and F. Merkl, Vol. 1, pp. 263–324, John Wiley & Sons, Hoboken, NJ, 2011.

2 Glossary of Terms Useful in Biochemistry and Biotechnology

ABBREVIATED NEW DRUG APPLICATION (ANDA)

An Abbreviated New Drug Application (ANDA)[1–3] is submitted to FDA for the review and ultimate approval of a generic drug product. A generic drug product is one that is comparable to an innovator drug product in dosage form, strength, route of administration, quality, performance characteristics and intended use. Generic drug applications are termed "abbreviated" because they are generally not required to include preclinical (animal) and clinical (human) data to establish safety and effectiveness. Instead, generic applicants must scientifically demonstrate that their product is bioequivalent (i.e. performs in the same manner as the innovator drug). The generic version must deliver the same amount of active ingredients into a patient's bloodstream in the same amount of time as the innovator drug.

1. Food and Drug Administration, HHS, Abbreviated New Drug Applications; https://www.fda.gov/Drugs/DevelopmentApprovalProcess/HowDrugsareDevelopedandApproved/ApprovalApplications/AbbreviatedNewDrugApplicationANDAGenerics/default.htm.
2. Food and Drug Administration, HHS, https://www.fda-help.us/abbreviated-new-drug-application.html.
3. Pramod, K., Tahir, M.A., Charoo, N.A., Ansari, S.H., and Ali, J., Pharmaceutical product development: A quality by design approach, *Int. J. Pharm. Investig.* 6, 129–138, 2016.

ABC TRANSPORTER

The ATP-binding cassette transporter (ABC transporter) family are complexes of membrane proteins responsible for the ATP-driven transport of a large variety of compounds across cell membranes.[1] ABC transporters are found in fungi, bacteria, plants, and animals.[2] ABC transporters can be divided into two general types, importer and exporters. Importers are found only in bacteria and plants[2] and can be divided into three types (I, II, III) on the basis of structure and function.[3,4] ABC exporters have a wider distribution than ABC importers and mediate the efflux of a variety of substances from cells[5,6] including drugs contributing to multi-drug resistance.[7] A defect in an ABC transporter is important in cystic fibrosis.[8]

1. Locher, K.P., Structure and mechanism of ABC transporters, *Curr. Opin. Struct. Biol.* 14, 426–431, 2004.
2. Rice, A.J., Park, A., and Pinkett, H.W., Diversity in ABC transporters: Type I, type II, and type III importers, *Crit. Rev. Biochem. Mol. Biol.* 49, 426–437, 2007.
3. Swier, L.J.Y.M., Slotboom, D-J., and Poolman, B., ABC importers, in *ABC Transporters—40 Years On*, ed. A.M. George, Cham Springer, Berlin, German, 2016.
4. Lewinson, O., and Livnat-Levanon, N., Mechanism of action of ABC importers: Conservation, divergence, and physiological adaptations, *J. Mol. Biol.* 429, 606–619, 2017.
5. Moeller, A., Lee, S.C., Tao, H., et al., Distinct conformational spectrum of homologous multidrug ABC transporters, *Structure* 23, 450–460, 2015.
6. Seeger, M.A., Bordignon, E., and Hohl, M., ABC exporters from a structural perspective, in *ABC Transporters—40 Years On*, ed. A.M. George, Cham Springer, Berlin, Germany, 2016.
7. Prasad, R., and Goffeau, A., Yeast ATP-binding cassette transporters conferring multidrug resistance, *Annu. Rev. Microbiol.* 66, 39–63, 2012.
8. Vauthier, V., Housset, C., and Faiguières, T., Targeted pharmacotherapies for defective ABC transporters, *Biochem. Pharmacol.* 136, 1–11, 2017.

ABLATION

Ablation is a multifunctional word derived from the Latin word *ablatus* (to carry away). In medicine, refers to the removal of tissue usually by a form of radiation.[1] Myoablative conditioning prior to hematopoietic stem cell transplantation results in the loss of a variety of cells and cell precursors, although considerable progress has been made in developing more selective approaches.[2] Immune ablation is the use of an antibody to deplete a specific cell population.[3] The term ablation has seen a broader use in medicine such as the removal of a class of biological compounds.[4] It can also refer to the reduction of particles into smaller sizes during erosion by other particles or the surrounding fluid[5] or as in aeronautic and aerospace technology to describe the dissipation of heat generated by atmospheric friction as, for example, in the reentry of a space vehicle.[6]

1. Saini, A., Hu, Y.L., Kasirajan, V., et al., Long term outcomes of minimally invasive surgical ablation for atrial fibrillation: A single center experience, *Heart Rhythm* 14, 1281–1288, 2017.
2. Buchmann, I., Meyer, R.G., Mier, W., and Haberkorn, U., Myeloablative radioimmunotherapy in conditioning prior to haematological stem cell transplantation: Closing the gap between benefit and toxicity? *Eur. J. Nucl. Med. Mol. Imaging* 36, 484–498, 2009.
3. Reiff, A., Shaham, B., Weinberg, K.I., Crooks, G.M., and Parkman, R., Anti-CD53 antibody-mediated immune ablation with autologous immune recovery for the treatment of refractory juvenile polymyositis, *J. Clin. Immuno.* 31, 615–622, 2011.
4. Velardi, E., Dudakov, J.A., and van den Brink, M.R., Sex steroid ablation: An immunoregenerative strategy for immunocompromised patients, *Bone Marrow Transplant* 50 (Suppl 2), S77–S81, 2015.
5. Lindner, H., Koch, J., Niema, K., Production of ultrafine particles by nanosecond laser sampling using orthogonal prepulse laser breakdown, *Anal. Chem.* 77, 7528–7533, 2005.
6. Duffa, *Ablative Thermal Protection Systems Modeling*, American Institute of Aeronautics and Astronautics, Reston, VA, 2013.

ABSCISIC ACID

Abscisic acid is a plant hormone.[1–4]

1. Leung, J., and Giraudet, J., Abscisic acid signal transduction, *Annu. Rev. Plant Physiol. Plant Mol. Biol.* 25, 199–221, 1998.
2. Finkelstein, R.R., Gampala, S.S., and Rock, C.D., Abscisic acid signaling in sees and seedlings, *Plant Cell* 14Suppl, S15–S45, 2002.
3. Bannerjee, A., and Roychoudhury, A., Abscissic-acid-dependent basic leucine zipper (bZIP) transcription factors in plant abiotic stress, *Protoplasma* 254, 3–16, 2017.
4. Yan, A., and Chen, Z., The pivotal role of abscisic acid signaling during transition from seed maturation to germination, *Plant Cell Rep.* 36, 689–703, 2017.

ABSORPTION

Absorption, in general, refers to the ability of one material to absorb another substance such the absorption of substances by skin[1,2] or to absorb energy or light such as in spectrophotometry.[3–5] Absorption is distinguished from adsorption, which refers more to an interaction of one substance with another such as physical interaction a material such as protein, with a surface.

1. Schmieder, S., Patel, P., and Krishnamurthy, K., Research techniques made simple: Drug delivery techniques, Part 1: Concepts in transepidermal penetration and absorption, *J. Invest. Dermatol.* 135, e38, 2015.
2. Li, J., Xu, W., Liang, Y., and Wang, H., The application of skin metabolomics in the context of transdermal drug delivery, *Pharmacol. Rep.* 69, 252–259, 2017.
3. Sommer, L., *Analytical Absorption Spectrophotometry in the Visible and Ultraviolet*, Elsevier, Amsterdam, the Netherlands, 1989.
4. Howell, J.A., and Hargis, L.G., Ultraviolet and light absorption spectrophotometry, *Anal. Chem.* 66, 445R–461R, 1994.
5. Stewart, K.K., and Ebel, R.E., *Chemical Measurements in Biological Systems*, Chapter 3, Ultraviolet and Visible Absorption Spectrophotometry and Photometry, pp. 39–63, Wiley-Interscience, New York, 2000. See adsorption.

ABSOLUTE OILS

See **essential oils**

ABZYMES

Abzymes are antibodies possessing catalytic activity similar to that of an enzyme.[1–4] The term catalytic antibody[5–7] is the more preferred term, although it was not possible to find a definitive statement from a recognized scholarly body. The term catalytic monoclonal antibody is also used as the abbreviation catmab.

1. Joron, L., Izadyar, L., Fribouet, A., et al., Antiidiotypic antibodies exhibiting an acetylcholinesterase abzyme activity, *Ann. N.Y. Acad. Sci.* 672, 216–223, 1992.
2. Friboulet, A., Izadyar, L., Avalle, B., Roseto, A., and Thomas, D., Abzyme generation using an anti-idiotype antibody as the "internal image" of an enzyme active site, *Appl. Biochem. Biotechnol.* 47, 229–237, 1994.
3. Nishi, Y., Enzyme/abzyme prodrug activation systems: Potential use in clinical oncology, *Curr. Pharm. Des.* 9, 2113–2130, 2003.
4. Pavlovic, M., Cavallo, M., Kats, A., et al., From Pauling's abzyme concept to the new era of hydrolytic anti-DNA autoantibodies: A link to rational vaccine design?—A review, *Int. J. Bioinform. Res.* 7, 220–238, 2011.
5. Hifumi, E., Matsumoto, S., Nakashima, H., et al., A novel method of preparing the monoform structure of catalytic antibody light chain, *FASEB J.* 30, 895–908. 2016.
6. Wenthur, C.J., Cai, X., Ellis, B.A., and Janda, K.D., Augmenting the efficacy of anti-cocaine catalytic antibodies through chimeric hapten design and combinatorial vaccination, *Bioorg. Med. Chem. Lett.* 27, 3666–3668, 2017.
7. Shahsavarian, M.A., Chaaya, N., Costa, N., et al., Multitarget selection of catalytic antibodies with β-lactamase activity using phage display, *FEBS J.* 284, 634–653, 2017.

ACCURACY

The difference between the measured value for an analyte and the true value.[1-3] Absolute error is the difference between the measured value and the true value while the relative error is that fraction that the absolute error is of the measured amount and is usually expressed as a percentage or at ppt/ppm. From the FDA, accuracy is the degree of closeness of the determined value to the nominal or known true value under prescribed conditions. This is sometimes termed trueness.[4]

1. *Handbook of Analytical Chemistry*, ed. L. Meites, McGraw-Hill, New York, 1963.
2. *Analytical Chemistry Handbook*, J.A. Dean, McGraw-Hill, New York, 1995.
3. *Dean's Analytical Chemistry Handbook,* McGraw-Hill, New York, 2005.
4. Food and Drug Administration, https://www.fda.gov/downloads/Drugs/Guidance/ucm070107.pdf.

ACTIVE PHARMACEUTICAL INGREDIENT

An active pharmaceutical ingredient (API) is any component of a final drug product that provides pharmacological activity or other direct effect in the diagnosis, cure, mitigation, treatment, or prevention of disease or to affect the structure on any function of the body of man or animals.[1-4] An API can be referred to as an active ingredient.

1. Food and Drug Administration, Guidance for Industry, Q7A Good Manufacturing Practice Guidance for Active Pharmaceutical Ingredients. https://www.fda.gov/ICECI/ComplianceManuals/CompliancePolicyGuidanceManual/ucm200364.htm.
2. Fujinuma, K., Ishii, Y., Yashihashi, Y., et al., Triboelectrification of active pharmaceutical ingredients: Weak acids and their salts, *Int. J. Pharm.* 493, 434–438, 2015.
3. Ticehurst, M.D., and Marziano, I., Integration of active pharmaceutical ingredient solid form selection and particle engineering into drug product design, *J. Pharm. Pharmacol.* 67, 782–802, 2015.
4. Caldwell, D.J., Mertens, B., Kappler, K., et al., A risk-based approach to managing active pharmaceutical ingredients in manufacturing effluent, *Environ. Toxicol. Chem.* 35, 813–822, 2016.

ACTIVITY-BASED PROTEOMICS

Activity-based proteomics is the identification of proteins in the proteome by the use of reagents that measure biological activity.[1-13] Frequently, the activity is measured by the incorporation of a "tag" into the active site of the enzyme. The earliest probes were derivatives of alkylflurophosphonates, which were well-understood inhibitors of serine proteases. The technical approach is related to enzyme histochemistry/histocytochemistry.

1. Berger, A.B., Willams, S.J., Hekmat, O., and Withers, S.G., Synthesis and testing of mechanism-based protein-profiling probes for retaining endo-glycosidases, *ChemBioChem* 7, 116–124, 2006.
2. Sieber, S.A., and Cravatt, B.F., Analytical platforms for activity-based protein profiling—Exploiting the versatility of chemistry for functional proteomics, *Chem. Commun.* 22, 2311–2318, 2006.
3. Schmidinger, H., Hermetter, A., and Birner-Gruenberger, R., Activity-based proteomics: Enzymatic activity profiling in complex proteomes, *Amino Acids* 30, 333–350, 2006.
4. Pan, Z., Jeffery, D.A., Chehade, K., et al., Development of activity-based probes for trypsin-family serine proteases, *Bioorg. Med. Chem. Lett.* 16, 2882–2885, 2006.
5. Gillet, L.C.J., Namoto, K., Ruchti, A., et al., In-cell selectivity profiling of serine protease inhibitors by activity-based proteomics, *Mol. Cell. Proteomics* 7, 1241–1253, 2008.
6. Serim, S., Haedke, U., and Verhelst, S.H.L., Activity-based probes for the study of proteases: Recent advances and developments, *ChemMedChem* 7, 1146–1159, 2012.
7. Stubbs, K.A., Activity-based proteomics probes for carbohydrate processing enzymes; current trends and future outlook, *Carbohydrate Res.* 390, 9–19, 2014.
8. Willems, L.I., Overkleeft, H.S., and van Kasteren, S.I., Current developments in activity based protein profiling, *Bioconjug. Chem.* 25, 1181–1191, 2014.
9. Sadler, N.C., and Wright, A.T., Activity-based protein profiling of microbes, *Curr. Opin. Chem. Biol.* 24, 139–144, 2015.
10. Yang, P., and Liu, K., Activity-based protein profiling: Recent advances in probe development and applications, *ChemBioChem* 16, 712–724, 2015.
11. Edgington-Mitchell, L.E., Barlow, N., Aurello, L., et al., Fluorescent diphenylphosphonate-based probes for detection of serine protease activity during inflammation, *Bioorg. Med. Chem. Lett.* 27, 254–260, 2017.
12. Roberts, A.M., Ward, C.C., and Nomura, D.K., Activity-based protein profiling for mapping and pharmacologically interrogating proteome-wide ligandable hotspots, *Curr. Opin. Biotechnol.* 43, 25–33, 2017.
13. Marques, A.R., Willems, L.I., Herrara Moro, D., et al., Specific activity-based probe to monitor family BH59 galactosylceramidase, the enzyme deficient in Krabbe disease, *ChemBioChem* 18, 402–412, 2017.

ACCURATE MASS TAG (AMT)

A peptide of sufficiently distinctive and accurate mass and elution time from liquid chromatography can be used a single identifier of a protein.[1-7]

1. Conrads, T.P., Anderson, G.A., Veenstra, T.D., et al., *Anal. Chem.* 72, 3349–3354, 2000.
2. Smith, R.D., Anderson, G.A., Lipton, M.S., et al., An accurate mass tag strategy for quantitative and high-throughput proteome measurements, *Proteomics* 2, 513–523, 2002.
3. Strittmatter, E.F., Ferguson, P.L., Tang, K., and Smith, R.D., Proteome analyses using accurate mass and elution time peptide tags with capillary LC time-of-flight mass spectrometry, *J. Am. Soc. Mass Spectrom.* 14, 980–991, 2003.
4. Shen, Y., Tolic, N., Masselon, C., et al., Nanoscale proteomics, *Anal. Bioanal. Chem.* 378, 1037–1045, 2004.
5. Zimmer, J.S., Monroe, M.E., Qian, W.J., and Smith, R.D., Advances in proteomics data analysis and display using an accurate mass and time tag approach, *Mass Spectrom. Rev.* 25, 450–482, 2006.
6. Izrael-Tomasevic, A., Phu, L., Phung, Q.T., Lill, J.R., and Arnott, D., Targeting interferon alpha subtypes in serum: A comparison of analytical approaches to the detection and quantitation of proteins in complex biological matrices, *J. Proteome Res.* 8, 3132–3140, 2009.
7. Brown, L.M., Quantitative shotgun proteomics with data independent acquisition and traveling wave ion mobility spectrometry: A versatile tool in the life sciences, *Adv. Exp. Med. Biol.* 806, 79–91, 2014.

ACTIVE SEQUENCE COLLECTION (ACS)

A collection of active protein sequences or protein fragments or subsequences, collected in the form of function-oriented databases.[1,2] There has been a related approach in the identification of substrate sequences for transglutaminase.[3] There have been no additions to the ACS database since 2005.

1. Fachiano, A.M., Facchiano, A., and Facchiano, F., Active sequence collection (ASC) database: A new tool to assign functions to protein sequences, *Nucl. Acids Res.* 31, 379–382, 2003.
2. http://bioinformatica.isa.cnr.it/ACS/.
3. Sugimrua, Y., Hosono, M., Kitamura, M., et al., Identification of preferred substrate sequences for transglutaminase 1—Development of a novel peptide that can efficiently detect cross-linking activity in the skin, *FEBS J.* 275, 5667–5677, 2008.

ACUTE-PHASE PROTEINS

Acute-phase proteins are proteins primarily of hepatic origin which are markedly elevated after challenge by infectious disease, inflammation or other challenges to homeostasis Notable acute-phase proteins include C-reactive protein, fibrinogen, α-1-antitrypsin, haptoglobin, serum amylase A, and α-1-acid glycoprotein.[1–3] It has been suggested that any protein increasing by 25% in concentration as a result of inflammation could be considered an acute-phase protein.[4] The production of acute-phase proteins in the liver is mediated by cytokines such as IL-1 and IL-6.[5,6] There is use of acute-phase proteins as biomarkers.[7–10] While the majority of acute-phase proteins are of hepatic origin, there are other tissue sources[11,12] including tumor cells.[13,14] The concentration of some protein such as albumin and transferrin decrease in the acute phase and are known as negative acute-phase proteins.[15] There are changes in the glycosylation patterns of acute-phase proteins.[16] See also **heat shock proteins**.

1. Mackiewicz, A., Kushner, I., and Baumann, A., *Acute Phase Proteins: Molecular Biology, Biochemistry, and Clinical Applications,* CRC Press, Boca Raton, FL, 1993.
2. Gabay, C., and Kushner, I., Acute-phase proteins and other systemic responses to inflammation, *New Engl. J. Med.* 330, 448–454, 1999.
3. Watterson, C., Lanevschi, A., Horner, J., and Louden, C., A comparative analysis of acute-phase proteins as inflammatory biomarkers in preclinical toxicology studies: Implications for preclinical to clinical translation, *Toxicol. Pathol.* 37, 28–33, 2009.
4. Kushner, I., The phenomenon of the acute phase response, *Ann. N.Y. Acad. Sci.* 389, 39–48, 1982.
5. Kampschmidt, R.F., Upchurch, H.F., and Pulliam, L.A., Characterization of a leukocyte-derived endogenous mediator responsible for increased plasma fibrinogen, *Ann. N.Y. Acad. Sci.* 389, 339–353, 1982.
6. Bode, J.G., Albrecht, U., Häussinger, D., Heinrich, P.C., and Schaper, F., Hepatic acute phase proteins–regulation by IL-6- and IL-1-type cytokines involving STAT3 and its crosstalk with NF-κB-dependent signaling, *Eur. J. Cell Biol.* 91, 496–505, 2012.
7. Armstrong, E.J., Morrow, D.A., and Sabatine, M.S., Inflammatory biomarkers in acute coronary syndromes: Part II: Acute-phase reactants and biomarkers of endothelial cell activation, *Circulation* 113, e152–e155, 2006.
8. Correale, M., Totaro, A., Abruzzese, S., Di Biase, M., and Brunetti, N.D., Acute phase proteins in acute coronary syndrome: An up-to-date, *Cardiovasc. Hematol. Agents. Med. Chem.* 10, 352–361, 2012.
9. Schrödl, W., Büchler, R., Wendler, S., et al., Acute phase proteins as promising biomarkers: Perspectives and limitations for human veterinary medicine, *Proteomics Clin. Appl.* 10, 1077–1092, 2016.
10. Piccardi, B., Giralt, D., Bustamante, A., et al., Blood markers of inflammation and endothelial dysfunction in cardioembolitc stroke: Systemic review and meta-analysis, *Biomarkers* 22, 200–209, 2017.
11. Sehgal, P.B., Interleukin-6: A regulator of plasma protein expression in hepatic and non-hepatic tissues, *Mol. Biol. Med.* 7, 117–130, 1990.

12. Steel, D.M., Donoghue, F.C., O'Neill, R.M., Uhlar, C.M., and Whitehead, A.S., Expression and regulation of constitutive and acute phase serum amyloid A mRNAs in hepatic and non-hepatic cell lines, *Scand. J. Immunol.* 44, 493–500, 1996.

13. Lee, S.Y., Lim, J.W., and Kim, Y.M., Effect of α1-acid glycoprotein expressed in cancer cells on malignant characteristics, *Mol. Cell.* 11, 341–345, 2001.

14. Malle, E., Sodin-Semrl, S., and Kovacevic, A., Serum amyloid A: An acute-phase protein involved in tumour pathogenesis, *Cell. Mol. Life. Sci.* 66, 9–26, 2009.

15. Ritchie, R.F., Palomaki, G.E., Neveus, L.M., and Navolotskaia, O., Reference distributions for the negative acute phase proteins, albumin, transferrin, and transthyretin: A large cohort to the world's literature, *J. Clin. Lab. Anal.* 13, 280–286, 1999.

16. McCarthy, C., Saldova, R., Wormald, M.R., et al., The role and importance of glycosylation of acute phase proteins with focus on alpha-1-antitrypsin in acute and chronic inflammatory conditions, *J. Proteome Res.* 13, 3131–3143, 2014.

A DISINTEGRIN AND METALLOPROTEINASE (ADAM)

A disintegrin and metalloproteinase (ADAM) protein family are characterized by the presence of a disintegrin domain and metalloproteinase domain, thus having the ability to bind to the cell surface integrins and degrade proteins.[1-4] ADAM proteins primarily function as membrane-bound proteases distinguishing from ADAMTS proteases, which are soluble. There are several members of the ADAM protease family that are soluble either from ectodomain cleavage or from secretion of the protein. ADAM proteases can be attached to a cell membrane with a transmembrane segment connected to a cytoplasmic tail. The ectodomain may contain an EGF-domain in addition to a cysteine-rich domain, a disintegrin domain, a metalloproteinase domain with an amino-terminal prodomain and signal peptide. Several of the ADAM protease family members are present in a soluble form (designated as s forms) as opposed to the membrane-bound form (designated as m forms).

1. White, J., Bridges, L., DeSimone, D., Tamczuk, M., and Wolfsberg, T., Introduction to the ADAM family, in *The ADAM Family of Proteases*, ed. N.M. Hooper and U. Lendeckel, Chapter 1, pp. 1–18, Springer, Dordrecht, the Netherlands, 2005.

2. *The ADAM Family of Proteases*, ed. N.M. Hooper and U.Lendeckal, Springer, Dordrecht, the Netherlands, 2006.

3. Wei, S., ADAM metalloproteinases, in *The Handbook of Proteolytic Enzymes*, ed. N.D. Rawlings and G.S. Salvesen, Chapter 248, pp. 1086–1194, Amsterdam, the Netherlands, 2013.

4. Pizzo, S.V., Lundblad, R.L., and Willis, M., *Proteolysis in the Interstitial Space*, Chapter 4, Proteolysis in the Interstitium, pp. 91–121, CRC Press/Taylor & Francis Group, Boca Raton, FL, 2016.

A DISINTEGRIN AND METALLOPROTEINASE WITH THROMBOSPONDIN (ADAMTS)

A disintegrin and metalloproteinase with thrombospondin (ADAMTS) proteinases are a group of multidomain metalloproteinases with a variety of biological activities distinct from the ADAM proteins.[1-3] There are 19 ADAMTS proteases (there is no ADAMTS11 as it was found to be identical with ADAMTS 5) and 7 secreted ADAMTS-like glycoproteins of undefined function. There are only limited studies on the activation of the zymogen forms of the ADAMTS proteases but it is likely that many are secreted as active enzymes with intracellular processing by furin-like enzymes, although further processing may occur after secretion. ADAMTS13 is involved in the processing of von Willebrand Factor may be the best-known member of this family.[4] Deficiency of plasma ADAMTS-13 activity results in a bleeding disorder known as thrombotic thrombocytopenic purpura.[5] Failure to process von Willebrand factor results in the presence of very-high-molecular-weight von Willebrand factor.[6]

1. Duball, J., and Apte, S.S., Insights on ADAMTS proteases and ADAMTS-like proteins from mammalian genetics, *Matrix Biol.* 44–46, 24–37, 2015.

2. Kelwick, R., Desanis, I., Wheeler, G.N., and Edwards, D.R., The ADAMTS (a disintegrin and metalloproteinase with thrombosponding motifs) family, *Genome Biol.* 16:113, 2015.

3. Takeda, S., ADAM and ADAMTS family proteins and snake venom metalloproteinases: A structural overview, *Toxins* (Basel) 8(5), E155, 2016.

4. Zheng, X.L., Structure-function and regulation of ADAMTS-13 protease, *J. Thromb. Haemost.* 11(Suppl 1), 11–23, 2013.

5. Zhou, Z., Nguyen, T.C., Guchhait, P., and Dong, J.F., Von Willebrand factor, ADAMTS-13, and thrombotic thrombocytopenic purpura, *Senin. Thromb. Hemost.* 36, 71–81, 2010.

6. Moake, J.L., von Willebrand factor, ADAMTS-13, and thrombotic thrombocytopenic purpura, *Semin. Hematol.* 41, 4–14, 2004.

ADAPTOR PROTEIN

An adaptor protein is a protein that does not have enzymatic activity but functions in combination with other proteins to exert an effect. Early examples include proteins with scr homology 2(SH2) and src homology 3 (SH3) domains.[1,2] Recently the term adaptor protein has been used for proteins involved in the development of clathrin-coated vesicles in the process of endocytosis.[3,4] The adaptor protein has been referred to as an **assembly protein**.[5,6] The term assembly protein has been used more frequently to describe proteins involved in the assembly of complexes such as ribonucleoproteins but are not part of the final product.[7]

1. Downward, J., The GRB2/Sem-5 adaptor protein, *FEBS Letters* 338, 113–117, 1994.
2. McCarty, J.H., The Nck SH2/SH3 adaptor protein: A regulator of multiple intracellular signal transduction events, *BioEssays* 20, 913–920, 1998.
3. Ahle, S., and Ungewickell, E., Identification of a clathrin binding subunit in the HA2 adaptor protein complex, *J. Biol. Chem.* 264, 20089–20093, 1989.
4. Yao, P.J., Zhang, P., Mattson, M.P., and Furukawa, K., Heterogeniety of endocytic proteins: Distribution of clathrin adaptor proteins in neurons and glia, *Neuroscience* 121, 25–37, 2003.
5. Keen, J.H., Chestnut, M.H., and Beck, K.A., The clathrin coat assembly polypeptide complex. Autophosphorylation and assembly activities, *J. Biol. Chem.* 262, 3864–3871, 1987.
6. Stavrou, I., and O'Halloran, T.J., The monomeric clathrin assembly protein, AP180, regulates contractile vacuole size in *Dictyostelium discoideum, Mol. Biol. Cell* 17, 5381–5389, 2006.
7. Singh, M., Wang, Z., Cascio, D., and Feigon, J., Structure and interactions of the CS domain of human H/ACA RNP assembly protein Shq1, *J. Mol. Biol.* 427, 807–823, 2015.

Arf FAMILY OF GTPases

The ADP-ribosylation family of GTP-binding proteins (Arf) are members of the RAS superfamily.[1] Members of the Arf family are small (20–30 kDa) proteins that bind GTP and have a role in the regulation of vesicular function via the regulation of vesicular traffic, microtubule dynamics, and other cellular processes.[2,3] The presence of a factor that enhanced the transfer of ADP ribose to an acceptor protein can be inferred from early studies on diphtheria toxin[4,5] and cholera toxin.[6] The Arf family is somewhat divergent and frequently includes the **Arf-like proteins**[7,8] and **Sar proteins**.[9] Arf proteins binding GTP in the active form has an allosteric effect on the target protein; hydrolysis of the GTP to GDP results in loss activity.[10,11] The hydrolysis of GTP on Arf proteins is regulated by **GTPase activating proteins** (GAP).[12]

1. Colicelli, J., Human RAS superfamily proteins and related GTPases, *Sci. STKE* 2004:RE13, 2004.
2. Goud, B., Small GTP-binding proteins as compartmental markers, *Semin. Cell Biol.* 3, 301–307, 1992.
3. Kahn, R.A., Yu, C., and Lee, F.J., Volpicelli-Daley, B., Boward, B., et al., Arf family GTPases: Roles in membrane traffic and microtubule dynamics, *Biochem. Soc. Trans.* 33, 1269–1272, 2005.
4. Collier, R.J., and Cole, H.A., Diphtheria toxin subunit active *in vitro, Science* 164, 1179–1181, 1969.
5. Goor, R.S., and Maxwell, E.S., The diphtheria toxin-dependent adenosine diphosphate ribosylation of rat liver aminoacyl transferase. II. General characteristics and mechanism of the reaction, *J. Biol. Chem.* 245, 616–623, 1970.
6. Welsh, C.F., Moss, J., and Vaughan, M., ADP-ribosylation factors: A family of ~20-kDa guanine nucleotide-binding proteins that activate cholera toxin, *Mol. Cell. Biochem.* 138, 157–166, 1994.
7. Burd, C.G., Strochlic, T.I., and Setty, S.R., Arf-like GTPases: No so Arf-like after all, *Trends Cell Biol.* 14, 1691–1699, 2004.
8. Yu, C.J., and Lee, F.J., Multiple activities of Arl1 GTPase in the *trans*-Golgi network, *J. Cell Sci.* 130, 1691–1699, 2017.
9. Li, Y., Kelly, W.G., Logsdon, J.M., Jr., et al., Functional genomic analysis of the ADP-ribosylation factor family of GTPases: Phylogeny among diverse eukaryotes and function in *C. elegans, The FASEB J.* 18, 1834–1850, 2017.
10. Szafter, E., Rotman, M., and Cassel, D., Regulation of GTP hydrolysis on ADP-ribosylation factor-1 at the Golgi membrane, *J. Biol. Chem.* 276, 47834–47839, 2001.
11. Chavier, P., and Ménétrey, J., Toward a structural understanding of Arf family: Effector spreading, *Structure* 18, 1552–1558, 2001.
12. Inoue, H., and Randazzo, P.A., Arf GAPs and their interacting partners, *Traffic* 8, 1465–1475, 2007.

ADJUVANT

A substance that increases an immune response. It is frequently a component of the excipients in the formulation of vaccine.[1-8]

1. Brown, L.E., and Jackson, D.C., Lipid-based self-adjuvating vaccines, *Curr. Drug Deliv.* 2, 283–393, 2005.
2. Gluck, R., Burri, K.G., and Metcalfe, I., Adjuvant and antigen delivery properties of virosomes, *Curr. Drug Deliv.* 2, 395–400, 2005.
3. *Topics in Vaccine Adjuvant Research*, ed. D.R. Spriggs and W.C. Koff, CRC Press, Boca Raton, FL, 1991.
4. *Vaccine Design: The Subunit and Adjuvant Approach*, ed. M.F. Powell, Plenum Press, New York, 1995.
5. *Therapeutic Proteins: Methods and Protocols*, ed. M.C. Smales and D.C. James, Humana Press, Totowa, NJ, 2005.
6. *Immunopotentiation in Modern Vaccines,* ed. V.E.J.C. Schijns and D.T. O'Hagan, Elsevier, Amsterdam, the Netherlands, 2006.

7. Chauhan, N., Tiwari, S., Type, T., and Jain, U., An over-view of adjuvants utilized in prophylactic vaccine formulation as immunomodulators, *Expert Rev. Vaccines* 16, 491–502, 2017.
8. Moreno-Mendieta, S., Guillén, D., Hernández-Pando, R., Sánchez, S., and Rodríguez-Sanoja, R., Potential of glucan as vaccine adjuvants: A review of the α-glucans case, *Carbohydrate Polym.* 165, 103–114, 2017.

ADSORPTION

The transfer of a substance from one medium to another such as the adsorption of a substance from a fluid onto (but into) a surface. The **adsorbent** is the substrate onto which a material is adsorbed. The **adsorbate** is the material adsorbed onto a matrix. Adsorption is usually considered to be a passive process resulting from the interaction between a solute such as a protein and a surface contrasted with immobilization which can be considered to be an active process with the formation of a covalent bond between a solute such as a protein and a surface.[1] Adsorption of proteins to surfaces is of importance in blood-implanted device interactions.[2] While adsorption is a passive process, there can be specificity provided by the nature of the surface and quality of the protein. Competitive adsorption provides insight into the specificity of the adsorption process.[3–5] The binding of proteins to surfaces can result in conformational change.[6] The adsorption of a protein to a surface can also result in the irreversible denaturation of the protein.[7]

1. Pivatal, J., Pereira, F.M., Barbosa, A.I., et al., Covalent immobilisation of antibodies in Teflon-FEB microfluidic devices for the sensitive quantification of clinically relevant protein biomarkers, *Analyst* 142, 959–968, 2017.
2. Vogler, E.A., Protein adsorption in three dimensions, *Biomaterials* 33, 1201–1037, 2012.
3. Lassen, B., and Malmsten, M., Competitive protein adsorption at plasma polymer surfaces, *J. Colloid Interface Sci.* 186, 9–16, 1997.
4. Holmberg, M., and Hou, X., Competitive protein adsorption—Multilayer adsorption and surface-induced protein aggregation, *Langmuir* 25, 2081–2089, 2009.
5. Song, S., Xie, T., Ravensbergen, K., and Hahm, J.L., Ascertaining effects of nanoscale polymeric interfaces on competitive protein adsorption at the individual protein level, *Nanoscale* 8, 3496–3509, 2016.
6. Zamarron, C., Ginsberg, M.H., and Plow, E.F., Monoclonal antibodies specific for a conformationally altered state of fibrinogen, *Thromb. Haemost.* 64, 41–46, 1990.
7. Edwards, R.A., and Huber, R.E., Surface denaturation of proteins: The thermal inactivation of β-galactosidase (*Escherichia coli*) on wall-liquid surfaces, *Biochem. Cell Biol.* 70, 63–69, 1992.

ADVANCED GLYCATION END PRODUCTS (AGE)

A heterogeneous group of products resulting from a series of chemical reactions starting with the formation of adducts between reducing sugars and protein nucleophiles such as nitrogen bases. Reaction with nucleic acid is also possible but has not been extensively described. The reactions in the formation of AGE are initially complex involving the formation of a Schiff base with rearrangement to form an Amadori product. The Amadori product can degrade through the Maillard reaction to form AGE. Some products include triosidines, N^{ε}-carboxymethyl-lysine, and pentosidine-adducts. These products can undergo further reactions to form cross-linked products; advanced glycation end products are involved in the generation of reactive oxygen species. The first step in the formation of these complex products is glycation.[1–3]

1. Fedorova, M., Frolov, A., and Hoffmann, R., Fragmentation behavior of Amadori peptides obtained by non-enzymatic glycosylation of lysine residues with ADP ribose in tandem mass spectrometry, *J. Mass Spectrom.* 45, 664–669, 2010.
2. Méndex, J.D., and Xie, J., Aguilar-Hernández, M., Méndez-Valenzuela, V., Molecular susceptibility to glycation and its implication in diabetes mellitus and related diseases, *Mol. Cell. Biochem.* 344, 185–193, 2010.
3. Bai, X., Wang, Z., Huang, C., Wang, Z., and Chi, L., Investigation of non-enzymatic glycosylation of human serum albumin using ion trap-time-of-flight mass spectrometry, *Molecules* 17, 8782–8794, 2012.

AERATION

The dispersion and/or dissolution of a gas into a liquid; generally refers to the process of dispersing air or an oxygen–gas mixture into a liquid such as culture media Aeration can also refer to the process of air dispersion in the pulmonary system, which can include both the inspiratory process and the exchange between the pulmonary system and the vascular bed; most frequently the latter.[1,2] The process of aeration is responsible for the concentration of oxygen in cell culture and fermentation systems affecting both the quantity and quality of proteins and glycoproteins expressed in such systems.[3–6]

1. Newman, B., and Oh, K.S., Abnormal pulmonary aeration in infants and children, *Radiol. Clin. North Am.* 26, 323–339, 1988.
2. Kothari, N.A., and Kramer, S.S., Bronchial diseases and lung aeration in children, *J. Thorac. Imaging* 16, 207–223, 2001.

3. Kamihari, M., Yoshida, H., Hjima, S., and Kobayashi, T., Effects of oxygen aeration on production of monoclonal antibody in immobilized hybridoma-cell bioreactor, *J. Fermentation Bioengineer.* 69, 311–312, 1990.

4. Kunkel, J.P., Jan, D.C.H., Jamieson, J.C., and Butler, M., Dissolved oxygen concentration in serum-free continuous culture affects N-linked glycosylation of a monoclonal antibody, *J. Biotechnol.* 62, 55–71, 1998.

5. Werner, R.G., Kopp, K., and Schlueter, M., Glycosylation of therapeutic proteins in different production systems, *Acta Paediatrica* 96, 17–22, 2007.

6. Rathore, A.S., Kumar, S., Sumit, P., et al., Fermentanomics: Related quality attributes of a monoclonal antibody to cell culture process variables and raw materials using multivariate data analysis, *Biotechnol. Progress* 31, 1586–1599, 2015.

AEROSOL

A colloid-like dispersion of a liquid or solid material into a gas. There is considerable interest in the use of aerosols for pulmonary drug delivery.[1–7]

1. Guilleminault, L., Azzopardi, N., Arnoult, C., et al., Fare of inhaled monoclonal antibodies after the deposition of aerosolized particles in the respiratory system, *J. Control. Release* 196, 344–354, 2014.

2. Respaud, R., Vecellio, L., Diot, P., and Heuzé-Vourc'h, Nebulization as a delivery method for mAbs in respiratory diseases, *Expert Opin. Drug. Deliv.* 12, 1027–1039, 2015.

3. Wanning, S., Süverkrüp, R., and Lamprecht, A., Pharmaceutical spray freeze drying, *Int. J. Pharm.* 488, 136–153, 2015.

4. Weers, J.G., and Miller, D.P., Formulation design of dry powders for inhalation, *J. Pharm.* 104, 3259–3288, 2015.

5. Hertel, S.P., Winter, G., and Friess, W., Protein stability in pulmonary drug delivery via nebulization, *Adv. Drug Deliv. Rev.* 93, 79–94, 2015.

6. Poursina, N., Vatranara, A., Rouini, M.R., Gilani, K., and Najafabadi, A.R., The effect of excipients on the stability and aerosol performance of salmon calcitonin dry powder inhalers via the spray freezing process, *Acta. Pharm.* 66, 207–218, 2016.

7. Ung, K.T., Rao, N., Weers, J.G., Huang, D., and Chan, H.K., Design of spray dried insulin microparticles to bypass deposition in the extrathoracic region and maximize total lung dose, *Int. J. Pharm.* 511, 1070–1079, 2016.

AFFIBODIES

Affibodies are small proteins with specific binding characteristics based on α-helical domain (Fc binding surface of the Z-domain) from staphylococcal protein A.[1,2] One could argue that affibodies are not proteins but rather large peptides. Affibodies can be selected for specific binding characteristics from combinatorial libraries using phage display technology.[3] There is considerable interest in the use of affibodies for **molecular imaging**.[4–8] The small size of affibodies has complicated therapeutic use but there has been interest in affibody conjugates with other proteins.[9,10]

1. Nord, K., Gunneriusson, E., Ringdahl, J., et al., Binding proteins selected from an α-helical bacterial receptor domain, *Nature Biotechnology* 15, 772–777, 1997.

2. Löfblom, J., Feldwisch, J., Tommachev, V., et al., Affibody molecules: Engineered proteins for therapeutic, diagnostic and biotechnological applications, *FEBS Letts.* 584, 2670–2680, 2010.

3. Friedman, M., Nordberg, E., Höidén-Guthenberg, I., et al., Phage display selection of affibody molecules with specific binding to the extracellular domain of the epidermal growth factor receptor, *Protein Eng. Des. Sel.* 20, 189–199, 2007.

4. Feldwisch, J., and Tolmache, V., Engineering of affibody molecules for therapy and diagnostics, *Methods Mol. Biol.* 899, 103–126, 2012.

5. Da Pieve, C., Allott, L., Martins, C.D., et al., Efficient [18F] AlF radiolabeling of $Z_{HER3:8698}$ affibody molecule for imaging of HER3 positive tumors, *Bioconjug. Chem.* 27, 1839–1849, 2016.

6. Andersson, K.G., Oroujeni, M., Garousi, J., et al., Feasibility of imaging of epidermal growth factor receptor expression with ZEGFR:2377 affibody molecule labeled with 99mTc using a peptide-based cysteine-containing chelator, *Int. J. Oncol.* 49, 2285–2293, 2016.

7. de Souza, A.L., Marra, K., Gunn, J., et al., Fluorescent affibody molecule administered *in vivo* at a microdose level labels EGFR-expressing glioma tumor regions, *Mol. Imaging Biol.* 19, 41–48, 2017.

8. Sandberg, D., Tolmachev, V., Velikyan, I., et al., Intraimage referencing for simplified assessment of HER2-expression in breast cancer metastases using the affibody molecule ABY-025 with PET and SPECT, *Eur. J. Nucl. Med. Mol. Imaging,* 44, 1337–1346, 2017.

9. Seijsling, J., Lindborg, M., Hölden-Guthenberg, I., et al., An engineered affibody molecule with pH-dependent binding FcRn mediates extended circulatory half-life of a fusion protein, *Proc. Natl. Acad. Sci. USA* 111, 17710–17715, 2014.

10. Dong, D., Zia, G., Li, Z., and Li, Z., Human serum albumin and HER2-binding affibody fusion proteins for targeted delivery of fatty acid-modified molecules and therapy, *Mol. Pharmaceutics* 13, 3370–3380, 2016.

AFFINITY CHROMATOGRAPHY

Affinity chromatography is a separation technology using the specific binding characteristics of a protein for a ligand bound to a backbone matrix such as polyacrylamide or dextran. Leonard Lerman published the first description of the affinity chromatography of a protein in 1963.[1]

The work described the use of *p*-azophenol derivatives (4,4-dihydroxyazobenzene derivatives) coupled to a cellulose matrix for the purification of mushroom tyrosinase. Some years later Donald McCormick at Cornell published a series of paper describing the affinity purification of flavokinase[2] and flavin mononucleotide-dependent enzymes.[3] McCormick also reported the purification of avidin on a biotin cellulose.[4] At the same time of these studies, Cuatrecasas, Wilchek, and Anfinsen presented a more practical approach using CNBr-mediated coupling to a cross-linked dextran matrix.[5] There are a number of modes of affinity chromatography.[6–11]

1. Lerman, L.S., A biochemically specific method for enzyme isolation, *Proc. Natl. Acad. Sci. USA* 39, 232–236, 1953.
2. Arsenis, C., and McCormick, D.B., Purification of liver flavokinase by column chromatography on flavin-cellulose compounds, *J. Biol. Chem.* 239, 3093–3097, 1964.
3. Arsenis, C., and McCormick, D.B., Purification of flavin mononucleotide-dependent enzymes by column chromatography on flavin phosphate cellulose compounds, *J. Biol. Chem.* 241, 330–334, 1966.
4. McCormick, D.B., Specific purification of avidin by column chromatography on biotin-cellulose, *Anal. Biochem.* 13, 194–198, 1965.
5. Cuatrecasas, P., Wilchek, M., and Anfinsen, C.B., Selective enzyme purification by affinity chromatography, *Proc. Natl. Acad. Sci.* 39, 636–643, 1968.
6. Schott, H., *Affinity Chromatography: Template Chromatography of Nucleic Acids and Protein*, Marcel Dekker, New York, 1984.
7. Mohr, P., and Pommerening, K., *Affinity Chromatography: Practical and Theoretical Aspects*, Marcel Dekker, New York, 1985.
8. *Affinity Chromatography: A Practical Approach*, ed. P.D.G. Dean, W.S. Johnson, and F.A. Middle, IRL Press at Oxford, Oxford, UK, 1985.
9. Turkova, J., *Bioaffinity Chromatography*, Elsevier, Amsterdam, the Netherlands, 1993.
10. *Handbook of Affinity Chromatography*, ed. D. Hage, CRC Press, Boca Raton, FL, 2006.
11. *Phage Display in Biotechnology and Drug Discovery*, ed. S.S. Sidhu and C.R. Geyer, CRC Press, Boca Raton, FL 2015.

AFFINITY LABELING

Affinity labeling is a process in which the covalent labeling of a macromolecule, usually a protein, at a unique site is accomplished with a reagent specific for binding at the site to be modified. The concept was originally advanced by Singer and coworkers.[1] The best-known examples are where an enzyme is modified at the active site with a reagent similar to a substrate as with the peptide chloromethyl ketones developed by Elliott Shaw and coworkers.[2] Factors important in the design of an affinity reagent have been reviewed by Bryce Plapp.[3] Affinity labeling continues as an active area of study with the development of novel reagents.[4–6] **Photoaffinity labeling** is a type of affinity labeling where the reactive group, usually a free radical, is generated by irradiation after binding to the target.[7–8] The possibility does exist as reagents not bound to the target site can react at other sites.[9] The concept of photoaffinity labeling dates to work on chymotrypsin from Frank Westheimer's laboratory more than 50 years ago.[10,11] Photoaffinity labeling has had considerable success with membrane proteins.[12–14] The work on affinity labeling with active-site-directed reagents provided the ground work for activity-based proteomics.[15] See **activity-based protein profiling**.

1. Wofsy, L., Metzger, H., and Singer, S.J., Affinity labeling—a general method for labeling the active sites of antibody and enzyme molecules, *Biochemistry* 1, 1031–1039, 1962.
2. Schoellmann, G., and Shaw, E., Direct evidence for the presence of histidine in the active center of chymotrypsin, *Biochemistry* 2, 252–255, 1963.
3. Plapp, B.V., Application of affinity labeling for studying structure and function of enzymes, *Methods Enzymol.* 87, 469–499, 1982.
4. Tomohiro, T., Nakabayshi, M., Sugita, Y., and Morimoto, S., Kinetic controlled affinity labeling of target enzyme with thioester chemistry, *Bioorg. Med. Chem.* 24. 3336–3341, 2016.
5. Ono, S., Nakai, T., Kuroda, H., et al., Site-selective chemical modification of chymotrypsin using peptidyl derivatives bearing optically active diphenyl-1-amino-2-phenylethylphosphonate: Stereochemical effect of the diphenyl phosphonate moiety, *Biopolymers* 106, 521–530, 2016.
6. Takaoka, Y., Nukadzuka, Y., and Ueda, M., Reactive group-embedded affinity labeling reagent for efficient intracellular protein labeling, *Bioorg. Med. Chem.* 25, 2888–2894, 2017.
7. *Photochemical Probes*, ed. P.E. Nielsen, Kluwer, Dordrecht, Boston, MA, 1989.
8. Kotzyba-Hibert, F., Kapfer, I., and Goeldner, M., Recent trends in photoaffinity labeling, *Angw. Chem. Int. Ed. Engl.* 34, 1299–1312, 1995.
9. Ruoho, A.E., Kiefer, H., Roeder, P.E., and Singer, S.J., The mechanism of photoaffinity labeling, *Proc. Natl. Acad. Sci. USA* 70, 2567–2571, 1973.
10. Singh, A., Thornton, E.R., and Westheimer, F.H., The photolysis of diazoacetylchymotrypsin, *J. Biol. Chem.* 237, PC3006–PC3008, 1962.
11. Shafer, J., Barnowsky, P., Lauren, R., Finn, F., and Westheimer, Products from the photolysis of diazoacetyl chymotrypsin, *J. Biol. Chem.* 241, 421–427, 1966.

12. Mezic, K.G., Cress, B.F., Koffas, M.A.B., et al., Identification of the binding sites for ubiquinone and inhibitors in the (NA+)-pumping NADH-ubiquinone oxidoreductase from *Vibrio cholera* by photoaffinity labeling, *J. Biol. Chem.* 292, 7727–7742, 2017.

13. Jiao, C.Y., Sachon, E., Alves, I.D., et al., Exploiting benzophenone photoreactivity to probe the phospholipid environment and insertion depth of the cell penetrating peptide Penetratin in model membranes, *Angew. Chem. Int. Ed. Engl.*, 56, 8226–8230, 2017.

14. Budelier, M.M., Cheng, W.W., Bergdoll, L., et al., Photoaffinity labeling with cholesterol analogues precisely maps a cholesterol-binding site in voltage-dependent anion channel-1, *J. Biol. Chem.* 292, 9294–9304, 2017.

15. Barglow, K.T., and Cravatt, B.F., Activity-based protein profiling for the functional annotation of enzymes, *Nat. Methods* 4, 822–827, 2007.

AFFINITY PROTEOMICS

Affinity proteomics is based on the isolation of proteins from complex mixtures coupled with a method for identification of the isolated proteins.[1] Isolation techniques include classical immunoaffinity methods with antibody-bead technologies.[2,3] Aptamers have proved to be useful affinity reagents.[4–6] The use of aptamer-based technology enables broader multiplexing (more than 1000 proteins) permitting genome-wide association studies (GWAS).[7] Affinity proteomics also includes the use of specific binding probes to identify cellular and tissue proteins.[8] See also **affinity labeling, activity-based proteomics**.

1. Smith, J.G., and Gerszten, R.E., Emerging affinity-based proteomic technologies for large-scale plasma profiling in cardiovascular disease, *Circulation* 135, 1651–1664, 2Lurid.

2. Lourido, L., Ayoglu, B., Fernández-Tajes, J., et al., Discovery of circulating proteins associated to knee radiographic osteoarthritis, *Sci. Rep.* 7(1), 137, 2017.

3. Byström, S., Fredolini, C., Edqvist, P.H., et al., Affinity proteomics exploration of melanoma identifies proteins in serum with association to T-stage and recurrences, *Trans. Oncol.* 10, 385–395, 2017.

4. Stoevesandt, O., and Taussig, M.J., Affinity reagent resources for human proteome detection: Initiatives and perspectives, *Proteomics* 7, 2738–2850, 2007.

5. Kinghorn, A.B., Dirkzwager, R.M., Liang, S., et al., Aptamer affinity maturation by resampling and microarray selection, *Anal. Chem.* 88, 6981–6985, 2016.

6. Pfeiffer, F., Rosenthal, Z.M., Siegl, J., Ewers, J., and Mayer, G., Customised nucleic acid libraries for enhanced aptamer selection and performance, *Curr. Opin. Biotechnol.* 48, 111–118, 2017.

7. Suhre, K., Arnold, M., Bhagwat, A.M., et al., Connecting genetic risk to disease end points through the human blood plasma proteome, *Nat. Commun.* 8, 14357, 2017.

8. Larsson, T., Bergstrom, J., Nilsson, C., and Karlsson, K.A., Use of an affinity proteomics approach for the identification of low-abundant bacterial adhesins as applied on the Lewis(b)-binding adhesin of *Helicobacter pylori*, *FEBS Lett.* 469, 155–158, 2000.

AGAR/AGAROSE

Agar is a heterogeneous natural product derived from algae/seaweed. It is used as a food additive,[1] and as a formed gel, a model system for food processing.[2,3] Agar has been used as a matrix for culturing bacterial cells for more than a century[4] and has seen increasing use in mammalian cell culture.[5] Soft agar colony formation assay is used to measure the ability of cells to proliferate in semi-solid matrices and is important in measuring cell proliferation in cancer studies.[6,7] Agar is composed of two primary components, **agarose** which is a gelling component and agaropectin which is a sulfated, non-gelling component. Agarose is used as a matrix for the electrophoretic separation of large molecules such as DNA[8–12] and is the matrix for the **comet assay** for DNA damage.[13–15] Agarose is also used as a matrix for 3-D culture of mammalian cells.[16–18]

1. Anon., *Fed. Register* 42(161), 41876–41878, 1977.

2. Fuchigami, M., and Teramoto, A., Changes in temperature and structure of agar gel as affected by sucrose during high-pressure freezing, *J. Food Sci.* 68, 528–533, 2003.

3. De Nobili, M.D., Rojas, A.M., Abrami, M., Lapasin, R., and Grassi, M., Structure characterization by means of rheological and NMR experiments as a first necessary approach to study the (L-(+)-ascorbic acid diffusion from pectin and pectin/alginate films to agar hydrogels that mimic food materials, *J. Food Engineer.* 165, 82–92, 2015.

4. Buerger, L., Studies of the *Pneumococcus* and allied organisms with reference to their occurrence in the human mouth, *J. Exp. Med.* 7, 497–546, 1905.

5. Mohamed, A., Sun, C., De Mello, V., et al., The Hippo effector TAX (WWTR1) transforms myoblasts and TAZ abundance is associated with reduced survival in embryonal rhabdomyosarcoma, *J. Pathol.* 240, 3–14, 2016.

6. Horibata, S., Vo, T.V., Subramanian, V., Thompson, P.R., and Coonrod, S.A., Utilization of the soft agar colony formation assay to identify inhibitors of tumorigenicity in breast cancer cells, *J. Vis. Exp.* (99), e52727, 2015.

7. Crowlye, L.C., and Waterhouse, N.J., Measuring survival of hematopoietic cancer cells with the colony-forming assay in soft agar, *Cold Spring Harbon Protoc.* 2016(8), pdb.prott087189, 2016.

8. *Electrophoresis in Practice: A Guide to Methods and Applications of DNA and Protein Separations*, Wiley-VCH, Berlin, Germany, 2001.

9. Stellwagen, N.C., and Stellwagen, E., Effect of the matrix on DNA electrophoretic mobility, *J. Chromatog. A* 1216, 1917–1929, 2009.

10. Stellwagen, N.C., Electrophoresis of DNA in agarose gels, polyacrylamide gels and in free solution, *Electrophoresis* Suppl 1, S188–S195, 2009.

11. Silva, S., Costa, E.M., Vicente, S., et al., DNA agarose gel electrophoresis for antioxidant analysis: Development of a quantitative approach for phenolic extracts, *Food Chem.* 233, 45–51, 2017.

12. Henno, L., Tombak, E.M., Geimanen, J., et al., Analysis of human papillomavirus genome replication using two- and three-dimensional agarose gel electrophoresis, *Curr. Protoc. Microbiol.* 45:14B.10.1-10.37, 2017.

13. Collins, A.R., Measuring oxidative damage to DNA and is repair with the comet assay, *Biochim. Biophys. Acta* 1840. 794–800, 2014.

14. Singh, N.P., The comet assay. Reflections on its development, evolution and applications, *Mutat. Res. Rev. Mutat. Res.* 767, 23–30, 2016.

15. Glei, M., Schneider, T., and Schlörmann, W., Comet assay: An essential tool in toxicological research, *Arch. Toxicol.* 90, 2315–2336, 2016.

16. Gruber, H.E., Hoelscher, G.L., Leslie, K., Ingram, J.A., and Hanley, E.N., Three-dimensional culture of human disc cells within agarose or a collagen sponge: Assessment of proteoglycan production, *Biomaterials* 27, 371–376, 2006.

17. Gorth, D.J., Lothstein, K.E., Chiaro, J.A., et al., Hypoxic regulation of functional extracellular matrix elaboration by nucleus pupposa cells in long-term agarose culture, *J. Ortho. Res.* 33, 747–754, 2015.

18. Tam, R.V., Smith, L.I., and Shoichet, M.S., Engineering cellular microenvironments with photo-and enzymatically responsive hydrogels: Toward biomimetic 3D cell culture models, *Acc. Chem. Res.* 50, 703–713, 2017.

AGGREGATION

Aggregation is the process of forming an ordered or a disordered group of particles, molecules, bubbles, drops, or other physical components that bind together in an undefined fashion; a common physical analogy is concrete. The item formed by such a process is referred to as an aggregate. Aggregation in biochemistry and biotechnology most often applies to macromolecules such as proteins or to cells such as platelets. Protein aggregation may occur as a result of protein denaturation.[1,2] Protein aggregation can occur as unwanted event in the processing of biopharmaceuticals[3–5] Systems have been proposed for the classification of protein aggregates.[6,7] Several techniques can be used to assess protein aggregation including analytical ultracentrifugation,[8] light scattering,[9] size-exclusion chromatography,[10] and electrophoresis.[11] Protein aggregates also occur *in vivo* with amyloid formation[12] and intracellular aggregation of p53 in cancer.[13] The aggregation of blood platelets is a critical part of blood coagulation and is measured by change in light transmittance upon aggregation.[14] **Agglutination** is a term used to described the aggregation or clumping of blood cells or bacteria caused by antibody or other biological or chemical factors.[15]

1. Tsai, A.M., van Zanten, J.H., and Betenbaugh, M.J., I. Study of protein aggregation due to heat denaturation: A structural approach using circular dichroism, spectroscopy, nuclear magnetic resonance, and static light scattering, *Biotechnol. Bioengineer.* 59, 273–280, 1998.

2. Oldfield, D.J., Singh, H., and Taylor, M.W., Kinetics of heat-induced whey protein denaturation and aggregation in skim milks with adjusted whey protein concentration, *J. Dairy Res.* 72, 369–378, 2005.

3. Shahrokh, Z., Stratton, P.R., Eberlein, G.A., and Wang, Y.S., Approaches to analysis of aggregates and demonstrating mass balance in pharmaceutical protein (basic fibroblast growth factor) formulation, *J. Pharmaceut. Sci.* 83, 1645–1650, 1994.

4. Roberts, C.L., Darrington, R.T., and Whitley, M.B., Irreversible aggregation of basic fibroblast growth factor (bG-CSF) and implications for predicting protein shelf-life, *J. Pharmaceut. Sci.* 92, 1095–1111, 2003.

5. Mahler, H-C., Freiss, W., Grauschopf, U., and Kiese, S., Protein aggregation: Pathways, induction factors and analysis, *J. Pharmaceut. Sci.* 98, 2909–2934, 2009.

6. Narhi, L.O., Schmit, J., Bechtold-Peters, K., and Sharma, D., Classification of protein aggregates, *J. Pharmaceut. Sci.* 101, 493–498, 2012.

7. D'Addio, S.M., Bothe, J.R., Neri, C., et al., New and evolving techniques for the characterization of peptide therapeutics, *J. Pharmaceut. Sci.* 105, 2989–3006, 2016.

8. Berkowitz, S.A., Role of analytical ultracentrifugation in assessing the aggregation of protein biopharmaceuticals, *AAPS J.* 8, E590–E605, 2006.

9. Hofmann, M., Winzer, M., Weber, C., and Gieseler, H., Prediction of protein aggregation in high concentration protein solutions utilizing protein-protein interactions determined by low-volume static light scattering, *J. Pharmaceut. Sci.* 105, 1819–1828, 2016.

10. Sahin, E., and Roberts, C.J. Size-exclusion chromatography with multi-angle light scattering for elucidating protein aggregation mechanisms, *Methods Mol. Biol.* 899, 403–423, 2012.

11. Mulcahy, E.M., Fargier-Lagrange, M., Mulvihill, D.M., and O'Mahoney, J.A., Characterization of heat-induced protein aggregation in whey protein isolate and the influence of aggregation on the availability of amino groups as measured the ortho-phthaldialdehyde (OPA) and trinitrobenzenesulfonic acid (TNBS) methods, *Food Chem.* 229, 66–74, 2017.

12. Lucato, C.M., Lupton, C.J., Halle, M.L., and Ellisdon, A.M., Amyloidogenicity at a distance: How distal protein regions modulate aggregation in disease, *J. Mol. Biol.* 429, 1289–3004, 2017.

13. Wang, C., and Ferscht, A.R., Multisite aggregation of p53 and implications for drug rescue, *Proc. Natl. Acad. Sci. USA* 114, E2534–E2543, 2017.
14. Breddin, H.K., Can platelet aggregometry be standardized, *Platelets* 16, 151–158, 2005.
15. El Kenz, H., and Corazza, F., Automated point-of-care testing for ABO agglutination test: Proof of concept and validation, *Vox Sang.* 109, 78–85, 2015.

AGONIST

An agonist is a compound or substance that binds to a receptor site, which could be on a cell membrane or a protein, and elicits a positive response.[1–4] Adenosine-5'-diphosphate promotes the aggregation of blood platelets by binding to several receptors including $P2Y_{12}$.[5] 2-Methylthio-adenosine-5-diphosphate is agonist of ADP. An agonist is the opposite of an antagonist. See also **antagonist**.

1. Deupi, X., and Standfuss, J., Structural insights into agonist-induced activation of G protein-coupled receptors, *Curr. Opin. Struct. Biol.* 21, 541–551, 2011.
2. Lebon, G., Warne, T., and Tate, C.G., Agonist-bound structures of G protein-coupled receptors, *Curr. Opin. Struct. Biol.* 22, 482–490, 2012.
3. Heifetz, A., Aldeghi, M., Chudyk, E.I., et al., Using the fragment molecular orbital method to investigate agonist-orexin-2 receptor interactions, *Biochem. Soc. Trans* 44, 574–581, 2016.
4. Ciancetta, A., and Jacobson, K.A., Structural probing and molecular modeling of the A_3 adenosine receptor: A focus on agonist binding, *Molecules* 22(3), 449, 2017.
5. Zhang, J., Zhang, K., Gao, Z-G., et al., Agonist-bound structure of the human $P2Y_{12}$ receptor, *Nature* 509, 119–122, 2014.

ALARMINS

Alarmins are a diverse group of proteins released during tissue trauma and inflammation that act on components of the immune system.[1,2] Alarmins are considered to function in pathogen-associated molecular patterns (PAMP) and damage-associated molecular patterns (DAMPs).[3] Alarmins include such proteins as IL-33 and HMGB1 (high-mobility group box 1),[4] certain S100 proteins,[5] and defensins.[6,7]

1. Raymond, S.L., Holden, D.C., Mira, J.C., et al., Microbial recognition and danger signals in sepsis and trauma, *Biochim. Biophys. Acta* 1863, 2564–2573, 2017.
2. Gard, A.D., and Agostinis, P., Cell death and immunity in cancer: From danger signals to mimicry of pathogen defense responses, *Immunol. Rev.* 280, 126–148, 2017.
3. Bianchi, M.E., DAMPs, PAMPs and alarmins: All we need to know about danger, *J. Leuk. Biol.* 81, 1–5, 2017.
4. Gougeon, M.-L., Alarmins and central nervous system inflammation in HIV-associated neurological disorders, *J. Int. Med.* 281, 433–447, 2017.
5. Bertheloot, D., and Latz, E., HMGB1, IL-1α, IL-33 and S100 proteins: Dual-function alarmins, *Cell. Mol. Immunol.* 14, 43–64, 2017; S100 proteins: Potential therapeutic targets for arthritis, *Expert Opin. Ther. Targets* 21, 738–750, 2017.
6. Oppenheim, J.J., and Yang D., Alarmins: Chemotactic activators of immune response, *Curr. Opin. Immunol.* 17, 359–366, 2005.
7. Holly, M.K., Diaz, K., and Smith, J.G., Defensins in viral infection and pathogenesis, *Annu. Rev. Virol.* 4, 369–301, 2017.

ALGORITHM

An algorithm is the underlying iterative method or mathematic theory for any particular computer programming technique; a precisely described routine process that can be applied and systematically followed through to a conclusion; a step-by-step procedure for solving a problem or accomplishing some end. An algorithm can be viewed as computational procedure that takes an input and processes the information into an output.[1]

1. Cormen, T.H., Leiserson, C.E., Rives, R.L., and Stein, C., *Algorithms Unlocked*, MIT Press, Cambridge, MA, 2014.

ALBUMIN

Albumin is a protein, most notably derived from plasma or serum and secondarily from egg (ovalbumin). Plasma albumin is the most abundant protein in blood/plasma constituting approximately half of the total plasma protein.[1–3] Albumin is a general designation to describe a fraction of simple proteins which are soluble in water and dilute salt solutions as opposed to the globulin fraction which is insoluble in water but soluble in dilute salt solutions. This is an old classification, which has many exceptions.[4] Albumins also migrate faster than globulins on electrophoresis, which results in the development of the classification of plasma proteins as albumins and globulins.[5] Plasma albumin functions in establishing plasma colloid strength preserves the fluid balance between the intravascular and extravascular space[6] and for the binding and transport of low molecular materials such as fatty acids.[7] The ability of albumin to bind drugs influences pharmacokinetics.[8] The ability of albumin to bind drugs has been used for specific drug delivery.[9] Albumin, particularly bovine serum albumin (BSA), has a long history of use as a model protein[10–12] and as a standard for the measurement of protein concentration.[13,14] Blood plasma albumin was the first protein biopharmaceutical[15,16] and is used for a variety of clinical indications.[17–19] It is recognized that there has been considerable discussion of the value of albumin and there is a study suggesting albumin quality is an issue.[20] The long circulatory half-life of albumin has stimulated the development of fusion proteins between albumin and therapeutic proteins.[21] Albumin has been used in an extracorporeal shunt device developed as a "bridge-to-transplant"[22,23] and is currently referred to as albumin dialysis.[24,25] Albumin is also noted for its ability to interact with various dyes and the binding of bromocresol green is an example of a clinical assay method for albumin.[26]

1. Foster, J.F., Plasma albumin, in *The Plasma Proteins*, Vol. 1 ed. F.W. Putnam, Academic Press, New York, Chapter 6, pp. 179–239, 1960.
2. Peters, T., *All about Albumin: Biochemistry, Genetics, and Medical Applications*, Academic Press, San Diego, CA, 1996.
3. Lundblad, R.L., *Biotechnology of the Plasma Proteins*, Albumin, Chapter 4, pp. 83–181, CRC Press/Taylor & Francis Group, Boca Raton, FL, 2013.
4. Taylor, J.F., The isolation of proteins, in *The Proteins. Chemistry, Biological Activity and Methods*, Volume I. Pt. A, ed. H. Neurath and K. Bailey, Chapter 1, pp. 1–85, 1953.
5. Cooper, G.R., Electrophoretic and ultracentrifugal analysis of normal human serum, in *The Plasma Proteins*, ed. F.W. Putman, Academic Press, New York, 1960, Chapter 3, pp. 51–103, 1960.
6. Starling, E.H., On the absorption of fluids from the connective tissue spaces, *J. Physiol.* 19, 312–326, 1896.
7. van der Vusse, G.J., Albumin as fatty acid transporter, *Drug. Metab. Pharmokinet.* 24, 300–307, 2009.
8. Jusko, W.J., and Gretch, M., Plasma and tissue protein binding of drugs in pharmacokinetics, *Drug. Metab. Rev.* 5, 43–140, 1976.
9. Larsen, M.T., Kuhlmann, M., Hvam, M.L., and Howard, K.A., Albumin-based drug delivery: Harnessing nature to cure disease, *Mol. Cell. Ther.* 4:3, 2016.
10. Tanford, C., Protein Denaturation, *Adv. Protein Chem.* 23, 121–282, 1968.
11. Yamakura, F., and Ikeda, K., Modification of tryptophan and tryptophan residues in proteins by reactive nitrogen species, *Nitric Oxide* 14, 152–161, 2006.
12. Yuan, D., Jacquier, J.C., and O'Riordan, E.D., Entrapment of protein in chitosan triphosphate beads its release in an in vitro digestive model, *Food Chem.* 229, 495–501, 2017.
13. Sapan, C.V., Lundblad, R.L., and Price, N.C., Colorimetric protein assay techniques, *Biotechnol. Appl. Biochem.* 29, 99–108, 1999.
14. Sapan, C.V., and Lundblad, R.L., Review of methods for determination of total protein and peptide concentration in biological samples, *Proteomics Clin. Appl.* 9, 268–276, 2015.
15. Newhauser, L.R., and Loznen, E.L., Studies on human albumin in military medicine: The standard Army-Navy package of serum albumin (concentrated), *U.S. Navy Med. Bull.* 40, 796–799, 1942.
16. Heyl, J.T., Gibson, J.G., 2nd, and Janeway, C.W., Studies on the plasma proteins. V. The effect of concentrated solutions of human and bovine serum albumin in man, *J. Clin. Invest.* 22, 763–773, 1943.
17. Caironi, P., Langer, T., and Gattinoni, L., Albumin in critically ill patients: The ideal colloid? *Curr. Opin. Crit. Care* 21, 302–308, 2015.
18. Spinella, R., Sawhney, R., and Jalan, R., Albumin in chronic liver disease: Structure, functions and therapeutic implications, *Heptaol. Int.* 10, 124–132, 2016.
19. Ellaiek, R., Heybroeck, C., and Dubois, M.J., Albumin administration for fluid resuscitation in burn patients: A systematic review and meta-analysis, *Burns* 43, 17–24, 2017.
20. Penn, A.H., Dubick, M.A., and Torres-Filho, I.P., Fatty acid saturation of albumin used in resuscitation fluids modulates cell damage in shock: In vitro results using a novel technique to measure fatty acid binding capacity, *Shock*, 48, 449–458, 2017.
21. Lyseng-Williamson, K.A, Coagulation factor IX (recombinant), albumin fusion protein (Albutrepenonacog alpha; idelvion®): A review of its use in haemophilia B, *Drugs* 77, 97–106, 2017.
22. Sen, S., and Williams, R., New liver support devices in acute liver failure: A critical evaluation, *Semin. Liver Dis.* 23, 283–294, 2003.
23. George, J., Barshes, N.R., Gay, A.N., Williams, B., et al., Support for the acutely failing liver: A comprehensive review of historic and contemporary strategies, *J. Am. Coll. Surg.* 201, 458–476, 2005.
24. Schmuck, R.B., Nawrot, G.H., Fikatas, P., et al., Single-pass albumin dialysis—A dose-finding study to define optimal albumin concentration and dialysate flow, *Artif. Organs* 41, 153–161, 2017.
25. Huber, W., Henschel, B., Schmid, R., and Al-Chalabi, A., First clinical experience in 14 patients treated with ADVOS: A study on feasibility, safety and efficacy of a new type of albumin dialysis, *BMC Gastroenterol.* 17, 32, 2017.
26. Rodkey, F.L., Direct spectrophotometric determination of albumin in human serum, *Clin. Chem.* 11, 478–487, 1965.

ALLELISM

Alleism refers to the presence of two or more variants of a gene in an outbred population.[1] The polymorphism in the HLA (human leukocyte antigen) family has been of particular interest.[2] Allotypes are examples of allelism in the expression of immunoglobulins.[3]

1. *Dictionary of Immunology*, ed. W.J. Herbert, P.C. Wilkinson, and D.I. Stott, Blackwell Scientific, Oxford, UK, 1985.
2. Sodoyer, R., Nguyen, C., Strachan, T., et al., Allelism in the HLA Class I multigene family, *Ann. Inst. Pasteur Immunol.* 136C, 71–84, 1985.
3. Jefferis, R., Allotypes, Immunoglobulins, in *Encyclopedia of Immunology*, ed. P.J. Delver and I.M. Roitt, pp. 74–77, Academic Press, San Diego, CA, 1998.

ALLOANTIBODY

An alloantibody is also referred to as an isoantibody and is an antibody directed against a material (e.g. a protein, cell, or tissue) from an individual of the same species.[1-5] Transplantation antibodies, transfusion antibodies and antibodies against blood coagulation factors such as factor VIII inhibitors are examples of alloantibodies.

1. Colvin, R.B., and Smith, R.N., Antibody-mediated organ-allograft rejection, *Nat. Rev. Immunol.* 5, 807–817, 2005.
2. Moll, S., and Pascual, M., Humoral rejection of organ allografts, *Am. J. Transplant.* 5, 2611–2618, 2005.
3. Pankewycz, O., Soliman, K., and Laftavi, M.R., The increasing importance of alloantibodies in kidney transplantation, *Immunol. Invest.* 43, 775–789, 2014.
4. Everly, M.J., Update on alloantibodies in solid organ transplantation, *Clin. Transpl.* 2014, 125–149, 2014.
5. Carta, P., Di Maria, L., Caroti, L., et al., Anti-human leukocyte antigen DQ antibodies in renal transplantation: Are we underestimated the most frequent donor specific alloantibodies? *Transplant. Rev.* (Orlando) 29, 135–138, 2015). See also **alleism**.

ALLOANTIGEN

Alleic forms of an antigen expressed at the same gene locus in all individuals of a species.[1,2] The histocompatibility antigens of importance in transplantation are a well-known example.[3,4]

1. *Dictionary of Immunology*, 3rd edn., ed. W.J. Herbert, P.C. Wilkinson, and D.I. Stott, *Blackwell Scientific,* Oxford, UK, 1985.
2. Misra, D.N., Kunz, H.W., and Gill, T.J.,III, Alloantigens, in *Dictionary of Immunology*, 2nd edn., ed. P.J. Delves and I.M. Roitt, pp. 70–74, Academic Press, San Diego, CA, 1998.
3. Yoshimura, Y., Yadav, R., Christianson, G.J., et al., Duration of alloantigen presentation and avidity of T-cell antigen recognition correlate with immunodominance of CTL response to minor histocompatibility antigens, *J. Immunol.* 172, 6666–6674, 2004.
4. Koyama, M., and Hill, G.R., Alloantigen presentation and graft-versus-host disease: Fuel for the fire, *Blood* 127, 2963–2970, 2016. See also **alleism**.

ALLOSTERIC

Allosteric is a term which described the interaction of small molecules with an enzyme or other protein at a site physically distant from the active site where such interaction influenced enzyme or other biological activity. The term is derived from the combination of allo (different or other) and steric (three-dimensional form of atoms)[1] was advanced by Monod and Jacob in 1961.[2] The original term was developed for enzymes but has been extended to other biological activities. The original concept was based on the regulation of a specialized pathway by inhibition of the first enzyme by the final product of the pathway, where such product was structurally unrelated to the starting material.[3] It was shown that this effect involved multi-subunit proteins such as aspartate transcarbamylase, where there is a catalytic subunit that contains the enzyme active site and a regulatory subunit that contains the binding site for the allosteric modifier.[4] There are several reviews that describe the progress in the understanding of allosterism.[5,6] More recently, the term allosteric has been used to describe the binding of a large or small molecule, which can be described as modifiers, to a site or sites distant from a functional site (orthosteric site) resulting in the modulation of the activity of a broader range of proteins in addition to enzymes. The effective of the allosteric modifier may stimulate activity (positive allosteric modified, PAM) or inhibitory (negative allosteric modifier, NAM). Examples include the allosteric regulation of heme binding by human serum albumin,[7] the allosteric effect of ATP on GroEl,[8] and the allosteric regulation of receptors.[9,10]

1. *Oxford Dictionary of the English Language,* Oxford University Press, Oxford, UK, 2017.
2. Monod, J., and Jacob, F., *Cold Spring Harbor Symposium on Quantitative Biology,* Cold Spring Harbor Press, Cold Spring Harbor, NY, 1961.
3. Mond, J., Changeux, J-P., and Jacob, F., Allosteric proteins and cellular control systems, *J. Mol. Biol.* 6, 306–329, 1963.
4. Gerhart, J.C., and Schachman, H.K., Distinct subunits for the regulation and catalytic activity of aspartate transcarbamylase, *Biochemistry* 4, 1054–1062, 1965.
5. Perutz, M., *Mechanisms of Cooperativity and Allosteric Regulation in Enzymes,* Cambridge University Press, Cambridge, UK, 1990.
6. Traut, T., *Allosteric Regulatory Enzymes*, Springer, New York, 2008.
7. Ascenzi, P., and Fasano, M., Allostery in a monomeric protein: The case of human serum albumin, *Biophys. Chem.* 148, 16–22, 2010.

8. Horovitz, A., and Willison, K.R., Allosteric regulation of chaperonins, *Curr. Opin. Struct. Biol.* 15, 645–651, 2005.

9. Claessens, F., Johlau, S., and Helsen, C., Comparing the rules of engagement of androgen and glucocorticoid receptors, *Cell. Mol. Life Sci.* 74, 2217–2228, 2017.

10. Hackos, D.H., and Hansen, J.E., Diverse modes of NMDA receptor positive allosteric modulation: Mechanisms and consequences, *Neurophramcology* 112, 34–45, 2017.

ALTERNATIVE READING FRAME (ARF) PROTEIN

A **reading frame** refers to the order in which nucleotide triplets are "read" in either translation or transcription. In reading a sense sequence, there are three distinct reading frames depending on the selection of the first nucleotide. The antisense sequence would also have three distinct reading frames providing six reading frames for a given DNA or RNA sequence.[1] As an example, a given mRNA could code for two different proteins (proteoforms) depending on the starting nucleotide.[2] Peptides derived from proteins expressed via alternative reading frame of a normal mRNA can be recognized as "nonself" as shown by studies in type I diabetes.[3] The term alternative reading frame protein is frequently used to describe a protein, p19[arf], which is encoded by the *INK4a* tumor suppressor gene and with p53 has a tumor suppressor function.[4,5] There are other uses of the term alternative reading frame protein.[6,7]

1. https://www.ncbi.nlm.nih.gov/Class/MLACourse/ Original8Hour/Genetics/readingframe.html.

2. Gawron, D., Gevaert, K., and Van Damme, P., The proteomic under translational control, *Proteomics* 14, 2647–2662, 2014.

3. Wei, J., and Yewdall, J.W., Autoimmune T cell recognition of alternative-reading-frame-encoded peptides, *Nature Med.* 21, 409–410, 2017.

4. Sherr, C.J., Bertwistle, D., DEN Besten, W., et al., p53-dependent and p53-independent functions of the Arf tumor suppressor, *Cold Spring Harbor Symp Quant. Biol.* 70, 129–137, 2005.

5. Carrascp-Garcia, E., Moreno, M., Moreno-Cugnon, I., and Matheu, A., Increased Arf/p53 activity in stem cells, aging and cancer, *Aging Cell* 16, 219–222, 2017.

6. Fiorucci, M., Foulant, S., Fournillier, A., et al., Expression of the alternative reading frame protein of Hepatitis C virus induces cytokines involved in hepatic injuries, *J. Gen. Virol.* 88, 1149–1162, 2007.

7. Qureshi, H., Qazi, R., Hamid, S., and Qureshi, S.A., Identification of immunogenic regions within the alternative reading frame protein of hepatitis C virus (genotype 3), *Eur. J. Clin. Microbiol. Infect. Dis.* 30, 1075–1083, 2011.

ALTERNATIVE SPLICING

Alternative splicing is a process by which biological diversity can be increased without change in DNA content. Alternative splicing is a mechanism by a single premRNA is processed is different ways (different splicing sites) to yield a diverse group of messenger RNA molecules. Alternative splicing is a mechanism by which the coding capacity of a genome can be increase by the generation of a large number of distinct messenger RNA molecules from a limited amount of DNA (number of genes).[1] Alternative splicing is of considerable importance in development[2] and cancer.[3,4] It has been suggested that only a small number of alternatively spliced transcripts result in expressed proteins.[5,6]

1. Fiszbein, A., and Kornblihtt, A.R., Alternative splicing switches: Important players in cell differentiation, *Bioessays* 39, 2017.

2. Baralle, F.E., and Giudice, J., Alternative splicing as a regulator of development and tissue identity, *Nat. Rev. Mol. Cell Biol.* 18, 437, 2017.

3. Narayanan, S.P., Singh, S., and Shukla, S., A saga of cancer epigenetics linking epigenetics to alternative splicing, *Biochem. J.* 474, 885–896, 2017.

4. Kozlovski, I., Siegfried, Z., Amar-Schwartz, A., and Karni, R., The role of RNA alternative splicing in regulating cancer metabolism, *Hum. Genet.* 136, 1113–1127, 2017.

5. Tress, M.L., Abascal, F., and Valencia, A., Alternative splicing may not be the key to proteome complexity, *Trends Biochem. Sci.* 42, 98–100, 2017.

6. Blencowe, B.J., The relationship between alternative splicing and proteomic complexity, *Trends Biochem. Sci.* 42, 407–408, 2017.

AMINOPHOSPHOLIPIDS

Amino-containing phospholipids such as phosphatidyl ethanolamine and phosphatidyl serine have important roles in cell biology. Phosphatidyl serine is involved in specific membrane function and changes in membrane distribution of phosphatidyl serine producing asymmetry are considered important for its function. There are enzymes described as flippases, floppases, transporters, scramblase, and aminophospholipid translocase that are responsible for this asymmetry which results in aminophospholipids on the cytoplasmic side of the membrane and cholines and sphingolipids on the outer surface.[1–6] The movement of phosphatidyl serine is of importance in the process of blood coagulation.[7–9]

1. Devaux, P.F., Protein involvement in transmembrane lipid asymmetry, *Annu. Rev. Biophys. Biomol. Struct.* 21, 417–439, 1992.

2. Schelgel, R.A., Callahan, M.K., and Williamson, *Ann. N.Y. Acad. Sci.* 926, 271–225, 2000.

3. Daleke, D.L., and Lyles, J.V., Identification and purification of aminophospholipid flippases, *Biochem. Biophys. Acta.* 1486, 108–127, 2000.

4. Balasubramanian, K., and Schroit, A.J., Aminophospholipid asymmetry: A matter of life and death, *Annu. Rev. Physiol.* 65, 701–734, 2003.

5. Daleke, D.L., Regulation of transbilayer plasma membrane phospholipid asymmetry, *J. Lipid. Res.* 44, 233–242, 2003.

6. Bevers, E.M., and Williamson, P.L., Getting to the outer leaflet: Physiology of phosphatidylserine exposure at the plasma membrane, *Physiol. Rev.* 96, 605–645, 2016.

7. Freysinet, J.M., and Toti, F., Formation of procoagulant microparticles and properties, *Thromb. Res.* 125(Suppl 1), S46–S48, 2010.

8. Gilbert, G.E., Novakovic, V.A., Shi, J., Rasmussen, J., and Pipe, S.W., Platelet binding sites for factor VIII in relation to fibrin and phosphatidylserine, *Blood* 126, 1237–1244, 2015.

9. Gao, C., Xie, R., Yu, C., et al., Thrombotic role of blood and endothelial cells in uremia through phosphatidylserine exposure and microparticle release, *PLoS One* 10(11), e0142835, 2015.

AMBISENSE

Single-stranded RNA viruses can be broadly classified into plus (positive) strand [(+)ss] viruses and minus (negative) strand [(−)ss] viruses. Ambisense viruses are frequently included in the negative strand viruses.[1,2] In **plus-strand single-strand RNA viruses**, genomic RNA is messenger RNA (5′→3′) which can directly serve as a template for synthesis of a polyprotein which is subsequently processed.[3] In **negative strand single-strand RNA viruses**, genomic RNA serves as a template (3′→5′) for the synthesis of the various messenger RNAs (**subgenomic RNAs**) required for viral replication.[4] In **ambisense viruses**, the genomic RNA contains both plus-sense sequence and minus-sense sequence and thus can direct serve as the template for protein synthesis with another region serving as the template for the synthesis of subgenomic messenger RNA.[5–8]

1. Lee, J.A., Fraenkel-Conrat, H., and Owens, R.A, *Virology*, 3rd edn., Prentice Hall, Englewood Cliffs, NJ, 1994.

2. Strauss, H.J., and Strauss, E.G., *Viruses and Human Disease*, Academic Press, San Diego, CA, 2002.

3. Paul, D., and Bartenschlager, R., Architecture and biogenesis of plus-strand RNA virus replication factories, *World J. Virol.* 2, 32–48, 2013.

4. Wu, B., and White, K.A., Uncoupling RNA virus replication from transcription via the polymerase: Functional and evolutionary insights, *EMBO J.* 26, 5120–5130, 2007.

5. Ihara, T., and Akashi, H., and Bishop, D.H.L., Novel coding strategy (ambisense genomic RNA) revealed by sequence analysis of Purta Toro phleoviru S RNA, *Virology* 136, 392–306, 1984.

6. Bishop, D.H., Ambisense RNA viruses: Positive and negative polarities combined in RNA virus genomes, *Microbiol. Sci.* 3, 183–187, 1986.

7. Ngugen, M., and Naenni, A.L., Expression strategies of ambisense viruses, *Virus Res.* 93, 141–150, 2003; van Knippenberg, I., and Elliott, R.M., Flexibility of Bunyavirus genomes: Creation of an Orthobunyavirus with an ambisense S segment, *J. Virol.* 89, 5525–5535, 2015.

8. Ciuffo, M., Nerva, L., and Turina, M., Full-length genome sequences of the topsovirus melon severe mosaic virus, *Arch. Virol.* 162, 1419–1422, 2017.

Genome Replication	Single-Strand Virus	Source of mRNA
(+)ss RNA ← (−)ss RNA ←	(+) ssRNA	Genomic RNA is mRNA
(−)ss RNA ← (+)ss RNA ←	(−) ssRNA	Genomic RNA produces mRNA
ss RNA ← cRNA ←	Ambisense ss RNA (ss RNA)	Genomic RNA produces mRNA and is mRNA

AMORPHOUS ICE

Amorphous ice (also known as amorphous water; glassy water)[1] is a frozen form of water that lacks a crystalline structure. Amorphous ice is formed from water frozen at −135°C but not from water frozen at −80°C; water frozen at −135°C lack Bragg peaks on X-ray diffraction and is characterized as an amorphous solid and not a crystalline material.[2] Amorphous ice, in form of high-density amorphous ice, has been suggested to be the most common form of water in the universe.[3] The formation of amorphous ice has been described as the **vitrification of water**.[4] Application of the vitrification of water in the preparation of samples for electron microscopy.[5] has resulted in cryo-electron microscopy. The temperature at which amorphous ice changes to the crystalline state is known as the glass transition temperature and is associated with the transient formation of a liquid form.[6] The glass transition temperature is of importance in the process of lyophilization and is influenced by additives.[7]

1. Mishima, O., and Stanley, H.E., The relationship between liquid, supercooled and glassy water, *Nature* 391, 328–335, 1998.

2. Burton, E.F., and Oliver, W.F., X-Ray diffraction patterns of ice, *Nature* 135, 505–506, 1935.

3. Jenniskens, P., Blake, D.F., Wilson, M.A., and Pohorille, A., High-density amorphous ice, the frost of intersteller grains, *Astrophysical J.* 455, 389–401, 1995.

4. Yannas, I., Vitrification temperature of water, *Science* 160, 298–299, 1968.

5. McDowall, A.W., Chang, J.J., Freeman, R., et al., Electron microscopy of frozen hydrated sections of vitreous ice and vitrified biological sections, *J. Microsc.* 131, 1–9, 1983.

6. Jenniskens, P., Barham, S.F., Blake, D.F., and McCoustra, M.R.S., Liquid water in the domain of crystalline ice I_c, *J. Chem. Phys.* 107, 1231–1241, 1997.

7. Jennings, T.A., *Lyophilization Introduction and Basic Principles*, Intepharm Press, Denver, CO, 1999.

AMORPHOUS POWDER

A solid form of a material that does not have a definite form such as a crystal structure. Differing from a crystal form, an amorphous form is thermodynamically unstable and does not have a defined melting point. The physical characteristics of an amorphous powder make it the desired physical state for drug after lyophilization.[1–5]

1. Jennings, T.A., *Lyophilization Introduction and Basic Principles,* Interpharm Press, Denver, CO, 1999.

2. Royall, P.G., Huang, C.Y., Tang, S.W., et al., The development of DMA for the detection of amorphous content in pharmaceutical powdered material, *Int. J. Pharm.* 301, 181–191, 2005.

3. Stevenson, C.L., Farber, L., Tardos, G.I., and Michaels, J.N., Micro-mechanical properties of drying material bridges of pharmaceutical excipients, *Int. J. Pharm.* 306, 41–55, 2005.

4. Tonnis, W.F., Amori, J.P., Vreeman, M.A., et al., Improved storage stability and immunogenicity of hepatitis B vaccine after spray-freeze drying in the presence of sugars, *Eur. J. Pharm. Sci.* 55, 36–45, 2014.

5. Trnka, H., Palou, A., Panouillet, P.E., et al., Near-infrared imaging for high-throughput screening of moisture induced changes in freeze dried formulations, *J. Pharm. Sci.* 103, 2839–2846, 2014.

AMPHIPATHIC (AMPHIPHILIC)

Amphipathic is a term that describes a compound which has both hydrophilic (lyophilic) and hydrophobic (lyophobic) properties such as sodium dodecyl sulfate (SDS).[1,2] There are proteins with amphipathic properties such as cytochrome b5[3] where the hydrophobic domain is in a membrane.[4] The amphipathic property of cell-penetrating peptides[5,6] is critical for the delivery of nucleic acid-based therapeutics.[7–9]

1. Helenius, A., and Simons, K., Solubilization of membranes by detergents, *Biochim. Biophys. Acta* 415, 29–79, 1975.

2. Jones, M.N., A theoretic approach to binding of amphipathic molecules globular proteins, *Biochem. J.* 151, 109–114, 1975.

3. Robinson, N.C., and Tanford, C., The binding of deoxycholate, Triton X-100, sodium dodecyl sulfate, and phosphatidylcholine vesicles to cytochrome b5, *Biochemistry* 14, 369–378, 1975.

4. Mulrooney, S.B., Meinhardt, D.R., and Waskell, L., The α-helical membrane spanning domain of cytochrome b5 interacts with cytochrome P450 via nonspecific interactions, *Biochim. Biophys. Acta* 1674, 319–326, 2004.

5. El-Andaloussi, S., Holm, T., and Langel, U., Cell-penetrating peptides: Mechanisms and applications, *Curr. Pharm. Des.* 11, 3597–3611, 2005.

6. Deshayes, S., Morris, M.C., Divita, G., and Heitz, F., Interactions of primary amphipathic cell penetrating peptides with model membranes: Consequences on the mechanism of intracellular delivery of therapeutics, *Curr. Pharm. Des.* 11, 3629–3638, 2005.

7. Majidi, A., Nikjkah, M., Sadeghian, F., and Hosseinkhani, S., Development of novel recombinant biomimetic chimeric MPG-based peptide as nanocarriers for gene delivery: Imitation of a real cargo, *Eur. J. Pharm. Biopharm.* 107, 191–204, 2016.

8. Juks, C., Lorents, A., Arukuusk, P., Langel, Ü., and Pooga, M., Cell-penetrating peptides recruit type A scavenger receptors to the plasma membrane for cellular delivery of nucleic acids, *FASEB J.* 31, 975–988, 2017.

9. Vaissière, A., Aldrain, G., Konate, K., et al., A retro-inverso cell-penetrating peptide for siRNA delivery, *J. Nanobiotechnol.* 15(1), 354, 2017.

AMPHIPOL

An amphipol is a linear amphipathic synthetic polymer used to keep membrane proteins in solution.[1,2] Amphipols are thought to bind to sites in membrane proteins different from detergent binding sites and maintain membrane proteins in native conformation.[3,4]

1. Tribet, C., Audebert, R., and Popot, J-L., *Proc. Natl. Acad. Sci. USA* 93, 15047–15050, 1996.

2. Byrne, B., and Jormakka, M., Solubilization and purification of membrane proteins, in *Structural Genomics of Membrane Proteins*, ed. K.H. Lundstrom, Chapter 11, pp. 179–198, CRC Press/Taylor & Francis Group, Boca Raton, FL, 2006.

3. Gorzelle, B.M., Hoffman, A.K., Keyes, M.H., et al., Amphipols can support the activity of a membrane enzyme, *J. Am. Chem. Soc.* 124, 11594–11595, 2002.

4. Watkinson, T.G., Calabrese, A.N., Ault, J.R., Radford, S.E., and Ashcroft, A.E., FPOP-LC-MS/MS suggests differences in interaction of sites of amphipols and detergents with outer membrane proteins, *J. Am. Soc. Mass Spectrom.* 28, 50–55, 2017.

AMPHOLYTE

An ampholyte is an amphoteric electrolyte defined as molecule with both acidic and basic groups.[1] This term is used here to describe the small multi-charged organic buffer(s) used to establish pH gradients for the separation of proteins by isoelectric focusing. The term ampholine® is a proprietary term used for ampholytes used in isoelectric focusing. Ampholytes have functional groups with closely space pKa and Pi values.[2–5] Ampholytes for use in isoelectric focusing can be carrier ampholytes that carry a charge and buffering capacity.[6] The development of ampholytes has been described.[7] See also **zwitterion**.

1. *Oxford English Dictionary*, Oxford, UK, 2017.
2. http://www.lkbprod.com/test/pdf/Electrophoresis.pdf.
3. Svensson, H., Isoelectric fractionation, analysis, and characterization of ampholytes in natural pH gradients. I. The differential equation of solute concentrations at a steady state and its solution for simple cases, *Acta Chem. Scand.* 15, 325–341, 1961.
4. Pettersson, E., Isoelectric fractionation, analysis, and characterization of ampholytes in natural pH gradients IX. A method for obtaining pH gradients in the region below pH 3.0 stable enough to permit isoelectric focusing of ampholytes, *Acta Chem. Scand.* 23, 2631–2635, 1969.
5. Vesterberg, O., Synthesis and isoelectric fractionation of carrier ampholytes, *Acta Chem. Scand.* 23, 2653–2666, 1969.
6. Berkelman, T., Generation of pH gradients, in *Handbook of Isoelectric Focusing and Proteomics,* ed. D. Garfin and S. Ahuja, Chapter 4, pp. 69–92, Elsevier, Amsterdam, the Netherlands, 2005.
7. Righetti, P.G., Incidents of travel in IEF and IPGS, in *Handbook of Isoelectric Focusing and Proteomics,* ed. D. Garfin and S. Ahuja, Chapter 4, pp. xvii–xxii, Elsevier, Amsterdam, the Netherlands, 2005.

AMPHOTERIC

The term amphoteric refers to a condition where a molecule such as protein, peptide, amino acid is capable of having a positive charge, negative charge, or zero net charge depending on solvent conditions.[1–3] Such molecule may be described as a **zwitterion** when at a zero net charge; an example would be an amino acid at its isoelectric point. The amphoteric nature of proteins and peptides is an attribute in their purification by large-scale electrophoresis.[4,5] The amphoteric nature of proteins is a major factor in separation by ion-exchange chromatography.[6] Amphoteric matrices may be of value in chromatographic separation of carbohydrates.[7] There is some use of the term amphoteric to describe herbs with a "balancing effect."[8]

1. Haynes, D., The action of salts and non-electrolytes upon buffer solutions and amphoteric electrolytes and the relation of these effects to the permeability of the cell, *Biochem. J.* 15, 440–461, 1921.
2. Akabori, S., Tani, H., and Noguchi, J., A synthetic amphoteric polypeptide, *Nature* 167, 1591–160, 1951.
3. Coway-Jacobs, A., and Lewin, L.M., Isoelectric focusing in acrylamide gels: Use of amphoteric dyes as internal markers for determination of isoelectric points, *Anal. Biochem.* 43, 294–400, 1971.
4. Akahoshi, A., Sato, K., Nawa, Y., et al., Novel approach for large-scale, biocompatible, and low-cost fractionation of peptides in proteolytic digest of food protein based on the amphoteric nature of peptides, *J. Agric. Food Chem.* 48, 1955–1959, 2000.
5. Hashimoto, K., Sato, K., Nakamura, Y., and Ohtsuki, K., Development of continuous type apparatus for ampholyte-free isoelectric focusing (autofocusing) of peptides in protein hydrolysates, *J. Agric. Food Chem.* 54, 650–655, 2006.
6. Grodzki, A.C., and Berenstein, E., Antibody purification: Ion-exchange chromatography, *Methods Mol. Biol.* 588, 27–32, 2010.
7. Sha, Y., Hasegawa, A., Aimoto, U., and Adachi, S., Distribution of saccharides and salts on amphoteric ion-exchange resin, *Biosci. Biotechnol. Biochem.* 81, 817–822, 2017.
8. Shantaram, P.G., Concept of *Rayasana Chikitsa* w.s.r. *Charaka Samhite, Int. J. Res. Indian Med.* 1, 32–38, 2017). See also **zwitterion**.

AMPLICON

An amplicon is the DNA product of a PCR reaction, usually an amplified segment of a gene or DNA.[1,2] The production of amplicons is important for some approaches to next-generation sequencing of DNA.[3–5] There are some earlier uses of the term amplicon that are not necessarily exclusive from the above.[6,7]

1. Espy, M.J., Smith, T.F., and Persing, D.H., Dependence of polymerase chain reaction product inactivation protocols on amplicon length and sequence composition, *J. Clin. Microbiol.* 31, 2361–2365, 1993.
2. Ikegawa, S., Mabuchi, A., Ogawa, M., and Ikeda, T., Allele-specific PCR amplification due sequence identity between a PCR primer and amplicon: Is direct sequencing reliable? *Hum. Genet.* 110, 606–608, 2002.
3. de la Cuestra-Zuluaga, J., and Escobar, J.S., Considerations for optimizing microbiome analysis using a marker gene, *Front. Nutr.* 3, 26, 2016.
4. Clark, B.E., Shooter, C., Smith, F.M., Brawand, D., and Thein, S.L., Next-generation sequencing as a tool for breakpoint analysis in rearrangement of the globin gene clusters, *Int. J. Lab. Hematol.* 39(Suppl 1), 111–120, 2017.
5. Morgan, H.H., du Toit, M., and Setati, M.E., The grapevine and wine microbiome: Insights from high-throughput amplicon sequencing, *Front. Microbiol.* 8, 820, 2017.

6. Lima-de-Faria, A., Gustafsson, T., and Jaworska, H., Amplification of ribosomal DNA in *Acheta* II. The number of nucleotide pairs of the chromosomes and chromomeres involved in amplification, *Hereditas* 73, 119–142, 1973.
7. Spaete, R.R., and Frankel, N., The herpes simplex virus amplicon: A new eukaryotic defective-virus cloning-amplifying vector, *Cell* 30, 295–304, 1982.

AMYLIN

Amylin is a 37-amino acid peptide hormone, which is a member of the calcitonin peptide family.[1] Amylin is produced in the pancreas has diverse actions but the primary effect is on glucose metabolism via action on the CNS to inhibit the release of glucagon.[2] Amylin acts by G-protein coupled receptors.[3] The amylin receptor has been suggested as pharmacological target for Alzheimer's disease.[4] Amylin was first described as "insulinoma amyloid polypeptide" in the islet amyoid in type 2 human diabetes mellitus,[5] purified from amyloid rich pancreas from type 2 diabetic patients as diabetes associated peptide (DAP)[6] and renamed as amylin in 1988.[7]

1. MacIntyre, I., The calcitonin family of peptides, *Ann. N.Y. Acad. Sci.* 657, 117–118, 1992.
2. Hay, D.L., Chen, S., Lutz, T.A., Parkes, D.G., and Roth, J.D., Amylin: Pharmacology, physiology, and clinical potential, *Pharmacol. Rev.* 67, 564–600, 2015.
3. Hay, D.L., Christopoulos, G., Christopoulos, A., and Sexton, P.M., Amylin receptors: Molecular composition and pharmacology, *Biochem. Soc. Trans.* 32, 865–867, 2004.
4. Qiu, W.C., Amylin and its G-protein-coupled receptor: A probable pathological process and drug target for Alzheimer's disease, *Neuroscience* 360, 44–51, 2017.
5. Westermark, P., Wernstedt, C., O'Brien, T.D., Hayden, D.W., and Johnson, K.H., Islet amyloid in type 2 human diabetes mellitus and adult diabetic cats contains a novel putative polypeptide hormone, *Am. J. Pathol.* 127, 414–417, 1987.
6. Cooper, G.J., Willis, A.C., Clark, A., et al., Purification and characterization of a peptide from amyloid-rich pancreases of type 2 diabetic patients, *Proc. Natl. Acad. Sci. USA* 84, 8628–8632, 1987.
7. Cooper, G.F., Leighton, B., Dimitriadis, G.D., et al., Amylin found in amyloid deposits in human type 2 diabetes mellitus may be a hormone that regulates glycogen metabolism in skeletal muscle, *Proc. Natl. Acad. Sci. USA* 85, 7763–7766, 1988.

AMYLOID

Amyloid was originally described as a starch-like translucent insoluble material, which had a composition similar to a protein found as an infiltrate in a variety of human tissues.[1,2]

Amyloid is now described as an extracellular deposit characterized by a fibrillar structure consisting of proteins that react with Congo Red (congophilic) which show green birefringence in a polarizing microscope.[3] Amyloid deposits, resulting from misfolded proteins, are derived from more than thirty different proteins.[4] The various diseases resulting from the deposition of amyloid, Systemic amyloidosis, are classified according to the protein contributing to the fibrillar deposit.[5] The most prevalent amyloidosis, immunoglobulin light chain amyloidosis, AL amyloidosis (systemic primary amyloidosis), results from misfolded monoclonal antibody light chains[6] while the less prevalent systemic AA amyloidosis (secondary amyloidosis) results from the deposition serum amyloid A.[7] Amyloid deposition is important in a number of neurological disorders, including Alzheimer's disease.[8,9]

1. Budd, G., Amyloid Degeneration, *Brit. Med. J.* 957, 659, 1879.
2. Tschermak, A., Ueber die Stellung der amyloiden Substanz unter den Eniweiss-körpern, *Zeitschrift Physiol. Chem.* 20, 343–356, 1885.
3. Cohen, A.S., Amyloid, in *Encyclopedia of Immunology*, ed. P.J. Delves, pp. 84–86, Elsevier, San Diego, CA, 1998.
4. Chiti, F., and Dobson, C.M., Protein misfolding, amyloid formation, and human disease: A summary of progress over the last decade, *Annu. Rev. Biochem.* 86, 27–68, 2017.
5. Khoor, A., and Colby, T.V., Amyloidosis of the lung, *Arch. Path. Lab. Med.* 141, 247–254, 2017.
6. Kastritis, E., and Dimopoulos, M.A., Recent advances in the management of AL amyloidosis, *Brit. J. Haemat.* 172, 170–186, 2016.
7. Westermark, G.T., Fändrich, M., and Westermark, P., AA amyloidosis: Pathogenesis and targeted therapy, *Annu. Rev. Pathol.* 10, 321–344, 2015.
8. *Alzheimer's Disease. Cellular and Molecular Aspects of Amyloid β*, ed. J.H. Harris and F. Fahrenholz, Springer Science, New York, 2005.
9. Müller, U.C., Deller, T., and Korte, M., Not just amyloid: Physiological functions of the amyloid precursor protein family, *Nat. Rev. Neuroscience* 18, 281–298, 2017.

ANAPHYLATOXIN

The term anaphylatoxin (from the Greek term meaning "without protection")[1] is of historical origin[2,3] and refers to the activities of large peptides/polypeptides released during the complement cascade.[4,5] There are two generally recognized anaphylatoxins, C3a and C5a, which bind to specific G-protein receptors on immune cells to elicit a physiological response.[6–9] C3a is a basic peptide with a molecular weight of approximately

9 kDa.[10] C5a is a glycopolypeptide with a molecular weight of approximately 15,000.[11,12] C4a is a somewhat less studied anaphylatoxin.[13-15] C4a is a somewhat unusual peptide of molecular of approximately 9000 and does not contain carbohydrate, histidine, or tryptophan.[16] There is one report challenging the role of C4a as an anaphylatoxin.[17] Anaphylatoxins are also known as split products.[18]

1. Hugli, T.E., Anaphylatoxin, in *Encyclopedia of Immunology*, ed. I.M. Raitt and P.J. Delves, pp. 63–67, Academic Press, London, UK, 1992.
2. Silverstein, A.M., *A History of Immunology*, p. 218, Academic Press, San Diego, CA, 1989.
3. Friedberger, E., and Valiardi, C., Ueber Anaphlaxie VIII. Mittelung. Die quantitativen Bezielhungen bei der Anaphylatoxinbildung, *Zeitschrift für Immunitaeisforschung under Experimentelle Therapie* 1. Originale 7, 94–157, 1910.
4. Hugli, T.E., and Müller-Eberhard, H.J., Anaphylatoxins: C3a and C5a, *Adv. Immunol.* 26, 1–53, 1978.
5. Mathern, D.R., and Heeger, P.S., Molecules great and small: The complement system, *Clin. J. Am. Soc. Nephrol.* 10, 1636–1650, 2015.
6. Sacks, S.H. Complement fragments C3a and C5a: The salt and pepper of the immune response, *Eur. J. Immunol.* 40, 668–670, 2010.
7. Kemper, C., and Köhl, J., Novel roles for complement receptors in T cell regulation and beyond, *Mol. Immunol.* 56, 181–190, 2013.
8. Quadros, A.U., and Cunha, T.M., C5a and development: An old molecule, a new target, *Pharmacol. Res.* 112, 58–67, 2010.
9. Afshar-Kharghan, V., The role of the complement system in cancer, *J. Clin. Invest.* 127, 780–789, 2017.
10. Hugli, T.E., Human anaphylatoxin (C3a) from the third component of complement. Primary structure, *J. Biol. Chem.* 250, 8293–8301, 1975.
11. Fernandez, H.N., and Hugli, T.E., Partial characterization of human C5a anaphylatoxin. I Chemical description of the carbohydrate and polypeptide portions of human C5a, *J. Immunol.* 117, 1688–1694, 1976.
12. Minta, J.O., and Man, D.P., Cleavage of human C5 by trypsin: Characterization of the digestion products by gel electrophoresis, *J. Immunol.* 119, 1567–1602, 1977.
13. Gorski, J.P., Hugli, T.E., and Müller-Eberhard, H.J., Characterization of human C4a anaphylatoxin, *J. Biol. Chem.* 256, 2707–2711, 1981.
14. Hugli, T.E., Gerard, C., Kawahara, M., et al., Isolation of three separate anaphylatoxins from complement-activated human serum, *Mol. Cell. Biochem.* 41, 59–66, 1981.
15. Lechner, J., Chen, M., Hogg, R.E., et al., Higher plasmas levels of complement C3a, C4a, and C5a increase the risk of subretinal fibrosis in neovascular age-related macular degeneration. Complement activation in AMD, *Immunity Aging* 13, 4, 2016.
16. Moon, K.E., Gorski, J.P., and Hugli, T.E., Complete primary structure of human C4a anaphylatoxin, *J. Biol. Chem.* 256, 8685–8692, 1981.
17. Barnum, S.R., C4a: An anaphylatoxin in name only, *J. Inate Immun.* 7, 333–339, 2015.
18. Stricker, R.B., Savely, V.R., Motanya, N.C., and Gioclas, P.C., Complement split products C3a and C4a in chronic lyme disease, *Scand. J. Immunol.* 69, 64–69, 2008.

ANERGY

Anergy is a term used most frequently to describe the lack of an immune response to an allergen and can refer to an individual immune cell, a tissue, or an intact organism. The term is used most often with respect to T-cells[1] or B-cells[2] but does see occasional use with other cell types.[3] The term clonal anergy is used to indicate that the unresponsive state is due to a single antigen. T-cell anergy is caused by the binding of an antigenic peptide to the T-cell receptor (TCR) without professional costimulation.[4,5] T-cell anergy is thought be different from another state of T-cell unresponsiveness described as T-cell exhaustion.[6] B-cell anergy is a condition of peripheral B cell different from the processes of clonal deletion and receptor editing that occur in the bone marrow. B-cell anergy is a complex process that is suggested to result from early exposure to antigen.[7] A condition similar to B-cell anergy can result from exposure to commercial intravenous immunoglobulin.[8,9]

1. Schwartz, R.H., Anergy, T cell, in *Encyclopedia of Immunology*, ed. P.J. Delves. Academic Press, San Diego, CA, 1998.
2. Tarlinton, D.M., Anergy, B cell, in *Encyclopedia of Immunology*, ed. P.J. Delves. Academic Press, San Diego, CA, 1998.
3. MacGlashan, D.W., Jr., Self-termination/allergic mechanisms in human basophils and mast cells, *Int. Arch. Allergy Immunol.* 150, 109–121, 2009.
4. Schwartz, R.H., T-cell clonal anergy, *Curr. Opin. Immunol.* 9, 351–357, 1997.
5. Koretzky, G.A., T lymphocyte signaling mechanisms and activation, in *Fundmental Immunology*, 6th edn., ed. W.E. Paul, Chapter 11, pp. 346–375, Lippincott/Kluwer, Philadelphia, PA, 2008
6. Pereira, R.M., Hogan, P.G., Rao, A., and Martinez, G.J., Transcriptional and epigenetic regulation of T cell hyporesponsiveness, *J. Leukoc. Biol.*, 102, 601–615, 2017.
7. Yarkoni, Y., Getahun, A., and Cambier, J.C., Molecular underpinning of B-cell anergy, *Immunol. Rev.* 237, 249–263, 2010.
8. Seite, J-F., Goutsmedt, C., Youinou, P., et al., Intravenous immunoglobulin induces a functional silencing program similar to anergy in human B cells, *J. Allergy Clin. Immunol.* 133, 181–188, 2014.

9. Mitrevski, M., Marrapodi, R., Camponeschi, A., et al., Intravenous immunoglobulin and immunomodulation of B-cell—*In vitro* and *in vivo* effects, *Front. Immunol.* 6, 4, 2015.

ANGIOPOIETINS

The angiopoietins are a family of secreted proteins with action on vascular growth and development.[1,2] The angiopoietins (1–4) have approximate molecular weights of 70 kDa but occur as dimers[3] with the exception of angiopoietin-1 that occurs as a tetramer (and larger).[4] Angiopotietin-1 binds to the Tie2 receptor (tyrosine kinase with immunoglobulin-like and EGF-like domain 2) with activation of a tyrosine kinase Angiopotietin-1 binds to the Tie2 receptor (tyrosine kinase with immunoglobulin-like and EGF-like domain 2) with activation of a tyrosine kinase.[5] Angiopotietin-1 contains substantial carbohydrate.[6] Angiopoietin-2 is more complex acting as an agonist and antagonist for the Tie2 receptor.[7] In addition to roles in vascular development, the angiopoietins have a role in tumor development and inflammation[8,9] providing an opportunity for therapeutic intervention.[10] There is a group of eight proteins with homology to the angiopoietins described as the angiopoietin-like proteins.[11] Some of these proteins are involved in the control of lipoprotein metabolism.[12,13]

1. Eklund, L., and Saharinen, P., Angiopoietin signaling in the vascular, *Exp. Cell Res.* 319, 1271–1280, 2013.
2. Eklund, L., Kangas, J., and Saharinen, P., Angiopoietin-Tie signaling in the cardiovascular and lymphatic systems, *Clin. Sci.* 131, 87–103, 2016.
3. Lee, H.J., Cho, C-H., Hwang, S-J., et al., Biological characterization of angiopoietin-3 and angiopoietin-4, *FASEB J.* 18, 1200–1208, 2004.
4. Davis, S., Papadopoulos, N., Aldrich, T.H., et al., Angiopoietins have distinct modular domains essential for receptor binding, dimerization and superclustering, *Nat. Struct. Biol.* 10, 38–44, 2003.
5. Yu, X., Seegar, T.C.M., Dalton, A.C., et al., Structural basis for angiopoietin-1-mediated signaling initiation, *Proc. Natl. Acad. Sci. USA* 110, 7205–7210, 2013.
6. Davis, S., Aldrich, T.H., Jones, P.F., et al., Isolation of angiopoietin-1, a ligand for the Tie2 receptor, by secretion-trap expression cloning, *Cell* 87, 1161–1169, 1996.
7. Thurston, G., and Daly, C., The complex role of angiopoietin-2 in the angiopoietin-Tie signaling pathway, *Cold Spring Harb. Perspect. Med.* 2, a006650, 2012.
8. Saharinen, P., Eklund, L., Pulkki, K., Bono, P., and Alitalo, K., VEGF and angiogenesis signaling in tumor angiogenesis and metastasis, *Trends Mol. Med.* 17, 347–362, 2011.
9. Scholz, A., Piale, K.H., and Reiss, Y., Angiopoietin-2: A multifaceted cytokine that functions in both angiogenesis and inflammation, *Ann. N.Y. Acad. Sci.* 1347, 45–51, 2015.
10. Saharinen, P., Eklund, P., and Alitalo, K., Therapeutic targeting of the angiopoietin-TIE pathway, *Nat. Rev. Drug Discov.* 16, 635, 2017.
11. Santulli, G., Angiopoietin-like proteins: A comprehensive look, *Front. Endocrinol.* 5, 4, 2014.
12. Tikka, A., and Jauhiainen, M., The role of ANGPTL3 in controlling lipoprotein metabolism, *Endocrine* 52, 187–193, 2016.
13. Andron, J.S., and Hegele, R.A., Genetics of triglycerides and the risk of atherosclerosis, *Curr. Atheroscler. Rep.* 19:31, 2017.

ANISOTROPY

Anisotropy, derived from the Greek word for turning, is the difference in values, when measured on different axes, obtained for a physical quantity of a material. The optical properties of a crystal are anisotropic; the value of the refractive index depends on the direction of light relative to crystallographic axes.[1] Anisotropy is (usually) only observed in solids; liquids, glasses and amorphous material are isotropic unless subject to external forces. Anisotropy is important for a variety of disciplines, including geology where the magnetic susceptibility in a mineral depends on direction which it is measured.[2] Anisotropy is also condition of seismic waves with different velocities in vertical and horizontal directions.[3] In botany, anisotropy is used for differential development of the cytoskeleton.[4,5] Anisotropy is of importance to two analytical techniques in biochemistry: fluorescence anisotropy and nuclear magnetic resonance. Fluorescence anisotropy is based on the principle of photoselective excitation of fluorophores by polarized light[6] and is of use in the study of protein structure.[7–9] Chemical shift anisotropy is observed when the magnitude of the chemical shift is dependent on the orientation of the molecule in the external magnetic field. Chemical shift anisotropy is of importance in solid-state NMR; chemical shift anisotropy is reduced to zero by random molecular motion.[10] Anisotropy is important in the nuclear magnetic resonance study of membranes.[11–13]

1. Fox, M., *Optical Properties of Solids*, Oxford University Press, Oxford, UK, 2010.
2. Collinson, D.W., *Methods in Rock Magnetism and Paleomagnetism. Techniques and Instrumentation*, Chapman and Hall, London, UK, 1983.
3. *Glossary of Geology*, ed. J.A. Jackson, American Geological Institute, Alexandria, VA, 1997.
4. Baskin, T.I., Anisotropic expansion of the plant cell wall, *Annu. Rev. Cell Dev. Biol.* 21, 203–222, 2005.
5. Wasteneys, G.O., and Fujita, M., Establishing and maintaining axial growth: Wall mechanical properties and the cytoskeleton, *J. Plant Res.* 119, 5–10, 2006.

6. Lakoowicz, J.R., *Principles of Fluorescence Spectroscopy*, Springer, New York, 2006.

7. Bucci, E., and Steiner, R.F., Anisotropy decay of fluorescence as an experimental approach to protein dynamics, *Biophys. Chem.* 30, 199–224, 1988.

8. Matozo, H.C., Santos, M.A, de Oliveira Neto, M., et al., Low-resolution structure and fluorescence anisotropy analysis of protein tyrosine phosphatase η catalytic domain, *Biophys. J.* 92, 4424–4432, 2007.

9. Goodrich, A.C., Meyers, D.J., and Frueh, D.P., Molecular impact of covalent modifications on nonribosomal peptide synthetase carrier protein communication, *J. Biol. Chem.* 292, 10002–10013, 2017.

10. http://www.protein-nmr.org.uk/general/chemical-shifts/chemical-shift-anisotropy/.

11. Gopinath, T., More, K.R., and Veglia, G., Sensitivity and resolution enhancement or oriented solid-state NMR: Application to membrane proteins, *Prog. Nucl. Mag. Res. Spectroscopy* 75, 50–68, 2013.

12. Zhang, L., Liu, L., Maltsev, S., Lorigan, G.A., and Dabney-Smith, C., Solid-state NMR investigations of peptide-lipid interactions of the transmembrane domain of a plant derived protein, Hct106, *Chem. Phys. Lipids* 175–176, 123–130, 2013.

13. De Simone, A., Mote, K.R., and Veglia, G., Structural dynamics and conformational equilibria of SERCA regulatory proteins in membranes by solid-state NMR restrained simulations, *Biophys. J.* 106, 2566–2576, 2014.

ANKYRIN REPEAT

The ankyrin repeat (less frequently referred to as the ankyrin domain) is a 30–34 amino acid sequence,[1] so named from the protein in which they were described.[2] Ankyrin was originally described as being critical for the binding of the spectrin in the cytoskeleton to the membrane in red blood cells. Subsequent work showed that ankyrin was also associated with Band 3 protein.[3] The role of ankyrin has continued to evolve.[4,5] Ankyrin repeat proteins are also found in *Drosophila*.[6,7] Current interest in ankyrin repeats is based on its role in mediating protein-protein interactions.[8] Designed ankyrin repeat proteins (DARPins) have been of particular interest as alternatives to antibodies in binding to therapeutic targets such as receptors[9] where binding is optimized by phage display, ribosomal display, or related technologies.[10–12]

1. Davis, L.H., and Bennett, V., Mapping the binding sites of human erythrocyte ankyrin for anion exchanger and spectrin, *J. Biol. Chem.* 265, 10589–10596, 1990.

2. Bennett, V., and Stenbuck, P.J., Identification and partial purification of ankyrin, the high affinity membrane attachment site for human erythrocyte spectrin, *J. Biol. Chem.* 254, 2533–2541, 1979.

3. Bennett, V., and Stanbuck, P.J., The membrane attachment protein for spectrin is associated with band 3 in human erythrocyte membranes, *Nature* 280, 468–473, 1979.

4. Baines, A.J., Evolution of spectrin function in cytoskeletal and membrane networks, *Biochem. Soc. Trans.* 37, 796–803, 2009.

5. Lux, S.E., IV, Anatomy of the red cell membrane skeleton: Unanswered questions, *Blood* 127, 187–199, 2016.

6. Gay, N.J., and Ntwasa, M., The *Drosophila* ankyrin protein cactus has a predominately α-helical secondary structure, *FEBS Lett.* 335, 155–160, 1993.

7. Domsch, K., Acs, A., Obermeier, C., Nguyen, H.T., and Reim, I., Identification of the essential protein domains for Mib2 function during the development of the *Drosophila* larval musculature and adult flight muscles, *PLoS One* 12(3), e1073733, 2017.

8. Li, J., Mahajan, A., and Tsai, M.-D., Ankyrin repeat: A unique motif mediating protein-protein interactions, *Biochemistry* 45, 15168–15178, 2006.

9. Stumpp, M.T., Binz, H.K., and Amstutz, P., DARPins: A new generation of protein therapeutics, *Drug Discov. Today* 13, 695–701, 2008.

10. Steiner, D., Forrer, P., and Plückthun, A., Efficient selection of DARPins with sub-nanomolar affinities using SRP phage display, *J. Mol. Biol.* 382, 1211–1227, 2008.

11. Plückthun, A., Designed ankyrin repeat proteins (DARPins): Binding proteins for research, diagnostics and therapy, *Annu. Rev. Pharmacol. Toxicol.* 55, 489–511, 2015.

12. Houlihan, G., Gatti-Lafraconi, P., Lowe, D., and Hollfelder, F., Directed evolution of anti-HER2 DARPins by SNAP display reveals stability/function trade-offs in the selection process, *Protein Eng. Des. Sel.* 28, 269–279, 2015.

ANNOTATION

The term annotation describes information added to a text after the initial overall entry. *Oxford English Dictionary* defines it as "to add notes to, to furnish with notes".[1] Most frequently used in molecular biology for the addition of information regarding function to the initial description of a gene/gene sequence in a genome.[2–5] However, as data acquisition becomes more complex in other areas, it has been applied, for example, to metabolomics.[6,7]

1. *Oxford English Dictionary*, Oxford University Press, Oxford, UK, 2019.

2. Engel, K.L., Mackiewicz, M., Hardigan, A.A., Myers, R.M., and Savic, D., Decoding transcriptional enhancers: Evolving from annotation to functional interpretation, *Semin. Cell Dev. Biol.* 57, 40–50, 2016.

3. Mudge, J.M., and Harrow, J., The state of play in higher eukaryote gene annotation, *Nat. Rev. Genet.* 17, 758–772, 2016.

4. Thomas, C.M., Thomson, N.R., et al., Annotation of plasmid genes, *Plasmid* 91, 61–67, 2017.

5. Steward, C.A., Parker, A.P.I., Minassian, B.A., et al., Genome annotation for clinical genomic diagnostics: Strengths and weaknesses, *Genome Med.* 9(1), 49, 2017.
6. Allard, P.M., Genta-Jouve, G., and Wolfender, J.L., Deep metabolome annotation in natural product research: Toward a virtuous cycle in metabolite identification, *Curr. Opin. Chem. Biol.* 36, 40–49, 2017.
7. Viant, M.R., Kurland, I.J., Jones, M.R., and Dunn, W.B., How close are we to complete annotation of metabolomes? *Curr. Opin. Chem. Biol.* 36, 64–69, 2017.

ANOIKIS

Anoikis is a term describing apoptosis (programmed cell death) following cell detachment from extracellular matrix.[1,2] Anoikis resistance is considered a critical step in tumor metastasis.[3,4]

1. Gilmore, A.P. Anoikis, *Cell Death Different* 12, 1473–1477, 2005.
2. Paoli, P., Giannoni, E., and Chiarugi, P., *Anoikis* molecular pathways and its role in cancer progression, *Biochem. Biophys. Acta* 1833, 3481–3498, 2013.
3. Geiger, T.R., and Peeper, D.S., The neutrotrophic receptor TrkB in anoikis resistance and metastasis: A perspective, *Cancer Res.* 65, 7033–7036, 2005.
4. de Sousa Mesquita, A.P., de Araújo Lopes, S., Pernambuco Filho, P.C.A., Nader, H.B., and Lopes, C.C., Acquisition of anoikis resistance promotes alterations in the Ras/ERK and PI3K/Akt signaling pathways and matrix remodeling in endothelial cells, *Apoptosis* 22, 1116–1137, 2017.

ANTH DOMAIN

Proteins containing the ANTH Domain (assembly protein 180 [AP180] N-terminal homology domain) bind to membranes and participate in the process of clathrin-mediated endocytosis.[1,2] The ANTH domain binds to phosphoinositol 4,5-diphosphate [Ptd(4,5)P_2] in the plasma membrane.[3] ANTH-containing proteins participate with ENTH-domain (epsin N-terminal homology domain) in clathrin-mediated endocytosis.[4] Proteins with the ANTH domain are involved in with the trafficking between the Golgi apparatus and endosomes.[5]

1. Silkov, A., Yoon, Y., Lee, H., et al., Genome-wide structural analysis reveals novel membrane binding properties of AP180 N-terminal homology (ANTH) domains, *J. Biol. Chem.* 286, 34155–34163, 2011.
2. Skruzny, M., Brach, T. Ciuffa, R., et al., Molecular basis for coupling the plasma membrane to the actin cytoskeleton during clathrin-mediated endocytosis, *Proc. Natl. Acad. Sci. USA* 109, E2533–E2542, 2012.
3. Sun, Y., Kaksonen, M., Madden, D.T., Sheckman, R., and Drubin, D.G., Interaction of Sla2p's ANTH domain with Ptd(4,5)P_2 is important for actin-dependent endocytotic internalization, *Mol. Biol. Cell* 16, 717–730, 2005.
4. Mann, P.T., Gadelha, C., Putlick, A.E., and Field, M.C., ENTH and ANTCH domain proteins participate in AP2-independent clathrin-mediated endocytosis, *J. Cell. Sci.* 128, 2130–2142, 2015.
5. Duncan, M.C., and Payne, G.S., ENTH/ANTH domains expand to the Golgi, *Trends Cell Biol.* 13, 211–215, 2003; Zouhar, J., and Sauer, M., Helping hands for budding prospects: ENTH/ANTH/VHS accessory proteins in endocytosis, vacuolar transport, and secretion, *Plant Cell* 26, 4232–4244, 2014.

ANTIBODY

Antibodies are synthesized and secreted by differentiated B cells (plasma cells) in response to an antigen which is usually a protein that may be present the cell wall of a bacterial or in the coat protein of a virus (the adaptive immune response). Antibodies are considered reasonably specific for reaction with a specific antigen. This specificity forms the basis for immunoassays such as ELISA and immunoprecipitation. The various classes of antibodies are IgM, IgG, IgA, IgD, and IgE. IgM is a pentamer of IgG, comprises about half of the adult IgM population and is thought to function in the initial response to pathogens.[1,2] IgG is the major immunoglobulin adult blood and the effector of the adaptive immune response and is their therapeutic product in intravenous immunoglobulin.[3] Therapeutic antibody preparations are polyclonal in that such preparations are derived from proteins produced by a population of plasma cells and found in the γ-globulin fraction of blood plasma.[4] Monoclonal antibodies are primarily IgG in nature and derived from a single plasma cell. A hybridoma is the product of the fusion of a tumor cell with a plasma cell.[5,6] IgA is responsible for mucosal defense.[7] Natural antibodies, IgM, IgA, and IgG, are produced in the apparent absence of exposure to external antigens.[8] Antibodies can be formed against self; such antibodies are referred to as autoantibodies. Disease resulting from the formation of antibodies are called autoimmune diseases.[9,10] There are unusual naturally occurring antibodies such as camelid antibodies[11,12] and artificial derivatives such as Fab' fragments and scFv fragments, which can be considered derivatives of IgG proteins.[13] Antibody quality for immunoassays is an issue.[14]

1. Klimovich, V.G., IgM and its receptors: Structural and functional aspects, *Biochemistry* 76, 534–549, 2011.

2. Grönwall, C., and Silverman, G.J., Natural IgM: Beneficial autoantibodies for the control of inflammatory and autoimmune disease, *J. Clin. Immunol.* 34(Suppl 1), S12–S21, 2014.

3. Schwab, I., and Nimmerjahn, F., Intravenous immunoglobulin therapy: How does IgG modulate the immune system? *Nat. Rev. Immunol.* 13, 176–189, 2013.

4. Wine, Y., Boutz, D.B., Lavinder, J.J., et al., Molecular deconvolution of the monoclonal antibodies that comprise the polyclonal serum response, *Proc. Natl. Acad. Sci.USA* 110, 2993–2998, 2013.

5. Kohler, G., and Milstein, C., Continuous cultures of fused cells secreted antibody of predefined specificity, *Nature* 256, 495–497, 1973.

6. Smith, S.A., and Crowe, J.E., Jr., Use of human hybridoma technology to isolate human monoclonal antibodies, *Microbiol. Spect.* 3(1), AID-0027-2014, 2015.

7. Heineke, M.H., and van Egmond, M., Immunoglobulin A: Magic bullet or Trojan horse? *Eur. J. Clin. Invest.* 47, 184–192, 2017.

8. Panda, S., and Ding, J.L., Natural antibodies bridge innate and adaptive immunity, *J. Immunol.* 194, 13–20, 2015.

9. Tan, E.M., Autoantibodies, autoimmune disease, and the birth of immune diagnostics, *J. Clin. Invest.* 122, 3835–3836, 2012.

10. Hu, Z.D., and Dend, A.M., Autoantibodies in pre-clinical autoimmune disease, *Clin. Chim. Acta* 437, 14–18, 2014.

11. Muyldermans, S., Single domain camel antibodies: Current status, *J. Biotechnol.* 74, 277–302, 2001.

12. Desmyter, A., Spinelli, S., Roussel, A., and Cambillau, C., Camelid nanobodies: Killing two birds with one stone, *Curr. Opin. Struct. Biol.* 32, 1–8, 2015.

13. Tiller, K.E., and Tessier, P.M., Advances in antibody design, *Annu. Rev. Biomed. Eng.* 17, 191–216, 2015.

14. Roncador, G., Engel, P., Maestre, L., The European antibody network's practical guide to finding and validating suitable antibodies for research, *MABs* 18, 27–36, 2016.

ANTIBODY-BASED PROTEOMICS

Antibody-based proteomics[1] is the use of antibodies for the analysis of the proteome. One example would be the use of an antibody-based protein microarrays.[2] Another approach is reverse-phase protein arrays (RPPAs).[3] Antibody-based proteomics can also be used in immunohistochemistry.[4,5] Antibody-based proteomics is a type of affinity proteomics.[6] The limiting factor in antibody-based proteomics and other immunoassay technologies is the lack of large numbers of validated antibodies.[7] While recombinant monoclonal antibodies are the reagent of choice, progress can be made with monospecific antibodies derived from polyclonal preparations.[8–10] Antibody-based proteomics can be distinguished from immunoproteomics as antibody-based proteomics is the use of antibodies in proteomics while immunoproteomics is based on the use of proteomic technologies to study the proteins involved in humoral and cellular immunology. See also **immunoproteomics**.

1. Wingren, C., Antibody-based proteomics, *Adv. Exp. Med. Biol.* 926, 163–179, 2016.

2. Delfani, P., Dexlin Mellby, L., Nordström, M., et al., Technical advances for the recombinant antibody microarray technology platform for clinical immunoproteomics, *PLoS One* 11(7), e159138, 2016.

3. Lu, Y., Ling, S., Hegde, A.M., et al., Using reverse-phase protein arrays as pharmacodynamic assays for functional proteomics, biomarker discovery, and drug development in cancer, *Sem. Oncology* 43, 476–483, 2016.

4. Lindskog, C., The potential clinical impact of the tissue-based map of the human proteome, *Expert Rev. Proteomics* 12, 213–215, 2015.

5. Zieba, A., Sjöstedt, E., Olovsson, M., et al., The human endometrium-specific proteome defined by transcriptomics and antibody-based profiling, *OMICS* 19, 659–668, 2015.

6. Olsson, N., Wingren, C., Mattsson, M., et al., Proteomic analysis and discovery using affinity proteomics and mass spectrometry, *Mol. Cell. Proteomics* 11: M110.003962, 2011.

7. Roncador, G., Engel, P., Maestre, L., The European antibody network's practical guide to finding and validating suitable antibodies for research, *MABs* 18, 27–36, 2016.

8. Agaton, C., Falk, R., Holden Guthenberg, I., et al., Selective enrichment of monospecific polyclonal antibodies for antibody-based proteomics efforts, *J. Chromatog. A* 1043, 33–40, 2004.

9. Hjelm, B., Forsström, B., Igel, U., et al., Generation of monospecific antibodies based on affinity capture of polyclonal antibodies, *Protein Science* 20, 1824–1835, 2011.

10. Edfors, F., Boström, T., Forsström, B., et al., Immunoproteomics using polyclonal antibodies and stable isotope-labeled affinity purified recombinant proteins, *Mol. Cell. Proteomics* 13: 1611–1624, 2014.

ANTIBODY-DEPENDENT CELLULAR CYTOTOXICITY (ADCC)

Antibody-dependent cellular cytotoxicity (ADCC) is the process by which a host organism destroys bacterial and viral pathogens[1,2] and also is used to describe the mechanism by which tumor cells are lysed secondary to treatment with antibodies.[3,4] The process involves the recognition of epitopes by the Fab region of the IgG on the target cell surface resulting in the binding of the antibody. The Fc domain is then recognized by a phagocytic cell such as a natural killer (NK) cell.[5] The Fc domain of the antibody is critical for ADCC.[6]

1. Lowell, G.H., Smith, L.F., Artenstein, M.S., Nash, G.S., and MacDermott, R.P., Jr., Antibody-dependent cell-mediated antibacterial activity of human mononuclear cells. I. K lymphocytes and monocytes are effective against meningococci in cooperation with human immune sera, *J. Exp. Med.* 150, 127–137, 1979.
2. Wren, L.H., Stratov, I., Kent, S.J., and Parsons, M.S., Obstacles to ideal anti-HIV antibody-dependent cellular cytotoxicity responses, *Vaccine* 31, 5506–5517, 2013.
3. Iannello, A., and Ahmad, A., Role of antibody-dependent cell-mediated cytotoxicity in the efficacy of therapeutic anti-cancer monoclonal antibodies, *Cancer Rev.* 24, 487–499, 2005.
4. Gül, N., and van Egmond, M., Antibody-dependent phagocytosis of tumor cells by macrophages: A potent effector mechanism of monoclonal antibody therapy of cancer, *Cancer Res.* 75, 5008–5013, 2015.
5. Wallace, P.K., Howell, A.L., and Fanger, M.W., Role of Fcγ receptors in cancer and infectious disease, *J. Leukoc. Biol.* 55, 816–826, 1994.
6. Boesch, A.W., Brown, E.P., and Ackerman, M.E., The role of the Fc receptors in HIV prevention and therapy, *Immunol. Rev.* 268, 296–310, 2015.

ANTIBODY VALENCE

Antibody valence refers to the number of antigen binding sites on a single antibody molecule. An IgG molecule that consists of two heavy chain and two light chains (a dimer of heterodimers) has two antibody-binding sites and hence it is bivalent and has a valency of two, although the observed valency can be influenced by the spacing of cognate epitopes.[1] IgM is a pentamer of IgG and thus should have a valency of 10; however, observed valency has been shown to vary with epitope (hapten) concentration[2] and antigen size.[3] An scFv fragment is monovalent as are some other IgG derivatives which contain only one paratope.[4] The scFv fragment can be combined with other scFV fragments to yield hetero- and homo diabodies and tribodies.[5,6]

1. Dimmock, N.J., and Hardy, S.A., Valency of antibody binding to virions and its determination by surface plasmon resonance, *Rev. Med. Virology* 14, 123–135, 2004.
2. Goldstein, B., Theory of hapten binding to IgM: The question of repulsive interactions between binding sites, *Biophys. Chem.* 3, 363–367, 1975.
3. Edberg, S.C., Bronson, P.M., and Van Oss, C.J., The valency of IgM and IgG rabbit anti-dextran antibody as a function of the size of dextran molecule, *Immunochemisry* 9, 273–288, 1972.
4. Li, K., Zettlitz, K.A., Lipianskaya, J., et al., A fully human scFv phage display library for rapid antibody fragment reformatting, *Protein Eng. Des. Selection* 28, 307–315, 2015.

5. Korti, A.A., Dolezal, O., Power, B.E., and Hudson, P.J., Dimeric and trimeric antibodies: High avidity scFvs for cancer targeting, *Biomol. Eng.* 18, 95–108, 2001.
6. Kamada, H., Taki, S., Nagano, K., et al., Generation and characterization of a bispecific diabody targeting both EPH receptor A10 and CD3, *Biochem. Biophys. Res. Commun.* 456, 908–912, 2015.

ANTIGEN

An antigen is a material such as protein, polysaccharide, or microorganism that elicits an immune response. An immune response can be the formation of an antibody directed against the antigen (humoral response; B-cell response) as well as a cellular response (T-cell response) or both. An epitope is a specific region on an antigen which can elicit an immune response; thus an antigen may have several epitopes. A humoral response to a single epitope can elicit a polyclonal response.[1] Antigens may be separated into immunogens which can elicit an immune response with antibody formation[2,3] and haptens which do not by themselves elicit an immune response but can react with antibodies.[4,5] Haptens require conjugation with a larger molecule such as protein to elicit antibody formation.[6,7]

1. Wine, Y., Boutz, D.R., Lavinder, J.J., et al., Molecular deconvolution of the monoclonal antibodies that comprise the polyclonal serum response, *Proc. Natl. Acad. Sci. USA* 110, 2993–2999, 2013.
2. Sattentau, Q.J., Immunogen design to focus the B-cell repertoire, *Curr. Opin. HIV AIDS* 9, 217–223, 2014.
3. Das, S., Boliar, S., Samal, S., et al., Identification and characterization of a naturally occurring, efficiently cleaved, membrane-bound, clade A HIV-1 Emv, suitable for immunogen design, with properties comparable to membrane-bound BG505, *Virology* 510, 22–28, 2017.
4. Avery, O.T., and Goebel, W.F., Chemo-immunological studies on conjugated carbohydrate-proteins; II. Immunological specificity of synthetic sugar antigens, *J. Exp. Med.* 50, 533–550, 1929.
5. Nishikawa, T., Nephelometric immunoassay for therapeutic drug level monitoring, *Pharm. Res.* 1, 105–109, 1984.
6. Hermanson, G.T., *Bioconugate Techniques*, Elsevier, Amsterdam, the Netherlands, 2013.
7. Fujiwara, K., Yasuno, M., and Kitagawa, T., Novel preparation method of immunogen for hydrophobic hapten, enzyme immunoassay for daunomycin and adrimycin, *J. Immunol. Methods* 45, 195–203, 1981.

ANTIGENIC DETERMINANT

An antigenic determinant or epitope is that portion of an immunogen that binds to an antibody.[1] An immunogen may have one or more antigenic determinants, each of which will elicit an immune response.[2,3] There are linear or continuous determinants that would be a continuous amino acid sequence in an antigenic determinant[4–6] or conformational or discontinuous determinants where, for example, with a protein, the epitope is formed by protein folding.[7–9] An immunogen may contain both continuous and discontinuous epitopes.[10] A linear determinant is recognized by T cells as well as B cell and antibodies, while a discontinuous determinant is recognized only by B cells and antibodies.[11,12]

1. Kabat, E.A., The nature of an antigenic determinant, *J. Immunol.* 97, 1–11, 1966.
2. Blondelle, S.E., Moya-Castro, R., Osawa, K., Schroeder, K., and Wilson, D.B., Immunogenically optimized peptides derived from natural mutants of HIV CTL epitopes and peptide combinatorial libraries, *Biopolymers* 90, 683–694, 2008.
3. Brinck-Jensen, N-S., Leutscher, P.D.C., Petersen, E., Vorup-Jensen, T., and Erikstrup, C., Immunogenicity of twenty-peptides representing epitopes of the hepatitis B core and surface antigens by IFN-γ response in chronic and resolved HBV, *BMC Immunology* 16, 65, 2015.
4. Lew, A.M., Langford, C.J., Anders, R.F., et al., A protective monoclonal antibody recognizes a linear epitope in the precursor to the major marozoite antigens of *Plasmodium chabaudi adami*, *Proc. Natl. Acad. Sci. USA* 86, 3768–3185, 1989.
5. Hansen, C.S., Dufva, M., Bøgh, K.L., et al., Linear epitope mapping of peanut allergens demonstrates individualized and persistent antibody-binding patterns, *J. Allergy Clin. Imnunol.* 138, 1728–1730, 2016.
6. Izac, J.C., Oliver, L.D., Jr., Earnhart, C.G., and Marconi, R.T., Identification of a defined linear epitope in the OSpA protein of the Lyme disease spirochetes that elicits bacterial antibody responses: Implications of vaccine development, *Vaccine* 35, 3178–3185, 2017.
7. Thiel, C., Weber, K., and Gerke, V., Characterization of a discontinuous epitope on annexin II by site-directed mutagenesis, *FEBS Lett.* 285, 59–62, 1991.
8. Hager-Braun, C., Hochleitner, E.O., Gorny, M.K., et al., Characterization of a discontinuous epitope of the HIV envelope protein gp120 recognized by a human monoclonal antibody using chemical modification and mass spectrometric analysis, *J. Am. Soc. Mass Specttrom.* 21, 1687–1698, 2016.
9. Werkhoven, P.R., Elwakiel, M., Meuleman, T.J., et al., Molecular construction of HIV-gp120 discontinuous epitope mimics by assembly of cyclic peptides on an orthogonal alkyne functionalized TAC-scaffold, *Org. Bioorg. Chem.* 14, 701–710, 2016.
10. Norek, A., and Janda, L., Epitopoe mapping of *Borrelia burgdorferi* OspC protein in homodimeric fold, *Protein Sci.* 26, 796–806, 2017.
11. Atassi, M.Z., Bixler, G.S., Jr., and Yokoi, T., Conformation-dependent recognition of a protein by T cells requires presentation with processing, *Biochem. J.* 259, 731–735, 1989.
12. Levine, T.P., and Chain, B.M., The cell biology of antigen processing, *Crit. Rev. Biochem. Mol. Biol.* 26, 439–473, 1991.

ANTI-IDIOTYPIC

Anti-idiotypic is a term used in reference to antibodies whose specificity is directed against the idiotypic region of an antibody (the region of the antibody that confers specificity, the CDR region or paratope); most frequently with naturally occurring antibodies including IgE.[1–4] An anti-idiotypic antibody has also been developed for the pharmacokinetic analysis of a therapeutic antibody.[5] An anti-idiotypic antibody against a pathogenic autoantibody has been isolated from intravenous immunoglobulin (IVIG).[6] Since receptors and antibodies share common binding characteristics,[7] the term anti-idiotypic is sometimes used to describe antibodies directed against receptors.[8–12] See **idiotypic**.

1. Hebert, J., and Boutin, Y., Anti-idiotypic antibodies in the treatment of allergies, *Adv. Exp. Med. Biol.* 409, 431–437, 1996.
2. Bobu, K.S., Arshad, S.H., and Holgate, S.T., Omalizumab, a novel anti-IgE therapy in allergic disorders, *Expert Opin. Biol. Ther.* 1, 1049–1058, 2001.
3. Nyborg, A.C., Zacco, A., Ettinger, R., et al., Development of an antibody that neutralized soluble IgE and eliminates IgE expressing B cells, *Cell. Mol. Immunol.* 13, 391–400, 2016.
4. Licari, A., Castagnoli, R., De Sando, E., and Maseglia, G.L., Development of a peptide conjugate vaccine for inducing therapeutic anti-IgE antibodies, *Expert. Opin. Biol. Ther.* 17, 429–434, 2017.
5. Lim, S.Y., Chan, C.E., Lisowska, M.M., Hanson, B.J., and MacAry, P.A., The molecular engineering of an anti-idiotypic antibody for pharmacokinetic analysis of a fully human anti-infective, *PLoS One* 10(12), e0145381, 2015.
6. Svetlicky, N., Kivity, S., Odeh, Q., et al., Anti-citrullinated-protein-antibody-specific intravenous immunoglobulin attenuates collagen-induced arthritis in mice, *Clin. Exp. Immunol.* 182, 241–250, 2015.
7. Englebienne, P., *Immune and Receptor Assays in Theory and Practice*, CRC Press, Boca Raton, FL, 2000.
8. Couraud, P.O., and Strosberg, A.D., Anti-idiotypic antibodies against hormone and neurotransmitter receptors, *Biochem. Soc. Trans.* 19, 147–151, 1991.
9. Erlanger, B.F., Antibodies to receptors by an auto-anti-idiotypic strategy, *Biochem. Soc. Trans.* 19, 138–143, 1991.

10. Jurzak, M., Jans, D.A., Hasse, W., Peters, R., and Fahrenholz, F., Generation of anti-idiotypic monoclonal antibodies recognizing vasopressin receptors in cultured cells and kidney sections, *Exp. Cell. Res.* 202, 182–191, 1992.
11. Christanson, C.J., Sun, V.Z., Akilesh, S., et al., Monoclonal antibodies directed against human FcRn and their applications, *MAbs* 4, 208–216, 2012.
12. Lan, H., Hong, P., Li, R., et al., Internal image anti-idiotypic antibody: A new strategy for the development a new category of protactin receptor (PRLR) antagonist, *Mol. Immunol.* 87, 86–93, 2017.

ANTISENSE NUCLEOTIDE (ANTISENSE OLIGONUCLEOTIDE)

The term antisense nucleotide refers a nucleotide sequence (oligonucleotide; either DNA or RNA) that is complementary (antisense) to a sequence of messenger RNA which is the product of the noncoding (antisense) sequence of DNA. There are some natural antisense RNA molecules that are antisense to DNA. The original work observed inhibition of protein synthesis in *E. coli* by antisense DNA oligonucleotide where the phosphodiester bond was replaced with a methylcarbamate linkage.[1] There are a variety of antisense nucleotide therapies that are mostly directed against RNA.[2] An antisense sequence will have therefore a sequence identical (with the exception of U for T with an RNA) to the noncoding DNA sequence and will bind, in principle, to mRNA and inhibit transcription. Antisense oligonucleotide is, for the most, Hud products of chemical synthesis. Since the naturally occurring phosphodiester bond linking the individual nucleotides is labile, other linkage technologies are used such as phosphoroamidate linkages join morpholino nucleic acids.[3,4] Antisense nucleotides are also referred to as complementary nucleotides.[5] While most antisense nucleotides are the product of chemical synthesis, there are some naturally occurring antisense products.[6–9] Antisense nucleotides differ from aptamers in that while both are nucleotides, the structure of an aptamer is not based on a natural oligonucleotide sequence; there are also peptide aptamers. Aptamers are selected on the basis of binding to a target molecule, usually a protein. See also **MicroRNA**, **siRNA**, **antisense peptides**, **aptamers**, **antisense peptide nucleotides**.

1. Rahman, M.A., Summerton, J., Foster, E., et al., Antibacterial activity and inhibition of protein synthesis in *Escherichia coli* by antisense DNA analogs, *Antisense Res. Dev.* 1, 319–327, 1991.
2. Lundin, K.E., Giseberg, O., and Smith, C.I.E., Oligonucleotide therapies: The past and the present, *Human Gene Therapy* 26, 475–485, 2015.
3. Hudziak, R.M., Barofsky, E., Barofsky, D.F., et al., Resistance of morpholino phosphorodiamidate oligomers to enzymatic degradation, *Antisense Nucleic Acid Drug Devel.* 6, 267–272, 1996.
4. Dirin, M., and Winkler, J., Influence of diverse chemical modifications on the ADME characteristics and toxicology of antisense oligonucleotides, *Expert Opin. Biol. Ther.* 13, 875–888, 2013.
5. Thoduka, S.G., Zaleski, P.A., Dabrowska, Z., et al., Analysis of ribosomal inter-subunit sites as targets for complementary oligonucleotides, *Biopolymers* 107, e23004, doi:10.1002/bip.23004, 2017.
6. Korneev, S., and O'Shea, M., Natural antisense RNAs in the nervous system, *Rev. Neurosci.* 16, 213–222, 2005.
7. Zong, X., Nakagawa, S., Freier, S.M., et al., Natural antisense RNA promotes 3′ end processing and maturation of MALAT1 lncRNA, *Nucleic Acids Res.* 44, 2298–2908, 2016.
8. Deniz, E., and Erman, B. Long noncoding RNA (lincRNA), a new paradigm in gene expression control, *Funct. Integr. Genomics* 17, 135–143, 2017.
9. Sun, Y., Li, D., Zhang, R., et al., Strategies to identify natural antisense transcripts, *Biochimie* 132, 131–151, 2017.

ANTISENSE PEPTIDES

An antisense peptide is a peptide derived from the translation/transcription of the antisense strand of DNA (the transcription product of antisense RNA). The transcription of the antisense (noncoding, template) DNA strand yields the mRNA which codes for the sense peptide. The mRNA is an exact replica (except for substitution of U for T) of the sense (coding, nontemplate) strand. An antisense peptide is a peptide, that would be coded for by an RNA molecule complementary to the mRNA coded by the antisense DNA strand. This mRNA would be an exact replica (except for the substitution of U for T) of the sense DNA strand.[1,2] This is hypothetical since it is not clear that this occurs *in vivo*, although it not absolutely clear that this does not happen. Below is shown the sense and antisense peptide for an exposed loop in IL-1β.[3]

AA	Gln	Gly	Glu	Glu	Ser	Asn	Asp	
5′	CAA	GGA	GGA	GAA	AGU	AAU	GAC	3′
3′	GUU	CCU	CUU	CUU	UCA	UUA	CUG	5′
AA	Leu	Ser	Phe	Phe	Thr	Ile	Val	

Some antisense peptides have been demonstrated to show affinity properties that appear to be unique to that sequence and not seen in scrambled sequences.[4–7] The term complementary peptide has been used to describe antisense peptides as the concept is extended beyond a single product of the transcription of an antisense RNA.[8,9] Antisense/complementary peptides are of interest in autoimmunity.[10,11] It should be noted that the term antisense peptide overlaps with antisense peptide nucleic acid; the term antisense peptide nucleic acid refers to antisense oligonucleotide sequence on a peptide back composed of aminoethyl glycine.[12,13] See also **peptide nucleic acid**, **scrambled peptide**, **antisense peptide nucleic acids**.

1. Bost, K.L., Smith, E.M., and Blalock, J.E., Similarity between the corticotrophin (ACTH) receptor and a peptide encoded by an RNA that is complementary to ACTH mRNA, *Proc. Natl. Acad. Sci. USA* 82, 1372–375, 1985.
2. Rasmussen, U.B., and Hesch, R.D., On the antisense peptides: The parathyroid hormone as an experimental example and a critical theoretical view, *Biochem. Biophys. Res. Commun.* 149, 930–938, 1987.
3. Heal, J.R., Bino, S., Roberts, G.W., Raynes, J.G., and Miller, A.D., Mechanistic investigation into complementary (antisense) peptide mini-receptor inhibitors of cytokine interleukin-1, *ChemBioChem.* 3, 76–85, 2002.
4. Chaiken, I., Interactions and uses of antisense peptides in affinity technology, *J. Chromatog.* 597, 29–36, 1992.
5. Root-Bernstein, R.S., and Holsworth, D.D., Antisense peptides: Critical mini-review, *J. Theoret. Biol.* 190, 107–1199, 1998.
6. Siemion, I.Z., Cebrat, M., and Kluczyk, A., The problem of amino acid complementarity and antisense peptides, *Curr. Protein Pept. Sci.* 5, 507–527, 2004.
7. Miller, A.D., Sense-antisense (complementary) peptide interactions and the proteomic code; potential opportunities in biology and pharmaceutical science, *Expert Opin. Biol. Ther.* 15, 245–267, 2015.
8. Bhakoo, A., Raynes, J.G., Heal, J.R., Keller, M., and Miller, A.D., De-novo design of complementary (antisense) peptide mini-receptor inhibitor of interleukin 18 (IL-18), *Mol. Immunol.* 41, 1217–1224, 2004.
9. Siemion, I.Z., Cebrat, M., and Khuczyk, A., The problem of amino acid complementarity and antisense peptides, *Curr. Prot. Pept. Sci.* 5, 507–527, 2004.
10. McGuire, K.L., and Holmes, D.S., Role of complementary proteins in autoimmunity: An old idea re-emerges with new twists, *Trends Immunol.* 26, 367–372, 2005.
11. Reynolds, J., Preston, G.A., Pressler, B.M., et al., Autoimmunity to the alpha 3 chain of type IV collagen in glomerulonephritis is triggered by "autoantigen complementarity". *J. Autoimmun.* 59, 8–18, 2015.
12. Nielsen, P.E., Egholm, M., Berg, R.H., and Burchardt, O. Sequence-selective recognition of DNA by strand displacement with a thymine-substituted polyamide, *Science* 254, 1497–1500, 1991.
13. Nielsen, P.E., Antisense peptide nucleic acids, *Curr. Opin. Mol. Ther.* 2, 282–287, 2000.

ANTISENSE PEPTIDE NUCLEIC ACID

An antisense peptide nucleic acid is an antisense nucleic acid on a peptide nucleic acid backbone instead of a phosphodiester or morpholino/phosphorodiamidate backbone.[1–3]

1. Yang, L., Liu, Y.F., Wu, G., et al., Blocking the CC chemokine receptor 5 pathway by antisense peptide nucleic acid prolongs islet allograft survival, *Transplant. Proc.* 39, 185–190, 2007.
2. Pandey, V.N., Upadhyay, A., and Chaubey, B., Prospects for antisense peptide nucleic acid (PNA) therapies for HIV, *Expert Opin. Biol. Ther.* 9, 975–989, 2009.
3. Montagner, G., Bezzerri, V., Cabrini, G., et al., An antisense peptide nucleic acid against *Pseudomonas aeruginosa* inhibiting bacterial-induced inflammatory response in the cystic fibrosis IB3-a cellular model system, *Int. J. Biol. Macromol.* 99, 492–498, 2017. See **antisense nucleotide, peptide nucleic acid (PNA)**.

APICAL

The term apical refers to that portion of a differentiated cell that is pointed toward the lumen.[1–3] In the case of endothelial cells, the apical protein is directed toward the circulatory system while the basolateral portion is directed toward the interstitial space. In the case of intestinal epithelial cells, the apical domain is facing the intestinal lumen and the basolateral domain facing the interstitial space. The membrane protein distribution is frequently different between the apical domain and the basolateral domain (polarized distribution). The secretion of proteins may differ between the two domains in a process described as vectorial secretion.[4,5] See **basolateral**.

1. Hubbard, A.L., Targeting of membrane and secretory proteins to the apical domain in epithelial cells, *Semin. Cell Biol.* 2, 365–374, 1991.
2. Ito, K., Suszuki, H., Horie, T., and Sugiyama, Y., Apical/basolater surface expression of drug transporters and its role in vectorial drug transport, *Pharm. Res.* 22, 1559–1577, 2005.
3. Vagin, O., Kraut, J.A., and Sachs, G., Role of *N*-glycosylation in trafficking of apical membrane proteins in epithelia, *Am. J. Physiol. Renal Physiol.* 296, F459–F469, 2009.
4. Hornung, D., Levovic, D.I. Shifren, J.L., Vigne, J.L., and Taylor, R.N., Vectorial secretion of vascular endothelial growth factor by polarized human endometrial epithelial cells, *Fertil. Steril.* 69, 909–915, 1998.
5. Zuehlke, J., Ebenau, A., Krueger, B., and Goppelt-Struebe, M., Vectorial secretion of CTGF as a cell-type specific response to LPA and TFG-β in human tubular epithelial cells, *Cell Comnun. Signal.* 10, 25, 2012.

APOPTOSIS

Apoptosis is a term derived from the Greek for falling off or away[1] to describe programmed cell death, a normal, organized process by which cell undergo degradation and elimination. Apoptosis is one the several mechanisms for cell death (type I cell death); other mechanisms are autophagy (type II cell death) and necrosis (type III cell death).[2] **Permeabilization** of the mitochondrial membrane[3,4] and formation of the **apoptosome**[5,6] are major processes in **intrinsic (mitochondrial) apoptosis**.[7] The **extrinsic apoptosis** pathway is initiated by occupancy of death receptors by member of the TNF family such as TRAIL (TNF-related apoptosis-induced ligand).[8] Both intrinsic and extrinsic pathways of apoptosis involved the activation of caspases.[9]

1. *Oxford English Dictionary*, Oxford University Press, Oxford, UK, 2019.
2. Green, D.R., and Llambi, F., Cell Death Signaling, *Cold Spring Harbor Perspect. Biol.* 7: pii:a006808; doi:10.1101/cshperspect.a006808, 2015.
3. Cosentino, K., and García-Sáez, A.J., Mitochondrial alterations in apoptosis, *Chem. Phys. Lipids* 181, 62–75. 2014.
4. Bonora, M., Wieckowski, M.R., Chinopoulos, C., et al., Molecular mechanisms of cell death: Central implications of ATP synthase in mitochondrial permeability transition, *Oncogene* 34, 1475–1486, 2015.
5. Salvesen, G.S., and Renatus, M., Apoptosome: The seven-spoked death machine, *Dev. Cell.* 2, 256–257, 2002.
6. Cain, K., Bratton, S.B., and Cohen, G.M., The Apaf-1 apoptosome: A large caspase-activating complex, *Biochemie* 84, 203–214, 2002.
7. Dejean, L.M., Martinez-Caballero, S., Guo, L., et al., Oligomeric Bax is a component of the putative cytochrome *c* release channel MAC, mitochondrial apoptosis-induced channel, *Mol. Biol. Cell* 16, 2424–2432, 2005.
8. Sayers, T.J., Targeting the extrinsic apoptosis signaling pathway for cancer therapy, *Cancer Immunol. Immunother.* 60, 1173–1180, 2011.
9. Kiraz, Y., Adan, A., Kartal, Y.M., and Baran, Y., Major apoptotic mechanisms and genes involved in apoptosis, *Tumour Biol.* 37, 8471–8486, 2016.

APOPTOSOME

The apoptosome is macromolecular structure composed of Apaf-1 (apoptosis protease activating factor-1) which serves as a platform for the activation of procaspases.[1–4] The formation of the apoptosome in the intrinsic apoptosis pathway is initiated by cytochrome c release from mitochondria.[5]

1. Adrain, C., and Martin, S.J., The mitochondrial apoptosome: A killer unleashed by the cytochrome seas, *Trends Biochem. Sci.* 26, 390–397, 2001.
2. Shi, Y., Apoptosome assembly, *Methods Enzymol.* 442, 141–156, 2008.
3. Yuan, S., and Akey, C.W., Apoptosome structure, assembly, and procaspase activation, *Structure* 21, 501–515, 2013.
4. Shakeri, R., Khelrollahi, A., and Davoodi, J., Apaf-1: Regulation and function in cell cell, *Biochemie* 135, 111–125, 2017.
5. Wu, C.C., and Bratton, S.B., Regulation of the intrinsic apoptosis pathway by reactive oxygen species, *Antioxid. Redox. Signal.* 19, 546–558, 2013.

APROTININ

Aprotinin (Trasylol®) is a small protein (single chain protein, MW 6.5 kDa; 58 amino acids) also known as basic pancreatic trypsin inhibitor (BPTI) or the Kunitz pancreatic trypsin inhibitor.[1,2] Aprotinin is best known as an inhibitor of tryptic-like serine proteases such as plasma kallikrein and plasmin[3,4] and has limited use as a therapeutic.[5] Aprotinin has also been used as model for protein folding.[6,7]

1. Kunitz, M., and Northrup, J.H., Isolation from bovine pancreas of crystalline trypsinogen, trypsin, a trypsin inhibitor, and an inhibitor-trypsin compounds, *J. Gen. Physiol.* 19, 991–1007, 1936.
2. Fritz, H., and Wunderer, G., Biochemistry and applications of aprotinin, the kallikrein inhibitor from bovine organs, *Arzneimittelforschung* 33, 479–494, 1983.
3. Sharpe, S., De Meester, I., Hendriks, D., et al., Proteases and their inhibitors: Today and tomorrow, *Biochimie* 73, 121–126, 1991.
4. Turkon, H., Toprak, B., Yalcin, H., Colak, A., and Ozturk, N., The effectiveness of temperature versus aprotinin in maintaining the preanalytical stability of adrenocortico-trophin, *Lab. Med.* 47, 279–282, 2016.
5. Royston, D., The current place of aprotinin in the management of bleeding, *Anaesthesia* 70(Suppl 1), 46–49, e17, 2015.
6. Creighton, T.E., Protein folding pathways determined using disulphide bonds, *Bioessays* 14, 195–199, 1992; Chang, J.Y., Diverse pathways of oxidative folding of disulfide proteins: Underlying causes and folding models, *Biochemistry* 50, 3414–3431, 2011.
7. Qin, M., Wang, W., and Thirumalai, D., Protein folding guides disulfide bond formation, *Proc. Natl. Acad. Sci. USA* 112, 11241–11246, 2015.

APTAMERS

Aptamers are relatively short (generally 20–90 bp) oligonucleotides, either DNA[1,2] or RNA[3,4] which have the property of acting as specific ligands to a broad range of targets including small molecules,[5] proteins,[6] and cells.[7,8] The binding of aptamers to cells has both diagnostic and therapeutic considerations.[9] Aptamers binding to cells have been used as drug delivery vehicles.[10,11] Aptamers labeled with a fluorophore have been developed to enhance sensitivity of detection.[12] Aptamers expressed inside of the cell are referred to as **intramers**.[13] Peptide aptamers which are short (20–30 amino acids) peptides with specific binding characteristics for protein targets obtained by combinatorial chemistry have been described.[14,15] While aptamers and antisense nucleotides are both synthetic oligonucleotides, they differ in that aptamers are selected by a process such as SELEX to optimize function, while antisense oligonucleotide structure is dictated by a complementary oligonucleotide sequence.

1. Tucker, W.O., Shum, K.T., and Tanner, J.A., G-quadruplex DNA aptamers and their ligands: Structure, function and application, *Curr. Pharm. Des.* 18, 2014–2026, 2012.

2. Volk, D.E., and Lokesh, G.L.R., Development of phosphorothioate DNA and DNA thioaptamers, *Biomedicines* 5(3), 41, doi:10.33io/biomedicines5040041, 2017.

3. Kang, K.N., and Lee, Y.S., RNA aptamers: A review of recent trends and applications, *Adv. Biochem. Eng. Biotechnol.* 131, 153–169, 2013.

4. Trachman, R.J., Truong, L., and Ferré-D'Amaré, Structural properties of fluorescent RNA aptamers, *Trends Pharmacol. Sci.* doi:10.1016/j.tips.2017.06.007, 2017.

5. Ruscito, A., and DeRosa, M.C., Small-molecule binding aptamers: Selection strategies, characterization, and applications, *Front. Chem.* 4, 14, 2016.

6. Deng, B., Lin, Y., Wang, C., et al., Aptamer binding assays for proteins: The thrombin example—A review, *Anal. Chim. Acta* 837, 1–15, 2014.

7. Jeong, S., Eom, T., Kim, S., Lee, S., and Yu, J., In vitro selection of the RNA aptamer against the Sialyl Lewix X and its inhibition of cell adhesion, *Biochem. Biophys. Res. Commun.* 281, 237–243, 2001.

8. Jaremko, W.J., Huang, Z., Wen, W., et al., Identification and characterization of RNA aptamers: A long aptamerblocks the AMPA receptor and a short aptamer blocks both AMPA and kainate receptors, *J. Biol. Chem.* 292, 7338–7347, 2017.

9. Mayer, S., Maufort, J.P., Nie, J., et al., Development of an efficient targeted cell-SELEX procedure for DNA aptamer reagents, *PLoS One* 8(8), e71798, 2013.

10. Yoon, S., Armstrong, B., Habib, N., and Rossi, J.J., Blind SELEX approach identifies RNA aptamers that regulate EMT and inhibit metastasis, *Mol. Cancer Res.* 15, 811–820, 2017.

11. Gopinath, S.C., Lakahmiipriya, T., Chen, Y., et al., Cell-targeting aptamers act as intracellular delivery vehicles, *Appl. Microbiol. Biotechnol.* 100, 6955–6669, 2016.

12. Yuan, B., Jiang, X., Chen, Y., et al., Metastatic cell and tissue-specific fluorescence imaging using a new DNA aptamer developed by cell-SELEX, *Talanta* 170, 56–62, 2017.

13. Famulok, M., Blind, M., and Mayer, G., Intramers as promising new tools in functional proteomics, *Chem. Biol.* 8, 931–939, 2001.

14. Colas, P., Cohen, P., Jessen, T., et al., Genetic selection of peptide aptamers that recognize and inhibit cyclin-dependent kinase 2, *Nature* 380, 585–550, 1996.

15. Colombo, M., Mizzotti, C., Masiero, S., Kater, M.M., and Pesaresi, P., Peptide aptamers: The versatile role of specific protein function inhibitors in plant biotechnology, *J. Integr. Plant Biol.* 57, 892–901, 2015. See **peptide aptamers, antisense nucleotides**.

AQUAPORINS

An aquaporin (AQP) is membrane pore which is reasonably specific for the transport of water.[1,2] There are several hundred AQPs[3,4] that are also referred to as membrane intrinsic proteins and water channel proteins.[5] The various AQP isoforms have a similar structure, tetramer with each monomer in the tetramer forming a separate water channel.[6–9] There is interest in AQPs as therapeutic targets.[10,11]

1. Li, C., and Wang, W., Molecular Biology of Aquaporins, *Adv. Expt. Med. Biol.* 969, 1–35, 2014.

2. *Aquaporins in Health and Disease. New Molecular Targets for Drug Discovery*, ed. G. Soveral, S. Nielsen, and A. Casani, CRC Press, Boca Raton, FL, 2016.

3. Abascal, F., Irisarri, I., and Zardoya, R., Diversity and evolution of membrane intrinsic proteins, *Biochim. Biophys. Acta* 1840, 1468–1481, 2014.

4. Benga, G., On the definition, nomenclature and classification of water channel proteins, aquaporins and relatives, *Mol. Aspects Med.* 33, 514–517, 2012.

5. Day, R.E., Kitchen, P., Owen, D.S., et al., Human aquaporins: Regulators of transcellular water flow, *Biochim. Biophys. Acta* 1840, 1492–1506, 2014.

6. Andrews, S., Reichow, S.L., and Tamir, G., Electron crystallography of aquaporins, *IUBMB Life* 60, 430–436, 2008.

7. Schenk, A.D., Hite, R.K., Engel, A., Fujiyoshi, Y., and Walz, T., Electron crystallography and aquaporins, *Methods Enzymol.* 483, 91–119, 2010.

8. Tani, K., and Fujiyoshi, Y., Water channel structures analyzed by electron crystallography, *Biochim. Biophys. Acta* 1840, 1605–1613, 2014.

9. Laforenza, U., Bottino, C., and Gastaldi, G., Mammalian aquaglyceroporin function in metabolism, *Biochim. Biophys. Acta* 1858, 1–11, 2016.
10. Beitz, E., Golldack, A., Rothert, M., and von Büllow, J., Challenges and achievements in the therapeutic modulation of aquaporin functionality, *Pharmacol. Ther.* 155, 22–35, 2015.
11. Tomita, Y., Dorward, H., Yool, A.J., et al., Role of aquaporin 1 signalling in cancer development and progression, *Int. J. Mol. Sci.* 10, E299, 2017.

ARABIDOPSIS THALIANA

Arabidopsis thaliana is a small plant in the mustard family that is extensively used for studies of plant biology[1-5] with approximately 68,000 citations on PubMed as of January 2019.

1. *Methods in Plant Molecular Biology and Biotechnology*, ed. B.R. Glick and J.E. Thompson, CRC Press, Boca Raton, FL, 1993.
2. *Aribidopsis*, ed. M. Anderson and J.A. Roberts, Sheffield Academic Press, Sheffield, UK, 1998.
3. *Arabidopsis A Practical Approach*, ed. Z.A. Wilson, Oxford University Press, Oxford, UK, 2000.
4. *Aribidopsis Protocols*, ed. J. Salinas and J.J. Sánchez-Serrano, Humana Press, Totowa, NJ, 2006.
5. *The Arabidopsis Book*, The American Society of Plant Biologists, Rockville, MD, 2002 to present.

ARRHENIUS EQUATION

The Arrhenius equation relates rate constants to temperature: $k = Ae^{-E_a/RT}$, where k is a rate constant; A is a constant (pre-exponential factor) having the same units as the rate constant; k, R is the gas constant; and T the absolute temperature. The logarithmic form of the equation can be written as $\ln k = \ln A - E_a/RT$. A plot of ln k vs 1/T (Arrhenius plot) yields the Arrhenius constant (Arrhenius energy of activation, E_a). The larger the value for E_a, the slower the reaction rate. Calculation of the Arrhenius constant for the rate of the loss of activity of catalase during spray drying permitted rational evaluation of the effect of excipients.[1] The Arrhenius equation has been used for the study of protein thermal denaturation. A one-step irreversible denaturation model shows Arrhenius behavior.[2] The assumption is that the final stage in irreversible denaturation, aggregation, is much faster than unfolding and not measured. Measurement of the aggregation process will show non-Arrhenius behavior for the overall denaturation process.[3]

Some examples of the Arrhenius constant for some proteins:

Protein	E_a (kJ/mol)	$t_{1/2}$ (Days at 37°C)
Maltodextrin glucosidase	571	68
Lentil lectin	357	1.2×10^4
Ovalbumin (chicken)	430	1.2×10^5
Glucose oxidase (*Aspergillus*)	280	0.8
Bovine rhodopsin	386	1.6
α-Amylase (*Bacillus*)	172	42

Source: Goyal, M., Chaudhuri, T.K., and Kuwajima, K., *PLoS One* 9(12), e115877, 2014.

A multistep process such as the unfolding/folding of globular proteins may show non-Arrhenius behavior.[4,5] The Arrhenius equation is of value in the stability studies required for the qualification of pharmaceutical products[6,7] as well as stability studies on food products[8] and analytes in biological fluids.[9,10]

1. Shaefer, J., and Lee, G., Arrhenius activation energy of damage to catalase during spray-drying, *Int. J. Pharm.* 489, 124–130, 2015.
2. Goyal, M., Chaudhuri, T.K., and Kuwajima, K., Irreversible denaturation of maltodextrin glucosidase studied by differential scanning calorimetry, circular dichroism, and turbidity measurements, *PLoS One* 9(12), e115877, 2014.
3. Nikolaidis, A., and Moschakis, T., Studying the denaturation of bovine serum albumin by a novel approach of difference-UV analysis, *Food Chem.* 215, 235–244, 2017.
4. Kuhlman, B., Luisi, D.L., Evans, P.A., and Raleigh, D.P., Global analysis of the effects of temperature and denaturant on the folding and unfolding kinetics of the N-terminal domain of the protein L9, *J. Mol. Biol.* 284, 1661–1670, 1998.
5. Matagne, A., Jamin, M., Chung, E.W., et al., Thermal unfolding of an intermediate is associated with non-Arrhenius kinetics in the folding of hen lyzozyme, *J. Mol. Biol.* 297, 193–210, 2000.
6. Rauk, A.P., Guo, K., Hu, Y., Cahya, S., and Weiss, W.F., Arrhenius time-scaled least squares: A simple robust approach to accelerated stability data analysis for bio-products, *J. Pharm. Sci.* 103, 2278–2286, 2014.
7. Fan, Z., and Zhang, L., One- and two-stage Arrhenius models for pharmaceutical shelf life prediction, *J. Biopharm. Stat.* 25, 307–316, 2015.
8. Jafari, S.M., Ganje, M., Dehnad, D., Ghanbari, V., and Hajitabar, J., Arrhenius equation modeling for the shelf life prediction of tomato paste containing a natural preservative, *J. Sci. Food. Agric.* in 97, 5216–5222, 2017.

9. Cruz Ruiz, M., Recio Quijano, F., López Cortés, L.F., Hebles Duvison, M., and Vásquez Rubio, R., Determination of shelf life and activation energy for tumor necrosis factor-α in cerebrospinal fluid samples, *Clin. Chem.* 42, 670–674, 1996.

10. Kenis, G., Teunissen, C., De Johgh, R., et al., Stability of interleukin 6, a soluble interleukin 6 receptor, interleukin 10 and CC16 in human serum, *Cytokine* 19, 228–235, 2002.

ASSEMBLY PROTEIN

The term assembly protein has several different applications which are related. In one context, an assembly protein, without enzymatic activity, participates in the formation of a macromolecular structure such as a ribonucleoprotein (RNP),[1] nucleosomes,[2–4] iron–sulfur clusters,[5–7] and viruses.[8,9] An assembly protein can be considered a **scaffold protein**.[10,11] In another context, an assembly protein has enzymatic activity which assembles a macromolecular structure such as a polysaccharide.[12] The concept of assembly protein has also been used in relation to the import of protein into mitochondria.[13,14]

1. Singh, M., Wang, Z., Cascio, D., and Feigon, J., Structure and interactions of the CS domain of human H/ACA RNP assembly protein Shq1, *J. Mol. Biol.* 427, 807–823, 2015.

2. Park, Y.J., and Luger, K., Structure and function of nucleosome assembly proteins, *Biochem. Cell Biol.* 84, 549–558, 2006.

3. Lòpez-Panadès, E., and Casacuberta, E., NAP-1, nucleosome assembly protein 1,a histone chaperone involved in *Drosophila* telomeres, *Insert Biochem. Mol. Biol.* 70, 111–115, 2016.

4. Gupta, N., Thakker, S., and Verma, S.C., KSHV encoded LANA recruits nucleosome assembly protein NAP1L1 for recruiting viral DNA replication and transcription, *Sci. Rep.* 6, 32633, 2017.

5. Wu, G., and Li, L., Biochemical characterization of iron-sulfur cluster assembly in the scaffold IseU of *Escherichia coli*, *Biochemistry* (Moscow) 77, 135–142, 2012.

6. Van Houten, B., Kuper, J., and Kisker, C., Role of XPD in cellular functions: To TFIIH and beyond, *DNA Repair* 44, 136–142, 2016.

7. Cory, S.A., Van Vranken, J.G., Brignole, E.J., et al., Structure of human Fe-S assembly subcomplex reveals unexpected cysteine desulfurase architecture and acy-ACP-ISD11 interactions, *Proc. Natl. Acad. Sci. USA* 114, E5325-E5334, 2017.

8. Preston, V.G., Rixon, F.J., McDougall, I.M., McGregor, M., and Al Kobaisi, M.F., Processing of the Herpes Simplex virus assembly protein ICP35 near the carboxyl terminal end requires the product of the whole of the UL26 reading frame, *J. Virol.* 186, 87–98, 1992.

9. Robertson, B.J., McCann, P.J., III, Matusick-Kumar, L., Preston, V.G., and Gao, M., Na, an autoproteolytic product of the Herpes Simples virus type 1 protease, can functionally substitute for the assembly protein ICP35, *J. Virol.* 71, 1685–1687, 1997.

10. Yang, K., and Baines, J.D., Domain within Herpes Simplex virus 1 scaffold proteins required for interaction with portal protein in infected cells and incorporation of the portal vertex into capsids, *J. Virol.* 82, 5021–5030, 2008.

11. Osinalde, N., Sánchez-Quiles, V., Blagoev, B., and Kratchimarova, I., Changes in Gab2 phosphorylation and interaction partners in response to interleukin (IL)-2 stimulation in T-lymphocytes, *Sci. Reports* 6, 23530, 2016.

12. Williams, D.M., Ovchinnikova, O.G., Koizumi, A., et al., Single polysaccharide assembly protein that integrates polymerization, termination, and chain-length quality control, *Proc. Natl. Acad. Sci. USA* 114, E1215-E1223, 2017.

13. Weidemann, N., and Pfanner, N., Mitochondrial machineries for protein import and assembly, *Annu. Rev. Biochem.* 86, 685–714, 2017.

14. Ellenrieder, L., Rampelt, H., and Becker, T., Connection of protein transport and organelle contact sites in mitochondria, *J. Mol. Biol.* 429, 2148–2160, 2017.

ATOMIC FORCE MICROSCOPY

Atomic force microscopy (AFM) is a high resolution form of microscopy which involves a probe or tip moving over a surface (alternatively the sample can move with a static tip; the detection method is the same) and as the probe changes position in response to sample topography, the movement is tracked deflection of a laser beam, which is recorded by a detector.[1–3] AFM has a broad range of applications in nanobiology, including the study of protein–DNA interactions,[4] the study of structural transitions in proteins,[5] the study of interaction of cells with extracellular matrix,[6] and the study of cell membranes.[7–9]

1. Gadegaard, N., Atomic force microscopy in biology: Technology and techniques, *Biotechnic Histochem.* 81, 87–97, 2006.

2. *Atomic Force Microscopy in Nanobiology*, ed. K. Takeyasu, CRC/Pan Stanford, Boca Raton, FL, 2015.

3. Voigtländer, B., *Scanning Probe Microscopy, Atomic Force Microscopy, and Scanning Tunneling Microscopy*, Springer, Berlin, Germany, 2015.

4. Kasas, S., and Dietler, G., DNA-protein interactions explored by atomic force microscopy, *Semin. Cell Dev. Biol.*, in press, doi: 10.1016/semcbd.2017.07.015, 2017.

5. Ando, T., Directly watching biomolecules in action by high-speed atomic force microscopy, *Biophy. Rev.*, 9, 421–429, 2017.

6. Alcaraz, J., Otero, J., Jorba, A., and Navajas, D., Bidirectional mechanobiology between cells and their local extracellular matrix probed by atomic force microscopy, *Semin Cell Dev. Biol.* 73, 71–81, 2018.

7. Braet, F., Taatjes, D., and Wisse, E., Probing the unseen structure and function of liver cells through atomic force microscopy, *Semin. Cell Dev. Biol.* 73, 13–30, 2018.
8. Bitler, A., Dover, R., and Shai, Y., Fractal properties of cell surface structures: A view from the AFM, *Semin. Cell Dev. Biol.* 73, 64–70, 2018.
9. Hasan, I.Y., and Mechler, A., Analytical approaches to study domain formation in biomimetic membranes, *Analyst* 142, 3062–3078, 2017.

AUTACOID/AUTOCOID

Autacoid and autocoid are both used to describe a biological factor which, while not defined as a hormone, has a variety of actions on different cells and tissues. The term autacoid will be used herein as it appears (based on PubMed search) to be the more commonly used of the two. The term autacoid was introduced early in the last century to describe the physiological action of largely unknown (at that time) substances obtained from various internal organs such as the pituitary and thyroid.[1,2] The term is attributed to E.S. Shafer (Sir Edward Albert Sharpley-Schafer, a distinguished physiologist at the University of Edinburgh).[3] As with today, there were sharp disagreements about nomenclature.[4,5] Adenosine is one of the better examples of an autacoid as, apart from its role as purine base in RNA and DNA, it has diverse physiologic functions.[6-8] Other examples include melatonin[9] and a derivative of arachidonic acid.[10,11]

1. Schafer, E.S., and Lim, R.K.S., The effects of adrenalin on the pulmonary circulation, *Quart. J. Exptl. Physiol.* 12, 157–198, 1919.
2. Larsen, J.A., Functional correlation of the hypophysis and the thyroid, *Am. J. Physiol.* 49, 55–89, 1919.
3. Mettam, A.E., and Craig, M.A., Diabetes mellitus, *J. Comp. Pathol. Therapeut.* 29, 1–25, 1916.
4. Schafer, E.A., The nomenclature of "internal secretion", *Lancet* 189, 80, 1917.
5. Bell, W.B., The nomenclature of "internal secretion", *Lancet* 189, 124, 1917.
6. Kelley, GF.G., Aassar, O.S., and Forrest, J.N., Jr., Endogenous adenosine is an autocoid feedback inhibitor of chloride transport in the shark rectal gland, *J. Clin. Invest.* 88, 1933–1939, 1991.
7. Maeda, Y., Terada, Y., Nonoguchi, H., and Knepper, M.A., Hormone and autacoid regulation of cAMP production in rat IMCD subsegments, *Am. J. Physiol.* 263, F319–F327, 1992.
8. Haskó, G., and Cronstein, B.N., Adenosine: An endogenous regulator of innate immunity, *Trends Immunol.* 25, 33–39, 2004.
9. Tan, D.X., Manchester, L.C., Hadeland, R., Lopez-Burillo, S., Mayo, J.C., Sainz, R.M., and Reiter, R.J., Melatonin: A hormone, a tissue factor, an autacoid, a paracoid, and an antioxidant vitamin, *J. Pineal Res.* 34, 75–78, 2003.
10. Pinckard, R.N., The "new" chemical mediators of inflammation, in *Current Topics in Inflammation and Infection*, ed. G. Majno, R.S. Cotran, and N. Kaufman, Chapter 3, pp. 38–53, Williams & Wilkins, Baltimore, MD, 1982.
11. Hall, W.L., The future for long chain n-3 PUFA in the prevention of coronary heart disease: Do we need to target non-fish-eaters? *Proc. Nutr. Soci.* 76, 408–418, 2017.

AUTOANTIGEN

An autoantigens is a component of self, usually a protein, which is able to elicit an immune response (an autoimmune reaction)[1,2] frequently with pathological complications such as the destruction of pancreatic beta cells (Islets of Langerhans) by T-cells resulting in Type 1 diabetes.[3-5] Some other autoantigens include citrullinated proteins in rheumatoid arthritis[6] and antineutrophilic cytoplasmic antibodies in a vasculitis (ANCA-mediated vasculitis).[7]

1. Wu, C.T., Gershwin, M.E., and Davis, P.A., What makes an autoantigen an autoantigen? *Ann. N.Y. Acad. Sci.* 1050, 134–1045, 2005.
2. Selmi, C., Autoimmunity in 2016, *Clin. Rev. Allergy Immunol.* 53, 126–139, 2017.
3. Hull, C.M., Peakman, M., and Tree, T.I.M., Regulatory T cell dysfunction in type 1 diabetes: What's broke and how can fix it? *Diabetologia*, 60, 1839–1850, 2017.
4. Fenalti, G., and Buckle, A.M., Structural biology of the GAD autoantigen, *Autoimmun. Rev.* 9, 148–152, 2010.
5. Nakayama, M., Insulin as a key autoantigen in the development of type diabetes, *Diabetes Metab. Res. Rev.* 27, 773–777, 2011.
6. Planta, A., Arvikar, S.L., Strle, K., et al., Two rheumatoid arthritis-specific autoantigens correlated microbial immunity with autoimmune responses in joints, *J. Clin. Invest.* 127, 2946–2956, 2017.
7. Jennette, J.C., and Falk, R.J., Pathogenesis of antineutrophil cytoplasmic autoantibody-mediated disease, *Nat. Rev. Rheumatol.* 10, 463–473, 2014.

AUTOCRINE

The term autocrine refers the action of a hormone or other biological effector such as a peptide growth factor or cytokine which on the cell or tissue responsible for the synthesis/secretion of the given hormone or biological effector. The term autocrine is used in differentiation from endocrine or paracrine. Autocrine stimulation of particular interest in oncology.[1,2] Autocrine factors demonstrated to be of importance in oncology includes vascular endothelial growth factor (VEGF),[3] IL-6,[4] and TGF-β.[5] Locally synthesized C1q has been demonstrated to have an autocrine function in the function of monocytes and other immune cells.[6] Notable is the autocrine phenomena in unicellular organisms.[7–9]

1. Gharbaran, R., Insights into the molecular roles of heparan sulfate proteoglycans (HSPGs syndecans) in autocrine and paracrine growth factor signaling in the pathogenesis of Hodgkin's lymphoma, *Tumour Biol.* 37, 11573–11586, 2016.
2. Butera, G., Pacchiana, R., and Dondelli, M., Autocrine mechanisms of cancer chemoresistance, *Semin. Cell Dev. Biol.*, in press, doi:10.1016/j.sercdb.2017.07.019, 2017.
3. Ohba, T., Cates, J.M., Cole, H.A., et al., Autocrine VEGF/VEFGR1 signaling in a subpopulation of cells associates with aggressive osteosarcoma, *Mol. Cancer Res.* 12, 1100–1111, 2014.
4. Matthes, T., Manfroi, B., Zeller, A., et al., Autocrine amplification of immature myeloid cells by IL-6 in multiple myeloma-infiltrated bone marrow, *Leukemia* 29, 1883–1890, 2015.
5. Papageorgis, P., and Stylianopoulos, T., Role of TGFβ in regulation of the tumor microenvironment and drug delivery, *Int. J. Oncol.* 46, 933–943, 2015.
6. Ghebrehiwet, B., Hosszu, K.H., and Peerschke, E.I., C1q as an autocrine and paracrine regulator of cellular function, *Mol. Immunol.* 84, 26–33, 2017.
7. Ortenzi, C., Miceli, C., Bradshaw, R.A., and Luporini, P., Identification and initial characterization of an autocrine pheromone receptor in the protozoan ciliate *Euplotes raikovi, J. Cell. Biol.* 111, 607–614, 1990.
8. Vallesi, A., Giuli, G., Bradshaw, R.A., and Luporini, P., Autocrine mitogenic activity of pheromones produced by the protozoan ciliate *Euplotes raikovi, Nature* 376, 522–524, 1995.
9. Luporini, P., Vallesi, A., Alimenti, C., and Ortensi, C., The cell type-specific signal proteins (pheromones) of protozoan ciliates, *Curr. Pharm. Des.* 12, 3015–3024, 2006.

AUTOFOCUSING

Autofocusing is a term with several different definitions relevant to biochemistry and molecular biology. Autofocusing was introduced a term to describe isoelectric focusing in the absence of added carrier ampholytes.[1,2] The technique has seen continuing use in this context.[3,4] Autofocusing is also used in optical systems such as microscopes[5,6] and in oncology therapy (modulated electro-hyperthermia).[7]

1. Sova, O., Autofocusing—A term for isoelectric focusing without carrier ampholytes, *J. Chromatog.* 320, 15–22, 1985.
2. Sova, O., Separation of antibiotics by autofocusing, *Electrphoresis* 11, 963–966, 1990.
3. Park, E.Y., Imazu, H., Matsumara, H., Nakamura, Y., and Sato, K., Effects of peptide fractions with different isoelectric points from wheat gluten hydrolysates on lipid oxidation in pork meat patties, *J. Agric. Food Chem.* 60, 7483–7488, 2012.
4. Taniguchi, M., Kameda, M., Namae, T., et al., Identification and characterization of multifunctional cationic peptides derived from peptic hydrolysates of rice bran protein, *J. Functional Food* 34, 287–296, 2017.
5. Ren, L., Li, Z., Yuhua, B., et al., The impact of the condenser on cytogenetic image quality in digital microscope system, *Anal. Cell. Pathol.* 36, 45–59, 2013.
6. Kang, B-H., STEM tomography imaging of hypertrophied Golgi stacks in mucilage-secreting cells, *Methods Mol. Biol.* 1496 (Golgi Complex), 55–62, 2016.
7. Tsang, Y-W., Huang, C-C., Yang, K-L., et al., Improving immunological tumor microenvironment using electro hyperthermia followed by dendritic cell immunotherapy, *BMC Cancer* 15, 708, 2015.

AUTOPHAGY

Autophagy is a normal process for the physiological degradation of intracellular macromolecules and subcellular structures.[1] This pathway of "self-destruction" or "self-eating" is considered a separate process from proteosome-mediated degradation of macromolecules internalized from outside the cell (heterophagy), although the two processes share a common degradative vehicle in the lysosome or other digestive vacuole.[2] Autophagy can be divided into three related but separate processes; macroautophagy, microautophagy, and chaperone-mediated autophagy. Macroautophagy is a process by which cytoplasmic contents (cytosol and organelles such as mitochondria) are sequestered into fluid-filled double-membrane sacs or vesicles described as autophagosomes. The contents of the autophagosome are transported to an intracellular organelle such a vacuole or lysosome (in mammals) for degradation.[3] Microautophagy is a process where the cytoplasmic contents are directly taken into the lysosome (in mammals) or digestive vacuole by invagination.[4] Both macroautophagy and microautophagy can be selective where damaged organelles are removed or non-selective in the random removal of cytoplasm. Chaperone-mediated autophagy is a third autophagocytic process where a cytoplasmic chaperone delivers a specific cytoplasmic protein to a lysosome.[5] Chaperone-mediated autophagy is only found in mammals. Macroautophagy is characterized by morphological change with the formation of the autophagosome while microautophagy and chaperone-mediated autophagy are not associated with morphological change.[5,6] Selective macroautophagy can be further defined by the target such as mitophagy (mitochondria), pexophagy (peroxysomes), nucleophagy (portions of the nucleus), reticulophagy (portions of the endoplasmic reticulum) and ribophagy (ribosomes).[7] The study of autophagy is complex[8] and the study of complex systems such as cells and organisms requires considerable care to obtain reproducible results in different laboratories.[9] The study of autophagy is of importance in human diseases such as neurodegenerative disease, cardiovascular disease and aging.[10]

1. Yang, Z., and Klionsky, D.J., An overview of the molecular mechanism of autophagy, in *Autophagy in Infection and Immunity*, ed. B. Levine, T. Yoshimori, and V. Deretic, chapter 1, pp. 1–32, Springer Verlag, Berlin, Germany, 2009.
2. Harnett, M.M., Pineda, M.A., Latte de Laté, P., et al., From Christian de Duve to Yoshinori Ohsumi: More to autophagy than just dining at home, *Biochem. J.* 40, 9–22, 2017.
3. Feng, Y., He, D., Yao, Z., and Klionsky, D.J., The machinery of macroautophagy, *Cell Res.* 24, 24–41, 2014.
4. Li, W-w., and Bao, J-k., Microautophagy: Lesser-known self-eating, *Cell. Mol. Life. Sci.* 69, 1125–1136, 2012.
5. Bejarano, E., and Cuervo, A.M., Chaperone-mediated autophagy, *Proc. Am. Thor. Soc.* 7, 29–39, 2010.
6. Kaushik, S., and Cuervo, A.M., Chaperone-mediated autophagy: A unique way to enter the lysosome world, *Trends Cell Biol.* 22, 407–417, 2012.
7. Galluzzi, L., Baehrecke, E.H., Bellabio, A., et al., Molecular definitions of autophagy and related processes, *EMBO J.* 36, 1811–1836, 2017.
8. Klionsky, D.J., Developing a set of guidelines for your research field: A practical approach, *Mol. Cell. Biol.* 27, 733–738, 2016.
9. Lithgow, J., Driscoll, M., and Phillips, P., A long journey to reproducible results, *Nature* 548, 387–388, 2017.
10. Choi, A.M., Ryter, S.W., and Levine, B., Autophagy in human health and disease, *N. Eng. J. Med.* 368, 651–662, 2013.

AUTOPHOSPHORYLATION

Autophosphorylation may be a university feature of protein kinases, both receptor and nonreceptor, by which a kinase/kinase domain catalyzes "self-phosphorylation" in another domain, usually a regulatory domain, in the same protein.[1,2] Phosphorylation may occur at serine, threonine or tyrosine residues and may be intramolecular (*cis*),[3] intermolecular (*trans*),[4] or both *cis* and *trans* autophosphorylation.[5] Autophosphorylation is a feature of many receptors such as EGF receptor,[6–8] fibroblast growth factor receptor,[9] as well as insulin receptor and insulin-like growth factor receptor.[10–12]

1. Smith, J.A., Francis, S.H., and Corbin, J.D., Autophosphorylation: A salient feature of protein kinases, *Mol. Cell. Biochem.* 127–128, 51–70, 1993.
2. Beenstock, J., Moonshayef, N., and Engelberg, D., How do protein kinases take a selfie (autophosphorylate)? *Trends Biochem. Sci.* 41, 938–953, 2016.
3. Joseph, R.E., Severin, A., Mil, L., Fulton, D.B., and Andreotti, A.H., SH2-dependent autophosphorylation within the Tec family kinase ltkm *J. Mol. Biol.* 391, 164–177, 2009.
4. Meng, Y., Pond, M.P., and Roux, B., Tyrosine kinase activation and conformational flexibility: Lessons from Src-family tyrosine kinases, *Acc. Chem. Res.* 50, 1193–1201, 2017.
5. Beenstock, J., Melamed, D., Moonshavef, N., et al., p38β mitogen activated protein kinase modulates its own basal activity by autophosphorylation of the activating residue Thr180 and the inhibitory residues Thr241 and Ser261, *Mol. Cell. Biol.* 36, 1540–1553, 2016.
6. Margolis, B.L., Lax, I., Kris, R., et al., All phosphorylation sites of epidermal growth factor (EGF) receptor and HER2/neu and located in their carboxyl-terminal tails. Identification of a novel site in EGF receptor, *J. Biol. Chem.* 264, 10667–10671, 1989.
7. Wolff, M., Tetzlaff, K., Nivens, M.C., In vivo inhibition of epidermal growth factor receptor autophosophorylation prevents receptor internalization, *Exp. Cell Res.* 317, 42–50, 2011.
8. Purba, E.R., Saito, E., and Maruyama, I.N., Activation of the EGF receptor by ligand binding and oncogenic mutations: The "rotation model", *Cell* 6, 13, 2017.
9. Loo, B-M., Kreuger, J., Jaikanen, M., Lindahl, U., and Salmivirta, M., Binding of heparin/heparan sulfate to fibroblast growth factor receptor 4, *J. Biol. Chem.*276, 16868–16876, 2001.
10. Cobb, M.H., Sang, B.-C., Gonzalez, R., Goldsmith, E., and Ellis, L., Autophosphorylation activates the soluble cytoplasmic domain of the insulin receptor in an intermolecular reaction, *J. Biol. Chem.* 264, 18701–18706, 1989.
11. Frattali, A.L., Treadway, J.L., and Pessin, J.E., Transmembrane signaling by the human insulin receptor kinase. Relationship between intramolecular β subunit *trans*- and *cis*- autophosphorylation and substrate kinase activation, *J. Biol. Chem.* 267, 19521–19528, 1992.
12. Cabail, M.X., Li., S., Lemmon, E., et al., The insulin and IGF1 receptor kinase domains are functional dimers in the activated state, *Nat. Commun.* 6, 6406, 2015.

B-LYMPHOCYTES

B-lymphocytes are also called B-cells. The name was derived from the original studies involving the cells from the bursa of chickens.[1,2] B-cells are best known as the precursors memory B cells and plasma cells which are responsible for the production of antibodies.[3–5]

1. *T and B Lymphocytes: Origins, Properties and Roles in Immune Responses,* ed. M.F. Greaves, J.J.T. Owen, and M.C. Raff, Excerpta Medica, New York, 1973.
2. Cooper, M.D., The early history of B cells, *Nat. Rev. Immunol.* 15, 191–197, 2015.
3. *Fundamental Immunology*, 6th edn., ed. W.E. Paul, Wolters Kluwer Health/Lippincott, Williams, and Wilkins, Philadelphia, PA, 2013.

4. Zabe, F., Mohanan, D., Bess, J., et al., Viral particles drive rapid differentiation of memory B cells into secondary plasma cells producing increased levels of antibodies, *J. Immunol.* 192, 5499–5508, 2014.
5. Ribatti, D., The discovery of plasma cells: An historical note, *Immunol. Lett.* 188, 64–67, 2017.

BACTERIAL ARTIFICIAL CHROMOSOME

A bacterial artificial chromosome (BAC) is a construct based on the fertility plasmid (F-plasmid) and is used for cloning of intermediate-sized genomic DNA.[1] While BACs cannot contain as much DNA as a yeast artificial chromosome (YAC), BAC libraries are considered to be more stable than YAC libraries[2] but YACs have been more useful in defines contigs in large genomes.[3]

1. Shizuya, H., Birren, B., Kim, U-Y., et al., Cloning and stable maintenance of 300-kilobase-pair fragments of human DNA in *Escherichia coli* using an F-factor based vector, *Proc. Natl. Acad. Sci. USA* 89, 8794–8797, 1992.
2. Shi, B.J., Gustafson, J.P., and Langridge, P., A simple TAE-based method to generate large insert BAC libraries from plant species, *Methods Mol. Biol.* 513, 57–80, 2009.
3. Schalkwyk, L.C., Francis, F., and Lehrach, H., Techniques in mammalian genome mapping, *Curr. Opin. Biotechnol.* 6, 37–43, 1995, *Acids Res.* 34, 445–450, 2006.

BASOLATERAL

The term basolateral denotes the bottom opposite from the apical end of a differentiated or polarized cell. As with an epithelial cell, the basolateral surface is toward the extracellular matrix while the apical surface (also referred to as luminal surface) is toward the lumen.[1] The development of cellular polarity (apico-basal polarity) is associated with asymmetric distribution of membrane constituents as well as cytoplasmic constituents.[2] There is polarity in the absorption and secretion of biological materials. Fat-soluble vitamins are adsorbed at the apical surface of enterocytes, transported through the cytoplasm, and secreted at the basolateral surface into the interstitial space/lymph.[3] See **apical**.

1. Treyer, A., and Müsch, A., Hepatocyte Polarity, *Compr. Physiol.* 3, 243–287, 2013.
2. Ebnet, K., Kumar, D., Steinbacher, T., et al., Regulation of cell polarity by cell adhesion receptors, *Semin. Cell. Dev. Biol.* 18, 2–12, 2018.
3. Reboul, E., and Borel, P., Proteins involved in uptake, intracellular transport and basolateral section of fat-soluble vitamins and carotenoids by mammalian enterocytes, *Prog. Lipid Res.* 50, 388–402, 2011.

BATHOCHROMIC SHIFT

A bathochromic shift in the absorption/emission of light by a chemical compound to a longer wavelength ($\lambda > \lambda_0$).[1–6] This phenomenon is also known as a "red" shift.

1. Waleh, A., and Ingraham, L.L., A molecular orbital study of the protein-controlled bathochromic shift in a model of rhodopsin, *Arch. Biochem. Biophys.* 156, 261–266, 1973.
2. Kliger, D.S., Milder, S.J., and Dratz, E.A., Solvent effects on the spectra of retinal Schiff bases—I. models for the bathochromic shift of the chromophore spectrum in visual pigments, *Photochem. Photobiol.* 25, 277–286, 1977.
3. Cannella, C., Berni, R., Rosato, N., and Finazzi-Agro, A., Active site modifications quench intrinsic fluorescence of rhodanese by different mechanisms, *Biochemistry* 25, 7319–7323, 1986.
4. Zagalsky, P.F., β-Crustacyanin, the blue-purple carotenoprotein of lobster carapace: Consideration of the bathochromic shift of the protein-bound astaxanthin, *Acta Chrystallogr. D Biol. Chrystallogr.* 59, 1529–1531, 2003.
5. Cheng, H.B., Huang, Y.D., Zhao, L., Li.,X., and Wu, H.C., A prominent bathochromic shift of indole-containing diarylethylene derivatives, *Org. Biomol. Chem*, 13, 3570–2475, 2015.
6. Velusamy, N., Binoy, A., Bobba, K.N., et al., A bioorthogonal fluorescent probe for mitochondrial hydrogen sulfide: A new strategy for cancer cell labeling, *Chem. Commun.* (Camb) 53, 8802–8805, 2017.

BETAINE

Betaine (2-(trimethylazaniumyl)acetate, glycine betaine, oxyneurine, lycine, Cystadane®) is derived from the oxidation of choline. The mammalian, plant, and the majority of bacteria use a two-step process with the intermediate formation of betaine aldehyde which is further oxidized to betaine. Certain bacteria use a single flavoprotein enzyme, choline oxidase, to obtain betaine from choline.[1] Betaine serves as methyl donor in synthesis of methionine from homocysteine[2] in the methionine cycle.[3] Betaine is also important in osmoregulation in the kidney in mammals[4] and in plants.[5] There is considerable interest in the potential therapeutic use of betaines in liver disease.[6]

1. Sakamoto, A., and Murata, N., Genetic engineering of glycinebetaine synthesis in plants: Current status and implications for enhancement of stress tolerance, *J. Exp. Botany* 51, 81–88, 2000.
2. Garrow, T.A., Purification, kinetic properties, and cDNA cloning of mammalian betaine-homocysteine methyltransferase, *J. Biol. Chem.* 271, 22831–22838, 1990.

3. Storch, K.J., Wagner, D.A., Burke, J.F., and Young, V.R., Quantitative study in vivo of methionine cycle in humans using [methyl -^{2}H$_3$] and [1–^{13}C] methionine, *Am. J. Physiol.* 255, E322–E331, 1988.

4. Kempson, S.A., and Montrose, M.H., Osmotic regulation of renal betaine transport: Transcription and beyond, *Pflugers Arch.* 449, 227–234, 2004.

5. Chen, T.H., and Murata, N., Glycinebetaine protects plants against abiotic stress mechanisms and biotechnological applications, *Plant Cell Environ.* 34, 1–20, 2011.

6. Day, C.R., and Kempson, S.A., Betaine chemistry, roles, and potential use in liver disease, *Biochim. Biophys. Acta.* 1860, 1098–1106, 2016.

BIBODY

A bibody is an immunoglobulin derivative where an scFv is fused with the C-terminus of the C$_{H1}$ domain (F$_d$ domain) of a Fab fragment.[1–3] A search of the literature suggests that there is little current use of bibodies with far more interest in diabodies. See also **tribody, diabody**.

1. Schoonjans, R., Willems, A., Schoonooghe, S., et al., Fab chains as an efficient heterodimerization scaffold for the production of recombinant bispecific and trispecific antibody derivatives, *J. Immunol.* 165, 7050–7057, 2000.

2. Schoonooghe, S., Burvenich, I., Vervoort, L., et al., PHI-derived bivalent bibodies and trivalent tribodies bind differentially to she and tumour-associated MUCI, *Protein Eng. Des. Sel.* 23, 21–728, 2010.

3. Kellner, C., Bruenke, J., Horner, H., et al., Heterodimeric bispecific antibody-derivatives against CD19 and CD16 induce effective antibody-dependent cellular cytotoxicity against B-lymphoid tumor cells, *Cancer Lett.* 303, 128–139, 2011.

BICOID PROTEIN

Bicoid protein is a morphogen[1] described in *Drosophila* that functions in development.[2,3] Bicoid protein is a regulator of transcription.[4] Bicoid mRNA is localized at the anterior end of the developing embryo and a concentration gradient is established toward the posterior and is thought to regulate the expression of 20 genes.[5,6] Bicoid protein is a homeobox protein (Hox protein)[7] and interacts with target DNA via the homeobox domain[8] with a lysine residue at position 9 in the homeodomain recognition helix critical for binding.[9] Additional specificity in binding is provided by multiple conformers of bicoid protein.[10] Bicoid has also been suggested to bind to RNA.[11] The **Pitx gene** family is related to bicoid[12] and is important in human development.[13,14]

1. Porcher, A., Dostatni, N., The bicoid morphogen system, *Curr. Biol.* 20, R249–R254, 2010.

2. Lawrence, P.A., Background to bicoid, *Cell* 54, 1–2, 1988.

3. Stephenson, E.C., and Pokrywka, N.J., Localization of bicoid message during Drosophila oogenesis, *Curr. Top. Dev. Biol.* 26, 23–34, 1992.

4. Johnstone, O., and Lasko, P., Translational regulation and RNA localization in Drosophila oocytes and embryos, *Annu. Rev. Genet.* 35, 365–406, 2001.

5. Liu, J., and Ma, J., Dampened regulates the activating potency of bicoid and the embryonic patterning outcome in *Drosophila*, *Nat. Commun.* 4, 2968, 2013.

6. Ipiña, E.P., and Dawson, S.P., The effect of reactions on the formation and readout of the gradient of bicoid, *Phys. Biol.* 14, 016002, 2017.

7. McGregor, A.P., How to get ahead: The origin, evolution and function of bicoid, *Bioessays* 27, 904–913, 2005.

8. Baird-Titus, J.M., Clark-Baldwin, K., Dave, V., et al., The solution structure of the native K50 bicoid homeodomain bound to the consensus TAATCC DNA-binding site, *J. Mol. Biol.* 356, 1351–1376, 2006.

9. Hanes, S.D., and Brent, R., DNA specificity of the bicoid activator protein is determined by homeodomain recognition helix residue 9, *Cell* 57, 1275–1283, 1989.

10. Adhikary, R., Tan, Y.X., Liu, J., et al., Conformational heterogeneity and DNA recognition by the morphogen bicoid, *Biochemistry* 56, 2787–2793, 2017.

11. Cassiday, L.A., and Maher, L.J., 3rd, Having it both ways: Transcription factors that bind DNA and RNA, *Nucleic Acids Res.* 30, 4118–4126, 2002.

12. Gage, P.J., Suh, H., and Camper, S.A., The bicoid-related Pitx gene family in development, *Mamm. Genome* 10, 197–200, 1999.

13. Wang, J., Zhang, D.F., Sun, Y.M., and Yan, Y.Q., A novel PITX2c loss-of-function mutations associated with familial atrial fibrillation, *Eur. J. Med. Genet.* 57, 25–31, 2014.

14. Seifi, M., Footz, T., Taylor, S.A., et al., Novel PITX2 gene mutations in patients with Axenfeld-Rieger syndrome, *Acta Opthalmol.* 94, e571–e579, 2016.

BIOACTIVE PEPTIDES

Many peptides such as kinins (bradykinin) have biological activity. In many cases, these peptides are derived from specific precursors such as kininogens, serving as sources of kinins.[1,2] However, a consideration of the recent literature suggests that bioactive peptide is a peptide derived by fragmentation of dietary proteins.[3–6]

1. *Kinins*, ed. M. Badder, Degruyter, Berlin, Germany, 2012.

2. Schmaier, A.H., The contact activation and kallikrein/kinin systems pathophysiologic and physiologic activities, *J. Thromb. Haemost.* 14, 28–39, 2016.

3. Daliri, E.B., Oh, D.H., and Lee, B.H., Bioactive peptides, *Foods* 6(5), 32, 2017.

4. Cicero, A.F.G., Fogacci, F., and Colletti, A., Potential role of bioactive peptides in prevention and treatment of chronic diseases: A narrative review, *Br. J. Pharmacol.* 174, 1378–1394, 2017.

5. Gaglione, R., Dell'Olmo, E., Bosso, a., et al., Novel human bioactive peptides identified in apoliprotein B: Evaluation of their therapeutic potential, *Biochem. Pharmacol.* 130, 34–50, 2017.
6. Bougle, D., and Bouhallab, S., Dietary bioactive peptides: Human studies, *Crit. Rev. Food Sci. Nutr.* 57, 335–343, 2017.

BIOASSAY (BIOLOGICAL ASSAY)

The term bioassay (biological assay) is defined as a procedure that determines the composition of or effect of a substance on a living organism. The term bioassay does not define a specific technology.[1] The term bioassay is usually used to identify an assay using *ex vivo* techniques with cells[2,3] while an assay that uses living animals may be identifies as an *in vivo* assay.[4,5] Regardless of *in vitro* or *in vivo* methodology, validation of bioassays requires considerable rigor.[6–8] Reproducibility (and hence validation) can be extremely challenging.[9,10]

1. https://www.fda.gov/AboutFDA/Transparency/track/ucm252974.htm.
2. Indelicato, S.R., Bradshaw, S.L., Chapman, J.W., and Weiner, S.H., Evaluation of standard and state of the art analytical technology-bioassays, *Dev. Biol.* (Basal) 122, 102–114, 2005.
3. Gupta, S., Indelicato, S.R., Jethwa, V., et al., Recommendations for the design, optimization, and qualification of cell-based assays used for the detection of neutralizing antibody responses elicited to biological therapeutics, *J. Immunol. Methods* 321, 1–18, 2007.
4. Tako, E., Bar, H., and Glahn, R.P., The combined application of the CaCo-2 cell bioassay coupled with in vivo (*Gallus gallus*) feeding trial represents an effective approach to predicting Fe availability in humans, *Nutrients* 8(11), 732, 2016.
5. Zwierzyna, M., and Overington, J.P., Classification and analysis of a large collection of in vivo bioassay descriptions, *PLoS Comput. Biol.* 13(7), e1005641, 2017.
6. Fallarero, A., Hanski, L., and Vurela, P., How to translate a bioassay into a screening assay for natural products: General considerations and implementation of antimicrobial screens, *Planta Med.* 80, 1182–1199, 2014.
7. Rebelo, S.P., Dehne, E.M., Brito, C., et al., Validation of bioreactor and human-on-a-chip devices for chemical safety assessment, *Adv. Exp. Med. Biol.* 856, 299–316, 2016.
8. Yu, B., and Yang, H., Evaluation of different estimation methods for accuracy and precision in biological assay validation, *PDA J. PharmSci. Technol.* 71, 297–305, 2017.
9. Freedman, L.P., Gibson, M.C., Ethler, S.P., et al., Reproducibility: Changing the policies and culture of cell line authentication, *Nature Methods* 12, 493–497, 2015.
10. Lithgow, J., Driscoll, M., and Phillips, P., A long journey to reproducible results, *Nature* 548, 387–388, 2017.

BIOEQUIVALENCE

Two drug substances (active pharmaceutical ingredients or final drug products) are said to be bioequivalent when they have the same pharmacological effect when administered at the same molar quantity.[1,2] Bioequivalence is the concept used in the characterization of pharmaceuticals to demonstrate therapeutic equivalence of a drug product.[3–5] The term biosimilarity is used to indicate bioequivalence in the biologics,[6] although there is conceptual difference in the application of the concept of bioequivalence to drugs and biologics.[7,8]

1. https://www.fda.gov/Drugs/GuidanceCompliance RegulatoryInformation/Guidances/ucm075207.htm.
2. https://www.fda.gov/downloads/Drugs/GuidanceCompliance RegulatoryInformation/Guidances/UCM389370.pdf.
3. Li, Z., Fang, L., Jiang, W., Kim, M.J., and Zhao, L., Risk-based bioequivalence recommendations of antiepileptic drugs, *Curr. Neurol. Neurosci. Rep.* 17, 82, 2017.
4. Sferrazza, G., Siviero, P.D., Nicotera, G., et al., Regulatory framework on bioequivalence criteria for locally acting gastrointestinal drugs: The case for oral modified release mesalamie formulations, *Expert Rev. Clin. Pharmacol.* 10, 1007–1019. 2017.
5. Usami, O.S., Molimard, M., Gaur, V., et al., Scientific rationale for determining the bioequivalence of inhaled drugs, *Clin. Pharmacokinet.* 56, 1139–1156, 2017.
6. Azevedo, V., Hassett, B., Forseca, J.E., et al., Differentiating biosimilarity and comparability in biotherapeutics, *Clin. Rheumatol.* 35, 2877–2886, 2016.
7. Karalis, V.D., From bioequivalence to biosimilarity: The rise of a novel regulatory framework, *Drug. Res.* (Stuttg.) 66, 1–6, 2016.
8. Kadam, V., Bagde, S., Karpe, M., and Kadam, V., A comprehensive overview on biosimilars, *Curr. Protein Pept. Sci.* 17, 756–761, 2016.

BIOINFORMATICS

Bioinformatics can be defined as the branch of science concerned with information and information flow in biological systems, especially the use of computational methods in genetics and genomics.[1–7]

1. *Oxford English Dictionary*, Oxford University Press, Oxford, UK, 2017.
2. Buehler, L.K., and Rashidi, H.H., *Bioinformatics Basics: Applications in Biological Sciences and Medicine*, Taylor & Francis Group, Boca Raton, FL, 2005.
3. Evans, W.J., *Statistical Methods in Bioinformatics: An Introduction*, Springer, New York, 2005.
4. Wang, J.T.L., *Data Mining in Bioinformatics*, Springer, London, UK, 2005.
5. Lesk, A.M., *Introduction to Bioinformatics*, Oxford, New York, 2005.

6. Hodgman, R.C., French, A., and Westhead, C.R., *Bioinformatics*, Taylor & Francis Group, Milton Park, Abington, UK, 2010.
7. Agostino, M.J., *Practical Bioinformatics*, Garland Science, New York, 2013: *Allergy Bioinformatics*, ed. A. Tao and E. Rax, Springer Science, Dordrecht, the Netherlands, 2015.

BIOISOSTERES

Bioisosteres are isosteres with similar or antagonist biological activity. The term bioisosteres (bio-isosteres) was advanced by Harris Friedman in 1951.[1] The development of the early concepts of bioisosterism were discussed by Thornber in 1979.[2] Bioisosteres of particular interest includes those bases on phosphate groups.[3–5] Other bioisosteres are based on carboxyl groups,[6] amino acids,[7] purines,[8] and pyrimidines.[9]

1. Freidman, H.L., Influence of isosteric replacements upon biological activity, in *First Symposium on Chemical-Biological Correlation*, pp. 295–395, National Research Council, National Academy of Sciences, Washington, DC, 1950.
2. Thornber, C.W., Isosterism and molecular modification in drug design, *Chem. Soc. Rev.* 39, 563–590, 1979.
3. Rye, C.S., and Baell, J.B., Phosphate isosteres in medicinal chemistry, *Curr. Med. Chem.* 12, 3127–3141, 2005.
4. Fuhrmann, J., Subramanian, V., and Thompson, P.R., Synthesis and use of a phosponate amidine to generate an anti-phosphoarginine-specific antibody, *Angewandte Chem. Int. Ed. Eng.* 54, 1475–1478, 2015.
5. Zhang, Y., Borrel, A., Ghemtio, L., et al., Structural isosteres of phosphate groups in the protein data bank, *J. Chem. Inf. Model.* 57, 499–516, 2017.
6. Ballatore, C., Huryn, D.M., and Smith, A.B., Carboxylic acid (bio)isoteres in drug design, *ChemMedChem.* 8, 385–395, 2013.
7. Poulie, C.B.M., and Bunch, L., Heterocycles as nonclassical bioisosteres of α-amino acids, *ChemMedChem.* 8, 205–215, 2013.
8. Jorda, R., Paruch, K., and Krystof, V., Cyclin-dependent kinase inhibitors inspired by rescovitine: Purine bioisosteres, *Curr. Pharm. Des.* 18, 2974–2980, 2012.
9. Abd El Razik, H.A., Mroueh, M., Faour, W.H., et al., Synthesis of new pyrazolo[3,4-d]pyrimidine derivatives and evaluation of their anti-inflammatory and anticancer activities, *Chem. Biol. Drug. Des.* 90, 83–96, 2017.

BIOLOGICALS

A biological is a regulatory definition encompassing any virus, serum, toxin, antitoxin, blood, blood component or derivative, allergenic product, or analogous product applicable to the prevention, treatment, or cure of diseases or injury.[1–6] A biological may be combined with a drug as with an antibody-drug conjugate.[7]

1. https://www.fda.gov/AboutFDA/CentersOffices/OfficeofMedicalProductsandTobacco/CBER/ucm133077.htm.
2. Stein, K.E., and Webber, K.O., The regulation of biologic products derived from bioengineered plants, *Curr. Opin. Biotechnol.* 12, 308–311, 2001.
3. Sobell, J.M., Overview of biologic agents in medicine and dermatology, *Semin. Cutan. Med. Surg.* 23, 2–9, 2005.
4. Portela, M.D.C.C., Sinogas, C., Alburquerque de Almeida, F., Baptista-Leitre, R., and Castro-Caldas, A., Biologicals and biosimilars: Safety issues in Europe, *Expert Opin. Biol. Ther.* 17, 871–877, 2017.
5. Schutte, K., Szczepanska, A., Halder, M., et al., Modern science for better quality control of medicinal products "Towards global harmonization of 3Rs in biologicals": The report of an EPAA workshop, *Biologicals* 48, 55–65, 2017.
6. Rein, P., and Mueller, R.B., Treatment with biologicals in rheumatoid arthritis: An overview, *Rheumatol. Ther.* 4, 247–261, 2017.
7. Singh, S.K., Luisi, D.L., and Pak, R.H., Antibody-drug conjugates: Design, formulation and physicochemical stability, *Pharm. Res.* 32, 3541–3571, 2015.

BIOMARKER

A change in response to an underlying pathology; current examples of molecular changes include C-reactive protein, fibrin D-dimer, and troponin.[1–3] The term biomarker is also used to describe higher-level responses such as changes in behavior,[4–6] anatomical changes such as those observed by magnetic resonance imaging,[7,8] or changes in physiology.[9,10] While not extensive, there is use of the term "wet biomarker,"[11] which is used to distinguished "wet" laboratory tests such as immunoassays from assays such as EKG and MRI measurements.[12,13] Biomarkers may be further classified by matrix and purpose:

Genomic Biomarker: A measurable DNA and/or RNA characteristic that is an indication of normal biologic processes, pathogenic processes, and/or response to therapeutic or other interventions.[14] The below classification is obtained from BEST.[15]

Biomarker is a defined characteristic that is measured as an indicator of normal biological processes, pathogenic processes, or responses to an exposure or intervention, including therapeutic interventions. Molecular, histologic, radiographic, or physiologic characteristics are types of biomarkers. A biomarker is not an assessment of how an individual feels, functions, or survives. Categories of biomarkers include:

Diagnostic Biomarker: A biomarker used to detect or confirm presence of a disease or condition of interest or to identify individuals with a subtype of the disease.

Monitoring Biomarker: A biomarker measured serially for assessing status of a disease or medical condition or for evidence of exposure to (or effect of) a medical product or an environmental agent.

Pharmacodynamic/Response Biomarker: A biomarker used to show that a biological response has occurred in an individual who has been exposed to a medical product or an environmental agent.

Predictive Biomarker: A biomarker used to identify individuals who are more likely that similar individuals without the biomarkers to experience a favorable or unfavorable effect from exposure to a medical product or environmental agent.

Prognostic Biomarker: A biomarker used to identify likelihood of a clinical event, disease recurrence or progression in patients who have the disease or medical condition of interest.

Safety Biomarker: A biomarker measured before or after an exposure to a medical product or an environment agent to indicate the likelihood, presence, or extent of toxicity as an adverse effect.

Susceptibility/Risk Biomarker: A biomarker that indicates the potential for developing a disease or medical condition in an individual who does not have clinically apparent disease or the medical condition.

Biomarkers in toxicology have a different consideration, where a biomarker of exposure is the presence of a chemical, its metabolite, or the product of the reaction of a chemical with a target molecule or macromolecule (e.g. albumin)[16] that is measured in the compartment or fluid or an organism.[17] The term biomarker was first used (and still is) in geology to describe a pattern of organic chemicals in oil which are unique to origin of the sample.[18]

1. *Toxicological Biomarkers*, ed. A.P. DeCaprio, Taylor & Francis Group, New York, 2006.
2. Lundblad, R.L., *Development and Application of Biomarkers,* CRC Press, Boca Raton, FL, 2011.
3. *Biomarker Validation. Technological, Clinical and Commercial Aspects*, ed. H. Seitz and S. Schumacher, Wiley-VCH, Berlin, Germany, 2015.
4. Tronick, E.Z., The neonatal behavioral assessment scale as a biomarker of the effects of environmental agents on the newborn, *Environ. Health Perspect.* 74, 185–189, 1987.
5. Yager, J., and Feinstein, R.E., Potential applications of the National Institute of Mental Health's Research Domain Criteria (RDoC) in clinical psychiatric practice: How RDoC might be used is assessment, diagnostic processes, case formulation, treatment planning, and clinical notes, *J. Clin. Psychiatry* 78, 423–432, 2017.
6. Freedman, E.G., and Foxe, J.J., Eye movements, sensorimotor adaption and cerebellar-dependent learning in autism: Toward potential biomarkers and subphenotypes, *Eur. J. Neurosci.* 42, 549–555, 2018.
7. Trivedi, A., Hall, C., Hoffman, E.A., et al., Using imaging as a biomarker for asthma, *J. Allergy Clin. Immunol.* 139, 1–10, 2017.
8. Tuite, P., Brain magnetic resonance imaging (MRI) as a potential biomarker for Parkinson's disease (PD), *Brain Sci.* 7, 68, 2017.
9. Murphey, P.B., Kumar, A., Reilly, C., et al., Neural respiratory drive as a physiological biomarker to monitor change during acute exacerbations of COPD, *Thorax* 66, 602–608, 2011.
10. Bronzwaer, A.S., Ouweneel, D.M., Stok, W.J., Westerhof, B.E., and van Lieshout, J.J., Arterial pressure variation as a biomarker of preload dependency in spontaneously breathing subjects-A proof of principle, *PLoS One* 10(9), e0136364, 2015.
11. Antoniades, C.A., and Barker, R.A., The search for biomarkers in Parkinson's disease: A critical review, *Expert Rev. Neurotherapeutics* 8, 1841–1851, 2008.
12. Ludolph, A.C., Brettschneider, J., and Weishaupt, J.H., Amylotrophic lateral sclerosis, *Curr. Opin. Neurol.* 25, 530–535, 2012.
13. Finsterer, J., and Drory, V.F., Wet, volatile, and dry biomarkers of exercise-induced muscle fatigue, *BMC Musculoskel. Dis.* 17, 40, 2016.
14. FDA Guidance of Industry. E15 Definitions of Genomic Biomarkers, Pharmacogenomics, Pharmacogenetics, Genomic Data and Sample Coding, ICH, 2008.
15. *(Biomarkers, Endpoints, and other tools)* Resource, FDA-NIH Working Group, Silver Spring/Bethesda, MD, 2016.
16. Sabbioni, G., and Turesky, R.J., Biomonitoring human albumin adducts: The past, the present, and the future, *Chem. Res. Toxicol.* 30, 332–366, 2017.
17. Anon, Biomonitoring for occupational health risk assessment (BOHRA), *Toxicol. Lett.* 192, 3–16, 2010.
18. Snowdon, L.R., Volkman, J.K., Zhang, A., Tao, G., and Liu, P., The organic geochemistry of asphaltenes and occluded biomarkers, *Org. Geochem.* 91, 3–15, 2016.

BIOMOLECULAR INTERACTION DATABASE (BIND)

To the best of this writer's knowledge, this database is no longer active.

Biopharmaceutical Classification System

Class I	High Permeability	High Solubility
Class II	High Permeability	Low Solubility
Class III	Low Permeability	High Solubility
Class IV	Low Permeability	Low Solubility

The biopharmaceutical classification system (BCS) provides a classification of drugs that is intended to be predictive of pharmacokinetic behavior of a drug including dissolutions and absorption.[1] This system was developed in 1995.[2] The BCS is used in drug development.[3–8] A BCS has been proposed for excipients.[9]

1. https://www.fda.gov/AboutFDA/CentersOffices/OfficeofMedicalProductsandTobacco/CDER/ucm128219.htm.
2. Amidon, G., Lennernas, H., Shah, V.P., and Crison, J.A., A theoretical basis for a biopharmaceutic drug classification: The correlation of *in vitro* drug product dissolution and *in vivo* bioavailability, *Pharm. Res.* 12, 413–420, 1995.
3. Ku, M.S., Use of the biopharmaceutical classification system in early drug development, *AAPS J.* 10, 208–212, 2008.
4. Cook, J., Addicks, W., and Wu, Y.H., Application of the biopharmaceutical classification system in clinical drug development–an industrial view, *AAPS J.* 10, 306–310, 2008.
5. Lohani, S., Cooper, H., Jin, X., et al., Physicochemical properties, form, and formulation selection strategy for a biopharmaceutical classification system II preclinical drug candidate, *J. Pharm. Sci.* 103, 3007–3021, 2014.
6. Papich, M.G., and Martinez, M.N., Applying biopharmaceutical classification system (BCS) criteria to predict oral adsorption of drugs in dogs: Challenges and pitfalls, *AAPS J.* 17, 948–964, 2015.
7. Shawahna, R., Pediatric biopharmaceutical classification system: Using age-appropriate initial gastric volume, *AAPS J.* 18, 728–736, 2016.
8. Bou-Chacra, N., Melo, K.J.C., Morales, I.A.C., et al., Evolution of choice of solubility and dissolution and dissolution media after two decades of biopharmaceutical classification system, *AAPS J.* 19, 989–1001, 2017.
9. Vasconcelos, T., Marques, S., and Sarmento, B., The biopharmaceutical classification system of excipients, *Ther. Deliv.* 8, 65–78, 2017.

BLOT/BLOTTING

The term blot/blotting refers to various technologies when analytes are transferred from a separation medium such as an electrophoretic gel or a thin-layer chromatographic medium to another matrix where specific detection is possible.

Blotting Technologies in the Characterization of Biological Polymers

Technology	Description
Southern blotting	Southern blotting is an analytical process by which regions of DNA immobilized on a membrane are identified with a specific probe.[1] Early work used radioactive probes[1,2] while more recent work uses non-radioactive probes such as biotin.[3,4]
Northern blotting	Northern blotting is an analytical process where RNA is immobilized on a membrane and specific probes, frequently a labeled DNA, is used to detect specific regions on the RNA.[5–7] The use of Northern blot peaks in the middle 1990s and has steadily decreased in use. RT-PCR is more sensitive than a Northern blotting.[8]
Western blotting	Western blotting is a technique where protein immobilized on nitrocellulose after transfer from polyacrylamide gel electrophoresis (PAGE) is detected with antibody.[9,10] The current work uses polyvinylidene fluoride (PDVF) membrane in addition to nitrocellulose.[11,12]
Far-Western blotting	Far-Western blotting is a technique related to western blotting where the protein (prey)[a] is immobilized on nitrocellulose[13–15] or polyvinylidene fluoride[15] after separation on PAGE. The prey[b] is then incubated with the bait protein to form a prey-bait complex which is then detected with an antibait antibody (e.g. rat monoclonal anti bait) which is the detected with secondary probe (e.g. peroxidase-labeled goat-anti-rat antibody).[13] GST fusion proteins are detect with anti-GST immunoblotting.[14]
Southwestern blotting	Southwestern blotting is a technique similar to Western blotting where the proteins are immobilized on a nitrocellulose or polyvinylidene membrane after separation on PAGE. Specific interactions are identified with labeled DNA oligonucleotide probes.[16–18] Since most DNA probes are based on radioactive phosphate (^{32}P DNA), the use of alkaline phosphatase permits repeated probing of an electrophoretogram.[18]

(*Continued*)

Blotting Technologies in the Characterization of Biological Polymers (*Continued*)

Technology	Description
Eastern blot	The term Eastern blotting describes an analytical process where an antibody, usually monoclonal in nature, is used to identify low-molecular-weight compounds transferred from thin-layer chromatography plates to nitrocellulose. The antibody is usually detected with a secondary antibody. A Far-Eastern blot[19–22] has been described, which appears to be similar to the Eastern blot using high-performance thin layer chromatography.[23] Double Eastern blotting refers to the use of two antibodies on the same blot.[24]

[a] A general article on blotting technology (Nicholas, M.W., and Nelson, K., *J. Invest. Dermatol.* 133, e10, 2013).

[b] The concept of a prey protein and a bait protein is derived from the yeast two-hybrid system where a bait protein is used to identify interactions with a number of potential binding partners referred to as prey proteins expressed in a yeast system. (McAliste-Henn, L., Gibson, N., and Panisko, E., *Methods* 19, 330–337, 1999; Fashena, S.J., Serebriski, I., and Golemis, E.A., *Gene* 250, 1–14, 2000).

REFERENCES

1. Southern, E.M., Detection of specific sequences among DNA fragments separated by gel electrophoresis, *J. Mol. Biol.* 98, 503–517, 1975.
2. Cariani, E., and Bréchet, C., Detection of DNA sequences by Southern blot, *Ric. Clini. Lab.* 18, 161–170, 1988.
3. Zavala, A.G., Kulkarni, A.S., and Fortunato, E.A., A dual color Southern blot visualize two genomics or genic regions simultaneously, *J. Virol. Methods* 198, 64–68, 2014.
4. Aravalli, R.N., Park, C.W., and Steer, C.J., Detection of *Sleeping Beauty* transposition in the genome of host cells by non-radioactive Southern blot analysis, *Biochem. Biophys. Res. Comnun.* 477, 317–328, 2016.
5. Alwine, J.C., Kemp, D.J., and Stark, G.R., Method for detection of specific RNAs in agarose gels by transfer to diazobenzylmethyl-paper and hybridization with DNA probes, *Proc. Natl. Acad. Sci. USA* 74, 5350–5354, 1977.
6. Rohde, W., and Sänger, H.L., Detection of complementary RNA intermediates of viroid replication by Northern blot hybridization, *Biosci. Rep.* 1, 327–336, 1981.
7. Ferrer, M., Henriet, S., Chamotin, C., Lainé, S., and Mougel, M., From cells to virus particles: Quantitative methods to monitor RNA packaging, *Viruses* 8(8), E239, 2016.
8. Chwetzoff, S., and d'Andrea, S., Ubiquitin is physiologically induced by interferons in luminal epithelium of porcine uterine endometrium in early pregnancy: Global RT-PCR cDNA in place of RNA for differential display screening, *FEBS Lett.* 405, 148–152, 1997.
9. Towbin, H., Staehelin, T., and Gordon, J., Electrophoretic transfer of protein from polyacrylamide gels to nitrocellulose sheets: Procedure and some applications, *Proc. Natl. Acad. Sci. USA* 76, 4350–4554, 1979.
10. Sixma, J.J., Schiphorst, M.E., Verhoeckx, C., and Jockusch, B.M., Peripheral and integral proteins of human blood platelet membranes α-Actinin is not identical to glycoprotein III, *Biochim. Biophys. Acta* 704, 333–344, 1982.
11. MacPhee, D.J., Methodological considerations for improving western blot analysis *J. Pharmacol. Toxicol. Methods* 61, 171–177, 2010.
12. Taylor, S.C., and Posch, A., The design of a quantitative western blot experiment, *Biomed. Res. Int.* 2014, 362590, 2014.
13. Grässer, F.A., Sauder, C., Haiss, P., et al., Immunological detection of proteins associated with Epstein–Barr virus nuclear antigen 2A, *Virology* 195, 550–560, 1993.
14. Duprez, V., Blank, U., Chrétien, S., Gisselbrecht, S., and Mayeux, P., Physical and functional interaction between p72^{syk} and erythropoietin receptor, *J. Biol. Chem.* 267, 10670–10675, 1998.
15. Wu, Y., Li, Q., and Chen, X.-Z., Detecting protein-protein interactions by far western blotting, *Nat. Protoc.* 2(12), 3278–3284, 2007.
16. Bowen, B., Steinberg, J., Laemmli, U.K., and Weintraub, H., The detection of DNA-binding proteins by protein blotting, *Nucleic Acids Res.* 8, 1–20, 1980.
17. Siu, F.K.Y., Lee, L.T.O., and Chow, B.K.C., Southwestern blotting in investigating transcriptional regulation, *Nat. Protoc.* 3, 51–58, 2008.
18. Jia, Y., Daifeng, J., and Jarrett, H.W., Repeated probing of southwestern blots using alkaline phosphatase stripping, *J. Chromatog. A* 1217, 7177–7181, 2010.
19. Bogdanov, M., Sun, J., Kaback, H.R., and Dowhan, W., A phospholipid acts as a chaperone in assembly of a membrane transport protein, *J. Biol. Chem.* 271, 11615–11618, 1996.
20. Shan, S., Tanaka, H., and Shoyama, Y., Enzyme-linked immunosorbent assay for glycyrrhizin using anti-glycyrrhizin monoclonal antibody and an eastern blotting technique for glucuronides of glycyrrhetic acid, *Anal. Chem.* 73, 5784–5790, 2001.
21. Li, X.W., Morinaga, O., Tian, M., et al., Development of an eastern blotting technique for the visual detection of aristolochic acids in *Aristolochia* and *Asarum* species by using a monoclonal antibody against aristolochoic acids I and II, *Phytochem. Anal.* 24, 645–653, 2013.
22. Taki, T., Gonzalez, T.V., Goto-Inoue, N., Hayasaka, T., and Setou, M., TLC-blot (Far-Eastern Blot) and its applications, *Methods Mol. Biol.* 536, 545–556, 2009.
23. Rabel, F., and Sherma, J., New TLC/HPTLC commercially prepared and laboratory prepared plates: A review, *J. Liquid Chromatog. Related Technol.* 39, 385–393, 2016.
24. Fujii, S., Morinaga, O., Uto, T., Nomura, S., and Yukihiro, S., Development of double eastern blotting for major licorice components, glycyrrhizin and liquiritin for chemical quality control of licorice using anti-glycyrrhizin and anti-liquiritin monoclonal antibodies, *J. Agricultural Food Chem.* 64, 1087–1093, 2016.

BONE MORPHOGENETIC PROTEIN(S) (BMP)

Bone morphogenetic proteins (BMPs), which were first identified in 1971,[1,2] are a family of proteins which are members of the TGFβ superfamily.[3] There are multiple forms of bone morphogenetic proteins which are best known as differentiation factors for the maturation of mesenchymal cells into chondrocytes and osteoblasts. The canonical assay for BMPs has been based on ectopic bone growth on a suitable matrix[4,5] but new assays have been developed[6] including ELISA assays.[7] Bone morphogenetic proteins are secreted as single proteins which are dimerized via formation of an interchain disulfide bond undergo further proteolytic processing. There are approximately 30 members of the BMP family, which can be classified into several smaller groups. Specificity of BMP action is determined by the time of expression (temporal) as well as location (spatial) as well as interaction with specific receptors.[8] BMPs have effects on systems other than bone.[9,10] There is interest in the clinical application of BMPs.[11,12]

1. Urist, M.R., and Strater, B.S., Bone morphogenetic protein, *J. Dent. Res.* 50, 1392–1400, 1971.
2. Urist, M.R., Iwata, H., and Strater, B.S., Bone morphogenetic protein and proteases in guinea pig, *Clin. Orthopaed. Rel. Res.* 85, 275–290, 1972.
3. Rider, C.C., and Mulloy, B., Heparin sulphate and the TGF-β superfamily, *Molecules* 22(5), E713, 2017.
4. Urist, M.R., Mikulski, A., and Lietze, A., Solubilized and insolubilized bone morphogenetic protein, *Proc. Natl. Acad. Sci. USA* 76, 1828–1832, 1979.
5. Pietrzak, W.S., Woodell-May, J., and McDonald, N., Assay of bone morphogenetic protein-2, -4, and -7 in human demineralized bone matrix, *J. Craniofac. Surg.* 17, 84–90, 2006.
6. Logeart-Avramoglou, D., Bourguignon, M., Oudina, K., Ten Dijke, P., and Petite, H., An assay for the determination of biologically active bone morphogenetic proteins using cells transfected with an inhibitor of differentiation promoter-luciferase construct, *Anal. Biochem.* 349, 78–86, 2006.
7. Penn, M., Mausner-Fainberg, K., Golan, M., and Karni, A., High serum levels of BMP-2 correlate with BMP-4 and BMP-5 levels and induce reduced neuronal phenotype in patients with relapsing-remitting multiple sclerosis, *J. Neuroimmunol.* 310, 120–128, 2017.
8. Kawabata, M., and Miyazuma, K., Bone morphogenetic proteins, in *Skeletal Growth Factors*, ed. E. Canalis, Chapter 19, pp. 269–290, Lippincott, Williams and Wilkins/Wolters Kluwer, Philadelphia, PA, 2000.
9. Ripamonti, U., Teare, J., and Petit, J.C., Pleiotropism of bone morphogenetic proteins: From bone induction to cementogenesis and periodontal ligament regeneration, *J. Int. Acad. Periodontol.* 8, 23–32, 2006.
10. Chen, W., and Ten Dijke, P., Immunoregulation by members of the TGFβ superfamily, *Nat. Rev. Immunol.* 15, 723–740, 2016.
11. *Bone Morphogenetic Proteins: From Local to Systemic Therapeutics*, ed. S. Vukicevic and K.T. Sampath, Birkhäuser Verlag, Basel, Switzerland, 2008.
12. Razzouk, S., and Sarkis, R., BMP-2: Biological challenges to its clinical use, *N.Y. State Dent. J.* 78, 37–39, 2012.

BOTTOM-UP PROTEOMICS

Bottom-up proteomics is a method for the Identification of proteins by mass spectrometric analysis of peptides obtained by enzymatic (usually trypsin) hydrolysis of a sample consisting of a mixture of proteins.[1–3] The bottom-up approach is in contrast to the top-down approach which is based on the mass spectrometric analysis of intact proteins. Bottom-up proteomics usually requires fractionation of the sample prior to mass spectrometric analysis[4] and sophisticated data analysis.[5] Bottom-up proteomics may be combined with top-down proteomics in the analysis of complex proteins mixtures such as membrane proteins.[6] See **top-down proteomics**, **middle-down proteomics**.

1. Brock, A., Horn, D.M., Peters, E.C., et al., An automated matrix-assisted laser desorption/ionization quadrupole Fourier transform ion cyclotron resonance mass spectrometer for "bottom-up" proteomics, *Anal. Chem.* 75, 3419–3428, 2003.
2. Wenner, B.R., and Lynn, B.C., Factors that affect ion trap data-dependent MS/MS in proteomics, *J. Am. Soc. Mass Spectrom.* 15, 150–157, 2004.
3. McDonald, L., Robertson, D.H.L., Hurst, J.L., and Benyon, R.J., Positional proteomics: Selective recovery and analysis of *N*-terminal proteolytic peptides, *Nat. Methods* 2, 955–957, 2005.
4. Mayne, J., Ning, Z., Zhang, X., et al., Bottom-up proteomics (2013–2015): Keeping up in the era of systems biology, *Anal. Chem.* 88, 95–121, 2016.
5. Blein-Nicolas, M., and Zivy, M., Thousand and one ways to quantify and compare protein abundances in label-free bottom-up proteomics, *Biochim. Biophys. Acta* 1864, 883–895, 2016.
6. Kar, U.K., Simonian, M., and Whitelegge, J.P., Integral membrane proteins: Bottom-up, top-down and structural proteomics, *Expert Rev. Proteomics* 14, 715–723, 2017.

BRAND NAME DRUGS

A brand name drug is a drug marketed under a proprietary, trademarked-protected name as opposed to generic drugs.[1] The term reference biologic is used to refer to brand name biologicals in discussions concerning follow-on biologics or biosimilars.[2,3]

1. Payette, M., and Grant-Kels, J.M., Brand name versus generic drugs: The ethical quandary in caring for our sophisticated patients while trying to reduce health-care costs: Facts and controversies, *Clin. Dermatol.* 31, 772–776, 2013.
2. Tomaszewski, D., Biosimilar naming conventions: Pharmacist perceptions and impact on confidence in dispensing biologics, *J. Manag. Care Spec. Pharm.* 22, 919–926, 2016.
3. Sarpatwari, A., Gagne, J.J., Levidow, N.L., and Kesselheim, A.S., Active surveillance of follow-on biologics: A Prescription for uptake, *Drug. Saf.* 40, 105–108, 2017.

BIOLUMINESENCE RESONANCE ENERGY TRANSFER (BRET)

BRET is conceptually similar to FRET in that BRET is a technique which can be used to measure physical interactions between molecules based on changes in fluorescence.[1] While in the case of FRET, fluorophores are attached to proteins, BRET uses protein with intrinsic fluorescence (bioluminescence) as seen with fluorescent proteins such as green fluorescent protein, and blue fluorescent protein. The original study used fusion proteins where one fusion partner, luciferase, was the donor and another fusion partner, green fluorescent protein, was the recipient.[2] Luciferase functions as a "donor" on the basis of radiation released on the action on a substrate.[3–6] BRET has the advantage of being able to identify *in vivo* interactions in living cells The use of quantum dots has permitted the use of NIR irradiation providing better access to tissues.[7] Improvement in the quality of the luciferase used in BRET has been a significant advance.[8–12] Interesting recent applications including the interaction of AP-1 and Afr1.[13,14]

1. Sun, S., Yang, X., Wang, Y., and Shen, X., In Vivo analysis of protein-protein interactions with bioluminescence resonance energy transfer (BRET): Progress and prospects, *Int. J. Mol. Sci.* 17(10), E1704, 2016.
2. Xu, Y., Piston, D.W., and Johnson, C.H., A bioluminescence resonance energy transfer (BRET) system: Application to interacting circadian clock proteins. *Proc. Natl. Acad. Sci. USA* 96, 151–156, 1999.
3. De, A., and Gambhir, S.S., Noninvasive imaging of protein-protein interactions from live cells and living subjects using bioluminescence resonance energy transfer, *FASEB J.* 19, 2017–2019, 2005.
4. De, A., Loening, A.M., and Gambhir, S.S., An improved bioluminescence resonance energy transfer strategy for imaging intracellular events in single cells and living subjects, *Cancer Res.* 67, 7175–7183, 2007.

5. Prinz, A., Reither, G., Diskar, M., and Schultz, C., Fluorescence and bioluminescence procedures for functional proteomics, *Proteomics* 8, 1179–1196, 2008.
6. Borroto-Escuela, D.O., Li, X., Tarakanov, A.O., et al., Existence of 5-HTLA-5-HT2A isoreceptor complexes with antagonistic allosteric receptor-receptor interactions regulating 5-HT1A receptor recognition, *ACS Omega* 2, 4779–4789, 2017.
7. Tsuboi, S., and Jin, T., Bioluminescence resonance energy transfer (BRET) coupled annexin V functionalized quantum dots for near-infrared optical detection of apoptotic cells, *Chembiochem* 19(20), 2242, 2018.
8. Hall, M.P., Unch, J., Binkowski, B.F., et al., Engineered reporter from a deep sea shrimp utilizing a novel imidazopyrazinone substrate, *ACS Chem. Biol.* 7, 1848–1857, 2012.
9. Stacer, A.C., Nyati, S., Moudgil, P., et al., Nanoluc reporter for dual luciferase imaging in living animals, *Mol. Imaging* 12, 1–13, 2013.
10. Yeh, H.W., Karmach, O. Ji, A., et al., Red-shifted luciferase-luciferin pairs for enhanced bioluminescence imaging, *Nat. Methods* 14, 971–974, 2017.
11. Johnsson, K., Hiblot, J., Yu, Q., et al., Luciferases with tunable emission wavelengths, *Angew. Chem. Int. Ed.* 56, 14556–14560, 2017.
12. Schwinn, M.K., Machleidt, T., Zimmerman, K., et al., CRISPR-mediated tagging of endogenous proteins with a luminescent peptide, *ACS Chem. Biol.* 13, 467–474, 2018.
13. Sauvageau, E., McCormick, P.J., and Lefrancois, S., *In vivo* monitoring of the recruitment and activation of AP-1 by Arf-1, *Sci. Rep.* 7(1), 7148, 2017.
14. Zou, J., Salarian, M., Chen, M., et al., Direct visualization of interaction between calmodulin and connexin45, *Biochem. J.* 474, 4035–4051, 2017.

BROWNIAN MOVEMENT

The random movement of small particles, a category that includes proteins and other molecules in a solvent. The movement of the particles, which is a stochastic process, is due to the collision of the particle with solution molecules and with other particles.[1–3] Brownian motion is a force in diffusion[4] important for dynamic light scattering.[5] Rotational Brownian motion is an important consideration in NMR.[6] Solid-state NMR mitigates the effect of Brownian motion (Brownian tumbing, Brownian rotation) to permit the observation of slower internal motion.[7] Brownian motion is affected by crowding changing the behavior of proteins as particle in the cell[8] and membranes.[9] Brownian motion of molecules in solution can be translational[10,11] or rotational.[12] Brownian rotation has an influence on measurement made by NMR[13] and fluorescence measurements.[14] The Brownian correlation time (the time required for a molecule to move through one radian) is used to calculate NMR data.[15] In the case of fluorescence measurements, if rotational correlation time is less than the fluorescence emission time, data will be isotropic instead of anisotropic. Rotational correlation time can be increased by decreased temperature or increased solvent viscosity. Robert Brown is given credit for the description of the phenomenon known today as Brownian motion, although Adolphe Brongniart is also given credit.[16] The concept of Brownian motion was refined over subsequent centuries including a seminal contribution by Albert Einstein.[17] Brownian motion has been of at least as much interest in the world of finance where the concept is used in equity futures.[18,19]

1. Uhlenbeck, G.E., and Ornstein, L.S., On the theory of the Brownian motion, *Physical Rev.* 36, 823–841, 1930.
2. Weber, G., Rotational Brownian motion and polarization of the fluorescence of solutions, *Adv. Protein Chem.* 8, 415–459, 1953.
3. Cecconi, F., Cencini, M., Falcioni, M., and Vulpiani, A., Brownian motion and diffusion: From stochastic processes to chaos and beyond, *Chaos* 15, 26102, 2005.
4. Saffman, P.G., and Delbrück, M., Brownian motion in biological membranes, *Proc. Natl. Acad. Sci. USA* 72, 3111–3113, 1975.
5. Hassan, P.A., Rana, S., and Verma, G., Making sense of Brownian motion: Colloid characterization by dynamic light scattering, *Langmuir* 31, 3–12, 2015.
6. d'Auvergne, E.J., and Gooley, P.R., Optimisation of NMR dynamic models I. Minimization algorithm and their performance within the model-free and Brownian rotational diffusion spaces, *J. Biomol. NMR* 40, 107–119, 2008.
7. Krushelnitsky, A., Reichert, D., and Saalwächter, K., Solid-state NMR approaches to internal dynamics of proteins: From picoseconds to microseconds and seconds, *Acc. Chem. Res.* 46, 2028–2036, 2013.
8. Ross, M., Ott, M., Hofmann, M., et al., Coupling and decoupling of rotational and translational diffusion of proteins under crowding conditions, *J. Am. Chem. Soc.* 138, 10365–10372, 2016.
9. Krapf, D., Mechanisms underlying anomalous diffusion in the plasma membrane, *Curr. Top. Membr.* 75, 167–207, 2015.
10. Grima, R., and Yaliraki, S.N., Brownian motion of an asymmetrical particle in a potential field, *J. Chem. Phys.* 127(8), 084511, 2007.
11. Cichocki, B., Ekiel-Jenzewska, M.L., and Wajnryb, E., Communication: Translational Brownian motion for particles of arbitrary shape, *J. Chem. Phys.* 136, 071102, 2012.
12. Eloi, J.C., Okuda, M., Jones, S.E., and Schwarzacher, W., Protein Brownian rotation at the glass transition temperature of a freeze-concentrated buffer probed by superparamagnetic nanoparticles, *Biophys. J.* 104, 2681–2685, 2013.
13. Rule, G.S., and Hitchens, T.K., *Fundamentals of NMR Spectroscopy*, Springer, New York, 2006.
14. Lakowicz, J., *Principles of Fluorescence Spectroscopy*, Springer, New York, 2006.
15. Krishnan, V.V., and Cosman, M., An empirical relationship between rotational correlation time and solvent accessible surface area, *J. Biomolecular NMR* 12, 177–182, 1998.
16. Haw, M.D., Colloidal suspensions, Brownian motion, molecular reality: A short history, *J. Phys. Condens. Matter* 14, 7769–7779, 2002.
17. Kubo, R., Brownian motion and nonequilibrium statistical mechanics, *Science* 233, 330–334, 1986.
18. Szpiro, G.G., *Pricing the Future: Finance, Physics, and the 300-Year Journey to Black-Scholes Equation*, Basic Books/Perseus, New York, 2011.
19. De Spiegeleer, J., Schoutens, W., and VanHalle, C., *The Handbook of Hybrid Securities: Convertible Bonds, CoCo Bonds, and Bail-In,* John Wiley & Sons, Chichester, UK, 2012.

BULK SOLUTION

Bulk solution is defined as any macroscopic volume or space of a substance such as blood plasma or a solution of another protein relative to another volume or space of the same solvent with a different concentration of a molecular species or mixtures of species. This definition would also include interstitial fluid and a cell culture supernatant (conditioned media). In the case of interstitial fluid, bulk solution would consist of the fluid excluded from hyaluronan, a concept known as interstitial exclusion.[1] The movement of coagulation proteins from bulk solution to a multiprotein complex is responsible for the catalytic efficiency of the "tenase" complex and the "prothrombinase" complex.[2] Proteins are attracted to air–water interfaces from bulk solution resulting in aggregation.[3] The term bulk solution is also used to describe the difference between water structure in the hydration layer immediately around a macromolecule such as protein and the bulk solvent[4,5] or that between a solution phase and the adsorbate.[6] There is also a difference in hydrogen concentration in the intestine where the pH on the luminal surface (mucus layer) is markedly higher (pH $\approx$ 6) that the bulk luminal contents.[7,8]

1. Wiig, H., Gyenge, C., Iversen, P.O., et al., The role of the extracellular matrix in tissue distribution of macromolecules in normal and pathological tissues: Potential therapeutic consequences, *Microcirculation* 15, 283–296, 2008.
2. Mann, K.G., Nesheim, M.E., Church, W.R., Haley, P., and Krishnaswamy, S., Surface-dependent reactions of the Vitamin K-dependent enzyme complexes, *Blood* 76, 1–16, 1990.

3. Ghazvini, S., Kalonia, C., Volkin, D.B., and Dhar, P., Evaluating the role of the air–solution interface on the mechanism of subvisible particle formation caused by mechanical agitation for an IgG1 mAb, *J. Pharm. Sci.* 105, 1643–1656, 2016.

4. Perticaroli, S., Ehlers, G., Stanley, C.B., et al., Description of hydration water in protein (Green Fluorescent Protein) solution, *J. Am. Chem. Soc.* 139, 1098–1105, 2017.

5. Ronsin O., Caroli, C., and Baumberger, T., Preferential hydration fully controls the renaturation dynamics of collagen in water-glycerol solvents, *Eur. Phys. J. E.Soft Matter* 40(5), 55, 2017.

6. Parhi, P., Golas, A., Barnthip, N., Noh, H., and Vogler, E.A., Volumetric interpretation of protein adsorption: Capacity scaling with adsorbate molecular weight and adsorbent surface energy, *Biomaterials* 30, 6814–6824, 2009.

7. Bahari, H.M.M., Ross, I.N., and Turnberg, L.A., Demonstration of a pH gradient across the mucus layer on the surface of human gastric mucosa *in vitro*, *Gut* 23, 513–516, 1982.

8. Engel, E., Guth, P.H., Nishizaki, Y., and Kaunitz, J.D., Barrier function of the gastric mucus gel, *Am. J. Physiol.* 269, G994–G999, 1995.

CAD

A multifunctional protein that initiates and regulates *de novo* pyrimidine biosynthesis. CAD consists of a complex of four separate enzymatic activities (glutaminase, carbamoyl phosphate synthetase II, aspartate transcarbamylase, and dihydroorotase) in an approximate 1.6 MDa complex.[1] Early work had demonstrated a linkage between the carbamoyl phosphate synthetase II and aspartate transcarbamylase.[2,3] The acronym CAD was derived from three of the enzymes originally described in the complex, carbamoyl phosphate synthetase II, aspartate transcarbamylase, and dihydro orotase.[4,5] Later work established the existence of glutaminase activity together with carbamoyl phosphate synthetase II in linked domains.[6–8] Rheb protein has been shown to influence CAD function;[9] association with mTOR results in stimulation of CAD activity via phosphorylation of the carbamoyl phosphate synthetase domain.[10] Carbamoyl phosphate synthetase is a substrate for caspase during apoptosis.[11] Carbamoyl phosphate synthetase II (glutamine-hydrolyzing) in CAD is distinct from carbamoyl phosphate synthetase in mitochondria (carbamoyl phosphate [ammonia]) responsible for urea synthesis.[12] Mutations in the CAD gene have been observed.[13,14] Confusion in literature searches can result from the use of the CAD acronym for at least one more enzyme, caspase-activated DNase.[15,16] CAD is also an acronym for coronary artery disease and for computer-aided design.

1. Moreno-Morcillo, M., Grande-García, A., Ruiz-Ramos, A., et al., Structural insight into the core of CAD, the multifunctional protein leading de novo pyrimidine biosynthesis, *Structure* 25, 912–923, 2017.

2. Hoogenraad, N.J., Levine, R.L., and Kretchmer, N., Copurification of carbamoyl phosphate synthetase and aspartate transcarbamoylase from mouse spleen, *Biochem. Biophys. Res. Commun.* 44, 981–988, 1971.

3. Shoaf, T.W., and Jones, M.E., Initial steps in pyrimidine synthesis in Ehrlich ascites carcinoma, *Biochem. Biophys. Res. Commun.* 45, 796–802, 1971.

4. Grayson, D.R., and Evans, D.R., The isolation and characterization of the aspartate transcarbamylase domain of the multifunctional protein, CAD, *J. Biol. Chem.* 258, 4123–4129, 1983.

5. Sperling, R., Sperlling, J., Levine, A.D., et al., Abundant ribonucleoprotein form of CAD RNA, *Mol. Cell. Biol.* 5, 569–575, 1985.

6. Carrey, E.A., and Hardie, D.G., Mapping of catalytic domains and phosphorylation sites in the multifunctional pyrimidine-biosynthetic protein CAD, *Eur. J. Biochem.* 171, 583–588, 1988.

7. Maley, J.A., and Davidson, J.N., Identification of the junction between the glutamine amidotransferase and carbamyl phosphate synthetase domains of the mammalian CAD protein, *Biochemi. Biophys. Res. Commun.* 154, 1047–1053, 1988.

8. Chaparian, M.G., and Evans, D.R., The catalytic mechanism of the amidotransferase domain of the Syrian hamster multifunctional protein CAD. Evidence for a CAD-glutamyl covalent intermediate in the formation of carbamoyl phosphate, *J. Biol. Chem.* 266, 3387–3395, 1991.

9. Sato, T., Akasu, H., Shimono, W., et al., Rheb protein binds CAD (carbamoyl-phosphate synthetase 2, aspartate transcarbamoylase, and dihydroorotase) protein in a GTP- and effector domain-dependent manner and influences its cellular localization and carbamoyl-phosphate synthetase (CPSase) activity, *J. Biol. Chem.* 290, 1096–1105, 2015.

10. Ben-Sahra, I., Howell, J.J., Asara, J.M., and Manning, B.D., Stimulation of *de novo* pyrimidine synthesis by growth signaling through mTOR and S6K1, *Science* 339, 1323–1328, 2013.

11. Huang, M., Kozlowski, P., Collins, M., et al., Caspase-dependent cleavage of carbamoyl phosphate synthetase II during apoptosis, *Mol. Pharmacol.* 61, 569–577, 2002.

12. Aoki, T., Morris, H.P., and Weber, G., Regulatory properties and behavior of carbamoyl phosphate synthetase II (glutamine-hydrolyzing) in normal and proliferating tissues, *J. Biol. Chem.* 257, 432–438, 1982.

13. Ng, B.G., Wolfe, L.A., Ichikawa, M., et al., Biallelic mutations in CAD, impair *de novo* pyrimidine biosynthesis and decrease glycosylation precursors, *Hum. Mol. Genet.* 24, 3050–3057, 2015.

14. Koch, J., Mayr, J.A., Alhaddad, B., et al., CAD mutations and uridine-responsive epileptic encephalopathy, *Brain* 140, 279–286, 2017.

15. Samehima, K., Tone, S., and Earnshaw, W.C., CAD/DFF40 nuclease is dispensable for high molecular weight DNA cleavage and stage I chromatin condensation in apoptosis, *J. Biol. Chem.* 276, 45427–45432, 2001.

16. Sánchez-Osuna, M., Garcia-Belinchón, M., Iglesias-Guimarais, V., et al., Capase-activated DNase is necessary and sufficient for oligonucleosomal DNA breakdown, but not for chromatin disassembly during caspase-dependent apoptosis of LN-18 glioblastoma cells, *J. Biol. Chem.* 289, 18752–18769, 2014.

CADHERINS

A superfamily of proteins that enable cells to interact with other cells and extracellular matrix components.[1–3] The canonical structure of cadherins consists of extracellular portion consisting of five linked extracellular cadherin immunoglobulin-like domains (EC1-EC5), a transmembrane segment linked to the cytoskeleton via cateinin.[4,5] The term cadherin is thought to be derived from "calcium-dependent adhesion protein," although it was not possible to find a citation for this designation. The term cadherin came into use during the period of 1984–1985.[6,7] Cadherins participate in cell-cell interactions through the formation of adherin junctions.[8] The process of forming the adherins junction with some cadherins uses "cadherin strand swapping" where the *N*-terminal segment of the EC1 domain.[9,10] Cadherin switching is a separate process from cadherin strand swapping and involves the differential expression of cadherins during development[11,12] and is important in cancer.[13,14] Desmogleins are members of the cadherin family. Desmogleins are cell-to-cell adhesion molecules found in desmosomes and are involved I the pathology of pemphigus.[15]

1. Hulpiau, P., and van Roy, F., Molecular evolution of the cadherin superfamily, *Int. J. Biochem. Cell Biol.* 41, 349–358, 2009.

2. van Roy, F., Beyond E-cadherin: Roles of other cadherin superfamily members in cancer, *Nat. Rev. Cancer* 14, 121–134, 2014.

3. Gul, I.S., Hulpiau, P., Saeys, Y., and van Roy, F., Evolution and diversity of cadherin and catenans, *Exptl. Cell Res.* 358, 3–9, 2017.

4. Shapiro, L., and Weis, W.I., Structure and biochemistry of cadherins and catenins, *Cold Spring Harb. Perspect. Biol.* 1(3), a003053, 2009.

5. Hoffman, B.D., and Yap, A.S., Towards a dynamic understanding of cadherin-based mechanobiology, *Trends Cell Biol.* 25, 803–814, 2015.

6. Yoshida-Nora, C., Suzuki, K., and Takeichi, M., Molecular nature of the calcium-dependent cell-cell adhesion system in mouse teratocarcinoma and embryonic cells studied with a monoclonal antibody, *Develop. Biol.* 101, 19–27, 1984.

7. Hatta, K., Okada, T.S., and Takeichi, M., a monoclonal antibody disrupting calcium-dependent cell-cell adhesion in brain tissue. Possible role of the target antigen in animal pattern formation, *Proc. Natl. Acad. Sci. USA* 82, 2789–2793, 1985.

8. Troyanovsky, S., Adherins junction assembly, in *Adherins Junctions: From Molecular Mechanisms to Tissue Development and Disease* (*Subcellular Biochemistry 60*), ed. T. Harris, Chapter 5, pp. 89–108, Springer Science + Business Media, Dordrecht, the Netherlands, 2012.

9. Vendome, J., Posy, S., Jin, X., et al., Molecular design principles underlying β-strand swapping in the adhesive dimerization of cadherins, *Nat. Struct. Mol. Biol.* 18, 693–700, 2011.

10. Li, Y., Altorelli, N.L., Bahna, F., et al., Mechanism of E-cadherin dimerization probed by NMR relaxation dispersion, *Proc. Natl. Acad. Sci. USA* 110, 16462–16467, 2013.

11. Wheelock, M.J., Shintani, Y., Maeda, M., Fukumoto, Y., and Johnson K.R., Cadherin switching, *J. Cell Sci.* 121, 727–735, 2008.

12. Priya, R., and Yap, A.S., Making a choice: How cadherin switching controls cell migration, *Dev. Cell.* 34, 383–384, 2015.

13. Bryan, R.T., Cell adhesion and urothelial bladder cancer: The role of cadherin switching and related phenomena, *Philos. Trans. R. Soc. Lond. B. Biol. Sci.* 370 (1661), 20140042, 2015.

14. Tarhan, Y.E., Kato, T., Jang, M., et al., Morphological changes, cadherin switching, and growth suppression in pancreatic cancer by GALNT6 knockdown, *Neoplasia* 18, 265–272, 2016.

15. Kasperkiewicz, M., Ellebrecht, C.T., Takahashi, H., et al., Pemphigus, *Nat. Rev. Dis. Primers* 3, 17026, 2017.

CAENORHABDITIS ELEGANS

Caenorhabditis elegans (*C. elegans*) is a free-living roundworm, which has been used extensively for a variety of biological studies.[1–4] *C. elegans* is notable for the discovery of RNA silencing/RNA interference.[5,6] *C. elegans* is used as a model organism for a wide variety of studies including viruses,[7,8] preclinical drug discovery[9] and toxicology.[10,11] There is great interest in the use of *C. elegans* in aging research.[12–16] While *C. elegans* has been valuable, considerable care is required in experimental technique.[17]

1. *C. elegans: Methods and Applications*, ed. K. Strange, Humana Press, Totowa, NJ, 2006.

2. Hall, D.H., and Altum Z.F., *C. elegans Atlas*, Cold Spring Harbor Laboratory Press, Cold Spring Harbor, New York, 2008.

3. *Caenorhabditis: Molecular Genetics and Development*, ed. J.H. Rothman and A. Simpson, Elsevier, Amsterdam, the Netherlands, 2011.

4. *Caenorhabditis elegans: Cell Biology and Physiology*, Academic Press, San Diego, CA, 2012.

5. Fire, A., Xu, S., Montgomery, M.K., et al., Potent and specific genetic interference by double-stranded RNA in *Caenorhabditis elegans*, *Nature* 391, 806–811, 1998.

6. Youngman, E.M., and Claycomb, J.M., From early lessons to new frontiers: The worm as a treasure trove of small RHA biology, *Front. Genet.* 5, 416, 2014.

7. Diego, J., and Bratanich, A., The nematode *Caenorhabditis elegans* as a model to study viruses, *Arch. Viriol.* 159, 2843–2851, 2014.

8. van Sluijs, L., Pijlman, G.P., and Kammenga, J.E., Why do individuals differ in viral susceptibility? A story told by model organisms, *Viruses* 30, E284, 2017.

9. Kim, W., Hendricks, G.L., Lee, K., and Mylonakis, E., An update on the use the *C. elegans* for preclinical drug discovery: Screening and identifying anti-infective drugs, *Expert Opin. Drug Discov.* 12, 625–633, 2017.

10. Tejeda-Benitez, L., and Olivero-Verbel, J., *Caenorhabditis elegans*: A biological model for research in toxicology, *Rev. Environ. Camon. Toxicol.* 237, 1–35, 2016.

11. Honnen, S., *Caenorhabditis elegans* as a powerful alternative model organism to promote research in genetic toxicology and biomedicine, *Arch. Toxicol.* 91, 2029–2044, 2017.

12. Labuschagne, C.F., and Brenkman, A.B., Current methods in quantifying ROS and oxidative damage in *Caenorhabditis elegans* and other model organisms of aging, *Aging Res.* 12, 918–930, 2013.

13. Gruber, J., Chen, C.B., Fong, S., et al., *Caenorhabditis elegans*: What we can and cannot learn from aging worms, *Antioxid. Redox Signal.* 23, 256–279, 2015.

14. Kim, D.K., Kim, T.H., and Lee, S.J., Mechanisms of aging-related proteinopathies in *Caenorhabditis elegans*, *Exp. Mol. Med.* 48(10), e263, 2016.

15. Gao, A.W., Ult de Bos, J., Sterken, M.G., et al., Forward and reverse genetics approaches to uncover metabolic aging pathways in *Caenorhabditis elegans*, *Biochim. Biophys. Acta* 1864, 2697–2706, 2018.

16. Birkenfeld, A.L., The longevity gene INDY (I'm not dead yet) in metabolic control: Potential as pharmacological target, *Pharmacol. Ther.* 185, 1–18, 2018.

17. Lithgow, G.J., Driscoll, M., and Phillips, P., A long journey to reproducible results, *Nature* 548, 387–388, 2017.

CALCINEURIN

Calcineurin is a protein phosphatase consisting to two dissimilar subunits.[1,2] Early studies referred to calcineurin as protein phosphatase 2B.[3] The heterodimer consists of a 57–59 kDa catalytic subunit (CnA) and a 19–20 kDa regulatory subunit (CnB). Calcineurin is activated by the binding of Ca^{2+}/calmodulin.[4] The term calcineurin was advanced in 1979[5] to describe a protein isolated in 1978 as an inhibitor of 3′,5′-nucleotide phosphodiesterase.[6] Early work had shown that cyclosporin in combination with an immunophilin[7] inhibited T-cell activation[8] in its role as an immunosuppression agent. It was shortly shown that the action of cyclosporin and FK-506 as immunosuppression drugs were mediated through direction action on calcineurin.[9] Subsequent work has shown that calcineurin, in response to increased intracellular calcium ion, is a critical mediator of T-cell activation.[10–12] While there has been much emphasis on the role of calcineurin in T-cells, there has also been considerable interest in the role of calcineurin in nervous tissue[13] and glucose metabolism.[14]

1. Guerini, D., Calcineurin: Not just a simple protein phosphatase, *Biochem. Biophys. Res. Commun.* 235, 271–275, 1997.

2. Rusnak, F., and Mertz, F., Calcineurin: Form and function, *Physiol. Rev.* 80, 1483–1521, 2000.

3. Stewart, A.A., Ingebritsen, T.S., and Cohen, P., The protein phosphatases involved in cellular regulation. 5. Purification and properties of a Ca^{2+}/calmodulin-dependent protein phosphatase (2B) from rabbit skeletal muscle, *Eur. J. Biochem.* 132, 289–295, 1983.

4. Yang, S.D., Tallant, E.A., and Cheung, W.Y., Calcineurin is a calmodulin-dependent protein phosphatase, *Biochem. Biophys. Res. Commun.* 106, 1419–1425, 1982.

5. Klee, C.B., Crouch, T.H., and Krinks, M.H., Calcineurin: A calcium- and calmodulin-binding protein of the nervous system, *Proc. Natl. Acad. Sci. USA* 76, 6270–6275, 1979.

6. Klee, C.B., and Krinks, M.H., Purification of cyclic 3′,5′-nucleotide phosphodiesterase inhibitory protein by affinity chromatography on activator protein coupled to Sepharose, *Biochemistry* 17, 120–126, 1978.

7. Friedman, J., and Weissman, I., Two cytoplasmic candidates for immunophilin action are revealed by affinity for a new cyclophllin: One in the presence and one in the absence of CsA, *Cell* 66, 799–806, 1991.

8. Thomson, A.W., Woo, J., and Coooper, M., Mode of action of immunosuppression drugs with particular reference to the molecular basis of macrolide-induced immunosuppression, in *The Molecular Biology of Immunosuppression*, ed. A.W. Thomson, Chapter 8, pp. 153–179, John Wiley & Sons, Chichester, UK, 1992.

9. Liu, J., Farmer, J.D., Jr., Lane, W.B., et al., Calcineurin is a common target of cyclophilin-cyclosporin A and FKBP-FK506 complexes, *Cell* 66, 807–815, 1991.

10. Crabtree, C.B., Calcium, calcineurin, and the control of transcription, *J. Biol. Chem.* 275, 2313–2316, 2001.

11. Cristillo, A.D., and Bierer, B.E., Immunophilins and the immunophilin-binding agents, in *Clinical Immunology Prnciples and Practice*, 2nd edn., ed. Rich, R.R., Fleisher, T.A., Shearer, W.T., Kotzin, B.L, and Schroeder, H.W., Jr., Section 111, Mosby, London, UK, 2001.

12. Hogan, P.G., Calcium-NFAT transcriptional signalling in T cell activation and T cell exhaustion, *Cell Calcium* 63, 66–60, 2017.

13. Woolfrey, K.M., and Dell'Acqua, M.L., Coordination of protein phosphorylation and dephosphorylation in synaptic plasticity, *J. Biol. Chem.* 290, 28604–28612, 2015.
14. Chalckera, H.A., Kudva, Y., and Kaplan, B., Calcineurin inhibitors: Pharmacologic mechanism impacting both insulin resistance and insulin secretion leading to glucose dysregulation and diabetes mellitus, *Clin. Pharmacol. Ther.* 101, 114–120, 2017.

CALCIUM TRANSIENT

A calcium transient is a temporal change in intracellular calcium concentration ($[Ca^{2+}]$)[1,2] resulting primarily from Ca^{2+} release from the sarcoplasmic reticulum[3] but also from outside the cells via specialized calcium channels. Intracellular calcium ions are regulators of a wide variety of cellular function including insulin release from the pancreas,[4,5] the action of cholangiocytes in the secretion of bile,[6] and muscle contraction.[7] The measurement of calcium transients is generally accomplished with microscopy and fluorescent dyes which are specific for calcium ions.[8]

1. Cannell, M.B., Berlin, J.R., and Lederer, W.J., Effect of membrane potential changes on the calcium transients in single rat cardiac muscle cells, *Science* 238, 1419–1473, 1987.
2. Barcenas-Ruiz, L., and Wier, W.G., Voltage dependence of intracellular $[Ca^{2+}]_i$ transients in guinea pig ventricular myocytes, *Circulation Research* 61, 148–154, 1987.
3. Hancox, J.C., and Levi, A.J., Na-Ca exchange tail current indicates voltage dependence of the Ca_i transition in rabbit ventricular myocytes, *J. Cardiovascular Electrophysiol.* 6, 455–470, 1995.
4. Nadal, A., and Soria, B., Glucose metabolism regulates cytosolic Ca^{2+} in the pancreas by three different mechanisms, *Adv. Exptl. Med. Biol.* 426 (*Physiology and Pathophysiology of the Islets of Langerhans*), 236–243, 1997.
5. Llanos, P., Contreras-Ferrat, A., Barrientos, G., et al., Glucose-dependent insulin secretion in pancreatic β-islets from male rates requires Ca^{2+} release via ROS-stimulated ryanodine receptors, *PLoS One* 10(6), e0129238, 2015.
6. Amaya, M.J., and Nathanson, M.H., Calcium signaling and the secretory activity of bile epithelia, *Cell Calcium* 55, 317–324, 2014.
7. Baylor, S.M., and Hollingwoth, S., Intracellular calcium movements during excitation-contraction coupling in mammalian slow-twitch and fast-twitch muscle fibers, *J. Gen. Physiol.* 139, 261–272, 2012.
8. Su, Z., and Barry, W.H., Isolated myocyte mechanics and calcium transients, in *Cardiovascular Physiology in the Genetically Engineered Mouse*, 2nd edn., ed. B.D. Hoit and R.A. Walsh, Chapter 6, pp. 71–89, Kluwer Academic, Boston, MA, 2002.

CALM PROTEIN

CALM is an acronym for clathrin assembly lymphoid myeloid leukemia used to identify a protein, CALM-protein.[1] CALM-protein is a 62 kDa protein with homology to AP-180, a protein unique to brain and also involved in clathrin-mediated endocytosis as an adaptor protein.[2,3] As a homolog of AP-180, an adaptor/accessory protein specific of the nervous system, CALM participates in synaptic vesicle formation.[4,5] CALM-protein participates in clathrin-mediated endocytosis by directing interaction with the clathrin lattice[6,7] via specific domains on both clathrin and the CALM-protein.[8–10] CALM-protein is also implicated in leukemia through a gene fusion *CALM-AF10*.[11] Other work has shown that the CALM-protein provides a nuclear export signal, which is essential for the development of leukemia (leukemogenesis).[12] CALM-protein has also been suggested to be involved in Alzheimer's disease through the regulation of γ-secretase.[13,14] The *CALM* gene is also known as the *PICALM* gene.[15] The expression of *PICALM* has been suggested to be involved in Alzheimer's disease.[16] CALM protein also interacts with inositol lipids.[17] CALM is also involved in the regulation of the transport of KIT receptor kinase in hematopoietic cells.[18] The use of the CALM acronym is pleiotropic with use also to denote calmodulin protein[19] and calmodulin gene.[20]

1. Dreyling, M.H., Martinez-Ciment, J.A., Zheng, M., et al., The (10,11)(p13q14) in the U937 cell line results in the fusion of the *AF10* gene and *CALM* encoding a new member of the AP-3 clathrin assembly protein family, *Proc. Natl. Acad. Sci. USA* 93, 4804–4819, 1996.
2. Tebar, F., Bohlander, S.K., and Sorkin, A., Clathrin assembly lymphoid myeloid leukemia (CALM) protein: Localization in the endocytic-coated pits interactions with clathrin and the impact of overexpression on clathrin-mediated traffic, *Mol. Biol. Cell* 10, 2667–2702, 1999.
3. Kusner, L., and Carlin, C., Potential role for a novel AP180-related protein during endocytosis in MDCK cells, *Amer. J. Physiol.* 295, C995–C1008, 2003.
4. Granseth, B., Odermatt, B., Royle, S.J., and Lagnado, L., Clathrin-mediated endocytosis: The physiology mechanism of vesicle retrieval at hippocampal synapses, *J. Physiol.* 585, 681–686, 2007.
5. Miller, S.E., Mathiasen, S., Bright, N.A., et al., CALM regulates clathrin-coated vesicle size and maturation by directly sensing and driving membrane curvature, *Develop. Cell* 33, 163–175, 2015.
6. Rappaport, J.Z., Kemal, S., Benmerah, A., and Simon, S., Dynamics of clathrin and adaptor proteins during endocytosis, *Am. J. Physiol. Cell Physiol.* 291, C1072–C1081, 2006.

7. Sochacki, K.A., Dickey, A.M., Strub, M.P., and Taraska, J.W., Endocytic proteins are partitioned to the edge of the clathrin lattice in mammalian cells, *Nat. Cell. Biol.* 19, 352–361, 2017.

8. Martizen, T., Kos, J.J., and Haucke, V., Turning CALM into excitement: AP180 and CALM in endocytosis and disease, *Biol. Cell* 104, 588–602, 2012.

9. Chen, L-S., Moshkanbaryans, L., Xue, J., and Graham, M.E., The ~16 kDa C-terminal sequence of clathrin assembly protein AP180 is essential for efficient clatrin binding, *PLoS One* 9(11), e110557, 2014.

10. Moshkanbaryans, L., Xue, J., Wark, J.R., Robinson, P.J., and Graham, M.E., A novel sequence in AP180 and CALM promotes efficient clathrin binding and assembly, *PLoS One* 11(8), e0162050, 2016.

11. Caudell, D., and Aplan, P.D., The role of *CALM-AF10* gene fusion in acute leukemia, *Leukemia* 22, 678–685, 2008.

12. Conway, A.E., Scotland, P.B., Lavau, C.P., and Wechsler, D.S., A CALM-derived nuclear export signal is essential for CALM-AF10-mediated leukemogenesis, *Blood* 121, 4758–4768, 2013.

13. Kanatsu, K., Morohashi, Y., Suzuki, M., et al., Decreased CALM expression reduces Aβ42 to total Aβ ratio through clathrin-mediated endocytosis of γ-secretase, *Nat. Commun.* 5, 3386, 2014.

14. Kanatsu, K., Hori, Y., Takatori, S., et al., Partial loss of CALM function reduces Aβ42 production and amyloid deposition *in vivo*, *Hum. Genet.* 25, 3988–3997, 2016.

15. https://www.ncbi.nlm.nih.gov/gene/8301.

16. Ando, K., Brion, J.P., Stygelbout, V., et al., Clathrin adaptor CALM/PICALM is associated with neurofibrillary tangles and is cleaved in Alzheimer's brains, *Acta Neuropathol.* 125, 861–878, 2013.

17. Balla, T., Inositol-lipid binding motifs: Signal integrators through protein-lipid and protein-protein interactions, *J. Cell Sci.* 15, 118, 2005.

18. Rai, S., Tanaka, H., Suzuki, M., et al., Clathrin assembly protein CALM plays a critical role in KIT signaling by regulating its cellular transport from early to late endosomes in hematopoietic cells, *PLoS One* 9(10), e109441, 2014.

19. Meng, H., Zhu, X., LI., L., et al., Identification of nasopharyngeal carcinoma using a mass spectrometer-based comparative proteomic approach, *Int. J. Mol. Med.* 40, 1152–1164, 2017.

20. Rocchetti, M., Sala, L., Dreizelhunter, L., et al., Elucidating arrhythmogenic mechanisms of long-QT syndrome CALM1-F153L mutation in patient-specific induced pluripotent stem cell-derived cardiomyocytes, *Cardiovasc. Res.* 113, 531–541, 2017.

CALNEXIN

Calnexin is a trans-membrane lectin and chaperone for glycoproteins with a molecular weight of 64–66 kDa.[1–3] Calnexin was originally described as p88, a 88 kDa protein, which was transiently associated with class I histocompatibility heavy chain in murine tumor cell lines.[4] p88 protein was subsequently shown to be identical with calnexin.[5] Calnexin was shown to have homology with **calreticulin**[6] and participates with calreticulin as a chaperone to maintain glycoprotein quality in export from the ER (endoplasmic reticulum).[7] Calnexin (and calreticulin) is described as lectins on the basis of their ability to bind to glycoproteins.[8–10] Calnexin also recruits processing enzymes such as protein disulfide isomerase.[11,12] Palmitoylation of calnexin serve to regulate the function of calnexin; palmitoylation shifts calnexin to calcium regulation while a decrease in palmitoylation shifts calnexin function to the better know chaperone function.[13,14] The function of calnexin is also regulated by phosphorylation.[15,16]

1. Tatu, U., and Helenius, A., Interactions between newly synthesized glycoproteins, calnexin and a network of resident chaperones in the endoplasmic reticulum, *J. Cell Biol.* 136, 555–565, 1997.

2. Yamashita, T., Kiyoki, E., Tomita, Y., and Taira, H., Immunoaffinity purification and identification of the molecular chaperone calnexin, *Biosci. Biotechnol. Biochem.* 63, 1491–1493, 1999.

3. Lamriben, L., Graham, J.B., Adams, B.M., and Herbert, D.N., *N*-Glycan-based ER molecular chaperone and protein quality control system: The calnexin binding cycle, *Traffic* 17, 306–326. 2016.

4. Degen, E., and Williams, D.B., Participation of a novel 88-kD protein in the biogenesis of murine class I histocompatibility molecules, *J. Cell Biol.* 112, 1099–1115, 1991.

5. Ahluwalia, N., Bergeron, J.J., Wada, I., Degen, E., and Williams, E.B., The p88 molecular chaperone is identical to the endoplasmic reticulum membrane protein, calnexin, *J. Biol. Chem.* 267, 10914–10918, 1992.

6. Bergeron, J.J.M., Brenner, M.B., Thomas, D.Y., and Willams, D.B., Calnexin: A membrane-based chaperone of the endoplasmic reticulum, *Trends Biochem. Sci.* 19, 124–129, 1994.

7. Wiliams, D.B., Beyond lectins: The calnexin/calreticulin chaperone system of the endoplasmic reticulum, *J. Cell. Sci.* 119, 615–523, 2006.

8. Hammond, C., Braakman, I., and Helenius, A., Role of N-linked oligosaccharide recognition, glucose trimming, and calnexin in glycoprotein folding and quality control, *Proc. Natl. Acad. Sci. USA* 91, 913–917, 1994.

9. Bergeron, J.J., Zapun, A., Ou, W.J., et al., The role of the lectin calnexin in conformation independent binding to *N*-linked glycoproteins and quality control, *Adv. Exp. Biol. Med.* 435, 105–116, 1998.

10. Hirano, M., Imagawa, A., and Totani, K., Stratified analysis of lectin-like chaperones in the folding disease-related metabolic syndrome rat model, *Biochem. Biophys. Res. Commun.* 478, 247–253, 2016.

11. Nakao, H., Seko, A., Ito, Y., and Sakono, M., PDI family protein ERp29 recognizes P-domain of molecular chaperone calnexin, *Biochem. Biophys. Res. Commun.* 487, 763–767, 2017.
12. Kozlov, G., Muñoz-Excobar, J., Castro, K., and Gehring, K., Mapping the ER interactome: The P domains of calnexin and calreticulin as plurivalent adaptors for foldases and chaperones, *Structure* 25, 1415–1422, 2017.
13. Lynes, E.M., Raturi, A., Shenkman, M., et al., Palmitoylation is the switch that assigns calnexin to quality control or ER Ca²⁺ signaling, *J. Cell Sci.* 126, 3893–3903, 2013.
14. Dallavilla, T., Abrami, L., Sandoz, P.A., et al., Model-driven understanding of palmitoylation dynamics: Regulated acylation of the endoplasmic reticulum chaperone calnexin, *PLoS Comput. Biol.* 12(2), e1004774, 2016.
15. Chevet, E., Smirle, J., Cameron, P.H., et al., Calnexin phosphorylation: Linking cytoplasmic signalling to endoplasmic reticulum luminal functions, *Semin. Cell Dev. Biol.* 21, 486–490, 2010.
16. Bollo, M., Paredex, R.M., Holstein, D., et al., Calcineurin interacts with PERK and dephosphorylates calnexin to relieve ER stress in mammals and frogs, *PLoS One* 5(8), e11925, 2010.

CALPONIN

Calponin is a protein with several isoforms that regulates actin function in smooth muscle and non-muscle cells.[1] Calponin was first identified as a 34 kDa protein characterized by binding to calmodulin and actin was isolated from chicken gizzard smooth muscle.[2] Protein preparation with similar properties was subsequently isolated from bovine aorta smooth muscle. This protein preparation consisted of several species with different molecular masses around 35 kDa and was termed as calponin (calcium-binding and calmodulin-binding troponin T-like protein).[3] The isoforms of calponin differ by the length of a C-terminal variable region. The calponin homology domain is found in the N-terminal region of the calponins and may have a role in the binding of actin. The calponin homology domain[4] is found in a number of other proteins such as utrophin and dystrophin where there is a defined function in binding actin.[5]

1. Liu, R., and Jin, J.B., Calponin isoforms CNN1, CNN2, and CNN3: Regulators for actin cytoskeleton functions in smooth muscle and non-smooth muscle cells, *Gene* 585, 143–153, 2016.
2. Takahashi, K., Hiwada, K., and Kokubu, T., Isolation and characterization of a 34,000-dalton calmodulin-and F-actin-binding protein from chicken gizzard smooth muscle, *Biochem. Biophys. Res. Commun.* 141, 20–26, 1986.
3. Takahashi, K., Hiwada, K., and Kokubu, T., Vascular smooth muscle calponin. A novel troponin T-like protein, *Hypertension* 11, 620–626, 1988.
4. Korenbaum, E., and Rivero, F., Calponin homology domains at a glance, *J. Cell. Sci.* 115, 3543–3545, 2002.
5. Singh, S.M., Bandi, S., and Mallela, K.M., The N- and C-terminal domains differentially contribute to the structure and function of dystrophin and utrophin tandem calponin-homology domains, *Biochemistry* 54, 6942–6950, 2015.

CALRETICULIN

Calreticulin is a soluble 50–60 kDa protein with a variety of functions.[1] Calreticulin was originally isolated as protein with a high affinity for calcium ions[2] and subsequently described as a calsequestrin-like protein in non-muscle cells.[3] Calreticulin has an important function as a calcium buffer in the lumen of the endoplasmic reticulum.[4] Calreticulin functions with calnexin as a chaperone in the endoplasmic reticulum to maintain quality control in collaboration with other factors such as protein disulfide isomerases.[5–10] Autophagy results in the surface exposure of calreticulin on tumor cells promoting phagocytosis by dendritic cells. There is interest in calreticulin as a therapeutic target. See **autophagy**, **calnexin**.

1. Michalak, M., Corbett, E.F., Mesaeli, N., Nakamura, K., and Opas, M., Calreticulin one protein, one gene, many functions, *Biochem. J.* 344, 281–292, 1999.
2. Ostwald, T.J., MacLennan, D.H., and Dorrington, K.J., Effects of cation binding on the conformation of calsequestrin and the high affinity calcium-binding protein of sarcoplasmic reticulum, *J. Biol. Chem.* 249, 5867–5871, 1974.
3. Treves, S., De Mattei, M., Landredi, M., et al., Calreticulinis a candidate for a calsquestrin-like function in Ca²⁺-storage compartments (calciosomes) of liver and brain, *Biochem. J.* 271, 473–480, 1990.
4. Dudek, E., and Michalak, M., Calnexin and calreticulin, in *Encyclopedia of Metalloproteihs*, ed. R.H. Kretsinger, V.N. Uversky, and Permayaken, E.A., pp. 555–562, Springer, New York, 2013.
5. Trombetta, E.S., and Helenius, A., Lectins as chaperones in glycoprotein folding, *Curr. Opin. Struct. Biol.* 8, 587–592, 1998.
6. Williams, D.B., Beyond lectins: The calnexin/calreticulin chaperone system of the endoplasmic reticulum, *J. Cell Sci.* 199, 615–623, 2006.
7. Tannous, A., Pisoni, G.B., Helbert, D.N., and Molinari, M., N-linked sugar-regulated protein folding and quality control in the ER, *Semin. Cell Dev. Biol.* 41, 79–89, 2015.
8. Bloy, N., Garcia, P., Laumont, C.M., et al., Immunogenic stress and death of cancer cells: Contribution of antigenicity vs adjuvanticity to immunosurveillance, *Immun. Rev.* 280, 165–174, 2017.

9. Vandenabeele, P., Vandecasteele, K., Bachert, C., et al., Immunogenic apoptotic cell death and anticancer immunity, *Adv. Exp. Med. Biol.* 930, 133–149, 2016.
10. Eggleton, P., Bremer, E., Dudek, E., and Michalak, M., Calreticulin, a therapeutic target? *Expert Opin. Ther. Targets* 20, 1137–1147, 2016.

CAMELID ANTIBODIES

Camelids are unique antibodies and members of the Camelidae family. The antibody structure consists of the variable region from the heavy chain (VHH) and the CH2 and CH3 domains from the Fc region of the antibody molecule but no light chain.[1–3] The VHH domain is the smallest antibody antigen binding domain (paratope) that can be derived from a naturally occurring immunoglobulin.[4] VHH and VHH derivates are known as nanobodies.[5,6] There is considerable interest in the VHH technology in diagnostics as imaging agents[7–9] and therapeteutics.[10–13] Sharks also have single-domain immunoglobulins.[14] There is a recent report of a human single-domain antibody derivative referred to "i-bodies" with properties similar to a camelid antibody.[15]

1. Hamers-Castleman, C., Atarhouch, T., Muyldermans, S., et al., Naturally occurring antibodies devoid of light chain, *Nature* 363, 446–448, 1993.
2. Muyldermans, S., Atarhouch, T., Saldanha, J., Barbosa, J.A., and Hamers, R., Sequence and structure of VH domain from naturally occurring camel heavy chain immunoglobulin lacking light chain, *Protein Eng.* 7, 1129–1135, 1994.
3. De Genst, E., Saerens, D., Muyldermans, S., and Conrath, K., Antibody repertoire development in camelids, *Dev. Comp. Immunol.* 30, 187–198, 2006.
4. Muyldermans, S., Single domain camel antibodies: Current status, *Rev. Mol. Biotechnol.* 74, 377–303, 2001.
5. Muyldermans, S., Nanobodies: Natural single domain antibodies, *Annu. Rev. Biochem.* 82, 775–797, 2013.
6. Schumacher, D., Helma, J., Schneider, A.F.L., Leonhardt, H., and Hackenberger, C., Chemical functionalization strategies and intracellular applications of nanobodies, *Angew. Chem. Int. Ed. Engl.* 57, 2314–2333, 2018.
7. Massa, S., Xavier, C., De Vos, J., et al., Site-specific labeling of cysteine-tagged single-domain antibody fragments for use in molecular imaging, *Bioconjug. Chem.* 25, 979–988, 2014.
8. Blykers, A., Schoonooghe, S., Xavier, C., et al., PET imaging of macrophage mannose receptor-expressing macrophages in tumor stroma using ^{18}F-radiolabeled camelid single-domain antibody fragments, *J. Nucl. Med.* 56, 1265–1271, 2015.
9. Vandesquille, M., Li, T., Po, C., et al., Chemically-defined camelid antibody bioconjugate for the magnetic reasoning imaging of Alzheimer's disease, *mAbs* 9, 1016–1027, 2017.
10. Revets, H., Baetseller, P., and Muyldermans, S., Nanobodies as novel reagents for cancer therapy, *Expt. Opin. Biol. Ther.* 5, 111–124, 2005.
11. Yardehnavi, N., Behdani, M., Bagheri, K.P., et al., A camelid antibody candidate for development against *Hemicarpus lepturus* envenomation, *FASEB J.* 28, 4004–4014, 2014.
12. Beirnaert, E., Desmyter, A., Spinelli, S., et al., Bivalent Llama single-domain antibody fragments against tumor necrosis factor have picomolar potencies due to intramolecular interactions, *Front. Immunol.* 8, 867, 2017.
13. Krasniqi, A., D'Huyvetter, M., Xavier, C., et al., Theranostic radiolabeled anti-CD20 sdAb for targeted radionuclide therapy of Non-Hodgkin Lymphoma, *Mol. Cancer Ther.* 16, 2828–2839, 2017.
14. Goldman, E.R., Liu, J.L., Zabetakis, D., and Anderson, G.F., Enhancing stability of camelid and shark single domain antibodies: An overview, *Front. Immunol.* 8, 865, 2017.
15. Griffiths, K., Dolezal, O., Cao, B., et al., i- bodies, human single domain antibodies that antagonize chemokine receptor CXCR4, *J. Biol. Chem.* 291, 12641–12657, 2016.

CATABOLITE ACTIVATOR PROTEIN (CYCLIC AMP RECEPTOR PROTEIN)

Catabolite activator protein (CAP) was originally defined as cAMP receptor protein in *Escherichia coli*, a dimer with a molecular weight of 45,000.[1,2] CAP is regulated by cyclic AMP and binds to DNA near or at promoter regions[3] activating RNA polymerase and the transcription process of a large number of proteins.[4–6] The term cAMP receptor protein (CRP) is still used to refer to this activity[7,8] and would appear to be the preferred term.[9] Although most of the work are on transcription repressors and activators related to bacterial systems, there are relevant human studies.[10]

1. Busby, S., Aiba, H., and de Crombrugghie, B., Mutations in the *Escherichia coli* operon that defines two promoters and the binding site of the cyclic AMP receptor protein, *J. Mol. Biol.* 154, 211–227, 1982.
2. Aiba, H., Fujimoto, S., and Ozaki, N., Molecular cloning and nucleotide sequence the gene for the *E. coli* cAMP receptor protein, *Nucleic Acids Res.* 10, 1345–1361, 1982.
3. Zhou, Y., Merkel, T.J., and Ebright, R.H., Characterization of the activating region of *Escherichia coli* catabolite gene activator protein (CAP). II. Role at Class I and class II CAP-dependent promoters, *J. Mol. Biol.* 243, 603–610, 1994,
4. Busby, S., and Ebright, R.H., Transcription activation by catabolite activator protein (CAP), *J. Mol. Biol.* 293, 199–213, 1999.
5. Benoff, B., Yang, H., Lawson, C.L., et al., Structural basis of transcription activation: The CAP-alpha CTD-DNA complex, *Science* 297, 1562–1566, 2002.

6. Swigon, D., and Olson, W.K., Mesoscale modeling of multi-protein-DNA assemblies: The role of the catabolic activator protein in Lac-repressor-mediated looping, *Int. J. Non Linear Mech.* 43, 1082–1993, 2008.

7. Harman, J.B., Allosteric regulation of the cAMP receptor protein, *Biochim. Biophys. Acta* 1547, 1–17, 2001.

8. Geng, H., and Jiang, R., cAMP receptor protein (CRP)-mediated resistance/tolerance in bacteria: Mechanism and utilization in biotechnology, *Appl. Microbiol. Biotechnol.* 99, 4533–4543, 2015.

9. Lee, D.J., Minchin, S.D., and Busby, S.J., Activating transcription in bacteria, *Annu. Rev. Microbiol.* 66, 125–152, 2012.

10. Liang, H., Mao, X., Olejniczak, E.T., et al., Solution structure of the ets domain of Fli-1 when bound to DNA, *Nat. Struct. Biol.* 1, 871–875, 1994.

CATHEPSINS

The term cathepsins define a family of 11 thiol proteases (MEROPS Clan CA, for example, cathepsin B, C01.060)[1,2] involved in lysosomal digestion of proteins.[3–6] Cathepsins have long been considered to be responsible for the intracellular degradation of proteins.[7–9] Cathepsins also have a well-documented role in the processing proteins in the antigenic response.[10–14] More recent studies show a role for cathepsins in programmed cell death.[15–17] There is work showing that cathepsins do have extracellular activity.[18,19] As work has shown more specificity to the action(s) of cathepsins, there has been increased interest in cathepsins as therapeutic targets.[20–23]

1. https://www.ebi.ac.uk/merops/cgi-bin/pepsum?id=C01.060.

2. Rawlings, N.D., Using the MEROPS database for investigation of lysosomal peptidases, their inhibitors, and substrates, *Methods Mol. Biol.* 1594, 213–226, 2017.

3. Ballard, F.J., Intracellular protein degradation, *Essays Biochem.* 13, 1–37, 1977.

4. Barrettt, A.J., and Kischeke, H., Cathepsin B, Cathepsin H, and Cathepsin L, *Methods Enzymol.* 80, 535–561, 198.

5. Stoka, V., Turk, B., and Turk, V., Lysosomes as "suicide bags" in cell death: Myth or reality, *J. Biol. Chem.* 284, 21783–21787, 2009.

6. Erickson, A.H., Isidero, C., Mach, L., and Mort, J.S., Cathepsins: Getting in shape for lysosomal proteolysis, in *Proteases: Structure and Function*, ed. K. Brit and W. Stöcker, Chapter 4, pp. 127–173, Springer, Vienna, Austria, 2013.

7. Bohley, P., and Seglen, P.O., Proteases and proteolysis in the lysosome, *Experentia* 48, 151–157, 1992.

8. Dice, J.F., *Lysosomal Pathways of Protein Degradation*, Landes Bioscience, Georgetown, TX, 2000.

9. Müller, S., Faulhaber, S., Sieber, C., et al., The endolysosomal cysteine cathepsins L and K are involved in macrophage-mediated clearance of *Staphylococcus aureus* and concomitant cytokine induction, *FASEB J.* 28, 162–175, 2014.

10. Honey, K., and Rudensky, A.Y., Lysosomal cysteine proteases regulate antigen presentation, *Nat. Rev. Immunol.* 3, 472–482, 2003.

11. Bryant, P., and Ploegh, H., Class II MHC peptide loading by the professionals, *Curr. Opin. Immunol.* 16, 96–102, 2004.

12. Burster, T., Macmillan, H., Hou, T., Boehm, B.O., and Mellins, E.D., Cathepsin G: Roles in antigen presentation and beyond, *Mol. Immunol.* 47, 658–665, 2010.

13. van Kasteren, S.I., and Overkleeft, H.S., Endo-lysosomal proteases in antigen presentation, *Curr. Opin. Chem. Biol.* 23, 8–14, 2014.

14. Unanue, E.R., Turk, B., and Neefjes, J., Variations in MHC Class II antigen processing and presentation in health and disease, *Annu. Rev. Immunol.* 34, 265–297, 2016.

15. Kroemer, G., and Jäätelä, M., Lysosomes and autophagy in cell death control, *Nat. Rev. Cancer* 5, 886–897, 2005.

16. Fehrenbacher, N., Gyrd-Hansen, M., Poulsen, B., et al., Sensitization to the lysosomal cell death pathway upon immortalization and transformation, *Cancer. Res.* 64, 5301–5310, 2004.

17. Alts, S., and Jäätelä, M., Lysosomal cell death at a glance, *J. Cell Sci.* 126, 1905–1912, 2013.

18. Fonović, M., and Turk, B., Cysteine cathepsins and extracellular matrix degradation, *Biochim. Biophys. Acta* 1840, 2560–2570, 2014.

19. Pišlar, A., Perišić Nanut, M., and Kos, J., Lysosomal cysteine peptidases—Molecules signaling tumor cell death and survival, *Semin. Cancer Biol.* 35, 168–179, 2015.

20. Reiser, J., Adair, B., and Reinhekel, T., Specialized roles for cysteine cathepsins in heath and disease, *J. Clin. Invest.* 120, 3421–3431, 2010.

21. Appelqvist, H., Wäster, P., Kågedal, K., and Öllinger, K., The lysosome: From waste bag to potential therapeutic target, *J. Mol. Cell Biol.* 5, 214–226, 2013.

22. Cocchiaro, P., DePasquale, V., Della Morte, R., et al., The multifaceted role of the lysosomal protease cathepsins in kidney disease, *Front. Cell Dev. Biol.* 5, 114, 2017.

23. Kramer, L., Turk, D., and Turk, B., The future of cysteine cathepsins in disease management, *Trends Pharmacol. Sci.* 38, 873–898, 2017.

CASPASES

Caspases are a family (MEROPS C14)[1] of intracellular cysteine proteases that are involved in the process of apoptosis.[2] It is recognized that the classification/separation of the pathways of cell death is complex.[3,4] Caspases are a family of cysteine endopeptidases with a specificity for cleavage after aspartyl residues. However, factors other than the sissle peptide bond contribute to the specificity of caspases.[5] Classification of the caspase has been based on putative function(s) and size of prodomains.[6] The canonical process of procaspase activation is initiated by an increase in mitochondrial membrane permeability with the concomitant release of cytochrome C.[7–9] The activation of the several caspases occurs in cascade manner.[10] While most of the interest in caspases has been in apoptosis, it is clear that other functions are being elucidated.[11,12]

1. https://www.ebi.ac.uk/merops/cgi-bin/famsum?family=C14.
2. Jenkins, V.K., Timmons, A.K., and McCall, K., Diversity of cell death pathways: Insight from the fly ovary, *Trends Cell Biol.* 23, 567–574, 2013.
3. Kroemer, G., Galluzi, L., Abrams, J., et al., Classification of cell death: Recommendations of the nomenclature committee on cell death, 2009, *Cell Death Differentiation* 16, 3–11, 2009.
4. Yeganeh, B., Ghavami, S., Rabim, Md. N., et al., Autophagy activation is required for influenza A virus-induced apoptosis and replication, *Biochim. Biophys. Acta* 1865, 354–378, 2018.
5. Pop, C., and Salvesen, G.S., Human caspases: Activation, specificity and regulation, *J. Biol. Chem.* 284, 21777–21781, 2009.
6. Li, J., and Yuan, J., Caspases in apoptosis and beyond, *Oncogene* 27, 6194–6206, 2008.
7. de Castro Damasio, C., Nolte, S., Polak, L.P., et al., The lectin BJcul induces apoptosis through TRAIL expression, caspase cascade activation and mitochondrial membrane permeability in a human colon adenocarcinoma cell line, *Toxicon* 90, 299–307, 2014.
8. Catalán, E., Jaime-Sánchez, P., Aguiló, N., et al., Mouse cytotoxic T cell-derived granzyme B activates the mitochondrial cell death pathway in a Bim-dependent fashion, *J. Biol. Chem.* 290, 6868–6877, 2015.
9. Kitt, J.P., Bryce, D.A., Minteer, S.D., and Harris, J.M., Raman spectroscopy reveals selective interactions of cytochrome C with cardiolipin that correlated with membrane permeability, *J. Am. Chem. Soc.* 139, 3851–3860, 2017.
10. Slee, E.A., Harte, M.T., Kluck, R.M., et al., Ordering the cytochrome c-initiated caspase cascade: Hierarchical activation of caspases-2,-3,-6,-7,-8, and -10 in a caspase-9-dependent manner, *J. Cell Biol.* 144, 281–292, 1999.
11. Connolly, P.F., Jäger, R., and Fearnhead, H.O., New roles for old enzymes: Killer caspases as the engine of cell behavior changes, *Front. Physiol.* 5, 149, 2014.
12. Nakajima, Y.I., and Kuranaga, E., Caspase-dependent non-apoptotic processes in development, *Cell Death Differ.* 24, 1422–1430, 2017.

CATALOMICS

As with other "omics," catalomics would be the study of all enzymes in an organism, tissue, or cell or perhaps more accurately from etymological considerations, catalomics is the study of catalysis in a proteome. Since an enzyme is identified by its active site, the diverse mechanisms of catalysis does not permit the identification of all enzymes with a single technical approach, although "click chemistry" will be most useful.[1–3] It has been possible to apply the catalomics concept to enzyme families such as serine proteases[4] and metalloproteases.[5] While there has been little activity in the specific area of catalomics as judged by a literature search, there has been substantial activity in the related field of activity-based proteomics.[6,7]

1. Kalesh, K.A, Shi, H., Ge, J., and Yao, S.Q., The use of click chemistry in the emerging field of catalomics, *Org. Biomol. Chem.* 8, 1749–1762, 2010.
2. Martell, J., and Weerapana, E., Applications of copper-catalyzed click chemistry in activity-based protein profiling, *Molecules* 19, 1378–1393, 2014.
3. Soriano, G.P., Overjkleeft, H.A., and Florea, B.I., Two-step activity-based protein profiling with the proteasome system as a model of study, *Methods Mol. Biol.* 1491, 205–215, 2017.
4. Kidd, D., Liu, Y., and Cravatt, B.F., Profiling serine hydrolase activities in complex proteomes, *Biochemistry* 40, 4005–4015, 2001.
5. Lee, W.L., Li, J., Uttamchandani, M., Sun, H., and Yao, S.Q., Inhibitor fingerprinting of metalloproteinases using microplate and microarray platforms: An enabling technology in Catalomics, *Nat. Protoc.* 2, 2126–2138, 2007.
6. Li, S., Diego-Limpin, P.A., Bajrami, B., et al., Scaling proteome-wide reactions of activity-based probes, *Anal. Chem.* 89, 6295–6299, 2017.
7. Smith, J.N., Tyrrell, K.J., Hansen, J.R., et al., Plasma protein turnover rates in rats using stable isotope labeling, global proteomics, and activity-based protein profiling, *Anal. Chem.* 89, 13559–13566, 2017.

CATALYTIC ANTIBODIES

Catalytic antibodies are antibodies which demonstrate catalytic activity (also referred to as abzymes, catalytic monoclonal antibody or catmab). A catalytic antibody is usually a monoclonal antibody, although polyclonal catalytic antibody preparations have been described.[1–3] The development of a catalytic monoclonal antibodies has been based on the use of haptens.[4,5] There has been considerable interest in catalytic antibodies in pathological processes and as potential therapeutic agents.[6–8] Catalytic antibodies continue to be an active area of research.[9–11]

1. Resmini, M., Brocklehurst, K., and Gallacher, G., Polyclonal catalytic antibodies, *J. Immunol. Methods* 269, 111–124, 2002.
2. Tolmacheva, A.S., Blinova, E.A., Ermakov, E.A., et al., IgG abzymes with peroxidase and oxidoreductase activities from the sera of healthy humans, *J. Mol. Recognit.* 28, 565–580, 2015.

3. Odintsova, E.S., Baranova, S.V., Dmitrenok, P.S., et al., Anti-integrase abzymes from the sera of HIV-infected patients specifically hydrolyze integrase but nonspecifically cleave short oligopeptides, *J. Mol. Recognit.* 25, 193–207, 2012.

4. Xu, Y., Yamamoto, N., and Janda, K.D., Catalytic antibodies: Hapten design strategies and screening methods, *Bioorg. Med. Chem.* 12, 5247–5268, 2004.

5. Smirnov, I., Belolgurov, A., Jr., Frieboulet, A., Strategies for the selection of catalytic antibodies against organophosphorous nerve agents, *Chem. Biol. Interact.* 203, 196–201, 2013.

6. Paul, S., Nishiyama, Y., Planque, S., et al., Antibodies as defensive enzymes, *Springer Semin. Immunopathol.* 26, 485–503, 2005.

7. Mahendra, A., Sharma, M., Rao, D.N., et al., Antibody-mediated catalysis. Induction and therapeutic relevance, *Autoimmune Rev.* 12, 648–652, 2013.

8. Bowen, A., Wear, M., and Casadevall, A., Antibody-mediated catalysis in infection and immunity, *Infect. Immun.* 85, e00202–e00217, 2017.

9. Padiolieau-Lefèvre, S., Ben-Naya, R., et al., Catalytic antibodies and their applications in biotechnology: State of the art, *Biotechnol. Lett.* 36, 1369–1379, 2014.

10. Ishikawa, F., Shirahashi, M., Hayakawa, H., Yamaguchi, A., et al., Site-directed chemical mutations on abzymes: Large rate accelerations in the catalysis by exchanging the functionalized small nonprotein components, *ACS Chem. Biol.* 11, 2803–2811, 2016.

11. Shahsavarian, M.A., Chaaya, N., Costa, N., et al., Multitarget selection of catalytic antibodies with β-lactamase activity using phage display, *FEBS J.* 284, 634–653, 2017.

CATH

CATH is a classification process for protein domain structures based on class (C), architecture (A), topology (T), and homology superfamily (H).[1–5]

1. Orengo, C.A., Michie, A.D., Jones, S., Jones, D.T., Swindells, M.B., and Thornton, J.M., CATH–a hierarchic classification of protein domain structures, *Structure* 5, 1093–1108, 1997.

2. Bray, J.E., Todd, A.E., Pearl, F.M., Thornton, J.M., and Orengo, C.A., The CATH dictionary of homologous superfamilies (DHS): A consensus approach for identifying distant structural homologues, *Protein Eng.* 13, 153–165, 2000.

3. Sun, X-D., and Huang, R-B., Prediction of protein structural classes using support vector machines, *Amino Acids* 30, 469–475, 2006.

4. Csaba, G., Birzele, F., and Zimmer, R., Systematic comparison of SCOP and CATH: A new gold standard for protein structure analysis, *BMC Struct. Biol.* 9, 23, 2009.

5. Dawson, N.L., Lewis, T.E., Das, S., et al., CATH: An expanded resource to predict protein function though structure and sequence, *Nucleic Acids Res.* 45(D1), D289–D295, 2017.

CELISA

The term CELISA (as determined by search) can have several meanings. The most common use either as CELISA or cELISA refers to the use of **competitive ELISA**.[1–3] A lesser use describes a cellular ELISA where a cell is the sample and the protein analyte is an intrinsic surface protein.[4,5] Cellular ELISA is also used to detect proteins bound to cell surface proteins such as HLA antigens.[6] CELISA has also seen a single use for complement-enzyme linked immune sorbent assay.[7]

1. Dahlfors, G., Stål, P., Hansson, E.C., et al., Validation of a competitive ELISA assay for the quantification of human serum hepcidin, *Scand. J. Clin. Invest.* 75, 652–658, 2015.

2. Schuster, I., Mertens, M., Köllner, B., et al., A competitive ELISA for species-independent detection of Crimean-Congo hemorrhagic fever virus specific antibodies, *Antiviral Res.* 134, 161–166, 2016.

3. Fukushi, S., Fukuma, A., Kurosu, T., et al., Characterization of novel monoclonal antibodies against the MERS-cornavirus spike protein and their application in species-independent antibody detection by competitive ELISA, *J. Virol. Methods* 251, 22–29, 2018.

4. Morandini, R., Boeynaems, J.M., Wérenne, J., and Ghanem, G., Tips and step-by-step protocol for the optimization of important factors affecting cellular enzyme-linked immunosorbent assay (CELISA), *J. Immunoassay Immunochem.* 22, 299–321, 2001.

5. Diaz-Romero, J., Kürsener, S., Kohl, S., and Nesic, D., S100B + A1 CELISA: A novel potency assay and screening tool for redifferentiation stimuli of human articular chondrocytes, *J. Cell Physiol.* 232, 1559–1570, 2017.

6. Morris, R.E., Thomas, P.T., and Hong, R., Cellular enzyme-linked immunospecific assay (CELISA). I. A new micromethod that detects antibodies to cell-surface antigens, *Hum. Immunol.* 5, 1–19, 1982.

7. Tandon, A., Zahner, H., and Lämmler, G., CELISA (complement-enzyme linked immune sorbent assay) a new method for the estimation of complement fixing antibodies; its use for Chagas' disease, *Tropenmed Parasitol.* 30, 189–193, 1979.

CELL-BASED ASSAYS

This is a broad classification for bioassays where cells are used as the substrate or indicator for an assay. Examples include gene expression assays,[1,2] receptor-ligand interactions,[3–5] toxicity,[6,7] and potency for an antitoxin.[8]

1. Edmondson, R., Broglie, J.J., Adcock, A.F., and Yang, L., Three-dimensional cell culture systems and their applications in drug discovery and cell-based biosensors, *Assay Drug Dev. Technol.* 12, 207–218, 2014.

2. Schulpen, S.H., de Jong, E., de la Fonteyne, L.J., de Klerk, A., and Piersma, A.H., Distinct gene expression responses of two anticonvulsant drugs in a novel human embryonic stem cell based neural differentiation assay protocol, *Toxicol. In Vitro* 29, 449–457, 2015.

3. Imai, J., Yamzoe, Y., and Yoshinari, K., Novel cell-based reporter assay system using epitope-tagged protein for the identification of agonistic ligands of constitutive androstane receptor (CAR), *Drug Metab. Pharmacokinet.* 28, 290–298, 2013.

4. Aihara, A., Abe, N., Srauhashi, K., Kanaki, T., and Nishino, T., Novel 3-D cell culture system for in vitro evaluation of anticancer drugs under anchorage-independent conditions, *Cancer Sci.* 107, 1858–1866, 2016.

5. Van Hout, A., D'huys, T., Oeyen, M., Schols, D., and Van Loy, T., Comparison of cell-based assays for the identification and evaluation of competitive CXCR4 inhibitors, *PLoS One* 12, e0176057, 2017.

6. Huang, J.X., Blaskovich, M.A., and Cooper, M.A., Cell- and biomarker-based assays for predicting nephrotoxicity, *Expert Opin. Drug Metab. Toxicol.* 10, 1621–1635, 2014.

7. Wagener, J., Cell-based microarrays for in vitro toxicology, *Annu. Rev. Anal. Chem.* 8, 335–358, 2015.

8. Torgeman, A., Diamant, E., Levin, L., et al., An *in vitro* cell-based potency assay for pharmaceutical type A botulinum antitoxins, *Vaccine* 35, 7213–7216, 2017.

CELL CULTURE

The maintenance of animal cells[1–4] of plant cells[5–8] in a specialized media.[9–11] The term *culture* is also used for the growth and maintenance of yeast organisms.[12,13] In biotechnology manufacturing, the term cell culture is used primarily for the production of protein biopharmaceuticals using cells such as Chinese hamster ovary (CHO) cells or baby hamster kidney (BHK) cells. The use of the term *cell culture* differentiates such a process from fermentation, which is the term used to describe the culture of bacteria which can also be used for the manufacture of biopharmaceutical products. Cell culture in the manufacturing of protein biopharmaceutical can use different platforms ranging from suspension culture to perfusion bioreactors. Cell culture can also be used for cell-based assays where there is increased interest in 3D culture assay systems.[14–16] The development of organoids is an extension of 3D culture technology.[17–19] There is current interest in the development of cell culture technology for stem cells for use, for example, in regenerative medicine.[20,21]

1. *Animal Cell Culture* (Volume 9, Cell Engineering), ed. M. Al-Rubeai, Springer, Cham, Switzerland, 2014.

2. Warnock, J.N., and Al-Rubeai, M., Bioreactor systems for the production of biopharmaceuticals from animal cells, *Biotechnol. Appl. Biochem.* 45, 1–12, 2006.

3. Zhang, Y., Approaches to optimizing animal cell culture process: Substrate metabolism regulation and protein expression improvement, *Adv. Biochem. Eng. Biotechnol.* 113, 177–215, 2009.

4. Yao, T., and Asayama, Y., Animal-cell culture media: History, characteristic, and current issues, *Reprod. Med. Biol.* 16, 99–117, 2017

5. Evans, D.E., *Plant Cell Culture*, BIOS Scientific Publishers, London, UK, 2003; *Plant Cell Culture Protocols* (Methods in Molecular Biology, Volume 318), ed. V.M. Loyola-Vargas and F. Vázquez-Flota, Humana, Totowa, NJ, 2006.

6. Georgiev, M.I., and Weber, J., Bioreactors for plant cells: Hardware configuration and internal environment optimization as tools for wider commercialization, *Biotechnol. Lett.* 36, 1359–1367, 2014.

7. Tekoah, Y., Shulman, A., Kizhner, T., et al., Large-scale production of pharmaceutical proteins in plant cell culture—The Protalix experience, *Plant Biotechnol. J.* 13, 1199–1208, 2015.

8. Ochoa-Villarreal, M., Howat, S., Hong, S., et al., *BMB Rep.* 49, 149–158, 2016.

9. van der Valk, J., Brunner, D., De Smet, K., et al., Optimization of chemically defined cell culture media – replacing fetal bovine serum in mammalian *in vitro* methods, *Toxicol. In Vitro* 24, 1053–1063, 2010.

10. Perry, J.D., A decade of development of chromogenic culture media for clinical microbiology in an era of molecular diagnostics, *Clin. Microbiol. Rev.* 30, 449–479, 2017.

11. McGillicuddy, N., Floris, P., Albrecht, S., and Bones, J., Examining the sources of variability in cell culture media used for biopharmaceutical production, *Biotechnol. Lett.* 40, 5–21, 2018.

12. Looser, V., Bruhlmann, B., Bumbak, F., et al., Cultivation strategies to enhance productivity of *Pichia pastoris*: A review, *Biotechnol. Adv.* 33, 1177–1193, 2015.

13. Cao, J., Perez-Pinera, P., Lowenhaupt, K., et al., Versatile and on-demand co-production in yeast, *Nat. Commun.* 9(1), 77, 2018.

14. McNamara, M.C., Sharifi, F., Wrede, A.H., et al., Microfibers as physiologically relevant platforms for creation of 3D cell cultures, *Macromol. Biosci.* 17, 201700279, 2017.

15. De Luca, A., Raimondi, L., Salamanna, F., et al., Relevance of 3d culture system to study osteosarcoma environment, *J. Exp. Clin. Cancer Res.* 37(1), 2, 2018.

16. Patel, M., Lee, H.J., Park, S., Kim, Y., and Jeong, B., Injectable thermogel for 3D culture of stem cells, *Biomaterials* 159, 91–107, 2018.

17. Yilmaz, C.O., Xu, Z.S., and Gracias, D.H., Curved and folded micropatterns in 3D cell culture and tissue engineering, *Methods Cell Biol.* 121, 121–139, 2014.

18. Tsakmaki, A., Fonseca Pedro, P., and Bewick, G.A., 3D intestinal organoids in metabolic research: Virtual reality in a dish, *Curr. Opin. Pharmacol.* 37, 51–58, 2017.

19. Beckwitt, C.H., Clark, A.M., Wheeler, S., et al., Liver 'organ on a chip', *Exp. Cell Res.*, 363, 15–25, 2018.

20. Yamamoto, Y., and Ochiya, T., Epithelial stem cell culture: Modeling human disease and applications for regenerative medicine, *Inflamm. Regen.* 37, 3, 2017.
21. Abdal Dayem, A., Lee, S., Choi, H.Y., and Cho, S-G., The impact of adhesion molecules on the in vitro culture and differentiation of stem cells, *Biotechnol. J.* 13(2), 1700575, 2018.

CELL PENETRATING PEPTIDE

Cell-penetrating peptides are relatively small peptides, usually less than 30 amino acids in length (majority are between 10 and 20 amino acids in length), which have the ability to pass through the cellular membrane in via mechanisms that appear to be both receptor-independent (translocation) as well an endocytotic process.[1] There has been particular interest in the use of peptides containing arginine.[2–4] The observation on the internalization of tat protein from human HIV virus[5] and subsequent study of peptides derived from tat sequence[6] resulted in the TAT peptide (to differentiate from tat protein).[7] While there are issues (e.g. stability, specificity), there is substantial interest in the use of cell-penetrating peptides to deliver drugs to the interior of the cell.[8–11]

1. Kauffman, W.B., Fuselier, T., He, J., and Wimley, W.C. Mechanism matters: A taxonomy of cell penetrating peptides, *Trends Biochem. Sci.* 40, 749–764, 2015.
2. Brock, R., The uptake of arginine-rich cell-penetrating peptides: Putting the puzzle together, *Bioconjug. Chem* 25, 863–868, 2014.
3. Meloni, B.P., Milani, D., Edwards, A.B., et al., Neuroprotective peptides fused to arginine-rich cell penetrating peptides; Neuroprotective mechanism likely mediated by peptide endocytic properties, *Pharmacol. Ther.* 153, 36–54, 2015.
4. Takeuchi, T., and Futaki, S., Current understanding of direct translocation of arginine-rich cell-penetrating peptides and its internalization mechanisms, *Chem. Pharm. Bull.* 64, 1431–1437, 2016.
5. Frankel, A.D., and Pabo, C.O., Cellular uptake of the tat protein from human immunodeficiency virus, *Cell* 55, 1189–1193, 1988.
6. Fawell, S., Seery, J., Daikh, Y., et al., Tat-mediated delivery of heterologous proteins into cells, *Proc. Natl. Acad. Sci. USA* 91, 664–668, 1994.
7. Futaki, S., and Nakase, I., Cell-surface interactions on arginine-rich cell-penetrating peptides allow for multiplex modes of internalization, *Acc. Chem. Res.* 50, 2449–2456, 2017.
8. Lehto, T., Ezzat, K., Wood, M.J.A., and El Andaloussi, S., Peptides for nucleic acid delivery, *Adv. Drug Deliv. Rev.* 106, 172–182, 2016.
9. Cerrato, C.P., Künnapuu, K., and Langel, Ü., Cell-penetrating peptides with intracellular organelle targeting, *Expert Opin. Drug Deliv.* 14, 245–255, 2017.
10. Dissanayake, S., Denny, W.A., Gamage, S., and Sarojini, V., Recent developments in anticancer drug delivery using cell penetrating and tumor targeting peptides, *J. Control. Release* 250, 62–76, 2017.
11. Bruce, V.J., and McNaughton, B.R., Inside job: Methods for delivering proteins to the interior of mammalian cells, *Cell Chem. Biol.* 24, 924–934, 2017.

CELLULOSOME

The cellulosome is a multienzyme complex used by bacteria to degrade cellulose.[1,2] The cellulosome complex is based on a scaffolding matrix[3] used by anaerobic bacterial to degrade plant cell walls.[4]

1. Bayer, E.A., and Lamed, R., The cellulose paradox: Pollutant par excellence and/or a reclaimable natural resource? *Biodegradation* 3, 171–188, 1992.
2. Felix, C.R., and Ljungdahl, L.G., The cellulosome: The exocellular organelle of Clostridium, *Annu. Rev. Microbiol.* 47, 791–819, 1993.
3. Smith, S.P., Bayer, E.A., and Czjzek, M., Continually emerging mechanistic complexity of the multi-enzyme cellulosome complex, *Curr. Opin. Struct. Biol.* 44, 151–160, 2017.
4. Artzi, L., Bayer, E.A., and Moraïs, S., Cellulosomes: Bacterial nanomachines for dismantling plant polysaccharides, *Nat. Rev. Microbiol.* 15, 83–95, 2017.

CENTIRAY

A centiRay (Cr) is a chromosomal span within which a break may be induced with a 1% probability by a specified dose of radiation, 1 Cr = 3×10^4 bp DNA.[1] Another source suggests the length of a Cr is 20–50 kb DNA.[2] The Cr is used in radiation hybrid mapping which measures the distance between genes on a chromosome.[3,4] Cr is used in aquaculture[5] and agriculture.[6]

1. *Encyclopedia of Genomics, Proteomics and Informatics*, Springer, Dordrecht, the Netherlands, 2008.
2. Warrington, J.A., Bailey S.K., Armstrong, E., et al., A radiation hybrid map of 18 growth factor, growth factor receptor, hormone receptor, or neurotransmitter receptor genes on the distal region of the long arm of chromosome 5, *Genomics* 13, 803–808, 1992.
3. van Ommen, G.J., and Pearson, P.L., Long-range mapping in the research and diagnosis of genetic disease, *Genome* 31, 730–736, 1989.
4. Cox, D.R., Burmeister, M., Price, E.R., Kim, S., and Myers, R.M., Radiation hybrid mapping: A somatic cell genetic method for constructing high-resolution maps of mammalian chromosomes, *Science* 250, 245–250, 1990.

5. Aoki, J-Y., Kai, W., Kawabata, Y., et al., Construction of a radiation hybrid panel and the first yellowtail (*Seriola quinqueradiata*) radiation hybrid map using a nanofluidic dynamic array, *BMC Genomics* 15, 165, 2014.

6. Kumar, A., Seetan, R., Mergoum, M., et al., Radiation hybrid maps of the D-genome of *Aegilops tauschii* and their application in sequence assembly of the large and complex plant genomes, *BMC Genomics* 16, 800, 2015.

CENTIMORGAN

A centimorgan (Cm) is a measure of genetic distance that tells how far apart physically two genes are based on the frequency of recombination or crossover between the two gene loci. A frequency of 1% recombination in meiosis is one centimorgan and equals about 1 million base pairs. A Cm is determined by natural recombination while a Cr (centiRay) is determined by separation of markers subsequent to chromosomal DNA cleavage by X-radiation.[1] Neither a Cm or a Cr has defined distance (e.g. a specific number of base pairs). Combination of Cm data and Cr data is very useful in mapping genetic loci on chromosomes.[2] The term centimorgan was advanced by J.B.S. Haldane in 1919[3] based on earlier work by Thomas Hunt Morgan.

1. Voigt, C., Möller, S., Ibrahim, S.M., and Serrano-Fernández, P., Non-linear conversion between genetic and physical chromosomal distances, *Bioinformatics* 20, 1966–1967, 2004.

2. Kumar, A., Seetan, R., Mergoum, M., et al., Radiation hybrid maps of the D-genome of *Aegilops tauschii* and their application in sequence assembly of the large and complex plant genomes, *BMC Genomics* 16, 800, 2015.

3. Haldane, J.B.S., The combination of linkage values and calculation of distances between the loci of linked factors, *J. Genetics* 8, 299–309, 1919.

CHALCONES

Chalcones are phytochemicals with a variety of suggested pharmacological actions[1,2] serving as Michael acceptors in the alkylation of cysteine thiol groups in proteins.[3,4] Reaction with cysteine thiol groups occurs via Michael addition to conjugated double bond.

1. Mahapatra, D.K., Bharti, S.K., and Asati, V., Anti-cancer chalcones: Structural and molecular target perspectives, *Eur. J. Med. Chem.* 98, 69–114, 2015.

2. Venturelli, S., Burkard, M., Biendi, M., et al., Prenylated chalcones and flavonoids for the prevention and treatment of cancer, *Nutrition* 32, 1171–1178, 2016.

3. Rücker, H., Al-Rifai, H., Rascle, A., et al., Enhancing the anti-inflammatory activity of chalcones by tuning the Michael acceptor site, *Org. Biomol. Chem.* 13, 3040–3047, 2015.

4. Huang, X., Huang, R., Li, L., Guo, S., and Wang, H., Synthesis and biological evaluation of novel chalcone derivatives as a new class of microtubule destabilizing agents, *Eur. J. Med. Chem.* 132, 11–25, 2017.

CHAMELEON SEQUENCES

Chameleon sequences are identical sequences in a protein which can adopt either an alpha helical conformation or a beta sheet conformation.[1–4]

1. Mezei, M., Chameleon sequences in the PDB, *Protein. Eng.* 11, 411–414, 1998.

2. Ghozlane, A., Joseph, A.P., Bornot, A., de Brevern, A.G., Analysis of protein chameleon sequence characteristics, *Bioinformation* 3, 367–369, 2009.

3. LI, W., Kinch, L.N., Karplus, P.A., and Grishin, N.V., ChSeq: A database of chameleon sequences, *Protein Sci.* 24, 1075–1086, 2015.

4. Kim, B., Do, T.D., Hayden, E.Y., et al., Aggregation of chameleon peptides: Implications of α-helicity in fibril formation, *J. Phys. Chem.* 120, 5874–5883, 2016.

CHAOTROPIC

The term chaotropic is derived from chaos, which in this sense means disorders and tropic meaning forming. As such, the term chaotropic means a result and not necessarily a chemical structure or a specific process. In biochemistry and molecular biology, the term chaotropic is used to describe a reagent which can disrupt the structure of macromolecules, particularly proteins. The *Oxford English Dictionary* defines chaotropic as "Designating a molecule or substance that disrupts hydrogen bonds, esp. with the effect of disordering the structure of proteins and membranes; (also) of or characterized by such disruption." The term chaotropic can define uncharged molecules such as urea or thiourea as well as reagents such as guanidine hydrochloride and sodium thiocyanate.[1–12] The effect of chaotropic salts on proteins is well accepted with current interest in "**chaotropic chromatography**." The use of chaotropic salts in reverse-phase chromatography is a form of ion-pair chromatography. **Ion-pair chromatography** most commonly uses a hydrophobic anion or cation to pair with a water-soluble analyte to improve behavior in reverse-phase chromatography. As an example, trimethylammonium ion is an ion pair for oligonucleotides.[13] Chaotropic salts, in fact, the anions, bind to basic analytes as a counter ion changing the charge density, polarizability, solvation, and degree of hydration allowing for increased retention. Chaotropic salts also influence the structure of water.[10] The effectiveness of chaotropic salts follows the Hofmeister series.[14]

There is a limited use of the term chaotropic chromatography.[15,16] Heat has also been described as a chaotropic agent.[17] The term charotropic is also used to describe effects of intrinsic and extrinsic agents on gene expression.[18,19] Chaotropic agents should be distinguished from **kosmotropic agents** which stabilize macromolecules[20,21] and Hofmeister (lyotropic) agents, which "salt out" or "salt in" proteins.[22,23]

1. *Oxford English Dictionary,* Oxford University Press, Oxford, UK, 2019.
2. Dandliker, W.B., Alonso, R., de Saussure, V.A., Kierszenbaum, F., et al., The effect of chaotropic ions on the dissociation of antigen-antibody complexes, *Biochemistry* 6, 1460–1467, 1967.
3. Hanstein, W.G., Davis, K.A., and Hatefi, Y., Water structure and the chaotropic properties of haloacetates, *Arch. Biochem. Biophys.* 147, 534–544, 1971.
4. Sawyer, W.H., and Puckridge, J., The dissociation of proteins by chaotropic salts, *J. Biol. Chem.* 248, 8429–8433, 1973.
5. Hatefi, Y., and Hanstein, W.G., Destabilization of membranes with chaotropic ions, *Methods Enzymol.* 31, 770–790, 1974.
6. McLaughlin, S., Bruder, A., Chen, S., and Moser, C., Chaotropic anions and the surface potential of bilayer membranes, *Biochim. Biophys. Acta* 394, 304–313, 1975.
7. Stein, M., Lazaro, J.J., and Wolsiuk, R.A., Concerted action of cosolvents, chaotropic anions and thioredoxin on chloroplast fructose-1,6-bisphosphatase. Reactivity to iodoacetate, *Eur. J. Biochem.* 185, 425–431, 1989.
8. Moelbert, S., Normand, B., and De Los Rios, P., Kosmotropes and chaotropes: Modelling preferential exclusion, binding and aggregate stability, *Biophys. Chem.* 112, 45–57, 2004.
9. Salvi, G., De Los Rios, P., and Vendruscolo, M., Effective interactions between chaotropic agents and proteins, *Proteins* 61, 492–499, 2005.
10. LoBrutto, R., and Kazakevich, Y.V., Chaotropic effects in RP-HPLC, *Adv. Chromatog.* 44, 291–315, 2006.
11. Katevatis, C., Fan, A., Klapperich, C.M., Low concentration DNA extraction and recovery using a silica solid phase, *PLoS One* 12(5), e0176848, 2017.
12. Shiraga, K., Ogawa, Y., Tanaka, K., et al., Coexistance of kosmotropic and chaotropic impacts of urea on water as revealed by terahertz spectroscopy, *J. Phys. Chem.* 122, 1268–1277, 2018.
13. Zhang, L., Majeed, B., Lagae, L., et al., Ion-pair reversed-phase chromatography of short double-stranded deoxyribonucleic acid in silicon micro-pillar array columns: Retention model and applications, *J. Chromatog. A* 1294, 1–9, 2013.
14. Checchi, T., Retention mechanism for ion-pair chromatography with chaotropic reagents: From ion-pair chromatography toward a unified salt chromatography, *Adv. Chromatog.* 49, 1–35, 2011.
15. Čolović, J., Kalinič, M., Vemič, A., Erič, S., and Malenović, A., Investigation into the phenomena affecting the retention behavior of basic analytes in chaotropic chromatography: Joint effects of the most relevant chromatographic factors and analytes' molecular properties, *J. Chromatog.* 1425, 150–157, 2015.
16. Čolović, J., Kalinič, M., Vemič, A. Erič, S., and Malenović, A., Influence of the mobile phase and molecular structure parameters on the retention behavior of protonated basic solutes in chaotropic chromatography, *J. Chromatog. A* 1511, 68–76, 2017.
17. Westphal, A.H., Geerke-Volmer, A.A., van Mierlo, C.P.M., and van Berkel, W.J.H., Chaotropic heat treatment resolves native-like aggregation of a heterologously produced thermostable laminarinase, *Biotechnol. J.* 12, 1700007, 2017.
18. Fedorova, A.A., Goncharova, E.P., Koroleva, L.S., et al., Artificial ribonucleases inactivate a wide range of viruses using their ribonuclease, membranolytic, and chaotropic-like activities, *Antiviral Res.* 133, 73–84, 2016.
19. Vincent, A.T., Freschi, L., Jeukens, J., et al., Genomic characterization of environmental *Pseudomonas aeruginosa* isolated from dental unit waterlines revealed the insertion sequence ISPa11 as a chaotropic element, *FEMS Microbiol. Ecol.* 93, fix106, 2017.
20. Palmer, A.S., and Muschol, M., Hydration and hydrodynamic interactions of lysozyme: Effects of chaotropic versus kosmotropic ions, *Biophys. J.* 97, 590–598, 2009.
21. Jas, G.S., Middaugh, C.R., and Kuczera, K., Probing the selection mechanism of the most favorable conformation of a a dipeptide in chaotropic and kosmostropic solution, *J. Phys. Chem. B.* 120, 6939–6950, 2016.
22. Cacace, M.G., Landau, E.M., and Ramsden, J.J., The Hofmeister series: Salt and solvent effects on interfacial phenomena, *Q. Rev. Biophys.* 30, 241–277, 1997.
23. Lee, E., Choi, J.H., and Cho, M., The effect of Hofmeister anions on water structure at protein surfaces, *Phys. Chem. Chem. Phys.* 19, 20008–20015, 2017.

CHAPERONE (MOLECULAR CHAPERONE)

The canonical definition of a molecular chaperone in biochemistry is an intracellular factor, most frequently a protein, which guides the intracellular folding/assembly of another protein in the endoplasmic reticulum.[1] In addition to this quality control function, molecular chaperones were shown to target misfolded proteins for lysosomal degradation.[2,3] The role of molecular chaperones in protein degradation was extended to an understanding of their role in autophagy.[4–6] Molecular chaperones are being shown to have diverse functions beyond intracellular protein degradation.[7–11] While most work on molecular chaperones has focused on intracellular action, chaperones do act at the membrane surface[12,13] as well as in the extracellular space.[14,15]

1. Ellis, R.J., The molecular chaperone concept, *Semin. Cell Biol.* 1, 1–9, 1990.
2. Chiang, H.L., Terlecky, S.R., Plant, C.P., and Dice, J.F., A role for a 70-kilodalton heat shock protein in lysosomal degradation of intracellular proteins, *Science* 246, 382–385, 1989.
3. Dice, J.F., Terlecky, S.F., Chiang, H.L., et al., A selective pathway for degradation of cytosolic proteins by lysozymes, *Semin. Cell Biol.* 1, 449–455, 1989.
4. Tang, Y., Wang, X.W., Liu, Z.H., et al., Chaperone-mediated autophagy substrate proteins in cancer, *Oncotarget* 8, 51970–51985, 2017.
5. Fernández-Fernández, M.R., Gragera, M., Ochoa-Ibarrola, L., Quintana-Gallardo, L., and Valpuesta, J.M., Hsp-70—a master regulator in protein degradation, *FEBS Lett.* 591, 2568–2660, 2017.
6. Catarino, S., Pereira, P., and Girão, H., Molecular control of chaperone-mediated autophagy, *Essays Biochem.* 61, 663–674, 2017.
7. Yadav, R.P., and Artemyev, N.O., A specialized chaperone for the phototransduction effector, *Cell Signal.* 40, 183–189, 2017.
8. Fries, G.R., Gasson, N.C., and Rein, T., The FKBP51 glucocorticoid receptor co-chaperone: Regulation, function, and implications in health and disease, *Int. J. Mol. Sci.* 18, E2614, 2017.
9. Kim, J.H., Lee, E., Friedline, R.H., et al., Endoplasmic reticulum chaperone GRP78 regulates macrophage function and insulin resistance in diet-induced obesity, *FASEB J.* 32, 2292–2304, 2018.
10. Dutkiewicz, R., and Nowak, M., Molecular chaperones involved in mitochondrial iron-sulfur protein biogenesis, *J. Biol. Inorg. Chem.*, 23, 569–579, 2018.
11. Sekiya, T., Hu., Y., Kato, K., et al., Assembly and remodeling of viral DNA and RNA replicons regulated by cellular molecular chaperones, *Biophys. Rev.*10, 445–452, 2018.
12. De Maio, A., Extracellular Hsp70: Export and function, *Curr. Protein Pept. Sci.* 15, 225–231, 2014.
13. Shevtsov, H., Huile, and G., Multhoff, G., Membrane heat shock protein 70: A theranostic target for cancer therapy, *Philos. Trans. R. Soc. Lond. B. Biol. Sci.* 373(1738), 20160526, 2018.
14. *The Biology of Extracellular Molecular Chaperones*, ed. D.J. Chadwick and J. Goode, John Wiley & Sons, Chichester, UK, 2008.
15. Edkins, A.L., Price, J.T., Pockley, A.G., and Blatch, G.L., Heat shock proteins as modulators and therapeutic targets of chronic disease: An integrated perspective, *Philos. Trans. R. Soc. Lord. B. Biol. Sci.* 373(1738), 20160521, 2018.

CHEMICAL BIOLOGY

The term chemical biology was first used in 1930.[1] Chemical biology, as a discipline, has undergone some changes since the first use and today can be the use of chemistry to study intracellular processes.[2] Current work in chemical biology involves imaging technology such as near-infrared spectroscopy,[3,4] metabolic labeling,[5,6] activity-based probes,[7,8] and bioorthoganol labeling.[9,10]

1. Leathes, J.B., The Harvien Oration on the birth of chemical biology, *British Med. J.* 2(3462), 671–676, 1930.
2. Lundblad, R.L., Chemical Biology, in *Encyclopedia of Cell Biology*, ed. R.A. Bradshaw and P.D. Stahl, Volume 1., pp. 128–134, Academic Press/Elsevier, Waltham, MA, 2016.
3. Guo, Z., Park, S., Yoon, J., and Shin, I., Recent progress in the development of near-infrared fluorescent probes for bioimaging applications, *Chem. Soc. Rev.* 43, 16–29, 2014.
4. Chu, T.S., Lü, R., and Liu, B.T., Reversibly monitoring oxidation and reduction events in living biological systems: Recent development of redox-responsive reversible NIR biosensors and their applications in *in vitro/in vivo* fluorescence imaging, *Biosens. Bioelectron.* 86, 643–655, 2016.
5. Buescher, J.M., Antoniewicz, M.R., Boros, L.G., et al., A roadmap for interpreting 13C metabolite labeling patterns from cells, *Curr. Opin. Biotechnol.* 34, 189–201, 2015.
6. Ovryn, B., Li, J. Hong, S., and Wu, P., Visualizing glycans on single cells and tissues-visualizing glycans on single cells and tissues, *Curr. Opin. Chem. Biol.* 39, 39–45, 2017.
7. Yang, P., and Liu, K., Activity-based protein profiling: Recent advances in probe development and applications, *Chembiochem* 16, 712–724, 2015.
8. Roberts, A.M. Ward, C.D., and Nomura, D.K., Activity-based protein profiling for mapping and pharmacologically interrogating proteome-wide ligandable hotspots, *Curr. Opin. Biotechnol.* 43, 25–33, 2017.
9. Shieh, P., and Bertozzi, C.R., Design strategies for biooorthogonal smart probes, *Org. Biomol. Chem.* 12, 9307–9320, 2014.
10. Carell, T., and Vrabel, M., Bioorthogonal chemistry-Introduction and overview, *Top. Curr. Chem.* 374(1), 9, 2016.

CHEMICAL GENOMICS

Chemical genomics can be described as a systematic search using a technique such as high-throughput screening to identify selective modulators of the components of the genome.[1,2] Chemical genomics address the entire genome, while **chemical genetics** is defined as the use of a small molecule to modulate a single gene. **Chemicogenomics** can be defined as the informatic component of chemical genomics. The concept of chemical genomics was advanced in 1969 to describe drug screening for protein-protein interactions.[3] Experimental approaches have included that utilize the selective binding of phage display products representing the proteome[4] to immobilized target small molecules.[5] Another approach used bead-based analysis of mRNA expression to identify small molecule repressors.[6] Chemical genomics can be used for the repurposing of drugs.[7,8]

1. Spring, D.R., Chemical genetics to chemical genomics: Small molecules offer big insights, *Chem. Soc. Rev.* 34, 472–482, 2005.
2. *Chemical Genomics and Proteomics*, ed. F. Darvas, A. Guttman, and G. Dormán, CRC Press/Taylor & Francis Group, Boca Raton, FL, 2013.
3. Vidal, M., and Endoh, H., Prospects for drug screening using the reverse two-hybrid system, *Trends Biotech.* 17, 374–381, 1999.
4. Taylor, P.C., Clark, A.J., Marsh, A., Singer, D.R.J., and Dilly, S.J., A chemical genomics approach to identification of interactions between bioactive molecules and alternative reading frame proteins, *Chem. Commun.* 49, 9588–9590, 2013.
5. Dilly, S.J., Bell, M.J., Clark, A.J., et al., A photoimmobilization strategy that maximizes exploration of chemical space in small molecule affinity selection and target discovery, *Chem. Commun.* 2007, 2008–2010, 2007.
6. Wei, G., Margolin, A.A., Haery, L., Chemical genomics identifies small-molecule *MCL1* repressors and BCL-xL as a predictor 4 of MCL1 dependency, *Cancer Cell* 21, 547–562, 2012.
7. Bisson, W.H., Drug repurposing in chemical genomics: Can we learn from the past to improve the future? *Curr. Top. Med. Chem.*12, 1883–1888, 2012.
8. Segura-Cabrera, A., Tripathi, R., Zhang, X., et al., A structure- and chemical genomics-based approach for repositioning of drugs against VCP/p97, *Sci. Rep.* 7, 44912, 2017.

CHEMICAL PROTEOMICS

Chemical proteomics can be described as the use of classical protein chemistry techniques such as chemical modification[1,2] combined with separation technologies such as gel electrophoresis and analytical techniques such as mass spectrometry in the study of the proteome.[3] Earlier work did have a focus on the identification of enzymes in the proteome and to identify signaling pathways,[4–7] and there is current work in this area.[8–10]

1. Yang, Y., Fonović, M., and Verhelst, S.H., Cleavable linkers in chemical proteomics applications, *Methods Mol. Biol.* 1491, 185–203, 2017.
2. Kang, K., Park, J., and Kim, E., Tetrazine ligation for chemical proteomics, *Proteome Sci.* 15, 15, 2017.
3. Leitner, A., A review of the role of chemical modification methods in contemporary mass spectrometry-based proteomics research, *Anal. Chim. Acta* 1000, 2–19, 2018.
4. Jeffery, D.A., and Bogyo, M., Chemical proteomics and its application to drug discovery, *Curr. Opin. Biotechnol.* 14, 87–95, 2003.
5. Daub, H., Godl, K., Brehmer, D., et al., Evaluation of kinase inhibitor selectivity by chemical proteomics, *Assay Drug Dev. Technol.* 2, 215–224, 2004.
6. Beillard, E and Witte, O.N., Unraveling kinase signaling pathways with chemical genetic and chemical proteomic approaches, *Cell Cycle* 4, 434–437, 2005.
7. Daub, H., Characterization of kinase-selective inhibitors by chemical proteomics, *Biochim. Biophys. Acta* 1754, 183–190, 2005.
8. Gyenis, L., Turowec, J.P., Bretner, M., and Litchfield, D.W., Chemical proteomics and functional proteomics strategies for protein kinase inhibitor validation and protein kinase substrate identification: Applications to protein kinase CK2, *Biochim. Biophys. Acta* 1834, 1352–1358, 2013.
9. Daub, H., Quantitative proteomics of kinase inhibitor targets and mechanism, *ACS Chem. Biol.* 10, 201–212, 2015.
10. McCloud, R.L., Franks, C.E., Campbell, S.T., et al., Deconstructing lipid kinase inhibitors by chemical proteomics, *Biochemistry* 57, 231–236, 2018.

CHEMOKINES

Chemokines are a large family (more than 50 members as of January 2018) of cytokines having a wide variety of biological actions but are generally associated with inducing mobilization and activation of immune cells (chemoattraction of leukocytes).[1–5] The term chemokine represents a contraction of chemotactic cytokines. There are several smaller groups or families of chemokines characterized by the location of conserved cysteine residues (CXC, where X is any amino acid; CC; C; and CXXXC, also CX3C).[6,7] Chemokines are small proteins, 8–12 kDa, with a tendency to form oligomers.[8] Chemokines bind to specific G-protein coupled receptors (GPCR) which are designed by ligand such as CXCR1 for a CXC chemokine.[9] Atypical chemokine receptors (not GPCR) serve to regulate chemokine function.[10]

1. Vaddi, K., Keller, M., and Newton, R.C., *The Chemokine Factbook*, Academic Press, San Diego, CA, 1997.
2. *Chemokine Protocols*, Humana Press, ed. Proudfoot, A.E.I., and Well, T.N.C., and Powers, C.A., Totowa, NJ, 2000.
3. Schwiebert, L.M., *Chemokines, Chemokine Receptors, and Disease*, Elsevier, Amsterdam, the Netherlands, 2005.
4. *Chemokines: Types, Functions, and Structural Characteristics*, ed. K.J. Walker, Nova Science Publishers, New York, 2011.
5. *Chemokines: Chemokines and Their Receptors in Drug Discovery*, ed. N.J. Tschammer, Springer, Cham, Switzerland, 2015.

6. Ward, S.G., and Westwick, J., Chemokines: Understanding their role in T-lymphocyte biology, *Biochem. J.* 333, 457–470, 1998.
7. Tüzün, Y., Engin, B., and Wolf, R., Chemokines: Types, functions, and structural characteristics, in *Chemokines: Types, Functions, and Structural Characteristics,* ed. K.J. Walker, Chapter 6, pp. 123–137, Nova Science Publishers, New York, 2011.
8. Miller, M.C., and Mayo, K.H., Chemokines from a structural perspective, *Int. J. Mol. Sci.* 18(10), E2088, 2017.
9. Bachelerie, F., Ben-Baruch, A., Burkhardt, A.M., et al., (International Union of Basic and Clinical Pharmacology) LXXXIV. Update on the extended family of chemokine receptors and introducing a new nomenclature for atypical chemokine receptors, *Pharmacol. Rev.* 66, 1–79, 2013.
10. Bonecchi, R., and Graham, G.J., Atypical chemokine receptors and their roles in the resolution of the inflammatory response, *Front. Immunol.* 7, 224, 2016.

CHEMOPROTEOMICS

Chemoproteomics is the use of small molecules as affinity materials for the discovery of specific binding proteins in the proteome.[1–4] Chemoproteomics is closely related to chemical proteomics[5] and may have more of an emphasis on "classical" chemical modification of proteins.[6–8] However, it is difficult to clearly separate chemoproteomics from chemical proteomics. Chemoproteomics was advanced in 2002 as chemical modification based on biological structure ("the use of biological information to guide chemistry").

1. Beroza, P., Villar, H.O., Wick, M.M., and Martin, G.R., Chemoproteomics as a basis for post-genomic drug discovery, *Drug Discov. Today* 7, 807–814, 2002.
2. Gagna, C.E., Winokur, D., Lambert, W.C., Cell biology, chemogenomics and chemoproteomics, *Cell Biol. Int.* 28, 755–764, 2004.
3. Shin, D., Heo, Y.S., Lee, K.J., et al., Structural chemoproteomics and drug discovery, *Biopolymers* 80, 258–263, 2005.
4. Hall, S.E., Chemoproteomics-driven drug discovery: Addressing high attrition rates, *Drug Discov. Today* 11, 495–502, 2006.
5. Moellering, R.E., and Cravatt, B.F., How chemoproteomics can enable drug discovery and development, *Chem. Biol.* 19, 11–22, 2012.
6. Zhou, Y., Li, W., Wang, M., et al., Competitive profiling of celastrol targets in human cervical cancer HeLa cells via quantitative chemical proteomics, *Mol. Biosyst.* 13, 83–91, 2016.
7. Sun, R., Fu, L., Liu, K., et al., Chemoproteomics reveals chemical diversity and dynamics of 4-oxo-2-nonenal modifications in cells, *Mol. Cell. Proteomics* 16, 1789–1800, 2016.
8. Tian, C., Liu, K., Sun, R., Fu, L., and Yang, J., Chemoproteomics reveals unexpected lysine/arginine-specific cleavage of peptide chains as a potential protein degradation machinery, *Anal. Chem.* 90, 794–800, 2018.

CHONDROCYTE

A chondrocyte is a cartilage cell.[1–8]

1. von der Mark, K., and Conrad, G., Cartilage cell differentiation: Review, *Clin. Orthop. Relat. Res.* 139, 195–205, 1979.
2. Serni, U., and Mannoni, A., Chondrocyte physiopathology and drug efficacy, *Drug Exp. Clin. Res.* 17, 75–79, 1991; Urban, J.P., The chondrocytes: A cell under pressure, *Br. J. Rheumatol.* 33, 901–908, 1994.
3. Urban, J.P., The chondrocytes: A cell under pressure, *Br. J. Rheumatol.* 33, 901–908, 1994.
4. Yates, K.E., Shortkroff, S., and Reish, R.G., Wnt influence on chondrocyte differentiation and cartilage function, *DNA Cell Biol.* 24, 446–457, 2005.
5. Wendt, D., Jakob, M., and Martin, I., Bioreactor-based engineering of osteochondral grafts: From model systems to tissue manufacturing, *J. Biosci. Bioeng.* 100, 489–494, 2005.
6. Goldring, M.B., Tsduchmochi, K., and Ijiri, K., The control of chondrogenesis, *J. Cell Biochem.* 97, 33–44, 2006.
7. Ruano-Ravina, A., and Diaz, M.J., Autologous chondrocytes implantation: A systematic review, *Osteoarthritis Cartilage* 14, 47–51, 2006.
8. Toh, W.S., Yang, Z., Heng, B.C., and Cao, T., New perspectives in chondrogenic differentiation of stem cells for cartilage repair, *Sci. World J.* 6, 361–364, 2006.

CHROMATIN

Chromatin consists of a repeating fundamental nucleoprotein complex, the nucleosome; DNA wrapped around histones where the histones mediate the folding of DNA into chromatin.[1–4] Chromatin functions to pack DNA into nucleus and provide structural support and regulation on the basis of DNA exposure for transcription. Techniques such as DNA footprinting and DNA fingerprinting are used to map areas on chromatin interaction. Chromatin immunoprecipitation (ChIP) is a method for obtaining histones and other components of the nucleosome.[5–7] The value of ChIP is extended by combination with deep sequencing of the isolated DNA.[8–10] See **chromatin remodeling, heterochromatin**.

1. Wolfe, A., *Chromatin. Structure and Function*, 3rd ed., Academic Press, San Diego, CA, 1998.
2. Woodcock, C.L., Chromatin architecture, *Curr. Opin. Struct. Biol.* 16, 213–220, 2006.

3. Blossey, R., *Chromatin: Structure, Dynamics, Regulation,* CRC Press/Chapman & Hall/Taylor & Francis Group, Boca Raton, FL, 2017.
4. *Chromatin Regulation and Dynamics,* ed. A. Göndör, Academic Press/Elsevier, London, UK, 2017.
5. Collas, P., The current status of chromatin immunoprecipitation, *Mol. Biotechnol.* 45, 87–100, 2010.
6. Rodríguez-Ubreva, J., and Ballestar, E., Chromatin immunoprecipitation, *Methods Mol. Biol.* 1094, 309–318, 2014.
7. Wardle, F.C., and Tan, H., A ChIP on the shoulder? Chromatin immunoprecipitation and validation strategies for ChIP antibodies, *F1000Res* 4, 235, 2015.
8. Myers, K.S., Park, D.M., Beauchene, N.A., and Kiley, P.J., Defining bacterial regulons using ChIP-seq, *Methods* 86, 80–88, 2015.
9. Pavesi, G., ChIP-seq data analysis of define transcriptional regulatory networks, *Adv. Biochem. Eng. Biotechnol.* 160, 1–14, 2017.
10. Audrey, G., and Mundlos, S., The three-dimensional genome: Regulating gene expression during pluripotency and development, *Development* 144, 3646–3658, 2017.

CHROMATIN REMODELING

The dynamic structural change in chromatin by nucleosome sliding[1] or post-translational modifications (acetylation, methylation) of the histones[2] via the action of chromatin remodeling complexes/chromatin remodeling enzymes[3] permitting the regulation of transcription.[4,5]

1. Becker, P.B., The chromatin accessibility complex: Chromatin dynamics through nucleosome sliding, *Cold Spring Harb. Symp. Quant. Biol.* 69, 281–287, 2004.
2. Suzuki, K., and Luo, Y., Histone acetylation and the regulation of major histocompatibility Class II gene expression, *Adv. Protein Chem. Struct. Biol.* 106, 71–111, 2017.
3. Saha, A., Wittmeyer, J., and Cairns, B.R., Chromatin remodelling: The industrial revolution of DNA around histones, *Nat. Rev. Mol. Cell Biol.* 7, 437–447, 2006.
4. Clapier, C.R., and Cairns, B.R., The biology of chromatin remodeling complexes, *Annu. Rev. Biochem.* 78, 273–804, 2009.
5. Blossey, R., and Sciessel, H., The latest twists in chromatin remodeling, *Biophys. J.* 114, 2255–2261, 2018.

CHROMATOGRAPHY

Chromatography has become an essential tool in biochemistry and molecular biology since the establishment of basic principles by Martin and Synge in 1941.[1]

The basic principle is the same for both liquid chromatography and gas chromatography; the specific distribution of a solute between a mobile phase and a stationary phase. This distribution process may be called partitioning or adsorption and there is an excellent collection of articles which provide basic information on chromatography.[2,3] The coupling of these various separation technologies with mass spectrometry resulting in "hyphenated technologies" (e.g. LC-MS [liquid chromatography-mass spectrometry], GC-MS [gas chromatography-mass spectrometry])[4,5] has been critical for progress in proteomics and metabolomics. Chromatography may be separated into two groups based on the physical nature of the mobile phase.

GAS CHROMATOGRAPHY

Gas Chromatography is an analytical system consisted a tube or column passing through a heated chamber. The sample is introduced in a volatile form which frequently requires a process referred to as derivatization to convert the analyte into a volatile form. An inert gas such as helium, argon or nitrogen is the mobile phase[6] and the stationary phase may either be a liquid on the luminal wall of the chromatography column, a liquid adsorbed onto a porous support on the luminal wall of the chromatography column, or liquid adsorbed onto a material packed into the column.[7]

LIQUID CHROMATOGRAPHY

Current liquid chromatography is dominated by instrumentation and the physical nature of the solid support. The development of HPLC (high-performance liquid chromatography; high pressure chromatography) was a major technical advance leading to current technologies such as uHPLC.[8,9] These advances in separation technology resulted in increased sensitivity and analysis speed, and together with advances in electrophoresis and mass spectrometry permitted the development of proteomics as a discipline. The early work of Martin and Synge[1] was based on the partition of solute between two liquids, a liquid deposited on a solid phase, defined as the stationary phase, and a liquid mobile phase with the intent the two liquids should be totally immiscible. This was not the case and resulted in the chemical bonding of the liquid stationary phase to the solid resulted in what is described as a bonded phase.[10,11] There are a variety of liquid chromatographic methods based on the type of matrix or resin and solvent.

This variety of solid supports allows multidimensional chromatographic approaches to serve as orthogonal methods of separation. The term multidimensional defines the use or two or more chromatographic columns such size-exclusion followed by reversed-phase chromatography.[12] Multimodal chromatography refers to one matrix demonstrating two or more two mechanisms of separation[13] such as HILIC, which can use both ion-exchange and reversed-phase processes. While not referred to such, gel filtration media can resolve on the basis of hydrophobicity and charge in addition to size and ion-exchanged media can also bind on the basis of hydrophobicity.

1. Martin, A.J., and Synge, R.L., A new form of chromatogram employing two liquid phases 1. A theory of chromatography.
2. Application to the microdetermination of the higher monoamino-acids in proteins, *Biochem. J.* 35, 1358–1368, 1941.
3. *Encyclopedia of Chromatography*, ed. J. Cazes, Marcel Dekker, New York,, 2001.
4. Sarker, S.U., and Nahar, L., Hyphenated Techniques, in *Natural Products Isolation*, ed. S.U. Sarkar and L. Nahar, pp. 223–267, Sprinter/Humana, Totowa, NJ, 2005.
5. Theodoridis, G., and Wilson, I.D., Hyphenated techniques for global metabolite profiling, *J. Chromatog. B*. 871, 141–142, 2008.
6. Berezkin, V.G., Carrier gas in capillary gas-liquid chromatography, *Adv. Chromatog.* 41, 337–377, 2001.
7. *Practical Gas Chromatography*, ed. K. Dettmer-Wilde and W. Engewald, Springer, Berlin, Germany, 2014.
8. Lippert, J.A., Xin, B., Wu, N., and Lee, M.L., Fast ultra-high-pressure liquid chromatography: On-column UV and time-of-flight mass spectrophotometric detection, *J. Microcolumn Sep.* 11, 631–643, 1999.
9. Wu, N., Collins, D.C., Lippert, J.A., Ziang, Y., and Lee, M.L., Ultrahigh pressure liquid chromatography/time-of-flight mass spectrometry for fast applications, *J. Microcolumn Sep.* 12, 462–469, 2000.
10. Majors, R.E., and Hopper, M.S., Studies of siloxane phases bonded to silica gel for use in high-performance liquid chromatography, *J. Chromatog. Sci.* 12, 767–778, 1974.
11. Cox, G.B., Practical aspects of bonded phase chromatography, *J. Chromatog. Sci.* 15, 385–397, 1977.
12. Horvatovich, P., Hoekman, B., Govorukhina, N., and Bischoff, R., Multidimensional chromatography coupled to mass spectrometry in analysing complex proteomics samples, *J. Sep. Sci.* 33, 1421–1437, 2010.
13. Wolfe, L.S., Barringer, C.P., Mostafa, S.S., and Shukla, A.A., Multimodal chromatography: Characterization of protein binding and selectivity enhancement through mobile phase modulators, *J. Chromatog. A* 1340, 151–156, 2014.

Comparison of Liquid Chromatographic Methods

Method	Matrix	Initial Solvent
Ion-exchange	Charged functional group on organic matrix such as polystyrene/divinyl-benzene crosslinked dextran, or silica	Usually aqueous dilute salt solution containing buffer to control pH
Normal-phase	Silica-alumina-bonded phases such as amino, nitro, cyano, and diol	Non-polar organic solvents such as *n*-hexane, nonpolar organic solvents containing small of a less polar solvent such as 2-propanol
Aqueous normal-phase chromatography (ANPC)	Most applications use a silica hydride solid phase; other solid phases have been used	Organic solvents such as acetonitrile with water; may contain an additive such as formic acid or ammonium formate
Reverse-phase chromatography (RPC)	Alkyl or aryl modified silica. The most common are C_4 (butyl) or C_{18} (octadecyl) hydrocarbon chains	Water with dilute weak acid such as 0.1% trifluoroacetic acid or 0.1% formic acid
Hydrophobic interaction chromatography (HIC)	Aryl (e.g. Phenyl) or Alkyl (Butyl) modified silica	High-salt such as 1–2 M $(NH_4)_2SO_4$
Hydrophilic interaction chromatography (HILIC)	Polar matrix such unmodified silica or a bonded phase such as cyanopropyl, amino, or diol	Polar organic solvent such as acetonitrile with H_2O or a buffer such as ammonium formate
Electrostatic repulsion-hydrophilic interaction chromatography (ERLIC)	Polar matrix such unmodified silica, anion- and cation-exchange matrix	Organic solvent such as used in HILIC with a buffer salt
Gel filtration	Cross-linked dextran, agarose, or polyacrylamide matrix	Aqueous solvent with physiological ionic strength
Gel permeation	crosslinked polystyrene divinylbenzene (Styragel®) is major matrix. Other supports can be used depending on stability in solvent	Organic solvent such as chloroform, dimethylsulfoxide, or dimethyl acetamide
Hydroxyapatite	Hydroxyapatite which can also less frequently be referred to as calcium phosphate or hydroxylapatite	Aqueous solvents most frequently containing sodium phosphate buffer, although other solvent systems can be used

(Continued)

Comparison of Liquid Chromatographic Methods (*Continued*)

Method	Matrix	Initial Solvent
Affinity chromatography.	A specific ligand attached to a matrix (usually dextran or agarose)	Usually aqueous with elution by change in solvent composition
Supercritical fluid chromatography	Original matrix was silica. Now many difference matrices with ligands such as 2-ethyl pyridine, fluorophenyl as well as ligands such as octadecyl and other matrices used for other forms of liquid chromatography	Supercritical fluids with CO_2 the most common with the addition of another solvent such as methanol

CIRCADIAN

The term is circadian is used to describe an event, usually a physiological activity,[1–6] which occurs approximately every 24 hours (diurnal).[7] A circadian clock controls these **diurnal** variations.[8] Current work shows an appreciation of circadian variation on biomarker expression.[9,10] A consideration of the literature suggests that the term circadian is used to refer to variation between days while diurnal more specially refers to a variation within a 24-hour period.

1. Mills, J.N., Human circadian rhythms, *Physiol. Rev.* 46, 128–171, 1966.
2. Brady, J., How are insect circadian rhythms controlled? *Nature* 223, 781–784, 1969.
3. Menaker, M., Takahashi, J.S., and Eskin, A., The physiology of circadian pacemakers, *Annu. Rev. Physiol.* 40, 501–526, 1978.
4. Lewy, A.J., Emens, J., Jackman, A., and Yuhas, K., Circadian uses of melatonin in humans, *Chronobiol. Int.* 23, 403–412, 2006.
5. Rosato, E., Tauber, E., and Kyriacou, C.P., Molecular genetics of the fruit-fly circadian clock, *Eur. J. Hum. Genet.* 14, 729–738, 2006.
6. Hardin, P.E., and Yu, W., Circadian transcription: Passing the HAT to CLOCK, *Cell* 125, 424–426, 2006.
7. *Oxford Dictionary of the English Language*, Oxford University Press, Oxford, UK.
8. Dierickz, P., Van Laake, L.W., and Geijsen, N., Circadian clocks: From stem cells to tissue homeostasis and regeneration, *EMBO Rep.* 19, 18–28, 2018.
9. Dominguez-Rodriguez, A., Abreu-Gonzalez, P., Sanchez-Sanchez, J.J., Kaski, J.C., and Reiter, R.J., Metatonin and circadian biology in human cardiovascular disease, *J. Pineal Res.* 49, 14–22, 2010.
10. Amar, A., Chtourou, H., and Souissi, N., Effect of time-of-day on biochemical markers in response to physical exercise, *J. Strength Cond. Res.* 31, 272–282, 2017.

CIS-ELEMENT

A *cis*-element is a regulatory sequence in DNA that can control a gene only on the same chromosome. In bacteria, *cis*-elements are adjacent or proximal to the gene, while such sequences may be quite distant from the gene in eukaryotes.[1] *Cis*-element are binding sites for transcription factors/transcription enhancers.[2–4] *Cis*-elements are also found in RNA viruses.[5–8]

1. Lodish, H., Berk, A., Zipursky, S.L., Matsudaira, P., Baltimore, D., and Darnell, J., *Molecular Cell Biology*, 4th edn., W.H. Freeman, New York, 2000.
2. Ezer, D., Zabet, N.R., and Adryan, B., Homotypic clusters of transcription factor binding sites: A model system for understanding the physical mechanism of gene expression, *Comput. Struct. Biotechnol. J.* 10, 63–69, 2014.
3. Buffrey, A.D., Mendes, C.C., and McGregor, A.P., The functionality and evolution of eukaryotic transcriptional enhancers, *Adv. Genet.* 96, 143–206, 2016.
4. Inukai, S., Kock, K.H., and Bulyk, M.L., Transcription factor-DNA binding: Beyond binding site motifs, *Curr. Opin. Genet. Dev.* 43, 110–119, 2017.
5. *Viral Genome Replication*, ed. C.E. Cameron, M. Götte, and K.D. Rainey, Springer Science, New York, 2009.
6. Pathak, K.B., Pogany, J., Xu, K., White, K.A., and Nagy, P.D., Defining the roles of *cis*-acting RNA elements in tombusvirus replicase assembly *in vitro*, *J. Virol.* 86, 156–171, 2012.
7. Newburn, L.R., and White, K.A., *Cis*-Acting RNA elements in positive-strand RNA plant virus genomes, *Virology* 479–480, 434–443, 2015.
8. Madhugiri, R., Fricke, M., Marz, M., and Ziebuhr, J., Coronavirus *cis*-acting RNA elements, *Adv. Virus Res.* 96, 127–163, 2016.

CIRCULAR DICHROISM

Circular dichroism (CD) represents the differential absorption of plane polarized light, which consists of two circularly polarized components, one rotating counter-clockwise and the other clockwise passing through a solution of a chiral substance and is expressed as ellipticity (θ) as function of wavelength.[1,2] CD has been extensively used of the study of the secondary and tertiary structures or proteins.[3–7] CD is used for the study of ligand binding to proteins either through changes in the conformation of protein as with triterpenoids with human serum albumin[8] or by the use of CD to study a prosthetic groups such as heme in hemoglobin.[9] CD is also used for the study of nucleic acids.[10–14] There is increasing use of synchrotron radiation for CD studies of proteins.[15] Another approach, vibrational circular dichroism, uses infrared radiation as opposed to UV-VIS in conventional circular dichroism.[16]

1. Kobayashi, N., and Muranaka, A., *Circular Dichroism and Magnetic Circular Dichroism Spectroscopy for Organic Chemists*, Royal Society of Chemistry, Cambridge, UK, 2011.
2. *Circular Dichroism: Theory and Spectroscopy*, Nova Scientific, New York, 2012.
3. Johnson, W.C., Jr., Protein secondary structure and circular dichroism: A practical guide, *Proteins* 7, 205–214, 1990.
4. Greenfield, N.J., Analysis of circular dichroism data. *Meth. Enzymol*, 383, 282–317, 2004.
5. Kelly, S.M., Jess, T.J., Price, N.C., How to study proteins by circular dichroism. *Biochim. Biophys. Acta* 1751, 119–139, 2005.
6. Heller, G.T., Aprile, F.A., and Vendruscolo, M., Methods of probing the interactions between small molecules and disorders proteins, *Cell. Mo. Life Sci.* 74, 3225–3243, 2017.
7. Yao, H., Wyendaele, E., Xu, X., Kosgei, A., and De Spiegeleer, B., Circular dichroism in functional quality evaluation of medicines, *J. Pharm. Biomed. Anal.* 50–64, 2018.
8. Abboud, R., Charcosset, C., and Greige-Gerges, H., Interaction of triterpenoids with human serum albumin: A review, *Chem. Phys. Lipids* 207, 260–270, 2017.
9. Nagai, M., Mizusawa, N., Kitagawa, T., and Nagotomo, S., A role of heme side-chains of human hemoglobin in its function revealed by circular dichroism and resonance Raman spectroscopy, *Biophys. Rev.* 10, 271–284, 2018.
10. Kypr, J., Kejnovská, I., Renciuk, D., and Vorlíčková, M., Circular dichroism and conformational polymorphism of DNA, *Nucleic Acids Res.* 37, 1713–1725, 2009.
11. Chang, Y.M., Chen, C.K., and Hou, M.H., Conformational changes in DNA upon ligand binding monitored by circular dichroism, *Int. J. Med. Sci.* 13, 3394–3413, 2012.
12. Konvalinová, H., Dvořáková, Z., Renčiuk, D., et al., Diverse effects of naturally occurring base lesions on the structure and stability of the human telomere DNA quadruplex, *Biochimie* 118, 15–25, 2015.
13. Peng, Z., Li, J., Li, S., et al., Quantification of nucleic acid concentration in the nanoparticle or polymer conjugate using circular dichroism spectroscopy, *Anal. Chem.* 90, 2255–2262, 2018.
14. Hao, G., Sun, J., and Wei, C., Studies on interactions of carbazole derivatives with DNA, cell image, and cytotoxicity, *Bioorg. Med. Chem.* 26, 285–294, 2018.
15. Kumagai, P.S., DeMarco, R., and Lopes, J.L.S., Advantages of synchrotron radiation circular dichroism spectroscopy to study intrinsically disordered proteins, *Eur. Biophys. J.* 46, 599–606, 2017.
16. Kurouski, D., Advances of vibrational circular dichroism (VCD) in bioanalytical chemistry. A review, *Anal. Chim. Acta* 990, 54–66, 2017.

CLASS SWITCH RECOMBINATION

A process by which one constant region gene segment is switched with another gene segment during B-cell development when immunoglobulin production changes from IgM to IgA, IgE, or IgG.[1–7]

1. Davis, M.M., Kim, S.K., and Hood, L.E., DNA sequences mediating class switching in alpha-immunoglobulin, *Science* 209, 1360–1365, 1980.
2. Geha, R.S., Jabara, H.H., and Brodeur, S.R., The regulation of immunoglobulin E class-switch recombination, *Nat. Rev. Immunol.* 3, 721–732, 2003.
3. Min, I.M., and Selsing, E., Antibody class switch recombination: Roles for switch sequence and mismatch repair proteins, *Adv. Immunol.* 87, 297–328, 2005.
4. Stavnezer, J., and Schrader, C.E., IgH chain class switch recombination: Mechanism and regulation, *J. Immunol.* 193, 5370–5378, 2014.
5. Vaidyanathan, B., and Chaudhuri, J., Epigenetic codes programming class switch recombination, *Front. Immunol.* 6, 405, 2015.
6. Methot, S.P., and Di Noia, J.M., Molecular mechanisms of somatic hypermutation and class switch recombination, *Adv. Immunol.* 133, 37–87, 2017.
7. Scott-Taylor, T.H., Axinia, S.C., Amin, S., and Pettengell, R., Immunoglobulin G: Structure and functional implications of different subclass modifications in initiation and resolution of allergy, *Immun. Inflamm. Dis.* 6, 13–33, 2018.

CLINOMICS

Clinomics refers to the application of data obtained from the various "omics" (proteomics, genomics, etc.) and clinical data for the treatment of disease.[1] The term is not extensively used and, when used, is focused on cancer therapy.[2,3] A literature search for clinomics yielded studies, while not including the term clinomics, contained studies combining multiple omic studies with clinical studies in oncology.[4] Clinomics can be considered to be a concept underlying precision medicine.[5]

1. Wenz, F., Clinomics-an underutilized resource? *Translat. Cancer Res.* 5, 206–207, 2016.
2. Workman, P., and Clarke, P.A., Innovative cancer drug targets: Genomics, transcriptomics, and clinomics, *Expert Opin. Pharmacother.* 2, 911–915, 2001.
3. Chang, W., Brohl, A.S., Patidar, R., et al., MultiDimensional clinOmics for precision therapy of children and adolescent young adults with relapsed and refractory cancer: A report from the Center for Cancer Research, *Clin. Cancer Res.* 22, 3810–3820, 2016.

4. Dimitrakopoulos, L., Prassas, I., Diamandis, E.P., and Charames, G.S., Onco-proteogenomics: Multi-omics level data integration for accurate phenotype prediction, *Crit. Clin. Lab. Sci.* 54, 414–432, 2017.
5. Niehr, F., Eder, T. Pilz, T., et al., Multilayered omics-based analysis of a head and neck cancer model of cis-platinin resistance reveals intratumoral heterogeneity and treatment-induced clonal selection, *Clin. Cancer Res.* 24, 158–168, 2018.

CLONAL SELECTION

Clonal selection is, literally, the selection of a clone. The term is used most often used to describe the process by which a B cell is challenged by a specific antigen to produce a committed plasma cell or the differentiation of T-cell by a specific antigen.[1–9]

1. Burnet, F.M., *The Clonal Selection Theory of Acquired Immunity*, Vanderbilt University Press, Nashville, TN, 1959.
2. Williamson, A.R., The biological origin of antibody diversity, *Annu. Rev. Biochem.* 45, 467–500, 1976.
3. D'Eustachio, P., Rutishauser, U.S., and Edelman, G.M., Clonal selection and the ontogeny of the immune response, *Int. Rev. Cytol. Suppl.* 5, 1–60, 1977.
4. Coutinho, A., Beyond clonal selection and network, *Immunol. Rev.* 110, 63–87, 1989.
5. Mazumdar, P.M.H., *Immunology 1930–1980: Essays on the History of Immunology*, Wall & Thompson, Toronto, 1989.
6. Podolsky, S.H., and Tauber, A.I., *The Generation of Diversity: Clonal Selection Theory and Their Rise of Molecular Immunology*, Harvard University Press, Cambridge, MA, 1997.
7. Cohen, I.R., Antigenic mimicry, clonal selection and autoimmunity, *J. Autoimmun.* 16, 337–340, 2001.
8. Steele, E.J., Reverse transcriptase mechanism of somatic hypermutation: 60 years of clonal selection theory, *Front. Immunol.* 8, 1611, 2017.
9. Gupta, R.G., and Somer, R.A., Intratumor heterogeneity: Novel approaches for resolving genomic architecture and clonal evolution, *Mol. Cancer Res.* 15, 1127–1137, 2017.

CLONE

Clone (noun) is the term used to describe a cell or organism descended from and genetically identical to a single common ancestor. Clone (noun) is also used to refer to a DNA sequence encoding a product or an entire gene sequence from an organism that is replicated by genetic engineering. Such material can be transferred to another organism for the expression of such cDNA or gene. Clone (verb) is the term used to describe the process of making a clone, most frequently with DNA sequences. It is used a title for a number of novels as well as the popular literature.

CLONOTYPE

Clonotype is the term used to describe both B-cell and T-cell function. The concept of B-cell clonality was advanced in a number of studies in the period of 1960–1970 to describe the singularity of B-cell function. The actual term can be attributed to work in 1975[1] where clonotype is defined as the B-cell population which is specific of a specific antigen. Another group[2] defined clonotype as an antibody derived from a B-cell clone. A more advanced definition is based on homology in the CDR-H3 (third complementary determining region in heavy chain) region.[3] It is estimated that there can be 30 clonotypes (IgG-cd = 30) for an epitope in rabbits.[4] Other work on the human serum antibody response to vaccination can consist of 80–130 clonotypes (IgG-cd = 80–120) for an epitope.[5,6] The clonotype concept extends to T cells refers to the antibody specificity of T cell receptors (TCR).[7]

1. Klinman, N.R., and Press, J.L., The characterization of tech B-cell repertoire specificity for the 2,4-dinitrophenyl and 2,4,6-tirnitrophenyl determinants in BALB /c mice, *J. Expt. Med.* 141, 1133–1146, 1975.
2. Frost, H., and Braun, D.G., Clonotype pattern of antibodies released by single lymph nodes, *Scand. J. Immunol.* 9, 563–567, 1979.
3. Lavinder, J.J., Horton, A.P., Georgiou, G., and Ippolito, G., Next-generation sequencing and protein mass spectrometry for the comprehensive analysis of human cellular and serum antibody repertoires, *Curr. Opin. Chem, Biol.* 24, 112–120, 2015.
4. Wine, Y., Boutz, D.P., Lavinder, J.J., et al., Molecular deconvolution of the monoclonal antibodies that comprise the polyclonal serum response, *Proc. Natl. Acad. Sci.* 110, 2993–2998, 2013.
5. Lavinder, J.J., Wne, Y., Gerecke, C., et al., Identification and characterization of the constituent human serum antibodies elicited by vaccination, *Proc. Natl. Acad. Sci. USA* 111, 2259–2264, 2014.
6. Lee, J., Boutz, D.R., Chromikova, V., et al., Molecular level analysis of the serum antibody repertoire in young adults before and after seasonal influenza vaccination, *Nature Med.* 22, 1456–1464, 2016.
7. Mahe, E., Pugh, T., and Kamel-Reid, S., T-cell clonality assessment: Past, present and future, *J. Clin. Pathol.* 71, 195–200, 2018.

COCRYSTALS (CO-CRYSTALS)

A cocrystals (co-crystal) can be defined as a multicomponent molecular crystal containing neutral molecules in a definite stoichiometric ratio.[1,2] A cocrystal differs from a salt in that a salt contains charged molecules. A cocrystal may be considered different from a solvate, which is a crystal containing molecules of solvent but not necessarily in a stoichiometric quantity. An active pharmaceutical ingredient (API) can be incorporated into a cocrystal to improve the properties of the API.[3-5]

1. Bond, A.D., Fundamental aspects of salts and co-crystals, in *Pharmaceutical Salts and Co-Crystals*, ed. J. Wolters and L. Quéré, Royal Society of Chemistry, Cambridge, UK, 2012.
2. Dalpiaz, A., Pavan, B., and Ferretti, V., Can pharmaceutical co-crystals provide an opportunity to modify the biological properties of drugs? *Drug Discov. Today* 22, 1134–1138, 2007.
3. *Regulatory Classification of Pharmaceutical Co-Crystals*, CDER, FDA, 2013.
4. Challener, C.A., "Rebirth" of cocrystals? *Pharm. Tech.* 2016, 26–27, 2016.
5. Suzuki, N., Kawahata, M., Yamaguchi, K., et al., Comparison of the relative stability of pharmaceutical cocrystals consisting of paracetamol and dicarboxylic acids, *Drug Dev. Ind. Pharm.* 13, 1–24, 2017.

COEFFICIENT OF LINEAR THERMAL EXPANSION (CLTE)

The coefficient of linear thermal expansion is the increase in the length of a solid as a function of temperature under isobaric conditions $\alpha = 1/L\left(\frac{\partial L}{\partial T}\right)\rho$.[1] CLTE is used for solids, while the coefficient of thermal expansion is used for liquids. As an approximation, the CLTE can be considered one-third that of the coefficient of thermal expansion.[2] CLTE has been used to describe changes in the structure of proteins and other polymers as a function of temperature. It has been suggested that CLTE is used to measure anisotropic substances.[3] Data for proteins is obtained from work of crystals or from computer simulation. A value of $115 \times 10^{-6} \text{ K}^{-1}$ was obtained for myoglobin[4] while a value of $1.2 \times 10^{-4} \text{ K}^{-1}$ was obtained for lysozyme crystals.[5] Computational studies gave a value of $1.13 \times 10^{-4} \text{ K}^{-1}$ for T4 lysozyme and $0.817 \times 10^{-4} \text{ K}^{-1}$ for barnase[6] and $1.5 \times 10^{-3} \text{ K}^{-1}$ for crystal structure of amyloidβ(1-42) peptide but $-0.8 \times 10^{-3} \text{ K}^{-1}$ in solution.[7] A negative value for the coefficient of thermal expansion is unusual but is also seen for water in the ice form.[8] There is use of the CLTE to describe the effect of thermal stress on bacteria where measurement was accomplished with a scanning electron microscope to measure the axial distortion of the z-axis.[9] See **coefficient of thermal expansion**.

1. Mortimer, R.G., *Physical Chemistry*, 2nd edn., Chapter 2, Harcourt Academic, San Diego, CA, 2001. CLTE can be confused with the coefficient of thermal expansion.
2. *Macmillan Encyclopedia of Physics*, ed. J.S. Rigden, pp. 189–190, Simon & Schuster Macmillan, New York, 1996.
3. Gel'man, E.B., Temperature coefficients of expansion, in *Handbook of Physical Quantities*, ed. I.S. Grigoriev and E.Z. Meilikhov, Chapter 10, pp. 283–321, CRC Press, Boca Raton, FL, 1997.
4. Frauenfelder, H., Hartmann, H., Karplus, M., et al., Thermal expansion of a protein, *Biochemistry* 26, 254–261, 1987.
5. Kurinov, I.V., and Harrison, R.W., The influence of temperature of lysozyme crystals, structure and dynamics of proteins and water, *Acta Cryst.* D51, 98–109, 1995.
6. Palma, R., and Curmi, P.M.G., Computational studies on mutant protein stability: The correlation between surface thermal expansion and protein stability, *Protein Sci.* 8, 913–920, 1999.
7. Brovchenko, I., Burri, R.R., Krukau, A., Oleinikova, A., and Winter, R., Intrinsic thermal expansivity and hydrational properties of amyloid peptide $A\beta_{42}$ in liquid water, *J. Chem. Phys.* 129, 195101, 2008.
8. Wang, Q., Jackson, J.A., Ge., Q., et al., Lightweight mechanical metamaterials with tunable negative thermal expansion, *Phys. Rev. Lett.* 117, 175901, 2016.
9. Nakanishi, K., Kojuri, A., Fuji, J., et al., With respect to coefficient of linear thermal expansion, bacterial vegetative cells and spores resemble plastics and metals, respectively, *J. Nanobiotechnology* 11, 33, 2013.

COEFFICIENT OF THERMAL EXPANSION

The coefficient of thermal expansion (CTE) is the volume change of a material at constant pressure and concentration as a function of temperature $\beta = 1/V\ (\delta V/\delta T)_p$.[1] The CTE is useful for liquids and materials including dental materials.[2] The value can be presented as obtained as a specific temperature as shown or over a temperature range where an average value is presented. The Greek letter β is used for the coefficient of thermal expansion while the Greek letter α is used for the coefficient of linear expansion.[3] The mercury thermometer is a practical example of the use of the coefficient of thermal expansion. The coefficient of linear expansion is not necessarily constant over a range of temperature but a property of the respective material.[4] See **coefficient of linear thermal expansion**.

1. Mortimer, R.G., *Physical Chemistry*, 2nd edn., Chapter 2, Harcourt Academic, San Diego, CA, 2001.
2. Alnazzawi, A., and Watts, D.C., Simultaneous determination of polymerization shrinkage, exotherm and thermal expansion coefficient of dental resin-composites, *Dent. Mater.* 28, 1240–1249, 2012.
3. *MacMillan Encyclopedia of Physics*, ed. J.S. Rigden, pp. 1589–1590, Simon and Schuster Macmillan, New York, 1996.
4. Gel'man, E.B., Temperature coefficients of expansion, in *Handbook of Physical Quantitites*, ed. I.S. Grigoriev and E.Z. Meilikhov, Chapter 10, pp. 283–321, CRC Press, Boca Raton, FL, 1997.

Coefficient of Thermal Expansion for Some Liquids

Substance	β ($\times 10^{-6}$°C^{-1})	Substance	B ($\times 10^{-6}$°C^{-1})
H_2O, -10°C	-294.73[a]	0.100 m NaCl, 0°C	-58[b]
H_2O, 0°C	-68.14[a]	1.000 m NaCl, 0°C	110[b]
H_2O, 4°C	0.26[a]	Acetic Acid, 20°C	1080[b]
H_2O, 20°C	206.61[a]	Ethylene Glycol, 20°C	626[b]
H_2O, 25°C	257.05[a]	Acetone, 20°C	1460[b]
H_2O, 25°C	256[b]	Ethanol, 20°C	1400[b]

[a] Data from Kell, G.S., Precise representation of volume properties of water at one atmosphere, *J. Chem. Eng. Data* 12, 66–69, 1967.
[b] Data from *CRC Handbook of Chemistry and Physics*, 86th edn., ed. D.R. Lide, pp. 6–117, CRC Press, Boca Raton, FL, 2005–2006.

COLD-CHAIN PRODUCT

A product or reagent that must be kept cold during transit and storage; most often between 2° and 8°C.[1–3] Maintenance of cold chain is of particular importance in the distribution of vaccines.[4–6]

1. Elliott, M.A., and Halbert, G.W., Maintaining the cold chain shipping environment for phase I clinical trial distribution, *Int. J. Pharm.* 299, 49–54, 2005.
2. Kartoğlu, U., Nelaj, E., and Maire, D., Improving temperature monitoring in the vaccine cold chain at the periphery: An intervention study using a 30-day electronic refrigerator temperature logger (Fridge-tag), *Vaccine* 28, 4065–4072, 2010.
3. Hatchett, R., The medicines refrigerator and the importance of the cold chain in the safe storage of medicines, *Nurs. Stand.* 32, 53–63, 2017.
4. Billah, M.M., Zaman, K., Estivariz, C.F., et al., Cold-chain adaptability during introduction of inactivated polio vaccine in Bangladesh, 2015, *J. Infect. Dis.* 216(Suppl 1), S114–S121, 2017.
5. Heyerdahl, L.W., Ngwira, B., Demolis, R., et al., Innovative vaccine delivery strategies in response to a cholera outbreak in the challenging context of Lake Chiwa. A rapid qualitative assessment, *Vaccine* 36, 6491–6496, 2018.
6. Azimi, T., Franzel, L., and Probst, N., Seizing market shaping opportunities for vaccine cold chain equipment, *Vaccine* 35, 2260–2264, 2017.

COLD SHOCK PROTEINS

Cold shock proteins (CSPs) are a family of proteins which are synthesized by plant cells, prokaryotic and eukaryotic cells in response to cold stress. It has been suggested that CSPs function as chaperones for mRNA to enable continued translation at low temperature,[1] although it is clear that CSPs have a role regulating other responses to stress.[2] CSPs in both prokaryotes and eukaryotes are relatively small proteins (65–70 amino acids) characterized by the presence of a domain, the cold shock domain, which binds to nucleic acids.[3] There are several CSPs that have been found to be important in humans for reasons other than cold shock response. These include Y-box protein-1,[4] cold inducible RNA-binding protein (CIRP),[5] and RNA binding motif protein-3 (RBM-3).[6]

1. Phadtari, S., and Inouye, M., Cold shock proteins, in *Psychrophiles: From Biodiversity to Biotechnology*, 2nd edn. ed. R. Margesin, Chapter 12, pp. 191–209, Springer Verlag, Berlin, Germany, 2011.
2. Keto-Timonen, R., Hietala, N., Palonen, E., et al., Cold shock proteins: A minireview with special emphasis on Csp-family of enteropathogenic *Yersenia*, *Front. Immunol.* 7, 1151, 2016.
3. Kljashtorny, V., Nikonov, S., Ovchinnikov, L., et al., The cold shock domain of YB-1 segregates RNA from DNA by non-bonded interactions, *PLoS One* 10(7), e09130318, 2015.
4. Raffetseder, U., Liehn, E.A., Weber, C., and Mertens, P.R., Role of cold shock Y-box protein-1 in inflammation, atherosclerosis and organ transplantation rejection, *Eur. J. Cell Biol.* 91, 567–575, 2012.
5. Zhong, P., and Huang, H., Recent progress in the research of cold-inducible RNA-binding protein, *Future Sci. OA* 3, FSO246, 2017.
6. Zhu, X., Zelmer, A., Kapfhammer, J.P., and Wellman, S., Cold-inducible RBM3 inhibits PERK phosphorylation through cooperation with NF90 to protect cells from endoplasmic reticulum stress, *FASEB J.* 30, 624–634, 2016.

COLLOID

The term colloid refers to a particle with dimensions between 1 nm and 1 μm, although it is not necessary for all three dimensions to be in this size range.[1] The original definition in 1861 described a material in a peculiar state of aggregation as opposed to a crystalloid which does not diffuse through a membrane.[2] A variety of materials can be classified as colloids including inorganic materials such as clays and silicates, organic materials such as large carbon particles ("soot"). Also included are biocolloids, which is a loosely defined category including adsorbed enzymes on beads[3] and bacteria.[4] Proteins such as albumin and fibrinogen are considered to be colloids with albumin considered the primary factor in colloid osmotic pressure.[5] The characterization of proteins as colloids versus crystalloids date at least to 1861.[6] Colloids were defined as substances which formed gelatinous masses and did not pass through a membrane while a crystalloid material forms crystals and pass through a membrane. This distinction persists today in transfusion medicine where there is a distinction between crystalloid therapeutics (e.g. salt solutions) and colloids (e.g. albumin, dextran).[7] A colloidal dispersion is a system where colloid particles are dispersed in a continuous phase of a different composition such as a suspension (particles in a liquid), a emulsion (colloids of one liquid are suspended in another liquid where the two liquids are immiscible such as oil and water), a foam (gas dispersed in a liquid or gel), or an aerosol (a colloid in a gas such as air; a fog is a liquid colloid dispersed in a gas). There is a long history of work on colloidal gold[8,9] and is of current interest in a variety of areas.[10,11] There is considerable use of colloidal gold in cytochemistry.[12,13]

1. Hofmann, T., Bauman, T., Bundschuh, T., et al., Aquatische Kolloide I. Übersichtsarbeit zur Definition, zu Systemen und zur Relevanz, *Grundwasser* 8, 203–212, 2003.
2. *Oxford English Dictionary*, Oxford, University Press, Oxford, UK, 2017.
3. Bajrami, B., Hvastkovs, E.G., Jensen, G.C., et al., Enzyme-DNA biocolloids for DNA adduct and reactive metabolite detection by chromatography-mass spectrometry, *Anal. Chem.* 80, 922–932, 2008.
4. Dzoibakiewicz, E., Hrynkiewicz, K., Walczyk, M., and Buszewski, B., Study of charge distribution on the surface of biocolloids, *Colloids Surf B Biointerfaces* 104, 122–127, 2013.
5. Hankins, J., The role of albumin in fluid and electrolyte balance, *J. Infus. Nurs.* 29, 260–265, 2006.
6. Graham quoted in Loeb, J., *Proteins and the Theory of Colloidal Behavior*, 2nd edn., p. 1, McGraw-Hill, New York, 1924.
7. Fodor, G.H., Babik, B., Czövek, D., Doras, C., et al., Fluid replacement and respiratory function: Comparison of whole blood with colloid and crystalloid: A randomized animal study, *Eur. J. Anaesthesiol.* 33, 34–41, 2016.
8. Whitney, W.R., and Blake, J.C., The migration of colloids, *J. Am. Chem. Soc.* 26, 1339–1387, 1904.
9. Bernsohn, J., and Borman, E.K., Proteins in the colloidal gold reaction, *J. Clin. Invest.* 26, 1026–1030, 1947.
10. Prati, L., and Villa, A., Gold colloids: From quasi-homogeneous to heterogeneous catalytic systems, *Acc. Chem. Res.* 47, 855–863, 2014.
11. Letzel, A., Gökce, B., Menzel, A., and Barcikowski, S., Primary particle diameter differentiation and bimodality identification by five analytical methods using gold nanoparticle size distributions synthesized by laser ablation in liquids, *Appld. Surface Sci.* 435, 743–751, 2018.
12. Goodman, S.L., Hodges, G.M., and Livingston, D.C., A review of the colloidal gold marker system, *Scan. Electron Microsc.* (Pt.2), 139–146, 1980.
13. Bendayan, M., A review of the potential and versatility of colloidal gold cytochemical labeling for molecular morphology, *Biotech. Histochem.* 75, 203–242, 2000.

COMBINATION PRODUCT

The term combination product is used by regulatory agencies such as the FDA to describe a product composed of two or more components which are subject to control by a regulatory agencies.[1,2] Examples include the combination of a biologic with a drug (antibody–drug conjugate) in oncology[3] and a delivery device with a product.[4]

1. https://www.fda.gov/combinationproducts/aboutcombinationproducts/ucm118332.htm.
2. Hunter, N.L., and Sherman, R.E., Combination products: Modernizing the regulatory paradigm, *Nature Rev. Drug Discovery* 16, 513–514. 2017.
3. Dinh, T.N., Onea, A.S., and Jazirehi, A.R., Combination of celecoxib (Celebrex®) and CD19 CAR-redirected CTL immunotherapy for the treatment of B-cell non-Hodgkin's lymphomas, *Am. J. Clin. Exp. Immunol.* 6, 27–42, 2017.
4. Anderson, D., Lium R., Anand Subramony, J., and Cammack, J., Design control considerations for biologic-device combination products, *Adv. Drug Deliv. Rev.* 112, 101–105, 2017.

COMET ASSAY

The comet assay (single cell gel electrophoresis) is a method for determining the integrity of DNA in a single cell or tissue using electrophoresis in an agarose gel. The comet assay was developed by Ostling and Johanson in 1984.[1] Cells or tissue is embedded in an agarose gel and then lysed with detergent and high salt. Breakage or relaxing of the supercoiled in DNA in the nucleoids results from cell lysis allows DNA strands be pulled toward the anode resulting in a comet like pattern when observed by fluorescence microscopy after staining with a DNA binding dye such as ethidium bromide or 4,6-diamidino-2-phenylindole. The amount of DNA detected in the tail is a measure of DNA breakage.[2–4] The comet assay has been of particular value in toxicology research.[5,6]

1. Ostling, O., and Johanson, K.J., Microelectrophoretic study of the radiation-induced DNA damage in individual mammalian cells, *Biochem. Biophys. Res. Commun.* 123, 291–298, 1984.
2. Collins, A.R., The comet assay for DNA damage and repair, *Mol. Biotechnol.* 26, 249–261, 2004.
3. Azqueta, A., and Collins, A.R., The essential comet assay: A comprehensive guide to measuring DNA damage and repair, *Arch. Toxicol.* 87, 949–968, 2013.
4. Singh, M.P., The comet assay: Reflections on its development, evolution and applications, *Mutat. Res. Rev. Mutat. Res.* 767, 23–30, 2016.
5. Collins, A.R., Measuring oxidative damage to DNA and its repair with the comet assay, *Biochim. Biophys. Acta* 1840, 794–800, 2014.
6. Glei, M., Schneider, T., and Schlörmann, W., Comet assay: An essential tool in toxicological research, *Arch. Toxicol.* 90, 2315–2336, 2016.

COMPLEMENT

The term complement describes several related processes or systems using the interaction of as many as 35 plasma and membrane proteins[1,2] which can interact to form a membrane attack complex resulting in the lysis of bacterial pathogens[3] and apoptotic and necrotic cells.[4] Complement is also important in inflammation through the production of anaphylatoxins (split products). Anaphylatoxins are derived from the proteolysis of complement components during the activation process. For example, proteolysis of complement component C3 yields Ca, an anaphylatoxin, which binds to a specific receptor and has a role in the inflammatory process and Cb, a larger fragment, which binds to other proteins in the complement activation process.[5] There are three pathways of complement activation: the classical pathway, the alternative pathway, and the MBlectin (mannose-binding lectin, a plasma protein) pathway. The classical pathway is activated by an antigen-antibody complex (free antibody does not activate or fix complement) via the Fc domain of the antibody; there are other mechanisms for classical pathway activation which make minor contributions. The alternative pathway is activated by direct recognition of foreign materials in an antibody-independent manner. The alternative pathway is thought the oldest of the three pathways is phyllogenetic development. The MBlectin pathway is initiated by the interaction of the MBlectin with a bacterial cell surface polysaccharide. The activation of complement component C3 is common to all three pathways. It is noted that there are similarities to the blood coagulation cascade. See **anaphylatoxins**, **complement fixation**.

COMPLEMENT FIXATION

Complement fixation refers to the binding of the first component of the complement pathway, C1, to an IgG- or IgM-antigen complex to initiate the class pathway of complement activation.[1–6] The antigen is usually a cell surface protein. Free antibody does not fix complement. Productive binding of the antigen-antibody complex (binding involves the Fc portion of the antibody and a minimum of two Fc domains is required, and thus two intact antibody molecules) results in complement activation. An antibody that activates complement is described as having fixed complement. The ability of antibody to fix complement is traditionally measured by the lysis of sheep red blood cells by the membrane attack complex.[7] The term **complement fixation** or **fixing complement** is used to describe the quality of an antigen-antibody complex in the initiation of the classic pathway[8] and bactericidal activity.[9]

1. Moore, F., Jr., Complement, in *Immunology, Infection, and Immunity,* ed. G.B. Pier, J.B. Lyczak, and L.M. Wetzler, Chapter 5, pp. 85–109, ASM Press, Washington, DC, 2004.
2. Speth, C., Prodinger, W.M., Würzner, R., Stoiben. H., and Dierich, M.P., Complement, in *Fundamental Immunology*, ed. W.E. Paul, pp. 1047–1078, Wolters Kluwer Lippincott, Williams & Wilkins, Philadelphia, PA, 2008.
3. Bayly-Jones, C., Bubeck, D., and Dunstone, M.A., The mystery behind membrane insertion: A review of the complement membrane attack complex, *Philos. Trans. R. Soc. Lond. B* 372(1726), 2106021, 2017.
4. Martin, M., and Blom, A.M., Complement in removal of the dead—Balancing inflammation, *Immunol. Rev.* 274, 281–232, 2016.
5. Ember, J.A., Complement factors and their receptors, *Immunopharmacology* 38, 3–15, 1997.
6. Laumonnier, Y., Karsten, C.M., and Köhl, J., Novel insights into the expression pattern of anaphylatoxin receptors in mice and men, *Mol. Immunol.* 89, 44–58, 2017.
7. Welch, R.J., Merrigan, S.D., and Delgado, J.C., A spectrophotometric method to precisely determine endpoint titers in complement fixation assays, *J. Clin. Lab. Anal.* 26, 190–193, 2012.

8. Carter, D., and Lieber, A., Protein engineering to target complement evasion in cancer, *FEBS Lett.* 588, 334–340, 2014.
9. Weiss, A.A., Mobberley, P.S., Fernandez, R.C., and Mink, C.M., Characterization of human bactericidal antibodies to *Bordetella pertussis*, *Infect. Immun.* 67, 1424–1431, 1999.

CONFOCAL MICROSCOPY

Confocal microscopy is a fluorescent microscopy technique which uses a highly focused beam of light with suppression of fluorescence above and below the point of optimum focus.[1–4] An image is obtained by moving the excitation beam and measurement aperture over the sample with point-by-point measurement. Reflectance confocal microscopy is a method used in dermatology[5] based on use of near-infrared laser (830 nm) light which is reflected back from a point within in the skin providing a resolution of approximately 1 μm equivalent to ×30 magnification; this can be performed *in vivo*.[6]

1. Miyashita, T., Confocal microscopy for intracellular co-localization of proteins, *Methods Mol. Biol.* 261, 399–410, 2004.
2. Heilker, R., Zemanova, L., Valler, M.J., and Nienhaus, G.U., Confocal fluorescence microscopy for high-throughput screening of G-protein coupled receptors, *Curr. Med. Chem.* 12, 2551–2559, 2005.
3. *Handbook of Biological Confocal Microscopy*, ed. J. Pawley, Springer, New York, 2006.
4. *Confocal Raman Microscopy*, ed. T. Dieling, OP. Hollrecher, and J. Toporski, Springer, Berlin, Germany, 2011.
5. Rajadhyaksha, M., Marghoob, A., Rossi, A., Halpern, A.C., and Nehal, K.S., Reflectance confocal microscopy of skin in vivo: From bench to bedside, *Lasers Surg. Med.* 49, 7–19, 2017.
6. Que, S.K., Fraga-Braghiroli, N., Grant-Kels, J.M., et al., Through the looking glass: Basics and principles of reflectance confocal microscopy, *J. Am. Acad. Dermatol.* 73, 276–284, 2015.

CONJUGATE VACCINE

A conjugate vaccine is prepared by the coupling of a weak immunogen, usually a polysaccharide, to a protein to improve/enhance immunogenicity of the polysaccharide.[1–6]

1. Edwards, M.S., Group B streptococcal conjugate vaccine: A timely concept for which the time has come, *Hum. Vaccin.* 4, 444–448, 2008.
2. Ahmad, T.A., Haroun, M., Hussein, A.A., El Ashry, el Sh., and El-Sayed, L.H., Development of a new trend conjugate vaccine for the prevention of Klebsiella pneumoniae, *Infect. Dis. Rep.* 4, e33, 2012.
3. Frasch, C.E., Kapre, S.V., Lee, C.H., and Préaud, J.M., Technical development of a new Meningococcal conjugate vaccine, *Clin. Infect. Dis.* 61(Suppl 5), S404–S409, 2015.
4. Dellepiane, N., Akanmori, B.D., Gairola, S., et al., Regulatory pathways that facilitated timely registration of a new group A Meningococcal conjugate vaccine for Africa's meningitis belt countries, *Clin. Infect. Dis.* 61(Suppl 5), S428–S433, 2015.
5. Kulkarni, P.S., Socquet, M., Jadhav, S.S., et al., Challenges and opportunities while developing a group A Meningococcal conjugate vaccine within a product development partnership: A manufacturer's perspective from the Serum Institute of India, *Clin. Infect. Dis.* 61(Suppl 5), S483–S488, 2015.
6. Bröker, M., Berti, F., Schneider, J., and Vojtek, I., Polysaccharide conjugate vaccine protein carriers as a "neglected valency"—Potential and limitations, *Vaccine* 35, 3286–3294, 2017.

CONNEXINS

Connexins are proteins which form gap junctions critical for intercellular communications.[1,2] There are at least 20 connexins.[3] Connexins assemble to form a hexamer forming a hemichannel referred to as connexon.[4,5] Connexons may be homomeric (composed of one specific connexin) or heteromeric (several different connexins).[6,7] An individual connexin protein (Cx) is classified by species of origin and molecular weight in kilodaltons as in rCX43, which would specify a rat connexin of 43 kDa.[8,9] Mutations in the connexins are referred to as connexinopathies[10] which are responsible for a diversity of diseases[11,12] including deafness,[13,14] skin disorders,[15] and idiopathic atrial fibrillation.[16,17]

1. *Connexins A Guide*, ed. A.L. Harris and D. Locke, Humana/Springer Science, New York, 2009.
2. Ul Hussain, M., *Connexins: The Gap Junction Proteins*, Springer India, New Delhi, India, 2014.
3. Beyer, E.C., and Berthoud, V.M., the family of connexin genes, in *Connexins A Guide*, ed. A.L. Harris and D. Locke, Chapter 1, pp. 3–29, Humana/Springer Science, New York, 2009.
4. Sosinsky, G.E., and Nicholson, B.J., Structural organization of a gap junction channels, *Biochim. Biophys. Acta* 1711, 99–125, 2005.
5. Wang, H., Wu, K., Yu, L., et al., A novel dominant *GJB2* (DFNA3) mutation in a Chinese family, *Sci. Reports* 7, 34425, 2017.
6. Sosinsky, G., Mixing of connexins in gap junction membrane channels, *Proc. Natl. Acad. Sci. USA* 92, 9210–9214, 1995.

7. Jiang, J.X., and Goodenough, D.A., Heteromeric connexons in lens gap junction channels, *Proc. Natl. Acad. Sci. USA* 93, 2387–1291, 1996.

8. John, S.A., and Revel, J.P., Connexon integrity is maintained by non-covalent bonds: Intramolecular disulfide bonds link the extracellular domains in rat connexin-43, *Biochem. Biophys. Res. Commun.* 178, 1312–1318, 1991.

9. Söhl, G., and Willecke, K., An update on connexin genes and their nomenclature in mouse and man, *Cell Commun. Adhes.* 10, 173–180, 2003.

10. García, I.E., Prado, P., Pupo, A., et al., Connexinopathies: A structural and functional glimpse, *BMC Cell Biol.* 17(Suppl 1), 17, 2016.

11. Anand, R.J., and Hackam, D.J., The role of gap junctions in health and disease, *Crit. Care Med.* 33(Suppl 12), S535–S535, 2005.

12. Retamal, M.A., Reyes, E.P., Garcia, I.E., et al., Diseases associated with leaky hemichannels, *Front. Cell. Neurosci.* 9, 267, 2015.

13. Petit, C., From deafness genes to hearing mechanisms: Harmony and counterpoint, *Trends Mol. Med.* 12, 57–64, 2006.

14. Jagger, D.J., and Forge, A., Connexins and gap junctions in the inner ear—It's not just about K^+ recycling, *Cell Tissue Res.* 360, 633–644, 2015.

15. Lilly, E., Sellitto, C., Milstone, L.M., and White, T.W., Connexin channels in congenital skin disorders, *Semin. Cell. Dev. Biol.* 50, 4–12, 2016.

16. Gollob, M.H., Cardiac connexins as candidate genes for idiopathic atrial fibrillation, *Curr. Opin. Cardiol.* 21, 155–158, 2006.

17. Jenning S, M.M., and Donahue, J.K., Connexin remodeling contributes to atrial fibrillation, *J. Atr. Fibrillation* 6, 839, 2013.

CONTIG

The term contig (for contiguous) was originally defined as a set of overlapping DNA sequences and has been expanded to include a set of overlapping DNA clones. The original definition refers to a set of gel bands which can be related to each other by overlapping sequences (reads).[1,2] As noted in the cited URL, there is some confusion on the meaning of contig. Regardless, contigs are used to establish the sequence of a genome and various programs are being developed to organize contigs into genome sequence.[3–6]

1. http://staden.sourceforge.net/contig.html.

2. Staden, R., A new computer method for the storage any manipulation of DNA gel reading data, *Nucleic Acids Res.* 8, 3673–3694, 1980.

3. Tomescu, A.I., and Medvedev, P., Safe and complete contig assembly through omnitigs, *J. Comput. Biol.* 24, 590–602, 2017.

4. Kono, N., Tomita, M., and Arakawa, K., eRP arrangement: A strategy for assembled genomic contig rearrangement based on replication profiling in bacteria, *BMC Genomics* 18, 784, 2017.

5. Jiang, Y., Ninwichian, P., Liu, S., et al., Generation of physical map contig-specific sequences useful for whole genome sequence scaffolding, *PLoS One* 24(10), e78872, 2013.

6. Chen, K.T., Liu, C.L., Huang, S.H., et al., CSAR: A contig scaffolding tool using algebraic rearrangements, *Bioinformatics* 34, 109–111, 2018.

CONTOUR LENGTH

Contour length is the distance end-to-end of a polymer stretched without chain rupture.[1–3] Contour length is an important characteristic of polymers.[4–6] Contour length is a characteristic of peptides,[7] proteins,[8,9] polysaccharides,[10,11] and nucleic acids.[12,13] The **persistence length** of a polymer is a measure of the "stiffness" of a polymer.[14,15] Persistence length and contour length are both used to characterize polymers such as polysaccharides.[16]

1. Case, L.C., Elastomer behavior. I. Rupture elongation, *Makcromolekulare Chemie* 37, 243–250, 1960.

2. Bemis, J.E., Akhremitchev, B.B., and Walker, G.C., Single polymer chain elongation by atomic force microscopy, *Langmuir* 15, 2799–2805, 1999.

3. Aguayo, S., Donos, N., Spratt, D., and Bozec, L., Probing the nanoadhesion of *Streptococcus sanguinis* to titanium implant surfaces by atomic force microscopy, *Int. J. Nanomedicine* 11, 1443–1450, 2016.

4. Young, R.J., *Introduction to Polymers*, Chapman and Hall, London, UK, 1983.

5. Sarraguca, J.M., and Pais, A.A., Polyelectrolytes in solutions with multivalent salt. Effects of flexibility and contour length, *Phys. Chem. Chem. Phys.* 8, 4233–4241, 2006.

6. Wu, D., Lenhardt, J.M., Black, A.L., Akhremitchev, B.B., and Craig, S.L., Molecular stress relief through a force-induced irreversible extension in polymer contour length, *J. Am. Chem. Soc.* 132, 15936–15938, 2010.

7. Marllo, R., Kastantn, M., Drews, L.B., and Tirrell, M., Peptide contour length determines equilibrium secondary structure in protein-analogous micelles, *Biopolymers* 99, 573–581, 2013.

8. Ainavarapu, S.R., Brujic, J., Huang, H.H., et al., Contour length and refolding rate of a small protein controlled by engineered bonds, *Biophys. J.* 92, 225–233. 2007.

9. Fernanez, V.I., Kosuri, P., Parot, V., and Fernandez, J.M., Extend Kalman filter estimates the contour length of a protein in single molecule atomic force microscopy experiments, *Rev. Sci. Instrum.* 80, 113104, 2009.

10. Cao, Z., Tsoufis, T., Svaldo-Lanero, T., et al., The dynamics of complex formation between amylose brushes on gold and fatty acids by QCM-D, *Biomacromolecules* 14, 3713–3722, 2013.

11. Wie, C.Y., Li, W.Q, Shao, S.S., et al., Structure and chain conformation of a neutral intracellular heteropolysaccharide from mycelium of *Paecilomyces cicadae*, *Carbohydr. Polym.* 136, 728–737, 2016.

12. Lang, D., Molecular weights of coliphages and coliphage DNA. 3. Contour length and molecular weight of DNA from bacteriophages T4, T5 and T7, and from bovine papilloma virus, *J. Mol. Biol.* 54, 557–565, 1970.

13. Revitti, C., DNA contour length measurements as tools for the structural analysis of DNA and nucleoprotein complexes, *Methods Mol. Biol.* 749, 235–254, 2011.

14. Manning, G.S., The persistence length of DNA is reached from the persistent length of its null isomer through an internal electrostatic stretching force, *Biophys. J.* 91, 3507–3716, 2006.

15. Hsu, H-P., Paul, W., and Binder, K., Standard definitions of persistence length do not describe the local "stiffness" of real polymer chains, *Macromolecues* 43, 3904–3912, 2010.

16. Abu-Lail, N.I., and Camesano, T.A., Polysaccharide properties probed with atomic force microscopy, *J. Microsc.* 212, 217–238, 2003.

CORE PROMOTER

The core promoter is an ~50 bp region containing specific sequence elements (e.g. TATAA boxTPIIB recognition element, downstream promoter element)[1] that is recognized by general transcription factors (pre-initiation complex, PIC) that dictates the correct transcription by RNA polymerase II (Pol II) in the process of gene expression.[2,3]

1. Roy, A.L., and Singer, D.S., Core promoters in transcription: Old problem, new insights, *Trends Biochem. Sci.* 40, 165–171, 2015.

2. Danino, Y.M., Even, D., Ideses, D., and Juven-Gershon, T., The core promoter: At the heart of gene expression, *Biochim. Biophys. Acta* 1849, 1116–1131, 2015.

3. Zabidi, M.A., and Stark, A., Regulatory enhancer-core-promoter communication via transcription factors and cofactors, *Trends Genet.* 32, 901–814, 2016.

CORIOLIS METER

A Coriolis meter is a device for measuring flow of liquids and gases. Coriolis meters measure mass flow, not fluid flow, past a point. Measurement of mass flow is of importance in supercritical fluid chromatography.[1,2]

1. Tarafder, A., Vajda, P., and Guiochon, G., Accurate on-line mass flow measurements in supercritical fluid chromatography, *J. Chromatog.* 1320, 130–137, 2013.

2. De Pauw, R., Shoykhet, K., Desmet, G., and Broeckhoven, K., Effect of reference conditions on flow rate, modifier fraction and retention in supercritical fluid chromatography, *J. Chromatog.* 1459, 129–135, 2016.

COSOLVENT

A cosolvent is a miscible solvent added to a primary solvent to enhance solvation or stability of a specific solute. Cosolvents include such liquids as ethyl alcohol[1] and chaotropic agents such as guanidine.[2] Cosolvents are extensively used in the measurement of enzymatic activity when a cosolvent is necessary to dissolve a component of the assay system such as the substrate. Cosolvents are important in the study of enzyme activity, where such solvents are required for substrate solubility resulting in a homogeneous system rather than a heterogeneous system[3] as well as influencing protein stability.[4,5] Cosolvents such as alcohols and chaotropic agents are important for the modulation of intercellular functions.[6,7] Cosolvents are suggested to be of great importance inside the cell where both solvents such as alcohol and chemicals such as urea are important in modulating hydrophobic interactions.[8,9] Cosolvents are also used in the formulation of pharmaceuticals[10,11] and in liquid chromatography.[12,13]

1. DiGuiseppi, D., Milorey, B., Lewis, G., et al., Probing the conformation-dependent preferential binding of ethanol to cationic glycylalanylglycine in water/ethanol by vibrational and NMR spectroscopy, *J. Phys. Chem.* 121, 5744–5758, 2017.

2. Cui, D., Ou, S.C., and Patel, S., Protein denaturants at aqueous-hydrophobic interfaces: Self-consistent correlation between induced interfacial fluctuations and denaturant stability at the interface, *J. Phys. Chem. B* 119, 164–178, 2015.

3. Viswanathan, K., Omorekbokhae, R., Li, G., and Gross, R.A., Protease-catalyzed oligomerization of hydrophobic amino acid ethyl esters in homogenous reaction media using 1-phenylalanine as a model system, *Biomacromolecules* 11, 2152–2160, 2010.

4. Luong, T.Q., and Winter, R., Combined pressure and cosolvent effects on enzyme activity- a high-pressure stopped-flow kinetic study on α-chymotrypsin, *Phys. Chem. Chem. Phys.* 17, 23273–23278, 2015.

5. Nazari-Robati, M., Golestani, A., and Asadikaram, G., Improvement of proteolytic and oxidative stability of chondroitinase ABC I by cosolvents, *Int. J. Biol. Maccromol.* 91, 812–817, 2016.

6. Gao, M., Held, C., Patra, S., et al., Crowders and cosolvents-major contributors to the cellular milleu and efficient means to counteract environmental stresses, *Chemphyschem* 18, 2951–2972, 2017.

7. van der Vegt, N.F.A., and Nayar, D., The hydrophobic effects and the role of cosolvents, *J. Phys. Chem. B* 121, 9986–9998, 2017.

8. vean der Vegt, N.F.A., and Nayar, D., The hydrophobic effect and the role of cosolvents, *J. Phys. Chem. B* 121, 9986–9998, 2017.

9. Gao, M., Held, C., Patra, S., et al., Crowders and cosolvents-major contributors to the cellular milieu and efficient means to counteract environments stresses, *Chemphyschem* 18, 2951–2972, 2017.

10. Mallick, S., Pattnaik, S., Swain, K., and De, P.K., Current perspectives of solubilization: Potential for improved bioavailability, *Drug Dev. Ind. Pharm.* 33, 865–873, 2007.

11. Chen, X., Fadda, H.M., Aburub, A., Mishra, D., and Pinal, R., Cosolvency approach for assessing the solubility of drugs in poly (vinylpyrrolidone), *Int. J. Pharm.* 494, 346–356, 2015.

12. Arakawa, T., Ejima, D., Li, T., and Philo, J.S., The critical role of mobile phase composition in size exclusion chromatography of protein pharmaceuticals, *J. Pharm. Sci.* 99, 1674–1692, 2010.

13. Pokrovskiy, O.I., Ustinovich, K.B., Usovich, O.I., et al., A case of Z/E-isomers elution order inversion caused by cosolvent percentage change in supercritical fluid chromatography, *J. Chromatog. A* 1479, 177–184, 2017.

COUPLED ENZYME SYSTEMS

A coupled enzyme system consists of a pathway with two or more enzymes, where the product of one reaction is the substrate for a second reaction. Most metabolic systems are composed of enzymes in a pathway where there is the sequential transformation of a substrate into a product through a series of separate enzyme-catalyzed reactions. One of the simpler coupled systems is the detoxification of ethyl alcohol[1] or more complex as in intermediary metabolism.[2] In the case of ethanol toxification, ethanol is converted to acetaldehyde by alcohol dehydrogenase; acetaldehyde, which is toxic, is converted into acetate. In intermediary metabolism, glucose is converted to acetate.

Coupled enzyme systems are also used extensively in clinical chemistry where they are also referred to an indicator enzyme systems.[3,4] One of the better known coupled enzyme assays in clinical chemistry is that for aspartate aminotransferase (AST; formerly known as serum glutamic-oxaloacetic transaminase, SGOT) where a transamination reaction forming oxaloacetate is coupled with the reduction of oxaloacetate to malate measured by absorbance change in NADH conversion to NAD. A coupled enzyme assay system is used in many solid-phase immunoassays such as ELISA assays.[5] There are other examples of coupled enzyme systems.[6,7] A recent example is said to measure protein in a single cell.[8]

1. Plapp, B.V., Rate-limiting steps in ethanol metabolism and approaches to changing these rates biochemically, *Adv. Expt. Biol. Med.* 56, 77–109, 1975.

2. Brooks, S.P.J., Enzymes in the cell. What's really going on? in *Function and Metabolism*, ed. K.B. Storey, Wiley-Liss, Hoboken, NJ, Chapter 3, pp. 55–86, 2004.

3. Russell, C.D., and Cotlove, E., Serum glutamic-oxaloacetic transaminase: Evaluation of a coupled-reaction enzyme assay by means of kinetic theory, *Clin. Chem.* 17, 1114–1122, 1971.

4. Bais, R., and Pateghini, M., Principles of clinical enzymology, in *Tietz Textbook of Clinical Chemistry and Molecular Diagnostics*, ed. C.A. Burtis, E.R. Ashwood, and D.E. Bruns, Elsevier/Saunders, St. Louis, MO, Chapter 9, pp. 191–218, 2006.

5. Kircks, LJ., Selected strategies for improving sensitivity and reliability of immunoassays, *Clin. Chem.* 40, 347–357, 1994.

6. Wimmer, M.C., Artiss, J.D., and Zak, B., Peroxidase-coupled method for kinetic colorimetry of total creatine kinase activity in serum, *Clin. Chem.* 31, 1616–1620, 1965.

7. Shin, T., Murao, S., and Matsumura, E., A chromogenic oxidative coupling reaction of laccase: Applications for laccase and angiotensin I converting enzyme assay, *Anal. Biochem.* 166, 380–388, 1987.

8. Watabe, S., Morikawa, M., Kaneda, M., et al., Ultrasensitive detection of proteins and sugars at single-cell level, *Commun. Integr. Biol.* 9(1), e1124201, 2016.

CREATINE

A nitrogenous compound which is synthesized from arginine, glycine and *S*-adenosylmethionine.[1–7] Creatine is used as a biomarker for erthyrocytes.[8–11] There is increased use of creatine as a nutritional supplement.[12–15]

1. Van Pilsum J.F., Stephens, G.C., and Taylor, D., Distribution of creatine, guanidinoacetate and the enzymes for their biosynthesis in the animal kingdom, *Biochem. J.* 126, 325–345, 1972.

2. Walker, J.B., and Hannan, J.K., Creatine biosynthesis during embryonic development. False feedback suppression of liver amidinotransferase by *N*-acetimdoylsarcosine and 1-carboxymethyl-2-iminoimdazolidine (cyclocreatine), *Biochemistry* 15, 2519–2522, 1976.

3. Walker, J.B., Creatine: Biosynthesis, regulation, and function, *Enzymes* 50 (ed. A. Meister, Academic Press, New York), 177–242, 1979.

4. Wyss, M., and Wallimann, T., Creatine metabolism and the consequences of creatine depletion in muscle, *Mol. Cell. Biochem.* 133–134, 51–66, 1994.

5. Wu, G., and Morris, S.M., Jr., Arginine metabolism: Nitric oxide and beyond, *Biochem. J.* 336, 1–17, 1998.

6. Brosnan, M.E., and Brosnan, J.T., Renal arginine metabolism, *J. Nutr.* 134 (Suppl 10), 2791S–2795S, 1994.

7. Morris, S.M., Jr., Enzymes of arginine metabolism, *J. Nutr.* Suppl. 10, 2743S–2747S, 1994.

8. Beyer, C., and Alting, I.H., Enzymatic measurement of creatine in erythrocytes, *Clin. Chem.* 42, 313–318, 1996.
9. Jiao, Y., Okumiya, T., Saibara, T., et al., An enzymatic assay for erythrocyte creatine as an index of the erythrocyte life time, *Clin. Biochem.* 31, 59–65, 1998.
10. Takemoto, Y., Okumiya, T., Tsuchida, K., et al., Erythrocyte creatine as an index of the erythrocyte life span and erythropoiesis, *Nephron* 86, 513–514, 2000.
11. Okumiya, T., Ishikawa-Nishi, M., Doi, T., et al., Evaluation of intravascular hemolysis with erythrocyte creatine in patients with cardiac valve prostheses, *Chest* 125, 2115–2120, 2004.
12. Korzun, W.J., Oral creatine supplements lower plasma homocysteine concentrations in humans, *Clin. Lab. Sci.* 17, 102–106, 2004.
13. Pearlman, J.P., and Fielding, R.A., Creatine monohydrate as a therapeutic aid in muscular dystrophy, *Nutr. Rev.* 64, 80–88, 2006.
14. Hespel, P., Maughan, R.J., and Greenhaff, P.L., Dietary supplements for football, *J. Sports Sci.* 24, 749–761, 2006.
15. Shao, A., and Hathcock, J.N., Risk assessment for creatine monohydrate, *Regul. Toxicol. Pharmacol.*, 45, 242–251, 2006.

CRITICAL ASSESSMENT OF STRUCTURE PREDICTION (CASP)

Critical Assessment of Structure Prediction (CASP) describes a process for the evaluation of protein model building.[1-6]

1. Martin, A.C., MacArthur, M.W., and Thorton, J.M., Assessment of comparative modeling in CASP2, *Proteins* 29(Supp 1), 14–28, 1997.
2. Moult, J., Predicting protein three-dimensional structure, *Curr. Opin. Biotechnol.* 10, 583–588, 1999.
3. Moult, J., Fidelis, K., Kryshtafovych, A., et al., *Proteins* 82 (Suppl 2), 1–6, 2014.
4. Kinch, L.N., Li, W., Schaeffer, R.D., et al., CASP11 target classification, *Proteins* 84(Suppl 1), 20–33, 2016.
5. Tamò, G.E., Abriata, L.A., Fonti, G., and Dal Peraro, M., Assessment of data-assisted prediction by inclusion of cross-linking/mass-spectrometry and small angle X-ray scattering data in the 12th Critical Assessment of protein structure prediction experiment, *Proteins*, 86(Suppl 1), 215–227, 2018.
6. Moult, J., Fidelis, K., Kryshtafovych, A., Swede, T., and Tranmontano, A., Critical assessment of methods of protein structure prediction (CASP)-Round XII, *Proteins*, 86(Suppl 1), 7–15, 2018.

CRITICAL PRESSURE

The minimum pressure required to condense gas to liquid at the critical temperature. There are other definitions not related to gases.

CRITICAL TEMPERATURE

The critical point (end of a vapor pressure curve in a phase diagram); above this temperature, a gas cannot be liquefied. As with critical pressure, there are other definitions unrelated to the behavior of gases.

CROWDING

A term used to describe general effect of polymers including proteins and polysaccharides on the behavior of compounds including enzyme in solution. Crowding of particular importance for intracellular function[1-7] and behavior in the interstitial space[8-10] where crowding can increase the local concentration of large molecules.[11]

1. Minton, A.P., Molecular crowding: Analysis of effects of high concentrations of inert cosolutes on biochemical equilibria and rates in terms of volume exclusion, *Methods Enzymol.* 295, 127–149, 1998.
2. Johansson, H.O., Brooks, D.E., and Haynes, C.A., Macromolecular crowding and its consequences, *Int. Rev. Cytol.* 192, 155–170, 2000.
3. Ellis, R.J., Macromolecular crowding: Obvious but underappreciated, *Trends Biochem. Sci.* 26, 597–604, 2001.
4. Grailhe, R., Merola, F., Ridard, J., et al., Monitoring protein interactions in the living cell through the fluorescence decays of the cyan fluorescent protein, *Chemphyschem.* 7, 1442–1454, 2006.
5. Tyrell, J., Weeks, K.M., and Pielak, G.J., Challenge of mimicking the influences of the cellular environment of RNA structure by PEG-induced macromolecular crowding, *Biochemistry* 54, 6447–6453, 2015.
6. Nishizawa, K., Fujiwara, K., Ikenaga, M., et al., Universal glass-forming behavior on *in vitro* and living cytoplasm, *Sci. Rep.* 7(1), 15143, 2017.
7. Tovato, F., and Fumigalli, G., Molecular simulations of cellular processes, *Biophys. Rev.* 9, 941–958, 2017.
8. Del Monte, U., and Caiani, E.G., From Kepler's conjecture and FCC lattice to modelling of crowding in living matter, *Ital. J. Anat. Embryol.* 118, 92–104, 2013.
9. Reitinger, S., and Lepperdinger, G., Hyaluronan, a ready choice to fuel regeneration: A mini-review, *Gerontology* 59, 71–76, 2013.
10. Dewavrin, J.V., Hamzavi, N., Shim, V.P., and Raghunath, M., Tuning the architecture of three-dimensional collagen hydrogels by physiological macromolecular crowding, *Acta Biomater.* 10, 4351–4359, 2014.
11. Cowman, M.K., Hyaluronan and hyaluronan fragments, *Adv. Carbohydr. Chem. Biochem* 74, 1–59, 2017.

CROWN GALL DISEASE/CROWN GALL TUMORS

Crown gall is caused by bacteria (*Agrobacterium tumefaciens*). These galls begin with tumor-like cell growth at or just below the soil's surface, near the base of the plant and commonly on bud unions. Galls usually begin as green, pliable tissue; then develop into dark, crusty growths. Crown gall disease has been used to study transformation with relevance to tumor formation.[1-6]

1. Zhu, J., Oger, P.M., Schrammeijer, B., et al., The bases of crown gall tumorigenesis, *J. Bacteriol.* 182, 3885–3895, 2000.
2. Escobar, M.A., and Dadekar, A.M., *Agrobacterium tumefaciens* as an agent of disease, *Trends Plant. Sci.* 8, 380–386, 2003.
3. Brencic, A., and Winans, S.C., Detection of and response to signals involved in host-microbe interactions by plant-associated bacteria, *Micobiol. Mol. Biol. Rev.* 69, 155–194, 2005.
4. Reader, J.S., Ordoukhanisn, P.T., Kim, J.G., et al., Major biocontrol of plant tumors targets tRNA synthetase, *Science* 309, 1533, 2005.
5. Yang, Q., Li, X., Tu, H., et al., Agrobacterium-delivered virulence protein VirE2 is trafficked inside host cells via a myosin XI-K-powered ER/actin network, *Proc. Natl. Acad. Sci. USA* 114, 2982–2987, 2017.
6. David, S., Mandabi, A., Uzi, S., Aharoni, A., and Meijler, M.M., Mining plants for bacterial quorum sensing modulators, *ACS Chem. Biol.* 13, 247–252, 2018.

Cryo ELECTRON MICROSCOPY (Cryo EM)

Cryo EM is a method for determining the structure of wide range of biological materials ranging from proteins of Mr = 38 kDa to intact cells.[1] Cryo-EM has the potential of providing structural information similar to that obtained with classical X-Ray crystallography and NMR. Cryo EM is not to be confused with cryosections which is a sample preparation technique using tissue sections cut from a frozen tissue sample. Cryo-EM used transmission electron microscopy to determine the structure of biological material in amorphous ice (also known as a glassy ice). Amorphous ice does not contain crystals so there is minimal damage to the objects being studied. The sample is quick-frozen in a cryogen such as ethane or ethane/propane cooled with liquid nitrogen to provide the amorphous ice matrix. In single particle analysis[2] the 2D data from a large number of molecules (there is an assumption of random conformations) is averaged requiring considerable skill in sample preparation.[3,4] As of this writing (December 2017), the majority of work is on protein complexes and cellular/subcellular organelles/membranes.[5] Cryo-electron tomography, which can obtain a 3D image, is being used to study cells and subcellular structures.[6,7]

1. Murata, K., and Wolf, M., Cryo-electron microscopy for structural analysis of dynamic biological macromolecules, *Biochim. Biophys. Acta* 1862, 324–334, 2018.
2. Cheng, Y., Grigorieff, N., Penczek, P.A., and Walz, T., A primer to single-particle cryo-electron microscopy, *Cell* 161, 438–339, 2015.
3. Thompson, R.F., Walker, M., Siebert, C.A., Muench, S.P., and Ranson, N.A., An introduction to sample preparation and imaging by cryo-electron microscopy for structural biology, *Methods* 100, 3–15, 2016.
4. Passmore, L.A., and Russo, C.J., Specimen preparation for high-resolution cryo-EM, *Methods Enzymol.* 579, 51–86, 2016.
5. Chanda, P., and Locker, J.K., The sleeping beauty kissed awake: New methods in electron microscopy to study cellular membranes, *Biochem. J.* 474, 1042–1053, 2017.
6. Irobalieva, R.N., Martins, B., and Medalia, O., Cellular structural biology as revealed by cryo-electron tomography, *J. Cell Sci.* 129, 469–476, 2016.
7. Wagner, J., Schaffer, M., Fernández-Busnadiego, R., Cryo-electron tomography-the cell biology that came in from the cold, *FEBS Lett.* 591, 2520–2533, 2017.

CRYOSECTION

A cryosection, also known as a frozen section, is a histological technique where a tissue sample, instead of be subjected to chemical fixation, is frozen quickly. Tissue for histological examination is usually subjected to fixation by chemical means such as formaldehyde[1-3] and embedding in paraffin before sections (the term section describes a thin slice of tissue cut on a microtome which is usually stained prior to microscopic examination) are prepared. This is a time-consuming process are there are surgical procedures which require "real-time" analysis of tissue samples as, for example in establishing margins.[4,5] Frozen sections (obtained from tissues frozen in liquid nitrogen) can be immediately subjected to histological analysis. Frozen sections can also be used directly for mass spectrometric analysis.[6] Frozen sections may also be prepared from "fixed" tissues.[7,8] It is possible that the use of frozen sections might avoid artifacts in the analysis of DNA.[9]

1. Grizzle, W.E., Special symposium: Fixation and tissue processing models, *Biotech. Histochem.* 26, 797–193, 2009.
2. Klopfleisch, R., Weiss, A.T., and Gruber, A.D., Excavation of a buried treasure—DNA, mRNA, miRNA and protein analysis in formalin fixed, paraffin embedded tissues, *Histol. Histopathol.* 26, 797–810, 2011.
3. Becker, K.F., Using tissue samples for proteomic studies—critical considerations, *Proteomics Clin. Appl.* 9, 257–267, 2015.
4. Esbona, K., Li, Z., and Wilke, L.G., Intraoperative imprint cytology and frozen section pathology for margin assessment in breast conservation surgery: A systematic review, *Ann. Surg. Oncol.* 19, 3236–3245, 2012.
5. Makris, E.A., and Poultsides, G.A., Surgical considerations in the management of gastric adenocarcinoma, *Surg. Clin. North Am.* 97, 95–316, 2017.

6. Chaurand, P., Cornett, D.S., and Caprioli, R.M., Molecular imaging of thin mammalian tissue sections by mass spectrometry, *Curr. Opin. Biotechnol.* 17, 431–436, 2006.
7. Bernhard, W., and Leduc, E.H., Ultrathin frozen sections. I. Methods and ultrastructural preservation, *J. Cell Biol.* 34, 757–771, 1967.
8. Liou, W., Geuze, H.J., and Slot, J.W., Improving structural integrity of cryosections for immunogold labeling, *Histochem. Cell Biol.* 100, 41–50, 1996.
9. Do, H., and Dobrovic, A., Sequence artifacts in DNA from formalin-fixed tissues: Causes and strategies for minimization, *Clin. Chem.* 61, 64–71, 2015.

C-TERMINOMICS

C-terminomics is proteome-wide study of C-terminal amino acid sequences.[1–5]

1. Schilling, O., Barré, O., Huesgen, P.F., and Overall, C.M., Proteome-wide analysis of protein carboxy termini: C-terminomics, *Nat. Methods* 7, 506–511, 2010.
2. Tanco, S., Tort, O., Demol, H., et al., C-terminomics screen for natural substrates of cytosolic carboxypeptide-1 reveals processing of acidic protein C termini, *Mol. Cell. Proteomics* 14, 177–190, 2015.
3. Tanco, S., Gevaert, K., and Van Damme, P., C-terminomics: Targeted analysis of natural and posttranslational modified protein and peptide C-terimini, *Proteomics* 15, 903–914, 2015.
4. Somasdumdaram, P., Koudelka, T., Linke, D., and Tholey, A., Terminal charge reversal derivatization and parallel use of multiple proteases facilitates identification of protein C termini by C-terminomics, *J. Proteome Res.* 15, 1369–1378, 2016.
5. Zhang, Y., Li, Q., Huang, J., et al., An approach to incorporate multi-enzyme digestion into C-TAILs for C-terminomics study, *Proteomics* 18(1), 1700034, 2018.

CYANINE DYES (CYDYES)

Cyanine dyes are a family of fluorescent polymethine dyes contain containing a −CH= group linking two nitrogen-containing heterocyclic rings, developed as sensitizer for photographic emulsions. Used in biochemistry and molecular biology for characterization of nucleic acids,[1,2] in DNA microarray analysis,[3,4] and for detecting proteins on electrophoretograms.[5–7] There is also use of these dyes for the measurement of membrane potential.[8–11] Cyanine derivatives are used to measure the formation of reactive oxygen species in cells.[12–14] A cyanine dye has been developed for the staining of RNA in cells.[15]

1. Bruijns, B.B., Tiggelaar, R.M., and Gardeniers, J.G., Fluorsecent cyanine dyes for the quantification of low amounts of dsDNA, *Anal. Biochem.* 511, 74–79, 2016.

2. Miranda, P., Oliveira, L.M., and Weber, G., Mesoscopic modelling of Cy3 and Cy5 dyes attached to DNA duplexes, *Biophys. Chem.* 230, 62–67, 2017.
3. Kim, Y., Rao, A.N., Rodesch, C.K., and Grainger, D.W., Real-time fluorescent image analysis of DNA spot hybridization kinetics to assess microarray spot heterogeneity, *Anal. Chem.* 84, 9379–9387, 2012.
4. Kim, Y., Seo, H.H., Jeong, M.S., et al., Method to minimize ozone effect on Cy5 fluorescent intensity in DNA microarrays, *Anal. Biochem.* 538, 1–4, 2017.
5. Bjerneld, E.J., Johansson, J.D., Laurin, Y., et al., Pre-labeling of diverse protein samples with a fixed amount of Cy5 for sodium dodecyl sulfate-polyacrylamide gel electrophoresis analysis, *Anal. Biochem.* 484, 51–57, 2015.
6. Hagner-McWhirter, Å., Laurin, Y., Larsson, A., Bjerneld, E.I., and Rönn, O., Cy5 total protein normalization in Western blot analysis, *Anal. Biochem.* 486, 54–61, 2015.
7. Wycisk, V., Achazi, K., Hirsch, O., et al., Heterobifunctional dyes: Highly fluorescent linkers based on cyanine dyes, *ChemistryOpen* 6, 437–446, 2017.
8. Johnstone, R.M., Laris, P.C., and Eddy, A.A., The use of fluorescent dyes to measure membrane potentials: A critique, *J. Cell Physiol.* 112, 298–300, 1982.
9. Andersen, A.Z., Poulsen, A.K., Brasen J.C., and Olsen, L.F. On-line measurements of oscillating mitochondrial membrane potential in glucose-fermenting *Saccharomyces cerevisiae*, *Yeast* 24, 731–739, 2007.
10. Onoe, S., Temma, T., Shimizu, Y., Ono, M., and Saji, H., Investigation of cyanine dyes for in vivo optical imaging of altered mitochondrial membrane potential in tumors, *Cancer Med.* 3, 775–786, 2014.
11. Zhang, H.K., Yan, P., Kang, J., et al., Listening to membrane potential: Photoacoustic voltage-sensitive dye recording, *J. Biomed. Opt.* 22, 45006, 2017.
12. Oushiki, D., Kojima, H., Terai, T., et al., Development and application of a near-infrared fluorescence probe for oxidative stress based on differential reactivity of linked cyanine dyes, *J. Am. Chem. Soc.* 132, 2795–2801, 2010.
13. Liu, F., Wu, T., Cao, J., et al., A novel fluorescent sensor for detection of highly reactive oxygen species, and for imaging such endogenous hROS in the mitochondria of living cells, *Analyst* 138, 775–778, 2013.
14. Zhdanov, A.V., Aveillo, G., Knaus, U.G., and Papkovsky, D.B., Cellular ROS imaging with hydro-Cy3 dye is strongly influenced by mitochondrial membrane potential, *Biochim. Biophys. Acta* 1861, 198–204, 2017.
15. Kovalska, V., Kuperman, M., Varzatskii, O., Kryvorotenko, D., et al., [1,10]Phenanthroline based cyanine dyes as fluorescent probes for ribonucleic acids in live cells, *Methods Appl. Fluoresc.* 5, 045002, 2017.

CYCLITOLS

Cyclitols are cycloalkanes containing hydroxyl groups on three or more of the ring carbons.[1] Cyclitols can be considered analogues of sugars where the endocyclic oxygen has been replaced with a carbon atom. Inositol (*myo*-inositol, cyclohexane, 1,2,3,4,5,6 hexol) is one of the better known cyclitols is found natural occurring in membranes as a derivative such as a glycosyl-phosphatidyl-inositol (GPI) anchors[2] and phosphatidyl inositides.[3] Inositol-1,4,5-triphosphate is an important biological regulator.[4] In addition to the phosphorylated inositol derivatives, the individual inositols have biological activity in carbohydrate metabolism.[5,6] **Carbasugars**, originally referred to as pseudo-sugars,[7] can be considered a subclass of cyclitols.[8,9] **Conduritols** are occasionally grouped with cyclitols but are cycloalkenes, not cycloalkanes.[10]

1. IUPAC Commission on the Nomenclature of Organic Chemistry (CNOC) and IUPAC-IUB Commission on Biochemical Nomenclature (CBN). Nomenclature of cyclitols. Recommendations, 1973, *Biochem. J.* 153, 23–31, 1976.
2. López-Cobo, S., Campos-Silva, C., and Valés-Gómez, M., Glyosyl-phosphatidyl-inositol (GPI)-anchors and metalloproteinases: Their roles in the regulation of exosome composition and NCG2D-mediated immune recognition, *Front. Cell. Dev. Biol.* 4, 97, 2016.
3. De Craene, J.O., Bertazzi, D.L., Bär, S., et al., Phosphoinositides, major actors in membrane trafficking and lipid signaling pathways, *Int. J. Mol. Sci.* 18, E634, 2017.
4. Parys, J.B., and Smedt, H., Inositol 1,4,5-triphosphate and its receptors *Adv. Exp. Med. Biol.* 740, 255–279, 2012.
5. Gao, Y., Zhang, M., Wu, T., et al., Effects of D-pinitol on insulin resistance through the P13K/Akt signaling pathway in type 2 diabetes mellitus rats, *J. Agr. Food Chem.* 63, 6019–6025, 2015.
6. Maurizi, A.R., Menduni, M., Del Toro, R., et al., A pilot study of D-*chiro*-inositol plus folic acid in overweight patients with type 1 diabetes, *Acta Diabetol.* 54, 361–365, 2017.
7. McCasland, G.E., and Furuta. Alicyclic carbohydrates. XXIX. The synthesis of a pseudo-hexose (2,3,4,5- tetrahydrocyclohexamethanol), *J. Org. Chem.* 31, 1516–1521, 1966.
8. Compain, P., and Martin, O.R., Carbohydrate mimetics-based glycosyltransferase inhibitors, *Bioorg. Med. Chem.* 9, 3077–3092, 2001.
9. Mondal, S., and Sureshan, K.M., Carbasugar synthesis via vinylogous ketal: Total synthesis of (+)-MY7607, (−)-MK7607, (−)-gabosine A, (−)-epoxydine B, (−)-epoxydine C, epi-(+)-gabosine E and epi-(+)-MK7607, *J. Org. Chem.* 81, 11635–11645, 2016.
10. Duchek, J., Adams, D.B., and Hudlicky, T., Chemoenzymatic synthesis of inositols, conduritols and cyclitol analogues, *Chem. Rev.* 111, 4223–4258, 2011.

CYTOCHROME P450 ENZYMES (CPY)

The cytochrome P450 superfamily consists of 57 enzymes involved in variety and expanding number of metabolic functions.[1,2] The P450 enzymes are best known for monooxygenase activity and are involved in the metabolism/catabolism of drugs.[3–7]

1. Nebert, D.W., and Russell, D.W., Clinical importance of the cytochrome P450, *Lancet* 360, 1155–1162, 2002.
2. Shalan, H., Kato, M., and Cheruzel, L., Keeping the spotlight on cytochrome P450, *Biochim. Biophys. Acta* 1866, 80–87, 2018.
3. Johnson, E.F., and Stout, C.D., Structural diversity of human xenobiotic-metabolizing cytochrome P450, *Biochem. Biophys. Res. Commun.* 338, 331–336, 2005.
4. Krishna, D.R., and Shekar, M.S., Cytochrome P450 3A: Genetic polymorphisms and inter-ethnic differences, *Methods Find. Exp. Clin. Pharmacol.* 27, 559–567, 2005.
5. Qi, G., Li, D., and Zhang, X., Genetic variation of cytochrome P450 in Uyghur Chinese population, *Drug Metab. Pharmacokinet* 33, 55–60, 2018.
6. Adiraju, S.K.S., Shekar, K., Fraser, J.F., Smith, M.T., and Ghassabian, S., Effect of cardiopulmonary bypass on cytochrome P450 enzyme activity: Implications for pharmacotherapy, *Drug Metab Rev.* 50, 109–124, 2018.
7. Gouws, C., and Hamman, J.H., Recent developments in our understanding of the implications of traditional African medicine on drug metabolism, *Expert Opin. Drug Metab. Toxicol.* 14, 161–168, 2018.

CYTOKERATIN

Cytokeratin describes intermediate filament keratins found in epithelial tissue.[1,2] There are two types of cytokeratins the acidic type I cytokeratins and the basic or neutral type II cytokeratins.[3,4] There are 20 known cytokeratins expressed at pairs, one type I and one type II, in tissues.[5] Cytokeratins are thought to play role in the activation of plasma prekallikrein[6,7] and plasminogen.[8–10]

1. Fraser, R.D., and Macrae, T.P., Molecular structure and mechanical properties of keratins, *Symp. Soc. Exp. Biol.* 34, 211–246, 1980.
2. Lazarides, E., Intermediate filaments: A chemically heterogeneous, developmentally regulated class of proteins, *Annu. Rev. Biochem.* 51, 219–250, 1982.
3. Moll, R., Franke, W.W., Schiller, D.L., et al., The catalog of human cytokeratins: Patterns for expression in normal epithelia, tumors and cultured cells, *Cell* 31, 11–24, 1982.
4. Nagle, R.B., Intermediate filaments: A review of the basic biology, *Am. J. Surg. Pathol.* 12(Suppl 1), 4–16, 1988.
5. Jacques, C., de Aquino, A.M., and Ramos e Silva, M., Cytokeratins and dermatology, *Skinmed* 4, 354–360, 2005.
6. Shariat-Madar, Z., Mahdi, F., and Schmaier, A.H., Assembly and activation of the plasma kallikrein/kinin system: A new interpretation, *Int. Immunopharmacol.* 2, 1841–1849, 2002.
7. Kaplan, A.P., and Joseph, K., Pathogenic mechanisms of bradykinin mediated diseases: Dysregulation of an innate inflammatory pathway, *Adv. Immnol.* 121, 41–89, 2014.

8. Gonias, S.L., Hembrough, T.A., and Sankovic, M., Cytokeratin 8 functions as a major plasminogen receptor in select epithelial and carcinoma cells, *Front. Biosci.* 6, D1403–D1411, 2001.

9. Ceruit, P., Principe, M., Capello, M., Cappello, P., and Novelli, F., Three are better than one: Plasminogen receptors as cancer theragnostic targets, *Exp. Hematol. Oncol.* 2, 12, 2013.

10. Kumari, S., and Malla, R., New insight on the role of plasminogen receptor in cancer progression, *Cancer Growth Metastasis* 8, 35–42, 2015.

CYTOKINES

Cytokines are proteins secreted by immune system cells such as neutrophils and have both autocrine and paracrine function. This is a large category and includes the various interleukins (Type 1 cytokines) and interferons (Type II cytokines).[1]

1. Leonard, W.J., Type I cytokines and interferons and their receptors, in *Fundamental Immunology*, 6th edn., ed. W.E. Paul, Wolters Kluwer/Lippincott, Williams and Wilkins, Philadelphia, PA, 2011.

CYTOKINESIS

Cytokinesis refers to the division of the cytoplasm of a cell as differentiated from karyokinesis, the process of the division of the nucleus.[1–3] Cytokinesis and karyokinesis are functions within mitosis.[4–7]

1. Robinson, D.N., and Spudich, J.A., Mechanics and regulation of cytokinesis, *Curr. Opin. Cell Biol.* 16, 181–188, 2004.

2. Mayer, U., and Jurgens, G., Cytokinesis: Lines of division taking shape, *Curr. Opin. Plant Biol.* 7, 599–604, 2004.

3. Albertson, R., Riggs, B., and Sullivan, W., Membrane traffic: A driving force in cytokinesis, *Trends Cell Biol.* 15, 92–101, 2005.

4. Juanes, M.A., and Piatti, S., The final cut: Cell polarity meets cytokinesis at the bud neck in *S. cerevisiae*, *Cell. Mol. Life Sci.* 73, 3115–3136, 2016.

5. McIntosh, J.F., Mitosis, *Cold Spring Harb. Perspect. Biol.* 8(9), a023218, 2016.

6. Fry, A.M., Bayliss, R., and Roig, J., Mitotic regulation by NEK kinase networks, *Front. Cell Dev. Biol.* 5, 102, 2017.

7. Mukhopadhyay, D., and Dasso, M., The SUMO pathway in mitosis, *Adv. Exp. Med. Biol.* 963, 171–184, 2017.

CYTOMICS

As will other "omics," cytomics is the study of the cytome, where the cytome was described as the 3D structure, function, and location of all cellular proteins, changes in subcellular localization, the phenotype of a single cell.[1,2] As cytomics is the study of single cells, it is the study of the heterogeneity of cytomes.[3] Current work in cytomics appears to be based on the combination of specific labeling of intracellular components and analysis by flow cytometry.[4–6]

1. Davies, E., Stankovic, B., Azama, K., et al., Novel components of the plant cytoskeleton: A beginning to plant "cytomices," *Plant Sci.* 160, 185–196, 2001.

2. Kriete, K., Cytomics in the realm of systems biology, *Cytometry Part A* 66A, 19–20, 2005; Bernas, T., Gregori, G., Asem, E.K., and Robinson, J.P., Integrating cytomics and proteomics, *Mol. Cell. Proteomics* 5, 2–13, 2006.

3. Herrera, G., Diaz, L., Martinez-Romero, A., et al., Cytomics: A multiparametric, dynamic approach to cell research, *Toxicol. In Vitro*, 21, 176–182, 2006.

4. Jehmlich, N., Hübschmann, T., Gesell Salazar, M., et al., Advanced tool for characterization of microbial cultures by combining cytomics and proteomics, *Appl. Microbiol. Biotechnol.* 88, 575–584, 2010.

5. Jaye, D.L., Bray, R.A., Gebel, H.M., Harris, W.A., and Waller, E.K., Translational applications of flow cytometry in clinical practice, *J. Immunol.* 188, 4715–4719. 2012.

6. Volovitz, I., Melzer, S., Amar, S., et al., Dendritic cells in the context of human tumors: Biology and experimental tools, *Int. Rev. Immunol.* 35, 116–135, 2016.

CYTOSKELETON

The cytoskeleton is the scaffold of fibers inside cell responsible for shape and movement. From a practical point of view, the cytoskeleton is the collection of components insoluble when a cell is delipidated with detergent in buffers of similar ionic composition to the intracellular fluid.[1] In eukaryotes, the cytoskeleton consists of a collection of actin filaments, intermediate filaments, and microtubles, which is acted on by motor proteins including myosin, kinesin, and dynein.[2] Prokaryotes do not have a formal cytoskeleton but do contain polymers similar to actin and tubulin but no motors. Bacteria also do not have a cytoskeleton but do contain proteins similar to intermediate filaments. The members of the spectrin superfamily such as actin, spectrin, and dystrophin are dominant factors in the structure and function of the cytoskeleton.[3–5]

1. Hartwig, J.H., An ultrastructural approach to understanding the cytoskeleton, in *The Cytoskeleton A Practical Approach*, ed. K.L. Carraway and C.A.C. Carraway, IRL Press at Oxford University Press, Oxford, UK, 1992.

2. Pollard, T.D., and Goldman, R.D., Overview of the cytoskeleton from an evolutionary perspective, in *The Cytoskeleton*, ed. T.D. Pollard and R.D. Goldman, Chapter 1, pp. 1–7, Cold Spring Harbor Press, Cold Spring Harbor, NY, 2017.
3. Speicher, D.W., and Ursitti, J.A., Spectrin motif: Conformation of a mammoth protein, *Curr. Biol.* 4, 154–157, 1994.
4. Liem, R.K., Cytoskeletal integrators: The spectrin superfamily, *Cold Spring Harb. Perspect. Biol.* 8(10); pii, a018259, 2016.
5. Delalande, O., Czogalla, A., Hubert, J.E., Sikorski, A., and Le Rumeur, E., Dystrophin and spectrin, two highly dissimilar sisters of the same family, *Subcell. Biochem.* 82, 373–403, 2017.

CYTOTOXIC T-CELLS; CYTOTOXIC T-LYMPHOCYTES

Cytotoxic T-cells/cytotoxic T-lymphocytes are also known as cytolytic T cells. The majority of cytolytic T-cells are CD8[+] cells that recognize and bind to peptides bound to antigenic/foreign peptides bound to MHC I complexes on antigen presenting cells induced apoptosis.[1] CD4[+] T cells are described as helped T cells but have been demonstrated to have a cytotoxic effect with MHC II specificity.[2] It is likely that cytolytic T-cells are identical with cytotoxic T-cells.[3] The T cell receptor (TCR) on T cells has been engineered to improve the cytotoxic effect toward tumor cells.[4–7] Cytotoxic CD8[+] cells are not identical to killer T cells. Killer T cells are more similar to T cells than B cells but do not expressed the T cell receptor which recognizes MHC I presented peptides.[8]

1. Noonen, J., and Murphy, B.M., Cytotoxic T lymphocytes and their granzymes: An overview, in *Resistance of Cancer Cells to CTL-Mediated Immunotherapy,* ed. B. Bonavida and S. Chouaib, Chapter 5, pp. 91–112, Springer International, Cham, Switzerland, 2015.
2. Mucida, D., Husain, M.M., Muroi, S., et al., Transcriptional reprogramming of mature CD4[+] helped T cells generates distinct MHC II-restricted cytotoxic T lymphocytes, *Nat. Immunol.*14, 281–289, 2013.
3. Rosen, F.S., Steiner, L.A., and Unanue, E.R., *Dictionary of Immunology*, Strockton Press, New York, 1989.
4. Levine, B.L., Performance-enhancing drugs: Design and production of redirected chimeric antigen receptor (CAR) T cells, *Cancer Gene Ther.* 22, 79–84, 2015.
5. Ager, A., Watson, H.A., Wehenkel, S.C., and Mohammed, R.N., Homing to solid cancers: A vascular checkpoint in adoptive cell therapy using CAR T-cells, *Biochem. Soc. Trans.* 44, 377–385, 2016.
6. Marcinkiewicz, K., The best spot to park a CAR, *Nat. Biotechnol.* 35, 341, 2017.
7. Pettit, D., Arshad, Z., Smith, J., et al., CAR-T cells: A systematic review and mixed method analysis of the clinical trial landscape, *Mol. Ther.* 26, 342–353, 2018.
8. Yokoyama, W.M., Natural Killer Cells, in *Fundamental Immunology*, ed. W.E. Paul, Chapter 16, pp. 483–517, Wolters Kluwer/Lippincott, Williams & Wilkins, Philadelphia, PA, 2008.

DARK MATTER

Dark matter in physics can be defined as that material in the universe that is thought to exist to account for the estimated mass or dynamic behavior of the universe. An early definition in physics referred to nonluminous material. The early definition of dark matter in cell biology, in analogy with physics, referred to the amount of genomic sequence could not be accounted for as coding DNA (or mRNA or tRNA). As early estimate of amount of DNA which might code for the expression of protein estimated to be 1%–2%[1] while other studies have suggested higher values.[2,3] Thus, the early work would suggest that there could be 90% "unknown" protein or RNA with the assumption that all genomic DNA was functional. Other early work defined short proteins without homology matches (dissimilar to any known protein) as dark matter.[4] Microbial dark matter is a term used to designate genetic information from uncultured bacterial phyla (candidate phyla).[5,6] It is estimated that there are 1,500 bacterial phyla of which less than 100 have been cultivated.[7] The concept of dark matter can be considerably expanding beyond genomic expression to include ionic species (e.g. metal ions) and weakly interacting systems forming transient complexes.[8] Another approach to dark matter is based on the number of possible protein folds relative to the number of such folds described.[9] It is noted that estimates of dark matter may reflect mRNA and protein with very fast catabolism.[10] The production of noncoding RNA has been shown to another genomic function separate from the production of coding RNA. The amount of noncoding RNA is equal to or larger than the amount of coding RNA (mRNA, polyA RNA). The production of noncoding RNA has been shown to another genomic function separate from the production of coding RNA. The amount of noncoding RNA is equal to or larger than the amount of coding RNA (mRNA, polyA RNA).[11] More recent work suggests that 75% of the genome is transcribed into RNA.[12] The investigation of various RNA species including long, noncoding RNA (lncRNA) as dark matter is of interest in oncology research.[13–16] See **dark proteome**.

1. Ponting, C.P., The functional repertoires of metazoan genomes, *Nat. Rev. Genet.* 9, 689–698, 2009.
2. Levitt, M., Nature of the protein universe, *Proc. Natl. Acad. Sci. USA* 106, 11079–11084, 2009.

3. Scaiewicz, A., and Levitt, M., The language of the protein universe, *Curr. Opin. Genet.* 35, 50–56, 2015.

4. Frith, M.C., Forrest, A.R., Nourbakhsh, E., et al., The abundance of short proteins in the mammalian proteome, *PLoS Genet.* 2, e52, 2006.

5. Rinke, C., Schwientek, P., Sczyrba, A., et al., Insights into the phylogeny and coding potential of microbial dark matter, *Nature* 499, 431–437, 2013.

6. Solden, L., Lloyd, K., and Wrighton, K., The bright side of microbial dark matter: Lessons learned from the uncultivated majority, *Curr. Opin. Microbiol.* 31, 217–226, 2016.

7. Yarza, P., Yilmaz, P., Pruesse, E., et al., Uniting the classification of cultured and uncultured bacteria and archaea using 16S rRNA gene sequences, *Nat. Rev. Microbiol.* 12, 635–645, 2014.

8. Ross, J.L., The dark matter of biology, *Biophys. J.* 111, 909–916, 2016.

9. Taylor, W.R., Chelliah, V., Hollup, S.M., et al., Probing the "dark matter" of protein fold space, *Structure* 17, 1244–1252, 2009.

10. Baboo, S., and Cook, P.R., "Dark matter" worlds of unstable RNA and protein, *Nucleus* 5, 281–286, 2014.

11. Kapronov, P., St. Laurent, G., Raz, T., et al., The majority of total nuclear-encoded non-ribosomal RNA in a human cell is "dark matter" un-annotated RNA, *BMC Biol.* 8, 149, 2010.

12. Djebali, S., Davis, C.A., Merkel, A., et al., Landscape of transcription in human cells, *Nature* 489, 101–108, 2012.

13. Evans, J.R., Feng, J.Y., and Chinnaiyan, A.M., The bright side of dark matter: lncRNAs in cancer, *J. Clin. Invest.* 126, 2775–2782, 2015.

14. Ling, H., Vincent, K., Pichler, M., et al., Junk DNA and the long noncoding RNA twist in cancer genetics, *Oncogene* 34, 5003–5011, 2015.

15. Diederichs, S., Bartsch, L., Berkmann, J.C., et al., The dark matter of the cancer genome: Aberrations in regulatory elements, untranslated regions, splice sites, noncoding RNA and synonymous mutations, *EMBO Mol. Med.* 6, 442–457, 2016.

16. Ling, H., Girnita, L., Buda, O., and Calin, G.A., Noncoding RNAs: The cancer genome dark matters? *Clin. Chem. Lab. Med.* 55, 705–714, 2017.

DARK PROTEOME

The term dark proteome has several definitions in the literature. One approach defines the dark proteome as the "un-annotated" protein sequences[1] within a cell or organism. The dark proteome (proteins for which sequence has not been determined) can represent 44%–54% of the total proteome in eukaryotes and 14% in the total proteome in archaea and bacteria.[2] Another approach defined the dark proteome as intrinsically discorded proteins.[3–5] See **dark matter**.

1. Bitard-Feildel, T., and Callebaut, I., Exploring the dark foldable proteome by considering hydrophobic amino acid topology, *Sci. Rep.* 7, 41425, 2017.

2. Perdigão, N., Heinrich, J., Stolte, C., et al., Unexpected features of the dark proteome, *Proc. Natl. Acad. Sci. USA* 112, 15898–15893, 2015.

3. Bhowmick, A., Brookes, D.H., Yost, S.R., et al., Finding our way in the dark proteome, *J. Am. Chem. Soc.* 138, 9730–9742, 2016.

4. Olson, M.A., On the helix propensity in generalized born solvent descriptions of modeling the dark proteome, *Front. Mol. Biosci.* 4, 3, 2017.

5. Stuchfield, D., France, A.P., Migas, L.G., et al., The use of mass spectrometry to examine IDPs: Unique insights and caveats, *Methods Enzymol.* 611, 459–502, 2018.

DATABASE OF INTERACTING PROTEINS (DIP)

The database of interacting proteins integrates the experimental evidence available on protein interactions into a single on-line resource.[1–6] There is a consistent pattern of use of this database with these recent applications.[7–12]

1. http://dip.doe-mbi.ucla.edu.

2. Xenarious, I., Fernandez, E., Salwinski, L., Duan, X.J., et al., DIP: The database of interacting proteins: 2001 update, *Nucleic Acids Res.* 29, 239–241, 2001.

3. Deane, C.M., Salwinski, L., Xenarios, I., and Eisenberg, D., Protein interactions: Two methods for assessment of the reliability of high throughput observations, *Mol. Cell Proteomics* 1, 349–356, 2002.

4. Salwinski, L., Miller, C.S., Smith, A.J., et al., *Nucleic Acids Res.* 32, D449–D451, 2004.

5. Han, D., Kim, H.S., Seo, J., and Jang, W., A domain combination based probabilistic framework for protein-protein interaction prediction, *Genome Inform. Ser. Workshop Genome Inform.* 14, 250–259, 2003.

6. Espadaler, J., Romero-Isart, O., Jackson, R.M., and Oliva, B., Prediction of protein-protein interactions using distant conservation of sequence patterns and structure relationships, *Bioinformatics* 21, 3360–3368, 2005.

7. Wang, J., LI, M., Wang, H., and Pan, Y., Identification of essential proteins based on edge clustering coefficient, *IEEE/ACM Trans. Comput. Biol. Bioinform.* 8, 1070–1080, 2014.

8. Chin, C., Chen, S-H., Wu, H-H., et al., *cytoHubba*: Identifying hub objects and sub-networks from complex interactome, *BMC Systems Biol.* 8(Suppl 4), S11, 2014.

9. Hamp, T., and Rost, B., Evolutionary profiles improve protein-protein interaction prediction from sequence, *Bioinformatics* 31, 1945–1950, 2015.

10. Lei, X., Wang, F., Wu, F-X., Zhang, A., and Pedrycz, W., Protein complex identification through Markov clustering with firefly algorithm on dynamic protein-protein interaction networks, *Information Sci.* 329, 303–316, 2016.

11. Burel, J.G., Apte, S.H., and Doolan, D.L., Systems approaches towards molecular profiling of human immunity, *Trends Immunol.* 37, 53–67, 2016.

12. Tran, L., Hamp, T., and Rost, B., ProfPPIdb: Pairs of physical protein-protein interactions predicted for entire proteomes, *PLoS One* 13(7), e0199988, 2018.

DECONVOLUTION

Deconvolution is the process of resolving a complex form into its constituent elements.[1] Deconvolving is the process of using an algorithm to resolve the complex data obtained in, for example, mass spectrometry[2] or spectroscopy.[3]

1. *Oxford English Dictionary*, Oxford University Press, Oxford, UK, 2018.
2. Smirnov, A., Jia, A., Walker, D.I., Jones D.P., and Du, X., ADAP-GC 3.2: Graphical software tool for efficient spectral deconvolution of gas chromatography-high-resolution mass spectrometry metabolomics data, *J. Proteome Res.* 17, 470–478, 2018.
3. Schenk, J., Nagy, G., Pohl, N.L.B., et al., Identification and deconvolution of carbohydrates with gas chromatography-vacuum ultraviolet spectroscopy, *J. Chromatog A* 1513, 210–221, 2017.

DENDRIMERS

Dendrimers are complex synthetic organic compounds characterized by core, multiple branches with a periphery of functional groups.[1,2] The early work on dendrimers has been reviewed.[1,3] The term dendrimer is derived from dendrite, a natural marking or figure of a branching form, like a tree or moss, found on or in some stones or minerals so marked.[4] The term dendrite is used to describe branched crystal growth[5] and the branched growth of protrusions from neurons.[6] Dendrimers are suggested for use for drug delivery[7–10] and diagnostic imaging.[11–14] The term dendriplex refers to the complex between a dendrimer and another compound which is frequently a drug such as a nucleic acid.[15–17]

1. Tomalia, D.A., Baker, H., Dewald, J., et al., A new class of polymers: Starburst dendritic macromolecules, *Polymer J.* 17, 117–132, 1985.
2. Myung, J.H., Hsu, H.J., Bugno, J., Tam, K.A., and Hong, S., Chemical structure and surface modification of dendritic nanoparticles tailor for therapeutic and diagnostic applications, *Curr. Top. Med. Chem.* 17, 1542–1554, 2017.
3. Tomalia, D.A., Naylor, A.M., and Goddard, W.A., III, Starburst dendrimers: Molecular level control of size, shape, surface chemistry, topology, and flexibility from atoms to macroscopic matter, *Angew. Chem. Int. Edn. Eng.* 29, 138–175, 1990.
4. *Oxford English Dictionary*, Oxford University Press, Oxford, UK, 2019.
5. Tong, X., Beckermann, C., and Karma, A., Velocity and shape selection of dendritic crystals in a forced flow, *Phys. Rev. E. Stat. Phys. Plasma Fluids Relat. Interdiscip. Topics* 61, R49–R62, 2000.
6. Bono, J., Wilmes, K.A., and Clopath, C., Modelling plasticity in dendrites: From single cells to networks, *Curr. Opin. Neurobiol.* 46, 136–141, 2017.
7. Shcharbin, D., Janaszewska, A., Klajnert-Maculewicz, B., et al., How to study dendrimers and dendriplexes III. Biodistribution, pharmacokinetics and toxicity *in vivo*, *J. Control. Release* 181, 40–52, 2014.
8. Palmerston Mendes, L., Pan, J., and Torchilin, V.P., Dendrimers as nanocarriers for nucleic acid and drug delivery in cancer therapy, *Molecules* 22, E1401, 2017.
9. Pitorre, M., Gondé, H., Haury, C., et al., Recent advances in nanocarrier-loaded gels: Which drug delivery technologies against which diseases? *J. Control. Release* 266, 140–155, 2017.
10. Elkin, I., Banquy, X., Barrett, C.J., and Hildgen, P., Non-covalent formulation of active principles with dendrimers: Current state-of-the-art and prospects for further development, *J. Control Release* 28, 264–305, 2017.
11. Kobayashi, H., and Brechbiel, M.W., Dendrimer-based macromolecular MRI contrast agents: Characteristics and application, *Mol. Imaging* 2, 1–10, 2003.
12. Li, D., Wen, S., and Shi, X., Dendrimer-entrapped metal colloids as imaging agents, *Wiley Interdiscip. Rev. Nanomed. Nanobiotechnol.* 7, 678–690, 2015.
13. Boreham, A., Brodwolf, R., Walker, K., Haag, R., and Alexiev, U., Time-resolved fluorescence spectroscopy and fluorescence lifetime imaging microscopy for characterization of dendritic polymer nanoparticles and applications in nanomedicine, *Molecules* 22, E17, 2016.
14. Kondo, T., Kimura, Y., Yamada, H., and Aoyama, Y. Polymer 1H MRI probes for visualizing tumor in vivo, *Chem. Rec.* 17, 555–568, 2017.
15. Shcharbin, D., Pedziwiatr, E., and Bryszwska, M., How to study dendriplexes I: Characterization, *J. Control. Release* 135, 186–197, 2009.
16. Lim, L.Y., Koh, P.Y., Somani, S., et al., Tumor regression following intravenous administration of lactoferrin- and lactoferricin-bearing dendriplexes, *Nanomedicine* 11, 1445–1454, 2015.
17. Li, J., Chen, L., Liu, N., et al., *Drug. Deliv.* 23, 1718–1725, 2016.

DESORPTION

Desorption is defined as "the liberation of a substance from the surface upon which is adsorbed or from the liquid in which it is dissolved."[1] The term desorption is widely used to describe the release of materials from surfaces as in gas chromatography[2] and mass spectrometry.[3,4]

1. *Oxford English Dictionary*, Oxford University Press, Oxford, UK, 2019.
2. Marcillo, A., Jakimovska, V., Widdig, A., and Birkemeyer, C., Comparison of two common adsorption materials for thermal desorption gas chromatography—Mass spectrometry of biogenic volatile organic compounds, *J. Chromatog. A*, 1514, 16–28, 2017.

3. Fan, W.T., Qin, T.T., Bi, R.R., et al., Performance of the matrix-assisted laser desorption ionization time-of-flight mass spectrometry for rapid identification of streptococci: A review, *Eur. J. Clin. Microbiol. Infect. Dis.* 36, 1005–1012, 2017.

4. van Belkum, A., Welker, M., Pincus, D., Charrier, J.P., and Girard, J.P., Matrix-assisted laser desorption ionization time-of-flight mass spectrometry in clinical microbiology: What are the current issues? *Ann. Lab. Med.* 37, 475–483, 2017.

DETERGENT

The term detergent is most commonly associated with cleansing. A formal definition of detergent is a cleansing agent. Current the term detergent is use to describe any of various synthetic solids or liquids which are soluble in or miscible with water, which resemble soap in their cleansing properties, but which differ from it in not combining with the salts present especially in hard water; also, any of various oil-soluble substances which have the property of holding dirt in suspension in lubricating oils—so detergent oil, an oil containing such a substance.[1] A detergent in biochemistry and molecular biology used interchangeably with the term surfactant.[2] A surfactant can be defined as a substance that reduces or otherwise affects the surface tension of water or other liquid, a surface-active agent.[1] Not all surfactants are detergents; consider pulmonary surfactants that are lipoproteins.[3] Detergents in biochemistry and molecular biology are a diverse group of organic compounds characterized by a moiety with hydrophobic properties and a polar head group. The hydrophobic moiety may be long-chain alkane or alkene, an aromatic ring(s) or a steroid while the polar head group can be anionic, cationic, or nonionic (hydrophilic). Laundry detergents contain surfactants in addition to other compounds such as soaps as well as other compounds.[4] Detergents have diverse use in medicine and biology with the majority of use related the study of membranes and solubilization of membrane proteins.[5–8] Early work on the effect of detergents on membranes lead to the concept of lipid rafts as membrane structures not soluble in cold, nonionic detergents.[9] This area evolved into the definition of detergent-resistant membranes.[10,11] Certain peptides have been described with detergent-like properties.[12] Detergents do disrupt lipid-enveloped viruses with the practical application in viral reduction in human blood plasma.[13] See **soap**.

1. *Oxford English Dictionary*, Oxford University Press, Oxford, UK, 2018.

2. Linke, D., Detergents: An overview, *Methods Enzymol.* 463, 603–617, 2009.

3. Olmeda, B., García-Álvarez, B., and Pérez-Gill, J., Structure-function correlations of pulmonary surfactant protein SP-B and the saposin-like family of proteins, *Eur. J. Biophys.* 42, 209–222, 2013.

4. Bajpai, D., and Tyagi, U.K., Laundry detergents: An overview, *J. Oleo Sci.* 56, 327–340, 2007.

5. Liu, S.H., and Guidotti, G., Purification of membrane proteins, *Methods Enzymol.* 463, 619–629, 2009.

6. Zhang, Q., Tao, H., and Hong, W.X., New amphiphiles for membrane protein structural biology, *Methods* 55, 318–323, 2011.

7. Nazari, M., Kurdi, M., and Heerklotz, H., Classifying surfactants with respect to their effect on lipid membrane order, *Biophys. J.* 102, 496–506, 2012.

8. Rawlings, A.E., Membrane proteins: Always an insoluble problem? *Biochem. Soc.* 44, 790–795, 2016.

9. Chamberlain, L.H., Detergents as tools for the purification and classification of lipid rafts, *FEBS Lett.* 559, 1–5, 2006.

10. Brown, D.A., Lipid rafts, detergent-resistant membranes, and raft targeting signals, *Physiology* 21, 430–439, 2006.

11. Caritá, A.C., Mattel, B., Dominguez, C.C., de Paula, E., and Riske, K.A., Effect of Triton X-100 on raft-like lipid mixtures: Phase separation and selective solubilization, *Langmuir* 31, 7312–7321, 2017.

12. Bechinger, B., and Lohner, K., Detergent-like actions of linear amphipathic cationic antimicrobial peptides, *Biochim. Biophys. Acta* 1758, 1529–1539, 2006.

13. Horowitz, B., Bonomo, R., Prince, A.M., et al., Solvent/detergent-treated plasma: A virus-inactivated substitute for fresh-frozen plasma, *Blood* 79, 826–831, 1992.

DETERMINISTIC

Deterministic is the effect of determinism which posits that everything that happens is determined by a necessary chain of causation.[1] When used in biochemistry and molecular biology, the term deterministics describes a series or model which contains no random or probabilistic elements.[2] Deterministic is contrasted with stochastic.[3–6]

1. *Oxford English Dictionary*, Oxford University Press, Oxford, UK, 2019.

2. *The Cambridge Dictionary of Statistics*, ed. B.S. Everitt, Cambridge University Press, Cambridge, UK, 1998.

3. Golestani, A., Jahed Motagh, M.R., Ahmadian, K., Omidvarnia, A.H., and Mozayani, N., A new criterion to distinguish stochastic and deterministic time series with the Poincaré section and fractal dimension, *Chaos* 19, 013137, 2009.

4. Sasai, M., Chikenji, G., and Terada, T.P., Cooperativity and modularity in protein folding, *Biophys. Physicobiol.* 13, 281–293, 2016.

5. Monachino, E., Spenkelink, L.M., and van Oijen, A.M., Watching cellular machinery in action, one molecule at a time, *J. Cell Biol.* 216, 41–51, 2017.

6. Adair, K.L., and Douglas, A.E, Making a microbiome: The many determinants for host-associated microbial community composition, *Curr. Opin. Microbiol.* 35, 23–29, 2017.

DIABODY

A diabody was originally developed as an engineered dimer of an scFv derivative ($V_H V_L$) which has two antigen binding sites which may be homologous or heterologous. Most of the derivatives are heterologous to yield a bispecific (heterologous) derivative.[1] The engineered scFv is composed of a heavy chain variable domain from antibody A linked to light chain variable domain from antibody with a different specificity (antibody B) which is coexpressed with an scFv with heavy chain variable domain from antibody B linked to a light chain variable domain from antibody A. When the two scFv derivatives are coexpressed, there is non-covalent association of the derivatives providing a bispecific antibody. The normal linker engineered between the V_H and V_L domains is 15 residues (usually glycine and serine to promote maximum flexibility) which yields as monomer; if the linker is reduced to 10 residues, a dimer (diabody) is formed while with no linker there is a trimer (tribody) or higher order polymer.[2-4] Stabilization of the diabody is accomplished by a disulfide at the C-terminal of the scFv chains.[5-8] It has been observed that if the order of the variable regions are switch in scFv construct (V_L-V_H instead of V_H-V_L), the engineered scFv with a zero-length linker formed a dimer (diabody) instead of the expected trimer.[9] There are other bispecific antibody derivatives that use chemistry different from diabody.[10,11] See **single chain Fv fragment**, **bibody**, and **triabody**.

1. Holliger, P., Prospero, T., and Winter, G., "Diabodies": Small bivalent and bispecific antibody fragments, *Proc. Natl. Acad. Sci.US* 90, 6444–6448, 1993.
2. Atwell, J.L., Breheney, K.A., Lawrence, L.J., et al., scFv multimers of the anti-neuraminidase antibody NC10: Length of the linker between V_H and V_L domains dictates precisely the transition between diabodies and triabodies, *Protein Eng.* 12, 597–604, 1999.
3. Todorovska, A., Roovers, R.C., Dolezal, O., et al., Design and application of diabodies, triabodies and tetrabodiese for cancer targeting, *J. Immunol. Methods* 248, 47–66, 2001.
4. Powers, G.A., Hudson, P.J., and Wheatcroft, M.P., Design and production of multimeric antibody fragments, focused of diabodies with enhanced clinical efficacy, *Methods Mol. Biol.* 907, 699–712, 2012.
5. Olafsen, T., Cheung, C.-w., Yazaki, P.J., et al., Covalent disulfide-linked anti-CEA diabody allows site-specific conjugation and radiolabeling for tumor targeting applications, *Prot. Eng. Des. Sel.* 17, 21–27, 2004.
6. Johnson, S., Burke, S., Huang, L., et al., Effector cell recruitment with novel Fv-based dual-affinity re-targeting protein leads to potent tumor cytolysis and *in Vivo* B-cell depletion, *J. Mol. Biol.* 399, 436–449, 2010.
7. Walseng, E., Nelson, C.G., Qi, J., et al., Chemically programmed bispecific antibodies in diabody format, *J. Biol. Chem.* 291, 19661–19673, 2016.
8. Cai, Y., Yao, S., Zhong, J., et al., Inhibition activity of a disulfide-stabilized diabody against basic fibroblast growth factor in lung cancer, *Oncotarget* 8, 20187–20197, 2017.
9. Arndt, M.A.E., Krauss, J., and Rybak, S.M., Antigen binding and stability properties of non-covalently linked anti-CD22 single-chain Fv dimers, *FEBS Lett.* 578, 257–261, 2004.
10. Kellner, C., Bruenke, J., Horner, H., et al., Heterodimeric bispecific antibody-derivatives against CD19 and CD16 induce effective antibody-dependent cellular cytotoxicity against B-lymphoid tumor cells, *Cancer Lett.* 303, 128–139, 2011.
11. Yu, S., Li, A., Liu, Q., et al., Recent advances of bispecific antibodies in solid tumors, *J. Hematol. Oncol.* 10, 155, 2017.

DIAPEDESIS

In a canonical sense, diapedesis refers to the migration or transit of immune system cells (leukocytes, monocytes) through the interendothelial junction space and the extracellular matrix/basement membrane to the site of tissue inflammation. Diapedesis can be regarded as a process driven by chemotaxis and preceded by margination or adherence of the cells to the luminal wall.[1] The term transendothelial cell migration is also used to describe the process of diapedesis.[2-4] While most diapedesis occurs across the endothelial luminal wall in the circulatory system, a process described as transepithelial migration occurs in the pulmonary bed.[5]

1. Yeh, Y.T., Serrano, R., Francois, J., et al., Three-dimension forces exerted by leucocytes and vascular endothelial cells dynamically facilitate diapedesis, *Proc. Natl. Acad. Sci. USA* 115, 133–138, 2018.
2. Mittal, M., Nepal, S., Tsukasaki, Y., et al., Neutrophil activation of endothelial cell-expressed TRPM2 mediates transendoethelial neutrophil migration and vascular injury, *Circ. Res.* 121, 1081–1091, 2017.
3. English, W.R., Siviter, R.J., Hansen, M., and Murphy, G., ADAM9 is present at endothelial cell-cell junctions and regulates monocyte-endothelial transmigration, *Biochem. Biophys. Res. Commun.* 493, 1057–1062, 2017.
4. Burn, T., and Alvarez, J.I., Reverse transendothelial cell migration in inflammation: To help or to hinder? *Cell. Mol. Life Sci.* 74, 1871–1881, 2017.
5. Yonker, L.M., Pazos, M.A., Lanter, B.B., et al., Neutrophil-derived cytosolic PLA2α contributes to bacterial-induced neutrophil transepithelial migration, *J. Immunol.* 199, 2873–2884, 2017.

DICER

Dicer is an RNAse III nuclease (class III) which is specific for double-stranded RNA and yields siRNAs.[1-6] Structurally it consists of an amino terminal helicase domain, a PAZ domain, two RNAse III motifs, and a dsRNA binding motif.[7]

1. Carmell, M.A., and Hannan, G.J., RNAse III enzymes and their initiation of gene silencing, *Nat. Struct. Mol. Biol.* 11, 214–218, 2004.
2. Hammond, S.M., Dicing and slicing. The core machinery of the RNA interference pathway, *FEBS Lett.* 579, 5822–5829, 2005.
3. Ha, M., and Kim, V.N., Regulation of microRNA biogenesis, *Nat. Rev. Mol. Cell. Biol.* 15, 509–524, 2014.
4. Kurzynska-Kokorniak, A., Koralewska, N., Pokornowska, M., et al., The many faces of Dicer: The complexity of the mechanisms regulating Dicer gene expression and enzyme activities, *Nucleic Acids Res.* 43, 4365–4380, 2015.
5. Burger, K., and Gullerova, M., Swiss army knives: Noncanonical functions of nuclear Drosha and Dicer, *Nat. Rev. Mol. Cell. Biol.* 16, 417–430, 2015.
6. Song, M.S., and Rossi, J.J., Molecular mechanisms of Dicer: Endonuclease and enzymatic activity, *Biochem. J.* 474, 1603–1618, 2017.
7. Liu, Z., Wang, J., Cheng, H., et al., Cryo-EM structure of human dicer and its complexes with a pre-miRNA substrate, *Cell* 173, 1191–1203, 2018.

DIFFERENTIAL SCANNING CALORIMETRY (DSC)

Differential Scanning Calorimetry (DSC) is a physical technique for the study of conformation of proteins, other polymers, and diverse materials based on measuring changes in heat capacity of a sample.[1,2] There is application of DSC to diverse samples.[3-8] There is considerable use of DSC to study proteins.[9-12] There are important applications of DSC in the characterization of biopharmaceutical products.[13-16] While the bulk of DSC work is associated with proteins, there is use in the characterization of nucleic acids[17-21] and polysaccharides.[22-25]

1. Bruylants, G., Wouters, J., and Michaux, C., Differential scanning calorimetry in life sciences, thermodynamics, stability, molecular recognition and application in drug design, *Curr. Med. Chem.* 12, 2011–2020, 2005.
2. Spink, C.H., Differential scanning calorimetry, *Methods Cell Biol* 84, 115–141, 2008: *Differential Scanning Calorimetry: Application in Fat and Oil Technology*, ed. E. Chiavaro, CRC Press/Taylor & Francis Group, Boca Raton, FL, 2015.
3. Garbett, N.C., Mekmaysy, C.S., Helm, C.W., Jenson, A.B., and Chaires, J.B., Differential scanning calorimetry of blood plasma for clinical diagnosis and monitoring, *Exp. Mol. Pathol.* 86, 186–191, 2009.
4. Pleitner, A., Zhai, Y., Winter, R., et al., Compatible solutes contributes to heat resistance and ribosome stability in *Escherichia coli* AW1.7, *Biochim. Biophys. Acta* 1824, 1351–1357, 2012.
5. Yennawar, N.H., Fecko, J.A., Schowalter, S.A., and Bevilacqua, P.C., A high-throughput biological calorimetry core: Steps to startup, run, and maintain a multiuser facility, *Methods Enzymol.* 567, 435–460, 2016.
6. Srivastava, Y., Semwal, A.D., Sajeevkumar, V.A., and Sharma, G.K., Melting, crystallization and storage stability of virgin coconut oil and its blends by differential scanning calorimetry (DSC) and Fourier transform infrared spectroscopy (FTIR), *J. Food Sci. Technol.* 54, 45–54, 2017.
7. Boguta, P., Sokolowska, Z., and Skic, K., Use of thermal analysis coupled with differential scanning calorimetry, quadrupole mass spectrometry and infrared spectroscopy (TG-DSC-QMS-FTIR) to monitor chemical properties and thermal stability of fluvic and humic acids, *PLoS One* 12(12), e0189653, 2017.
8. Veber, A., Cicconi, M.R., Reinfelder, H., and de Ligny, D., Combined differential scanning calorimetry, Raman and Brillouin spectroscopies: A multiscale approach for materials investigation, *Anal. Chim. Acta* 998, 37–44, 2018.
9. Zecchinon, L., Oriol, A., Netzel, U., et al., Stability domains, substrate-induced conformational changes, and hinge-bending motions in a psychrophilic phosphoglycerate kinase. A microcalorimetric study, *J. Biol. Chem.* 280, 41307–41314, 2005.
10. Levitsky, D.I., Pivovarova, A.V., Mikhailova, V.V., and Nikolaeva, O.P., Thermal unfolding and aggregation of actin, *FEBS J.* 275, 4280–4295, 2008.
11. Johnson, C.M., Differential scanning calorimetry as a tool for protein folding and stability, *Arch. Biochem. Biophys.* 531, 100–109, 2013.
12. Sasahara, K., and Goto, Y., Application and use of differential scanning calorimetry in studies of thermal fluctuation associated with amyloid fibrin formation, *Biophys. Rev.* 5, 259–269, 2013.
13. Jorgensen, L., Moeller, E.H., van de Weert, M., Nielsen, H.M., and Frokjaer, S., Preparing and evaluating delivery systems for proteins, *Eur. J. Pharm. Sci.* 29, 174–182, 2006.
14. van der Walle, C.F., Sharma, G., and Ravi Kumar, M., Current approaches to stabilizing and analyzing proteins during microencapsulation in PLGA, *Expert Opin. Drug Deliv.* 6, 177–186, 2009.
15. Manta, B., Obal, G., Ricciardi, A., Pritsch, O., and Denicola, Tools to evaluate the conformation of protein products, *Biotechnol. J.* 6, 731–741, 2011.
16. Pansare, S.K., and Patel, S.M., Practical considerations for determination of glass transition temperature of a maximally freeze concentrated solution, *AAPS PharmSciTech* 17, 805–819, 2016.

17. Kump, H., Calorimetric studies of the interaction between DNA and poly-L-lysine, *Biophys. Chem.* 5, 363–367, 1976.
18. Mikulecky, P.J., and Feig, A.L., Heat capacity changes associated with nucleic acid folding, *Biopolymers* 82, 38–58, 2006.
19. Kumar, G.S., and Basu, A., The use of calorimetry in the biophysical characterization of small molecule alkaloids binding to RNA structures, *Biochim. Biophys. Acta* 1860, 930–944, 2016.
20. Reiling-Steffensmeier, C., and Marky, L.A., The complementarity of the loop to the stem in DNA pseudoknots gives rise to local TAT base-triplets, *Methods Enzymol.* 567, 413–432, 2016.
21. Reiling-Steffensmeier, C., and Marky, L.A., Structural insight into the unbound state of the DNA analogue of the PreQ₁ riboswitch: A thermodynamic approach, *Biochemistry* 56, 6231–6239, 2017.
22. Cascone, M.G., Barbani, N., Cristallini, C., et al., Bioartificial polymeric materials based on polysaccharides, *J. Biomater. Sci. Polym. Ed.* 12, 267–281, 2001.
23. Zhang, Y., Rempel, C., and Liu, Q., Thermoplastic starch processing and characteristics—A review, *Crit. Rev. Food Sci. Nutr.* 54, 1353–1370, 2014.
24. Mura, P., Analytical techniques for characterization of cyclodextrin complexes in the solid state: A review, *J. Pharm. Biomed. Anal.* 113, 226–238, 2015.
25. Hu, S., Zhao, G., Zheng, Y., et al., Effect of drying procedures on the physicochemical properties and antioxidant activities of polysaccharides from *Crassostrea gigas*, *PLoS One* 12(11), e0188536, 2017.

DIPOLAR COUPLINGS

Dipolar coupling (also known as residual dipolar couplings) measures the interaction between nuclei in an applied magnetic field as used in nuclear magnetic resonance. Measurement of dipolar coupling is used for the determination of the solution structure of peptides, proteins, nucleic acids, and carbohydrates.[1–7] Study of dipolar coupling is also for the study of ligand binding.[8–11]

1. Bush, C.A., Martin-Pastor, M., and Imberty, A., Structure and conformation of complex carbohydrates of glycoproteins, glycolipids, and bacterial polysaccharides, *Ann. Rev. Biophys. Biomol. Struct.* 28, 269–293, 1999.
2. MacDonald, D., and Lu, P., Residual dipolar couplings in nucleic acid structure determination, *Curr. Opin. Struct. Biol.* 12, 337–343, 2002.
3. Marion, D., An introduction to biological NMR spectroscopy, *Mol. Cell. Proteomics* 12, 3006–3025, 2013.
4. Huster, D., Solid-state NMR spectroscopy to study protein-lipid interactions, *Biochim. Biophys. Acta* 1841, 1146–1160, 2014.
5. Pomin, V.H., Solution NMR conformation of glycosaminoglycans, *Prog. Biophys. Mol. Biol.* 114, 61–68, 2014.
6. Battistel, M.D., Azurmendi, H.F., Yu, B., and Freedberg, D.I., NMR of glycans: Shedding new light on old problems, *Prog. Nucl. Magn. Reson. Spectrosc.* 79, 48–68, 2014.
7. Gopinath, T., and Veglia, G., Probing membrane ground and conformationally excited states using dipolar- and J-coupling mediated MAS solid state NMR experiments, *Methods* 148, 115–122, 2018.
8. Post, C.B., Exchange-transferred NOE spectroscopy and bound ligand structure determination, *Curr. Opin. Struct. Biol.* 13, 581–588, 2003.
9. Kang, M., Eichhorn, C.D., and Feigon, J., Structural determinants for ligand capture by a class II preQ1 riboswitch, *Proc. Natl. Acad. Sci. USA* 111, E663–E671, 2014.
10. Atkinson, J., Clarke, M.W., Warnica, J.M., Boddington, K.F., and Graether, S.P., Structure of an intrinsically disordered stress protein along and bound to a membrane surface, *Biophys. J.* 111, 480–491, 2016.
11. Gao, Q., Yang, Y.F., Moremen, K.W., Flanagan, J.G., and Prestdgard, J.H., Structural characterization of a heparan sulfate pentamer interacting with LAR-Ig1–2, *Biochemistry* 57, 2189–2199, 2018.

DIRECTED LIBRARY

A directed library (also focused library) is a library of chemical compounds which may be prepared by parallel synthesis, combinatorial chemistry, phage display or similar multiplexed technologies most often for the synthesis of potential drugs. A directed library may be "directed" from the use of a complete template to introduce diversity of structure.[1,2] or the screening of a groups of compounds (potential inhibitors) against a library of potential target enzymes.[3]

1. Siegel, M.G., Shaker, A.J., Droste, C.A., et al., The use of high-throughput synthesis and purification in the preparation of a directed library of adrenergic agents, *Molecular Diversity* 3, 113–116, 1988.
2. Subramanian, T., Wang, Z., Troutman, J.M., et al., Directed library of anilinogeranyl analogues of farnesyl diphosphate via mixed solid- and solution-phase synthesis, *Org. Lett.* 7, 2109–2112, 2005.
3. Bachovchin, D.A., Koblan, L.W., Wu, W., et al., A high-throughput, multiplexed assay for superfamily-wide profiling of enzyme activity, *Nat. Chem. Biol.* 10, 656–663, 2014.

DISTRIBUTED ANNOTATION SYSTEM (DAS)

The distributed annotation system is a communication protocol for the exchange of biological annotations. (In genetics, the process of identifying the locations and coding regions of genes in a genome and determining what those genes do. An annotation is note added with comment on the function of the gene and/or coding region.)[1–11]

1. Hubbard, T., Biological information: Making it accessible and integrated (and trying to make sense of it), *Bioinformatics* 18(Suppl 2), S140, 2002.
2. Olason, P.I., Integrating protein annotation resources through the Distributed Annotation System, *Nucleic Acids Res.* 33, W468–W470, 2005.
3. Prlic, A., Down, T.A., and Hubbard, J.T., Adding some SPICE to DAS, *Bioinformatics* 21(Suppl 2), ii40–ii41, 2005.
4. Stamm, S., Riethovan, J.J., Le Texier, V., Gopalakrishnan, C., Kumanduri, V., Tang, Y., Barbosa-Morais, N.L., and Thanaraj, T.A., ASD: A bioinformatics resource on alternative splicing, *Nucleic Acids Res.* 32, D46–D55, 2006.
5. Gel Moreno, B., and Messeguer Peypoch, X., GenExp: An interactive web-based genomic DAS client with client-side data rendering, *PLoS One* 6(7), e21270, 2011.
6. Salazar, G.A., Jimenez, R.C., Garcia, A., et al., DAS writeback: A collaborative annotation system, *BMC Bioinformatics* 12, 143, 2011.
7. Salazar, G.A., García, L.J., Jones, P., et al., MyDas, an extensible Java DAS server, *PLoS One* 7(9), e44180, 2012.
8. Speier, W., and Ochs, M.F., Updating annotations with the distributed annotation system and the automated sequence annotation pipeline, *Bioinformatics* 28, 2858–2859, 2012.
9. Schmidt, E.E., Pelz, O., Buhlmann, S., et al., GenomeRNAi: A database for cell-based and in vivo RNAi phenotypes, 2013 update, *Nucleic Acids Res.* 41(Database issue), D1021–D1026, 2013.
10. Falk, M.J., Shen, L., Gonzalez, M., et al., Mitochondrial disease sequence data resource (MSeqDR): A global grass-roots consortium to facilitate deposition, curation, annotation, and integrated analysis of genomic data for the mitochondrial disease clinical and research communities, *Mol. Genet. Metab.* 114, 288–396, 2015.
11. Chrystostomou, C., and Brookes, A.J., Extension to distributed annotation system: Summary and summary plot commands, *Conf. Proc. IEEE Eng Med. Biol. Soc.* 2015, 7655–7658, 2015.

DIVISOME

A divisome is a contractile ring of proteins involved in bacterial cell division (cytokinesis).[1–3] Since a number of proteins are involved in the divisome, there is reference to a cell division interactome.[4] The elucidation of the role of bacterial cell protein FtsZ in cell division occurred in 1991[5] with the term divisome appearing in the same year.[6] A similar ring formation is suggested to occur in eukaryotes.[7]

1. den Blaauwen, T., Hamoen, L.W., and Levin, P.A., The Divisome at 25: The road ahead, *Curr. Opin. Microbiol.* 36, 85–94, 2017.
2. Söderstrom, B., and Daley, D.O., The bacterial Divisome: More than a ring? *Curr. Genet.* 63, 161–164, 2017.
3. Du, S., and Lutkenhaus, J., Assembly and activation of *Escherichia coli* Divisome, *Mol. Microbiol.* 105, 177–187, 2017.
4. Zou, Y., Li, Y., and Dillon, J.R., The distinctive cell division interactome of *Neisseria gonorheae*, *BMC Microbiol.* 17, 232, 2017.
5. Bi, E.F., and Lutkenhaus, J., FtsZ ring structure associated with division in *Escherichia coli*, *Nature* 354, 161–164, 1991.
6. Nanninga, N., Cell division and peptidoglycan assembly in *Escherichia coli*, *Mol. Microbiol.* 5, 791–795, 1991.
7. Cheffings, T.H., Burroughs, N.J., and Balasubramanian, M.K., Actomyosin ring formation and tension generation in eukaryotic cytokinesis, *Curr. Biol.* 26, R719–R737, 2016.

DNA FINGERPRINTING

DNA fingerprinting was designed as a process where DNA is cleaved by a restriction endonuclease (restriction enzyme). The resulting DNA fragments are separated by gel electrophoresis and detected by specific and non-specific probes (Southern Blotting).[1] Subsequent work used PCR with arbitrary (random) primers.[2–4] DNA fingerprinting is extensively used for forensic purposes.[5–8] DNA fingerprinting is also used for the identification of plants[9,10] and bacteria.[11,12] PCR amplification is also used to detect DNA fragments after cleavage with restriction endonucleases.[13] The term fingerprinting is derived from the use of this term to describe two-dimensional separation of peptides on paper following by detection by staining with ninhydrin.[14]

1. Carter, R.E., Wetton, J.H., Parkin, D.T., Improved genetic fingerprinting using RNA probes, *Nucleic Acids Res.* 17, 5867, 1989.
2. Rollo, F., Salvi, R., Amici, A., and Anconetani, A., Polymerase chain reaction fingerprints, *Nucleic Acids Res.* 15, 9094, 1987.
3. Welsh, J., and McClelland, M., Fingerprinting genomes using PCR with arbitrary primers, *Nucleic Acids Res.* 18, 7213–7218, 1990.
4. Mazurier, S., van de Giessen, A., Heuvelman, K., and Wernars, K., RAPD analysis of *Campylobacter* isolates: DNA fingerprinting without the need to purify DNA, *Lett. Appl. Microbiol.* 14, 260–262, 1992.
5. Roewer, L., DNA fingerprinting in forensics: Past, present, future, *Invest. Genet.* 4, 22, 2013.

6. Zoppis, S., Muciaccia, B., D'Alessio, A., et al., DNA fingerprinting secondary transfer from different skin areas: Morphological and genetic studies, *Forensic Sci. Int. Genet.* 11, 137–143, 2014.
7. *Forensic DNA Typing Protocols*, ed. W. Goodwin, Springer Science, New York, 2016.
8. *Forensic DNA Evidence Interpretation*, ed. J.S. Bodulton, J.-A. Bright and D. Taylor, CRC Press, Boca Raton, FL2016.
9. Sucher, N.J., Hennell, J.R., and Carles, M.C., DNA fingerprinting, DNA barcoding, and next generation sequencing technology in plants, *Methods Mol. Biol.* 862, 13–22, 2012.
10. El Hawary, S., El Sayed, A., Helmy, M.W., et al., DNA fingerprinting, biological and chemical investigation of certain Yucca species, *Nat. Prod. Res.*, 32, 2617–2620, 2018.
11. van Belkum, A., DNA fingerprinting of medically important microorganisms by use of PCR, *Clin. Microbiol. Rev.* 7, 174–184, 1994.
12. Thanos, M., Schonian, G., Meyer, W., et al., Rapid identification of *Candida* species by DNA fingerprinting with PCR, *J. Clin. Microbiol.* 34, 615–621 1996.
13. Di Lodovico, S., Del Vecchio, A., Cataldi, V., et al., Microbial contamination of smartphone touchscreens of Italian university students, *Curr. Microbiol.* 75, 336–342, 2018.
14. Ingram, V., A specific chemical difference between the globins of normal human and sickle-cell anaemia, *Nature* 178, 792–794, 1956.

DNA FOOTPRINTING

DNA footprinting is a method for determining a region in a DNA molecule that interacts with a protein or macromolecule as, for example, in the nucleosome.[1,2] A reagent, such as dimethyl sulfate or hydroxyl radical, which reacts with an exposed sequence of DNA but not with a sequence which, for example, is interacting with the histone, is added to a sample and the modified DNA subsequently can be cleaved at the modified guanine residue.[3,4] Dimethyl sulfate modification is also used to identify G-quadruplex structures.[5–7] DNA footprinting can also be achieved by the use of DNAse I.[8–10] The utility of DNAse I in footprinting is extended by the concept of DNAse-seq which used PCR driven sequence analysis of cleaved DNA fragments (cleavage at DNAse hypersensitivity sites).[11] DNA footprinting can also be accomplished by reaction with hydroxyl radicals.[12,13] Footprinting is also used to identify regions on RNA that interact with proteins as well as for the study of RNA conformation.[14–16]

1. Brown, P.M., and Fox, K.R., Footprinting studies with nucleosome-bound DNA, *Methods Mol. Biol.* 90, 81–93, 1997.
2. Jeltsch, A., Jurkowska, R.Z., Jurkowski, T.P., et al., Application of DNA methyltransferases in targeted DNA methylation, *Appl. Microbiol. Biotechnol.* 75, 1233–1240, 2007.
3. Shaw, P.E., and Stewart, A.F., Identification of protein/DNA contacts with dimethyl sulfate: Methylation protection and methylation interference, *Methods Mol. Biol.* 543, 97–104, 2009.
4. He, G., Tolic, A., Bashkin, J.K., and Pool, G.M., Heterologous dynamics in DNA site discrimination by the structural homologous DNA-binding domains of ETS-family transcription factors, *Nucleic Acids Res.* 43, 4322–4331, 2015.
5. Sun, D., and Hurley, L.H., Biochemical techniques for the characterization of G-quadruplex structures: EMSA, DMS footprinting, and DNA polymerase stop assay, *Methods Mol. Biol.* 608, 65–79, 2010.
6. Sun, D., Guo, K., and Shin, Y.J., Evidence of the formation of G-quadruplex structures in the promoter region of the human vascular endothelial growth factor gene, *Nucleic Acids Res.* 39, 1256–1265, 2011.
7. Sekibo, D.A.T., and Fox, K.R., The effects of DNA supercoiling on G-quadruplex formation, *Nucleic Acids Res.* 45, 120969–12079, 2017.
8. Ellis, T., Evans, D.A., Martin, C.R., and Hartley, J.A., A 96-well DNase I footprinting screen for drug-DNA interactions, *Nucleic Acids Res.* 35(12), e89, 2007.
9. Gusmao, E.G., Allhoff, M., Zenke, M., and Costa, I.G., Analysis of computational footprinting methods for DNase sequencing experiments, *Nat. Methods* 13, 303–309, 2016.
10. Baraquet, C., and Harwood, C.S., Use of nonradiochemical DNAse footprinting to analyze c-di-GMP modulation of DNA-binding proteins, *Methods Mol. Biol.* 1657, 303–315, 2017.
11. He, H.H., Meyer, C.A., Hu, S.S., et al., Refined DNase-seq protocol and data analysis reveals intrinsic bias in transcription factor footprint identification, *Nat. Methods* 11, 73–78, 2014.
12. He, G., Vasilieva, E., Bashkin, J.K., and Dupureur, C.M., Mapping small DNA ligand hydroxyl radical footprinting and affinity cleavage of products for capillary electrophoresis, *Anal. Biochem.* 439, 99–101, 2013.
13. Shaytan, A.K., Xiao, H., Armeev, G.A., et al., Hydroxyl-radical footprinting combined with molecular modeling identifies unique features of DNA conformation and nucleosome positioning, *Nucleic Acid Res.* 45, 9229–9243, 2017.
14. Jørgensen, T., Siboska, G.E., Wikman, F.P., and Clark, B.F., Different conformations of tRNA in the ribosomal P-site and A-site, *Eur. J. Biochem.* 153, 283–289, 1985.
15. Gracia, B., Xue, Y., Bisaria, N., et al., Structural modules control the rate and pathway of RNA folding and assembly, *J. Mol. Biol.* 428, 3972–3985, 2016.
16. Fay, M.M., Lyons, S.M., and Ivanov, P., RNA G-quadruplexes in biology: Principles and molecular mechanisms, *J. Mol. Biol.* 429, 2127–2147, 2017.

DNA METHYLATION

DNA Methylation is one of the more common epigenetic modification.[1] The methylation of DNA is catalyzed by DNA methyltransferase enzymes with modification occurring primarily at cytosine in a CpG doublet.[2] The DNAse methylation product has been referred to as the DNA methylome.[3–5] The methylation of DNA has a wide variety of effects on normal growth and development as well as in the etiology of various pathologies.[6] Methylation of cytosine residues in DNA is important in oncology,[7–9] psychology,[10] biological rhythms,[11] viral infections,[12] metabolic disorders,[13] development of handedness,[14] and coronary artery disease.[15] DNA methyltransferases have been used to label DNA.[16]

1. *DNA Methylation and Complex Human Disease*, ed. M. Neidhart, Academic Press/Elsevier, San Diego, CA, 2016.
2. Jeltsch, A., and Jurkowska, R.Z., New concepts in DNA methylation, *Trends Biochem. Sci* 39, 310–318, 2014.
3. Wilson, I.M., Davies, J.J., Weber, M., et al., Epigenomics: Mapping the methylome, *Cell Cycle* 5, 155–158, 2006.
4. Seymour, D.K., and Becker, C., The causes and consequences of DNA methylome variation in plants, *Curr. Opin. Plant Biol.* 36, 56–63, 2017.
5. Madakshira, B.P., and Sadler, K.C., DNA methylation, nuclear organization, and cancer, *Front. Genet.* 8, 76, 2017.
6. *DNA Methyltransferases—Role and Function* (volume 945 in Advances in Experimental Biology and Medicine), ed. E. Jeltsch and R.Z. Jurkowska, Springer, Cham, Switzerland, 2016.
7. Levine, A.J., The p53 protein plays a central role in the mechanism of action of epigenetic drugs that alter the methylation of cytosine residues in DNA, *Oncotarget* 8, 7228–7230, 2017.
8. El Bairi, K., Tariq, K., Himri, I., et al., Decoding colorectal cancer epigenomics, *Cancer Genet.* 220, 49–76, 2018.
9. Lapinska, K., Faria, G., McGonagle, S., et al., Cancer progenitor cells: The result of an epigenetic event? *Anticancer Res.* 38, 1–6, 2018.
10. Kader, F., Ghai, M., and Maharaj, L., The effects of DNA methylation on human psychology, *Behav. Brain Res.* 346, 47–65, 2018.
11. Stevenson, T.J., Epigenetic regulation of biological rhythms: An evolutionary ancient molecular timer, *Trends Genet.* 34, 90–100, 2018.
12. Balkrishnan, L., and Milavetz, B., Epigenetic regulation of viral biological processes, *Viruses* 9, E346, 2017.
13. Cheng, Z., Zheng, L., and Almeida, F.A., Epigenetic reprogramming in metabolic disorders: Nutritional factors and beyond, *J. Nutr. Biochem.* 54, 1–10, 2017.
14. Schmitz, J., Metz, G.A.S., Güntürkün, O., and Ocklenburg, S., Beyond the genome—Towards an epigenetic understanding of handedness ontogenesis, *Prog. Neurobiol.* 159, 68–89, 2017.
15. Duan, L. Hu, J., Xiong, X., Liu, Y., and Want, J., The role of DNA methylation in coronary artery disease, *Gene*, 646, 91–97, 2018.
16. Tomkuvienė, M., Kriukienė, E., and Klimašauskas, S., DNA labeling using DNA methyltransferases, *Adv. Exp. Med. Biol.* 945, 511–535, 2016.

DNAse HYPERSENSTIVITY SITE

A DNAse hypersensitivity site is an exposed region of native DNA, which can be cleaved by DNAse I. This is typically a region where clusters of transcriptional activators bind to DNA and usually reflect a change in chromatin structure.[1–4]

1. McGinnis, W., Shermoen, A.W., Heemskerk, J., and Beckendorf, S.K., DNA sequence changes in an upstream DNAse I-hypersensitive region are correlated with reduced gene expression, *Proc. Nat. Acad. Sci. USA* 80, 1063–1067, 1983.
2. Cereghini, S., Saragosti, S., Yaniv, M., and Hamer, D.H., SV40-alpha-globulin hybrid minichromosomes. Differences in DNase I hypersensitivity of promoter and enhancer sequences, *Eur. J. Biochem.* 144, 545–553, 1984.
3. Rothenberg, E.V., and Ward, S.B., A dynamic assembly of diverse transcription factors integrates activation and cell-type information for interleukin 2 gene regulation, *Proc. Nat. Acad. Sci. USA* 93, 9358–9365, 1996.
4. Hermann, B.P., and Heckert, L.L., Silencing of Fshr occurs through a conserved, hypersensitive site in the first intron, *Mol. Endocrinol.* 19, 2112–2131, 2005.

DNAzymes

DNAzymes (also referred to as deoxyribozymes) are small, synthetic DNA molecules that were initially shown to have catalytic activity in the intramolecular cleavage and subsequently the intermolecular cleavage of a ribonucleotide phosphodiester bond.[1] The early studies required the presence of lead ions with subsequent studies showing that magnesium ions would support the reaction.[2] The development of DNAzymes used the SELEX process developed for the selection of aptamers[3] where a functional DNAzyme would catalyze its own release from the matrix.[4] Other early work showed the catalysis of porphyrin metalation by a small synthetic DNA in the absence of divalent cations but enhanced by potassium ions with little effect of sodium ions with a stabilizing effect of Tris.[5] There is continued emphasis on the development of DNAzymes that act on RNA.[6] It has been suggested that there is therapeutic use for DNAzymes[7] but there are challenges.[8] There is current used of DNAzyme technology for the development of sensors.[9–11]

1. Silverman, S.K., Catalytic DNA: Scope, applications, and biochemistry of deoxyribozymes, *Trends Biochem. Sci.* 41, 595–609, 2016.
2. Breaker, R.R., and Joyce, G.F., A DNA enzyme with Mg^{2+}-dependent RNA phosphodiesterase activity, *Chem. Biol.* 1, 655–660, 1995.
3. Drolet, D.W., Jenison, R.D., Smith, D.E., Pratt, D., and Hicke, B.J., A high throughput platform for systematic evaluation of ligands by exponential enrichment (SELEX), *Comb. Chem. High Throughput Screen* 2, 271–278, 1999.
4. Breaker, R.R., and Joyce, G.F., A DNA enzyme that cleaves RNA, *Chem. Biol.* 1, 223–229, 1994.
5. Li, Y., and Sen, D., Toward an efficient DNAzyme, *Biochemistry* 36, 5589–5599, 1997.
6. Hollenstein, M., DNA catalysis: The chemical repertoire of DNAzymes, *Molecules* 20, 20777–20804, 2015.
7. Dass, C.R., Choong, P.F., and Khachigian, L.M., DNAzyme technology: Cleave and let die, *Mol. Cancer Ther.* 7, 243–251, 2008.
8. Victor, J., Steger, G., and Riesner, D., Inability of DNAzymes to cleave RNA in vivo is due to limited Mg^{2+} concentration in cells, *Eur. J. Biophys.* 47, 333–343, 2018.
9. Chang, D., Zakaria, S., Deng, M., et al., Integrating deoxyribozymes into colorimetric sensing platforms, *Sensors* (Basal) 16(12), 2061, 2016.
10. McGhee, C.E., Loh, K.Y., and Lu, Y., DNAzyme sensors for detection of metal ions in the environment and imaging them in living cells, *Curr. Opin. Biotechnol.* 45, 191–201, 2017.
11. Zhou, W., Saran, R., and Liu, J., Metal sensing by DNA, *Chem. Rev.* 117, 8272–8325, 2017.

DOMAIN

A domain is a contiguous group of monomer units (amino acids in proteins; nucleic acid bases in nucleic acids; monosaccharide in oligosaccharides/polysaccharides). The term domain is most often associated with proteins where a domain can be defined as a structurally independent region with its own hydrophobic core.[1] A domain can be continuous or discontinuous[2,3] and is usually identified by a unique function such as catalysis or binding.[4] Domains may be identified by homology and can be used to group proteins into families.[5–8]

1. *Structural Bioinformatics*, ed. P.E. Bourne and H. Weissig, Wiley-Liss, Hoboken, NJ, 2003.
2. Xue, Z., Jang, R., Govindarajoo, B., Huang, Y., and Wang, Y., Extending protein domain boundary predictors to detect discontinuous domains, *PLoS One* 10(10), e0141541, 2015.
3. Berezovsky, I.N., Guarnera, E., and Zheng, Z., Basic units of protein structure, folding, and function, *Prog. Biophys. Mol. Biol.* 128, 85–99, 2017.

4. Rack, J.G., Perina, D., and Ahel, I., Macrodomains: Structure, function, evolution, and catalytic activities, *Annu. Rev. Biochem.* 85, 431–454, 2016.
5. Hinck, A.P., Mueller, T.D., and Springer, T.A., Structural biology and evolution of the TGF-β family, *Cold Spring Harb. Perspect. Biol.* 8(12), a022103, 2016.
6. Bloudoff, K., and Scheing, T.M., Structural and functional aspects of the nonribosomal peptide synthetase condensation domain superfamily: Discovery, dissection and diversity, *Biochim. Biophys. Acta.* 1865, 1587–1604, 2017.
7. Arnolds, O., Zhong, Z., Tuo Yip, K., et al., Implications for the MIA protein family, *Curr. Med. Chem.* 24, 1788–1796, 2017.
8. Pang, S.W., Lahiri, C., Poh, C.L., and Tan, K.O., PNMA family: Protein interaction network and cell signaling pathways implicated in cancer and apopotosis, *Cell Signal.* 45, 54–62, 2018.

DOMAIN ANTIBODIES (SINGLE DOMAIN ANTIBODIES)

A fragment that contains a single antigen-binding domain representation the variable region of the heavy chain or the highly variable regions from both the heavy chain and light chain of an IgG protein. These proteins are naturally occurring in camelids (members of the order Camelidae which includes llamas and camels).[1,2] The small size of these proteins have attracted interest for therapeutic use.[3–8]

1. Dick, H.M., Single domain antibodies, *BMJ* 300, 959, 1990.
2. Riechman, L., and Muyldermans, S., Single domain antibodies: Comparison of camel VH and camelized human VH domains, *J. Immunol. Methods* 231, 25–38, 1999.
3. Stockwin, L.H., and Holmes, S., Antibodies as therapeutic agents: Vive la renaissance! *Expert Opin. Biol. Ther.* 3, 1133–1152, 2003.
4. Holt, L.J., Herring, C., Jespers, L.S., Woolven, B.P., and Tomlinson, I.M., Domain antibodies: Proteins for therapy, *Trends Biotechnol.* 21, 484–490, 2003.
5. Kijanka, M., Dorresteijn, B., Oliveira, S., and van Bergen en Henegouwen, P.M., Nanobody-based cancer therapy of solid tumors, *Nanomedicine* (London) 10, 161–174, 2015.
6. Wu, Y., Jiang, S., and Ying, T., Single-domain antibodies as therapeutics against human viral diseases, *Front. Immunol.* 8, 1802, 2017.
7. Böldicke, T., Single domain antibodies for the knockdown of cytosolic and nuclear proteins, *Protein Sci.* 26, 925–945, 2017.
8. Fernandes, C.F.C., Pereira, S.D.S., Luiz, M.B., et al., Camelid single-domain antibodies as an alternative to overcome challenges related to the prevention, detection, and control of neglected tropical diseases, *Front. Immunol.* 8, 653, 2017.

DROSHA

Drosha, an enzyme with a molecular mass of approximately 150 kDa, is a member of the RNAse III family of double-stranded specific endonucleases. Drosha is defined in Class II in the RNAse III family in which each member contains tandem RNAse III catalytic motifs and one C-terminal dsRNA-binding domain. Class I proteins contain only one RNAse III catalytic domain and a dsRNA binding domain. Class III (see Dicer) contains a PAZ domain, a DUF283 domain, the tandem nuclease domains, and a dsRNA-binding domain.[1,2] Drosha in combination with DGCR8 (DiGeorge syndrome critical region 8 gene) participates in the nuclear phase of microRNA formation (processing of the primary microRNA) by the formation of the microprocessor where Drosha is the ds-nuclease (double strand nuclease) and DGCR8 recognizes the nucleic acid.[3–5] Final processing of the microRNA is accomplished with Dicer, a Class III member of the RNAase III family.[6,7] The presence of Drosha was likely demonstrated by early work on tissue ribonuclease activity.[8] A homologue for the Drosha nuclease in *Drosophila* was suggested in 2000[9] and human protein was cloned the same year.[10]

1. Carmell, M.A., and Hannan, G.J., RNAse III enzymes and their initiation of gene silencing, *Nat. Struct. Mol. Biol.* 11, 214–218, 2004.
2. Aguado, L.C., and tenOever, B.R., RNAase III nuclease and the evolution of antiviral systems, *BioEssays* 40, 170173, 2018.
3. Gregory, R.I., Yan, K.P., Amuthan, G., et al., The microprocessor complex mediates the genesis of microRNAs, *Nature* 432, 235–240, 2004.
4. Macias, S., Cordiner, R.A., and Cáceres, J.F., Cellular function of the microprocessor, *Biochem. Soc. Trans.* 41, 838–843, 2013.
5. Partin, A.C., Ngo, T.C., Herrell, E., et al., Heme enables proper positioning of Drosha and DGCR8 on primary microRNAs, *Nat. Commun.* 8(1), 1737, 2017.
6. Roberts, T.C., The microRNA machinery, in *microRNA: Basic Science (Advanced in Experimental Biology and Medicine vol 887)*, Chapter 2, pp 15–30, Springer International, Cham, Switzerland, 2015.
7. Song, M.S., and Rossi, J.J., Molecular mechanisms of Dicer: Endonuclease and enzymatic activity, *Biochem. J.* 474, 1603–1618, 2017.
8. Roth, J.F, Ribonuclease. III. Ribonuclease activity in rat liver and kidney, *J. Biol. Chem.* 208, 181–194, 1954.
9. Filippov, V., Solovyev, V., Filippova, M., and Gill, S.S., A novel type of RNase III family proteins in eukaryotes, *Gene* 245, 213–221, 2000.
10. Wu., H., Xu, H., Miraglia, L.J., and Crooke, S.T., Human RNase III is a 160-kDa protein involved in preribosomal RNA processing, *J. Biol. Chem.* 275, 36957–36965, 2000.

DRUG

A drug is defined as (1) a substance recognized by an official pharmacopoeia or formulary; (2) a substance intended for use in the diagnosis, cure, mitigation, treatment, or prevention of disease; (3) a substance (other than food) intended to affect the structure or any function of the body; (4) a substance intended for use as a component of a medicine but not a device or a component, part or accessory of a device; (5) biological products that are included within this definition and are generally covered by the same laws and regulations, but differences exist regarding their manufacturing processes (chemical processes vs. biological processes). The statutory (FDA) definition is Section 201(g) of the FD&C Act (21 USC 321(g)) provides that the term "drug" means (1) articles recognized in the official United States Pharmacopoeia, official Homoeopathic Pharmacopoeia of the United States, or official National Formulary, or any supplement to any of them; (2) articles intended for use in the diagnosis, cure, mitigation, treatment, or prevention of disease in man or other animals; (3) articles (other than food) intended to affect the structure or any function of the body of man or other animals; and (4) articles intended for use as a component of any articles specified in clause (1), (2), or (3).[1] There are differences in the regulation of drugs and biological but some biological products such as monoclonal antibodies are regulated as drugs.

1. https://www.fda.gov/regulatoryinformation/guidances/ucm258946.htm.

DRUG MASTER FILE

A Drug Master File (DMF) contains information on the processes and facilities used in drug or drug component manufacture and storage and are submitted to the FDA for examination and approval. Per FDA, "A Drug Master File (DMF) is a submission to the Food and Drug Administration (FDA) that may be used to provide confidential detailed information about facilities, processes, or articles used in the manufacturing, processing, packaging, and storing of one or more human drugs."[1] The presence of a Drug Master File for a material or device used in the manufacturing of a drug product is very useful, if not essential.

1. https://www.fda.gov/drugs/guidancecomplianceregulatory information/guidances/ucm122886.htm.

DRUG PRODUCT

It is the final dosage form which contains a drug substance (active pharmaceutical ingredient) or drug substances as well as inactive materials which are also considered as excipients. The drug product is differentiated from the drug substance but may or may not be the same as the drug substance. FDA definition from FDA (from ICH): **Active Pharmaceutical Ingredient (API)** *(or Drug Substance)*: Any substance or mixture of substances intended to be used in the manufacture of a drug (medicinal) product and that, when used in the production of a drug, becomes an active ingredient of the drug product. Such substances are intended to furnish pharmacological activity or other direct effect in the diagnosis, cure, mitigation, treatment, or prevention of disease or to affect the structure and function of the body. The above is taken from Guidance for Industry, Q7A Good Manufacturing Practice Guidance for Active Pharmaceutical Ingredients.[1]

1. https://www.fda.gov/iceci/compliancemanuals/compliance policyguidancemanual/ucm200364.htm#P1422_111232.

DRUG TARGETING (TARGETED DRUG DELIVERY)

Drug targeting is the ability to target a compound to a specific organ or cell type within an organism. The compound can be a drug/pharmaceutical[1,2] or it can be a compound, such as a radioisotope, which can be used as a diagnostic.[3] Antibody-drug conjugates (ADCs) are examples of specific drug targeting in cancer.[4-6] It should be noted that oncology drugs are quite expensive and can have significant off-target effects so delivery to target cells/tissue is extremely important for both economic and drug safety considerations.

1. Muzykantov, V.R., Biomedical aspects of targeted delivery of drugs to pulmonary endothelium, *Expert Opin. Drug Deliv.* 2, 909–926, 2005.
2. Weissig, V., Targeted drug delivery to mammalian mitochondria in living cells, *Expert Opin. Drug Deliv.* 2, 89–102, 2005.
3. Hilgenbrink, A.R., and Low, P.S., Folate-receptor-mediated drug targeting: From therapeutics to diagnostics, *J. Pharm. Sci.* 94, 2135–2146, 2005.
4. Wolska-Washer, A., Robak, P., Smolewkski, P., and Robak, T., Emerging antibody-drug conjugates for treating lymphoid malignancies, *Expert Opin. Emerg. Drugs* 22, 259–273, 2017.
5. Joubert, N., Denevault-Sabourin, C., Brydin, F., and Viaud-Massuard, M.C., Towards antibody-drug conjugates and prodrug strategies with extracellular stimuli-responsive drug delivery in the tumor microenvironment for cancer therapy, *Eur. J. Med. Chem.* 142, 393–415, 2017.
6. Malik, P., Phipps, C., Edgjnton, A., and Blay, J. Pharmacokinetic considerations for antibody-drug conjugates against cancer, *Pharm. Res.* 34, 2579–2595, 2017.

DYE

A dye is a chemical compound with a structure which yields a color (a chromophore) which can be coupled either covalently or noncovalently to a substrate matrix.[1-9] The ability of the compound to yield color is based on its ability to absorb light in the visible spectrum (400–700 nm). Dyes can be classified by various characteristics including mechanism/chemistry (e.g. basic dyes, acid dyes; acid/base indicators/redox dyes), structure (nitroso, acridine dyes, thiazole dyes) and process use (e.g. vat dyes). A dye is a colorant (a substance which yields color) as are pigments. A dye is chemically different from a pigment, which is a particle suspended in a medium as particles in paint. More recently, the term dye has expanded to include fluorescent compounds.[10-13]

1. Venkataraman, K., *The Chemistry of Synthetic Dyes*, Academic Press, New York, NY, 1952.
2. Conn, H.J., *Biological Stains: A Handbook on the Nature and Uses of the Dyes Employed in the Biological; Handbook*, Williams & Wilkins, Baltimore, MD, 1961.
3. Gurr, E., *Synthetic Dyes in Biology, Medicine, and Chemistry*, Academic Press, London, UK, 1971.
4. Venkataraman, K., *The Chemistry of Synthetic Dyes*, Academic Press, New York, NY, 1978.
5. Egan, H., and Fishbein, L., *Some Aromatic Amines and Azo Dyes in the General and Industrial Environment*, International Agency for Research on Cancer, Lyon, France, 1981.
6. Clark, G., and Koastan, F.H., *History of Staining*, 3rd edn., Williams & Wilkins, Baltimore, MD, 1983.
7. Zollinger, H., *Color Chemistry. Syntheses, Properties, and Applications of Organic Dyes and Pigments*, 2nd edn., VCH, Weiheim, Germany, 1991.
8. *Physico-Chemical Principles of Color Chemistry*, ed. A.T. Peters and H.W. Freeman, Blackie Academic and Professional, London, UK, 1996.
9. *Conn's Biological Stains. A Handbook of Dyes, Stains, and Fluorochromes for Use in Biology and Medicine*, 10th edn., ed. R.W. Horobin and J.A. Kiernan, Bios, Oxford, UK, 2002.
10. Mason, W.T., *Fluorescent and Luminescent Probes for Biological Activity: A Practical Guide to Technology for Quantitative Real-Time Analysis*, Academic Press, San Diego, CA, 1999.
11. Kalyanraman, B., Oxidative chemistry of fluorescent dyes: Implications in the detection of reactive oxygen and nitrogen species, *Biochem. Soc. Trans.* 39, 1221–1225, 2011.
12. Fardel, O., Le Vee, M., Jouan, E., Denizot, C., and Parmentier, Y., Nature and uses of fluorescent dyes for drug transporter studies, *Expert Opin. Drug. Metab. Toxicol.* 11, 1233–1251, 2015.
13. Minoshima, M., and Kikuchi, K., Photostable and photoswitching fluorescent dyes for super-resolution imaging, *J. Biol. Inorg. Chem.* 22, 639–652, 2017.

DYNAMIC LIGHT SCATTERING

Dynamic light scattering (DLS) (photon correlation spectroscopy; quasi-elastic light scattering) is a method for determining the translational and rotational diffusion of particles, such as a protein in solution.[1,2] Dynamic light scattering measures the fluctuations in the intensity of the scattered light that is caused by Brownian motion of the particles. The diffusion constant can be used to determine the hydrodynamic radius and frictional coefficient for a particle. DLS permits the evaluation of homogeneity of macromolecules and the effect of interactions on conformation as well protein aggregation.[3] Other techniques such as Fabry-Perot interferometry are included on occasion with DLS.[4,5]

1. Schmitz, K.S., *An Introduction to Dynamic Light Scattering by Macromolecules*, Academic Press, Harcourt Bruce Javanovich, Boston, MA, 1990.
2. Stetefeld, J., McKenna, S.A., and Patel, T.R., Dynamic light scattering: A practical guide and applications in biomedical sciences, *Biophys. Rev.* 8, 409–427, 2016.
3. Zhou, C., Qi, W., Lewis, E.N., and Carpenter, J.F., Characterization of sizes of aggregates of insulin analogs and the conformations of the constituent protein molecules: A concomitant dynamic light scattering and Raman spectroscopy study, *J. Pharm. Sci.* 105, 551–558, 2016.
4. Percora, R., Dynamic light scattering from macromolecules, *Static and Dynamic Light Scattering in Medicine and Biology*, ed. R.J. Nossal, R. Pecora, and A.V. Priezzhev, *Proceedings of SPIE*, 1884, 2–15, 1993.
5. Olmsted, I.R., Xiao, Y., Cho, M., et al., Measurement of aptamer-protein interactions with back-scattering interferometry, *Anal. Chem.* 83, 8867–8870, 2011.

ECTODOMAIN

An ectodomain is the extracellular domain of a transmembrane protein having specific function and is released by limited proteolysis in a processing referred to as ectodomain shedding.[1–3] Ectodomain shedding is mediated by ADAMs (a disintegrin and metallo) proteinases and matrix metalloproteinases (MMPs).[4,5] There is particular interest in the role of ADAM10[6,7] and ADAM 17 which is also known as tumor necrosis factor-alpha-converting enzyme.[8] Ectodomain shedding is involved in the genesis of Alzheimer's disease.[9,10] Ectodomain shedding is a critical factor in the function of cells such as the participation of neutrophils in inflammation.[11,12] The term extracellular domain is also used to describe the portion of a transmembrane protein outside of the cell such as a receptor which may be released by proteolysis but as part of a process different from ectodomain shedding.[13–15]

1. Arribas, J., and Borroto, A., Protein ectodomain shedding, *Chem. Rev.* 102, 4627–4638, 2002.
2. Hartmann, M., Herrlich, A., and Herrlich, P., Who decides to cleave an ectodomain? *Trends Biochem. Sci.* 38, 111–120, 2013.
3. Tien, W.S., Chen, J.H., and Wu, K.P., Sheddome DB: The ectodomain shedding database for membrane-bound shed markers, *BMC Bioinformatics* 18(Suppl 3): 42, 2017.
4. Higashiyama, S., and Nanba, D., ADAM-mediated ectodomain shedding of HB-EGF in receptor cross-talk, *Biochim. Biophys. Acta* 1751, 110–117, 2005.
5. Clark, P., Protease-mediated ectodomain shedding, *Thorax* 69, 682–684, 2014.
6. Wetzel, S., Seipold, L., and Saftig, P., The metalloproteinase ADAM10: A useful therapeutic target?, *Biochim. Biophys. Acta* 1864, 2071–2081, 2017.
7. Peron, R., Vatanabe, I.P., Mazine, P.R., Camins, A., and Cominetti, M.R., *Pharmaceuticals* (Basal) 11(1), 12, 2018.
8. Rego, S.L., Helms, R.S., and Dréau, D., Tumor necrosis factor-alpha-converting enzyme activities and tumor-associated macrophages in breast cancer, *Immunol. Res.* 58, 87–100, 2014.
9. Zhang, H., Ma, Q., Zhang, Y.W., and Xu, H., Proteolytic processing of Alzheimer's β-amyloid precursor protein, *J. Neurochem.* 120(Suppl. 1), 9–21, 2012.
10. Saftig, P., and Lichtenthaler, S.F., The alpha-secretase ADAM10: A metalloprotease with multiple functions in the brain, *Prog. Neurobiol.* 135, 1–20, 2015.
11. Garton, K.J., Gough, P.J., and Raines, E.W., Emerging roles for ectodomain shedding in the regulation of inflammatory responses, *J. Leukoc. Biol.* 79, 1105–1116, 2006.
12. Mishra, H.K., Ma, J., and Walcheck, B., Ectodomain shedding by ADAM17: Its role in neutrophil recruitment and the impairment of the process during sepsis, *Front. Cell Infect. Microbiol.* 7, 138, 2017.
13. Tsé, C., Gauchez, A.S., Jacot, W., and Lamy, P.J., HER2 shedding and serum HER2 extracellular domain: Biology and clinical utility in breast cancer, *Cancer Treat. Rev.* 38, 133–142, 2012.
14. Zarei, O., Benvenuti, S., Ustun-Alkan, F., Hamzeh-Mivehroud, M., and Dastmalchi, S., Strategies of targeting the extracellular domain of RON tyrosine kinase receptor for cancer therapy and drug delivery, *J. Cancer Res. Clin. Oncol.* 142, 2429–2446, 2016.
15. Riquelme, M.A, Kar, R., Gu, S., and Jiang, J.S., Antibodies targeting extracellular domain of connexins for studies of hemichannels, *Neuropharmacology* 75, 525–532, 2013.

ELECTRODE POTENTIAL ($E°$)

The electrode potential is electrical potential with two electrodes with an electrode of the left is a standard hydrogen electrode and the electrode of the right is measured with an electrode in contact with a solution of its ions.[1,2] The IUPAC definition is "Electromotive force of a cell in which the electrode on the left is a standard hydrogen electrode and the electrode on the right is the electrode in question."[3] Electrode potential values will predict whether a substance will be reduced or oxidized. Values are usually expressed as a reduction potential ($M^{n+} \rightarrow M$). A positive electrode potential would indicate that reduction is spontaneous. A negative potential for this reaction would suggest that the oxidation reaction ($M \rightarrow M^{n+}$) would be spontaneous. A common application of the electrode potential is the measurement of pH[4] and the concept is extended on system that measure glucose concentration by glucose oxidase.[5]

1. Milazzo, G., *Tables of Standard Electrode Potentials*, John Wiley and Sons, New York, 1977.
2. Compton, R.G., and Sanders, G.H.W., *Electrode Potentials*, Oxford University Press, Oxford, UK, 1993.
3. Lehmann, H.P., Fuentes-Arderiu, X., and Bertello, L.F., Glossary of terms in quantities and terms in clinical chemistry (IUPAC-IFCC Recommendations, 1996), *Pure Applied Chem.* 68, 957–1000, 1996.
4. Kohler, H.H., Haider, C., and Woelski, S., Selectivity and dynamic behavior of glass electrodes, *Adv. Colloid Interface Sci.* 114–115, 281–290, 2005.
5. Harpter, A., and Anderson, M.R., Electrochemical glucose sensors—developments using electrostatic assembly and carbon nanotubes for biosensor construction, *Sensors* (Basel) 10, 8248–1074, 2010.

ELECTRONEGATIVITY

Electronegativity is the tendency of an atom to attract electron forming a negative ion. The difference in electronegativity between atoms in a molecule results in polarity such as that seen in nucleophilic substitution reactions with compounds (e.g. bromoacetamide) with a primary halogen alpha to an electronegative function such as carbonyl group.[1]

1. Roberts, D.W., Schultz, T.W., Wolf, E.M., and Aptula, A.O., Experimental reactivity parameters for toxicity modeling: Application to the acute aquatic toxicity of SN2 electrophiles to *Tetrahymena pyriformis*, *Chem. Res. Toxicol.* 23, 228–234, 2010.

ELECTROPHORESIS

Electrophoresis is the separation of chemicals ranging from ions to very large DNA molecules based on their migration in an electric field. Electrophoresis may be performed without a supporting matrix such as free boundary electrophoresis or on a supporting matrix such as paper or polyacrylamide gel.[1] Capillary electrophoresis is used in combination with mass spectrometry for protein characterization.[2,3]

1. Westermeier, R., *Electrophoresis in Practice: A Guide to Methods and Applications of DNA and Protein Separations*, 5th edn., Wiley-VCh Verlag, Weinheim, Germany, 2016.
2. *Capillary Electrophoresis-Mass Spectrometry: Therapeutic Protein Characterization*, ed. J.Q. Xia and L. Zhang, Springer, Cham, Switzerland, 2016.
3. *Capillary Electrophoresis: Trends and Developments in Pharmaceutical Research,* ed. K. Suvardhan, Pan Stanford Publishing, Singapore, 2017.

ELISA

ELISA is an extensively used acronym for Enzyme-Linked Immunosorbent Assay which is an assay based on the reaction of an analyte, most often a protein, with a specific antibody. There are direct, indirect, direct sandwich, and indirect sandwich assay.[1–9] There is increasing use of aptamers in the place of protein antibodies in ELISA-based assays.[10–12]

1. Maggio, E.T., *Enzyme-Immunoassay*, CRC Press, Boca Raton, FL, 1980.
2. Kemeny, D.M., and Challacombe, S.J., *ELISA and Other Solid Phase Immunoassays: Theoretical and Practical Aspects,* Wiley, Chichester, UK, 1988.
3. Kemeny, D.M., *A Practical Guide to ELISA,* Pergamon Press, Oxford, UK, 1991.
4. Kerr, M.A., and Thorpe, R., *Immunochemistry LabFax*, Bios Scientific Publishers, Oxford, UK, 1994.
5. Law, B., *Immunoassay: A Practical Guide*, Taylor & Francis, London, UK, 1996.
6. Crowther, J.R., *The ELISA Guidebook*, Humana Press, Totowa, NJ, 2001.
7. Burns, R., *Immunochemical Protocols*, Humana Press, Totowa, NJ, 2005.
8. *The Immunoassay Handbook. Theory and Applications of Ligand Binding, ELISA and Related Techniques*, 4th edn., ed. D. Wild, Elsevier, Oxford, UK, 2013.
9. Tighe, P.J., Ryder, R.R, Todd, I., and Fairclough, L.C., ELISA in the multiplex era: Potentials and pitfalls, *Proteomics Clin. Appl.* 9, 406–422, 2017.
10. Li, P., Zhou, L., Wei, J., et al., Development and characterization of aptamer-based enzyme-linked apta-sorbent assay for the detection of Singapore grouper iridovirus infection, *J. Appl. Microbiol.* 121, 634–643, 2016.
11. Lee, K.H., and Zeng, H., Aptamer-based ELISA assay for highly specific and sensitive detection of Zika NS1 protein, *Anal. Chem.* 89, 12743–12748, 2017.
12. Shan, S., He, Z., Mao, S., et al., Quantitative determination of VEGF165 in cell culture medium by aptamer sandwich based chemiluminescence assay, *Talanta* 171, 197–203, 2017.

ELISPOT

The use of membranes to measure cells secreting a specific product such as an antibody or a cytokine.[1–11] A membrane (nitrocellulose or PDVF) containing an antibody or other specific binding protein is placed in a microtiter plate. Cells secreting a product, such as a cytokine, are grown in this plate and the secretion of the specific product evaluated in response to stimuli. As product is secreted from an individual cell, it is captured immediately by the antibody or other specific binding protein on the membrane and subsequently detected with a probe. An individual spot then corresponds to the secretion from a single cell. There are a number of instruments designed to measure such spots.

1. Kalyuzhny, A., *Handbook of ELISPOT: Methods and Protocols*, Totowa, NJ, 2005.
2. Stot, D.I., Immunoblotting, dot-blotting, and ELISPOT assay: Methods and applications, in *Immunochemistry*, ed. C.J. van Oss and M.H.V. van Regenmortel, Marcel Dekker, New York, Chapter 35, pp. 925–948, 1994.
3. Kalyuzhny, A.E., Chemistry and biology of the ELISPOT system, *Methods Mol. Biol.* 302, 15–31, 2005.
4. Periwal, S.B., Spagna, K., Shahabi, K., et al., Statistical evaluation for detection of peptide specific interferon-gamma secreting T-cells induced by HIV vaccine determined by ELISPOT assay, *J. Immunol. Methods* 305, 128–134, 2005.
5. Slota, M., Lim, J.B., Dang, Y., and Disis, M.L., ELISpot for measuring human immune responses to vaccines, *Expert Rev. Vaccines* 10, 299–306, 2011.
6. Lehman, P.V., and Zhang, W., Unique strengths of ELISPOT for T cell diagnostics, *Methods Mol. Biol.* 792, 3–23, 2012.
7. Weiss, A.J., Overview of membranes and membrane plates used in research and diagnostic ELISPOT assays, *Methods Mol. Biol.* 792, 243–256, 2012.
8. Augustine, J.J., and Hricik, D.E., T-cell immune monitoring by the ELISPOT assay for interferon gamma, *Clin. Chim. Acta* 413, 1359–1363, 2012.
9. Neubauer, J.C., Sébastien, I., Germann, A., et al., Towards standardized automated immunomonitoring: An automated ELISpot assay for safe and parallelized functionality analysis of immune cells, *Cytotechnology* 69, 57–73, 2017.
10. Conos, S.A., Lindqvist, M., and Vince, J.E., Simultaneous detection of cellular viability and interleukin-1β secretion from single cells by ELISpot, *Methods Mol. Biol.* 1714, 229–236, 2018.
11. Lehmann, A., Megyesi, Z., Przybyla, A., and Lehmann, P.V., Reagent tracker dyes permit quality control for verifying plating accuracy in ELISPOT tests, *Cells* 7(1), 3, 2018.

EMBEDDING

Embedding is frequently the infiltration of a tissue specimen with a liquid medium such as paraffin[1–6] that can be solidified/polymerized to form a matrix to support the tissue for subsequent manipulation, usually by microscopy. There are a variety of media used for embedding tissues depending on analytical need.

1. Hance, R.T., A new paraffin embedding mixture, *Science* 77, 353, 1933.
2. Popham, R.A., The importance of controlling cooling temperatures during embedding in paraffin, *Science* 106, 475–476, 1947.
3. Bell, A.W., On paraffin embedding, *Science* 107, 166, 1948.
4. Do, H., and Dobrovic, A., Sequence artifacts in DNA from formalin-fixed tissues: Causes and strategies for minimization, *Clin. Chem.* 61, 64–71, 2015.
5. McClelland, K.S., Ng, E.T., and Bowles, J., Agarose/gelatin immobilization of tissues or embryo segments for orientated paraffin embedding and sectioning, *Differentiation* 91, 68–71, 2016.
6. Guo, Z., and Lloyd, R.V., Use of monoclonal antibodies to detect specific mutations in formalin-fixed, paraffin-embedded tissue sections, *Hum. Pathol.* 53, 168–177, 2016.

ENDOCRINE

The term endocrine is usually in reference to a hormone or other biological effector such as peptide growth factor or cytokine such as insulin which has a systemic effect frequently distant from the site of synthesis and secretion. The term endocrine is in contrast to the term paracrine where an effector acts on an adjacent cell or cells[1] or autocrine where the effector acts on the cell of effector synthesis.[2]

1. Mayourian, J., Ceholski, D.K., Gonzalez, D.M., et al., Physiologic, pathologic, and therapeutic paracrine modulation of cardiac excitation-contraction coupling, *Circ. Res.* 122, 167–183, 2018.
2. Butera, G., Pacchiana, R., and Donadelli, M., Autocrine mechanisms of cancer chemoresistance, *Semin. Cell Dev. Biol.*, 78, 3–12, 2018.

ENDOPLASMIC RETICULUM-ASSOCIATED PROTEIN DEGRADATION (ERAD)

ERAD is a highly specific pathway for the degradation of misfolded proteins in the endoplasmic reticulum, which serves as a control mechanism for protein synthesis and secretion.[1–6]

1. Werner, E.D., Brodsky, J.L., and McCracken, A.A., Proteasome-dependent endoplasmic reticulum-associated protein degradation: An unconventional route to a familiar fate, *Proc. Natl. Acad. Sci. USA* 93, 13797–13801, 1996.

2. Meusser, B., Hirsch, C., Jarosch, E., and Sommer, T., ERAD: The long road to destruction, *Nature Cell Biol.* 7, 766–772, 2005.
3. Needham, P.G., and Brodsky, J.L., How early studies on secreted and membrane protein quality control gave rise to the ER associated degradation (ERAD) pathway: The early history of ERAD, *Biochim. Biphys. Acta* 1833, 2447–1457, 2013.
4. Goder, V., Roles of ubiquitin in endoplasmic reticulum-associated protein degradation (ERAD), *Curr. Protein Pept. Sci.* 13, 425–435, 2012.
5. Römisch, K., A case for Sec61 channel involvement in ERAD, *Trends Biochem. Sci.* 42, 171–179, 2017.
6. Roth, J., and Zuber, C., Quality control of glycoprotein folding and ERAD: The role of *N*-glycan handling, EDEM1 and OS-9, *Histochem. Cell Biol.* 147, 269–284, 2017.

ENDOSOME

The endosome is an intracellular vesicle or process functioning in the process of endocytosis. It provides a pathway for transport of ingested materials to the lysosome.[1] The endosome can be separated into two compartments or phases; the early endosome and late endosome. Materials taken in by endocytosis may be returned to the plasma membrane by a process referred to as recycling endocytosis.[2] Recycling endosomes are responsible for the sorting of endocytosed materials[3] via the *trans*-Golgi network.[4] Endosomes are important in the process of antigen presentation.[5–7]

1. Elkin, S.R., Lakoduk, A.M., and Schmid, S.L., Endocytotic pathways and endosomal trafficking: A primer, *Wien Med. Wochenschr.* 166, 196–204, 2016.
2. Scott, C.C., Vacca, F., and Grudenberg, J., Endosome maturation, transport and functions, *Semin. Cell Dev. Biol.* 31, 2–10, 2014.
3. Glendenning, J.R., Recycling endosomes, *Curr. Opin. Cell Biol.* 35, 117–122, 2015.
4. Makaraci, P., and Kim, K., *trans*-Golgi network-bound cargo traffic, *Eur. J. Cell Biol.*, 97. 137–149, 2018.
5. Heit, A., Schmitz, F., and Bauer, S., Targeting split vaccines to the endosome improves vaccination, *Curr. Opin. Biotechnol.* 15, 538–542, 2004.
6. Li, P., Gregg, J.L., Wang, N., Zhou, D., O'Donnell, P., Blum, J.S., and Crotzer, V.L., Compartmentalization of class II antigen presentation: Contribution of cytoplasmic and endosomal processing, *Immunol. Rev.* 207, 206–217, 2005.
7. Gleeson, P.A., The role of endosomes in innate and adaptive immunity, *Semin. Cell Dev. Biol.* 31, 64–72, 2014.

ENHANCER ELEMENTS

Enhancer elements are DNA sequences which increase transcription from a linked promoter region independent of operation and position (in contrast to proximal promoter elements).[1–4] Enhancer elements are located at varying distances upstream and downstream of the linked gene. There is recent interest in the role of **eRNA**, noncoding RNA encoded by enhancer sequences.[5–7]

1. Marand, A.P., Zhang, T., Zhu, B., and Jiang, J., Towards genome-wide prediction and characterization of enhancers in plants, *Biochim. Biophys. Acta.* 1860, 131–139, 2017.
2. Reiter, F., Wienerroither, S., and Stark, A., Combinatorial function of transcription factors and cofactors, *Curr. Opin. Genet. Dev.* 43, 73–81, 2017.
3. Hu, Z., and Tee, W.W., Enhancers and chromatin structures: Regulatory hubs in gene expression and diseases, *Biosci. Rep.* 37(2), BSR20160183, 2017.
4. Chatterjee, S., and Ahituv, N., Gene regulatory elements, major drivers of human disease, *Annu. Rev. Genomics Hum. Genet.* 18, 45–63, 2017.
5. Takemata, N., and Ohta, K., Role of noncoding RNA transcription around gene regulatory elements in transcription factor recruitment, *RNA Biol.* 14, 1–5, 2017.
6. Rothschild, G., and Basu, U., Lingering questions about enhancer RNA and enhancer transcription-coupled genomic instability, *Trends Genet.* 33, 143–154, 2017.
7. Liu, F., Enhancer-derived RNA: A primer, *Genomics Proteomics Bioinformatics* 15, 196–200, 2017.

ENSEMBL

Ensembl is a database[1] maintained by the European Bioinformatics Institute (EMBL-EBI).[2–6] This database organizes large amounts of biological information around the sequences of large genomes. The database is at http://useast.ensembl.org/index.html (February 14, 2018).

1. http://www.ensembl.org.
2. Birney, E., Andrews, T.D., Bevan, P., et al., An overview of Ensembl, *Genome Res.* 14, 925–928, 2004.
3. Baxevanis, A.D., Using genomic databases for sequence-based biological discovery, *Mol. Med.* 9, 185–192, 2003.
4. Stabenau, A., McVicker, G., Melsopp, C., Procter, G., Clamp, M., and Birney, E., The Ensembl core software libraries, *Genome Res.* 14, 929–933, 2004.
5. Yanai, I., Korbel, J.O., Boue, S., McWeeney, S.K., Bork, P., and Lercher, M.J., Similar gene expression profiles do not imply similar tissue functions, *Trends Genet.* 22, 132–138, 2006.
6. Galante, P.A., Sandhu, D., de Sousa Abreu, R., et al., A comprehensive in silico expression analysis of RNA binding proteins in normal and tumor tissue: Identification of potential players in tumor formation, *RNA Biol.* 6, 426–433, 2009.

EOXINS

Eoxins were originally described as a class of oxygenated derivatives formed from arachidonic acid by the initial action of 15-lipoxygenase-1 in human eosinophils and mass cells to form 14,15-epoxy-eicosatetraenoic acid (LTA_4; eoxin A_4) which is subsequently conjugated with glutathione form 14,15-LTC_4(eoxin C_4).[1-3] Eoxamides are related derivatives formed from an andamide.[4] Eoxins have been included in a larger group of oxidation products referred to as oxylipids.[5] It is noted that eoxin is used infrequently.

1. Feltenmark, S., Gautam, N., Brunnström, Å., et al., Eoxins are proinflammatory arachidonic acid metabolites produced via the 15-lipoxygenase-1 pathway in human eosinophils and mass cells, *Proc. Natl. Acad. Sci.* 105, 680–685, 2008.
2. Ono, E., Mita, H., Taniguchi, M., et al., Concentration of 14,15-leukotriene C4 (eoxin C4) in bronchoalveolar lavage fluid, *Clin. Exp. Allergy* 39, 1348–1352, 2009.
3. Brunnström, Å., Tryselius, Y., Feltenmark, S., et al., On the biosynthesis of 14-HETE and eoxin C4 by human airway epithelial cells, *Prostaglandins Other Lipid Mediat.* 121, 83–90, 2015.
4. Forsell, P.K.A., Brunnström, Å., Johannesson, M., and Claesson, H.-E., Metabolism of anandamide into eoxamides by 15-lipoxygenase-1 and glutathione transferase, *Lipids* 47, 781–791, 2012.
5. Gabbs, M., Leng, S., Devassy, J.G., Monirujjaman, M., and Aukema, H.M., Advances in our understanding of oxylipins derived from dietary PUFAs, *Adv. Nutr.* 6, 513–540, 2015.

Eph RECEPTORS/EPHRIN

Eph (erythropoietin-producing-hepatocellular carcinoma) receptors (*eph*, the largest known family of putative growth factor receptors)[1] are a family of receptor tyrosine kinases encoded by the *eph* gene.[2,3] The structure of Eph receptor is comprised of an extracellular domain, an intracellular domain containing a tyrosine kinase domain which are linked by a transmembrane segment.[4] Eph receptor bind to ephrin (ephrin family receptor interacting proteins).[5] Eph receptors and ephrin ligand are integral components of cell surfaces and their interactions mediate growth and development. There has been use of Eph to describe "edema-proteinuria-hypertension" in EPH-gestosis, better known as pre-eclampsia.[6,7]

1. Barquilla, A., and Pasquale, E.B., Eph receptors and ephrins: Therapeutic opportunities, *Annu. Rev. Pharmacol. Toxicol.* 55, 465–487, 2015.
2. Hirai, H., Maru, Y., Hagiwara, K., Nishida, J., and Takaku, F., A novel putative tyrosine kinase receptor encoded by the eph gene, *Science* 238, 1717–1720, 1987.
3. Letwin, K., Yee, S.P., and Pawson, T., Novel protein-tyrosine kinase cDNA related to fps/fes and eph cloned using anti-phosphotyrosine antibody, *Oncogene* 2, 621–627, 1988.
4. Kania, A., and Klein, R., Mechanism of ephrin-Eph signalling in development, physiology and disease, *Nat. Rev. Mol. Cell Biol.* 17. 240–256, 2016.
5. Eph nomenclature committee, Unified nomenclature for Eph family receptors and their ligands, the ephrins, *Cell* 90, 403–404, 1997.
6. Döderlein G., EPH-Gestosis Ophthaloskopie und Eklampsia Verhültung, *Munch. Med. Wochenschr.* 114, 745–748, 1972.
7. Galewska, Z., Bańkowski, E., Romanowicz, L., and Jaworski, S., Pre-eclampsia (EPH-gestosis)-induced decrease of MMP-s content in the umbilical cord artery, *Clin. Chim. Acta* 335, 109–115, 2003.

EPIGENOME

The epigenome is the sum of the various factors separate from the DNA backbone composed of nucleic acid bases which influence transcription.[1] **DNA methylation**[2] is the most highly studied process in the epigenome as the modification can be studied reliably in large number of samples.[3] Other factors in the epigenome are **histone modification**[4,5] and **associated acetylation reader domain** (bromodomain)[6-8] and **noncoding RNA interaction with DNA**.[9,10] The epigenome has been referred to as the second dimension to the genome.[11] See also **methylome**.

1. Susiarjo, M., Introduction to epigenetic mechanisms: The probable common thread for various developmental origins of health and disease effects, in *The Epigenome and Developmental Origins of Health and Disease,* ed. C.S. Rosenfeld, Academic Press/Elsevier, London, UK, 2016.
2. Cloverdale, L.E., and Cristofre, M.C., Epigenomics-genome-wide modifications of cytosine and new dimensions in our understanding of differentiation and disease, *Curr. Genomics* 6, 491–500, 2005.
3. Teschendorff, A.E., and Relton, C.L., Statistical and integrative system-level analysis of DNA methylation data, *Nat. Rev. Genet.* 19, 129–147, 2018.
4. Acharya, M.R., Sparreboom, A., Venitz, J., and Figg, W.D., Rational development of histone deacetylase inhibitors as anticancer agents, *Molec. Pharmacol.* 68, 917–932, 2005.
5. Fraga, M.F., and Esteller, M., Towards the human cancer epigenome: A first draft of histone modifications, *Cell Cycle* 4, 1377–1381, 2005.
6. Sanchez, R., Meslamani, J., and Zhou, M.M., The bromodomain: From epigenome reader to druggable target, *Biochim. Biophys. Acta* 1839, 676–685, 2014.
7. Gong, F., Chiu, L.Y., and Miller, K.M., Acetylation reader proteins: Linking acetylation signaling to genome maintenance and cancer, *PLoS Genet.* 12(9), e1006272, 2016.

8. Zaware, N., and Zhou, M.M., Chemical modulators for epigenome reader domains as emerging epigenetic therapies for cancer and inflammation, *Curr. Opin. Chem. Biol.* 39, 116–125, 2017.
9. Bhan, A., Soleimani, M., and Mandal, S.S., Long noncoding RNA and cancer: A new paradigm, *Cancer Res.* 77, 3965–3981, 2017.
10. Mathy, M., and Chen, X.M., Long noncoding RNAs (lncRNAs) and their transcriptional control of inflammatory responses, *J. Biol. Chem.* 292, 12375–12382, 2017.
11. Rivera, C.M., and Ron, B., Mapping human epigenomes, *Cell* 155, 39–55, 2013.

EPIGENETIC

Epigenetic refers to processes which influence the transcription of DNA separate from the genomic sequence of deoxyribonucleotides.[1,2] Examples of epigenetic modification include the formation of 5-methylcytosine and derivatives form such as 5-hydroxymethylcytosine and 5-formylcytosine,[3] the action of noncoding RNA,[4] and the chemical modification of histones such as acetylation, ADP-ribosylation, and phosphorylation.[5] See **epigenome, DNA methylation**.

1. Armstrong, L., *Epigenetics*, Garland Science/Taylor & Francis, New York, 2014.
2. Dawson, M.A., The cancer epigenome: Concepts, challenges, and therapeutic opportunities, *Science* 355, 1147–1152, 2017.
3. Plongthongkum, N., Diep, D.H., and Zhang, K., Advances in the profiling of DNA modifications: Cytosine methylation and beyond, *Nat. Rev. Genet.* 15, 647–661, 2014.
4. Peschansky, V.J., and Wahlestedt, C., Noncoding RNAs as direct and indirect modulators of epigenetic regulation, *Epigenetics* 9, 3–12, 2014.
5. Andreoli, F., and Del Rio, A., Physicochemical modifications of histones and their impact on epigenomics, *Drug Discov. Today* 19, 1372–1379, 2014.

EPITRANSCRIPTOME

The epitranscriptome is the sum of post-transcriptional modifications of RNA which affect the process of translation.[1–5]

1. Wetzel, C., and Limbach, P.A., Mass spectrometry of modified RNAs: Recent developments, *Analyst* 141, 16–23, 2016.
2. Schwartz, S., Cracking the epitranscriptome. *RNA* 22, 169–174, 2016.
3. Gilbert, W.W., Bell, T.A., and Schaening, C., Messenger RNA modifications: Form, distribution, and function, *Science* 352, 1408–1412, 2016.

4. Zhao, B.S., Roundtree, I.A., and He, C., *Nat. Rev. Mol. Cell. Biol.* 18, 31–42, 2017.
5. Eisenstein, M., Epitranscriptomics: Mixed messages, *Nat. Methods* 14, 15–17, 2017.

EPISTASIS

Epistasis can be defined as the effect or one or more genes on the expression of another gene or the effects of mutations on the phenotype caused by other mutations.[1] Epistasis analysis can be used to define order of gene expression in a genetic pathway.[2–5]

1. Segrè, D., Deluna, A., Church, G.M., and Kishony, R., Modular epistasis in yeast metabolism, *Nat. Genet.* 37, 77–83, 2005.
2. Starr, T.N., and Thornton, J.W., Epistasis in protein evolution, *Protein Sci.* 25, 1204–1218, 2016.
3. Storz, J.F., Compensatory mutations and epistasis for protein function, *Curr. Opin. Struct. Biol.* 50, 18–25, 2017.
4. Bendixsen, D.P., Østman, B., and Hayden, E.J., Negative epistasis in experimental RNA fitness landscapes, *J. Mol. Evol.* 85, 159–168, 2017.
5. Hook, M., Roy, S., Williams, E.G., et al., Genetic cartography of longevity in humans and mice: Current landscape and horizons, *Biochim. Biophys. Acta Mol. Basis Dis.* 1864, 2718–2732, 2018.

EPITOME

The epitome can be defined as all epitopes present in the antigenic universe[1–3] but the term is not extensively used. Epitome is also defined as example, paradigm; a brief presentation or statement.[4]

1. Schessinger, A., Ofran, Y., Yachdav, G., and Rost, B., Epitome: Database of structure-inferred antigenic epitopes, *Nucleic Acids Res.* 34, D777–D780, 2006.
2. Molero-Abraham, M., Glutting, J.P., Flower, D.R., Lafuente, E.M., and Reche, P.A., EPIPOX: Immunoinformatic characterization of the shared T-cell epitome between Variola virus and related pathogenic Orthopoxviruses, *J. Immunology. Res.* 2015, 738020, 2015.
3. Xu, W.X., Wang, J., Tang, H.P., Epitomics: IgG-epitome decoding of E6, E7 and L1 proteins from oncogenic human papillomavirus type 58, *Sci. Rep.* 6:34686, 2016.
4. *Oxford English Dictionary*, Oxford University Press, Oxford, UK, 2018.

ERK 1/2

Erks (extracellular signal-regulated kinases)[1] are serine-threonine protein kinases participating as the terminal effector in the Ras-Raf-MEK-ERK cascade/pathway (also known as the MAPK [mitogen-activated protein kinase pathway]).[2,3] There are two ERKs, ERK1 and ERK2, which are usually described as ERK 1/2 in the literature.[4-6] ERK 1/2 which show 84% sequence homology are converted to active forms by phosphorylation catalyzed by MEK (MAP/ERK kinase) kinases and in turn phosphorylate a large number of nuclear and cytoplasmic substrates.[7] The ERK kinases and related kinases are of great interest as drug targets in oncology.[8]

1. Boulton, T.G., and Cobb, M.H., Identification of multiple extracellular signal-regulated kinases (ERKs) with anti-peptide antibodies, *Cell Regul.* 2, 357–371, 1991.
2. De Luca, A., Maiello, M.R., D'Alessio, A., Pergameno, M., and Normanno, N., The RAS/RAF/MEK/ERK and the P13K/AKT signalling pathways: Role in cancer pathogenesis and implications for therapeutic approaches, *Expert Opin. Ther. Targets* 16(Suppl 2), S17–S27, 2012.
3. Roskowski, R., Jr., A historical overview of protein kinases and their targeted small molecule inhibitors, *Pharmacol. Res.* 100, 1–23, 2015.
4. Mehdizadeh, A., Somi, M.H., Darabi, M., and Jabbarpour-Bonyadi, M., Extracellular signal-regulated kinase 1 and 2 and cancer therapy: A focus on hepatocellular carcinoma, *Mol. Biol. Rep.* 43, 107–116, 2016.
5. Gonsalvez, D., Ferner, A.H., Peckham, H., Murray, S.S., and Xiao, J., The roles of extracellular related-kinases 1 and 2 signaling in CNS myelination, *Neuropharmacology* 110, 586–593, 2016.
6. Luo, F. Shi, J., Shi, Q., et al., Mitogen-activated protein kinases and hypoxic/ischemic neuropathy, *Cell Physiol. Biochem.* 39, 1051–1067, 2016.
7. Roskoski, R., Jr., ERK1/2 MAP kinases: Structure, function, and regulation, *Pharmacol. Res.* 66, 105–143, 2012.
8. Mandal, R., Becker, S., and Strebhardt, K., Stamping out RAF and ERK1/2 pathway: An emerging threat to anticancer therapy, *Oncogene* 35, 2457–2461, 2016.

ESSENTIAL OILS

Essential oils[1-3] describe a heterogeneous mixture of lipophilic substances originally obtained by steam distillation from a plant; also referred to as absolute oils. Steam distillation is still the preferred method of extraction of essential oils from plant biomass, although it is more carefully controlled to avoid decomposition of product.[4] The production of raw material (plant biomass) is also much more sophisticated.[5] Essential oils have a long history of use as aromatic products and in to what today would be referred to as alternative medicine.[6] There is extensive use of essential oils as a drug,[7] in transdermal drug delivery,[8] as an insecticide,[9] and in dermatology.[10] It is noted that there is a vast literature in the use of essential oils of which that cited herein is very small sample.

1. Gildenmeister, E., and Kremer, E., *The Volatile Oils*, 2nd edn., John Wiley & Sons, New York, 1913–1922.
2. *Bioessential Oils and Cancer*, ed. S.P. de Sousa, Springer, Cham, Switzerland, 2015.
3. *Handbook of Essential Oils Science, Technology and Applications,* ed. K. Husnu Can Baser and G. Buchbauer, CRC Press, Boca Raton, FL, 2015.
4. Schmidt, E., Production of essential oils, in *Handbook of Essential Oils Science, Technology and Applications,* ed. K. Husnu Can Baser and G. Buchbauer, Chapter 5, pp. 122–164, CRC Press, Boca Raton, FL, 2015.
5. Franz, C., and Novak, J., sources of essential oils, in *Handbook of Essential Oils Science, Technology and Applications,* ed. K. Husnu Can Baser and G. Buchbauer, Chapter 3, pp. 43–86, CRC Press, Boca Raton, FL, 2015.
6. Kubeczka, K.-H., History and sources of essential oil research, in *Handbook of Essential Oils Science, Technology and Applications,* ed. K. Husnu Can Baser and G. Buchbauer, Chapter 2, pp. 33–42, CRC Press, Boca Raton, FL, 2015.
7. Pina, L.T.S., Ferro, J.N.S., Rabelo, T.K., et al., Alcoholic monoterpenes found in essential oil of aromatic spices reduce allergic inflammation by the modulation of inflammatory cytokines, *Nat. Prod. Res.*, 33, 1773–1777, 2019.
8. Eid, R.K., Essa, E.A., and El Maghraby, G.M., Essential oils in niosomes for enhanced transdermal delivery of delodipine, *Pharm. Dev. Technol.* 24, 157–165, 2019.
9. Candy, K., Nicolas, P., Andriantsanirina, V., Izri, A., and Durand, R., In vitro efficacy of five essential oils against *Pediculus humanus captitus*, *Paristol. Res.* 117, 603–609, 2018.
10. Zeichner, J.A., Berson, D., and Donald, A., The use of an over-the-counter hand cream with sweet almond oil for the treatment of hand dermatitis, *J. Drug. Dermatol.* 17, 78–82, 2018.

EUROFAN

EUROFAN (European Functional Analysis Network) was established to elucidate the physiological and biochemical functions of open reading frames in yeast.[1-7] It is not clear that EUROFAN is still an active network.

1. http://mips.gsf.de/proj/eurofan/.
2. Sanchez, J.C., Golaz, O., Frutiger, S., et al., The yeast SWISS-2DPAGE database, *Electrophoresis* 17, 556–565, 1996.
3. Dujon, B., European Functional Analysis Netword (EUROFAN) and the functional analysis of the *Saccharomyces cerevisiae* genome, *Electrophoresis* 19, 617–624, 1998.
4. Bianchi, M.M., Ngo, S., Vandenbol, M., et al., Large-scale phenotypic analysis reveals identical contributions to cell functions of known and unknown yeast genes, *Yeast* 18, 1397–1412, 2001.

5. Avaro, S., Belgareh, N., Sibella-Arguelles, C., et al., Mutants defective in secretory/vacuolar pathways in the EUROFAN collection of yeast disruptants, *Yeast* 19, 351–371, 2002.
6. Castrillo, J.I., Hayes, A., Mohammed, S., Gaskell, S.J., and Oliver, S.G., An optimized protocol for metabolome analysis in yeast using direct infusion electrospray mass spectrometry, *Phytochemistry* 62, 929–937. 2003.
7. Davydenko, S.G., Juselius, J.K., Munder, T., Bogengruber, E., Jantti, J., and Keranen, S., Screening for novel essential genes of *Saccharomyces cerevisiae* involved in protein secretion, *Yeast* 21, 463–471, 2004.

EUTECTIC

A eutectic is a mixture of components in such proportions that said mixture melts and solidifies as a single temperature lower than the melting points of the constituents or any other mixture of the components; usually depicted a point in diagram.[1] This is an issue with cryobiology and therapeutic protein processing processes such as lyophilization.[2–5] A **deep eutectic solvent** is formed from a mixture of Brønsted or Lewis acids or bases to form a eutectic containing a mixture of anionic and/or cationic species.[6,7] Examples of deep eutectic solvents are a mixture of choline chloride and ethylene glycol, known as ethaline[8] and a mixture of choline chloride and 1,2,3-propanetriol(glycerol), known as glyceline.[9] There is considerable interest the use of deep eutectic solvents in green chemistry.[10–12] There are studies on the stability of proteins in deep eutectic solvents[13] supporting application in bioprocessing.[14,15]

1. *Oxford English Dictionary*, Oxford University Press, Oxford, UK.
2. Gutierrez-Merino, C., Quantitation of the Forster energy transfer for two-dimensional systems. II. Protein distribution and aggregation state in biological membranes, *Biophys. Chem.* 14, 259–266, 1981.
3. Gatlin, L.A., and Nail, S.L., Protein purification process engineering. Freeze drying: A practical overview, *Bioprocess Technol.* 18, 317–367, 1994.
4. Nail, S.L., Jiang, S., Chongprasert, S., and Knopp, S.A., Fundamentals of freeze-drying, *Pharm. Biotechnol.* 14, 281–360, 2002.
5. Han, B., and Bischof, J.C., Thermodynamic nonequilibrium phase change behavior and thermal properties of biological solutions for cryobiology applications, *J. Biomech. Eng.* 126, 196–203, 2004.
6. Patel, K., Munjal, B., and Bansal, A.K., Effect of cyclophosphamide on the solid form of mannitol during lyophilization, *Eur. J. Pharm. Sci.* 101, 251–257, 2017.
7. Li, X., and Row, K.H., Development of deep eutectic solvents applied in extraction and separation, *J. Sep. Sci.* 39, 3505–3520, 2016.
8. Prasad, K., Mondal, D., Sharma, M., et al., Stimuli responsive ion gels based on polysaccharides and other polymers prepared using ionic liquids and deep eutectic solvents, *Carbohydrate Polym.* 180, 328–336, 2018.
9. de La Harpe, K., Kohl, F.R., Zhang, Y., and Kohler, B., Excited state dynamics of a DNA duplex in a deep eutectic solvent probed by femtosecond time-resolved IR spectroscopy, *J. Phys. Chem. A*, 122, 2437–2444, 2018.
10. Kim, K.-S., and Heung, B., Volumetric properties of solutions of choline chloride+glycerol deep eutectic solvent with water, methanol, ethanol, and iso-propanol, *J. Mol. Liquids* 254, 272–279, 2018.
11. Zhu, S., Liu, D., Zhu, X., et al., Extraction of illegal dyes from red chili peppers with cholinium-based deep eutectic solvents, *J. Anal. Methods Chem.* 2017, 2753752, 2018.
12. Fernández, M.L.Á., Espino, M., Gomez, F.J.V., and Silva, M.F., Novel approaches mediated by tailor-made green solvents for the extraction of phenolic compounds from agro-food industrial by-products, *Food Chem.* 239, 671–678, 2018.
13. Morais, E.S., Mendonca, P.V., Coelho, J.F.J., et al., Deep eutectic solvents aqueous solutions as efficient media for the solubilization of hardwood xylans, *ChemSusChem.* 11, 753–776, 2018.
14. Monhemi, H., Housaindokht, M.R., Moosavi-Movahedi, A.A., and Bozorgmehr, M.R., How a protein can remain stable in a solvent with high content of urea: Insights from molecular dynamics simulation of *Candida anartica* lipase B in urea:choline chloride deep eutectic solvent, *Phys. Chem. Chem. Phys.* 16, 14882–14893, 2014.
15. Chen, Z., and Wan, C., Ultrafast fractionation of lignocellulosic biomass by microwave-assisted deep eutectic solvent pretreatment, *Biosour. Technol.* 250, 532–547, 2017.

EXON

An exon is that region of a genomic DNA sequence that is encoded into a primary RNA transcript and codes for a protein. Exons are separated by introns in eukaryotes and the combination of introns and exons is referred to as a transcriptional unit. There is an average of 10.4 exons per gene in the human genome.[1] The primary RNA transcript is processed by spicing to yield the final mRNA product.[2] Alternative splicing of a primary RNA transcript can yield different protein products.[3] See **intron**.

1. Alberts, B., Johnson, A., Lewis, J., Raff, M., Roberts, K., and Walter, P., *Molecular Biology of the Cell*, 5th edn., Chapter 2, Garland Science/Taylor & Francis Group, New York, 2008.
2. Shi, Y., Mechanistic insights into precursor messenger RNA splicing by the spliceosome, *Nat. Rev. Mol. Cell Biol.* 18, 655–670, 2017.

3. Naftelberg, S., Schor, I.E., Ast, G., and Kornblihtt, A.R., Regulation of alternative splicing through coupling with transcription and chromatin structure, *Annu. Rev. Biochem.* 84, 165–198, 2015.

11. Gurbaxanin, B., Dostalek, M., and Gardner, I., Are endosomal trafficking parameters better targets for improving mAB pharmacokinetics than FcRn binding affinity? *Mol. Immunol.* 56, 660–674, 2013.

EXOSOME

Exosomes are analogous to **endosomes** in being intracellular vesicles which participate in the process of exocytosis, that is the process of exporting materials from the cell[1,2] and are of considerable interest in cancer and other pathologies.[3,4] Exosomes can be biomarkers[5,6] and facilitate the immune response.[7,8] Exosomes are likely involved in the mechanisms by which binding to FcRn extend IgG circulatory half-life.[9–11]

1. Stoorvogel, W., Kleijmeer, M.J., Geuze, H.J., and Raposo, G., The biogenesis and functions of exosomes, *Traffic* 3, 321–330, 2002.
2. Février, B., and Raposo, G., Exosomes: Endosomal derived vesicles shipping extracellular messages, *Curr. Opin. Cell Biol.* 16, 415–421, 2004.
3. Barile, L., Milano, G., and Vassalli, G., Beneficial effects of exosomes secreted by cardiac-derived progenitor cells and other cell types in myocardial ischemia, *Stem Cell Investig.* 4, 93, 2017.
4. Bjørge, I.M., Kim, S.Y., Mano, J.F., Kalionis, B., and Chrzanowski, W., Extracellular vesicles, exosomes and shedding vesicles in regenerative medicine—A new paradigm for tissue repair, *Biomater. Sci.* 6, 60–78, 2017.
5. Caradec, K., Kharmate, G., Hosseini-Beheshti, E., Adomat, H., et al., Reproducibility and efficiency of serum-derived exosome extraction methods, *Clin. Biochem.* 47, 1286–1292, 2014.
6. Reclusa, P., Taverna, S., Pucci, M., et al., Exosomes as diagnostic and predictive biomarkers in lung cancer, *J. Thorac. Dis.* 9(Suppl 13), S1737–S1382, 2017.
7. Martin, R.K., Brooks, K.B., Henningsson, F., Heyman, B., and Conrad, D.H. Antigen transfer from exosomes to dendritic cells as an explanation for the immune enhancement by IgE immune complexes, *PLoS One* 9(10), 110609, 2014.
8. Lindenbergh, M.F.S., and Stoorvogel, W., Antigen presentation by extracellular vesicles from professional antigen-presenting cells, *Annu. Rev. Immunol.*, 36, 435–459, 2018.
9. Lencer, W.I., and Blumberg, R.S., A passionate kiss, then run: Exocytosis and recycling of IgG by FcRn, *Trends Cell Biol.* 15, 5–9, 2005.
10. Suzuki, T., Ishii-Watabe, A., Tada, M., et al., Importance of neonatal FcR in regulating the serum half-life of therapeutic proteins containing the Fc domain of human IgG1: A comparative study of the affinity of monoclonal antibodies and Fc-fusion proteins to human neonatal FcR, *J. Immunol.* 184, 1968–1976, 2010.

EXPANSINS

Expansins are small (20–30 kDa) plant proteins that induce the cell wall loosening essential for plant growth described in 1992[1] and cloned/sequenced in 1994.[2] The nonezymatic mechanism of cell wall expansion results from the loosening of interactions of cellulose with matrix components such as pectin or with cellulose microfibrils.[3] There are microbial and fungal expansins, which have pathological and mutualistic symbiotic relationships.[4]

1. McQueen-Mason, S., Durachko, D.M., and Cosgrove, D.J., Two endogenous proteins that induce cell wall extension in plants, *Plant Cell* 4, 1425–1433, 1992.
2. Shcherban, T.Y., Shi, J., Durachko, D.M., et al., Molecular cloning and sequence analysis of expansins—A highly conserved multigene family of proteins that mediate cell wall extension in plants, *Proc. Natl. Acad. Sci. USA* 92, 9345–9249, 1995.
3. Cosgrove, D.J., Plant expansins: Diversity and interactions with plant cell walls, *Curr. Opin. Plant Biol.* 25, 162–172, 2015.
4. Cosgrove, D.J., Microbial expansins, *Annu. Rev. Microbiol.* 71, 479–497, 2017.

EXPRESSED SEQUENCE TAG

An expressed sequence tag (EST) is a short sequence of DNA (approximately 200 base pairs long) which located in cDNA (coding DNA); cDNA is the product of "reverse translation" (catalyzed by reverse transcriptase) of mRNA. Thus, as EST is a product which may or may not code for a functional protein. ESTs were developed as an approach to sequencing the human genome[1,2] and therefore can be used to identify the parent gene for the product expressed by the DNA and thus map the position of that gene in a genome.[3–6] There are a number of uses of ESTs.[7] ESTs are used with simple sequence repeats (microsatellites, short tandem repeats in population genetics[8] including the speciation of olive trees.[9]

1. Adams, M.D., Kelley, J.M., Gocayne, J.D., et al., Complementary DNA sequencing expressed sequence tags and human genome project, *Science* 252, 1651–1666, 1991.
2. Adams, M.D, Dubnick, M., Kerlavage, A.R., et al., Sequence identification of 2,375 human brain genes, *Nature* 355, 632–634, 1992.

3. Polymeropoulos, M.H., Xiao, H., Glodek, M., et al., Chromosomal assignment of 46 brain cDNAs, *Genomics* 12, 492–496, 1992.

4. Claverie, J.M., Hardelin, J.P., Legouis, R., et al., Characterization and chromosomal assignment of a human cDNA encoding a protein related to the murine 102-kDa cadherin-associated protein (α-catenin), *Genomics* 15, 13–20, 1993.

5. Gerhold, D., and Caskey, C.T., It's the genes! EST access to human genome content, *Bioessays* 18, 973–981, 1996.

6. Hoffman, M., Gene expression patterns in human and mouse B cell development, *Curr. Top. Microbiol. Immunol.* 294, 19–29, 2005.

7. Wilson, A.K, Expression sequence tags, in *Encyclopedia of Molecular Biology*, ed. T.E. Creighton, John Wiley & Sons, New York, 1999.

8. Khimoun, A., Ollivier, A., Faivre, B., and Garnier, S., Level of genetic differentiation affects relative performance of expressed sequence tag and genomic SSRs, *Mol. Ecol. Resour.* 17, 893–903, 2017.

9. Mousavi, S., Mariotti, R., Regni, L., et al., The first molecular identification of an olive collection applying standard simple sequence repeats and novel expressed sequence tag markers, *Front. Plant. Sci.* 8, 1283, 2017.

GENE EXPRESSION PROFILING

Gene expression profiling is the measurement or determination of DNA (cDNA) expression by the measurement of mRNA (transcriptomics) or by determination of protein expression as determined by proteomic technology. Specific gene expression can be evaluated by a variety of techniques[1] including **microarray analysis**[2] and **RNA-Seq**.[3] A gene signature is the expression profiling under specific physiologic conditions.[4] Proteomics is being used for gene expression profiling.[5-7]

1. Melouane, A., Ghanemi, A. Aubé, S., Yoshioka, M., and St-Amand, J., Differential gene expression analysis in ageing muscle and drug discovery perspectives, *Ageing Res. Rev.* 41, 53–63, 2018.

2. Kappelhoff, R., Puente, X.S., Wilson, C.H., et al., Overview of transcriptomic analysis of all human proteases, non-proteolytic homologs and inhibitors: Organ, tissue and ovarian cancer cell line expression profiling of the human protease degradome by the CLIP-CHIP™ DNA microarray, *Biochim. Biophys. Acta* 1864, 2210–2219, 2017.

3. Costa-Silva, J., Domingues, D., and Lopes, F.M., RNA-Seq differential expression analysis: Ana extended review and a software tool, *PLoS One* 12(12), 0190152, 2017.

4. Xu, J., Gong, B., Wu, L., et al., Comprehensive assignments of RNA-seq by the SEQC Consortium: FDA-led efforts advance precision medicine, *Pharmaceutics* 8(1), 8, 2016.

5. Ciuffa, R., Caron, E., Leitner, A., et al., Contribution of mass spectrometry-based proteomics to the understanding of TNF-α signaling, *J. Proteome Res.* 16, 14–33, 2017.

6. Fels, U., Gevaert, K., and Van Damme, P., Proteoegenomics in aid of host-pathogen interaction studies: A bacterial perspective, *Proteomes* 5(4), 26, 2017.

7. Mardamshina, M., and Geiger, T., Next-generation proteomics and its applications top clinical breast cancer research, *Am. J. Pathol.* 187, 2175–2184, 2017.

EXPRESSION LEAKAGE

Expression leakage is a concept where the functionally important expression of one gene can result in the ectopic expression of a neighboring gene resulting in apparent expression similarity between tissues (ectopic expression).[1-3]

1. Yanai, I., Korbel, J.O., Boue, S., McWeeney, S.K., Bork, P., and Lercher, M.J., Similar gene expression profiles do not imply similar tissue functions, *Trends Genet.* 22, 132–138, 2006.

2. Dashkoff, J., Lerner, E.P., Truong, N., et al., Tailored transgene expression to specific cell types in the central nervous system after peripheral injection with AAV9, *Mol. Ther. Methods Clin. Dev.* 3, 16081, 2016.

3. Agahonov, M.O., Improvement of a yeast self-excising integrating vector by prevention of expression leakage of the intronated Cre recombinase gene during plasmid maintenance in *Escherichia coli*, *FEMS Microbiol. Lett.* 364, fnx222, 2017.

FAMILIES OF STRUCTURALLY SIMILAR PROTEINS (FSSP)

Families of structurally similar proteins (FSSP) is a database based on three-dimensional comparisons of protein structures.[1-6] It was not possible to find recent use of this database.

1. http://ekhidna.biocenter.helsinki.fi/dali/start.

2. Holm, L., Ouzounis, C., Sander, C., Tuparev, G., and Vriend, G., A database of protein structure families with common folding motifs, *Protein Sci.* 1, 1691–1698, 1992.

3. Holm, L., and Sander, C., The FSSP database: Fold classification based on structure alignment of proteins, *Nucleic Acids Res.* 24, 206–209, 1996.

4. Notredame, C., Holm, L., and Higgins, D.G., COFFEE: An objective function for multiple sequence alignments, *Bioinformatics* 14, 407–422, 1998.

5. Hadley, C., and Jones, D.T., A systematic comparison of protein structure classifications: SCOP, CATH and FSSP, *Structure* 7, 1099–1112, 1999.

6. Getz, G., Vendruscolo, M., Sachs, D., and Domany, E., Automated assignment of SCOP and CATH protein structure classifications from FSSP scores, *Proteins* 46, 405–415, 2002.

9. Gutteridge, J.M.C., Iron promoters of the Fenton reaction and lipid peroxidation can be release from haemoglobin by peroxides, *FEBS Lett.* 201, 291–295, 1986.
10. Goldstein, S., Meyerstein, D., and Czapski, G., The Fenton reagents, *Free Radic. Biol. Med.* 15, 435–445, 1993.

FENTON REACTION

The Fenton Reaction is a ferrous ion-dependent formation of hydroxyl radical from hydrogen peroxide which can be coupled with the oxidation of hydroxyl function to ketone/aldehydes.[1–4] The photo-Fenton reaction where light ($\lambda > 320$ nm) is used irradiate an aqueous solution of Fe^{2+} and H_2O_2 oxidizes substrates much faster than a similar reaction in the dark.[5] Subsequent work has shown that oxygen can partially replace H_2O_2 in the photo-Fenton reaction.[6] The Fenton reaction is used for the removal of toxic materials from wastewater.[7] There is use of heterogeneous catalysis in the treatment of wastewater.[8] There are examples of Fenton reactions *in vivo* where small amounts of iron become available either from leakage from ferroproteins such as hemoglobin.[9] While the canonical interpretation of the oxidation mechanism of Fenton reaction is based on the hydroxyl radical, there are other interpretations.[10]

1. Fenton, H.J.H., Oxidation of certain organic acids in the presence of ferrous salts, *Proc. Chem. Soc.* 15, 224–228, 1899.
2. Goldstein, S., Meyerstein, D., and Czapski, G., The Fenton reagents, *Free Rad. Biol. Med.* 15, 435–445, 1993.
3. Odyuo, M.M., and Sharan, R.N., Differential DNA strand breaking abilities of ·OH and ROS generating radiomimetic chemicals and γ-rays: Study of plasmid dNA, pMTa4, *in vitro*, *Free Rad. Res.* 39, 499–505, 2005.
4. Stadtman, E.R., Role of oxidized amino acids in protein breakdown and stability, *Meth. Enzymol.* 258, 379–393, 1995.
5. Ruppert, G., and Bauer, R., The photo-Fenton reaction— An effective photochemical wastewater treatment process, *J. Photochem. Photobiol.* 73, 75–78, 1993.
6. Utset, B., Garcia, J., Casado, J., Domènech, X., and Peral, J., Replacement of H_2O_2 by O_2 in Fenton and photo-Fenton reactions, *Chemosphere* 41, 1187–1192, 2000.
7. Wen, D., Wu, Z., Tang, Y., Li, M., and Qiang, Z., Accelerated degradation of sulfamethazine in water by VUV/UV photo-Fenton process: Impact of sulfamethazine concentration on reaction mechanism, *J. Hazard Mater.* 344, 1181–1187, 2018.
8. Mirzaei, A., Chen, Z., Haghighat, F., and Yerushalmi, L., Removal of pharmaceuticals from water by homo/heterogonous Fenton-type processes—A review, *Chemosphere* 174, 665–688, 2017.

FERMENTATION

The controlled aerobic or anaerobic process where a product is produced by yeast, molds, or bacteria from a substrate. Historically, fermentation was used to describe the action of a leavan (yeast) on a carbohydrate (saccharine) as in the production of beers and wines or a dough such as in making bread. The term **fermentation** is used to describe the use of yeast or bacteria while the term **cell culture** is used to describe the use of animal cells or plants cells.[1–5] Fermentation technology is of particular value in the production of specialized biochemicals[6] including amino acids.[7] Fermentation technology is used for the production of biopharmaceutical products.[8–10]

1. Wiseman, A., *Principles of Biotechnology*, Chapman and Hall, New York, 1983.
2. Sinclair, C.G., Kristiansen, B., and Bu'Lock, L.D., *Fermentation Kinetics and Modelling*, Open University Press, New York, 1987.
3. *The Encyclopedia of Bioprocess Technology*, ed. M.C. Flickinger and S.W. Drew, Wiley, New York, 1999.
4. *Molecular Biology and Biotechnology*, ed. J.M. Walker and R. Rapley, Royal Society of Chemistry, Cambridge, UK, 2000.
5. *Fermentation Biotechnology*, ed. S.C. Badal, American Chemical Society, Washington, DC, 2003.
6. Dai, K., Wen, J.L., Zhang, F., and Zeng, R.J., Valuable biochemical production in mixed culture fermentation: Fundamentals and process coupling, *Appl. Microbiol. Biotechnol.* 101, 6575–6586, 2017.
7. *Amino Acid Fermentation*, ed. A. Yokota and M. Ikeda, Springer, Tokyo, Japan, 2017.
8. Altman, R.D., Bedi, A., Karlsson, J., Sancheti, P., and Schemitsch, E., Product differences in intra-articular hyaluronic acids for osteoarthritis of the knee, *Am. J. Sports Med.* 44, 2158–2165, 2016.
9. Wang, J., Xiao, H., Qian, Z.G., and Zhong, J.J., Bioproduction of antibody-drug conjugate payload precursors by engineered cell factories, *Trends Biotechnol.* 35, 466–478, 2017.
10. Gupta, S.K., and Shukla, P., Sophisticated cloning, fermentation, and purification technologies for an enhanced therapeutic protein production: A review, *Front. Pharmacol.* 8, 419, 2017.

FERREDOXIN

Ferredoxin is a small protein (6 kDa in bacteria, 12 kDa in chloroplasts) which functions in the transport of electrons (reducing potential) in a variety of organisms.

There are several classes of ferredoxins based on the nature of the chemistry of iron binding: Fe_2S_2, Fe_3S_4, Fe_4S_4.[1-4] Ferredoxin is a critical component of photosystem I in plants.[5-8] Adrenodoxin is mammalian protein (Mr = 14.4 kDa)[9] which interacts with cytochrome P450 proteins.[10]

1. Orme-Johnson, W.H., and Holm, R.H., Identification of iron-sulfur clusters in proteins, *Methods Enzymol.* 53, 268–274, 1978. The iron is bound to cysteine residues in a cluster which also contains inorganic sulfur.
2. Orme-Johnson, W.H., and Orme-Johnson, N.R., Overview of iron—Sulfur proteins, *Methods Enzymol.* 53, 259–268, 1978.
3. Fox, N.G., Chakrabarti, M., McCormick, S.P., Lindahl, P.A., and Barondeau, D.P., The human iron-sulfur assembly complex catalyzes the synthesis of [2Fe-2S] clusters on ISCU2 that can be transferred to acceptor molecules, *Biochemistry* 54, 3871–3879, 2015.
4. Boniecki, M.T., Freibert, S.A., Mühlenhoff, U., Lilli, R., and Cygler, M., Structure and functional dynamics of the mitochondrial Fe/S cluster synthesis complex, *Nat. Commun.* 8(1), 1287, 2017.
5. San Pietro, A., A personal historical introduction of photosystem I: Ferredoxin + FNR, the key to NADP+ reduction, in *Photosystem I: The Light-Driven Photosystem: Ferredoxin Reductase*, ed. J.H. Goldbeck, Chapter 1, pp. 1–8, Springer, Dordrecht, the Netherlands, 2006.
6. Hanke, G., and Mulo, P., Plant type ferredoxins and ferredoxin-dependent metabolism, *Plant Cell Environ.* 36, 1071–1084, 2013.
7. Pierella Karlusish, J.J., and Carrillo, N., Evolution of the acceptor side of photosystem I: Ferredoxin, flavodoxin, and ferredoxin-NADP+ oxidoreductase, *Photosynth. Res.* 134, 235–250, 2017.
8. Mulo, P., and Medina, M., Interaction and electron transfer between ferredoxin-NADP+ oxidoreductase and its partners: Structural, functional, and physiological implications, *Photosynth. Res.* 134, 265–280, 2017.
9. Grinberg, A.V., Hannemann, F., Schiffler, B., et al., Adrenodoxin: Structure, stability, and electron transfer properties, *Proteins: Structure, Function, and Generics* 40, 598–612, 2000.
10. Ewen, K.M., Ringle, M., and Bernhardt, R., Adrenodoxin—A versatile ferredoxin, *IUBMB Life* 64, 506–512, 2012.

FERET DIAMETER

The ferret diameter is the perpendicular distance between two tangents touching opposite sides of a profile of a particle.[1] It also referred to as the caliper diameter in reference to the instrument frequently used for measurement of the feret diameter. The Feret diameter is a value used in characterization of particles[2] and irregular biological objects.[3-5]

1. Walton, W.H., Feret's statistical diameter as a measure of particle size, *Nature* 162, 329–330, 1948.
2. Levin, M., Particle characterization—Tools and Methods, *Laboratory Equipment*, November, 2005.
3. Xia, C., and Xia, Z., Nuclear volume estimation using different sampling, measurement and calculation methods, *Anal. Quant. Cytol. Histol.* 22, 258–262, 2000.
4. Thakur, G., Mitra, A., Basak, A., and Sheet, D., Characterization and scanning electron microscopic investigation of crosslinked freeze dried gelatin matrices for study of drug diffusivity and release kinetics, *Micron* 43, 311–320, 2012.
5. Nghiem, P.P., Kornegay, J.N., Uaesoontrachoon, K., et al., Osteopontin is linked with AKT, Fox01, and myostatin in skeletal muscle cells, *Muscle Nerve* 56, 1119–1127, 2017.

FERTILITY PLASMID

The fertility plasmid (F-plasmid) in bacteria contains the *tra* gene (a transfer gene)[1] and is capable of conjugation (contact-dependent DNA transfer) in bacterial sexual expression (horizontal gene transfer).[2,3] The F-plasmid is of importance in the use of bacterial artificial chromosomes for genomic cloning.[4] **Bacterial artificial chromosomes** are built on the fertility plasmid.[5,6]

1. Johnson, D.A, and Willetts, N.S., λ-Transducing phages carrying transfer genes isolated from an abnormal prophage insertion into the traY gene of F-plasmid, *Plasmid* 9, 71–85, 1983.
2. Koraimann, G., and Wager, M.A., Social behavior and decision making in bacterial conjugation, *Front. Cell. Infect. Microbiol.* 4, 54, 2014.
3. Johnson, C.M., and Grossman, A.D., Integrative and conjugative elements (ICEs): What do they do and how do they work), *Annu. Rev. Genet.* 49, 577–601, 2015.
4. Schalkwyk, L.C., Francis, F., and Lehrach, H., Techniques in mammalian genome mapping, *Curr. Opin. Biotechnol.* 6, 37–43, 1995.
5. Schalkwyk, L.C., Francis, F., and Lehrach, H., Techniques in mammalian genome mapping, *Curr. Opin. Biotechnol.* 6, 37–43, 1995.
6. Kurnaz, I.A., *Techniques in Genetic Engineering*, CRC/Taylor & Francis Group, Boca Raton, FL, 2015.

FIBRILLATION

Fibrillation is the process of forming fibers (fibrillar material from small, soluble polymeric materials which have distinct properties.[1-3] The term fibrillation is used to describe the process responsible for the formation of amyloid fibrils in Alzheimer's disease.[4] Fibrillation of pharmaceutical proteins and peptides has been of interest.[5-8] There has been specific interest in the fibrillation of insulin.[9-11] Fibrillation is a property of misfolded/

intrinsically disordered proteins.[12–15] The term fibrillation was used in the nineteenth century to describe the physical changes in blood as a result of clotting before the elucidation of the process of fibrinogen clotting. The term fibrillation is also used to describe physical changes in structural materials such as ligaments and tendons[16] as well cardiovascular events.[17]

1. *Amyloid Fibrils and Profibrillare Aggregates: Molecular and Biological Properties,* ed. D.E. Otzen, Wiley, Weinheim, Germany, 2013.
2. Kurouski, D., Van Duyne, R.P., and Lednev, I.K., Exploring the structure and formation mechanism of amyloid fibrils by Raman spectroscopy: A review, *Analyst* 140, 4967–4980, 2015.
3. *Protein Amyloid Aggregates: Methods and Protocols*, ed. D. Eliezer, Humana/Springer, New York, 2015.
4. Luo, J., Wärmländer, S.K., Gräslund, A., and Abrahams, J.P., Cross-interactions between the Azlheimer disease amyloid-β peptide and other amyloid proteins: A further aspect of the amyloid cascade hypothesis, *J. Biol. Chem.* 291, 16485–16493, 2016.
5. Ricci, C., Spinnozzi, F., Mariani, P., and Ontore, M.G., Protein amyloidogenesis investigated by small angle scattering, *Curr. Pharm. Des.* 22, 3937–3949, 2016.
6. Mahmoudi, M., Kalhor, H.R., Laurent, S., and Lynch, I., Protein fibrillation and nanoparticle interactions: Opportunities and challenges, *Nanoscale* 5, 2570–2588, 2013.
7. Wang, S., Zhang, X., Wu., G., Tian, Z., and Qian, J., Optimization of high-concentration endostatin formulation: Harmonization of excipients' contributions on colloidal and conformational stabilities, *Int. J. Pharm.* 530, 173–186, 2017.
8. Shang, H., Chen, X., Liu, Y., et al., Cucurbit [7]-assisted sustained release of human calcitonin from thermosensitive block copolymer hydrogel, *Int. J. Pharm.* 527, 52–60, 2017.
9. Brange, J., and Langkjoer, L., Insulin structure and stability, *Pharm. Biotechnol.* 5, 315–350, 1993.
10. Groenning, M., Frokjaer, S., and Vestergaard, B., Formation mechanism of insulin fibrils and structural aspects of the insulin fibrillation process, *Curr. Protein Pept. Sci.* 10, 509–528, 2009.
11. Alam, P., Beg, A.Z., Siddiqi, M.K., et al., Ascorbic acid inhibits human insulin aggregation and protects against amyloid induced cytotoxicity, *Arch. Biochem. Biophys.* 621, 54–62, 2017.
12. Jesús-Kim, L.D., Hernández-Rivera, S., Zagorevski, D., et al., Hydrogen sulfide inhibits amyloid formation, *J. Phys. Chem. B* 119, 1265–1274, 2015.
13. Jarosz, D.F., and Khurana, V., Specification of physiologic and disease states by distinct proteins and protein conformations, *Cell* 171, 1001–1014, 2017.
14. Khan, M.V., Zakariya, S.M., and Khan, R.H., Protein folding, misfolding and aggregation: A tale of constructive to destructive assembly, *Int. J. Biol. Macromol.* 112, 217–229, 2018.
15. Rosario-Alomar, M.R., Quiñones-Ruiz, T., Kurouski, D., et al., Insights into the molecular mechanisms of Alzheimer's and Parkinson's diseases with molecular simulations in intrinsically disordered proteins related to pathology, *Int. J. Mol. Sci.* 19, 336, 2018.
16. Cohen, M.S., Turner, T.M., and Urban, R.M., Effects of implant material and plate design on tendon function and morphology, *Clin. Orthop. Relat. Res.* 445, 81–90, 2006.
17. *Atrial Fibrillation*, ed. P. Kowey and G.V. Maccarelli, Marcel Dekker, New York, 2006.

FIBROBLAST GROWTH FACTOR

Fibroblast growth factors (FGFs) are a large family of peptide growth factors which regulate cell growth and proliferation.[1] There is an excellent review of the initial work on FGFs.[2] Early work demonstrated the presence of basic fibroblast growth factor and acidic growth factor.[3] FGFs interact with heparin-like molecules.[4] The number FGFs rapidly increased to six in 1991[5] expanding to at least 22 by 2017.[6] FGFs consist of five families of paracrine FGFs and one endocrine FGF family. The endocrine FGF family has three members and is notable for lack of interaction of heparin.[7,8] FGFs binding to a group of tyrosine kinase receptors known as the fibroblast growth factor receptors.[9] See also **fibroblast growth factor receptors**.

1. Folkman, J., and Klagsbrun, M., Angiogenic factors, *Science* 235, 442–447, 1987.
2. Baird, A., and Walicke, P.A., Fibroblast growth factors, *Brit. Med. Bull.* 45, 438–452, 1989.
3. Gospodarowicz, D., Neufeld, G., and Schweigerer, L., Fibroblast growth factor, *Mol. Cell. Endocrinol.* 46, 187–204, 1986.
4. Yayon, A., Klagsbrun, M., Esko, J.D., Leder, P., and Ornitz, D.M., Cell surface, heparin-like molecules are required for binding basic fibroblast growth factor to its high affinity receptor, *Cell* 64, 841–848, 1991.
5. Anon., The fibroblast growth factor family. Nomenclature meeting report and recommendations, *Ann. N.Y. Acad. Sci.* 638, xiii–xvi, 1991.
6. Maddaluno, L., Urwyler, C., and Werner, S., Fibroblast growth factors: Key players in regeneration and tissue repair, *Development* 144, 4047–4060, 2017.
7. Fernandes-Freitas, I., and Owen, B.M., Metabolic roles of endocrine fibroblast growth factors, *Curr. Opin. Pharmacol.* 25, 30–35, 2015.
8. Degirolamo, C., Sabbà, C., and Moschetta, A., Therapeutic potential of the endocrine fibroblast growth factors FGF19, FGF21, and FGF23, *Nat. Rev. Drug Discov.* 15, 51–59, 2016.
9. Eswarakumar, V.P., Lax, I., and Schlessinger, J., Cellular signaling by fibroblast growth factor receptors, *Cytokine Growth Factor Rev.* 16, 139–149, 2005.

FIBROBLAST GROWTH FACTOR RECEPTOR(S)

There are four canonical paracrine fibroblast growth factor receptors (FGFR1, FGFR2, FGFR3, and FGFR4) coupled to tyrosine kinase with a fifth (FGFRL1) lacking an intracellular tyrosine kinase.[1] The FGFRs are single-chain transmembrane proteins with an extracellular segment consisting of three immunoglobulin (Ig)-like domains, a transmembrane domain, and intracellular tyrosine kinase which dimerizes on forming a ternary complex with FGF and a cell-surface heparan sulfate proteoglycan.[2] Intracellular signal transduction is mediated through the action of the tyrosine kinase.[3] The canonical paracrine FGFRs require the participation of heparan-sulfate proteoglycan while the endocrine FGFs require the presence of cell surface proteins designated klothos (α-klotho; β-klotho).[4,5]

1. Carter, E.P., Fearon, A.E., and Grose, R.P., Careless talk costs lives: Fibroblast growth factor receptor signalling and the consequences of pathway malfunction, *Trends Cell Biol.* 25, 221–233, 2015.
2. Pelegrini, L., Burke, D.F., von Delft, F., Mulloy, B., and Blundell, T.L., Crystal structure of fibroblast growth factor receptor ectodomain bound to ligand and heparin, *Nature* 407, 1029–1034, 2000.
3. Ornitz, D.M., and Itoh, N., The fibroblast growth factor signaling pathway, *WIREs Dev. Biol.* 4, 215–266, 2015.
4. Kurosu, H., Kuro-o, m., The Klothogene family as regulator of endocrine fibroblast growth factors, *Mol. Cell. Endocrinol.* 299, 72–78, 2009.
5. Li, X., Wang, C., Xiao, J., McKeehan, W.L., and Wang, F., Fibroblast growth factors, old kids on the new block, *Semin. Cell Dev. Biol.* 53, 155–167, 2016.

FixJ-FixL

FixJ-FixL is a two-component system which is a regulator of nitrogen fixation by serving as a sensitive oxygen sensor.[1–3]

1. Kahn, D., and Ditta, G., Modular structure of FixJ: Homology of the transcriptional activator domain with the -35 binding domain of sigma factors, *Mol. Microbiol.* 5, 987–997, 1991.
2. Sousa, F.H.S., Gonzalez, G., and Gilles-Gonazalez, M.-A., Oxygen blocks the reaction of FixL-FixJ complex with ATP but does not influence binding of FixJ or ATP to FixL, *Biochem.* 44, 15359–15365, 2005.
3. Wright, G.S.A., Saeki, A., Hikima, T., et al., Architecture of the complete oxygen-sensing FixL-FixJ two-component signal transduction system, *Sci. Signal.* 11(525), eaaq0825, 2018.

FLAG™

FLAG™ is an affinity "tag" which has the sequence of AspTyrLysAspAspAspAspLys which includes an enterokinase cleavage site.[1] This epitope tag is used as fusion partner for purification of proteins.[2–4] FLAG peptide has also been used to measure protein expression.[5–7]

1. Knappik, A., and Plückthun, A., An improved affinity tag based on the FLAG peptide for the detection and purification of recombinant antibody fragments, *Biotechniques* 17, 754–761, 1994.
2. Einhauer, A., and Jungbauer, A., The FLAG™ peptide, a versatile fusion tag for the purification of recombinant proteins, *J. Biochem. Biophys. Methods* 49, 455–465, 2001.
3. Terpe, K., Overview of tag protein fusions: From molecular and biochemical fundamentals to commercial systems, *Appl. Microbiol. Biotechnol.* 60, 523–533, 2003.
4. Lichty, J.J., Malecki, J.L., Agnew, H.D., Michelson-Horowitz, D.J., and Tan, S., Comparison of affinity tags for protein purification, *Protein Exp. Purif.* 41, 98–105, 2005.
5. Xiong, X., Zhang, Y., Yan, J., et al., A scalable epitope tagging approach for high throughput ChIP analysis, *ACS Synth. Biol.* 6, 1034–1042, 2017.
6. Hayashi, K., Yamashita, R., Takami, R., et al., Strategy for identification of phosphorylation levels of low abundance proteins *In vivo* for which antibodies are not available, *J. Cardiobvasc. Dev. Dis.* 4, 17, 2017.
7. Jiaravuthisan, P., Maeda, A., Takakura, C., et al., A membrane-type surfactant protein D (SP-D) suppresses macrophage-mediated cytotoxicity in swine endothelial cells, *Transpl. Immunol.* 47, 44–48, 2018.

FLAP ENDONUCLEASE (FEN1)

Flap endonuclease (FEN-1) is a nuclease encoded by the *FEN1* gene.[1,2] FEN1 was originally described as an enzyme which cleaved DNA "flap" resulting from nucleotide excision repair.[3,4] Work has been shown that FEN1 is involved in a spectrum of activities in DNA processes including Okazaki fragment maturation, telomere maintenance, and stalled replication fork repair.[5] The overexpression of FEN1 is associated with poor prognosis in lung cancer[6] and is a drug target in oncology.[7]

1. Kim, I.S., Lee, M.Y., Lee, I.H., Shin, S.L., and Lee, S.Y., Gene expression of flap endonuclease-1 during cell proliferation and differentiation, *Biochim. Biophys. Acta* 1496, 333–340, 2000.
2. Finger, L.D., Atack, J.M., Tsutakawa, S., et al., The wonders of flap endonucleases: Structure, function, mechanism and regulation, *Subcell. Biochem.* 62, 301–326, 2012.

3. Harrington, J.J., and Lieber, M.R., The characterization of a mammalian DNA structure-specific endonuclease, *EMBO J.* 13, 1235–1246, 1994.

4. Harrington, J.J., and Lieber, M.R., Functional domains within FEN-1 and RAD2 define a family of structure-specific endonucleases: Implications for nucleotide excision repair, *Genes Dev.* 8, 1344–1355, 1994.

5. Balakrishnan, L., and Bambara, R.A., Flap endonuclease 1, *Annu. Rev. Biochem.* 82, 119–138, 2013.

6. Zhang, K., Keymeulen, S., Nelson, R., et al., Overexpression of Flap endonuclease proliferation and poor prognosis of non-small-cell lung cancer, *Am. J. Pathol.* 188, 242–251, 2018.

7. Deshmukh, A.L., Chandra, S., Singh, D.K., Siddiqi, M.I., and Banerjee, D., Identification of human flap endonuclease 1 (FEN1) inhibitors using a machine learning based consensus virtual screening, *Mol. Biosyst.* 13, 1630–1639, 2017.

FLUX

Flux is the continuous flow of a substance. Flux can occur with electrons[1] and protons[2] as well and ions and other substances.[3–8] Flux is defined in several ways: Unidirectional influx is defined as the molar quantity of a solute passing across 1 cm^2 membrane in a unit period of time; unidirectional efflux is defined as the molar quantity of a solute crossing 1 cm^2 membrane outward from a cell in a unit period of time. Net flux is the difference between unidirectional influx and unidirectional efflux in a unit period of time. Understanding net flux is of importance in the design and interpretation of dialysis studies used to measure protein binding of small molecules.[9]

1. Gutman, M., Electron flux through the mitochondrial ubiquinone, *Biochim. Biophys. Acta* 594, 53–84, 1980.

2. Wang, J.H., Coupling of proton flux to the hydrolysis and synthesis of ATP, *Annu. Rev. Biophys. Bioeng.* 12, 21–34, 1983.

3. Schwartz, A., Cell membrane Na$^+$, K$^+$-ATPase and sarcoplasmic reticulum: Possible regulators of intracellular ion activity, *Fed. Proc.* 35, 1279–1282, 1976.

4. Meissner, G., Monovalent ion and calcium ion fluxes in sarcoplasmic reticulum, *Mol. Cell. Biochem.* 55, 65–82, 1983.

5. Jones, D.P., Intracellular diffusion gradients of O$_2$ and ATP, *Am. J. Physiol.* 250, C663–C675, 1986.

6. Hunter, M., Kawahara, K., and Giebisch, G., Calcium-activated epithelial potassium channels, *Miner. Electrolyte Metab.* 14, 48–57, 1988.

7. *Cation Flux across Biomembranes*, ed. Y. Mukohata, and L. Packer, Academic Press, New York, 1979.

8. Weir, E.K., and Hume, J.R., *Ion Flux in Pulmonary Vascular Control*, Plenum Press, New York, NY, 1993.

9. Kalvass, J.C., Phipps, C., Jenkins, G.J., Stuart, P., et al., Mathematical and experimental validation of flux dialysis method: An improved approach to measure unbound fraction for compounds with high protein binding and other challenging properties, *Drug Metab. Dispos.* 46, 458–469, 2018.

FOCAL ADHESION

Focal adhesion, also known as focal contact, is a membrane area/cell junction that is responsible for adhesion of cells to the extracellular matrix transmitting signals from the extracellular matrix (ECM) to the interior of the cell providing the basis for cell adhesion and motility.[1–3] Cell surface integrins such as fibronectin interact with ECM and bind with components of the focal adhesion complex including focal adhesion kinase (FAK) which is a tyrosine kinase.[3] Focal adhesion results from the clustering of receptors forming fibrillar structures.[4] Focal adhesion kinase, together with Src kinase, phosphorylate proteins such as paxillin[5] resulting effects beyond cell migration.[6,7]

1. Garrod, D., Focal Contact, in *Encyclopedia of Molecular Biology*, ed. T. Creighton, John Wiley & Sons, New York, 1999.

2. Jahed, Z., Shams, H., Mehrbod, M., and Mofrad, M.R., Mechanotransduction pathways linking the extracellular matrix to the nucleus, *Int. Rev. Cell. Mol. Biol.* 310, 171–220, 2014.

3. Burridge, K., Focal adhesions: A personal perspective on a half century of progress, *FEBS J.* 284, 3355–3361, 2017.

4. Digiacomo, G., Tusa, I., Bacci, M., et al., Fibronectin induces macrophage migration through a SFK-FAK/CSF-1R pathwy, *Cell. Adh. Migr.* 11, 327–337, 2017.

5. Leube, R.E., Moch, M., and Windoffer, R., Intermediate filaments and the regulation of focal adhesion, *Curr. Opin. Cell Biol.* 32, 13–30, 2015.

6. López-Colomé, A.M., Lee-Rivera, I., Benavides-Hidalgo, R., and López, E., Paxillin: A crossroad in pathological cell migration, *J. Hematol. Oncol.* 10, 50, 2017.

7. Kleinschmidt, E.G., and Schlaepfer, D.D., Focal adhesion kinase signaling in unexpected places, *Curr. Opin. Cell. Biol.* 45, 24–30, 2017.

FOK1 RESTRICTION ENDONUCLEASE

A type II restriction endonuclease isolated from *Flavobacterium okeanokoites,* which has been used to identify DNA polymorphisms.[1–9] While CRISPR/Cas 9-based approaches have come to dominate the field of gene editing, Fok1 nuclease has served as the nuclease portion of other approaches to gene editing such as zinc-finger nuclease and TALENS (transcription activator-like effector nucleases).[10–15]

1. Sugisaki, H., and Kanazawa, S., New restriction endonucleases from Flavobacterium okeanokoites (FokI) and Micrococcus luteus (MluI), *Gene* 16, 73–78, 1981.
2. Kato, A., Yakura, K., and Tanifuji, S., Sequence analysis of Vicia faba repeated DNA, the FokI repeat element, *Nucleic Acids Res.* 24, 6415–6426, 1984.
3. Kita, K., Kotani, H., Sugisaki, H., and Tanami, M., The foci restriction-modification system. I. Organization and nucleotide sequences of the restriction and modification genes, *J. Biol. Chem.* 264, 5751–5756, 1989.
4. Posfai, G., and Szybalski, W., A simple method for locating methylated based in DNA using class-IIS restriction enzymes, *Gene* 74, 179–181, 1988.
5. Aggarwal, A.K., and Wah, D.A., Novel site-specific DNA endonucleases, *Curr. Opin. Struct. Biol.* 8, 19–25, 1998.
6. Kovall, R.A., and Matthews, B.W., Type II restriction endonucleases: Structural, functional and evolutionary relationships, *Curr. Opin. Chem. Biol.* 3, 578–583, 1999.
7. Akar, A., Orkunoglu, F.E., Ozata, M., Sengul, A., and Gur, A.R., Lack of association between vitamin D receptor FokI polymorphism and alopecia areata, *Eur. J. Dermatol.* 14, 156–158, 2004.
8. Guy, M., Lowe, L.C., Bretherton-Watt, D., et al., Vitamin D receptor gene polymorphisms and breast cancer risk, *Clin. Cancer Res.* 10, 5472–5481, 2004.
9. Claassen, M., Nouwen, J., Fang, Y., et al., *Staphylococcus aureus* nasal carriage is not associated with known polymorphism in the vitamin D receptor gene, *FEMS Immunol. Med. Microbiol.* 43, 173–176, 2005.
10. Bolu, S.E., Orkunoglu Suer, F.E., Deniz, F., et al., The vitamin D receptor foci start codon polymorphism and bone mineral density in male hypogonadotrophic hypogonadism, *J. Endocrinol. Invest.* 28, 810–814, 2005.
11. Collin, J., and Lako, M., Concise review: Putting a finger on stem cell biology: Zinc finger nuclease-driven targeted genetic editing in human pluripotent stem cells, *Stem Cells* 29, 1021–1033, 2011.
12. Sun, N., and Xhao, H., Transcription activator-like effector nucleases (TALENs): A highly efficient and versatile tool for genome editing, *Biotechnol. Bioeng.* 110, 1811–1821, 2013.
13. Varshney, G.K., and Burgess, S.M., DNA-guided genome editing using structure-guided endonucleases, *Genome Biol.* 17(1), 187, 2016.
14. Mahata, B., and Biswas, K., Generation of stable knockout mammalian cells by TALEN-mediated locus-specific gene editing, *Methods Mol. Biol.* 1498, 107–120, 2017.
15. Bak, R.O., Gomez-Ospina, N., and Porteus, M.N., Gene editing on center stage, *Trends Genet.* 34, 600–611, 2018.

FOLDAMERS

Foldamers are single-chain polymers that can adopt secondary structure in solution and thus mimic biopolymers such as proteins, nucleic acids, and polysaccharides.[1] Foldamers have polymeric backbones which are designed to have well-defined and predictable folding properties.[2–5] Many foldamers are prepared from peptoids and β-amino acids.[6,7]

1. *Foldamers*, ed. S. Hecht and I. Huc., Wiley-VCH Verlag, Weinheim, Germany, 2007.
2. Cheng, R.P., Beyond de novo protein design—de novo design of non-natural folded oligomers, *Curr. Opin. Struct. Biol.* 14, 512–520, 2004.
3. Stone, M.T, Heemstra, J.M., and Moore, J.S., The chain-length dependence test, *Acc. Chem. Res.* 39, 11–20, 2006.
4. Guichard, G., and Huc, I., Synthetic foldamers, *Chem. Commun.* 47, 5933, 5941, 2011.
5. Hegedüs, Z., Wéber, E., Kriston-Pál, É., et al., Foldameric α/β-peptide analogs of the β-sheet-forming antiangiogenic anginex: Structure and bioactivity, *J. Am. Chem. Soc.* 135, 16578–16584, 2013.
6. Mándity, I.M., and Fülip, F., An overview of peptide and peptoid foldamers in medicinal chemistry, *Expert Opin. Drug Discov.* 10, 1163–1177, 2015.
7. Cabrele, C., Martinek, T.A., Reiser, O., and Berliki, L., Peptides containing β-amino acid patterns: Challenges and successes in medicinal chemistry, *J. Med. Chem.* 57, 9718–9739, 2014.

FRAGONOMICS

Fragonomics is a term that describes the use of smaller molecules (fragments) as a starting point in the drug discovery process.[1,2] An algorithm (fragment topology-activity landscapes (FRAGTAL) for encoding molecular descriptors for fragonomics into a database has been described.[3]

1. Zartler, E.R., and Shapiro, M.J., Fragonomics: Fragment-based drug discovery, *Curr. Opin. Chem. Biol.* 9, 366–370, 2005.
2. Zartler, E.R., Fragonomics: The -omics with real impact, *ACS Med. Chem. Lett.* 5, 952–953, 2014.
3. Bak, A., Magdziarz, T., Kurczyk, A., Serafin, K., and Polanski, J., Probing a chemical space for fragmental topology-activity landscapes (FRAGTAL): Application for diketo acid and catechol HIV integrase inhibitor offspring fragments, *Comb. Chem. High Throughput Screen.* 16, 274–287, 2013.

FRASS

Frass is debris or excrement produced by insects. Proteases present in cockroach frass is thought to be involved in the development of asthma.[1,2] Specific allergens present in frass are also thought to be involved in the development of asthma.[3] There are specific interactions between frass and plant hosts.[4,5]

1. Page, K., Hughes, V.S., Bennett, G.W., and Wong, H.R., German cockroach proteases regulate matrix metalloproteinase-9 in human bronchial epithelial cells, *Allergy* 61, 988–995, 2006.

2. Day, S.B., Ledford, J.R., Zhou, P., Lewkowich, I.P., and Page, K., German cockroach proteases and protease-activated receptor-2 regulate chemokine production and dendritic cell recruitment, *J. Innate Immun.* 4, 100–110, 2012.

3. Mueller, G.A., Pedersen, L.C., Lih, F.B., et al., The novel structure of the cockroach allergen Bla g 1 has implications for the allergenicity and exposure assessment, *J. Allergy Clin. Immunol.* 132, 1420–1426, 2013.

4. Chen, H., Gonzales-Vigil, E., Wilkerson, C.G., and Howe, G.A., Stability of plant defense proteins in the gut of insect herbivores, *Plant Physiol.* 143, 1952–1967, 2007.

5. Ray, S., Alves, P.C., Ahmad, I., Turnabout in fair play: Herbivory-induced plant chitinases excreted in Fall Armyworm frass suppress herbivore defenses in maize, *Plant Physiol.* 171, 694–706, 2016.

FREE RADICAL

A free radical is fragment containing an unpaired valence electron.[1] Free radicals may be created by the homolytic cleavage of a molecule.[2] One of the better known current examples of a free radical in biology is the generation of 5′-deoxyadenosyl radical.[3–5] Free radical chemistry is also used for modification of proteins (protein mapping) via hydroxyl radicals produced by the radiolysis of water ($H_2O \rightarrow H_2O\bullet + e^-$; $H_2O\bullet + e^- + H_2O \rightarrow\rightarrow H_3O^+ + \bullet OH$).[6,7] Nitric oxide is a free radical resulting in the formation of peroxynitrite ($NO\bullet + O_2^- \rightarrow ONOO^-$) resulting in tyrosine nitration[8] and carbonate radical formation.[9] The Fenton reaction ($Fe^{3+} + H_2O_2 \rightarrow Fe^{2+} + H_2O + \bullet OH$) is well known for the formation of hydroxyl radical. See **Fenton reaction**.

1. Perkins, J., *Radical Chemistry: The Fundamentals*, Oxford University Press, Oxford, UK, 2000.

2. *Oxford Dictionary of Chemistry*, ed. R. Rennie, Oxford University Press, Oxford, UK, 2019.

3. Kempmeier, J.A., Regioselectivity in the hemolytic cleavage of S-adenosylmethionine, *Biochemistry* 49, 16397–16405, 2010.

4. Horitani, M., Byer, A.S., Shisler, K.A., Broderick, J.B., and Hoffman, B.M., Why nature uses radical SAM enzymes so widely: Electron nuclear double resonance studies of lysine 2,3-aminomutase show the 5′-dAdo• "free radical" is never free, *J. Am. Chem. Soc.* 137, 7111–7121, 2015.

5. Latham, J.A., Barr, I., and Klinman, J.P., At the confluence of ribosomally synthesized peptide modification and radical S-adenosylmethione (SAM) enzymology, *J. Biol. Chem.* 292, 16397–16405, 2017.

6. Takamoto, K., and Chance, M.R., Radiolytic protein fingerprinting with mass spectrometry to probe the structure of macromolecular compounds, *Annu. Rev. Biophys. Biomol. Struct.* 35, 251–276, 2005.

7. Kiselar, J.G., and Chance, M.R., Future directions of structural mass spectrometry using hydroxyl radical footprinting, *J. Mass Spectrom.* 45, 1373–1382, 2010.

8. Bartesaghi, S., and Radi, R., Fundamentals on the biochemistry of peroxynitrite and protein tyrosine nitration, *Redox Biol.* 14, 618–625, 2018.

9. Augusto, O., Bonini, M.G., Amanso, A.M., et al., Nitrogen dioxide and carbonate radical anion: Two emerging radicals in biology, *Free Radic. Biol. Med.* 32, 841–859, 2002.

FRET (FLUORESCENCE RESONANCE ENERGY TRANSFER)

Fluorescence resonance transfer (FRET; also known as Förster resonance transfer) is a technique for assaying the proximity of regions in a protein or other macromolecule or larger subcellular assembly by observed energy transfer between two fluorophores, a donor fluorophore and an acceptor fluorophore, initially at some distance from one another. The donor fluorophore absorbs a photon and transfers this energy to an acceptor molecule in a radiationless process. The extent of the observed effect (quenching of donor fluorescence and enhancement of acceptor fluorescence) is a measure of the distance between the donor and acceptor.[1,2] FRET can be used to measure interactions between two different molecules or in single-molecule FRET where donor and acceptor fluorophores are placed on a molecule to measure protein folding[3] and mature protein conformational change.[4,5] Genetically encoded fluorophores have been developed to study intracellular interactions.[6]

1. Clegg, R.M., Fluorescence resonance energy transfer and nucleic acids, *Methods Enzymol.* 211, 353–388, 1992.

2. Mátyus, L., Fluorescence resonance energy transfer measurement on cell surfaces. A spectroscopic tool for determining protein interactions, *J. Photochem. Photobiol. B* 12, 323–337, 1992.

3. Chung, H.S., and Eaton, W.A., Protein folding transition path times from single molecule FRET, *Curr. Opin. Struct. Biol.* 48, 30–39, 2018.

4. Gomes, G.N., and Gradinaru, C.C., Insights into the conformation and dynamics of intrinsically disordered proteins using single-molecule fluorescence, *Biochim. Biophys. Acta* 1865, 1696–1706, 2017.

5. von Voithenberg, V., and Lamb, D.C., Single pair Förster resonance energy transfer: A versatile tool to investigate protein conformational dynamics, *Bioessays* 40 (3), 1700078, 2018.

6. Halls, M.L., and Canals, M., Genetically encoded FRET biosensors to illuminate compartmentalized GPCR signalling, *Trends Pharmacol. Sci.* 39, 148–157, 2018.

FREUND'S ADJUVANT

Freund's adjuvant[1-3] is a mixture of killed/lyophilized *Mycobacterium bovis* or *Mycobacterium tuberculosis* cells and oil resulting in an emulsion (referred to as Complete Freund's adjuvant) used with an antigen to improve the immune response (antibody formation secondary to B-cell activation).[4-13] **Incomplete Freund's adjuvant** does not contain the bacterial cells and is used to avoid an inflammatory response.[14,15]

1. Freund, J., and McDermott, K., Sensitization by means of adjuvants, *Proc. Soc. Expt. Biol. Med.* 49, 548–553, 1942.
2. Freund, J., and Walter, A.W., Saphrophytic acidfast bacteria and paraffin oil as adjuvants for immunization, *Proc. Soc. Expt. Biol. Med.* 56, 42–50, 1944.
3. Freund, J., and Bonanto, M.V., The effect of paraffin oil, lanolin-like substances and killed tuberculi bacilli on immunization with diphtheria-toxoid and bact. typhosum, *J. Immunol.* 48, 325–334, 1944.
4. White, R.G., Factor affecting the antibody response, *Br. Med. Bull.* 19, 207–213, 1963.
5. White, R.G., Antigen adjuvants, *Mod. Trends Immunol.* 2, 28–52, 1967.
6. Myrvik, Q.N., Adjuvants, *Ann. N. Y. Acad. Sci.* 221, 324–330, 1974.
7. Osebold, J.W., Mechanisms for action by immunologic adjuvants, *J. Am. Vet. Med. Assoc.* 181, 983–987, 1982.
8. Warren, H.S., Vogel, F.R., and Chedid, L.A., Current status of immunological adjuvants, *Annu. Rev. Immunol.* 4, 369–388, 1986.
9. Claassen, E., de Leeuw, W., de Greeve, P., Hendriksen, C., and Boersma, W., Freund's complete adjuvant: An effective but disagreeable formula, *Res. Immunol.* 143, 478–483, 1992.
10. Billiau, A., and Matthys, P., Modes of action of Freund's adjuvants in experimental models of autoimmune diseases, *J. Leukoc. Biol.* 70, 849–860, 2001.
11. Stills, H.F., Jr., Adjuvants and antibody production: Dispelling the myths associated with Freund's complete and other adjuvants, *ILAR J.* 46, 280–293, 2005.
12. *Vaccine Adjuvants: Methods and Protocols*, ed. G. Davies, Humana/Springer, New York, 2010.
13. Melén, K., Kakkola, L., He, F., et al., Production, purification and immunogenicity of recombinant Ebola virus proteins—A comparison of Freund's adjuvant and adjuvant system 03, *J. Virol. Methods* 242, 35–45, 2017.
14. Miller, L.H., Saul, A., and Mahanty, S., Revisiting Freund's incomplete adjuvant for vaccines in the developing world, *Trends Paristol.* 21, 412–414, 2005.
15. Jagessar, S.A., Heijmans, N., Blezer, E.L., et al., Immune profile of an atypical EAE model in marmoset monkeys immunized with recombinant human myelin oligodendrocyte glycoprotein in incomplete Freund's adjuvant, *J. Neuroinflammation* 12, 169, 2015.

FUNCTIONAL GENOMICS

Functional genomics refers to the establishment of a verifiable link between gene expression and cell/organ/tissue function/dysfunction.[1-8]

1. *PCR Applications: Protocols for Functional Genomics*, ed. J.J. Sminsky, M.A. Innis, and D.H. Gelfand, Academic Press, San Diego, CA, 1999.
2. Hunt, S.P., and Livesey, R., *Functional Genomics: A Practical Approach*, Oxford University Press, Oxford, UK, 2000.
3. *Functional Genomics Methods and Protocols*, ed. M.J. Brownstein and A.B. Khodursky, Humana Press, Totowa, NJ, 2003.
4. Grotewold, E., *Plant Functional Genomics*, Humana Press, Totowa, NJ, 2003.
5. Zhou, J., *Microbial Functional Genomics*, Wiley-Liss, Hoboken, NJ, 2004.
6. Luca, F., Kupfer, S.S., Knights, D., Khoruts, A., and Blekhman, R., Functional genomics of host-microbiome interactions in humans, *Trends Genet.* 34, 30–40, 2018.
7. Roman, T.S., and Mohlke, K.L., Functional genomics and assays of regulatory activity detect mechanisms at loci for lipid traits and coronary artery disease, *Curr. Opin. Genet. Dev.* 50, 52–59, 2018.
8. Winter, D.R., Thinking BIG rheumatology: How to make functional genomics data work for you, *Arthritis Res. Ther.* 20, 29, 2018.

FUNCTIONAL PROTEOMICS

Functional proteomics represents a broad area of enquiry encompassing the study of the function of proteins in the proteome, study of changes in protein expression within the proteome, and the use of reactive chemical probes to identify enzymes in the proteome.[1-3] As should be obvious, there are disciplines such as **activity-based proteomics**[4] and **transcriptomics/gene expression profiling**[5,6] that fit within functional proteomics.

1. *Posttranslational Modifications of Proteins: Tools for Functional Proteomics*, ed. Kannicht, C.I., Humana Press, Totowa, NJ, 2002.
2. *Functional Proteomics: Methods and Proteomics*, ed. Schaeffer-Reiss, C.I., Thompson, J.D., and Uefling, M.I., Humana Press, Totowa, NJ, 2008.
3. *Functional and Structural Proteomics of Glycoproteins*, ed. Nettleship, J.E., and Owens, R.J., Springer, Dordrecht, the Netherlands, 2011.
4. Fonović, M., and Bogyo, M., Activity-based probes as a tool for functional proteomic analysis of proteases, *Expert Rev. Proteomics* 5, 721–730, 2008.
5. D'Agostino, P.M., Woodhouse, J.N., Makower, A.K., et al., Advances in genomics, transcriptomics and proteomics of toxin-producing cyanobacteria, *Environ. Microbiol. Rep.* 8, 3–13, 2016.

6. Aslam, B., Basit, M., Nisar, M.A., Khurshid, M., and Rasool, M.H., Proetomics: Technologies and their applications, *J. Chromatog. Sci.* 55, 182–196, 2017.

FURIN/PROPROTEIN CONVERTASES

Furin is a subtilisin-like regulatory protease described as one several proprotein convertases[1] located in the trans-Golgi network, which function in processing precursor proteins in the secretory pathway.[2–4] Furin is a therapeutic target in several pathologies including cancer and cardiovascular disease.[5] Engineering of furin is used to improve the expression of recombinant proteins.[6–9] Other proprotein convertases include subtilisin/kexin type 9 (PCSK9).[10] Subtilisin/Kexin type 9 is of particular interest in cardiovascular disease[11] because of its role in the modulation of the hepatic low-density lipoprotein receptor.[12,13]

1. Jaaks, P., and Bernasconi, M., The proprotein converatase furin in tumor progression, *Int. J. Cancer* 141, 654–663, 2017.

2. Rockwell, N.C., and Thorner, J.W., The kindest cuts of all: Crystal structures of kex2 and furin reveal secrets of precursor processing, *Trends Biochem. Sci.* 29, 80–87, 2004.

3. Seidah, N.G., The proprotein convertases, 20 years later, *Methods Mol. Biol.* 768, 23–57, 2011.

4. Seidah, N.G. Sadr, M.R., Chrétien, M., and Mbikay, M., The multifaceted proprotein convertases: Their unique, redundant, complementary, and opposite functions, *J. Biol. Chem.* 288, 21473–21481, 2013.

5. Constam, D.B., Regulation of TGFβ and related signals by precursor processing, *Semin. Cell Dev. Biol.* 32, 85–97, 2014.

6. Klein-Szanto, A.J., and Bassi, D.E., Proprotein convertase inhibition: Paralyzing the cell's master switches, *Biochem. Pharmacol.* 140, 8–15, 2017.

7. Lind, P., Larsson, K., Spira, J., et al., Novel forms of B-domain-deleted recombinant factor VIII molecules. Construction and biochemical characterization, *Eur. J. Biochem.* 232, 19–27, 1995.

8. Demasi, M.A., de S., Molina, E., Bowman-Colin, C., et al., Enhanced proteolytic processing of recombinant human coagulation factor VIII B-domain variantsby recombinant furins, *Mol. Biotechnol.* 58, 404–414, 2016.

9. Nguyen, G.N., George, L.A., Siner, J.I., et al., Novel factor VIII variants with a modified furin cleavage site improve the efficiency of gene therapy for hemophilia A, *J. Thromb. Haemost.* 15, 110–121, 2017.

10. Hussain, H., Fisher, D.I., Abbott, W.M. Roth, R.G., and Dickson, A.J. Use of a protein engineering strategy to overcome limitations in the production of "difficult to express" recombinant proteins, *Biotechnol. Bioeng.* 114, 2348–2359, 2017.

11. Durairaj, A., Sabates, A., Nieves, J., Moraes, B., and Baum, S., Proprotein convertase subtilisin/kexin type 9 (PCSK9) and its inhibitors: A review of physiology, biology, and clinical data, *Curr. Treat. Options Cardiovasc. Med.* 19, 58, 2017.

12. Seidah, N.G., Abifadel, M., Prost, S., Boileau, C., and Prat, A., The proprotein convertases in hypercholesterolemia and cardiovascular diseases: Emphasis of proprotein convertase subilisin/kexin 9, *Pharm. Rev.* 69, 33–52, 2017.

13. Baragetti, A., Grejtakova, D., Casula, M., et al., Proprotein convertase subtilisin-Kexin type-9 (PCSK9) and triglyceride-rich lipoprotein metabolism: Facts and gaps, *Pharmacol. Res.*130, 1–11, 2018.

GAMMA(γ)-SECRETASE

γ-Secretase is a membrane-bound regulatory protease responsible for the cleavage of amyloid precursor protein and notch protein. Gamma(γ)-secretase is composed of four subunits, presenilin, nicastrin, Aph-1 and Pen-2. Presenilin is responsible for the catalytic gamma(γ)-secretase activity and nicastrin and Aph-2 have a function in substrate recognition and complex stabilization while Pen-2 assists in catalytic function.[1–7] Gamma(γ)-secretase is a therapeutic target for Alzheimer's disease.[8–11]

1. Mundy, D.L., Identification of the multicatalytic enzyme as a possible γ-secretase for the amyloid precursor protein, *Biochem. Biophys. Res. Commun.* 204, 333–341, 1994.

2. Wolfe, M.S., and Haass, C., The role of presenilins in gamma-secretase activity, *J. Biol. Chem.* 276, 5413–5416, 2001.

3. Kimberly, W.T., and Wolfe, M.S., Identify and function of gamma-secretases, *J. Neurosci. Res.* 74, 353–360, 2003.

4. Iwatsubo, T., The gamma secretase complex: Machinery for intramembrane proteolysis, *Curr. Opin. Neurobiol.* 14, 379–383, 2004.

5. Wolfe, M.S., The γ-secretase complex: Membrane-embedded proteolytic ensemble, *Biochemistry* 45, 7931–7939, 2006.

6. Sun, L., Li, X., and Shi, Y., Structural biology of intramembrane proteases: Mechanistic insights from rhomboid to γ-secretase, *Curr. Opin. Struct. Biol.* 37, 97–107, 2016.

7. Yang, G., Zhou, R., and Shi, Y., Cryo-EM structures of human γ-secretase, *Curr. Opin. Struct. Biol.* 46, 55–64, 2017.

8. Churcher, I., and Beher, D., Gamma-secretase as a therapeutic target for the treatment of Alzheimer's disease, *Curr. Pharm. Des.* 11, 3363–3382, 2005.

9. Barten, D.M., Meredith, J.E.,Jr., Zaczek, R., et al., Gamma-secretase inhibitors for Alzheimer's disease: Balancing efficacy and toxicity, *Drugs R&D* 7, 87–97, 2006.

10. Kumar, D., Ganeshpurkar, A., Kumar, D., Secretase inhibitors for the treatment of Alzheimer's disease: Long road ahead, *Eur. J. Med. Chem.* 148, 436–452, 2018.

11. Sadhukhan, P., Saha, S., Dutta, S., Mahalanobish, S., and Sil, P.C., Nutraceuticals: An emerging therapeutic approach against the pathogenesis of Alzheimer's disease, *Pharmacol. Res.* 129, 100–114, 2018.

G PROTEIN (GUANINE NUCLEOTIDE-BINDING PROTEIN)

G protein (guanine nucleotide-binding protein) is a heteromeric protein which functions in signal transduction by binding and hydrolyzing guanosine triphosphate (GTP) with via modulation by G protein-coupled receptors (GPCRs). G protein function is controlled by regulation via G-protein coupled receptors.[1–5] Gα-protein (G-alpha protein), a member of the Ras superfamily of GTP-binding proteins, is a subunit of the heterotrimeric G protein which dissociates from the heterotrimer on when bound GDP is replaced by GTP in a process regulated by the GPCR.[6] The β and γ subunits of G protein serve to bind the heterotrimer to the cytoplasmic membrane. The dissociated Gα protein is a GTPase,[7] and hydrolysis of GTP to GDP (slow turnover rate, 2–4 seconds) is associated with a conformation change in the Gα protein permitting binding to the βγ dimer.[8] Both Gα-GTP and Gβγ can interact with effector proteins to initiate intracellular events.[9] PDZ proteins are important for G-protein interactions.[10]

1. Naccache, P.H., *G Proteins and Calcium Signaling,* CRC Press, Boca Raton, FL, 1990.
2. Johnson, R.A., and Corbin, J.D., *Adenyl Cyclase, G Proteins, and Guanylyl Cyclase,* Academic Press, San Diego, CA, 1991.
3. Ravi, I., *Heterotrimeric G Proteins,* Academic Press, San Diego, CA, 1994 *G Proteins: Techniques of Analysis,* ed. D.R. Manning, CRC Press, Boca Raton, FL, 1999.
4. Siderovski, D.P., *G Proteins and Calcium Signaling,* Elsevier Academic Press, Amsterdam, the Netherlands, 2004.
5. *G Protein Signaling: Methods and Protocols,* ed. Smrcka, A.V., Humana Press, Totowa, NJ, 2004; *Integrated G Protein Signaling in Plants,* ed. F.I. Baluška, A.M. Jones, and S.I. Yalovsky, Springer, Berlin, Germany, 2010.
6. Herrman, R., Heck, M., Henklein, P., et al., Signal transfer from GPCRs to G proteins: Role of the Gα N-terminal region in rhodopsin-transducin coupling, *J. Biol. Chem,* 281, 30234–30241, 2006.
7. *The GTPase Superfamily,* ed. J. March and J. Goode, Wiley, Chichester, UK, 1993.
8. Sprang, S.R., Activation of G proteins by GTP and the mechanism of Gα-catalyzed hydrolysis, *Biopolymers* 105, 449–462, 2016.
9. Wu, G., *Assay Development Fundamentals and Practices,* Chapter 10, Assays with GPCRs, pp. 265–288, Wiley, Hoboken, NJ, 2010.
10. Dunn, H.A., and Ferguson, S.S., PDZX protein regulation of G protein-coupled receptor trafficking and signalling pathways, *Mol. Pharmacol.* 88, 624–639, 2015.

G-PROTEIN COUPLED RECEPTOR (GPCR)

The G-protein coupled receptor (GPCR)[1–3] may be the most common human protein with more than 800 reported sequences. GPCRs are one of the two major families of membrane receptors, the other being the tyrosine kinase receptor.[4] G-protein coupled receptors are characterized by the presence of seven transmembrane segments and can be grouped into five families by the GRAFS (glutamate, rhodopsin, adhesion, frizzled/taste2, and secretin).[5] As the name implies, the signal passed from ligand binding to GPCR is mediated inside the cell by the activation of a trimeric G protein complex (G protein) resulting in the dissociation of bound GDP and subsequent binding of GTP by the alpha subunit (Gα). The Gα with bound GTP can then initiate other intracellular events such the activation of adenyl cyclase. See **G proteins**. The Gα protein, while a member of the Ras superfamily of GTP-binding proteins, is distinct from other members of that superfamily of protein and is designated as a heterotrimeric GTP-binding protein while other members of the Ras family are designated as small GTP-binding proteins.[6,7] The heterotrimeric GTP-binding proteins and the small GTP-binding proteins share common mechanism in the hydrolysis of GTP and their interaction with their GTPase-activating proteins (GAPs).[8] PDZ proteins are important in G protein-coupled receptor function.[9]

1. Watson, S.P., and Arkinstall, S., *The G-Protein Linked Receptor Factbooks,* Academic Press, London, UK, 1994.
2. *The G Protein-Coupled Receptor Handbook,* ed. A.L. Devi, Humana Press, Totowa, NJ, 2005.
3. *G-Protein Receptor Dimers,* ed. K. Herrick-Davis, G. Miligan, and G. Di Giovanni, Humana/Springer, Cham, Switzerland, 2017.
4. *Receptor Tyrosine Kinases: Family and Subfamilies,* ed. D.L. Wheeler and Y.Yarden, Humana/Springer, Cham, Switzerland, 2015; *Receptor Tyrosine Kinases: Structure, Functions and Role in Human Disease,* ed. D.L. Wheeler and Y. Yarden, Humana/Springer, Cham, Switzerland, 2015.
5. Fredriksson, R., Lagerström, M.C., Ludin, L-G., and Schiöth, H.B., The G-protein-coupled receptors in the human genome form five main families, phylogenetic analysis, paralogon groups, and fingerprints, *Molec. Pharmacol.* 63, 1256–1272, 2003.

6. Welsh, G.I., Hers, I., Wherlock, M., and Tavaré, J.M, Regulation of small GTP-binding proteins by insulin, *Biochem. Soc. Trans.* 34, 209–212, 2008.

7. Lezoualc'h, F., Métrich, M. Hmitou, I., et al., Small GTP-binding proteins and their regulators in cardiac hypertrophy, *J. Mol. Cell. Cardiol.* 44, 623–632, 2008.

8. Gerwert, K., Mann, D., and Kötting, C., Common mechanisms of catalysis in small and heterotrimeric GTPases and their respective GAPs, *Biol. Chem.* 398, 523–533, 2017.

9. Dunn, H.A., and Ferguson, S.S., PDZ protein regulation of G protein-coupled receptor trafficking and signaling pathways, *Mol. Pharmacol.* 88, 624–639, 2015.

GELSOLIN; GELSOLIN-LIKE DOMAINS, GELSOLIN FAMILY OF PROTEINS

Gelsolin is signature protein for the gelsolin family of proteins which interact with actin and influence the structure of the cytoskeleton.[1–3] Gelsolin has molecular weight of approximately 90 kDa.[4] Gelsolin contains six domains of ~15 kDa, which bind calcium ions resulting in a conformational change. The conformational change allows gelsolin to bind actin polymers resulting the separation of monomers in the process described as actin severing. Following the separation of the actin monomers, gelsolin bind to the "barbed" end of the actin filament in a process described as capping prevent further extension of the filaments. The gelsolin cap is modulated by interaction with phosphatidyl inositol 4,5-diphosphate (PIP2)[5] permitting extension of the actin filaments. In addition to its roles in modulating the formation of actin filaments, gelsolin has a role in regulation of transcription.[6,7] Gelsolin is also important in apoptosis.[5]

1. Yin, H.L., and Stossel, T.P., Control of cytoplasmic actin gel-sol transformation by gelsolin, a calcium-dependent regulatory protein, *Nature* 281, 583–586, 1979.

2. McGough, A.M., Staiger, C.J. Min, J-K., and Simonetti, K.D., The gelsolin family of actin regulatory proteins: Modular structures, versatile functions, *FEBS Lett.* 552, 75–81, 2003.

3. Nag, S., Larsson, M., Robinson, R.C., and Burtnick, L.D., Gesolin: The tail of a molecular gymnast, *Cytoskeleton* 70, 360–384, 2013.

4. Brady, R.J., Allen, R.D., Yin, H.L., and Stossel, T.P., Gelsolin inhibition of fast axonal transport indicates a requirement for actin microfilaments, *Nature* 310, 56–58, 1984.

5. Li, G.H., Arora, P.D., Chen, Y., McCulloch, C.A., and Liu, P., Multifunctional roles of gelsolin in health and diseases, *Med. Res. Rev.* 32, 999–1025, 2012.

6. Archer, S.K., Ciaudianos, C., and Campbell, H.D., Evolution of the gelsolin family of actin-binding proteins as novel transcriptional coactivators, *BioEssays* 27, 4, 2005.

7. Lu, M., Muers, M.R., and Lu, X., Introducing STRaNDs: Shuttling transcriptional regulators that are non-DNA binding, *Nat. Rev. Mol. Cell Biology* 17, 523–532, 2016.

GENERAL TRANSCRIPTION FACTORS

General transcription factors (also known as basal transcription factors) were identified as proteins which were required for the transcription of DNA by RNA polymerase II (Pol II) to produce messenger RNA (mRNA).[1] These factors bind to core promoter regions such at the TATA box which is upstream from the transcription initiation site.[2–4] General transcription factors are distinct from specific promoters or enhancers.[5–7] While there has been more work on the interaction of general transcription factors with Pol II, general transcription factors do interact with RNA polymerase I (Pol I) which is responsible for synthesis of ribosomal RNA (rRNA)[8] and RNA polymerase III which is responsible for synthesis of small RNA molecules.[9]

1. Matsui, T., Segall, J., Weil, A., and Roeder, R.G., Multiple factors required for accurate initiation of transcription by purified RNA polymerase II, *J. Biol. Chem.* 255, 11992–11996, 1980.

2. Weinmann, R., The basic RNA polymerase II transcriptional machinery, *Gene. Expr.* 2, 81–91, 1992.

3. Conaway, R.C., and Conaway, J.W., General initiation factors for RNA polymerase II, *Annu. Rev. Biochem.* 62, 161–190, 1993.

4. Orphanides, G., Lagrange, T., and Reinberg, D., The general transcription factors of RNA polymerase, *Genes Dev.* 10, 2657–2683, 1996.

5. Carey, M., and S.T. Smale, *Transcriptional Regulation in Eurkaryotes*, Cold Spring Harbor Press, Cold Spring Harbor, NY, 2000.

6. Rana, R., Surapureddi, S., Kam, S., Ferguson, S., and Goldstein, J.A., Med25 is required for RNA polymerase II recruitment to specific promoters, thus regulating xenobiotic and lipid metabolism in human liver, *Mol. Cell Biol.* 31, 466–481, 2011.

7. Plank, J.L., and Dean, A., Enhancer function: Mechanistic and genome-wide insights come together, *Mol. Cell* 55, 5–14, 2014.

8. Knutson, B.A., and Hahn, S., TFIIB-related factors in RNA polymerase I transcription, *Biochim. Biophys. Acta* 1829, 265–273, 2013.

9. Graczyk, D., Cieśla, M., and Boguta, M., Regulation of tRNA synthesis by the general transcription factors of RNA polymerase III -TFIIIB and TFIIIC, and by the MAF1 protein, *Biochim. Biophys. Acta Gene Regul. Mech.* 1861, 320–329, 2018

GENE EXPRESSION DOMAIN

The gene expression domain is a genomic region that contains a gene and all of the *cis*-acting elements that are required to obtain the homeostatic level and timing of gene expression *in vivo*.[1,2] Gene expression domains are generally defined by their ability to function independently of the site of integration into a transgene. This term is seldom used; a PubMed search found 24 total reference when "gene expression domain" was used as the search term.

1. Macedo, D.C., Isihikawa, E.C., Santos, C.B., et al., Proposed method for dimensionality reduction based on framework in gene expression domain, *Genet. Mol. Res.* 13, 10582–10591, 2014.
2. Koshikawa, S., Enhancer modularity and the evolution of new traits, *Fly*(Austin) 9, 155–159, 2015.

GENERIC DRUG

A generic drug is assumed to be the same as a brand name drug in dosage, safety, strength, administration, quality, and intended use. The suitability of a generic drug is based on the concept of "therapeutic equivalence." By law, a generic product must contain the identical amounts of the same active ingredient(s) as the brand name product.[1,2] The FDA definition is "A generic drug is the same as a brand name drug in dosage, safety, strength, how it is taken, quality, performance, and intended use. Before approving a generic drug product, FDA requires many rigorous tests and procedures to assure that the generic drug can be substituted for the brand name drug. The FDA bases evaluations of substitutability, or "therapeutic equivalence," of generic drugs on scientific evaluations. By law, a generic drug product must contain the identical amounts of the same active ingredient(s) as the brand name product. Drug products evaluated as "therapeutically equivalent" can be expected to have equal effect and no difference when substituted for the brand name product."[3] The term generic is used for substances defined as drugs as opposed to biologics such as proteins or nucleic acids where such products are defined as biosimilars[4,5] or follow-on biologics.[6,7] Follow-on biologics are products similar to existing products as are biosimilars but regulated by CDER (Center for Drug Evaluation and Research) with a regulatory filing through an NDA (New Drug Application) while biosimilars are regulated by CBER (Center for Biologic Evaluation and Research) with a regulatory filing through a Biological License Application (BLA). Some products such as insulin and human growth hormone which have properties similar to biologics are regulated by CDER providing the basis for regulation by NDA.

1. Verbeeck, R.K., Kanfer, I., and Walker, R.B., Generic substitution: The use of medicinal products containing different salts and implications for safety and efficacy, *Eur. J. Pharm. Sci.* 28, 1–6, 2006.
2. Devine, J.W., Cline, R.R., and Farley, J.F., Follow-on biologics: Competition in the biopharmaceutical marketplace, *J. Am. Pharm. Assoc.* 46, 193–201, 2006.
3. https://www.fda.gov/Drugs/InformationOnDrugs/ucm079436.htm.
4. Kirchhoff,C.F.,Wang,X.M.,Conlon,H.D.,et al.,Biosimilars: Key regulatory considerations and similarity assessment tools, *Biotechnol. Bioeng.* 114, 2696–2705, 2017.
5. McKinnon, R.A., Cook, M., Liauw, W., et al., Biosimilarity and interchangeability: Principles and evidence: A systematic review, *BioDrugs* 32, 27–52, 2018.
6. Sarpatwari, A., Avorn, J., and Kesselheim, A.S., Progress and hurdles for follow-on biologics, *N. Engl. J. Med.* 372, 2380–2382, 2015.
7. Dolinar, R., Lavernia, F., and Edelman, S., A guide to follow-on biologics and biosimilars with a focus on insulin, *Endocr. Pract.* 24, 195–204, 2018.

GENOME

The complete gene complement of any organism, contained in a set of chromosomes in eukaryotes, a single chromosome in bacteria, or a DNA or RNA molecule in viruses; the complete set of genes inside the cell or virus.[1-6]

1. DePamphilis, M.L., and Bell, S.D., *Genome Duplications*, Garland Science, New York, NY, 2011.
2. *Mitochondrial Genome Evolutiion*, ed. L. Maréchal-Dorouard, L.I., Academic Press/Elsevier, Amsterdam, the Netherlands, 2012.
3. Soh, J., *Genome Annotation*, Chapman & Hall/CRC Press, Boca Raton, FL, 2013.
4. Haber, J.E., *Genome Stability: DNA Repair and Recommendation*, Garland Science, New York, 2014.
5. *Genome Stability: From Virus to Human Application*, ed. I. Kovalchuk, Academic Press, London, UK, 2017.
6. Meneely, P.M., *Genetics: Genes, Genomes, and Evolution*, Oxford University Press, Oxford, UK, 2017.

GENOME-BASED PROTEOMICS

Gene-based approach to proteomics where the final product is a catalogue or encyclopedia of each protein coded by the genome.[1] There is limited interest in this concept as stated.[2-4] A closely related concept is the development of a human protein atlas.[5-8]

1. Agaton, C., Uhlén, M., and Hober, S., Genome-based proteomics, *Electrophoresis* 25, 1280–1288, 2004.
2. Wisz, M.S., Suarez, M.K., Holmes, M.R., and Giddings, M.C., GFSWeb: A web tool for genome-based identification of proteins from mass spectrometric samples, *J. Proteome Res.* 3, 1292–1295, 2004.
3. Falk, R., Ramström, M., Ericksson, C., et al., Targeted protein pullout from human tissue samples using competitive elution, *Biotechnol. J.* 6, 28–37, 2011.
4. Ku, T., Swaney, J., Park, J.Y., et al., Multiplexed and scalable super-resolution imaging of three-dimensional protein localization in size-adjusted tissues, *Nat. Biotechnol.* 34, 973–981, 2016.
5. Persson, A., Hober, S., and Uhlén, M., A human protein atlas based on antibody proteomics, *Curr. Opin. Mol. Ther.* 8, 185–190, 2006.
6. Hober, S., and Uhlén, M., Human protein atlas and the use of microarray technologies, *Curr. Opin. Biotechnol.* 19, 30–35, 2008.
7. Asplund, A., Edqvist, P.H., Schwenk, J.M., and Pontén, F., Antibodies for profiling the human proteome—The human protein atlas as a resource for cancer research, *Proteomics* 12, 2067–2077, 2012.
8. Thul, P.J., and Lindskog, C., The human protein atlas: A spatial map of the human proteome, *Protein Sci.* 27, 233–244, 2018.

GENOMIC DATABASES

There are a large number of genomic databases collectively referred to as the genomic commons.[1] Genomic databases include Genome[2] maintained by the National Center for Biotechnology Information and GOLD.[3] HUGO (Human Genetics Organization) has a list of genomic databases[4] (curated by the HUGO Gene Nomenclature Committee). An online tutorial for the use of genomic databases is available from the NIH.[5]

1. Contreras, J.L., and Knoppers, B.M., The genomic commons, *Ann. Rev. Genomics Human Genetics* 191, 1.1–1.25, 2018.
2. Genome, https://www.ncbi.nlm.nih.gov/genome/.
3. Genomes Online Directory; https://gold.jgi.doe.gov/).
4. https://www.genenames.org/seful/genome-databases-and-browsers.
5. https://www.genome.gov/27530225/free-online-tutorials-teach-anyone-how-to-use-genome-databases/.

GENOMICS

The study of the structure and function of the genome, including information about the sequence, mapping, and expression, and how genes and their products work in the organism; the study of the genetic composition of organisms.[1–6]

1. Chemical Genomics, ed. F. Darvas, A. Guttman, and G. Dormán, Marcel Dekker, New York, 2004.
2. *Genomics*, ed. I. Rigoutsos and G. Stephanopoulos, Oxford University Press, Oxford, UK, 2007.
3. *Comparative Genomics*, ed. N.H. Bergman, Humana Press, Totowa, NJ, 2007.
4. *Chemical Genomics*, ed. H. Fu., Cambridge University Press, New York, 2012.
5. *Comparative Genomics*, ed. X. Xia, Springer, Berlin, Germany, 2013.
6. *Clinical Genomics*, ed. Kulkami, S., and Pfeifer, J.D., Academic Press/Elsevier, London, UK, 2015.

GENOTYPE

The genetic information contained in an organism which would consist of all of the genes present in an organism. The genotype is separate from the phenotype which can be defined as the result of the expression of genotype and interaction with the environment; the observable characteristics of an organism.[1] The relationship of genotype and phenotype can be complex.[2,3]

1. *Oxford English Dictionary*, Oxford, UK, 2019.
2. Fisch, G.S., Whither the genotype-phenotype relationship? An historical and methodological appraisal, *Am. J. Med. Genet. C Semin. Med. Genet.* 175, 343–353, 2017.
3. Romanowska, J., and Joshi, A., From genotype to phenotype: Through chromatin, *Genes* (Basal) 10(2), E76, 2019.

GLASS

A glass may be best defined as a noncrystalline (amorphous) solid characterized by a lack of long range periodic atomic arrangement, high viscosity (approximately 10^{15} poises), and is energetically unstable relative to the crystalline state.[1–3] The formation of a glass is referred to as vitrification.[4,5] A glass is formed from a supercooled liquid and is associated with a decrease in enthalpy and an increase in viscosity. The formation of a glass from a melt requires rapid cooling to avoid crystallization.[6] While the term glass is most commonly associated with that formed from inorganic materials such as silicates,[7] glasses can be formed from other substances such as sugars,[8–10] and water.[11] It is suggested that most of the water in the universe is in the glassy state.[12] An intracellular glass state is suggested to occur in anhydrobiotic organisms.[13,14] The creation of an intracellular glass state is important for the cryopreservation of cells and tissues. The creation of a glass (vitrification) is critical in cryo-EM.[15]

1. Doremus, R.H., *Glass Sciences,* 2nd edn., John Wiley & Sons, New York, 1994.
2. Pfaender, H.G., *Schott Guide to Glass*, Chapman & Hall, London, UK, 1996.

3. Shelby, J.E., *Introduction to Glass Science and Technology*, Royal Society of Chemistry, Cambridge, UK, 1997.
4. Movy, G.W. *The Properties of Glass*, American Chemical Society/Rheinhold, New York, 1938.
5. Gutzow, I., and Schmelzer, J., *The Vitreous State. Thermodynamics, Structure, Rheology, and Crystallization*, Springer, Berlin, Germany, 1995.
6. Hilden, L.R., and Morris, K.R., Physics of amorphous solids, *J. Pharm. Sci.* 93(1), 3–12, 2004.
7. Zanotto, E.D., and Mauro, J.C., The glassy state of matter: Its definition and ultimate fate, *J. Non-Crystalline Solids* 171, 490–495, 2017.
8. Parks, G.S., Huffman, H.M., and Cattoir, F.R., Glass II. The transition between the glassy and liquid state in the case of glucose, *J. Phys. Chem.* 32, 1366–1379, 1928.
9. Teekamp, N., Tian, Y., Visser, J.C., et al., Addition of pullulan to trehalose glasses improves the stability of β-galactosidase at high moisture conditions, *Carbohydrate Polymers* 176, 374–380, 2017.
10. Sydykov, S., Olderhof, H., Sieme, H., and Wolkers, W.F., Hydrogen bonding interactions and enthalpy relaxation in sugar/protein glasses, *J. Pharm. Sci.* 106, 761–769, 2017.
11. Yannas, I., Vitrification temperatures of water, *Science* 160, 298–299, 1968.
12. Velkov, V., Borick, S., and Angeli, C.A., The glass transition of water, based on hyperquenching experiments, *Science* 294, 2235–2238, 2001.
13. Crowe, J.H., Carpenter, J.F., and Crowe, L.M., The role of vitrification in anhydrobiosis, *Annu. Rev. Physiol.* 60, 73–103, 1998.
14. Huebinger, J., Han, H.M, Hofnagel, O., et al., Direct measurement of water states in cryopreserved cells reveals tolerance toward ice crystallization, *Biophys. J.* 110, 840–849, 2016.
15. Passmore, L.A., and Russo, C.J., Specimen preparation for high-resolution cryo-em, *Methods Enzymol.* 579, 51–86, 2016.

GLASS TRANSITION/GLASS TRANSITION TEMPERATURE

"Glass transition" can best be described as marked changes in the physical properties of a substance over a usually narrow temperature range (glass transition temperature).[1,2] In the case of inorganic materials such as silicates, "glass transition" is associated with a marked increase in viscosity and decrease in enthalpy.[3] It was suggested that the glass transition temperature is 2/3 that of the melting temperature (temperature liquidus). With the production of glass from a melt, the material in the "glass transition" must be rapidly quenched to avoid crystallization (devitrification).[4] The term "glass transition" has also been used to refer to change of a polymer from an amorphous glass to rubber-like material.[5]

The "glass transition" temperature is a critical parameter during lyophilization of protein biopharmaceutical.[6,7] Independent of the "glass transition" of proteins cited above, there is at least one other "glass transition" or proteins occurring a lower temperatures (160–200 K).[8,9] The effect of water of these transitions is not clear; the "glass transition" of an anhydrous protein is suggested to occur at a higher temperature.[10] The glass transition temperature of water has been shown to be 165 K.[11] Earlier work had suggested a value of 134 K.

1. Richards, W.T., Remarks concerning the formation and crystallization of vitreous media, *J. Chem. Physics* 4, 449–457, 1936.
2. Doremus, R.H., *Glass Sciences*, 2nd edn., John Wiley, New York, 1994.
3. Sakata, S., and Mackenzie, J.D., Relation between apparent glass transition temperature and liquidus temperature for inorganic glasses, *J. Non-Crystalline Solids* 6, 145–162, 1971.
4. Hilden, L.R., and Morris, K.R., Physics of amorphous solids, *J. Pharm. Sci.* 93, 3–12, 2004.
5. Halley, P.J., and George, G.A., *Chemorheology of Polymers; From Fundamental Principles to Reactive Processing*, Cambridge University Press, Cambridge, UK, 2009.
6. Jennings, T.A., *Lyophilization: Introduction and Basic Principles.*, Interpharm Press, Englewood, CO, 1999.
7. Horn, J., Schanda, J., and Friess, W., Impact of fast and conservative freeze-drying on product quality of protein-mannitol-sucrose-glycerol lyophilizates, *Eur. J. Pharm. Biopharm.*127, 342–354, 2018.
8. Ringe, D., and Petsko, G.A., The "glass transition" in protein dynamics: What it is why it occurs, and how to exploit it, *Biophys. Chem.* 105, 667–680, 2003.
9. Coronel, L.G., Acierno, J.P., and Ermácora, M.P., Ultracompact states of native proteins, *Biophys. Chem.* 230, 36–44, 2017.
10. Monkos, K., Determination of the glass-transition temperature of proteins from a viscometric approach, *Int, J. Biol. Macromolecules* 74, 1–4, 2015.
11. Giovambattista, N., Angeli, C.A., Sciortino, F., and Stanley, H.E., Glass-transition temperature of water: A simulation study, *Phys. Rev. Lett.* 93(4), 047801, 2004.

GLOBAL PROTEOMICS

Global proteomics is a term used to describe the proteomic analysis of all proteins in a cell, tissue, organism, or in a specific pathology such as cancer.[1–4]

1. Yang, S., Chen, L., Chan, D.W., Li, Q.K., and Zhang, H., Protein signatures of molecular pathways in non-small cell lung carcinoma (NSCLC): Comparison of glycoproteomics and global proteomics, *Clin. Proteomics* 14, 31, 2017.

2. Ali, M., Khan, S.A., Wennerberg, K., and Aittokallio, T., Global proteomics profiling improves drug sensitivity prediction: Results from a multi-omics, pan-cancer modeling approach, *Bioinformatics* 34, 1353–1362, 2018.
3. Smith, J.N., Tyrrell, K.J., Hansen, J.R., et al., Plasma protein turnover rates in rats using stable isotope labeling, global proteomics, and activity-based protein profiling, *Anal. Chem.* 89, 13559–13556, 2017.
4. Vasaikar, S.V., Straub, P., Wang, J., and Zhang, B., LinkedOmics: Analyzing multi-omics data within and across 32 cancer types, *Nucleic Acids Res.* 46(D1), D956—D963, 2018.

GLOBULIN

The term globulin is a canonical definition for proteins which are insoluble in water but soluble in dilute salt solutions[1,2] and which migrate more slowly than albumin on free-boundary electrophoresis.[3] The globulins can be separated into several fractions including the γ-globulin fraction which contains the various immunoglobulin fractions and were defined as the most slowly moving protein fraction on electrophoresis at pH 8.6.[4–6] The term globulin is still occasionally used as a descriptor of proteins.[7,8] It is recognized that the term globulin is used to refer to specific therapeutic immunoglobulins such anti-thymocyte globulin.[9]

1. Osborne, T.B., and Harris, I.F. The solubility in salt solution, *Am. J. Physiol.* 14, 151–171, 1905.
2. Kodama, K., On the solubility of globulin in neutral salt solution, *J. Biochem.* 1, 419–432, 1922.
3. Cooper, G.R., Electrophoretic and ultracentrifugal analysis of normal human serum, in *The Plasma Proteins*, ed. F.W. Putnam, Academic Press, New York, Chapter 3, pp. 51–103, 1960.
4. Porter, H.R., γ-Globulins and antibodies, in *The Plasma Proteins*, ed. F.W. Putnam, Academic Press, New York, Chapter 7, pp. 241–277, 1960.
5. *Immunoglobulins*, ed. G.W. Litman and R.A. Good, Plenum Press, New York, 1978,
6. Lundblad, R.L., *Biotechnology of Plasma Proteins*, Plasma Immunoglobulins, Chapter 6, pp. 183–232, CRC Press, Boca Raton, FL, 2013.
7. Magni, C., Sessa, F., Capraro, J., et al., Structural and functional insights into the basic globulin 7S of soybean seeds by using trypsin as a molecular probe, *Biochem. Biophys. Res. Commun.* 496, 89–94, 2018.
8. Ji, X.G., Huang, J.H., Hui, M., Zhang, Y.Q., and Zhao, Y., Proteomic analysis and immunoregulation mechanism of wheat germ globulin, *Protein Pept. Lett.* 24, 1148–1165, 2018.
9. Mohty, M., Bacifalupo, A., Saliba, F., et al., New directions for rabbit antithymocyte globulin (Thymoglobuln®) in solid organ transplants, stem cell transplants and autoimmunity, *Drugs* 74, 1605–1634, 2014.

GLUCAN

A glucan is a polymer of D-Glucose produced by bacteria,[1] fungi,[2] and yeast.[3] β-Glucans are of medical interest.[4–6] A glucan is not be confused with a glycan. See **glycan**.

1. Xu, L., and Zhang, J., Bacterial glucans: Production, properties, and applications, *Appl. Microbiol. Biotechnol.* 100, 9023–9036, 2016.
2. Yoshimi, A., Miyazawa, K., and Abe, K., Function and biosynthesis of cell wall α-1,3-glucan in fungi, *J. Fungi* 3(4), 63, 2017.
3. Klis, F.M., Mol, P., Hellngwerf, K., and Brul, S., Dynamics of cell wall structure in *Saccharomyeces cerevisiae, FEMS Microbiol. Rev.* 26, 239–256, 2002.
4. Barton, C., Vigor, K., Scott, R., et al., Beta-glucan contamination of pharmaceutical products: How much should we accept? *Cancer Immunol. Immunother.* 65, 1289–1381, 2016.
5. Baldassano, S., Accardi, G., and Vasto, S., Beta-glucans and cancer. The influence of inflammation and gut peptide, *Eur. J. Med. Chem.* 142, 486–492, 2017.
6. Bashir, K.M.I., and Choi, J.S., Clinical and physiological perspective of β-glucans: The past, present, and future, *Int. J. Mol. Sci.* 18, 1906, 2017.

GLUCOSE OXIDASE

Glucose oxidase is a flavoprotein (FAD) enzyme (EC 1.1.3.4; β-D-glucose:oxygen 1-oxidoreductase), which catalyzes the oxidation of β-D-glucose to glucolactone/gluconic acid and hydrogen peroxide. The enzyme is highly specific for this form of glucose.[1–3] Glucose oxidase was discovered the early 1900s and originally described an antibacterial factor derived from molds such as *Pencilliium notatum* and *Aspergillus niger*.[4] Glucose oxidase was subsequently identified as the antibacterial/antibiotic activity in honey producing hydrogen peroxide.[5,6] The production of hydrogen peroxide by glucose oxidase was the basis for many assays for glucose in blood and bioreactors.[7–9] While glucose oxidase is still used for the direct measurement of glucose in biological fluids, there are new methods for measurement of glucose.[10,11] Glucose oxidase is also involved in herbivore offense in plants.[12,13]

1. Keilin, D., and Hartree, E.F., The use of glucose oxidase (Notatin) for the determination of glucose in biological material and for the study of glucose-producing systems by mannometric methods, *Biochem. J.* 42, 230–238, 1942.
2. Sols, A., and de la Fuente, G., On the substrate specificity of glucose oxidase, *Biochim. Biophys. Acta* 24, 206–207, 1957.

3. Wurster, B., and Hess, B., Anomeric specificity of enzymes for D-glucose metabolism, *FEBS Lett.* 40(Suppl), S112–S118, 1974.

4. Coulthard, C.E., Michaealis, R., Short, W.F., et al., Notatin: An antibacterial glucose aerodehydrogenase from *Penicillium notatum* and *Penicillium resitculosum* sp. nov, *Biochem. J.* 39, 24–36, 1945.

5. White, J.W., Jr., Subers, M.H., and Schepartz, A.I., The identification of inhibine, the antibacterial factor in honey, as hydrogen peroxide and its origin in a honey glucose-oxidase system, *Biochim. Biophys. Acta* 73, 57–70, 1963.

6. Bang, L.M., Bunting, C., and Molan, P., The effect of dilution on the rate of hydrogen peroxide production in honey and its implications for wound healing, *J. Alternative Complementary Med.* 9, 267–273, 2003.

7. Kiang, S.W., Kuan, J.W., Kuan, S.S., and Guilbault, G.G., Measurement of glucose in plasma, with use of immobilized glucose oxidase and peroxidase, *Clin. Chem.* 22, 1378–1382, 1976.

8. Chua, K.S., and Tan, I.K., Plasma glucose measurement with the Yellow Springs glucose analyzer, *Clin. Chem.* 24, 150–152, 1978.

9. Artiss, J.D., Strandbergh, D.R., and Zak, B., On the use of a sensitive indicator reaction for the automated glucose oxidase-peroxidase coupled reaction, *Clin. Biochem.* 1, 334–337, 1983.

10. Soni, A., and Jha, S.K., Smartphone based noninvasive salivary biosensor, *Anal. Chim. Acta* 996, 54–63, 2017.

11. Acciarioli, G., Vettoretti, M., Facchinetti, A., and Sparacino, G., Calibration of minimally invasive continuous glucose monitoring sensors: State-of-the-art and current perspectives, *Biosensors* 8(1), 24, 2018.

12. Musser, R.O., Cipollini, D.F., Hum-Musser, S.M., et al., Evidence that the caterpillar salivary enzyme glucose oxidase provides herbivore offense in solanaceous plants, *Archs. Insect Biochem. Physiol.* 58, 128–137, 2005.

13. Tian, D., Peiffer, M., Shoemaker, E., et al., Salivary glucose oxidase from caterpillars mediates the induction of rapid and delayed-induced defenses in the tomato plant, *PLoS One* 7(4), e36168, 2012.

GLUCOSE REGULATED PROTEIN 78, Grp78, BiP

Grp78 (glucose-regulated protein 78; BiP; immunoglobulin heavy-chain-binding protein) is an intracellular chaperone protein located in the endoplasmic reticulum.[1,2] As an intracellular chaperone, Grp78 assists in the correct folding of proteins and in the unfolded protein response.[3,4] GRP78 is a member the heat-shock protein 70 family (HSP 70)[5] and is found on the plasma membrane surface under stress conditions[6] where it has a variety of functions including the regulation of tissue factor activity and a receptor for angiogenic peptides.[7]

1. Munro, S., and Pelham, H.R., An Hsp70-like protein in the ER: Identity with the 78 kd glucose-regulated protein and immunoglobulin heavy chain binding protein, *Cell* 46, 291–300, 1986.

2. Hendershot, L.M., Ting, J., and Lee, A.S., Identity of the immunoglobulin heavy-chain-binding protein with the 78,000 dalton glucose-regulated protein and the role of posttranslational modifications in its binding function, *Mol. Cell Biol.* 8, 4250–4256, 1988.

3. Okudo, H., Kato, H., Arakaki, Y., and Urade, R., Cooperation of ER-60 and BiP in the oxidative refolding of denatured proteins in vitro, *J. Biochem.* 138, 773–780, 2005.

4. Sorgjerd, K., Ghafouri, B., Jonsson, B.H., et al., Retention of misfolded mutant transthyretin by the chaperone BiP/GRP78 mitigates amyloidogenesis, *J. Mol. Biol.* 356, 469–482, 2006.

5. Behnke, J., Feige, M.J., and Hendershot, L.M., BiP and its nucleotide exchange factors Grp170 and Sil1: Mechanisms of action and biological functions, *J. Mol. Biol.* 427, 1589–1608, 2015.

6. Panayi, G.S., and Corrigall, V.M., Immunoglobulin heavy-chain-binding protein (BiP): A stress protein that has the potential to be a novel therapy for rheumatoid arthritis, *Biochem. Soc. Trans.* 42, 1752–1755, 2014.

7. Gonzalez-Gronow, M., Pizzo, S.V., and Misra, U.K., GRP78 (BiP): A multifunctional cell surface receptor, in *Cellular Trafficking of Cell Stress Protein in Health and Disease*, ed. B. Henderson and A.G. Pockley, Springer Science, Dordrecht, the Netherlands, 2012.

GLUCOSYLTRANSFERASE

Transferases are a class of enzymes that transfer of moiety from a donor molecule to an acceptor. Glucosyltransferases can be considered to be glycosyltransferases. Glycosyltransferases are a group of enzymes which transfer a monosaccharide moiety from a donor to an acceptor where the acceptor could be protein-bound glycan, a protein, or another sugar.[1] UDP-glucose glycoprotein glucotransferase (UGGT) is located in endoplasmic reticulum and functions as quality control in the folding of proteins.[2,3] Protein O-glucosyltransferase (POGLUT) catalyzes the transfer of glucose from UDP-glucose to a serine residue in a polypeptide.[4,5] Protein O-glucosyltransferase also catalyzed the transfer xylose from UDP-zylose to a protein. A third type of glucosyl transfers glucose from a donor such as sucrose to form glucans.[6,7]

1. Coutinho, P.M., Deleury, E., Davies, G.J., and Henrissat, B., An evolving hierarchical family classification for glycosyltransferases, *J. Mol. Biol.* 326, 307–317, 2003.

2. Taylor, S.C., Ferguson, A.D., Bergeron, J.J.M., and Thomas, D.Y., The ER protein folding sensor EDP-glucose glycoprotein-glucosyltransferase modifies substrates distant to local changes in glycoprotein conformation, *Nature Struct. Mol. Biol.* 11, 128–134, 2004.

3. D'Alessio, C., Caramelo, J.J., and Parodi, A.J., UDP-GlC:protein glucosyltransferase-glucosidase II, the ying-yang of ER quality control, *Sem. Cell Dev. Biol.* 21, 491–499, 2010.

4. Takeuchi, H., Kantharia, J., Sethi, M.K., Bakker, H., and Haliwanger, R.S., Site-specific O-glucosylation of the epidermal growth factor-like (EGF) repeats of notch: Efficiency of glycosylation is affected by the proper folding and amino acid sequence of individual EGF repeats, *J. Biol. Chem.* 287, 33934–33944, 2012.

5. Li, Z., Fischer, M., Satkunarajah, M., Zhou, D. Withers, S.G., and Rini, J.M., Structural basis of Notch O-glycosylation and O-xylosylation by mammalian protein-O-glucosyltransferase 1 (POGLUT1), *Nat. Commun.* 8, 185, 2017.

6. Ciardi, J.E., Beaman, A.J., and Wittenberger, C.L., Purification, resolution, and interaction of the glucosyltransferases of *Streptococcus mutans* 6715, *Infect. Immun.* 18, 236–246, 1977.

7. Koo, H., Rosalen, P.L., Cury, J.A., Park, J.K., and Bowen, W.H., Effect of compounds found in propolis on *Streptococcus mutans* growth and on glucosyltransferase activity, *Antimicrobial Agents Chemother.* 46, 1302–1309, 2002.

GLUCOSE TRANSPORTER (GLUT)

The glucose transporter protein (GLUT) family are uniporters which facilitates the transport of glucose into the cell.[1] There are 14 members of human GLUT family which are encoded by the *SLC2* genes which show differences in tissue distribution and transport specificity.[2] The overexpression of GLUT1 in ovarian cancer is associated with a poor prognosis.[3] GLUT-1 expression is increased in other tumors suggesting that it might be a drug target but there are some complications.[4]

1. Gould, G.W., and Holman G.D., The glucose transporter family—Structure, function and tissue-specific expression, *Biochem. J.* 295, 329–341, 1993.

2. Mueckler, M., and Thorens, B., The SLC2 (GLUT) family of membrane transporters, *Molec. Aspects Med.* 34, 121–138, 2013.

3. Cho, H., Lee, Y.S., Kim, J., Chung, J.Y., and Kim, J.H., Overexpression of glucose transporter-1 (GLUT-1) predicts poor prognosis in epithelial ovarian cancer, *Cancer Invest.* 31, 607–615, 2013.

4. Oh, S., Kim, H., Nam, K., and Shin, I., Silencing of Glut1 induces chemoresistance via modulation of Akt/GSK-3β/β-catenin/survivin signaling pathway in breast cancer cells, *Arch. Biochem. Biophys.* 636, 110–122, 2017.

GLYCAN

A glycan is a polysaccharide chain that is covalently linked to a protein.[1–4] A glycan is not to be confused with glucan which is a polymer of glucose synthesized by bacteria, fungi, and yeast.

1. Lopez Aguilar, A., Briard, J.G., Yang, L., et al., Tools for studying glycans: Recent advances in chemoenzymatic glycan labeling, *ACS Chem. Biol.* 12, 611–621, 2017.

2. Johannsen, T., and Lepenies, B., Glycan-based cell targeting to modulate immune responses, *Trends Biotechnol.* 35, 334–346, 2017.

3. Shanker, S., Hu, L., Ramani, S., Atmar, R.L., et al., Structural features of glycan recognition among viral pathogens, *Curr. Opin. Struct. Biol.* 44, 211–218, 2017.

4. Manz, C., and Pagel, K., Glycan analysis by ion mobility-mass spectrometry and gas-phase spectroscopy, *Curr. Opin. Chem. Biol.* 42, 16–24, 2018.

GLYCATION

Glycation is a term used to the describe the non-enzymatic covalent linking of a reducing sugar such as glucose or product of metabolism such as methyl glyoxal with a primary amino group on a protein or nucleic acid.[1] Glycation is mechanistically different from glycosylation and yields a different product.[2] **Glycosylation** is a process catalyzed by a series of enzymes resulting in complex glycan covalently attached to a protein.[3] Lysine is the primary site of glycation in proteins while guanosine is the primary target in nucleic acids.[4] There has been a much greater emphasis on the study of the non-enzymatic glycation of proteins than nucleic acids. Glycation can be considered the initial step in the process of formation of more complex products (see Advanced Glycation End Products). The best-known glycation product is hemoglobin A1c which is the product of the reaction of glucose with the α-amino group of *N*-terminal valine of the β-chain of hemoglobin.[5] Hemoglobin A1c is a biomarker for diabetes.[6–8]

1. Shuck, S.C., Wuenschell, G.E., and Termini, J.S., Product studies and mechanistic analysis of the reaction of methylglyoxal with deoxyguanosine, *Chem. Res. Toxicol.* 31, 105–115, 2018.

2. Taniguchi, N., Takahashi, M., Kizuka, Y., et al., Glycation vs. glycosylation: A tale of two different chemistries and biology in Alzheimer's disease, *Glycoconj. J.* 33, 487–497, 2016.

3. *Essentials of Glycobiology*, ed. A. Varki, R. Cummings, J. Esko, H. Freeze, G. Hart, and J. Marth, Cold Spring Harbor Laboratory Press, Cold Spring Harbor, NY, 1999.

4. Krantz, S., Lober, M., and Henschel, L., The non-enzymatic glycation of proteins and nucleic acids, their importance for the development of diabetic complications, possible molecular basis of aging and autoimmunolgical processes, *Exp. Clin. Endocrinol.* 88, 257–269, 1986.

5. Holmquist, W.R., and Schroeder, W.A., Properties and partial characterization of adult human hemoglobin A1c, *Biochim. Biophys. Acta.* 82, 639–641, 1964.

6. Lyons, T.J., and Basu, A., Biomarkers in diabetes: Hemoglobin A1c, vascular and tissue markers, *Translational Res.* 159, 303–312, 2012.
7. Sandler, C.N., and McDonnell, M.E., The role of hemoglobin A1c in the assessment of diabetes and cardiovascular risk, *Cleveland Clin. J. Med.* 83(5 suppl 1), S4–S10, 2016.
8. Lenters-Westra, E., and English, E., Understanding the use of Sigma metrics in hemoglobin A1c analysis, *Clin. Lab. Med.* 37, 57–71, 2017.

GLYCOME

By analogy to the proteome, the glycome is the total polysaccharide, including glycans, content of an organism, tissue, or system.[1–8]

1. Ribeiro, J.P., and Mahal, L.K., Dot by dot: Analyzing the glycome using lectin microarrays, *Curr. Opin. Chem. Biol.* 16, 827–831, 2013.
2. Zoldoš, V., Novokmet, M., Bečeheli, I., and Lauc, C., Genomics and epigenomics of the human glycome, *Glycoconj. J.* 30, 41–50, 2013.
3. Glavey, S.V., Huynh, D., Reagan, M.R., et al., The cancer glycome: Carbohydrates as mediators of metastasis, *Blood Rev.* 29, 269–279, 2015.
4. Kavanaugh, D., O'Callaghan, J., Kilcoyne, M., et al., The intestinal glycome and is modulation by diet and nutrition, *Nutr. Rev.* 73, 359–375, 2015.
5. Lauc, G., Pezer, M., Rudan, I., and Campbell, H., Mechanisms of disease: The human *N*-glycome, *Biochim. Biophys. Acta* 1860, 1574–1582, 2016.
6. Bard, F., and Chia, J. Cracking the glycome encoder: Signaling, trafficking, and glycosylation, *Trends Cell Biol.* 26, 379–388, 2016.
7. Gerlach, J.Q., and Griffin, M.D., Getting to the know the extracellular vesicle glycome, *Mol. Biosyst.* 12, 1071–1081, 2016.
8. Alocci, D., Ghraichy, M., Barletta, E., et al., Understanding the glycome: An interactive view of glycosylation from glycocomposition to glycoepitopes, *Glycobiology* 28, 349–362, 2018.

GLYCOMICS

Glycomics is the study of the structure, function, and interactions of carbohydrates including polysaccharides and glycans within the glycome.[1–7] See also **glycoproteomics**.

1. Drake, R.R., Glycosylation and cancer: Moving Glycomics to the foretront, *Adv. Cancer Res.* 126, 1–10, 2015.
2. Moh, E.S., Thaysen-Andersen, M., and Packer, N.H., Relaive versus absolute quantitation in disease gycomics, *Proteomics Clin. Appl.* 9, 368–382, 2015.
3. Springer, S.A., and Gagneux, P., Glycomics revealing the dynamic ecology and evolution of sugar molecules, *J. Proteomics* 135, 90–100, 2016.

4. Chandler, K.B., and Costello, C.E., Glycomics and glycoproteomics of membrane proteins and cell surface receptors: Present trends and future opportunities, *Electrophoresis* 37, 1407–1419, 2016.
5. Miura, Y., and Endo, T., Glycomics and glycoproteomics focused on aging and age-related diseases-Glycans as a potential biomarker for physiological alterations, *Biochim. Biophys. Acta* 1860, 1608–1614, 2016.
6. Bennun, S.V., Hizal, D.B., Heffner, K., et al., Systems glycobiology: Integrating glycogenomics, glycoproteomics, glycomics, and other 'omics data sets to characterize cellular glycosylation processes, *J. Mol. Biol.* 428, 3337–3352, 2016.
7. Smith, J., Mittermayr, S., Váradi, C., and Bones, J., Quantiative glycomics using liquid phase separations coupled to mass spectrometry, *Analyst* 142, 700–720, 2017.

GLYCOPEGYLATION

Glycopegylation is a method by which a polyethylene glycol (PEG) chain may be attached to a serine or threonine residue in a protein.[1,2] The initial step involves the introduction of an *N*-acetylgalactosamine to a serine residue or threonine residue in a nonglycosylated recombinant protein by the action of a polypeptide *N*-acetylgalactosamine transferase. A PEG chain attached to sialic acid residue can be coupled to cytidine monophosphate forming a derivative which can be coupled to the protein-bound *N*-acetylgalactoseamine. Alternatively, a galactose residue can be added to the *N*-acetylgalactoseamine and the CMP-sialic acid-PEG derivative coupled to the disaccharide. Glycopegylation has been used to extend the circulatory half-life of blood coagulation factor VIII.[3]

1. DeFrees, S., Wang, Z-G., Xing, R., et al., GlycoPEGylation of recombinant therapeutic proteins produced in *Escherichia coli*, *Glycobiology* 16, 833–843, 2006.
2. Giorgi, M.E., Agusti, R., and de Lederkremer, R.M., Carbohydrate PEGylation, an approach to improve pharmacological potency, *Beilstein J. Org. Chem.* 10, 1433–1444, 2014.
3. Tiede, A., Brand, B., Fischer, R., et al., Enhancing the pharmacokinetic properties of recombinant factor VIII: First-in-human trial of glycoPEGylated recombinant factor VIII in patients with hemophilia A, *J. Thromb. Haemost.* 11, 670–678, 2013.

GLYCOPROTEOMICS

Glycoproteomics is a discipline within glycomics focuses on the study of glycans and the attachment of glycans to proteins.[1–3] See **glycans**.

1. Thaysen-Andersen, M., Packer, N.H., and Schulz, B.L., Maturing glycoproteomics technologies provide unique structural insights into the *N*-glycoproteome and its regulation in health and disease, *Mol. Cell. Proteomics* 15, 1773–1790, 2016.
2. Plomp, R., Bondt, A., de Haan, N., Rombouts, Y., and Wuhrer, M., Recent advances in clinical glycoproteomics of immunoglobulins (Igs), *Mol. Cell. Proteomics* 15, 2217–2228, 2016.
3. Halim, A., and Anonsen, J.H., Microbial glycoproteomics, *Curr. Opin. Struct. Biol.* 44, 143–150, 2017.

GLYCOSIDASE

An enzyme that hydrolyzes glycosidic bonds; most often in oligosaccharides and polysaccharides.[1–4] Glycosidases are important in the processing of glycoproteins in the endoplasmic reticulum.[5,6]

1. Allen, H.J., and Kisailus, E.C., *Glycoconjugates: Composition, Structure, and Function*, Dekker, New York, 1992.
2. *Guide to Techniques in Glycobiology*, ed. W.J. Lennarz and G.W. Hart, Academic Press, San Diego, CA, 1994.
3. Bucke, C., *Carbohydrate Biotechnology Protocols*, Humana Press, Totowa, NJ, 1999.
4. Himmel, M.E., and Baker, J.O., *Glycosyl Hydrolases for Biomass Conversion*, American Chemical Society, Washington, DC, 2001.
5. Harding, S.E., *An Introduction to Polysaccharide Biotechnology*, 2nd edn., CRC Press/Taylor & Francis Group, Boca Raton, FL, 2017.
6. Stigliano, I.D., Alculumbre, S.G., Labriola, C.A., et al., Glucosidase II and *N*-glycan mannose content regulate the half-life of monoglucosylated species *in vivo*, *Mol. Biol. Cell* 22, 1810–1823, 2011.

GLYCOSYLTRANSFERASE

A glycosyltransferase is an enzyme which synthesizes compounds with glycosidic bonds by catalyzing the transfer of glycosyl groups from a donor to an acceptor. Much emphasis is placed on the synthesis of glycan moieties of glycoproteins[1] but there are other glycosylated products[2] including steryl glycosides,[3] sucrose,[4] and dolichol phosphate derivatives.[5,6]

1. *Handbook of Glycosyltransferases and Related Genes*, 2nd edn., ed. N. Taniguchi, K. Honke, M. Fukuda, H. Narimatsu, Y. Yamaguchi, and T. Angata, Springer, Tokyo, Japan, 2014.
2. Heath, E.C., Complex polysaccharides, *Annu. Rev. Biochem.* 40, 29–56, 1971.)
3. Singh, G., Dhar, Y.V., Asif, M.H., and Misra, P., Exploring the functional significance of sterol glycosyltransferase enzymes, *Prog. Lipid Res.* 69, 1–10, 2018.
4. Schmölzer, K., Gutmann, A., Diricks, M., Desmet, M., and Nidetzky, B., Sucrose synthase: A unique glycosyltransferase for biocatalytic glycosylation process development, *Biotechnol. Adv.* 34, 88–111, 2016.
5. Maeda, Y., and Kinoshita, T., Dolichol-phosphate mannose synthase structure, function and regulation, *Biochim. Biophys. Acta* 1780, 861–868, 2008.
6. Banerjee, D.K., Zhang, Z., Baksi, K., and Serrano-Negrón, J.E., Dolichol phosphate mannose synthase: A glycosyltransferase with unity in molecular diversities, *Glycoconj. J.* 34, 467–479, 2017.

GOBLET CELL

Goblet cells are a specialized cell found in the epithelium with high occurrence in respiratory and digestive tracts. The goblet cells are among the specialized cells in the epithelium which also includes clara cells, ciliated cells, basal cells as well as dendritic cells.[1,2] Goblet cells secrete mucus which is composed of water, ionic species and macromolecules forming a functional layer on the epithelium in the pulmonary bed and digestive tract.[3] Mucus secretion by epithelium occurs in other sites such as the eye, trachea, and nasal passage. There is interaction between the microbiome and goblet cells.[4,5] There is evidence to suggest that the goblet cells is an antigen presenting cells to dendritic cells in the intestinal epithelia.[6]

1. Breeze, R.G., and Wheeldon, F.B., The cells of the pulmonary airways, *Am. Rev. Respir. Dis.* 116, 705–719, 2015.
2. Chang, M.M-J., Shih, L., and Wu, K., Pulmonary epithelium—cells types of functions, in *The Pulmonary Epithelium in Health and Disease,* ed. D. Proud, Chapter 1, pp. 1–26, John Wiley & Sons, Chichester, UK, 2008.
3. Palaseyed, T., Bergström, J.H., Gustafsson, J.K., et al., The mucus and mucins of goblet cells and enterocytes provide the first line of defense line of gastrointestinal tract and interact with the immune system, *Immunol. Rev.* 260, 8–20, 2014.
4. Knoop, K.A., McDonald, K.G., McCrate, S., McDole, J.R., and Newberry, R.D., Microbial sensing by goblet cells controls immune surveillance of luminal antigens in the colon, *Mucosal Immunol.* 8, 198–210, 2015.
5. Sicard, J-F., Le Bihan, G., Vogeleer, P., Jachques, M., and Harel, J., Interactions of intestinal bacteria with components of the intestinal mucus, *Front. Cell. Infect. Microbiol.* 7, 387, 2017.
6. McCauley, H.A., an Guasch, G., Three cheers for the goblet cell: Maintaining homeostasis in the mucosal epithelia, *Trends Mol. Med.* 21, 492–500, 2015.

GOLGI APPARATUS

The Golgi apparatus (also referred to as the Golgi complex) is a subcellular organelle consisting of a series of membrane structures referred to as cisternae.[1-6] The Golgi has a *cis*-side facing the endoplasmic reticulum and a *trans*-side which interfaces with the plasma membrane via the formation of secretory vesicles and also with components of the endocytotic pathway.[7] The Golgi apparatus functions in the protein secretory pathway by transporting and packing of proteins for distribution either elsewhere in the cell or for secretion is what is described as anterograde, *cis* to *trans*.[8-10] Transport through the Golgi is bidirectional with a selective retrograde transport, *trans* to cis, of some toxins and membrane components.[11,12] ARF (ADP ribosylation factor) proteins are involved in the retrograde transport process.[13,14] There are two concepts regarding transport through the Golgi; vesicular fusion and cisternal maturation.[15] Rab proteins (members of Ras GTPase family are involved in Golgi transport in either model).[16] Also, either model for transport through the Golgi apparatus involves the organized fusion of the vesicular structures regulated by SNARE proteins (SNARE, SNAP receptors).[17,18] See **golgins**.

1. Whaley, W.B., *The Golgi Apparatus*, Springer-Verlag, New York, 1975.
2. Pavelka, M., *Functional Morphology of the Golgi Apparatus*, Springer-Verlag, Berlin, Germany, 1987.
3. *The Golgi Apparatus*, ed. E.G. Berger and J. Roth, Birkhäuser Verlag, Basel, 1997.
4. Loh, Y.P., *Mechanisms of Intracellular Trafficking and Processing of Preproteins*, CRC Press, Boca Raton, FL, 1993.
5. Han, H.M., Bouchet-Marquis, C., Huebinger, J., and Grabenbauer, M., Golgi apparatus analyzed by cryo-electron microscopy, *Histochem. Cell Biol.* 140, 369–381, 2013.
6. Dunlop, M.H., Ernst, A.M., Schroeder, W., et al., Land-locked membrane Golgi reveals cargo transport between stable cisternae, *Nat. Commun.* 18, 432, 2017.
7. Prydz, K., Dick, G., and Tveit, H., How many ways through the Golgi maze? *Traffic* 9, 299–304, 2008.
8. *Guidebook to the Secretory Pathway*, ed. J. Rothblatt and Novak, P., Oxford University Press, Oxford, UK, 1997.
9. Robinson, D.G., *The Golgi Apparatus and the Plant Secretory Pathway*, CRC Press, Boca Raton, FL, 2003.
10. Witkos, T.M., and Lowe, M., Recognition and tethering of transport vesicles at the Golgi apparatus, *Curr. Opin. Cell Biol.* 47, 16–23, 2017.
11. Lord, J.M., and Roberts, L.M., Toxin entry: Retrograde transport through the secretory pathway, *J. Cell Biol.* 140, 733–736, 1998.
12. Bonifacino, J.S., and Roajas, R., Retrograde transport from exosomes to the *trans*-Golgi network, *Nat. Rev. Mol. Cell Biol.* 7, 568–579, 2006.
13. Souza-Schorey, C., and Chavrier, P., ARF proteins: Roles in membrane traffic and beyond, *Nat. Rev. Mol. Cell Biol.* 7, 347–358, 2006.
14. Huang, L.-H., Lee, W.-C., You, S-T., and Yu, C-J., Arfaptin-1 negatively regulates Arl1-mediated retrograde transport, *PLoS One* 10(3), 118743, 2015.
15. Alberts, B., Johnson, A., Lewis, J., Raff, M., Roberts, K., and Walter, P., *Molecular Biology of the Cell*, 5th edn., Garland Science, New York, 2008.
16. Goud, B., Liu, S., and Storrie, B. Rab proteins as major determinants of the Golgi complex structure, *Small GTPases* 9, 66–75, 2018.
17. Malsam, J., and Sollner, T.H., Organization of SNAREs within the Golgi stack, *Cold Spring Harb Perspectives Biology* 3, a005249, 2011.
18. Anderson, N.S., Mukherjee, I., Bentivoglio, C.M., and Barlowe, C., The golgin protein Coyl functions in intra-Golgi retrograde transport and interacts with the COG complex and Golgi SNAREs, *Mol. Biol. Cell* 28, 2686–2700, 2017.

GOLGINS

Golgins are a family of proteins associated with the Golgi apparatus.[1-3] Members of the golgin family are characterized by the presence of a long region of coiled-coil forming long rod-like structures which serve to tether components of the Golgi apparatus such as Rab GTPase responsible for vesicular transport.[4,5] The golgin also provide binding sites for SNARE proteins which are responsible for membrane fusion during transport through the Golgi apparatus.[6,7]

1. Kjer-Nielsen, L., Teasdale, R.D., van Vliet, C., and Gleeson, P.A., A novel Golgi-localization domain shared by a class of coiled-coil peripheral membrane proteins, *Curr. Biol.* 9, 385–388, 1999.
2. Munro, S., and Nichols, B.J., The GRIP domain—A novel Golgi-targeting domain found in several coiled-coil proteins, *Curr. Biol.* 9, 377–380, 1999.
3. Barinaga-Rementeria Ramirez, I., and Lowe, M., Golgins and GRASPs: Holding the Golgi together, *Sem. Cell Develop. Biol.* 20, 770–779, 2009.
4. Wilkins, T.M., and Lowe, M., The golgin family of coiled-coil tethering proteins, *Front. Cell Devel. Biol.* 3, 86, 2015.
5. Gillingham, A.K., and Munro, S., Finding the Golgi: Golgin coiled-coil proteins show the way, *Trends Cell Biol.* 26, 399–408, 2016.
6. Wang, T., Grabski, R., Sztul, E., and Hay, J.C., p115-SNARE interactions: A dynamic cycle of p115 binding monomeric SNARE motifs and releasing assembled bundles, *Traffic* 16, 148–171, 2015.
7. Cheung, P.Y., and Pfeffer, S.R., Transport vesicle tethering at the trans Golgi network: Coiled coil proteins in action, *Front. Cell. Dev. Biol.* 4, 18, 2016.

GRANZYMES

Granzymes are serine proteases that are contained in cytoplasmic granules in cytotoxic T cells and natural killer cells.[1,2] Granzymes enter the target cell through pores created by perforin[3,4] and induce apoptosis through a variety of mechanisms including caspase-dependent and caspase-independent pathways.[5,6] There are five human granzymes (there are a total of 12 identified granzymes) differentiated on the basis of specificity for peptide bond cleavage.[7-9]

1. Jenne, D.E., and Tchopp, J., Granzymes, a family of serine proteases released from granules of cytolytic T lymphocytes upon T cell receptor stimulation, *Immunol. Rev.* 103, 53–71, 1988.
2. Smyth, M.J., and Trapani, J.A., Granzymes: Exogenous proteinases that induce target cell apoptosis, *Immunol. Today* 16, 202–206, 1995.
3. Voskoboinik, I., Whisstock, J.D., and Trapani, J.A., Perforin and granzymes: Function, dysfunction and human pathology, *Nat. Rev. Immunol.* 15, 388–400, 2015.
4. Spicer, B.A., Conroy, P.J., Law, R.H.P., Voskovoinik, I., and Whisstock, J.C., Perforin-A key (shaped) weapon in the immunological arsenal, *Semin. Cell Dev. Biol.* 72, 117–123, 2017.
5. Ashton-Rickardt, P.G., The granule pathway of programmed cell death, *Crit. Rev. Immunol.* 25, 161–182, 2005.
6. Bleackely, R.C., A molecular view of cytotoxic T lymphocyte induced killing, *Biochem. Cell Biol.* 83, 747–751, 2005.
7. *Handbook of Proteolytic Enzymes,* ed. N.D. Rawlings and G. Salvesen, Elsevier, Amsterdam, the Netherlands, 2013.
8. Plasman, K., Mauer-Stroh, S., Gevaert, K., and Van Damme, P., Holistic view of the extended substrate specificities of orthologous granzymes, *J. Proteome Res.* 13, 1785–1793, 2014.
9. Arias, M., Martinez-Lostao, L., Santiago, L., et al., The untold story of granzymes in oncoimmunology: Novel opportunities with old acquaintances, *Trends Cancer* 3, 407–422, 2017.

GTP-BINDING PROTEINS (SMALL GTP-BINDING PROTEINS; SMALL GTPases)

Small GTP-binding proteins (G proteins) are intracellular proteins which bind GTP and have a wide variety of functions including signal transduction and in turn protein synthesis and cell proliferation. The small GTP-binding proteins are members of the Ras superfamily and are usually distinguished from the heterotrimeric GTP-binding protein (Gα) that is associated with the G-protein-coupled receptor (GPCR).[1] These proteins are "active" when GTP is bound; on hydrolysis of the GTP to GDP, "activity" is lost. The nature of the "activity" is poorly defined but involves interaction with other proteins, frequently protein kinases, which can be designated as effector proteins.[2] The exchange of GDP to GTP (transition from inactive form to active form) is regulated by guanine nucleotide exchange factor (GEF) and GTPase activity (transition from active form to inactive form is enhanced by GTPase-activating protein (GAP).[3,4] Transglutaminase II has been described as a GTP-binding proteins.[5-7]

1. Sprang, S.R., Activation of G proteins by GTP and the mechanism of Gα-catalyzed GTP hydrolysis, *Biopolymers* 105, 449–462, 2015.
2. Erijman, A. an Shifman, J.M., RAS/effector interactions from structural and biophysical perspective, *Mini Rev. Med. Chem.* 16, 370–375, 2016.
3. Autonny, B., Chardin, P., Roux, M., and Chabre, M., GTP hydrolysis mechanisms in ras p21 and the ras-GAP complex studied by fluorescence measurements on tryptophan mutants, *Biochemistry* 30, 8287–8295, 1991.
4. Corbett, K.D., and Alber, T., The many faces of Ras: Recognition of small GTP-binding proteins, *Trends Biochem. Sci.* 26, 710–716, 2001.
5. Russell, M.A., and Feng, J.F., Transglutaminase II: A new class of GTP-binding protein with new biological functions, *Cell Signal.* 9, 477–482, 1997.
6. Iismaa, S.E., Wu, M.J., Nanda, N., Church, W.B., and Graham, R.M., GTP binding and signaling by Gh/transglutaminase II involves distinct residues in a unique GTP-binding pocket, *J. Biol. Chem.* 275, 18259–18265, 2000.
7. Akbar, A., McNeil, N.M.R., Albert, M.R., et al., Structure-activity relationships of potent, targeted covalent inhibitors that abolish both the transamidation and GTP binding activities of human tissue transglutaminase, *J. Med. Chem.* 60, 7910–7927, 2017.

HABER–WEISS REACTION

The Haber–Weiss reaction was developed in 1934.[1] Previously, Fenton observed that the presence of iron salts increased the oxidizing power of hydrogen peroxide as observed by the oxidation of tartaric acid.[2]

$$O_2 + H_2O_2 \rightarrow OH^{\cdot} + O_2 + OH^{-} \quad Haber-Weiss$$

$$Fe^{2+} + H_2O_2 \rightarrow Fe^{3+} + OH^{-} + OH^{\cdot} \quad Fenton\ Reaction$$

It has been noted that Haber and Weiss did not reference Fenton in their 1934 paper.[3] Superoxide is generated as a consequence of normal metabolic activity.[4] The reaction is quite slow (possibly insignificant) in the absence of metal ions but the rate of hydroxyl radical formation is markedly enhanced by metal ions.[5-7] See **Fenton reaction**.

1. Haber, F., and Weiss, J., The catalytic decomposition of hydrogen peroxide by iron salts, *Proc. R. Soc. London Series A* 147, 332–351, 1934.
2. Fenton, H.J.H., Oxidation of tartaric acid in the presence of iron, *J. Chem. Soc. Trans* 65, 899–910, 1894.
3. Koppenol, W.H., The Haber–Weiss cycle—70 years later, *Redox Report* 6, 229–234, 2001.
4. Munro, D., and Tieberg, J.R., A radical shift in perspective: Mitochondria as regulator of reactive oxygen species, *J. Exp. Biol.* 220, 1170–1180, 2917.
5. Kehrer, J.P., The Haber–Weiss reaction and mechanisms of toxicity, *Toxicology* 149, 43–40, 2000.
6. Xu, D. Liu, D., Wang, B., et al., *In situ* generation from O_2^- and H_2O_2 plays a critical role in plasma-induced cell death, *PLoS One* 10(6), e128205, 2015.
7. Saporito-Magriñá, C., Musacco-Sebio, R., Acosta, J.M., et al., Copper (II) and iron (III) ions inhibit respiration and increase free radical-mediated phospholipid peroxidation in rat liver mitochondria: Effect of antioxidants, *J. Inorg. Biochem.* 172, 94–99, 2017.

HEAT CAPACITY (*C*)

Heat capacity as defined by IUPAC: Heat capacity (*C*) defined as heat brought to a system to increase its temperature divided by that temperature increase. At constant volume $C_V = \left(\frac{\partial U}{\partial T}\right)_V$ at constant pressure $C_P = \left(\frac{\partial H}{\partial T}\right)_P$, where U is the internal energy and H the enthalpy of the system.[1] Heat capacity in proteins[2-5] and other macromolecules including nucleic acids[6,7] is measured with techniques such as differential scanning calorimetry and isothermal titration calorimetry. An understanding of heat capacity of biopharmaceutical products is an important factor in the processing of biopharmaceutical products.[8,9] See **differential scanning calorimetry**.

1. *Compendium of Chemical Terminology* (*The Gold Book*), 2nd edn., compiled by A.D. McNaught and A. Wilkinson, Blackwell Scientific Publications, Oxford, UK, 1997 (http://goldbook.iupac.org).
2. Prabhu, N.V., and Sharp, K.A., Heat capacity in proteins, *Annu. Rev. Phys. Chem.* 56, 521–548, 2005.
3. Lemaster, D.M., Heat capacity-independent determination of differential free energy of stability between structurally homologous proteins, *Biophys. Chem.* 119, 94–100, 2006.
4. Johnson, C.M., Differential scanning calorimetry as a tool for protein folding and stability, *Arch. Biochem. Biophys.* 531, 100–109, 2013.
5. Sasahara, K., and Goto, Y., Application and use of differential scanning calorimetry in studies of thermal fluctuation associated with amyloid fibril formation, *Biophys. Rev.* 5, 259–269, 2013.
6. Rozners, E., Pilch, D.S., and Egli, M., Calorimetry of nucleic acids, *Curr. Protoc. Nucleic Acid Chem.* 63, 7.4, 1–12, 2015.
7. Samatanga, B., Clery, A., Barraud, P., Allain, F.H., and Jelesarov, I., Comparative analyses of the thermodynamic RNA binding signatures of different types of RNA recognition motifs, *Nucleic Acids Res.* 45, 6037–6050, 2017.
8. Pikal, M.J., Rigsbes, D.R., and Roy, M.L., Solid state chemistry of proteins. I. Glass transition behavior in freeze dried disaccharide formulations of human growth hormone (hGH), *J. Pharm. Sci.* 96, 2765–2776, 2007.
9. Pansare, S.K., and Patel, S.M., Practical considerations for determination of glass transition temperature of a maximally freeze concentrated solution, *AAPS PharmSciTech* 17, 805–819, 2016.

HEAT SHOCK PROTEINS

Heat shock proteins (HSPs), also known as stress proteins, are, with several exceptions, intracellular proteins with chaperone activity. There is evidence for the surface expression of heat shock proteins and the release of heat shock proteins has been reported.[1,2] Although HSPs are commonly associated with prokaryotes eukaryotes, HSPs are found in plants.[3] HSPs can be traced back to an observation of puffy chromosomes in *Drosophila* in 1962.[4] Subsequent work showed that the puffs were associated with markedly increased RNA synthesis[5] and increased synthesis of unique proteins.[6] Subsequent work showed that there were a number of HSPs expressed in response to cell stress and had complex functions.[7-9] HSPs are classified into families by molecular size.[10,11] Glucose-regulated protein 78 kDA (GRP78), which is also known as immunoglobulin heavy chain binding protein (BiP) is one of the better known members of this family and is constitutively expressed in the endoplasmic reticulum (ER) in a wide variety of cell types. The function of GRP78 beyond the ER is of interest in cancer.[12]

1. Graner, M.W., Cumming, R.I., and Bigner, D.D., The heat shock response and chaperones/heat shock proteins in brain tumors: Surface expression, release, and possible immune consequences, *J. Neurosci.* 27 11214–11227, 2007.
2. Gonzalez-Gronow, M., Selim, M., Papalas, J., and Pizzo S.V., GRP78: A multifunctional receptor on the cell surface, *Antioxid. Redox. Signal.* 11, 2299–2306, 2009.

3. *Heat Shock Proteins in Plants*, ed. A.S.S. Asca, S.K. Calderwood, and P. Kaur, Springer, Cham, Switzerland, 2016.
4. Ritossa, F., A new puffing pattern induced by temperature shock and DNP in Drosophila, *Experientia* 18, 571–573, 1962.
5. Ritossa, F., Behavior of RNA and DNA synthesis at the puff level in salivary gland chromosomes of *Drosophila*, *Exp. Cell Res.* 36, 515–523, 1964.
6. Tissières, A., Mitchell, H.K., and Tracy, V.M., Protein synthesis in salivary glands of *Drosophila melanogaster*. Relation to chromosome puffs, *J. Mol. Biol.* 84, 389–379, 1974.
7. Craig, E.A., The heat shock response, *CRC Crit. Rev. Biochem.* 18, 239–280, 1985.
8. Lindquist, S., The heat-shock response, *Annu. Rev. Biochem.* 55, 1151–1191, 1986.
9. Georgopolous, C., and Welch, W.J., Role of the major heat shock proteins as molecular chaperones, *Annu. Rev. Cell Biol.* 9, 601–634, 1993.
10. Kampinga, H.H., Hageman, J. Vos, M.J., et al., Guidelines for the nomenclature of the human heat shock proteins, *Cell Stress Chaperones* 14, 105–111, 2009.
11. Jee, H., Size dependent classification of heat shock proteins: A mini-review, *J Exerc. Rehabil.* 12, 255–259, 2016.
12. Casas, C., GRP78 at the centre of the stage in cancer and neuroprotection, *Front. Neurosci.* 11, 177, 2017.

HEDGEHOG

The term hedgehog (*hedgehog*, hh) was developed to defined a gene/protein required for normal development in *Drosophila*.[1] Mutation in *hedgehog* results in anterior-posterior patterning defects resulting a spikey-hedgehog appearance. Subsequent work resulted in the identification of mammalian proteins with homology to hedgehog which are important during embryonic development.[2–4] There are three mammalian hedgehog proteins, Desert Hedgehog (Dhh), Indian Hedgehog (Dhh) and Sonic Hedgehog (Shh). The term "sonic hedgehog" is derived from the name of a character in a video game to reflect its broad scope of activity.[5] Shh is a signaling molecule of critical importance in embryonic development.[6] Shh undergoes a complicated processing pathway on its transit from the ER to the cell surface. Shh is synthesized as 45 kDa precursor protein which undergoes autocatalytic cleavage to yield two fragments of approximately equal size. The C-terminal fragment is degraded in the ER. A cholesterol moiety is added to the carboxyl-terminal portion of the N-terminal fragment in the ER while a palmitoyl moiety is added to the amino-terminal portion. Subsequently there is cleavage in the amino-terminal portion of the bilipidated with the formation of a fragment retaining the cholesterol moiety. The cholesterol-containing fragment then undergoes multimerization before

secretion into the extracellular space. The processing of sonic hedgehog for release into the extracellular space is facilitated by dispatched.[7] Dispatched is a 12-pass trans-membrane protein.[8] Surface-bound heparan sulfate is also involved in the processing of sonic hedgehog.[9]

1. Nüsslein-Volhard, C., and Wieschaus, E., Mutations affecting segment number and polarity in *Drosophila*, *Nature* 287, 795–801, 1980.
2. Riddle, R.D., Johnson, R.L., Laufer, E., and Tabin, C., *Sonic hedgehog* mediates the polarizing activity of the ZPA, *Cell* 75, 1401–1416, 1993.
3. Echelard, Y., Epstein, D.J., St.-Jacques, B., et al., Sonic hedgehog, a member of a family of putative signaling molecules, is implicated in the regulation of CNS polarity, *Cell* 75, 1417–1430, 1993.
4. Borycki, A.G., Sonic hedgehog and Wnt Signaling pathways during development and evolution, in *Modularity in Development and Evolution*, ed. G. Schlosser and G.P. Wagner, Chapter 6, pp. 101–131, University of Chicago Press, Chicago, IL, 2004.
5. Rennie, J., Super sonic, *Scientific American* April, 1994, p. 20, 1994.
6. Ryan, K., and Chiang, C., Sonic hedgehog (Shh), in *Encyclopedia of Signaling Molecules,* 2nd edn., ed. S. Choi, Springer Nature, Cham, Switzerland, 2018.
7. Stewart, D.P., Marada, S., Bodeen, W.J., et al., Cleavage activates dispatched for sonic hedgehog ligand release, *eLife* 7, 31678, 2018.
8. Burke, R., Nellen, D., Bellotto, M., et al., Dispatched, a novel sterol-sensing domain protein dedicated to the release of cholesterol-modified hedgehog from signaling cells, *Cells* 99, 803–815, 1999.
9. Ortmann, C., Prickhinke, U., Exner, S., Sonic hedgehog processing and release are regulated by glypican heparan sulfate proteoglycans, *J. Cell Sci.* 128, 2374–2385, 2015.

HETEROCHROMATIN

Chromatin is complex in the nucleus of the cell composed of protein and DNA and can be divided into two populations, which have different configurations, euchromatin (*eu* = good) and heterochromatin (*hetero* = other). The classical histochemical definition of heterochromatin is a darkly staining "Condensed" or modified chromatin which is not conducive to gene transcription as compared to the more diffuse, lightly staining euchromatin.[1,2] Subsequent work has supported the concept that coding DNA is found in euchromatin while heterochromatin is important for genomic stability.[3] Noncoding RNAs (RNAi) are important for the formation of heterochromatin.[4–6] Heterochromatin was first described by histochemical techniques as material which remained condensed during interphase while retaining the staining properties of metaphase.[7]

1. Ham A.W., *Histology*, 7th edn., The Nucleus, Chapter 2, pp. 23–64, J.B. Lippincott, Philadelphia, PA, 1977.
2. Lewin, B., Chromatin and chromosomes, in *Cells*, ed. B. Lewin, L. Cassimeris, V.R. Lingappa, and G. Plopper, Chapter 6, pp. 253–315, Jones and Bartlett, Sudbury, MA, 2007.
3. Allshire, R.C., and Madhani, H.D., Ten Principles of heterochromatin formation and function, *Nature Rev. Mol. Cell Biol.* 19, 229–244, 2018.
4. Cam, H.P., Chen, E.S., and Grewal, S.L.S., Transcriptional scaffolds for heterochromatin assembly, *Cell* 136, 610–614, 2009.
5. Grewal, S.I.S., RNAi-dependent formation of heterochromatin and its diverse functions, *Curr. Opin. Genet. Develop.* 20, 134–141, 2010.
6. Meller, V.H., Joshi, S.S., and Deshpande, N., Modulation of chromatin by noncoding RNA, *Annu. Rev. Genet.* 49, 673–695, 2015.
7. Heitz, E., Das Heterochromatin der Moose, *Jahrb. wiss. Bot.* 69, 762–818, 1928.

HETEROGENEOUS CATALYST/ HETEROGENEOUS CATALYSIS

The term heterogeneous catalyst refers to a catalyst which is not present in bulk solution but present in a solid phase such as a surface.[1] An example is the use of metal oxide nanoparticles (Fe_3O_4) for supporting Fenton reaction for the treatment of waste water[2] instead of soluble metal salts.[3] Heterogeneous catalysts have been used for reactions of biochemical interest including the synthesis of a fluorescent probe inside of a cell.[4] Insoluble enzymes[5] can be considered heterogeneous catalysts.[6] Since heterogeneous catalysis is defined by catalyst and reactants/substrates in different phases, heterogeneous catalysis can also include a soluble catalyst (enzyme) and an insoluble substrates.[7,8]

1. Bligaard, T., and Nørskov, J.K., Heterogeneous catalysis, in *Chemical Bonding at Surfaces and Interfaces*, ed. A. Nilsson, L.G.M. Pettersson, and J.K. Nørskov, Chapter 4, pp. 255–321, Elsevier, Amsterdam, the Netherlands, 2008.
2. Dhakshinamoorthy, A., Navalon, S., Alvaro, M., and Garcia, H., Metal nanoparticles as heterogenous Fenton catalysts, *ChemSusChem.* 5, 46–64, 2012.
3. Neyens, E., and Baeyens, J., A review of classic Fenton's peroxidation as an advanced oxidation technique, *J. Hazard. Mater.* 98, 33–59, 2003.
4. Wang, F., Zhang, Y., Du, Z., Ren, J., and Qu, X., Designed heterogeneous palladium catalysts for reversible light-controlled biorthogonal catalysis in living cells, *Nat. Commun.* 9, 1209, 2018.
5. Silman, I., and Katchalski, E., Water-insoluble derivatives of enzymes, antigens, and antibodies, *Annu. Rev. Biochem.* 35, 873–908, 1966.
6. Xu, F., and Ding, H., A new kinetic model for heterogeneous (or spatially confined) enzymatic catalysis: Contributions from the fractal and jamming (overcrowding) effects, *Applied Catalysis A General* 317, 70–81, 2007.
7. Carvalho, A.L., Dias, F.M.V., Nagy, T., et al., Evidence for a dual binding mode of dockerin modules to cohesion, *Proc. Natl. Acad. Sci. USA* 104, 3089–3094, 2007.
8. Andersen, M., Kari, J., Burch, K., and Westh, P., Michaelis-Menten equation for degradation of insoluble substrate, *Math. Biosci.* 296, 93–97, 2018.

HETEROLYTIC CLEAVAGE, HETEROLYSIS

A heterolytic cleavage is a term describing an uneven division (heterolysis) of a molecule during a chemical reaction such as which usually generates ions such as a carbocation in contrast to a homolytic reaction, which generates free radicals. There are examples of enzyme-catalyzed heterolytic reactions including the hydrogenase reaction. Hydrogenase enzymes use hydrogen as an energy source via the heterolytic cleavage of H_2 to yield a proton (H^+) and a hydride ion (H^-).[1] Heterolytic cleavage is a mechanism in the cleavage of peroxy intermediates with non-heme iron enzymes.[2–4]

1. Liu, T., Wang, X., Hoffman, C., DuBois, D.L., and Bullock, R.M., Heterolytic cleavage of hydrogen by an iron hydrogenase model: An Fe-H•••H-N dihydrogen bond characterized by neutron diffraction, *Angewandte Chem. Int. Edn.* 53, 5300–5304, 2014.
2. Borowski, I., and Siegbahn, P.E.M., Density functional theory studies on non-heme iron enzymes, in *Iron-Containing Enzymes: Versatile Catalysts of Hydroxylation Reactions In Nature*, ed S.P. de Visser and D. Kumar, Chapter 4, pp. 88–118, RSC Publishing, Cambridge, UK, 2011.
3. Company, A., Gómez, L., and Costas, M., Bioinspired non-heme iron catalysts in C-H and C=C oxidation reactions, in *Iron-Containing Enzymes. Versatile catalysts of hydroxylation reactions In nature*, ed S.P. de Visser and D. Kumar, Chapter 4, pp. 88–118, RSC Publishing, Cambridge, UK, 2011.
4. Yokata, S., and Fujii, H., Critical factors in determining the heterolytic versus homolytic bond cleavage of terminal oxidants by Iron (III) porphyrin complexes, *J. Amer. Chem. Soc.* 140, 5127–5137, 2018.

HIS-TAG

The term his-tag refers to a hexahistidine sequence[1] which can be attached to the carboxyl-terminal or amino-terminal end of an expressed protein. The his-tag or hexahis-tag was developed for the purification of recombinant proteins[2,3] based on early work on metal cation affinity chromatography.[4,5] A his-tag is one of several "tags" which can be attached during the expression of a recombinant protein for purposes of purification. Other "tags" include FLAG™ sequence, DYKDDDDK,[6,7] and maltose-binding protein (MBP).[8,9] There are other tags available.[10] Fusion proteins with the his-tag retain biological activity.[11] The his-tag also permits the identification of binding partners by a "pull-down" method.[12]

1. Hengen, P., Purification of His-Tag fusion proteins from *Escherichia coli*, *Trends Biochem. Sci.* 20, 285–286, 1995.
2. Müller, K.M., Arndt, K.M., Bauer, K., and Plückthun, A., Tandem immobilized metal-ion affinity chromatography/immunoaffinity purification of His-tagged proteins-evaluation of two anti-his-tag monoclonal antibodies, *Anal. Biochem.* 259, 54–61, 1998.
3. Hochuli, E., Bannwarth, Döbeli, H., Gentz, R., and Stober, D., Genetic approach to facilitate purification of recombinant proteins with a novel metal chelate adsorbent, *Bio/Technology* 6, 1321–1325, 1988.
4. Porath, J., Carlsson, J., Olsson, I., and Belfrage, G., Metal chelate affinity chromatography, a new approach to protein purification, *Nature* 258, 598–599, 1975.
5. Hochuli, E., Döbeli, H., and Schacter, A., New metal chelate adsorbent selective for proteins and peptides containing neighboring histidine residues, *J. Chromatog.* 411, 177–184, 1987.
6. Knappik, A., and Plückthun, A., An improved affinity tag based on the FLAG peptide for the detection and purification of recombinant antibody fragments, *Biotechniques* 17, 754–761, 1994.
7. Han, M.J., Kim, H.T., O'Reilly, C., and Kim, C.H., Purification of functional reprogramming factors in mammalian cell using FLAG-Tag, *Biochem. Biophys. Res. Commun.* 492, 154–160, 2017.
8. di Guan, C., Li, P., Riggs, P.D., and Inouye, H., Vectors that facilitate the expression and purification of foreign peptides in *Escherichia coli* by fusion to maltose-binding protein, *Gene* 67, 21–30, 1988.
9. Maina, C.V., Riggs, P.D., Grandea, A.G., 3rd, et al., An *Escherichia coli* to express and purify foreign proteins by fusion to and separation from maltose-binding protein, *Gene* 74, 365–373, 1988.
10. Terpe, K., Overview of tag protein fusions: From molecular and biochemical fundamentals to commercial systems, *Appl. Microb. Biotechnol.* 60, 523–533, 2003.
11. Gupta, R., Soares da Costa, T.P., Faou, P., Dogovski, C., and Perugini, M.A., Comparison of untagged and his-tagged dihydrodipicolinate synthase from the enteric pathogen *Vibrio cholerae*, *Protein Expr. Purif.* 145, 85–93, 2018.
12. Ling, S., Luo, M., Jiang, S., et al., Cellular Hsp27 interacts with classical swine fever virus NS5A protein and negatively regulates viral replication by the NF-κB signaling pathway, *Virology* 518, 202–209, 2018.

HOFMEISTER SERIES

The Hofmeister series also known as the lyotropic series described the order of certain ions to "salt out" or precipitate certain hydrophilic materials from aqueous solution. For example, polyvalent anions such as citrate and sulfate tend to precipitate proteins from solution (i.e. ammonium sulfate) while monovalent anions such as chloride and thiocyanate tend to solubilize. A similar series exists for cations, although the effect is more pronounced for ionic liquids. The Hofmeister series was advanced to rationalize the effect of inorganic ions on the solubility of egg albumin.[1] A further characterization of the series is obtained by a separation of those anions which can have a chaotropic effect and those which have a kosmotropic effect; chloride ion is considered "neutral."[2] The early work on the Hofmeister series suggested that the differences in the effect of ions in the Hofmeister series was based on the effect of the anions on water but more recent work supported a direct effect on proteins or other polymers.[3–6] While it should be intuitively obvious, the ability of the Hofmeister series to predict solution behavior depends on solvent conditions (i.e. pH) and the isoelectric point of a protein or other charged polymer.[7] As an example, the crystallization of a protein occurs as a result of carefully reducing the solubility of a protein to foster the formation of a crystalline product as opposed to an amorphous precipitate. It has been shown that the effectiveness of anions to promote crystallization followed a "reverse" Hofmeister series when pH < pI and a "normal" Hofmeister series when pH > pI.[8] The effect of pH on the phenomenology of the Hofmeister series was observed in 1920.[9] There is interest by rationalizing the effect of anions on enzyme activity by position in the Hofmeister series.[10–12]

$$CO_3^{-2} > SO_4^{-2} > S_2O_3^{-2} > H_2PO_4^{-1} > F^{-1} > Cl^{-1}$$
$$> Br^{-1} \approx NO_2^{-1} > I^{-1} > ClO^{-1} > SCN^{-1}$$

Kosmotropic	Chaotropic

1. Hofmeister, F., Zur von der Wirkung der Salze. Ueber Regelmässigkeiten in der einweissfällenden Wirkung der Salze unde ihre Beziehung zum physiologischen Verhalten der selben, *Arkiv. Experiment. Pathol. Pharmakol.* 24, 247–260, 1988.
2. Garagová, K., Balogová, A., Dušeková, E., et al., Correlation of lysozyme activity and stability in the presence of Hofmeister series anions, *Biochim. Biophys. Acta* 1865, 281–288, 2017.
3. Zhang, Y., and Cremer, P.S., Interactions between macromolecules and ions: The Hofmeister series, *Curr. Opin. Chem. Biol.* 10, 658–663, 2006.

4. Zhang, Y., Furyk, S., Bergbreiter, D.E., and Cremer, P.S., Specific ion effects on the water solubility of macromolecules: PNIPAM and the Hofmeister series, *J. Amer. Chem. Soc.* 127, 14505–14510, 2005.
5. Schwierz, N., Hovinek, D., and Netz, R.P., Reverse anionic Hofmeister series: The interplay of surface change and surface polarity, *Langmuir* 407, 217–222, 2010.
6. Okur, H.J., Hladíková, J., Rembert, K.B., et al., Beyond the Hofmeister series; Ion-specific effects on proteins and their biological functions, *J. Phys. Chem. B.* 121, 1997–2014, 2017.
7. Lyklema, J., Simple Hofmeister series, *Chem. Phys. Lett.* 467, 217–222, 2009.
8. Boström, M., Tavares, F.W., Finet, S., et al., Why forces between proteins follow different Hofmeister series for pH above and below pI, *Biophys. Chem.* 117, 217–224, 2005.
9. Loeb, J., Ion series and the physical properties of proteins, II., *J. Gen. Physiol.* 3, 247–269, 1920.
10. Wondrak, E.M., Louis, J.M., and Oroszlan, S., The effect of salt on the Michaelis-Menton kinetics of the HIV-1 protease correlated with the Hofmeister series, *FEBS Lett.* 280, 344–346, 1991.
11. Zhao, H., Campbell, S.M., Jackson, C.L., Song, Z., and Olubajo, O., Hofmeister series of ionic liquids: Kosmotropic effects of ionic liquids on the enzymatic hydrolysis of enantiomeric phenylalanine methyl ester, *Tetrahedron Asymmetry* 17, 377–383, 2006.
12. Carucci, C., Salis, A., and Magner, E., Electrolyte effect on enzyme electrochemistry, *Curr. Opin. Electrochem.* 5, 158–164, 2017.

HOLLIDAY JUNCTION

The Holliday junction[1,2] is an intermediate structure composed of two double-stranded DNA molecules during homologous recombination providing for the transfer of DNA sequence between the adjacent strands.[3,4] There are single and double Holliday junctions which are "resolved" by selective endonucleases.[5-7] Cruciform DNA has a structure similar to the Holliday junction.[8,9]

1. Holliday, R., A mechanism for gene conversion in fungi, *Genet. Res.* 5, 282–304, 1964.
2. Holliday, R., The history of the DNA heteroduplex, *BioEssays* 12, 133–142, 1990.
3. Ho, P.S., and Eichman, B.F., The crystal structures of DNA Holliday junctions, *Curr. Opin. Struct. Biol.* 11, 302–308, 2001.
4. Bates, A.D., and Maxwell, A., *DNA Topology*, Oxford University Press, Oxford, UK, 2005.
5. Symington, L.S., and Kolodner, R., Partial purification of an enzyme from *Saccharomyces cerevisiae* that cleaves Holliday junctions, *Proc. Natl. Acad. Sci. USA* 82, 7247–7251, 1985.
6. Bizard, A.H., and Hickson, D., The dissolution of double Holliday junction, *Cold Spring Harb. Perspect. Biol.* 6(7), a16477, 2014.
7. Punator, R.S., Martin, R.J., Wyatt, H.D.M., Chan, Y.W., and West, S.C., Resolution of single and double Holliday junction recombination intermediate by GEN 1, *Proc. Natl. Acad. Sci. USA* 114, 443–450, 2017.
8. Kurahashi, H., Inagaki, H., Yamada, K., et al., Cruciform DNA structure underlies the etiology for palindrome-mediated human chromosomal translocation, *J. Biol. Chem.* 279, 35377–35383, 2004.
9. Etefanosky, V.Y., and Moss, T., The cruciform DNA mobility shift assay: A tool to study proteins that recognized bent DNA, *Methods Mol. Biol.* 1334, 195–203, 2015.

HOLOENZYME

The term holoenzyme is used to describe functional assembly of the various components of an enzyme where there are constituent components such as metal ions or coenzymes which are required for activity. The term apoenzyme is used to describe the protein component. This term was originally used to describe the combination of a coenzyme or other low-molecular-weight cofactor such as metal ion with a protein component designated as the apoenzyme to form the holoenzyme.[1-3] More recently, the term holoenzyme is used to describe DNA and RNA polymerases which are multiprotein complexes.[4,5] A similar concept of a multiprotein complex is extended to the telomerase complex.[6]

1. Weissbach, H., Redfield, B.G., Dickerman, H., and Brot, N., Studies of alkylcobamide derivatives on the formation of holoenzyme, *J. Biol. Chem.* 240, 856–862, 1965.
2. Tong, L., Striking diversity in holoenzyme architecture and extensive conformational variability in biotin-dependent carboxylases, *Adv. Protein Chem. Struct. Biol.* 109, 161–194, 2017.
3. He, D., Lorenz, R., Kim, C., Herberg, F.W., and Lim, C.J., Switching cyclic nucleotide-selective activation of cyclic adenosine monophosphate-dependent protein kinase holozyme reveals distinct roles of tandem cyclic nucleotide-binding domains, *ACS Chem. Biol.* 12, 3057–3066, 2017.
4. Kelman, Z., and O'Donnell, M., DNA polymerase III holoeyzme: Structure and function of a chromosomal replication machine, *Annu. Rev. Biochem.* 64, 171–200, 1995.
5. Koleske, A.J., and Young, R.A., The RNA polymerase II holoenzyme and its implications for gene regulation, *Trends Biochem. Sci.* 20, 113–116, 1995.
6. Hukezalie, K.R., and Wong, J.M., Structure-function relationship and biogenesis regulation of the human telomerase holoenzyme, *FEBS J.* 280, 3194–3204, 2013.

HOLOTYPE

The term holotype is used to describe the single specimen or illustration designated as the single type for naming a species or subspecies.[1] A holotype could also be the first individual of a species or subspecies used for study by an investigator.[2] The term holotype has also been used to designate proteins from a family or group used for structural analysis[3] and for an particular enzyme selected from a protein species, family or clan.[4]

1. Jønsson, K.A., Blom, M.P.K., Päckert, M., Ericson, P.G.P., and Irestedt, M., Relicts of the lost arc: High-throughput sequencing of the *Eutrichomyias rowleyi* (Aves: Passerifomes) holotype uncovers an ancient biogeographic link between the Philippines and Fiji, *Mol. Phylogenet. Evol.* 120, 28–43, 2018.
2. Pecher, W.T., Robledo, J.A., and Vasta, G.R., Identification of a second rRNA gene unit in the *Parkinsus andrewsi* genome, *J. Eukaryot. Microbiol.* 51, 234–245, 2004.
3. Crickmore, N., Zeigler, D.R., Feitelson, J., et al., Revision of the nomenclature for the *Bacillus thuringiensis* pesticidal crystal proteins, *Microbiol. Mol. Biol. Rev.* 62, 807–813, 1998.
4. Rawlings, N.O., Barrett, A.J., and Finn, R., Twenty years of the MEROPS database of proteolytic enzymes, their substrates and inhibitors, *Nucleic Acids Res.* 44, D343–D350, 2016.

HOMEOBOX

The term homeobox describes a highly conserved nucleotide sequence of nucleotides (ca 180 bp) in a gene[1,2] encodes an approximate 60 amino sequence referred to as homeodomain in regulatory protein (homeotic proteins). Homeodomain proteins are transcription factors which can serve as activators or repressors of expression. See **homeodomain**.

1. Gardinar, D.M., and Bryant, S.V., Homeobox-containing genes in limb regeneration, in *HOX Gene Expression*, ed. S. Papageogriou, Chapter 7, pp. 102–110, Landis Bioscience/Springer Science+Business, New York, 2007.
2. Holland, P.W., Evolution of homeobox genes, *Wiley Interdiscip Rev. Dev. Biol.* 2, 31–45, 2013.

HOMEODOMAIN

A homeodomain is a region in a protein (homeodomain protein) that is encoded for by a homeobox.[1] Homeodomain proteins are transcription factors. The homeodomains are approximately 60 amino acids in length with a high conserved sequence that binds to a common motif in DNA.[2] Homeodomain domain regulate transcription and can be either activators or repressors.[3] Six3 is homeodomain protein important in eye development vertebrates is a repressor[4] and more recently has shown to be important in carcinogenesis.[5]

1. Bürglin, T.R., and Affolter, M., Homeodomain protein: An update, *Chromosoma* 125, 497–512, 2016.
2. Treisman, J., Harris, E., Wilson, D., and Desplan, C., The homeodomain: A new face for the helix-turn-helix? *Bioessays* 14, 145–150, 1992.
3. Bobola, N., and Merabet, S., Homeodomain proteins in action: Similar DNA binding preferences, highly variable connectivity, *Curr. Opin. Genetics Dev.* 43, 1–6, 2017.
4. Zhu, C.C., Dyer, M.A., Uchikawa, M., et al., Six3-mediated auto repression and eye development requires its interaction with members of the Groucho-relaetd family of co-repressors, *Development* 129, 2835–2849, 2002.
5. Zheng, Y., Zeng, Y., Qiu, R., et al., The homoeotic protein Six3 suppresses carcinogenesis and metastasis through recruiting the LSD1/NuRD(MTA3) complex, *Theranostics* 8, 972–989, 2010.

HOMEOTIC GENE

A homeotic gene is a gene that regulates the development of a specific anatomic feature.[1–6] A mutation in homeotic gene function causes cells/tissue in one region of the body to behave as if located in another region.[7–9] Homeotic gene encode homeodomain proteins.[10] See **Hox genes**.

1. Dessain, S., and McGinnis, W., Regulating the expression and function of homeotic genes, *Curr. Opin. Genet. Dev.* 1, 275–282, 1991.
2. Mann, R.S., The specificity of homeotic gene function, *Bioessays* 17, 855–863, 1995.
3. Hayashi, S., Yamagata, H., and Shiga, V., Changing roles of homeotic gene functions in arthropod limb development, in *Morphogenesis and Pattern Development in Biological Systems: Experiments and Models*, Chapter 7, pp. 81–90, Springer-Verlag, Tokyo, Japan, 2003.
4. Zubko, M.K., Mitochondrial tuning fork in nuclear homeotic functions, *Trends Plant Sci.* 9, 61–64, 2004.
5. Liu, Z., and Mara, C., Regulatory mechanisms for floral homeotic gene expression, *Semin. Cell Dev. Biol.* 21, 80–86, 2010.
6. Matharu, N.K., Dasan, V., and Mishra, R.K., Homeotic gene regulation: A paradigm for epigenetic mechanisms underlying organismal development, *Subcell. Biochem.* 61, 177–207, 2013.
7. Morata, G., and Lawrence, P.A., The development of wingless, a homeotic mutation of *Drosophila*, *Dev. Biol.* 56, 227–240, 1977.

8. Hall, B.K., *Evolutionary Developmental Biology*, 2nd edn., Chapman & Hall, London, UK, 1998.
9. Ingle, E.K., and Gilmartin, P.M., Molecular characterization of four double-flowered mutants of *Silane dioica* representing four centuries of variation, *J. Exp. Bot.* 66, 3297–3307, 2015.
10. Mann, R.S., The specificity of homeotic gene function, *Bioessays* 17, 855–863, 1995.

HOMOLYTIC CLEAVAGE

A homolytic cleavage is an even division of the bonding electrons in a molecule which generates free radicals.[1,2] The most common hemolytic cleavage in biological systems is the cleavage of the peroxide bond.[3–6] A homolytic cleavage mechanism has also been proposed for chlorite dismutase,[7] in the enzymatic oxidation of methane to methanol,[8] and for the cleavage of a cobalt-carbon bond in the generation of the a carbene intermediate in glutamate mutase.[9] A homolytic mechanism is also proposed for the degradation of *N*-chloro derivatives of heparan sulfate[10] and *S*-nitroso derivatives.[11,12]

1. Ingold, C.K., *Structure and Mechanism in Organic Chemistry*, Cornell University Press, Ithaca, NY, 1953.
2. Harris, J.M., and Wamser, C.C., *Fundamentals of Organic Reaction Mechanisms*, John Wiley and Sons, New York, 1976.
3. White, R.E., Sligar, S.G., and Coon, M.J., Evidence for a homolytic mechanism of peroxide oxygen—oxygen bond cleavage during substrate hydroxylation by cytochrome P-450, *J. Biol. Chem.* 255, 11108–11011, 1980.
4. Barr, D.P., Martin, M.V., Guengerich, F.P., and Mason, R.P., Reaction of cytochrome P450 with cumene hydroperoxide: ESR spin-trapping evidence for the homolytic scission of the peroxide O-O bond by ferric cytochrome P450 1A2, *Chem. Res. Toxicol.* 9, 318–325, 1996.
5. Lymar, S.V., Khairutdinov, R.F., and Hurst, J.K., Hydroxyl radical formation by O-O bond homolysis in peroxynitrous acid, *Inorg. Chem.* 42, 5259–5266, 2003.
6. Araujo, J.C., Prieto, T., Prado, F.M., et al., Peroxidase catalytic cycle of MCM-14-entrapped microperoxidase-11 as a mechanism for phenol oxidation, *J. Nanosci. Nanotechnol.* 7, 3643–3652, 2007.
7. Schaffner, I., Mlynek, G., Flego, N., et al., Molecular mechanism of enzymatic chlorite detoxification: Insights from structural and kinetic studies, *ACS Catal.* 7962–7976, 2017.
8. Banerjee, R., Proshlyakov, V., Lipscomb, J.D., and Proshlyakov, D.A., Structure of the key species in the enzymatic oxidation of methane to methanol, *Nature* 518, 431–434, 2015.
9. Marsh, E.N.G., and Ballou, D.P., Coupling of cobalt-carbon bond homolysis and hydrogen bond abstraction in adenosylcobalamin-dependent glutamate mutase, *Biochemistry* 37, 11864–11872, 1998.
10. Rees, M.D., and Davies, M.J., Heparan sulfate degradation via reductive homolysis of its *N*-chloro derivatives, *J. Am. Chem. Soc.* 128, 3085–3097, 2006.
11. Nikitovic, D., and Holmgren, A., *S*-Nitrosoglutathione is cleaved by the thioredoxin system with liberation of glutathione and redox regulating nitric oxide, *J. Biol. Chem.* 271, 19180–19185, 1996.
12. Pfeiffer, S., Schrammel, A., Schmidt, K., and Mayer, B., Electrochemical determination of *S*-nitrosothiols with a Clark-type nitric oxide electrode, *Anal. Biochem.* 258, 68–73, 1998.

HOMOTYPE/HOMOTYPIC

A homotype is a "a part or organ having the same type of structure as another, a homologue: applied *esp.* to serially or laterally homologous parts in the same organism."[1] A homotype can be a structure having the same general/function as another which may or may not be opposing. For example, the left arm is a homotype of the right arm. The concept of homotype/homotypic has been extended to cells,[2,3] subcellular organelles,[4,5] proteins,[6,7] nucleoproteins,[8,9] and nucleic acids.[10]

1. *Oxford English Dictionary*, Oxford University Press, Oxford, UK, 2018.
2. Sander, L.M., and Deisboeck, T.S., Growth patterns of microscopic brain tumors, *Phys. Rev. E* 66, 051901, 2002.
3. Castro, M., Molina-Paris, C., and Deisboeck, T.S., Tumor growth instability and the onset invasion, *Phys. Rev. E* 72, 041907, 2005.
4. Sackmann, E., Endoplasmatic reticulum shaping by generic mechanisms and protein-induced spontaneous curvature, *Adv. Colloid Interface Sci.* 208, 153–160, 2014.
5. Wang, L., Kim, J.Y., Liu, H.M., et al., HCV-induced autophagosomes are generated via homotypic fusion of phagophores that mediate HCV RAN replication, *PLoS Pathog.* 13(9), 1006609, 2017.
6. Sawma, P., Roth, L., Blanchard, C., et al., Evidence for new homotypic and heterotypic interactions between transmembrane helices of proteins involved in receptor tyrosine kinase and neutrophil signaling, *J. Mol. Biol.* 426, 4099–4111, 2014.
7. Mondal, A., Potts, G.K., Dawson, A.R., Coon, J.J., and; Park, Y.H., Jeong, M.S, and Jang, S.B., Structural insights of homotypic interactions domains in the ligand-receptor signal transduction of tumor necrosis factor (TNF), *BMS Rep.* 49, 159–166, 2016.
8. Kawashima, S., and Imahori, K., Studies on histone oligomers. III. Effects of salt concentration and pH on the stability of histone oligomers in chicken erythrocyte chromatin, *J. Biochem.* 91, 959–966, 1982.
9. Mehle, A., Phosphorylation at the homotypic interface regulates nucleoproteins oligomerization and assembly of the influenza virus replication machinery, *PLoS Pathog.* 11(4), 1004826, 2015.

10. Trcek, T., Grosch, M., York, A., *Drosophila* germ granules are structured and contain homotypic mRNA clusters, *Nat. Commun.* 6, 7962, 2015.

HOOGSTEEN BASE PAIRING

Hoogsteen base pairing in DNA differs from the canonical Watson-Crick model of base pairing of nucleic acid bases.[1] Hoogsteen base pairing is important in the formation of DNA triple helixes.[2-5] The potential importance of Hoogsteen base-pairing beyond triple-helix formation is recognized.[6-8] Nucleoside derivatives have been developed to enhance triple-helix formation by Hoogsteen base pairing.[9,10] There are variations on the original Hoogsteen pairing including triplet base pairing in triple helix formation.[11] Hoogsteen base pairing has been used in PCR technology to recognize guanine oxidation as an epigenetic modification.[12]

1. Hoogsteen, K., The crystal and molecular structure of a hydrogen-bonded complex between 1-methythymine and 9-methyladenine, *Acta Cryst.* 16, 907–916, 1963.
2. Raghunathan, G., Miles, H.T., and Sasisekharan, V., Symmetry and structure of RNA and DNA triple helices, *Biopolymers* 36, 333–343, 1995.
3. Soliva, R., Luque, F.J., and Orozco, M., Can G-C Hoogsteen-wobble pairs contribute to the stability of d(G, C-C) triplexes, *Nucleic Acids Res.* 27, 2248–2255, 1999.
4. Kawai, K., and Maruyama, A., Triple helix conformation-specific blinking of Cy3 in DNA, *Chem. Commun.* (Camb) 51, 4861–4864, 2015.
5. Maldonado, R., Filarsky, M., Grummt, I.,and Längst, G., Purine- and pyrimidine triple-helix-forming oligonucleotides recognize qualitatively different target sites at the ribosomal DNA locus, *RNA* 24, 371–380, 2018.
6. Searle, M.S., and Wickham, G., Hoogsteen versus Watson-Crick A-T base pairing in DNA complexes of a new group of "quinomycin-like" antibiotics, *FEBS Lett.* 272, 171–174, 1990.
7. Chakraborty, D., and Wales, D.J., Energy landscape and pathways for transition between Watson-Crick and Hoogsteen base pairing in DNA, *J. Phys. Chem. Lett.* 9, 229–241, 2018.
8. Geena, V., Carloni, P., and De Vivo, M., A strategically located Arg/Lys residue promotes correct base pairing during nucleic acid biosynthesis in polymerases, *J. Am. Chem. Soc.* 140, 3312–3321, 2018.
9. Li, J.S., Shikiya, R., Marky, L.A., and Gold, B., Triple helix forming TRIPside molecules that target mixed purine/pyrimidine DNA sequences, *Biochemistry* 43, 1440–1448, 2004.
10. Li, J.S., and Gold, B., Synthesis of C-nucleosides designed to participate in triplex formation with native DNA: Specific recognition of an A:T base pair in DNA, *J. Org. Chem.* 70, 8764–8771, 2005.
11. Gowers, D.M., and Fox, K.R., Toward mixed sequence recognition by triple helix formation, *Nucleic Acids Res.* 27, 1569–1577, 1999.
12. Park, J., Park, J.W., Oh, H., et al., Gene-specific assessment of guanine oxidation as an epigenetic modulator for cardiac specification of mouse embryonic stem cells, *PLoS One* 11(6), e155792, 2016.

HORMONOLOGY

The term hormonology is used to describe the study of hormones and has been proposed as a substitute for the term endocrinology.[1-6] There is limited current use of this term mostly in reference to the academic affiliation of an author.[7,8]

1. Ross, J.W., Hormonology in obstetrics, *J. Natl. Med. Assoc.* 46, 19–21, 1954.
2. Swain, C.T., Hormonology, *N. Engl. J. Med.* 280, 388–389, 1969.
3. Kulinskii, V.I., and Kolesnichenko, L.S., Current aspects of hormonology, *Biochemistry(Mosc.)* 62, 1171–1173, 1997.
4. Holland, M.A., Occam's razor applied to hormonology (Are cytokines produced by plants?), *Plant Physiol.* 115, 865–868, 1997.
5. Hadden, D.R., 100 years of hormonology: A view from No. 1 Wimpole Street, *J. R. Soc. Med.* 98, 325–326, 2005.
6. Hsueh, A.J.W., Bouchard, P., and Ben-Shlomo, I., Hormonology: A genomic perspective on hormonal research, *J. Endocrinol.* 187, 333–338, 2005.
7. Maione, L., Dwyer, A.A., Francou, B., et al., Genetic conseling for congenital hypogonadotropic hypogonadism and Kalliman syndrome: New challenges in the era of oligogenism and next-generation sequencing, *Eur. J. Endocrinol.* 178, R55–R80, 1918.
8. Cavalier, E., Salsé, M., Dupuy, A.M., et al., Establishment of reference values in a healthy population and interpretation of serum PTH concentrations in hemodialyzed patients according to the KDIGO guidelines using the Lumipulse® G whole PTH (3rd generation) assay, *Clin. Biochem.* 54, 119–122, 2018.

HOT-START POLYMERASE CHAIN REACTION

A hot-start polymerase chain reaction describes an assay, where the DNA polymerase reaction in the PCR does not start until the temperature has reached a value at which the oligonucleotide primers no longer bind the template. This technique is intended to reduce non-specific amplification and primer dimer formation. There are a number of approaches to the application of hot-start technology to the PCR. The technical approaches to a hot-start PCR include the use of a wax barrier to separate component of the PRC reaction until the temperature is hot enough to melt the wax,[1,2] the reactivation of citraconylated polymerase at high temperature,[3] the dissociation of an Taq polymerase-antibody complex,[4] and the use of engineered DNA polymerases.[5,6] A different approaches uses thermally sensitive primers.[7] Sources of engineered polymerase include Solis Biodyne[8] and Promega.[9]

1. Simpson, L.H., Battlegay, M., Hoofnagle, J.H., et al., Hepatitis delta virus RNA in serum of patients with chronic delta hepatitis, *Dig. Dis. Sci.* 39, 2650–2655, 1994.
2. Medina, E., Rogerson, B.J., and North, R.J., The *Nramp I* antimicrobial resistance gene segregates independently of resistance to virulent *Mycobacterium tuberculosis*, *Immunology* 88, 479–481, 1996.
3. Louwrier, A., and van der Valk, A., Thermally reversible inactivation of *Taq* polymerase in an organic solvent for application in hot start PCR, *Enzyme Microb. Technol.* 36, 947–952, 2005.
4. Dahiya, R., Deng, G., Chen, K., et al., Terms and techniques: New approach to hot start polymerase chain reaction using Taq DNA polymerase antibody, *Urol. Oncol.* 1, 42–46, 1995.
5. Kermekchiev, M.B., Tzekov, A., and Barnes, W.M., Cold-sensitive mutants of Taq DNA polymerase provide a hot start for PCR, *Nucl. Acids Res.* 31, 6139–6147, 2003.
6. Stevens, A.J., Appleby, S., and Kennedy, M.A., Many commercial hot-start polymerases demonstrate activity prior to thermal activation, *Biotechniques* 61, 292–295, 2016.
7. Ashrafi, E.H., and Paul, N., Yee, J., et al., Hot start PCR with heat-activatable primers: A novel approach for improved PCR performance, *Nucl. Acids Res.* 36, e131, 2008.
8. https://www.sbd.ee/EN/products/pcr/firepol/.
9. https://www.promega.com/products/pcr/hot-start-pcr/gotaq-hot-start-polymerase/.

HOX GENES

The *Hox* genes[1,2] are homeobox genes but not all homeobox genes are *Hox* genes.[3] *Hox* genes encode transcription factors (homeoproteins) which are activators and repressor of expression during vertebrate development.[4] The *HOX* genes are located in clusters (nested).[5–8] It is apparent that increased metazoan complexity is a consequence of more complex gene regulation, in particular *cis* factors, and not an increased number of genes.[9] The expression of Hox genes (39 in human) is mediated or controlled by the Hox-code.[10–13] Knowledge of the Hox code of donor cells is important in tissue transplantation[14] and other areas of regenerative medicine where Hox expression patterns are determined by reverse transcription-polymerase chain reaction.[15] RNA-seq has also been used to measure HOX gene expression.[16] Hox gene expression is important in cancer research.[17,18] HOTAIR is a long noncoding RNA that regulates HOX gene expression.[19]

1. Morgan, S., *HOX* genes: A continuation of embryonic patterning? *Trends in Genetics* 22, 67–69, 2006.
2. Gehring, W.J., Kloter, U., and Suga, H., Evolution of the *Hox* gene complex from an evolutionary ground state, *Curr. Topics Develop. Biol.* 88, 35–61, 2009.
3. Deutsch, J.S., Homeosis and beyond. What is the function of Hox genes? in Hox Genes studies from the 20th to the 21st Century, ed. J.S. Deutsch, Landes Bioscience/Springer Science + Business, New York, 2010.
4. Merabet, S., Sambrani, N., Pradel, J., and Graba, Y., Regulation of Hox activity: Insights from protein motifs, in *Hox Genes: Studies from the 20th to the 21st Century*, ed. J.S. Deutsch, Chapter 1, pp. 3–16, Landes Bioscience and Springer Science+Business, New York, 2010.
5. Hoegg, S., and Meyer, A., HOX clusters as models for vertebrate genome evolution, *Trends Genet.* 21, 421–424, 2005.
6. Duboule, D., The rise and fall of Hox gene clusters, *Development* 134, 2549–2560, 2007.
7. Nolte, C., Jinks, T., Wang, X., Martinez Pastor, M.T., and Krumlauf, R., Shadow enhancers flanking the HoxB cluster direct dynamic Hox expression in early heart and endoderm development, *Dev. Biol.* 383, 158–173, 2013.
8. Mallo, M., Reassessing the role of hox genes during vertebrate development and evolution, *Trends Genet.* 34, 209–217, 2018.
9. Erwin, D.H., The developmental origins of animal bodyplans, in *Neoproterozoic Geobilogy and Paleobiology*, ed. S. Xiao and A.J. Kaufman, Chapter 6, pp. 159–197, Springer, Dordrecht, the Netherlands, 2006.
10. Lewis, S.A., A gene complex controlling segmentation in *Drosophila, Nature* 276, 565–570, 1978.
11. Hunt, P., and Krumlaw, R., Deciphering the Hox code: Clues to patterning branchial regions of head, *Cell* 66, 1075–1078, 1991.
12. Sekimoto, T., Yoshinobu, K., Yoshida, M., et al., Region-specific expression of murine *Hox* genes implies the *HOX* code-mediated patterning of the digestive tract, *Genes Cells* 3, 51–64, 1998.
13. Wellik, D.M., *Hos* genes and the vertebrate skeleton, *Curr. Top. Develop. Biol.* 88, 257–273, 2009.
14. Foissac, R., Villageois, P., Chignon-Sicard, B., et al., Homeotic and embryonic gene expression in breast adipose tissue and in adipose tissues used as donor sites in plastic surgery, *Plast. Reconstr. Surg.* 139, 685e–692e, 2017.
15. Liedtke, S., Sacchetti, B., Laitinen, A., et al., Low oxygen tension reveals distinct HOX codes in human cord blood-derived stromal cells associated with specific endochondral ossification capacities *in vitro* and *in vivo, J. Tissue Eng. Regen. Med.* 11, 2725–2736, 2017.
16. Knight, J.M., Kim, E., Ivanov, I., et al., Comprehensive site-specific whole genome profiling of stromal and epithelial colonic gene signatures in human sigmoid colon and rectal tissue, *Physiol. Genomics* 48, 651–659, 2016.
17. Bhatlekar, S., Fields, J.Z., and Boman, B.M., HOX genes and their role in the development of haman cancers, *J. Mol. Med.* (Berl.) 92, 811–823, 2014.

18. HOTAIR-mediated reciprocal regulation of EZH2 and DNMT1 contribute to polyphyllin I-inhibited growth of castration-resistant prostate cancer cells *in vitro* and *in vivo*, *Biochim. Biophys. Acta* 1862, 589–599, 2018.

19. Woo, C.J., and Kingston, R.E., HOTAIR lifts noncoding RNAs to new levels, *Cell* 129, 1257–1259, 2007.

HYDROGELS

A hydrogel is an easily deformed pseudo-solid mass formed from largely hydrophilic colloids dispersed in an aqueous medium (dispersion medium or continuous phase). The term hydrogel (hydro + gel) is derived from the large water content. The content of water can range from 30% to nearly 100%, but the gel is insoluble in water.[1–3] The term hydrogel was first applied inorganic materials.[4] Inorganic materials are still of interest in hybrid hydrogels.[5] Early work on hydrogels used gelatin and other biological polymers.[6–8] The development of organic polymers as hydrogels can be traced to work in 1960[9] with the use of a copolymer of 2-hydroxyethyl methacrylate (glycol methacrylate) and ethylene dimethylacylate.[10] Current work on hydrogels uses a variety of matrices including polysaccharides,[11–13] polysaccharide-protein composites,[14,15] collagen,[16,17] and fibrin.[18,19] In addition to therapeutic uses such as drug delivery[20] and tissue regeneration,[21] hydrogel technology serves as the basis for 3-D tissue culture.[22–24] Intelligent hydrogels are responsible to environmental changes.[25–27]

1. Jhon, M.S., and Andrade, J.D., Water and hydrogels, *J. Biomed. Mat. Res.* 7, 509–522, 1973.

2. Roorda, W., Do hydrogels contain different classes of water, *J. Biomater. Sci. Polym. Ed.* 5, 383–395, 1994.

3. Gun'ko, V.M., Savina, I.N., and Mikhalovsky, S.V., Properties of water bound in hydrogels, *Gels* 3, 37, 2017.

4. Foote, H.W., and Saxton, B., Effect of freezing on certain inorganic hydrogels, *J. Amer. Chem, Soc.* 38, 588–609, 1916.

5. Finetti, F., Terzuoli, E., Donnini, S., et al., Monitoring endothelial and tissue responses to cobalt ferrite nanoparticles and hybrid hydrogels, *PLoS One* 11(12), e0168727, 2016.

6. Hardy, W.B., On the mechanism of gelation in reversible colloidal systems, *Proc. Royal Soc. London* 66, 95–109, 1900.

7. Bradford, S.C., X. On the theory of gels. II. The crystallization of gelatin, *Biochem. J.* 14, 91–93, 1920.

8. Pallman, H., and Deuel, H., Über die Wasserdurchlässigkeit von Hydrogelen, *Experentia* 1, 325–326, 1945.

9. Wichterele, O., and Lim, D., Hydrophilic gels for biological use, *Nature* 185, 117–118, 1960.

10. Kopocek, I., Swell Gels, *Nature* 417, 388–391, 2002.

11. Catanzano, O., D'Esposito, V., Acierno, S., et al., Alginate-hyaluronan composite hydrogels accelerate wound healing process, *Carbohydrate Polymers* 131, 407–414, 2015.

12. *Polysaccharide Hydrogels: Characterization and Biomedical Application*, ed. P. Mastricardi, F. Alhaique, and T. Caviello, CRC Press, Boca Raton, FL, 2016.

13. Naseri-Nosar, M., and Ziora, Z.M., Wound dressing from naturally occurring polymers: A review on homopolysaccharide-based composites, *Carbohyd. Polym.* 189, 379–398, 2018.

14. Calderon, L., Collin, E., Velasco-Bayon, D., et al., Type II collagen-hyaluronan hydrogel—A step towards a scaffold for intervertebral disc tissue engineering, *Eur. Cell Mater.* 20, 134–148, 2010.

15. Ketabat, F., Karkhaneh, A., Mehdinavaz Aghdam, and Hossein Ahmadi Tafti, S., Injectable conductive collagen/alginate/polypyrrole hydrogels as a biocompatible system for biomedical applications, *J. Biomater. Sci. Polym. Ed.* 28, 794–805, 2017.

16. Côté, M-F., Laroche, G., Gagnon, E., Chevallier, P., and Doillon, C.J., Denatured collagen as support for FGF-2 delivery system: Physicochemical characterizations and in vitro release kinetics and bioactivity, *Biomaterials* 25, 3761–3772, 2004.

17. Gao, Y., Kong, W., Li, B., et al., Fabrication and characterization of a collagen-based injectable and self-crosslinkable hydrogels for cell encapsulation, *Colloids Surf B. Biointerfaces* 167, 448–456, 2018.

18. Ho, S.T.B., Gool, S.M., Hui, J.H., and Hutmacher, D.W., The influence of fibrin based hydrogels on the chrondrogenic differentiation of human bone marrow stromal cells, *Biomaterials* 31, 38–47, 2010.

19. Noori, A., Ashrafi, S.J., Vaez-Ghaemi, R., Haramian-Zaremi, A., and Webster, T.J., A review of fibrin and fibrin composites for bone tissue engineering, *Int. J. Nanomedicine* 12, 4937–4961, 2017.

20. *Functional Hydrogels in Drug Delivery*, ed. U.G. Spizzirri and G. Cirillo, CRC Press, Boca Raton, FL, 2017.

21. *Hydrogels in Cell-Based Therapies*, ed. C.J. Connon and I.W. Hamley, Royal Society of Chemistry, Cambridge, UK, 2014.

22. Prestwich, G.D., Simplifying the extracellular matrix for 3-D cell culture and tissue engineering: A pragmatic approach, *J. Cell. Biochem.* 101, 1370–1383, 2007.

23. Bränvall, K., Bergman, K., Wallenquist, U., et al., Enhanced neuronal differentiation in a three-dimensional collagen-hyaluronan matrix, *J. Neurosci. Res.* 85, 2138–2146, 2007.

24. Diekjürgen, D., and Grainger, D.W., Polysaccharide matrices used in 3D in vitro cell culture systems, *Biomaterials* 141, 96–115, 2017.

25. *Intelligent Hydrogels*, ed. G. Sadowski and W. Richtering, Springer, Cham, Switzerland, 2013.

26. Siegel, R.A., Stimuli sensitive polymers and self regulated drug delivery systems: A very partial review, *J. Control Release* 190, 337–351, 2014.

27. *Polymeric Hydrogels as Smart Biomaterials*, ed. S. Kalia, Springer, Cham, Switzerland, 2016.

HYDROPHOBICITY, HYDROPHOBIC, HYDROPHOBIC EFFECT, HYDROPHOBIC FORCES

Hydrophobicity is, literally, the tendency of a molecular structure to avoid water which results in an association or clustering of hydrophobic groups. Thus, the hydrophobic effect is a product of the structure of water rather than of a particular solute.[1] However, the definition of hydrophobicity has been[2] and continues to be elusive.[3,4] Hydrophobicity is frequently measured by the change in free energy on the transfer of a solute from an organic solvent to water and these measurements are used to studies in protein folding[5] in process which can be described as hydrophobic solvation.[6] The term nonpolar, describing the absence of function groups such as a carboxylate function, is frequently used to describe hydrophobic molecules. Polar and nonpolar groups or functions can exist in the same molecule as for example in arginine.[7] It is noted that the term hydrophobia, literally the fear of water, can be a symptom of rabies in humans.[8–10]

1. Tanford, C., *The Hydrophobic Effect: Formation of Micelles and Biological Membranes*, John Wiley & Sons, New York, 1980.
2. Dill, K.A., The meaning of hydrophobicity, *Science* 250, 297–298, 1990.
3. Gibb, B.C., Hydrophobia! *Nat. Chemistry* 21, 512–513, 2010.
4. Sun, Q., The physical origin of hydrophobic effects, *Chem. Phys. Lett.* 672, 21–25, 2017.
5. Baldwin, R.L., Temperature dependence of the hydrophobic interaction in protein folding, *Proc. Natl. Acad. Sci. USA* 83, 8069–8072, 1986.
6. Southall, N.T., and Dill, K.A., The mechanism of hydrophobic solvation depends on solute radius, *J. Phys. Chem. B* 104, 1325–1331, 2000.
7. Dasgupta, S., Lyer, G.H., Bryant, S.H., Lawrence, C.E., and Bell, J.A., Extent and nature of contacts between protein molecules in crystal lattices and between subunits of protein oligomers, *Proteins* 28, 494–514, 1997.
8. Prince, C.L., The employment of the Lichen *Cinereus terrestris* (of Ray) as a preventive against hydrophobia and rabies, *Brit. Med. J.* 2(616), 439–440, 1872.
9. Sharp, D., Hydrophobia phobia as social history, *Lancet* 371(9615), 797–798, 2008.
10. Kim, Y.R., Prophylaxis of human hydrophobia in South Korea, *Infect. Chemother.* 46, 143–148, 2014.

HYDROPHOBINS

Hydrophobins are small proteins (large peptides) with a molecular mass of 7–10 kDa, while having a relative large content of cysteine (8 residues, approximately 10%) present as disulfide bonds.[1] Hydrophobins are divided into two classes: class I hydrophobins and class II hydrophobins.[2] Hydrophobins are secreted proteins which function in the pathogenicity of fungi by promoting adhesion to tissues.[3,4] Hydrophobins are secreted as soluble monomers and form insoluble oligomers (amphipathic membranes) on contact with an interface (e.g. water/air; water/surface).[5] There are physical differences in the membrane structures form by the two classes of hydrophobins.[6] The secreted product derived from class I hydrophobins is soluble only in formic acid or trichloroacetic acid while those derived from class II hydrophobins are somewhat more soluble (2% SDS, 60% EtOH).[7] It has been suggested that hydrophobins could be the basis of biological adhesives.[8] Previous work has suggested that hydrophobins could convert hydrophobic surfaces to hydrophilic surfaces.[9] Hydrophobins adsorb unto hydrophobic surfaces/particles enhancing the solubility ("wet-in") of such particles (e.g. Teflon™).[10] Conversely, hydrophilic surfaces can be converted to hydrophobic surfaces.[11] There is interest in the expression of recombinant hydrophobins.[12,13]

1. Sunde, M., Kwan, A.H.Y., Teimpleton, M.D., Beever. R.D., and Mackey, J.P., Structural analysis of hydrophobins, *Micron* 39, 773–784, 2008.
2. Askolin, S., Linder, M., Scholtmeijer, K., et al., Interaction and comparison of a class I hydrophobin from *Schizophyllum commune* and class II hydrophobins from *Trichoderma reesei*, *Biomacromolecules* 7, 1295–1301, 2006.
3. Valsecchi, I., Dupress, V., Stephen-Victor, E., et al., Role of hydrophobins in *Asperigillus fumigatus*, *J. Fungi.* (Basel), 4(1), 2, 2017.
4. Moonjely, S., Keyhani, N.O., and Bidochka, M.J., Hydrophobins contribute to root colonization and stress responses in the rhizosphere-competent insect pathogenic fungus *Beauveria bassiana*, *Microbiology* 164, 517–528, 2018.
5. Askolin, S., Linder, M., Scholtmeijer, K., et al., Interaction and comparison of a class I hydrophobin from *Schizophyllum commune* and class II hydrophobins from *Trichoderma reesei*, *Biomacromolecules* 7, 1295–1301, 2006.
6. Paananen, A., Vuorimaa, E., Torkkeli, M., et al., Structural hierarchy in molecular films of two class II hydrophobins, *Biochemistry* 42, 5253–5258, 2003.
7. Wösten, H.A.B., and de Vocht, M.L., Hydrophobins, the fungal coat unraveled, *Biochim. Biophys. Acta* 1469, 79–86, 2000.
8. Li, B., Wang, X., Li, Y., et al., Single-molecule force spectroscopy reveals self-assembly enhanced surface binding of hydrophobins, *Chemistry* 24, 9224–9228, 2018.

9. Scholtmeijer, K., Janssen, M.I., van Leeuwen, M.B., et al., The use of hydrophobins to functionalize surfaces, *Biomed. Mater. Eng.* 14, 447–454, 2004.

10. Lumsdan, S.O., Green, J., and Stieglitz, B., Adsorption of hydrophobic proteins at hydrophobic and hydrophilic surfaces, *Colloid Surf. B. Biointerfaces* 44, 172–178, 2005.

11. Wösten, H.A., and Scholtmeijger, K., Applications of hydrophobins: Current state and perspectives, *Appl. Microbiol. Biotechnol.* 99, 1587–1597, 2015.

12. Przylucka, A., Akcapinar, G.B. Bonazza, K., et al., Comparative physiochemical analysis of hydrophobins produced in *Escherichia coli* and *Pichia pastoris*, *Colloids Surf. B Biointerfaces* 159, 913–923, 2017.

13. Gandier, J.A., and Master, E.R., *Pichia postoris* is a suitable host for the heterologous expression of predicted class I and class II hydrophobins for discovery, study, and application in biotechnology, *Microorganisms* 6, 9, 2018.

HYPSOCHROMIC

The term hypsochromic describes a shift of light absorption or emission to a shorter wavelength ($\lambda < \lambda_0$).[1] A hypsochromic shift is often referred to as a blue shift.[2] The term hypsochromic has also been used to describe a lightening of color.[3]

1. Zhao, N., Xuan, S., Fronczek, F.R., Smith, K.M., and Vicente, M.G., Enhanced hypsochromic shifts, quantum yield, and π-π interactions in a meso, β-heteroaryl-fused BODIPY, *J. Org. Chem.* 82, 3880–3885, 2017.

2. Mazumdar, P., Das, D., Sahoo, G.P., Salgado-Morán, G., and Misra, A., Aggregation induced emission enhancement of 4,4'-bis(disethylamino)benzophenone with an exceptionally large blue shift and its potential use as glucose sensor, *Phys. Chem. Chem. Phys.* 17, 3343–3354, 2015.

3. *Oxford English Dictionary*, Oxford University Press, Oxford, UK, 2018.

IDIOTYPIC

Idiotypic as in referring to immunologically detectable differences in the variable region of an antibody idiotype where idiotype is that portion of the variable region of an antibody which can be immunologically different and elicit an immunological response.[1-3] The idiotype is composed of individual determinants referred to as idiotopes; the idiotype represents the combined antigenic determinants (idiotopes).[4] Public idiotypes are found on the variable regions of immunoglobulins derived from the same germline.[5,6] Anti-idiotypic antibodies are directed again idiotopes and when such idiotopes directly bind paratopes, the anti-idiotypic antibody is referred to as internal or mirror image.[7,8]

1. Oudin, J., and Michel, M., Une nouvelle forme de l'allotype des globulin du serum de Lapin, apparemment Ile à le function e à spécificité anticorps, *Comp. Rend. Hebd. Seances Acad. Sci.* 257, 805–808, 1963.

2. Sher, A., and Cohn, M., Effect of haptens on the reaction of anti-idiotype antibody with a mouse anti-phosphorylcholine phasmacytoma protein, *J. Immunol.* 108, 176–178, 1972.

3. Greenspan, N.S., and Bona, C.A., Idiotypes: Structure and immunogenicity, *Faseb J.* 7, 437–444, 1993.

4. Bona, C., Idiotypes, in *Encyclopedia of Immunology*, ed. I.M. Roitt and P.J. Delves, pp. 723–726, Academic Press, London, UK, 1992.

5. Miller, A., Ch'ng, L-K., Benjamin, C., and Sercarz, E., Detailed analysis of the public idiotype of anti-hen egg-white lysozyme antibodies, *Ann. N.Y. Acad. Sci.* 418, 140–150, 1983.

6. Wong, Y.H., Goh, B.C., Lim, S.Y., et al., Structural mimicry of the Dengue virus envelope glycoprotein revealed by the crystallographic study of an idiotype-anti-idiotype Fab complex, *J. Virol.* 91, e00406–17, 2017.

7. Dalgleish, A.G., and Kennedy, R.C., Anti-idiotypic antibodies as immunogens: Idiotype-based vaccines, *Vaccine* 6, 215–220, 1985.

8. Roitt, I.M., Thanavala, Y.M., Male, D.K., and Hay, F.C., Anti-idiotypes as surrogate antigens: Structural considerations, *Immunol. Today* 6, 265–267, 1985.

IMAC (IMMOBILIZED METAL AFFINITY CHROMATOGRAPHY)

IMAC is a chromatographic procedure which uses a matrix consisting of a metal ion tightly bound to a matrix.[1,2] There was extensive use of IMAC for the purification of His-tag proteins on nickel affinity columns.[3] The IMAC concept has been used to immobilize proteins on surfaces.[4] Recently IMAC has focused on the purification of phosphopeptides.[5-7] While Fe^{3+} has been extensively used for IMAC purification of phosphopeptides, recent work has suggested the metal ions such as Ti^{4+} may be more useful.[8,9]

1. Porath, J., and Olin, B., Immobilized metal ion affinity adsorption and immobilized metal ion affinity chromatography of biomaterials. Serum protein affinities for gel-immobilized iron and nickel ions, *Biochemistry* 23, 1621–1630, 1982.

2. Porath, J., Immobilized metal ion affinity chromatography, *Protein Expr. Purif.* 3, 263–281, 1992. Separation of proteins and other materials is based on relative affinity for the bound metal ions.

3. Block, H., Maertens, B., Spriestersbach, A., et al., Immobilized-metal affinity chromatography (IMAC): Areview, *Methods Enzymol.* 463, 439–473, 2009.

4. Giusti, F., Kessler, P., Della Pia, E.A., et al., Synthesis of polyhistidine-bearing amphipol and its use of immobilizing membrane proteins, *Biomacromolecules* 16, 3751–3761, 2015.

5. Thingholm, T.E., Jensen, O.N., Robinson, P.J., and Larsen, M.R., SIMAC (Sequential Elution from IMAC), a phosphoproteomics strategies for the rapid separation of monophosphorylated from multiply phosphorylated peptides, *Mol. Cell. Proteomics* 7, 661–771, 2008.

6. Villén, J., and Gygi, S.P., The SCX/IMAC enrichment approach for global phosphorylation analysis by mass spectrometry, *Nat. Protoc.* 3, 1630–1638, 2008.

7. Potel, C.M., Lin, M-H., Heck, A.J.R., and Lemeer, S., Defeating major contaminants in Fe³⁺-immobilized metal ion affinity chromatography (IMAC) phosphopeptide enrichment, *Mol. Cell. Proteomics* 17, 1028–1934, 2018.

8. Yao, Y., Dong, J., Dong, M., et al., An immobilized titanium (IV) ion affinity chromatography adsorbent for solid phase extraction of phosphopeptides for phosphoproteome analysis, *J. Chromatog.* 1498, 22–28, 2017.

9. Jiang, J., Sun, X., Li, Y., Dong, C., and Duan, G., Facile synthesis of Fe₃O₄@PDA core-shell microspheres functionalized with various metal ions: A systematic comparison of commonly-used metal ions for IMAC enrichment, *Talanta* 178, 600–607, 2018.

IMINOSUGARS

Iminosugars are a class of carbohydrate mimetics which contain nitrogen in the place of oxygen in the ring. Iminosugars inhibit glycosidases.[1–3] Iminosugars have been shown to have antiviral activity.[4–7] Iminosugars do occur as natural products and have been used in traditional medicine.[8]

1. Neverova, I., Scaman, C.H., Srivastava, O.P., et al., A spectrophotometric assay for glucosidase I, *Anal. Chem,* 222, 190–195 1994.

2. Brás, N.F., Cerqueira, N.M., Ramos, M.J., and Fernandes, P.A., Glycosidase inhibitors: A patent review (2008–2013), *Expert Opin. Ther. Pat.* 24, 857–874, 2014.

3. Wadood, A., Ghufran, M., Khan, A., et al., Selective glycosidase inhibitors: A patent review (2012-present), *Int. J. Biol. Macromol.* 111, 82–91, 2018.

4. Jacob, J.R., Mansfield, K., You, J.E., Tennant, B.C., and Kim, Y.H. Natural iminosugar derivatives of 1-deoxynojirimycin inhibit glycosylation of hepatitis viral envelope proteins, *J. Microbiol.* 45, 431–440, 2007.

5. Hussain, S., Miller, J.L., Harvey, D.J., et al., Strain-specific antiviral activity of Iminosugars against human influenza A viruses, *J. Antimicrobial. Chemother.* 70, 136–152, 2015.

6. Sayce, A.C., Alonzi, D.S., Killingbeck S.S., et al., Iminosugars inhibit Dengue virus production via inhibition of ER alpha-glucosidases-not glycolipid processing enzymes, *PloS Negl. Trop. Dis.* 10(3), 0004524, 2016.

7. Tyrrell, B.E., Sayce, A.C., Warfield, K.L., Miller, J.L., and Zitzmann, N., Iminosugars: Promising therapeutics for influenza infection, *Crit. Rev. Microbiol.* 43, 521–545, 2017.

8. Gao, K., Zheng, C., Wang, T., et al., 1-Deoxynojirimycin: Occurrence, extraction, chemistry, oral pharmacokinetics, biological activities and in silico target fishing, *Molecules* 21, 1600, 2016.

IMMUNOBLOTTING

Immunoblotting is a mature technique used most frequently for the identification of proteins on a matrix[1,2] and has a variety of applications. Immunoblotting as a technique was introduced in 1979.[3,4] This work was extended to the development of western blotting.[5] Immunoblotting was adapted for the quantitative measurement of specific analytes in complex biological samples.[6] The use of immunoblotting for the quantitative measurement of protein analytes in complex mixtures continues to be of value.[7] The **dot-blot** method is used for protein quantitation.[8–10] The analysis of poorly antigenic materials such as peptides can be improved by the use of more potent antibodies obtained by the use of immunogens with increase epitope density.[11] This approach has been used for the immunoblot measurement of low molecular weight allergens from citrus fruits.[12] Another approach to the immunoblotting of peptides is based on chemical fixation of the analyte to a membrane.[13] Antibody specificity can be an issue with immunoblotting and other immunoassays.[14] Validation procedures for antibody specificity have been proposed.[15–17]

1. *CRC Handbook of Immunoblotting of Proteins*, ed. O.J. Bjerrum and N.H.H. Heegaard, CRC Press, Boca Raton, FL, 1988.

2. *Protein Blotting*, ed. B.S. Dunbar, IRL Press at Oxford University Press, Oxford, UK, 1994.

3. Renart, J., Reiser, J., and Stark, G.R., Transfer of proteins from gels to diazobenzyloxymethyl-paper and detection with antisera: A method for studying antibody specificity and antigen structure, *Proc. Natl. Acad. Sci. USA* 76, 3116–3120, 1979.

4. Towbin, H., Staehlin, T., and Gordon, J., Electrophoretic transfer of proteins from polyacrylamide gels to nitrocellulose sheets: Procedure and some applications, *Proc. Natl. Acad. Sci. USA* 76, 4350–4354, 1979.

5. Burnette, W.N., "Western blotting": Electrophoretic transfer of proteins from sodium dodecyl sulfate-polyacrylamide gels to unmodified nitrocellulose and radiographic detection with antibody and radioiodinated protein A, *Anal. Biochem.* 112, 195–203, 1981.

6. Howe, J.G., and Hershey, W.B., A sensitive immunoblotting method for measuring protein synthesis initiation factor levels in lysates of *Escherichia coli*, *J. Biol. Chem.* 256, 12836–12839, 1981.

7. McDonough, A.A., Veiras, L.C., Minas, J.N, and Ralph, D.L., Considerations when quantitating protein abundance by immunoblot, *Am. J. Physiol. Cell Physiol.* 308, C426–C433, 2015.

8. Wehr, N.B., and Levine, R.L., Quantitation of protein carbonylation by dot blot, *Anal. Biochem.* 423, 241–245, 2012.

9. Kovács, A., Patai, Z., Guttman, A., et al., Fractionation of the human plasma proteome for monoclonal proteomics-based biomarker discovery 2: Antigen identification by dot-blot array screening, *Electrophoresis* 34, 3064–3071, 2013.

10. Tian, G., Tang, F., Yang, C., et al., Quantitative dot blot analysis (QDB), a versatile high throughput immunoblot method, *Oncotarget* 8, 58553–55856, 2017.

11. Liu, W., and Chen, Y.-H., High epitope density in a single protein molecule significantly enhances antigenicity as well as immunogenicity: A novel strategy for modern vaccine development and a preliminary investigation about B cell discrimination of monomeric proteins, *Eur. J. Immunol.* 35, 505–514, 2005.

12. Wu, J., Deng, W., Lin, D., Deng, X., and Ma, Z., Immunoblotting quantification approach for identifying potential hypoallergenic citrus cultivars, *J. Agric. Food Chem.* 661964–1973, 2018.

13. Davey, L., Halperin, S.A., and Lee, S.F., Immunoblotting conditions for small peptides from streptococci, *J. Microbiol. Methods* 114, 40–42, 2015.

14. Baker, M., Antibody anarchy: A call to order, *Nature* 527, 545–551, 2015.

15. Uhlen, M., Bandrowski, A., Carr, A., et al., A proposal for validation of antibodies, *Nature Methods* 13, 823–827, 2016.

16. Vanli, G., Cuesta-Marban, A., and Widmann, C., Evaluation and validation of commercial antibodies for the detection of Shb, *PLoS One* 12(12), 186311, 2017.

17. Weller, M.G., Ten basic rules of antibody validation, *Anal. Chem. Insights* 13, 1–15, 2018.

IMMUNOGLOBULIN (Ig)

Immunoglobulins (Igs) are a family of primarily plasma proteins (globulins)[1] which are synthesized by plasma cells (activated B-cells) which are derived from B-cells (B-lymphocytes). B-cells (so named because of their origin the bursa of chicken) originate in the liver and mature in the bone marrow. Activation of B-cell occurs when a specific immunoglobulin (Ig) receptor is cross-linked by binding to an antigen such as a virus or bacteria. B-cell activation also occurs by interaction with a helper T-cell in a process called cognate activation after processing of the antigen, usually a protein, and expression on the B-cell surface as a class II MHC-peptide complex. There are five general classes of immunoglobulins: IgA, IgE, IgD, IgG, and IgM. With the exception of some unique immunoglobulins such as camelids, immunoglobulins are based on a structure of dimers or heterodimers where the heterodimers are composed of a light chain and a heavy chain. IgM is a pentamer of this basic building

block while IgA can be a monomer, dimer or trimer of the basic building block. The basic building block is bivalent in that each heterodimer can bind an antigen; IgA may be bivalent, tetravalent, or hexavalent while IgM is decavalent. While the bulk of the immunoglobulins are found in blood plasma, IgA can be found in saliva[2] and other biological fluids and in the intestinal tract.[3] These are known as secretory immunoglobulins and with IgA, referred to as sIgA.[4] Immunoglobulins are found in the interstitial space[5] and current antibody therapeutics is based on distribution through the interstitial space.[6]

1. Lundblad, R.L., *Biotechnology of the Plasma Proteins*, Chapter 5, Plasma Immunoglobulins, pp. 183–232, CRC Press, Boca Raton, FL, 2013.

2. Feller, L., Altini, M., Khammissa, R.A., et al., Oral mucosal immunity, *Oral Surg. Oral. Med. Oral Pathol. Oral Radiol.* 116, 576–583, 2013.

3. Jiang, H.Q., Thurnheer, M.C., Zuercher, A.W., et al., Interactions of commensal gut microbes with subsets of B- and T-cells in the murine host, *Vaccine* 22, 895–811, 2004.

4. Bienenstock, J. The significance of secretory immunoglobulins, *Can. Med. Assoc. J.* 103, 39–43, 1970.

5. Rossing, N., and Worm, A.M., Interstitial fluid: Exchange of macromolecules between plasma and skin interstitium, *Clin. Physiol.* 1, 275–284, 1981.

6. Boswell, C.A., Bumbaca, D., Fiedler, P.J., and Khawli, L.A., Compartmental tissue distribution of antibody therapeutics: Experimental approaches and interpretations, *AAPS J.* 14, 612–618, 2012.

Immunoglobulins Found in Human Plasma[a]

Immuno-globulin	MW[b] (kDa)	T$_{1/2}$ (Days)	(mg/dL)[c,d]	Comment
IgG	150	24	700–1600[e]	The most common immunoglobulin in plasma. Major function is protection against pathogens and facilitating opsonization of viral and bacterial pathogens.[f] The action can be either bacteriostatic or bacteriocidal or both. IgG in plasma is comprised of various subclasses; IgG1, IgG2, IgG3, and IgG4. These subclasses have various characteristics. IgG1 is the major subclass with somewhat less IgG2; there are relatively small amounts of IgG3 and IgG4. Comprises 80+% of plasma immunoglobulin.

(Continued)

Immunoglobulins Found in Human Plasma[a]
(Continued)

Immuno-globulin	MW[b] (kDa)	T$_{1/2}$ (Days)	(mg/dL)[c,d]	Comment
IgA	160	6	70–400	Provides protection against pathogens, primarily viral or bacterial,[f] with emphasis on mucosal secretion (mucosal immunity). Subclasses IgA1, IgA2. The plasma form is a monomer while the mucosal secretory product is a dimer or tetramer with an associated J chain of molecular mass 15 kDa containing one N-linked glycan. More IgA is synthesized per day than IgG but approximately one-half is catabolized in the liver and the remainder is transported to external secretion.
IgM	900	5	30–360	Early protection[f] against pathogens; a polymeric form (pentamer; closed ring including five IgG and a J chain) of IgG. Considered to be an early immunoglobulin with function linked to IgD; IgM may be the most ancient of the immunoglobulins. As with IgA. there is a secretory form of unknown function.
IgD	190	2.8[g]	N/A	Increasing evidence suggests a relationship to IgM and importance in immuno-modulation. There is also involvement in mucosal immunity.[h]
IgE	175	2.4g	N/A	Associated with mast cells; responsible for allergic responses such as hypersensitivity and anaphylaxis.

[a] The material in this table has been adapted from Lundblad, R.L., *Biotechnology of the Plasma Proteins*, Chapter 5, Plasma Immunoglobulins, pp. 183–232, CRC Press, Boca Raton, FL, 2013.

[b] Approximate values

[c] Concentration in plasma (reference interval)

[d] Adult values given

[e] Further data on IgG subclass values can be obtained from Schauer, U., Stemberg, F., Rieger, C.H., et al., IgG subclass concentrations in certified reference material 470 and reference values of children and adults determined with the binding site reagents, *Clin. Chem.* 49, 1924–1929, 2003.

[f] Resistance is frequently used to describe the innate ability of an organism to neutralize (resist) a pathogen or toxin produced in a disease (adapted from *Dorland's Illustrated Medical Dictionary*, 32nd edn., Elsevier/Saunders, Philadelphia, PA, 2012). In the above, resistance refers to the ability of an immunoglobulin to neutralize (bacteriostatic) or kill (bacteriocidal) pathogens or toxins.

[g] From Salonen, E.-M., Hovi, T., Meurman, O., et al., Kinetics of specific IgA, IgD, IgE, IgG., and IgM antibody responses in Rubella, *J. Med. Virol.* 16, 1–9, 1985.

[h] Gutzeit C, Chen K, Cerutti A. The enigmatic function of IgD: Some answers at last, *Eur. J. Immunol.* 48, 1101–1113, 2018.

IMMUNOGLOBULIN SUPERFAMILY

The finding of homology in the heavy and light chains in the constant domains of immunoglobulins[1] led to the postulate of common origin, and the finding of structures in proteins other than immunoglobulins resulted in the organization of the immunoglobulin superfamily.[2] The immunoglobulin superfamily is diverse but in most cases are cell surface glycoproteins which contain an extracellular domain homologous to immunoglobulin (Ig), a transmembrane component, and a cytoplasmics extension which interact with other cell adhesion molecules such as integrins in homotypic interactions.[3] Recent work has focused on junctional adhesion molecules (JAMs).[4–7]

1. Hill, R.L., Delaney, R., Fellows, R.E., Jr., and Hebovitz, H.E., The evolutionary origins of the immunoglobulins, *Proc. Natl. Acad. Sci. USA* 56, 1762–1769, 1966.
2. Williams, A.F., and Barclay, A.N., The immunoglobulin superfamily-domains for cell surface recognitions, *Annu. Rev. Immunol.* 6, 381–405, 1988.
3. Matthäus, C., Langhorst, H., Schütz, L., Jüttner, R., and Rathjen, F.G., Cell-cell communication mediated by the CAR subgroup of immunoglobulin cell adhesion molecules in health and disease, *Mol. Cell. Neursci.* 81, 34–40, 2017.
4. Mandell, K.J., and Parkos, C.A., The JAM family of proteins, *Adv. Drug. Deliv. Rev.* 57, 857–867, 2005.
5. Aricescu, A.R., and Jones, E.Y., Immunoglobulin superfamily cell adhesion molecules: Zippers and signals, *Curr. Opin. Cell Biol.* 19, 543–550, 2007.
6. Zinn, K., and Özkan, E., Neural immunoglobulin superfamily interaction networks, *Curr. Opin. Neurobiol.* 45, 99–105, 2017.
7. Kummer, D., and Ebnet, K., Junctional adhesion molecules (JAMs): The JAM-integrin connection, *Cells* 7, 25, 2018.

IMMUNOMICS

Immunomics is the study of the cellular and humoral response (the immunome) of a host to a specific pathogen such using omics technologies.[1] The concept of immunomics is also used in the study of tumors.[2] Work in immunomics has been dominated by proteomic approaches such as that for the immunome of colon cancer[3] and parasites.[4,5] There has been extensive use of peptide microarrays in immunomics.[6,7] Immunomics is useful for rational vaccine design.[8–10]

1. Holfreter, S., Kolata, J., Stentzel, S., et al., Omics approaches for the study of adaptive immunity to *Staphylococcus aureus* and the selection of vaccine candidates, *Proteomes* 4, 11, 2016.
2. Bulman, A., Neagu, M., and Constantin, C., Immunomics in skin cancer—Improvement in diagnosis, prognosis and therapy monitoring, *Curr. Proteomics* 10, 202–217, 2013.
3. Coronell, J.A.L., Sergelen, K., Hofer, P., et al., The immunome of colon cancer: Functional *in silico* analysis of antigenic proteins deduced from IgG microarray profiling, *Genom. Proteom. Bioinf.* 16, 73–84, 2018.
4. Gaze, S., Driguez, P., Pearson, M.S., et al., An immunomics approach to Schistosome antigen discovery: Antibody signatures of naturally resistant and chronically infected individuals from endemic areas, *PLoS Pathog.* 10(3), 1004033, 2014.
5. Kassegne, K., Abe, E.M., Chen, J.-H., and Zhou, X.-N., Immunomic approaches to antigen discovery of human parasites, *Expt. Rev. Proteomics* 13, 1091–1101, 2016.
6. Carmone, S.J., Nielsen, M., Schafer-Nielsen, C., et al., Towards high-throughput immunomics for infectious diseases. Use of next generation peptide microarrays for rapid discovery and mapping of antigenic determinants, *Mol. Cell. Proteomics* 14, 1871–1884, 2015.
7. Delfani, P., Dexlin-Mellby, L., Norström, M., et al., Technical advances of the recombinant antibody microarray technology platform for clinical immunoproteomics, *PLoS One* 11(7), eo159138, 2016.
8. Masignani, V., Rappuoli, R., and Pizza, M., Reverse vaccinology: A genome-based approach for vaccine development, *Expert. Opin. Biol. Ther.* 2, 895–905, 2002.
9. DeSousa, K.P., and Doolan, D.L., Immunomics: A 21st century approach to vaccine development for complex pathogens, *Parasitology* 143, 236–244, 2016.
10. Liao, W., Zhang, T.T., Gao, L., et al., Integration of novel materials and advanced "omics" technologies into new vaccine design, *Curr. Top. Med. Chem.* 17, 2286–2301, 2017.

IMMUNOPROTEOMICS

Immunoproteomics is the study of the cellular and humoral immune response using the proteomic techniques such as microarray analysis and mass spectrometry.[1–3] Immunoproteomics can be distinguished from antibody-based proteomics in that immunoproteomics is the use of proteomic technology to study the proteins of the humoral and cellular immune response while antibody-based proteomics is the use of antibodies to in proteomics (see antibody-based proteomics). Immunoproteomics is one of the several techniques used in immunomics.

1. Hoppes, R., Ekkebus, R., Schumacher, T.N., and Ovaa, H., Technologies for MHC class I immunoproteomics, *J. Proteomics* 73, 1945–1953, 2010.
2. Fulton, K.M., and Twine, S.M., Immunoproteomics: Current technology and applications, *Method Mol. Biol.* 1061, 21–57, 2013.
3. Edfors, F., Boström, T., Forsström, B., et al., Immunoproteomics using polyclonal antibodies and stable isotope-labeled affinity-purified recombinant proteins, *Mol. Cell. Proteomics* 13, 1611–1624, 2014.

IMMUNO PROTEASOME (IMMUNOPROTEOSOME)

An immune proteosome (preferred over immunoproteosome by PubMed) is 20S proteasome isoform responsible for the degradation of proteins to provide peptides for MHC class I antigen presentation.[1,2] The immune proteasome is one the several proteasomes; the other proteasomes are the standard proteasome and the intermediate proteasome.[3] Immunoproteasomes are suggested to have qualitative[4] and quantitative[5] differences in proteolytic specificity in the peptides provided to the MHC class I site. The peptides processed by the immune proteasome have been described as the **immunopeptidome**.[6]

1. Akiyama, K., Kagawa, S., Tamura, T., et al., Replacement of proteasome subunits X and Y by LMP7 and LMP2 induced by interferon-γ for acquirement of the functional diversity responsible for antigen processing, *FEBS Lett.* 343, 85–88, 1994.
2. Aki, M., Shimbara, N., Takashina, M., et al., Interferon-gamma induces different subunit organizations and functional diversity of proteasomes, *J. Biochem.* 115, 257–269, 1994.
3. Dahlmann, B., Mammalian proteasome subtypes: Their diversity in structure and function, *Arch. Biochem. Biophys.* 591, 132–140, 2016.
4. Winter, M.B., La Greca, F., Arastu-Kapur, S., et al., Immunoproteosome functions explained by divergence in cleavage specificity and regulation, *eLife* 6, e27364, 2017.
5. Mishto, M., Liepe, J., Textoris-Taube, K., et al., Proteosome isoforms exhibit only quantitative differences in cleavage and epitope generation, *Eur. J. Immunol.* 44, 3508–3521, 2014.
6. Chong, C., Marino, F., Pak, H., et al., High-throughput and sensitive immunopeptidomics platform reveals profound interferon γ-mediated remodeling of the human leukocyte antigen (HLA) ligandome, *Mol. Cell. Proteomics* 17, 533–548, 2018.

IMMUNOSTIMULATORY PEPTIDE

There is a peptide sequence (VQGEESNDK) in human IL-1β which can increase the antigenicity of proteins.[1] There has been limited use of this approach.[2,3] There are other peptides which have been characterized as immunostimulatory.[4–7]

1. Beckers, W., Villa, L., Gonfloni, S., et al., Increasing the immunogenicity of protein antigens through the genetic insertion of VOGEESNDK sequence of human IL-1β into their sequence, *J. Immunol.* 151, 1757–1764, 1993.
2. Boraschi, D., and Tagliabue, A., Interleukin-1 and interleukin-1 fragments as vaccine adjuvants, *Methods* 19, 108–113, 1999.
3. Gor, D.O., Ding, X., Li, Q., et al., Enhanced immunogenicity of Pneumococcal surface adhesin A by genetic fusion to cytokines and evaluation of protective immunity in mice, *Infect. Immun.* 70, 5589–5595, 2002.
4. Campbell, D.F., Saenz, R., Bharati, I.S., et al., A novel fusion protein-based vaccine comprising a cell penetrating and immunostimulatory peptide linked to human papillomavirus (HPV) type 16 E7 antigen generates potent immunologic and anti-tumor responses in mice, *Vaccine* 29, 920–930, 2011.
5. Saenz, R., Meemer, B., Futalan, D., et al., Activity of the HMGB1-derived immunostimulatory peptide Hp91 resides in the helical C-terminal portion and is enhanced by dimerization, *Mol. Immunol.* 57, 191–199, 2014.
6. Garg, R., Latimer, L., Gerdts, V., et al., Vaccination with the RSV fusion protein formulated with a combination adjuvant induces long-lasting protective immunity, *J. Gen. Virol.* 95, 1043–1054, 2014.
7. Larsson, M., and Messmer, D., Enhanced anti-tumor immune responses and delay of tumor development in human epidermal growth factor receptor-2 mice immunized with an immunostimulatory peptide in poly(D, L-lactic-co-glycolic) acid nanoparticles, *Breast Cancer Res.* 17, 48, 2015.

IMMUNOSTIMULATORY SEQUENCE OLIGODEOXYNUCLEOTIDE (ISS-ODN)

Host defense can be separated into innate processes and adaptive processes. Innate processes are relatively nonspecific involving various mechanisms including the participation of various receptors.[1] Adaptive processes are more specific with the production of specific antibodies and dedicated immune cells. Toll-like receptors[2] were shown to recognize certain DNA sequences in bacteria and other pathogens in the innate immune response.[3,4] This process of recognition is referred to as pathogen-associated molecular recognition (PAMP; also danger-associated molecular patterns, DAMP) using pattern-recognition receptors (PRRs).[5] Subsequent work established that oligodeoxyribonucleotides containing unmethyated CpG sequences had potent immunostimulatory properties.[6,7] More recent work has seen the use of an oligodeoxynucleotide containing substantial CpG sequence in whole tumor cell vaccine[8] and in a nanoparticle vaccine.[9]

1. De Nardo, D., Activation of the innate immune receptors: Guardians of the micro galaxy. Activation and functions of the innate immune receptors, in *Regulation of Inflammatory Signaling in Health and Disease* (*Advances in Experimental Biology and Medicine*, V.1024), ed. D. Xu, Chapter 1, 1–35, Springer Nature, Singapore, 2017.
2. Medzhitov, R., Toll-like receptors and innate immunity, *Nature Rev. Immunol.* 1, 135–145, 2001.
3. Tokunaga, T., Yamamoto, H., Shimada, S., et al., Antitumor activity of deoxyribonucleic acid fraction from *Mycobacterium bov* BCG. I. Isolation, physicochemical characterization, and antitumor activity, *J. Natl. Cancer Inst.* 72, 955–962, 1984.
4. Shimosato, T., and Kitazawa, H., Immunogenics: Immunostimulatory oligonucleotides from probiotics, in *Probiotics, Immunobiotics, and Immunogenics*, ed. H. Kitazawa, J. Villena, and S. Alvarez, CRC Press, Boca Raton, FL, 2013.
5. Akira, S., Uematsu, S., and Takeuchi, O., Pathogen recognition and innate immunity, *Cell* 124, 783–801, 2006.
6. Weiner, G.J., Liu, H-M., Wooldridge, J.E., Dahle, C.E., and Krieg, A.M., Immunostimulatory oligodeoxynucleotides containing the CpG motif and effective as immune adjuvants in tumor antigen immunization, *Proc. Natl. Acad. Sci. USA* 94, 10833–10837, 1997.
7. Klinman, D.M., Yamshchikov, G., and Ishigatsubo, Y., Contribution of CpG motifs to the immunogenicity of DNA vaccines, *J. Immunol.* 158, 3635–3639, 1997.
8. Goldstein, M.J., Varghese, B., Brody, J.D., et al., A CpG-loaded tumor cell vaccine induces antitumor CD4+T cells that are effective in adoptive therapy for large and established tumors, *Blood* 117, 118–127, 2011.
9. Wilson, J.T., Keller, S., Manganiello, M.J., et al., pH-Responsive nanoparticle vaccines for dual delivery of antigens and immunostimulatory oligonucleotides, *ACS Nano* 7, 3912–3924, 2013.

INFLAMMASOME

The inflammasome is a cytoplasmic heteromeric complex of proteins formed response to signaling from surface pattern recognition receptors which functions in the inflammatory response by activating caspase-1 and processing IL-1β and IL-8 which are cytokines involved in the inflammatory response.[1] The autocatalytic activation of caspase-1 occurs during the formation of the inflammasome upon interaction with an adaptor protein, ASC (apoptosis-associated speck-like protein containing a caspase recruitment domain; CARD). There is subsequent interaction with an intracellular PRP protein, NLR (nucleotide-binding domain and leucine-rich repeat) protein. This provides a scaffold for the function of caspase-1 in interaction with cytokines. The inflammasome is involved in a special type of cell death referred to as pyroptosis.[2]

1. Pétrilli, V., and Marinon, E., Molecular definitions of inflammasomes, in *The Inflammasomes*. ed. F. Couillin, V. Pétrilli, and F. Martinon, Chapter 1, pp. 1–16, Springer Basel, Cham, Switzerland, 2011 (Dubois, H., Wullert, A., and Lamkanfi, M., General strategies in inflammasome biology, in *Inflammation Signaling and Bacterial Infections*, ed. S. Backert, pp. 1–22, Springer International, Cham, Switzerland, 2016.)

2. Man, S.M., Karki, R., and Kanneganti, T.D., Molecular mechanisms and functions of pyroptosis, inflammatory caspases and inflammasomes in infectious diseases, *Immunol. Rev.* 277, 61–75, 2017.

INFRARED SPECTROSCOPY

Classification of Infrared spectra

Classification	Wavelength/Wavenumber[a]
Near-Infrared (NIR)	800–2500 nm/12,500–4000 cm^{-1}
Mid-Infrared (MIR)	2.5–25 μm/4000–400 cm^{-1}
Far-Infrared (THz)[b]	25–300 μm/400–33.3 cm^{-1}

[a] The wavenumber is the reciprocal of the wavelength. The SI unit is m^{-1} but the convention is cm^{-1} (wave number, cm^{-1} = 10,000/λ (μm)).

[b] Far infrared is also referred as tetrahertz (https://www.nist.gov/programs-projects/far-infrared-spectroscopy-biomolecules).

The common range for infrared spectroscopy is 10–12,800 cm^{-1} (780–10^6 nm). Absorption spectra are described as function of the wavenumber of the incident; the wavenumber is the reciprocal of the wavelength and has the advantage of being linear with energy. The infrared region can be divided into the near-infrared, the mid-infrared, and far-infrared regions. Infrared spectroscopy is vibrational spectroscopy as compared to UV-Vis spectroscopy which is adsorption spectroscopy. Infrared spectroscopy is related to Raman spectroscopy.[1]

NEAR-INFRARED SPECTROSCOPY

Near-infrared spectroscopy (NIR)[2] is of value for the study of tissues and biological fluids.[3,4] The presence of water does not interfere with NIR spectroscopy permitting a wide application. A common application of NIR spectroscopy uses a pulse oximetry to measure the extent of hemoglobin oxygen saturation in blood.[5] This method has been adapted to the measurement of hemoglobin oxygenation in tissues.[6] This work has been extended to what is known as functional near-infrared spectroscopy (fNIRs) to measure brain function.[7–9] NIR spectroscopy has been used for the *in vivo* measurement of glucose.[10,11] NIR spectroscopy has broad application in biopharmaceutical manufacturing[12]

including the monitoring of the composition of cell culture media.[13] As stated above, absorbance by water is less of an issue in NIR spectroscopy than it is in mid-range infrared. However, water has a definite spectrum in the NIR range with major absorbance bands at 760, 970, 1190, 1450, and 1940 nm.[14] The absorbance bands of water can be used to determine the content and quality of water in lyophilized materials.[15,16] NIR spectroscopy does permit analysis of final product in glass vials.[17–19] Quantitation of water by NIR spectroscopy is validated with the Karl Fischer method for determination of water.[20]

MID-INFRARED SPECTROSCOPY

The mid-infrared range is likely the most commonly used in organic chemistry and has been used extensively in the study of lipids as organic solvents can be used.[21] There has been use of mid-infrared spectroscopy of the study of proteins.[22–26] Spectroscopy in the mid-infrared range is complicated by high absorbance of water in this range of the spectrum.[23,27] Attenuated total reflectance infrared spectroscopy has been applied for the spectral analysis of proteins.[28,29] Quantitative measurement in mid-range infrared spectroscopy is more difficult because of band interpretation and instrument issues.[30]

FAR-INFRARED SPECTROSCOPY

There is less use of far-infrared spectroscopy for the study of biopolymers. Water does absorb in the far-infrared range.[31] Far-infrared spectroscopy has seen use in the study of lipids in membranes[32] and proteins.[33,34]

1. Baker, M.J., Byrne, H.J., Chalmers, J., et al., Clinical applications of infrared and Raman spectroscopy: State of play and future challenges, *Analyst* 143, 1735–1757, 2018.

2. *Near-Infrared Spectroscopy: Principles, Instruments, Applications*, ed. H.W. Seisler, Y. Ozaki, S. Kawata, and H.M. Heise, Wiley-CH, Weinheim, Germany, 2002.

3. *Application of Near Infrared Spectroscopy in Biomedicine,* T. Jue and K. Masuda, Springer, New York, 2013.

4. Ciurczak, E.W., and Inge, B., *Pharmaceutical and Medical Applications of Near-Infrared Spectroscopy*, CRC Press, Boca Raton, FL, 2015.

5. Taylor, M.B., and Whitman, J.G., The current status of pulse oximetry. Clinical value of continuous noninvasive oxygen saturation monitoring, *Anesthesia* 41, 943–949, 1986.

6. Ferrari, M., Wilson, D.A., Hanley, D.F., et al., Noninvasive determination of hemoglobin saturation in dogs by derivative near-infrared spectroscopy, *Am. J. Physiol. Heart Circ. Physiol.* 256, H1493–H1499, 1989.

7. Villringer, A., and Chance, B., Non-invasive optical spectroscopy and imaging of human brain function, *Trends Neurosci.* 20, 435–442, 1997.

8. Kim, H.Y., Seo, K., Jeon, H.J., Lee, U., and Lee, H., Application of functional near-infrared spectroscopy to the study of brain function in humans and animal models, *Mol. Cells* 40, 523–532, 2017.

9. Soltanlou, M., Sitrikova, M.A., Nuerk, H-C., and Dresler, T., Applications of functional near-infrared spectroscopy (FNIRS) in studying cognitive development: The case of mathematics and language, *Front. Physcol.* 9, 277, 2018.

10. Tura, A., Maran, A., and Pacini, G., Non-invasive glucose monitoring: Assessment of technologies and devices according to quantitative criteria, *Diabetes Res. Clin. Pract.* 77, 16–40, 2007.

11. Jiantao, X., Liming, Y., Yufei, L., Chunyan, L., and Han, C., Noninvasive and fast measurement of blood glucose *in vivo* by near infrared (NIR) spectroscopy, *Spectrochim. Acta A Mol. Biomol. Spectrosc.* 179, 250–254, 2017.

12. Reich, G., Near-infrared spectroscopy and imaging: Basic principles and pharmaceutical applications, *Adv. Drug Deliv. Rev.* 57, 1109–1143, 2005.

13. Rhiel, M., Cohen, M.B., Murhammer, D.W., and Arnold, M.A., Nondestructive near-infrared spectroscopic measurement of multiple analytes in undiluted samples of serum-based cell culture media, *Biotechnol. Bioeng.* 77, 73–82, 2002.

14. Curcio, J.A., and Petty, C.C, The near-infrared absorption spectrum of liquid water, *J. Opt. Soc. America* 44, 302–304, 1951.

15. Brülls, M., Folestad, S., Sporén, A., and Rasmusun, A., *In-situ* near-infrared spectroscopy monitoring of the lyophilization process, *Pharm. Res.* 20, 494–499, 2003.

16. Cao, W., Mao, O., Chen, W., et al., Differentiation and quantitative determination of surface and hydrate water in lyophilized mannitol using NIR spectroscopy, *J. Pharm. Sci.* 90, 2077–2084, 2006.

17. Kamat, M.S., Lodder, R.A., and Deluca, P.P., Near-infrared spectroscopic determination of residual moisture in lyophilized sucrose through intact glass vials, *Pharm. Res.* 6, 961–965, 1989.

18. Lin, T.P., and Hsu, C.C., Determination of residual moisture in lyophilized protein pharmaceuticals using a rapid and non-invasive method: Near infrared spectroscopy, *PDA J. Pharm. Sci. Technol.* 56, 196–205, 2002.

19. Kauppinen, A., Toiviainen, M. Korhonen, O., et al., In-line multipoint near-infrared spectroscopy for moisture content quantification during freeze-drying, *Anal. Chem.* 85, 2377–2384, 2013.

20. Clavaud, M., Roggo, Y., Dégardin, K., et al., Global regression model for moisture content determination using near-infrared spectroscopy, *Eur. J. Pharm. Biopharm.* 119, 343–352, 2017.

21. Chapman, D., Goni, F.M., and Gunstone, F.D., Physical properties: Optical and spectral characterization, in *The Lipid Handbook*, 2nd edn., ed. F.D. Gunstone, J.L. Harwood, and F.B. Padley, Chapter 9, pp. 487–560, Chapman & Hall, London, UK, 1994.

22. Slayton, R.M., and Anfinrud, P.A., Time-resolved mid-infrared spectroscopy: Methods and biological applications, *Curr. Opin. Struct. Biol.* 7, 717–721, 1997.

23. Barth, A., Infrared spectroscopy of proteins, *Biochim. Biophys.* Acta 1767, 1073–1101, 2007.

24. Rich, P.R., and Maréchal, A., Carboxyl group functions in the heme-copper oxidases: Information from mid-IR vibrational spectroscopy, *Biochim. Biophys. Acta* 1777, 912–918, 2008.

25. Carbonaro, M., and Nucara, A., Secondary structure of food proteins by Fourier transform spectroscopy in the mid-infrared region, *Amino Acids* 38, 679–690, 2010.

26. López-Lorente, Á.I., and Mizaikoff, B., Mid-infrared spectroscopy for protein analysis: Potential and challenges, *Anal. Bioanal. Chem.* 408, 2875–2889, 2016.

27. Campbell, I.D., and Dwek, R.A., *Biological Spectroscopy*, Chapter 3, Infrared spectroscopy, pp. 27–60, Benjamin Cummings, Menlo Park, CA, 1984.

28. Perez-Guaita, D., Ventura-Gayete, J., Pérez-Rambla, C., et al., Protein determination in serum and whole blood by attenuated total reflectance infrared spectroscopy, *Anal. Bioanal. Chem.* 404, 649–656, 2012.

29. Shai, Y., ATR-FTIR studies in pore forming and membrane induced fusion peptides, *Biochim. Biophys Acta* 1828, 2306–2313, 2013.

30. Smith, B., *Infrared Spectral Interpretation: A Systematic Approach*, CRC Press, Boca Raton, FL, 1999.

31. Draegert, D.A., Stone, N.W.B., Curnette, B., and Williams, D.A, Far infrared spectrum of liquid water, *J. Opt. Soc. America* 56, 64–69, 1966. Srour, B., Erhard, B., Süss, R., and Hellwig, P., Monitoring the pH triggered collapse of liposomes in the far IR hydrogen bonding continuum, *J. Phys. Chem. B* 120, 4047–4052, 2016.

32. D'Angelo, G., Conti Nibali, V., Crupi, C., et al., Probing intermolecular interactions in phospholipid bilayers by far-infrared spectroscopy, *J. Phys. Chem. B* 121, 1204–1210, 2017.

33. Falconer, R.J., Zakaria, H.A., Fan, Y.Y., Bradley, A.P., and Middelberg, A.P., Far-infrared spectroscopy of protein higher-order structures, *Appl. Spectrosc.* 64, 1259–1264, 2010.

34. Stehle, C.U., Abuillan, W., Gompf, B., and Dressel, M., Far-infrared spectroscopy on free-standing protein films under defined temperature and hydration control, *J. Chem. Phys.* 136(7), 075102, 2012.

INHIBIN

Inhibin has a long history starting with a hypothesis in 1923 and experimental confirmation in the 1960s.[1] Inhibin is a heterodimeric glycoprotein which is a member of the TGFβ superfamily and best known for the inhibition of the synthesis/secretion of follicle stimulating hormone (FSH). Inhibin is considered to be nonsteroidal gonadal hormone which also functions in other organs by autocrine, paracrine, and endocrine mechanisms.[2] Inhibin is pleotropic with one example being the inhibition of bone morphogenetic protein (BMP) function.[3] Inhibin exists in two forms, inhibin A which contains the common α subunit (20 kDa) and the βA subunit (13 kDa) and inhibin B which contains the common α subunit (20 kDa) and the βB unit (13 kDa). The activity of inhibin is modulated by betaglycan which can be considered as an accessory receptor (co-receptor) for the tyrosine/kinase receptors responsible for signal transduction by members of the TGFβ superfamily.[4] The action of inhibin as a non-steroidal hormone is based on the antagonism of activin which stimulates FSH synthesis/secretion.[5] Activin, also a member of the TGFβ superfamily, has structural similarity to inhibin in that activin is either a heterodimer of βA and αB subunits or homodimer of the βB subunits.[6] Activins have activity outside of reproductive biology as seen in hepatic cells[7] and adipose tissue.[8]

1. Chappel, S., The physiological significance, in *Inhibins: Isolation, Estimation and Physiology,* ed. A.R. Sheth, Chapter 5, pp. 17–29, CRC Press, Boca Raton, FL, 1987.
2. Makanji, Y., Zhu, J., Mishro, R., et al., Inhibition at 90: From discovery to clinical application, *Endocrine Rev.* 35, 747–794, 2014.
3. Winter, E., and Vale, W., Inhibin is an antagonist of bone morphogenetic protein signaling, *J. Biol. Chem.* 278, 7934–7941, 2000.
4. Bilandzic, M., and Stenvers, K.L., Betaglycan: A multifunctional accessory, *Mol. Cell. Endocrinol.* 339, 180–189, 2011.
5. Bernard, D.J., and Tran, S., Mechanisms of activin-stimulated FSH synthesis: The story of a pig and a FOX, *Biol. Reprod.* 88(3), 78, 2013.
6. Wijayarathna, R., and de Kretser, D.M., Activins in reproductive biology and beyond, *Hum. Reprod. Update* 22, 342–357, 2016.
7. Chabicovsky, M., Herkner, K., and Rossmanith, W., Overexpression of activinβ_c or activin β_E in the mouse liver inhibits regenerative deoxyribonucleic acid synthesis of hepatic cells, *Endocrinology* 144, 3497–3504, 2003.
8. Zaragosi, L.E., Wdziekonski, B., Villageois, P., et al., Activin A plays a critical role in proliferation and differentiation of human adipose progenitors, *Diabetes* 59, 2513–2521, 2010.

INSULIN RECEPTOR

The insulin receptor (a tyrosine kinase receptor) is a dimer of two extracellular α-subunits disulfide-bonded to two β-subunits. The β subunits contain a transmembrane domain and an intracellular domain containing a tyrosine kinase domain.[1] The tyrosine kinase activity serves to phosphorylate a variety of insulin receptor substrates[2] affecting glucose transport and a variety of other functions.[3]

The insulin receptor is structurally similar to fibroblast growth factor receptors and the epidermal growth factor receptor and there may be overlap between IFG-1 receptor function and insulin receptor function.[4] There are two isoforms of the insulin receptor, A and B. Insulin growth factor II also binds to insulin receptor A and it is suggested that insulin receptor A is more important for growth and development[5] while insulin receptors B is more important for metabolic effects including glucose uptake.[6] Insulin resistance, which is an important part of the metabolic syndrome, is thought to be a problem with signaling by the insulin receptor and not insulin binding to the receptor,[7] although it is a complicated problem.

1. Croll, T.I., Smith, B.J., Margetts, M.B., et al., Higher-resolution structure of the human insulin receptor ectodomain: Multi-modal inclusion of the insert domain, *Structure* 24, 469–476, 2016.
2. Kim, J.J., and Accili, D., Signalling though IGF-1 and insulin receptors: Where is the specificity? *Growth Hormone IGF Res.* 12, 84–90, 2002.
3. Haeusler, R.A., McGraw, T.E., and Acili, D., Biochemical and cellular properties of insulin receptor signaling, *Nature Rev. Mol. Cell. Biol.* 19, 31–44, 2017.
4. Holly, J., Physiology of the IGF systems, in *Biology of IGF-1: Its Interaction with Insulin in Health and Malignant States,* ed. G. Bock and J. Goode, pp. 19–35, John Wiley & Sons, Chichester, UK, 2004.
5. Janssen, J.A., and Varewijck, A.J., IGF-IR targeted therapy: Past, present, and future, *Front. Endocrinol.* 5, 224, 2014.
6. Haeusler, R.A., McGraw, T.E., and Acili, D., Biochemical and cellular properties of insulin receptor signaling, *Nature Rev. Mol. Cell. Biol.* 19, 31–44, 2017.
7. Czech, M.P., Insulin action and resistance in obesity and type 2 diabetes, *Nature Med.* 23, 804–814, 2017.

INTEGRINS

The term integrin was used to describe an anti-anxiety drug used in the 1970s.[1] Oxypertine is in current use[2] but apparently no longer referred to as integrin. The term integrin was introduced in its current context in 1986[3] to describe a mechanism by which actin in the cytoskeleton interacts with the extracellular matrix. The discovery of integrin provides a link between the ECM and the cytoskeleton as well for the interaction of soluble proteins such as fibrinogen with platelets.[4] The interaction between integrins and ECM ligands is based on the recognition of an RGD (Arg-Gly-Asp) sequence. Integrins have been shown to be noncovalent heterodimers with an α subunit and a β subunit with cytoplasmic, transmembrane, and short cytoplasmic domains. The type α subunit and a β subunit are both type I transmembrane glycoproteins.[5] There are a large number of individual integrins derived from the combination of as many as 18 individual α subunits and 8 β subunits.[6,7] Accessory proteins such as talins modulate integrin function.[8] There are number of other proteins which linked integrins to the cytoskeleton or, in addition to talins, modulate integrin expression; collectively these have been referred to as the integrin adhesome.[9]

1. Norris, W., and Wallace, P.G., Oxpertine (Integrin): A study of its use in premedication, *Br. J. Anaesth.* 45, 1222–1225, 1973.
2. Saini, T., Kumar, S., and Narashimhan, B., Central nervous system activities of indole derivatives: An overview, *Cent. Nerv. Syst. Agents Med. Chem.* 16, 19–28, 2015.
3. Tamkun, J.W., DeSimone, D.W., Fonda, D., et al., Structure of integrin, a glycoprotein involved in the transmembrane linkage between fibronectin and actin, *Cell* 46, 271–282, 1986.
4. Hynes, R.O., Integrins: A family of cell surface receptors, *Cell* 48, 549–554, 1987.
5. Arcangeli, A., and Becchetti, A., Integrin structure and functional relation with ion channels, in *Integrins and Ions Channels: Molecular Complexes and Signaling*, ed. A. Becchetti and A. Archangeli, Chapter 1, pp. 1–7, Landis Bioscience/Springer Science + Business, New York, 2010.
6. Srichai, M.B., and Zent, R., Integrin structure and function, in *Cell-Extracellular Matrix Interactions in Cancer*, ed. R. Zent and A. Pozzi, Chapter 2, pp. 19–41, Springer Science + Business, New York, 2010.
7. Hemler, M.E., Weitzman, J.B., Pasqualini, R., et al., in *Integrins: The Biological Problem*, ed. Y. Takada, CRC Press, Boca Raton, FL, 2017.
8. Gough, R.E., and Goult, B.T., The tale of two talins—Two isoforms to fine tune integrin signalling, *FEBS Lett.* 592, 2108–2125 2018.
9. Geiger, T., and Zaidel-Bar, R., Opening the floodgates: Proteomics and the integrin adhesome, *Curr. Opin. Cell Biol.* 24, 562–568, 2012.

INTEIN

An intein is an intervening protein sequence which is removed by post-translational self-splicing; analogous to intron splicing in RNA.[1] Its sequences are surrounded by an *N*-terminal extein and a *C*-terminal extein.[2] The identification of the intein arose from the observation that the product of *VMA1* gene was smaller than the gene isolated from genomic library suggesting that there was post-translation excision of an internal region which was predicted from the genomic sequence.[3] Subsequent work on another gene (*TFP1*) showed that protein splicing occurred to form the "mature" 69-kD subunit of vacuolar H$^+$-adenosine triphosphatase.[4] Protein splicing has subsequently been shown to be a common process.[5] The concept of intein ligation has been used in expressed protein ligation where the amino

terminal cysteine of an intein is engineered to form a peptide bond with a recombinant protein or fragment. Thiolysis of this with a thiol such as thiophenol (benzenethiol) which can be coupled to a peptide by native chemical ligation.[6] Expressed protein ligation used the methods developed for native chemical ligation.[7,8] Intein-mediated cleavage has been used to separate the desired protein from an affinity tag during purification.[9,10]

1. Pavankumar, T.L., Inteins: Localized distribution, gene regulation, and protein engineering for biological applications, *Microorganisms* 6, 19, 2018.
2. Perler, F.B., Davis, E.O., Dean, G.E., et al., Protein splicing elements: Inteins and exteins—a definition of terms and recommended nomenclature, *Nucleic Acids Res.* 22, 1125–1127, 1994.
3. Hirata, R., Ohsumi, Y., Nakano, A., et al., Molecular structure of a gene, *VMA1*, encoding the catalytic subunit of H$^+$-translocating adenosine triphosphatase from vacuolar membranes of *Saccharomyces cerevisiae*, *J. Biol. Chem.* 265, 6726–6733, 1990.
4. Kane, P.M., Yamashiro, C.T., Wolczyk, D.E., et al., Protein splicing converts yeast *TFP1* gene product to the 69-kD subunit of the vacuolar H$^+$-adenosine triphosphatase, *Science* 250, 651–657, 1990.
5. Mills, K.V., Johnson, M.A., and Perler, F.B., Protein splicing: How inteins escape from precursor proteins, *J. Biol. Chem.* 289, 14495–14503, 2014.
6. Muir, T.W., Sondhi, D., and Cole, P.A., Expressed protein ligation: A general method for protein engineering, *Proc. Natl. Acad. Sci. USA* 95, 6705–6710, 1998.
7. Severinov, K., and Muir, T.W., Expressed protein ligation, a novel method for studying protein-protein interactions in transcription, *J. Biol. Chem.* 273, 16205–16209, 1998.
8. Englehard, M., Quest for the chemical synthesis of proteins, *J. Pept. Sci* 22, 246–251, 2016.
9. Wu, W., Wood, D.W., Bellfort, G., et al., Intein-mediated purification of cytotoxic endonuclease I-TevI by insertional inactivation and pH-controllable splicing, *Nucleic Acids Res.* 30, 4864–4871, 2002.
10. Mills, K.V, Connor, K.R., Dorval, D.M., and Lewandowski, K.T., Protein purification via temperature-dependent, intein-mediated cleavage from an immobilized metal affinity resin, *Anal. Biochem.* 356, 86–93, 2006.

INTERCALATION

The formal definition of intercalation is "the insertion of any addition between the members of an existing or recognized series...."[1] In specific application to molecular biology, the canonical description is the insertion of a planar, heteroaromatic compound in between DNA base pairs in a double-stranded DNA.[2] Intercalation can also occur in RNA.[3-5] The concept of intercalation was advanced in 1961 to describe the interaction of DNA with acridine, proflavine, and acridine orange.[6] It was observed that a small amount of these compounds, which had been shown to be mutagenic, increased the viscosity of the DNA and increased the sedimentation coefficient. It is now known that intercalation causes unwinding of the DNA helix with resulting changes in transcriptional fidelity.[7] This unwinding is not as significant with circular DNA resulting in the binding of less dye.[8] Intercalating dyes with increased binding affinity and slow dissociation kinetics are being developed as therapeutics with the concept of threading through the disrupted DNA base pairs.[9,10] The concept of intercalation is of importance in the process of base excision repair where the recognition of DNA damage by alkyladenine DNA glycosylase where an aromatic residue is inserted between DNA base pairs.[11,12]

1. *Oxford English Dictionary*, Oxford, UK, 2019.
2. Long, E.C., and Barton, J.K., On demonstrating DNA intercalation, *Accts. Chem. Res.* 23, 271–273, 1990.
3. Isalm, S.A., and Neidle, S., Nucleic acid binding drugs. X. A theoretical study of proflavine intercalation into RNA and DNA fragments: Comparison with crystallographic results, *Act Cryst.* B40, 424–429, 1984.
4. Jamison, J.M., Gilloteaux, J., and Summers, J.L., The antiviral activity of RNA-dye combinations, *Prog. Mol. Subcell. Biol.* 14, 89–113, 1994.
5. Ranjan, N., and Arya, D.P., Linker dependent intercalation of bisbenzimidazole-aminosugars in an RNA duplex: Selectively in RNA vs. DNA binding, *Bioorg. Med. Chem. Lett.* 26, 5989–5994, 2016.
6. Lerman, L.S., Structural considerations in the interaction of DNA and acridines, *J. Mol. Biol.* 3, 18–30, 1961.
7. Bates, A.D., and Maxwell, A., *DNA Topology*, Oxford University Press, Oxford, UK, 2005.
8. Adams, R.L.P., Knowler, J.T., and Leader, D.P., *The Biochemistry of Nucleic Acids*, pp. 218–219, Chapman & Hall, London, UK, 1986.
9. Almagwashi, A.A., Andersson, J., Lincoln, P., et al., DNA intercalation optimized by two-step molecular lock mechanism, *Sci. Rep.* 6, 37993, 2016.
10. Clark, A.G., Naufer, M.N., Westerlund, F., et al., Reshaping the energy landscape transforms the mechanism and binding kinetics of DNA threading intercalation, *Biochemistry* 57, 614–619, 2018.
11. Hendershot, J.M., and O'Brien, P.J., Critical role of DNA intercalation I enzyme-catalyzed nucleotide flipping, *Nuc. Acid Res.* 42, 12681–12690, 2014.
12. Hendershot, J.M., and O'Brien, P.J., Search for DNA damage by human alkyladenine DNA glycosylase involves early intercalation by an aromatic residue, *J. Biol. Chem.* 292, 16070–16080, 2017.

INTERACTOME

The term interactome refers to the sum of the various protein-protein interactions within a proteome. Presumably the concept could be extended to included interactions of proteins with lipids, polysaccharides, and nucleic acids, although other interactions appear to be generating additional nomenclature. For example, the study of the interaction of proteins (and other materials) with the surface of extracellular vesicles is referred to as the extracellular vesicle surface interactome.[1] The interactome described here is concerned only with protein-protein interactions within a defined proteome. The yeast two-hybrid system is a popular technique used to define an interactome.[2-5] The use of cDNA libraries to express proteins for use in protein arrays (affinity purification) is another approach.[6-8] A related approach uses a target, such as a receptor, to "pull-down" interacting proteins.[9] Chemical crosslinking (photochemical) is a somewhat more limited approach.[10] Chemical crosslinking (photoactivation) is useful for identifying RNA-protein interactions[11,12] as is crosslinking with formaldehyde.[13] An interactome may be explored at the organelle level[14,15] or at the system level.[16] Other work explores the interactome for receptors[17] and cell function.[18,19]

1. Buzás, E.I., Tóth, E.Á., Sóder, B.W., and Szabó-Taylor, K.É., Molecular interactions at the surface of extracellular vesicles, *Semin. Immunopathol.*, 40, 453–464, 2018.
2. Ito, T., Chiba, T., and Yoshida, M., Exploring the protein interactome using comprehensive two-hybrid projects, *Trends Biotechnol.* 19(Suppl 10), S23–S27, 2001.
3. Ito, T., Ota, K., Kubota, H., et al., Roles for the two-hybrid system in exploration of the yeast protein interactome, *Mol. Cell. Proteomics* 1, 561–566, 2002.
4. Trigg, S.A., Garza, R.M., MacWilliams, A., et al., CrY2H—Seq: A massively multiplexed assay for deep-coverage interactome mapping, *Nat. Methods* 14, 819–825, 2017.
5. Woodsmith, J., Apelt, L., Casado-Medrano, V., et al., Protein interaction perturbation profiling at amino-acid resolution, *Nat. Methods* 14, 1213–1221, 2017.
6. *Protein Array Methods and Protocols*, ed. E.T. Fung, Human Press, Totowa, NJ, 2004.
7. Schweppe, D.K., Huttlin, E.L., Harper, J.W., and Gygi, S.P., Biopex display: An suite for large-scale AP-MS protein-protein interaction data, *J. Proteome Res.* 17, 722–726, 2018.
8. Yang, F. Lei, Y., Zhou, M., et al., Development and application of a recombination-based library versus library high-throughput yeast two-hybrid (RLL-Y2H) screening system, *Nucleic Acids Res.* 46, e17, 2018.

9. Acharya, K.D., Nettles, S.A., Sellers, K.J., et al., The Progestin receptor interactome in the female mouse hypothalamus: Interactions with synaptic proteins are isoform specific and ligand dependent, *eNeuro* 4(5), 271–317, 2017.

10. Chojnacki, M., Mansour, W., Hameed, D.S., et al., Polyubiquitin-photoactivatable crosslinking reagents for mapping ubiquitin interactome identify Rpn1 as a proteasome ubiquitin-associating subunit, *Cell Chem. Biol.* 24, 443–457, 2017.

11. Bach-Pages, M., Castello, A., and Preston, G.M., Plant RNA interactome capture: Revealing the plant RBPome, *Trends Plant Sci.* 22, 449–451, 2017.

12. Kastelic, N., and Landthaler, M., mRNA interactome capture in mammalian cells, *Methods* 126, 38–43, 2017.

13. Kroener, R.A., Becker, J.T., Scalf, M., Sherer, N.M., and Smith, L.M., Elucidating the *in vivo* interactome of HIV-1 by hybridization capture and mass spectrometry, *Sci. Rep.* 7(1), 16965, 2017.

14. Valm, A.M., Cohen, S., Legant, W.R., et al., Applying systems-level spectral imaging and analysis to reveal the organelle interactome, *Nature* 546, 162–167, 2017.

15. Simsek, D., Tiu, G.C., Flynn, R.A., et al., The mammalian ribo-interactome reveals ribosome functional diversity and heterogeneity, *Cell* 169, 1051–1065, 2017.

16. Huttlin, E.L., Bruckner, R.J., Paulo, J.A., et al., Architecture of the human interactome defines protein communities and disease networks, *Nature* 545, 505–509, 2017.

17. Eden, G., Archinti, M., Furlan, F., Murphy, R., and Degryse, B., The urokinase receptor interactome, *Curr. Pharm. Des.* 17, 1874–1889, 2011.

18. Zou, Y., Li, Y., and Dillon, J.R., The distinctive cell division interactome of *Neisseria gonorrhoeae*, *BMC Microbiol.* 17, 232, 2017.

19. Pires, H.R., and Boxem, M., Mapping the polarity interactome, *J. Mol. Biol.* 430, 3521–3544, 2018.

INTERLEUKIN

Interleukins are a category of cytokines (mainly type I cytokines) that are a functionally defined group of small proteins which "communicate" between various immune cell types (inter + leukocytes = interleukin).[1–5] This term was developed to rationalize the nomenclature for these materials as the different terms/names were selected on the basis of activity in a particular assay system rather than an intrinsic physical or biological property; this situation is not unlike that which occurred in blood coagulation somewhat earlier. Thus, lymphocyte activating factor (LAF; mitogenic protein, B-cell differentiation factor) is IL-1.[6] The term interleukin-1 describes a family of cytokines.[7,8] Thymocyte stimulating factor (TSF, T-cell growth factor, killer cell helper factor) became known as IL-2.[9–12] There are a large number of interleukins in the cytokine family.[5,13–17]

1. Aardem, L.A., Brunner, T.K., Creottini, J.C., et al., Revised nomenclature for antigen-nonspecific T-cell proliferation and helper factors, *J. Immunol.* 123, 2928–2929, 1979.

2. Paul, W.E., Kishimoto, T., Melchers, F., et al., Nomenclature for secreted regulatory proteins of the immune system (interleukins), *Clin. Immunol. Immunopathol.* 64, 3–4, 1992.

3. Oppenheim, J.J., and Gery, I., From lymphodrek to interleukin 1, *Immunol. Today* 14, 232–243, 1994.

4. IUIS/WHO Standing Committee on Interleukin Designation, Nomenclature for secreted regulatory proteins of the immune system (interleukins): Update, *Bull. World Health Org.* 75, 175, 1997.

5. Leonard, W.J., Type I cytokines and interferons and their receptors, in *Fundamental Immunology*, 6th edn., ed. W.E. Paul, Chapter 25, pp. 601–538, Wolters Kluwer, Philadelphia, PA, 2013.

6. Durum, S.K., Schmidt, J.A., and Oppenheim, J.J., Interleukin 1: An immunological perspective, *Annu. Rev. Immunol.* 3, 263–287, 1985.

7. Southcombe, J.H., Redman, C.W., Sargent, I.L., and Granne, I., Interleukin-1 family cytokines and their regulatory proteins in normal pregnancy and pre-eclampsia, *Clin. Exp. Immunol.* 181, 480–490, 2015.

8. Palomo, J., Dietrich, D., Martin, P., Palmer, G., and Gabay, C., The interleukin (IL)-1 cytokine family-balance between agonists and antagonists in the inflammatory diseases, *Cytokine* 76, 25–37, 2015.

9. Watson, J., and Mochizuki, D., Interleukin 2: A class of T cell growth factors, *Immunol. Rev.* 51, 287–278, 1980; Mizel, S.B., Interleukin 1 and T cell activation, *Immunol. Rev.* 63, 51–72, 1982.

10. Wagner, H., Hardt, C., Heeg, K., et al., The in vivo effects of interleukin 2 (TCGF), *Immunobiology* 161, 139–156, 1982.

11. Farrar, J.J., Benjamin, W.R., Hilfiker, M.L., et al., The biochemistry, biology, and role of interleukin 2 in the induction of cytotoxic T cell and antibody-forming B cell responses, *Immunol. Rev.* 63, 129–166, 1982.

12. *Interleukin-2 and Killer Cells in Cancer*, ed. R.B. Herberman and E. Lotzováa, CRC Press, Boca Raton, FL, 2018.

13. Kimball, E.S., *Cytokines and Inflammation*, CRC Press, Boca Raton, FL, 1991.

14. *The Cytokine Factsbook*, ed. K.A. Fitzgerald, L.A.J. O'Neill, A.J.H. Gearing, and R.E. Callard, Elsevier/Academic, San Diego, CA, 2001.

15. Vilček, J., The cytokines: An overview, in *The Cytokine Handbook*, ed. A.W. Thomson, and M.T. Lotze, 4th edn., Elsevier/Academic, London, UK, 2003.

16. Taga, T., and Kishimoto, T., GP130 and the Interleukin-6 family of cytokines, *Annu. Rev. Immunol.* 15, 797–819, 1997.

17. Cruse, J.M., Lewis, R.F., and Wang, H., *Immunology Guidebook*, Elsevier, Amsterdam, the Netherlands, 2004.

INTERNAL STANDARD

An internal standard is a compound or material which is not an analyte but is included in an unknown or standard to correct for issues in the processing or analysis of an analyte or analytes. An internal standard is not a calibration standard.[1] An example is the inclusion of an abnormal amino acid such as norleucine in classical amino acid analysis.[2] Another example is the inclusion of an isotopically labeled form of the analyte, such as deuterated *S*-methylmethionine, for analysis by mass spectrometry.[3] A similar approach in proteomics uses the inclusion of an isotopically labeled peptide.[4] Stable isotope coding is an approach to an internal standard in proteomics.[5] Stable isotope labeling is also used to provide internal standards in metabolomics.[6,7]

1. Coleman, D., and Vanatta, L., Statistics in Analytical Chemistry, Part 19-Internal Standards, *American Laboratory*, 2005.
2. Fauconnet, M., and Rochemont, J., A single-column amino acid analysis method which resolves hexosamines and several cysteine derivatives, *Anal. Biochem.* 91, 403–409, 1978.
3. Loscos, N., Séqurel, M., Dagan, L., Identification of *S*-methylmethionine in Petit Manseng grapes as dimethyl sulphide precursor in wine, *Anal. Chim. Acta* 621, 24–29, 2008.
4. Bronstrup, M., Absolute quantification strategies in proteomics based on mass spectrometry, *Expert Rev. Proteomics* 1, 503–512, 2004.
5. Julka, S., and Regnier, F., Quantification in proteomics through stable isotope coding: A review, *J. Proteome Res.* 3, 350–363, 2004.
6. Iglesias, J., Sleno, L., and Volmer, D.A., Isotopic labeling of metabolites in drug discovery applications, *Curr. Drug Metab.* 13, 1213–1225, 2012.
7. Hermann, G., Schwaiger, M., Volejnik, P., and Koellensperger, G., 13C-labelled yeast as internal standard for LC-MS/MS and LC high resolution MS based amino acid quantification in human plasma, *J. Pharm. Biomed. Anal.* 155, 329–334, 2018.

INTRABODIES

Intrabodies are (most frequently) functional recombinant antibody fragments which are expressed inside the cell.[1] Intrabodies can be used to study intracellular proteins.[2,3] Targets for intrabodies include the intracellular aspects of G-protein coupled receptors[4,5] and the endoplasmic reticulum.[6,7] There is considerable interest in the therapeutic application of intrabodies.[8–11]

1. Lo, A.S., Zhu, Q., and Marasco, W.A., Intracellular antibodies (intrabodies) and their therapeutic potential, *Handb. Exp. Pharmacol.* (181), 343–373, 2008.
2. Marschall, A.L., Dübel, S., and Böldicke, T., Specific *in vivo* knockdown of protein function by intrabodies, *MAbs* 7, 1010–1035, 2015.
3. Traenkle, B., and Rothbauer, U., Under the microscope: Single-domain antibodies for live-cell imaging and super-resolution microscopy, *Front. Immunol.* 8, 1030, 2017.
4. Staus, D.P., Wingler, L.M., Strachan, R.T., et al., Regulation of β2-adrenergic receptor function by conformationally selective single-domain intrabodies, *Mol. Pharmcol.* 85, 472–481, 2014.
5. Chaturvedi M., Schilling, J., Beautrait, A., et al., Emerging paradigm of intracellular targeting of G protein-coupled receptors, *Trends Biochem. Sci.* 43, 533–546, 2018.
6. Böldicke, T., Blocking translocation of cell surface molecules from the ER to the cell surface by intracellular antibodies targeted to the ER, *J. Cell. Mol. Med.* 11, 54–70, 2007.
7. Marschall, A.L., Dübel, S., Böldicke, T., Recent advances with ER targeted intrabodies, *Adv. Exp. Med. Biol.* 917, 77–93, 2016.
8. Sudol, K.L., Mastranglo, M.A., Narrow, W.C., et al., Generating differentially targeted amyloid-beta specific intrabodies as a passive vaccination for Alzheimer's disease, *Mol. Ther.* 17, 2031–2040, 2009.
9. Maleki, L.A., Baradaran, B., Majidi, J., Mohammadian, M., and Shahneh, F.Z., Future prospects of monoclonal antibodies as magic bullets in immunotherapy, *Hum. Antibodies* 22, 9–13, 2013.
10. Butler, D.C., Snyder-Keller, A., De Genst, E., and Messer, A., Differential nuclear localization of complexes may underlie *in vivo* intrabody efficacy in Huntington's disease, *Protein Eng. Des. Sel.* 27, 359–363, 2014.
11. Suzuki, R., Saito, K., Matsuda, M., et al., Single-domain intrabodies against hepatitis C virus core inhibit viral propagation and core-induced NFκB activation, *J. Gen. Virol.* 97, 887–892, 2016.

INTRON

The term intron refers to a sequence (an intervening sequence) in genomic DNA, which is not represented in the final RNA product (mRNA, tRNA, rRNA). The intron sequence is encoded into the primary RNA transcript, but it is not present in the final RNA product. The introns separate exon sequences; the combination of exons and introns comprise a transcriptional unit. Introns are common in eukaryotes and to a lesser extent in prokaryotes.[1] In eukaryotes, the primary nuclear RNA transcripts are processed (spliced) with the removal of introns to yield the final product by action of a spliceosome.[2–4] Group I introns[5,6] and Group II introns[7,8] are self-splicing with the mechanism involving RNA sequences known as ribozymes. tRNA introns (archaeal introns) are removed by a mechanism involving ATP and a splicing endonuclease.[9,10]

1. Alberts, B., Johnson, A., Lewis, J., Raff, M., Roberts, K., and Walter, P., *Molecular Biology of The Cell*, 5th edn., Chapter 2, Garland Science/Taylor & Francis Group, New York, 2008.
2. Roy, S.W., and Irimia, M., Mystery of intron gain: New data and new models, *Trends Genet.* 25, 67–73, 2009.
3. Matera, A.G., and Wang, Z., A day in the life of the spliceosome, *Nat. Rev. Mol. Cell Biol.* 15, 108–121, 2014.
4. Shi, Y., Mechanistic insights into precursor messenger RNA splicing by the spliceosome, *Nat. Rev. Mol. Cell. Biol.* 18, 655–670, 2017.
5. Haugen, P., Simon, D.M., and Bhattacharya, D., The natural history of group I introns, *Trends Genet.* 21, 111–119, 2005.
6. Nielsen, H., and Johansen, S.D., Group I introns. Moving in new directions, *RNA Biol.* 6, 373–383, 2009.
7. Bonen, L., and Vogel, J., The ins and outs of group II introns, *Trends Genet.* 17, 322–331, 2001.
8. Zhao, C., and Pyle, A.M., Structural insights into the mechanism of group II intron splicing, *Trends Biochem. Sci.* 42, 470–482, 2017.
9. Mair, B., Popow, J., Mechtler, K., Weitzer, S., and Martinez, J., Intron excision from precursor tRNA molecules in mammalian cells requires ATP hydrolysis and phosphorylation of tRNA-splicing endonuclease components, *Biochem. Soc. Trans.* 41, 831–837, 2013.
10. Yoshihisa, T., Handling tRNA introns, archaeal way and the eukaryotic way, *Front. Genet.* 5, 213, 2014.

INTRON DENSITY

The intron density is the average number of introns per gene over an entire genome.[1,2] There is data that suggests that increases in intron density promotes protein diversity.[3–5]

1. Roy, S.W., Fedorov, A., and Gilbert, W., The signal of ancient introns in obscured by intron density and homolog number, *Proc. Natl. Acad. Sci. USA* 99, 15513–15517, 2002.
2. Farlow, A., Meduri, E., and Schlötterer, C., DNA doubled-strand break repair and the evolution of intron density, *Trends Genet.* 27, 1–6, 2011.
3. Wu, X., and Hurst, L.D., Why selection might be stronger when populations are small: Intron size and density predict within the between-species usage of exonic splice associated *cis*-motifs, *Mol. Biol. Evol.* 32, 1847–1861, 2015.
4. Zhu, F.Y., Chen, M.X., Ye, N.H., et al., Proteogenomic analysis reveals alternative splicing and translation as part of the abscisic acid response in *Arabidopsis* seedlings, *Plant J.* 91, 518–533, 2017.
5. Vanichkina, D.P., Schmitz, U., Wong, J.J.-L., and Rasko, J.E.J., Challenges in defining the role of intron retention in normal biology and disease, *Sem. Cell Dev. Biol.* 75, 40–49, 2018.

INVADOSOME

The term invadosome is used to refer to podosomes and invadopodia.[1,2] Podosomes and invadopodia are both cellular protrusions derived from actin in the cytoskeleton which remain linked to the cell membrane[3,4] which participates in matrix degradation associated with cell motility.[5–8] Podosomes are associated with normal cells such as macrophages[9,10] and dendritic cells[11] while invadopodia are associated with tumor cells.[12] Invadopodia are therapeutic targets in oncology.[13,14] While there is considerable similarity between the action of podosomes and the action of invadopodia, there are differences in mechanism.[15] The podosome is a specialized cell-matrix contact point which is structural distinct from focal adhesion complexes.[16–18]

1. Génot, E., and Gligorijevic, B., Invadosomes in their natural habitat, *Eur. J. Cell Biol.* 93, 367–379, 2014.
2. Ponceau, A., Albigés-Rizo, C., Colin-Aronovicz, Y., Destaing, O., and Lecomte, M.C., αII-Spectrin regulates invadosome stability and extracellular matrix degradation, *PLoS One* 10(4), E0120781, 2015.
3. Murphy, D.A., and Courtneidge, S.A., The "ins" and "out" of podosomes and invadopodia: Characteristics, formation and function, *Nat. Rev. Cell Biol.* 12, 413–426, 2011.
4. Veittet, V., Spuul, P., Daubon, T., et al., Podosomes: Multipurpose organelles? *Int. J. Biochem. Cell Biol.* 65, 52–60, 2015.
5. Artym, V.V., Zhang, Y., Seillier-Maiseiwitsch, F., Yamada, K.M., and Mueller, S.C., Dynamic interactions of cortactin and membrane type I matrix metalloproteinase at invadopodia: Defining the stages of invadopodia formation and function, *Cancer Res.* 66, 3034–3043, 2006.
6. Hoshino, D., Branch, K.M., and Weaver, A.M., Signaling inputs to invadopodia and podosomes, *J. Cell. Sci.* 26, 2979–2989, 2013.
7. Seano, G., and Primo, L., Podosomes and invadopodia: Tools to breach vascular basement membrane, *Cell Cycle* 149, 1370–1374, 2015.
8. Spruul, P., Daubon, T., Pitter, B., et al., VEGF-A/Notch-induced podosomes proteolyse basement membrane collagen-IV during retinal sprouting angiogenesis, *Cell Reports* 17, 484–500, 2016.
9. Meddens, M.B., van den Dries, K., and Cambi, A., Podosomes revealed by advanced bioimaging: What did we learn? *Eur. J. Cell Biol.* 93, 380–387, 2014.
10. Baruzzi, A., Remelli, S., Lorenzetto, E., et al., Sos1 regulates macrophage podosomes assembly and macrophage invasive capacity, *J. Immunol.* 195, 4900–4012, 2015.
11. Cougoule, C., Lastrucci, C., Guiet, R., et al., Podosomes, but not the maturation status, determine the protease-dependent 3D migration in human dendritic cells, *Front. Immunol.* 9, 846, 2018.
12. Eddy, R.J., Weidmann, M.D., Sharma, V.P., and Condeelis, J.S., Tumor cell invadopodia: Invasive protrusions that orchestrate metastasis, *Trends Cell Biol.* 27, 585–607, 2017.

13. Stoletov, K., and Lewis, J.D., Invadopodia: A new thera-
    peutic target to block cancer metastasis, *Expert Rev.
    Anticancer Ther.* 15, 733–735, 2015.
14. Meirson, T., and Gil-Henn, H., Targeting invadopodia for
    blocking breast cancer metastasis, *Drug Resist. Updat.*
    39, 1–17, 2018.
15. Artym, V.V., Matsumoto, K., Mueller, S.C., and Yamada,
    K.M., Dynamic membrane remodeling at invadopodia
    differentiates invadopodia from podosomes, *Eur. J. Cell
    Biol.* 90, 172–180, 2011.
16. Linder, S., and Aepfelbacher, M., Podosomes: Adhesion
    hot-spots of invasive cells, *Trends Cell Biol.* 13, 376–385,
    2003.
17. McNiver, M.A., Baldassarre, M., and Buccione, R.,
    The role of dynamin in the assembly and function of
    podosomes and invadopodia, *Front. Biosci.* 9, 1944–
    1953, 2004.
18. Linder, S., and Kopp, P., Podosomes at a glance, *J. Cell
    Sci.* 118, 2079–2082, 2005.

ION CHANNEL

An ion channel is an integral membrane protein(s) providing for the regulated transport of ions across a membrane via the formation of a pore-like structure where
there can be specific interaction between an ion such as
potassium and charged groups in pore as well as a very
specific size limitation.[1] Ion channels may be either voltage gated[2-4] where a "gate" for the channel responds to
changes in membrane polarization (electrical potential
across the membrane or ligand (chemical) gated where
permeability is controlled by binding of a specific ligand
such as acetylcholine.[5-7] There are nomenclature systems
for ion-channels.[8-11]

1. Hille, B., *Ion Channels of Excitable Membranes*, 3rd
   edn., Sinauer Associates, Sunderland, MA, 2001.
2. Catterall, W.A., Voltage-gated sodium channels at 60:
   Structure, function and pathophysiology, *J. Physiol.* 590,
   2577–2589, 2012.
3. Groome, J.R., The voltage sensor module in sodium
   channels, *Handb. Exp. Pharmacol.* 222, 7–31, 2014.
4. Sahoo, N., Hoshi, T., and Heinemann, S.H., Oxidative
   modulation of voltage-gated potassium channels,
   Antioxid. Redox Signal. 21, 933–952, 2014.
5. Auerbach, A., The energy and work of a ligand-gated ion
   channel, *J. Mol. Biol.* 425, 1461–1475, 2013.
6. Comitani, F., Melis, C., and Moleteni, C., Elucidating
   ligand binding and channel gating mechanisms in pen-
   tameric ligand-gated ion channels by atomistic simulations, *Biochem. Soc. Trans.* 43, 151–156, 2015.
7. Cecchini, M., and Changeux, J.P., The nicotinic acetylcholine receptor and its prokaryotic homologues:
   Structure, conformational transitions & allosteric modulation, *Neuropharmacology* 96, 137–149, 2015.
8. Clapham, D.E., Julius, D., Montell, C., and Schultz,
   G., International Union of Pharmacology XLIX.
   Nomemclature and structure-function relationships of
   transient receptor potential channels, *Pharmacol. Rev.*
   57, 427–450, 2005.
9. Traynelis, S.F., Woomurth, L.P., McBain, C.J., et al.,
   Glutamate receptor ions channels: Structure, regulation,
   and function, *Pharmacol. Rev.* 62, 405–496, 2010.
10. Benga, G., On the definition, nomenclature, and classi-
    fication of water channel proteins (aquaporins and rela-
    tives), *Mol. Aspects Med.* 33, 514–517, 2012.
11. Kaczmarek, L.K., Aldrich, R.W., Chandy, K.G., et al.,
    International Union of Basic and Clinical Pharmacology
    C. Nomenclature and properties of calcium-activated and
    sodium-activated potassium channels, *Pharmacol. Rev.*
    69, 1–11, 2017.

IONIZATION ENERGY
(IONIZATION POTENTIAL)

The ionization energy is the energy required to remove
a given electron from its atomic orbital[1] resulting in the
formation of a cation (e.g. $Na \rightarrow e^- + Na^+$). The value is
usually expressed in electron volts (eV) (in physics for a
single atom) or kilojoules per mole (in chemistry for a
mole of the substance). Proton irradiation induced gly-
coside bond breakage in nucleosides is correlated with
ionization energy.[2] Work to correlate ionization energy
with antioxidant potential have instead shown that the
antioxidant activity is more closely associated with direct
transfer of a hydrogen atom.[3,4] A correlation between ionization energy and protein affinity has been suggested
for oxygen-containing molecules.[5] Later work has shown
that correlation between proton affinity and ionization
energy is restricted to similar compounds.[6] The ionization energy for nitric oxide has been reported.[7]

1. Ahrens, L.H., The use of ionization potentials. Part I
   The ionic radii of the elements, *Geochim. Cosmochim.*
   3, 155–169, 1952.
2. Pouilly, J.-C., Miles, J., De Canilis, S., Cassimi, A., and
   Greenwood, J.B., Protein irradiation of DNA nucleosides
   in the gas phase, *Phys. Chem. Chem. Phys.* 17, 7172–
   7180, 2012.
3. Fouegue, A.D.T., Ghogmu, J.N., Mama, D.B., Nkunli,
   N.K., and Younang, E., Structural and antioxidant
   properties of compounds obtained from Fe^{2+} chelation
   by juglone and two of its derivatives: DFT, QTAIM,
   and NBO studies, *Bioorg. Chem. Appl.* 2016, 8636409,
   2016.
4. Mendes, R.A., Almeida, S.K.C., Soares, J.N., et al.,
   A computational investigation on the antioxidant potential of myrcetin 3,4'-di-*O*-α-*L*-rhamnopyranoside, *J.
   Mol. Model.* 24, 133, 2018.

5. Benoit, F.M., and Harrison, A.G., Predictive value of proton affinity. Ionization energy correlations involving oxygenated molecules, *J. Am. Chem. Soc.* 99, 3980–3894, 1977.
6. Maksić, Z.B., Kovačević, B., and Vianello, R., Advances in determining the absolute proton affinities of neutral organic molecules in the gas phase and their interpretation: A theoretical account, *Chem. Rev.* 112, 5240–5270, 2012.
7. Reiser, G., Habenicht, W., Müller-Dethlefs, K., and Schlag, E.W., The ionization energy of nitric oxide, *Chem. Phys. Lett.* 152, 119–123, 1988.

IONOPHORE

An ionophore is a chemical compound that can bind a specific metal ion or forms an ion channel for transport across a biological/lipid membrane.[1] The term ionophore came from early work on antibiotic-mediated ion transport.[2,3] An early example was valinomycin which specifically binds potassium ions form a hydrophobic complex which is transported across a lipid membrane.[4] Another antibiotic, gramicidin A, functions as an ionophore by forming an ion channel.[5] Characterization of ionophores led to the development of ion-specific electrodes.[6,7] Valinomycin absorbed onto a porous membrane was the basis for a potassium-specific electrode which was used for measuring potassium efflux from human red blood cells.[8] A24187 is an antibiotic obtained from *Streptomyces chartreusensis* which has been very useful in cell biology.[9] A23187 can "activate" neutrophils in a manner similar to natural activators such as C5a.[10]

1. Dobler, M., *Ionophores and Their Structures*, John Wiley & Sons, New York, 1981.
2. Pressman, B.C., Harris, E.J., Jagger, W.S., and Johnson, J.H., Antibiotic-mediated transport of alkali ions across lipid barriers, *Proc. Natl. Acad. Sci. USA* 58, 1949–1955, 1967.
3. Pressman, B.C., The discovery of ionophores: An historical perspective, in *Metal Ions in Biological Systems*, Vol. 19, ed. H. Sigel, Chapter 1, pp. 1–18, Marcel Dekker, New York, 1985.
4. Franklin, T.J., and Snow, C.P., *Biochemistry of Antimicrobial Action,* 4th edn., pp. 65–67, Chapman & Hall, London, UK, 1989.
5. *Gramicidin and Related Ion Channel-Forming Peptides*, ed. D.J. Chadwick and C. Cardew, John Wiley & Sons, Chichester, UK, 1999.
6. Thomas, A.P., Viviani-Nauer, A., Arvantis, S., Morf, W.E., and Simon, W., Mechanism of neutral carrier mediated ion transport though ion-selective bulk membranes, *Anal. Chem.* 49, 1567–1576, 1977.
7. Arnold, M.A., and Meyerhoff, M.E., Ion-selective electrodes, *Anal. Chem.* 58, 20R–48R, 1984.

8. Morel, F.M., A study of passive potassium efflux from human red blood cells using ion-specific electrodes, *J. Membrane Biol.* 12, 69–88, 1973.
9. Reed, P.W., and Lardy, H.A., A23187: A divalent cation ionophore, *J. Biol. Chem.* 247, 6970–6977, 1972.
10. McDonald, P.P., McColl, S.R., Naccache, P.H., and Borgeat, P., Studies on the activation of neutrophil 5-lipoxygenase induced by natural agonists and Ca^{2+} ionophore A23187, *Biochem. J.* 280, 379–385, 1991.

IQ MOTIF

The IQ motif is a linear sequence of amino acids in proteins that were shown to bind protein in the cytoskeleton. The IQ motif was identified in an "unconventional" myosin which was suggested to bind myosin light chain and calmodulin.[1] Six tandem motifs of approximate 23 amino acids with a consensus sequence of IQXXXRGXXXR were identified as the IQ motifs. Subsequent work identified a cDNA sequence (*IQGAP*) which encoded as IQGAP protein of 1651 proteins.[2] The term IQGAP is derived from IQ motif and GAP (GTPase-activating protein). IQGAP proteins, which contain multiple domains, have been shown to have a variety of functions as a scaffold proteins[3] which link signaling cascades.[4–6] It has been suggested that proteins containing the IQ motif might have antimicrobial activity.[7]

1. Cheney, R.E., and Mooseker, M.S., Unconventional myosins, *Curr. Opin. Cell Biol.* 4, 27–35, 1992.
2. Weissbach, L., Settlemani, J., Kalady, M.F., et al., Identification of a human RasGAP-related protein containing calmodulin-binding motif, *J. Biol. Chem.* 269, 20517–20521, 1994.
3. Hedman, A.C., Smith, J.M., and Sacks, D.B., The biology of IQGAP proteins: Beyond the cytoskeleton, *EMBO Rep.* 16, 427–446, 2015.
4. Brown, M.D., and Sacks, D.B., IQGAP1 in cellular signaling: Bridging the GAP, *Trends Cell Biol.* 16, 242–249, 2006.
5. Brown, M.D., and Sacks, D.B., Protein scaffolds in MAP kinase signalling, *Cell. Signal.* 21, 462–469, 2009.
6. Choi, S., and Anderson, R.A., IQGAP1 is a phosphoinositide effector and kinase scaffold, *Adv. Biol. Regul.* 60, 29–35, 2016.
7. McLean, D.T.F., Lundy, F.T., and Timson, D.J., IQ-motif peptides as novel anti-microbial agents, *Biochimie* 95, 875–880, 2013.

ISOBAR

An isobar can be defined as an atomic species of approximately the same mass number but different chemical properties.[1,2] Isobaric compounds (isobars) are used for quantitation in mass spectrometry.[3–5] An isobar is also a line drawn on a map connecting points where barometric pressure is equal.[6]

1. Sharp, D.W.A., *Penguin Dictionary of Chemistry*, 2nd edn., Penguin Books, London, UK, 1990.
2. Dickel, T., Plaß, W.R., Lippert, W., et al., Isobar separation in a multiple-reflection time-of-flight mass spectrometer by mass-selective re-trapping, *J. Am. Soc. Mass Spectrom.* 28, 1079–1090, 2017.
3. Thompson, A., Schäfer, J., Kuhn, K., et al., Tandem mass tags: A novel quantification strategy for comparative analysis of complex protein mixtures by MS/MS, *Anal. Chem.* 75, 1895–1904, 2003.
4. Chong, P.K., Gan, C.S., Pham, T.K., and Wright, P.C., Isobaric tags for relative and absolute quantitation (iTRAQ) reproducibility: Implications of multiple injections, *J. Proteome Res.* 5, 1232–1240, 2006.
5. Rauniyar, N., and Yates, J.R., III, Isobaric labeling-based relative quantification in shotgun proteomics, *J. Proteome Res.* 13, 5293–5309, 2014.
6. *Oxford English Dictionary*, Oxford University Press, Oxford, UK, 2019.

ISOBARIC

A process or reaction can be considered isobaric if performed under constant pressure.[1] The measurement of isobaric heat capacity of fluids is an important metric.[2] The term isobaric is also used to refer to spinal anesthesia.[3] An isobaric anesthetic has the same specific gravity as cerebrospinal fluid (CSF) while a hyperbaric anesthetic has a higher specific gravity that CSF, a hypobaric anesthetic has a lower specific gravity than CSF. Isobaric is also used to the use of an isobar in mass spectrometry.[4]

1. Yoshidome, T., and Kinoshita, M., Hydrophobicity at low temperatures and cold denaturation of a protein, *Phys. Rev. E* 79, 939895(R), 2009.
2. Troncoso, J., The isobaric heat capacity of liquid water at low temperatures and high pressures, *J. Chem. Phys.* 147, 094501, 2017.
3. van Egmond, J.C., Verburg, H., Derks, E.A., et al., Optimal dose of intrathecal isobaric bupivacaine in total knee arthroplasty, *Can. J. Anaesth.* 65, 1004–1011, 2018.
4. Bai, B., Tan, H., Pagala, V.R., et al., Deep profiling of proteome and phosphoproteome by isobaric labeling, extensive liquid chromatography, and mass spectrometry, *Methods Enzymol.* 585, 377–395, 2017.

ISOCRATIC

Isocratic is a term used in chromatography to describe a stepwise elution process as opposed to a gradient elution.[1–6]

1. Wang, N.W., Ion exchange in purification, *Bioprocess Technol.* 9, 359–400, 1990.
2. Frey, D.D., Feedback regulation in preparative elution chromatography, *Biotechnol. Prog.* 7, 213–224, 1991.
3. Coffman, J.L., Roper, D.K., and Lightfoot, E.N., High-resolution chromatography of proteins in short columns and adsorptive membranes, *Bioseparation* 4, 183–200, 1994.
4. Marsh, A., Clark, B.J., and Altria, K.D., A review of the background, operating parameters and applications of microemulsion liquid chromatography, *J. Sep. Sci.* 28, 2023–2032, 2005.
5. Peris-García, E., Ortiz-Bolsico, C., Baeze-Baeza, J.J., and García-Alvarez-Coque, M.C., Isocratic and gradient elution in micellar liquid chromatography with Brij-35, *J. Sep. Sci.* 38, 2059–2067, 2015.
6. Zhang, M.T., Ye, X.X., Lan, W., et al., Strategic combination of isocratic and gradient elution for simultaneous separation of polar compounds in traditional Chinese medicines by HPLC, *J. Anal. Methods Chem.* 2018, 7569283, 2018.

ISOELECTRIC FOCUSING (IEF)

Isoelectric focusing is an electrophoretic method for separating amphoteric molecules, usually proteins, in a pH gradient which used ampholytes to establish a pH gradient. Early work used carrier ampholytes to establish a pH gradient stabilized in a polyacrylamide gel.[1–6] More recent work has used immobilized pH gradients (IPG) to address the technical problems with pH gradients established with ampholytes in solutions.[7] Immobilized pH gradients are prepared by mixing covalently bound ampholytes by gradient mixing to prepare the gel. Current matrices for immobilized pH gradient isoelectric focusing are obtained from commercial sources. While the use of this technology decreasing, it continues to be a useful technology as an orthogonal method in the electrophoretic analysis of proteins.[8–12]

1. Righetti, P.G., and Drysdale, J.W., Isoelectric focusing in polyacrylamide gels, *Biochim. Biophys. Acta* 236, 17–28, 1971.
2. Haglund, H., Isoelectric focusing in pH gradients—A technique for fractionation and characterization of ampholytes, *Methods Biochem. Anal.* 19, 1–104, 1971.
3. Righetti, P.G., and Drysdale, J.W., Small-scale fractionation of proteins and nucleic acids by isoelectric focusing in polyacrylamide gels, *Ann. N. Y. Acad. Sci.* 209, 163–186, 1973.
4. Righetti, P.G., Molarity and ionic strength of focused carrier ampholytes in isoelectric focusing, *J. Chromatog.* 190, 275–282, 1980.
5. Righetti, P.G., Tudor, G., and Gianazza, E., Effect of 2-mercaptoethanol on pH gradients in isoelectric focusing, *J. Biochem. Biophys. Methods* 6, 219–227, 1982.

6. Righetti, P.G., Isoelectric focusing theory, methodology and application, Volume 11, in *Laboratory Techniques in Biochemistry and Molecular Biology*, Elsevier, Amsterdam, the Netherlands, 1983.

7. Righetti, P.G., *Immobilized pH gradients: Theory and Methodology*, Elsevier, Amsterdam, the Netherlands, 1990.

8. Görg, A., Obermaler, C., Boguth, G., and Weiss, W., Recent developments in two-dimensional gel electrophoresis with immobilized pH gradients: Wide pH gradients up to pH 12, longer separation distances and simplified procedures, *Electrophoresis* 20, 712–717, 1999.

9. Wildgruber, R., Harder, A., Obermaier, C., et al., Towards higher resolution: Two-dimensional electrophoresis of *Saccharomyces cerevisiae* proteins using overlapping narrow immobilized pH gradients, *Electrophoresis* 21, 2610–2616, 2000.

10. Towbin, H., Blotting from immobilized pH gradient gels: Application to total cell lysates, *Methods Mol. Biol.* 1238, 321–326, 2015.

11. Dada, O.O., Jaya, N., Valliere-Douglas, J., and Salas-Solano, O., Characterization of acidic and basic variants of IgG1 therapeutic monoclonal antibodies based on non-denaturing IEF fractionation, *Electrophoresis* 26, 2695–2702, 2015.

12. Grochalová, M., Konečná, H., Stejskal, K., et al., Deep coverage of the beer proteome, *J. Proteomics* 162, 119–124, 2017.

4. Canaves, J.M., Page, R., Wilson, I.A., and Stevens, R.C., Protein biophysical properties that correlate with crystallization success in *Thermotoga maritime*: Maximum clustering strategy for structural genomics, *J. Mol. Biol.* 344, 977–991, 2004.

5. Kirkwood, J., Hargreaves, D., O'Keefe, S., and Wilson, J., Using isoelectric point to determine the pH for initial protein crystallization trials, *Bioinformatics* 31, 1444–1451, 2015.

6. Audain, E., Ramos, Y., Hermijakob, H., Flower, D.R., and Perez-Riverol, Y., Accurate estimation of isoelectric point of protein and peptide based on amino acid sequences, *Bioinformatics* 32, 821–827, 2016.

7. Kozlowski, L.P., IPC-Isoelectric point calculator, *Biol. Direct* 11(5), 55, 2016.

8. Lin, F.-Y., Chen, C.-S., Chen, W.-Y., and Yamamoto, S., Microcalorimetric studies of the interaction mechanisms between proteins and Q-Sepharose at pH near the isoelectric point (pI) effects of NaCl concentration, pH value, and temperature, *J. Chromatog. A* 912, 281–289, 2001.

9. Kittelmann, J., Lang, K.M.H., Ottens, M., and Hubbuch, J., Orientation of monoclonal antibodies in ion-exchange chromatography: A predictive quantitative structure-activity relationship modeling approach, *J. Chromatog. A.* 1510, 33–39, 2017.

10. Fenton, J.W., 2nd, Olson, T.A., Zabinski, M.P., and Wilner, G.D., Anion-binding exosite of human α-thrombin and fibrin(ogen) recognition, *Biochemistry* 27, 7106–7112, 1988.

ISOELECTRIC POINT (I_p)

The isoelectric point is the pH at which an amphoteric molecule such as a protein has a net charge of zero. This pH is frequently associated with a decrease in solubility of proteins and has been used for purification.[1] The isoelectric point of a protein can present a challenge for therapeutic proteins.[2] Knowledge of the isoelectric point has been shown to be a useful tool in crystallization of proteins.[3–5] Methods have been reported for the calculation of the isoelectric point of protein.[6,7] However, it is possible for a protein at the isoelectric point to have localized areas or patches of positivity or negativity[8,9] which can be described a exosites.[10]

1. Naqvi, M.A., Singh, J., Han, E., Farshad, K., and Rousseau, D., Purification and identification of β-casein phosphopeptide (1–25), *J. Dairy Sci.* 99, 7803–7808, 2016.

2. Luo, S., and Zhang, B., Dextrose-mediated aggregation of therapeutic monoclonal antibodies in human plasma: Implications of isoelectric precipitation of complement proteins, *MAbs* 7, 1094–1103, 2015.

3. Kantaardjieff, K.A., and Rupp, B., Protein isoelectric point as a predictor for increased crystallization screening efficiency, *Bioinformatics* 20, 2162–2168, 2004.

ISOPEPTIDE BOND

An isopeptide bond is an amide bond between a carboxyl group of one amino acid and an amino group of another amino acid, where either the carboxyl or amino groups or both are not α in position. An example is provided by the peptide bond formed between glutamine and lysine in a transamidation reaction.[1] Isopeptide bonds between alkyl amino groups such as the ε-amino groups of lysine and either carboxyl groups (amidation) or amides (transamidation) have been shown to be useful in the preparation of conjugates.[2] The formation of an isopeptide between asparagine and lysine by a transamidation mechanism has been reported[3]—as has the formation of an isopeptide between lysine and aspartic acid by an amidation mechanism.[4] An isopeptide bond can be derived from asparagine and the proximate amino group in peptides or proteins as result of the deamidation.[5,6] The reaction of asparagine to form an isoaspartyl derivative is influenced by adjacent amino acid sequence[7] and is importance in the processing of therapeutic proteins.[8,9] Isopeptide bond formation is also observed in the conjugation between ubiquitin and ubiquitin-like modifiers and substrate proteins.[10–12] An analogous process referred to as pupylation occurs in a prokaryotic system.[13] While not an isopeptide bond in analogy with the above, the reaction of homoserine lactone arising from CNBr cleavage of proteins with amines can yield a similar product.[14] Glutathione[15] contains an isopeptide bond; γ-glutamyl transpeptidase is important in regulation of cysteine concentration.[16]

1. Chen, J.S., and Mehta, K., Tissue transglutaminase: An enzyme with a split personality, *Int. J. Biochem. Cell Biol.* 31, 817–836, 1999.
2. Brune, K.D., Buldun, C.M., Li, Y., et al., Dual plug-and-display synthetic assemble using orthogonal reactive proteins for twin antigen immunization, *Bioconj. Chem.* 28, 1544–1551, 2017.
3. Hu, X., Hu, H., Melvin, J.A., et al., Autocatalytic intramolecular isopeptide bond formation in gram-positive bacterial Pili: A QM/MM simulation, *J. Am. Chem. Soc.* 133, 478–485, 2011.
4. Hagan, R.M., Björnsson, R., McMahon, S.A., et al., NMR spectroscopic and theoretical analysis of a spontaneously formed Lys-Asp isopeptide bond, *Angewandte Chem. Int. Ed. Engl.* 49, 8421–8425, 2010.
5. Geiger, T., and Clarke, S., Deamidation, isomerization, and racemization at asparaginyl and aspartyl residues in peptides, *J. Biol. Chem.* 262, 785–794, 1987.
6. Di Donato, A., Ciardiello, M.A., de Nigris, M., Piccoli, R., Mazzarella, L., and D'Alessio, G., Selective deamidation of ribonuclease A. Isolation and characterization of the resulting isoaspartyl and aspartyl derivatives, *J. Biol. Chem.* 268, 4745–4751, 1993.
7. Brennan, T.V., and Clarke, T., Effect of adjacent histidine and cysteine residues on the spontaneous degradation of asparaginyl- and aspartyl-containing peptides, *Int. J. Peptide Protein Res.* 45, 547–555, 1995.
8. Connolly, B.D., Tran, B., Moore, J.M.R., Sharma, V.K., and Kosky, A., Specific catalysis of asparaginyl deamidation by carboxylic acids: Kinetic, thermodynamic, and quantitative structure-property relationship analyses, *Molec. Pharmaceutics* 11, 1345–1354, 2014.
9. Phillips, J.J., Buchanan, A., Andrews, J., et al., Rate of asparagine deamidation in a monoclonal antibody correlating with hydrogen exchange rate at adjacent downstream residues, *Anal. Chem.* 89, 2361–2368, 2017.
10. Pickart, C.M., Mechanisms underlying ubiquitination, *Annu. Rev. Biochem.* 70, 502–533, 2001.
11. Eletr, Z.M., and Wilkinson, K.D., Regulation of proteolysis by human deubiquitinating enzymes, *Biochim. Biophys. Acta* 1843, 114–128, 2014.
12. Yang, R., and Liu, C.F., Chemical methods for protein ubiquitination, *Top. Curr. Chem.* 362, 89–106, 2015.
13. Bonten, M., Vahlensieck, C., Lipp, C., et al., Depupylase Dop requires inorganic phosphate in the active site for catalysis, *J. Biol. Chem.* 292, 4044–4053, 2017.
14. Fricke, T., Mart, R.J., Watkins, C.L., et al., Chemical synthesis of cell-permeable apoptotic peptides from *in Vivo* produced proteins, *Bioconjug. Chem.* 22, 1763–1767, 2011.
15. *Glutathione Chemical Biochemical and Medical Aspects*, ed. D. Dolphin, R. Pouson and O. Avramović, John Wiley & Sons, New York, 1989.
16. Hanigan, M.H., Gamma-glutamyl transpeptidase: Redox regulation and drug resistance, *Adv. Cancer Res.* 122, 103–141, 2014.

ISOSTERES

The term isostere was introduced by Langmuir in 1919 to describe "comolecules" which contained the same number and arrangement of electrons. Carbon dioxide and nitrous oxide were advanced as examples of isosteres.[1] In what Langmuir described as the equivalent of today's "Dummies" series,[2] he extended the concept to include "similarly formed molecules." There is far more interest in bioisosteres which can be defined as compounds which have structural and chemical similarities and similar or antagonistic biological properties.[3] The term isostere appears to be used in broader context with considerable overlap with bioisostere where the latter seems more applicable to function than structure.[4]

1. Langmuir, I., Isomorphism, isosterism and covalence, *J. Am. Chem. Soc.* 41, 1543–1539, 1919.
2. Langmuir, I., The structure of atoms and the octet theory of valence, *Proc. Natl. Acad. Sci. USA* 5, 253–259, 1919.
3. Thornber, C.W., Isosterism and molecular modification in drug design, *Chem. Soc. Rev.* 39, 563–590, 1979.
4. Zhang, Y., Jumppanen, M., Maksimainen, M.M., et al., Adenosine analogs bearing phosphate isosteres as human MDO1 ligands, *Bioorg. Med. Chem.* 26, 1588–1597, 2018.

ISOTACHOPHORESIS

Isotachophoresis is an electrophoretic method for separating a broad range of analytes ranging from metal ions to proteins.[1,2] Isotachophoresis was originally described as displacement electrophoresis.[3] The current status of isotachophoresis date to the early 1970s with the work of Everaerts and coworkers.[4] The separation is based on the differing mobilities of the analytes in an electric field. The experimental variables can be complex but there is the advantage that an analyte is increased in concentration during analysis.[5] The ability to concentrate the analyte using isotachophoresis has been shown to be useful in immunoassays.[6–8]

1. Cui, H., and Ivory, C.F., Isotachophoresis, http://www.aesociety.org/areas/isotachophoresis.php.
2. Kosobucki, P., and Buszewski, B., Isotachophoresis, in *Electromigration Techniques,* Chapter 3, pp. 93–117, Springer Verlag, Heidelberg, Germany, 2013.

3. Martin, A.J.P., and Everaerts, F.M., Displacment electro-phoresis, *Anal. Chim. Acta* 38, 233–237, 1967.
4. Everaerts, F.M., Beckers, J.L., and Verheggen, Th. P.E.M., Some theoretical and practical aspects of iso-tachophoretical analysis, *Ann. N. Y. Acad. Sci.* 209, 412–444, 1973.
5. Bottenus, D., Jubery, T.Z., Dutta, P., and Ivory, C.F., 10,000-fold concentration in proteins in a cascade micro-chip using anionic ITP by a 3-D numerical simulation with experimental results, *Electrophoresis* 32, 550–562, 2011.
6. Khnouf, R., Goet, G., Baier, T., and Hardt, S., Increasing the sensitivity of microfluidics based immunoassays using isotachophoresis, *Analyst* 139, 4564–4571, 2014.
7. Moghadam, B.Y., Connelly, K.T., and Posner, J.D., Two orders of magnitude improvement in detection limit of lateral flow assays using isotachophoresis, *Anal. Chem.* 87, 1009–1017, 2015.
8. Paratore, F., Zeidman-Kalman, T., Rosenfeld, T., Kaigala, G.V., and Bercovici, M., Isotachophoresis-based surface immunoassay, *Anal. Chem.* 89, 7373–7378, 2017.

ISOTHERM

The term isotherm (based on the Greek word for equal) has diverse definitions which are based on phenomena occurring as the same temperature.[1] The most common example for isotherm is in meteorology where an iso-therm is a line on a map connecting points of identical temperature.[2] In the physical sciences, an isotherm is a plot of a substance bound to a surface as a function of concentration at constant temperature. The temperature is 25°C under standard conditions. The concept was devel-oped by Langmuir in 1981 for the adsorption of a gas to solid surfaces[3] and is referred to as the Langmuir iso-therm in application to chromatography.[4,5] The Langmuir isotherm is an empirical isotherm based on a postulated kinetic mechanism describing an equilibrium process for the process of adsorption based on several assumptions; assumptions include absolute uniformity of the absorbent service, all adsorption occurs by the same mechanism, and adsorbate molecules adsorb in a uniform monolayer on the absorbent. An isotherm can be developed for the interaction of a gas with a surface, a solute in a liquid with a surface or a solid solute adsorption.[6] A distribu-tion or partition coefficient can be developed from the isotherm which may be linear, concave, or convex.[7] Frontal chromatography can be used for the determina-tion of equilibrium isotherms,[8] although there are issues with this technical approach.[9] There are other approaches to the determination of an isotherm for chromatography.[10] The mode of binding of proteins to a matrix has an effect on the isotherm.[11,12]

1. *Oxford English Dictionary*, Oxford University Press, Oxford, UK, 2019.
2. Unger, J., Sümeghy, Z., Gulyás, Á., and Bottyán, Z., Land-use and meteorological aspects of the urgan heat island, *Meteorol. Appl.* 8, 189–194, 2001.
3. Langmuir, I., The adsorption of gases on plane surfaces of glass, mica, and platinum, *J. Am. Chem. Soc.* 40, 1361–1403, 1918.
4. Di Giovanni, O., Mazzotti, M., Morbidell, M., et al., Supercritical fluid simulated moving bed chromatogra-phy II. Langmuir isotherm, *J. Chromatog. A.* 919, 1–12, 2001.
5. Jacoson, J., Frenz, J., and Horváth, C., Measurement of adsorption isotherms by liquid chromatography, *J. Chromatog.* 316, 53–68, 1984.
6. Giles, C.H., and Smith, D., A general treatment and classification of the solute adsorption. I. Theoretical, *J. Colloid Interface Sci.* 47, 755–765, 1974.
7. Caude, M., and Jordy, A., Distribution coefficient, in *Encyclopedia of Chromatography*, ed. J. Cozes, pp. 257–258, Marcel Dekker, New York, 2001.
8. Sajarz, P., Frontal chromatography, in *Encyclopedia of Chromatography*, ed. J. Cozes, pp. 359–361, Marcel Dekker, New York, 2001.
9. Gritti, F., and Guiochon, G., Systematic errors in the measurement of adsorption isotherms by front analysis. Impact of choice of column hold-up volume, range and density of the data points, *J. Chromatog. A* 1097, 98–115, 2005.
10. Creasy, A., Reck, J., Pabst, T., et al., Systematic interpo-lation method predicts antibody monomer-dimer separa-tion by gradient elution chromatography at high protein loads, *Biotechnol. J.* 14, e1800132, 2019.
11. Finette, G.M.S., Mao, Q.-M., and Hearn, M.T.W., Comparative studies on the isothermal characteristics of proteins adsorbed under batch equilibrium conditions to ion-exchange, immobilized metal ion affinity and dye affinity matrices with different ionic strength and tem-perature conditions, *J. Chromatog. A* 761, 71–90, 1997.
12. Latour, R.A., The Langmuir isotherm: A commonly applied but misleading approach for the analysis of pro-tein adsorption behavior, *J. Biomed. Mater. Res. A* 103, 949–958, 2015.

ISOTHERMAL TITRATION CALORIMETRY (ITC)

Isothermal titration calorimetry is a physical method which directly measure the heat of interaction of two or more substances. Changes in temperature are measured as one substance is added another and molar heat (kcal/mol) is determined as function of the amount of mate-rial added. This information is used to calculate changes in enthalpy (ΔH). ITC is used for the study of the inter-actions of macromolecules such as that of proteins with small molecules,[1,2] protein-protein interactions,[3–5] and membrane proteins.[6–8] ITC has also been useful for the study of the interaction of proteins with surfaces such as chromatography matrices.[9]

1. Ciulli, A., and Abell, C., Biophysical tools to monitor enzyme-ligand interactions of enzymes involved in vitamin biosynthesis, *Biochem. Soc. Trans.* 33(4), 767–771, 2005.
2. Holdgate, G.A., and Ward, W.H.J., Measurements of binding thermodynamics in drug discovery, *Drug Discov. Today* 10, 1543–1550, 2005.
3. Velazquez-Campoy, A., Leavitt, S.A., and Freire, E., Characterization of protein-protein interactions by isothermal titration calorimetry, *Methods Mol. Biol.* 1276, 183–204, 2014.
4. Wang, F., Wang, X., Zhang, M., Huang, A., and Ma, L., Conformational change of lysozyme on the interaction with gene carrier, polyethyleneimine, *Int. J. Biol. Macromol.* 117, 532–537, 2018.
5. Dalton, S.R., Vienneau, A.R., Burstein, S.R., et al., Cyanylated cysteine reports sites-specific changes at protein-protein-binding interfaces without perturbation, *Biochemistry* 57, 3702–3712, 2018.
6. Rudolph, M.G., Luz, J.G., and Wilson, I.A., Structural and thermodynamic correlates of T cell signaling, *Ann. Rev. Biophys. Biomol. Struct.* 31, 121–149, 2002.
7. Draczkowski, P., Matosiuk, D., and Jozwiak, K., Isothermal titration calorimetry in membrane protein research, *J. Pharm. Biomed. Anal.* 87, 313–325, 2014.
8. Rajarathnam, K., and Rösgen, J., Isothermal titration calorimetry of membrane proteins—progress and challenges, *Biochim. Biophys. Acta* 1838, 69–77, 2014.
9. Rodler, A., Beyer, B., Ueberbacher, R., Hahn, R., and Jungbauer, A., Hydrophobic interaction chromatography of proteins: Studies of protein unfolding upon adsorption by isothermal calorimetry, *J. Sep. Sci.* 41, 3069–3080, 2018.

ISOTROPY

Isotropy defines a situation when a specific physical measurement of an item such as a crystal is identical when measured in different principal directions.[1] The concept is extended to function[2–4] and is applied in radiology.[5] The antonym, anisotropy, is of more significance in the study of crystals,[6] in fluorescence studies of macromolecules,[7] and the assembly of supramolecular structures.[8] See **anisotropy**.

1. Awad, W., Svensson Birkedal, G., Tunnissen, M.M., Mani, K., and Logan, D.T., Improvements in the order, isotropy and electron density of glypican-1 crystals by controlled dehydration, *Acta Crystallogr. D Biol. Crystallogr.* 69, 2524–2533, 2013.
2. Henderson, J.A., and Robinson, P.A., Using geometry to uncover relationships between isotropy, homogeneity, and modularity in cortical connectivity, *Brain Connect.* 3, 423–437, 2013.

3. Sassi, M., Ali, O., Boudon, F., et al., An auxin-mediated shift toward growth isotropy promotes organ formation at the shoot meristem in *Arabidopsis*, *Curr. Biol.* 24, 2335–2342, 2014.
4. Armezzani, A., Abad, U., Ali, O., et al., Transcriptional induction of cell wall remodeling genes in coupled to microtubule-driven growth isotropy at the shoot apex in *Arabidoposis*, *Development* 4, 145, 2018.
5. Hayes, J.W., Gomez-Cardona, D., Zhang, R., et al., Low-dose cone-beam CT via raw counts domain low-signal correction: Performance assessment and task-based parameter optimization (Part I: Assessment of spatial resolution and noise performance), *Med. Phys.* 45, 1942–1956, 2018.
6. Hadjittofis, E., Isbell, M.A., Karde, V., et al., Influences of crystal anisotropy in pharmaceutical process development, *Pharm. Res.* 35, 100, 2018.
7. Huang, H., Wei, H., Zou, M., et al., Modulating fluorescence anisotropy of terminally labeled double-stranded DNA via the interaction between dye and nucleotides for rational design of DNA recognition based applications, *Anal. Chem.* 87, 2748–2754, 2015.
8. Bianchi, E., Capone, B., Coluzza, I., Rovigatti, L., and van Oostrum, P.D.J., Limiting the valence: Advancements and new perspectives on patchy colloids, soft functionalized nanoparticles and biomolecules, *Phys. Chem. Chem. Phys.* 19, 19847–19858, 2017.

ISOTYPE

Iso (Gr. equal). The term isotype usually refers to an immunoglobulin group as defined by the chemical and antigenic characteristics of the constant region.[1] The primary immunoglobulin isotypes are IgA, IgD, IgG, IgM, and IgE. IgG isotype can be further divided into subclasses, IgG1, IgG2, IgG3, and Ig4.[2] In a broader sense, an isotype is a biological specimen that is a duplicate of a holotype. In biochemistry, the concept of isotype extends to other proteins such as tubulin[3,4] where isotypes (α-tubulin, β-tubulin) are important for function. A library search revealed that isotope is also an acronym (International System of Typographical Picture Education).[5]

1. Brezski, R.J., and Georgiou, G., Immunoglobulin isotype knowledge and application to Fc engineering, *Curr. Opin. Immunol.* 40, 62–69, 2016.
2. Irani, V., Guy, A.J., Andrew, D., et al., Molecular properties of human IgG subclasses and their implications for designing therapeutic monoclonal antibodies against infectious diseases, *Mol. Immunol.* 67, 171–182, 2015.
3. Minoura, I., Towards an understanding of the isotype-specific functions of tubulin in neurons: Technical advances in tubulin expression and purification, *Neurosci. Res.* 122, 1–8, 2017.

4. Gadadhar, S., Bodakuntla, S., Natarajan, K., and Janke, C., The tubulin code at a glance, *J. Cell Sci.* 130, 1347–1353, 2017.
5. Neurath, M., and Kimross, R., *The Transformer: Principles of Making Isotype Charts*, Hyphen, London, UK, 2009.

ISOTYPE SWITCHING

Isotype switching is the process by which antibody class expression changes as in the rearrangement of genes in B cells resulting from the exposure of the B cell to its antigen.[1,2] Isotype switching is also referred to as antibody class switching.[3–12] This is a process separate from that of somatic hypermutation, which involves the variable regions of the immunoglobulins and is responsible for antibody functional diversity.[13,14]

1. Maity, P.C., Datta, M., Nicolò, A., and Jamaa, H., Isotype specific assembly of B cell antigen receptors and synergism with chemokine receptor CXCR4, *Front. Immunol.* 9, 2988, 2018.
2. Ten Hacken, E., Gounari, M., Ghia, P., and Burger, J.A., The importance of B cell receptor isotypes and stereotypes in chronic lymphocytic leukemia, *Leukemia* 33, 287–298, 2019.
3. Rothman, P., Li, S.C., and Alt, F.W., The molecular events in heavy chain class-switching, *Semin. Immunol.* 1, 65–77, 1989.
4. Vercelli, D., and Geha, R.S., Regulation of isotype switching, *Curr. Opin. Immunol.* 4, 794–797, 1992.
5. Rothman, P., Interleukin 4 targeting of immunoglobulin heavy chain class-switch recombination, *Res. Immunol.* 144, 579–583, 1993.
6. Snapper, C., and Mond, J.J., Towards a comprehensive view of immunoglobulin class switching, *Immunol. Today* 14, 15–17, 1993.
7. Fiset, P.O., Cameron, L., and Hamid, Q., Local isotype switching to IgE in airway mucosa, *J. Allergy Clin. Immunol.* 116, 233–236, 2005.
8. Min, I.M., and Selsing, E., Antibody class switch recombination: Roles for switch seqences and mismatch repair proteins, *Adv. Immunol.* 87, 297–328, 2005
9. Salfeld, J.B., Isotype selection in antibody engineering, *Nat. Biotechnol.* 25, 1369–1372, 2007.
10. Jefferis, R., Antibody therapeutics: Isotype and glycoform selection, *Expert Opin. Biol. Ther.* 7, 1401–1413, 2007.
11. Chow, S.K., and Casadevall, A., Monoclonal antibodies and toxins—A perspective on function and isotype, *Toxins* (Basel) 4, 430–454, 2012.
12. Senger, K., Hackney, J., Payandeh, J., and Zarrin, A.A., Antibody isotype switching in vertebrates, *Results Probl. Cell. Differ.* 57, 295–324, 2015.
13. Methot, S.P., and Di Noia, J.M., Molecular mechanism of somatic hypermutation and class switch recombination, *Adv. Immunol.* 133, 37–87, 2017.
14. Zuo, T., Gautam, A., and Wesemann, D.R., Affinity war: Forging immunoglobulins, *Curr. Opin. Immunol.* 57, 32–39, 2019.

JAK (JANUS-ASSOCIATED KINASE)

JAK kinases (Janus-associated kinases) are a family of tyrosine kinases involved in signal transduction through cytokine receptors.[1–3] The term Janus is derived from the Roman god for beginnings, ends, transitions, doors, and pathways frequently depicted with two faces looking in opposite directions. There are four JAK family members, JAK1, JAK2, JAK3, and TYK2. JAK1 and JAK2 are involved in type II interferon (interferon-gamma) signaling, whereas JAK1 and TYK2 are involved type I interferon signaling.[4–6] The term Jaks-Stats refers to the interaction of Janus kinases (Jaks) with signal transducers and activators of transcriptions (STATs).[7]

1. Ihle, J.N., The Janus protein tyrosine kinase family and its role in cytokine signaling, *Adv. Immunol.* 60, 1–35, 1995.
2. Silvennoinen, O., and O'Shea, J.J., The Janus kinases (Jaks), *Genome Biol.* 5, 253(epub), 2004.
3. Clark, J.D., Flanagan, M.E., and Telliez, J.B., Discovery and development of Janus kinase (JAK) inhibitors for inflammatory diseases, *J. Med. Chem.* 57, 5023–5038, 2014.
4. Watanabe, S., Itoh, T., and Arai, K., Roles of JAK kinases in human GM-CSF receptor signal transduction, *J. Allergy Cllin. Immunol.* 98, A183–A191, 1996.
5. Leonard, W.J., Role of JAK kinases and STATs in cytokine signal transduction, *Int. J. Hematol.* 73, 271–277, 2001.
6. Wilks, A.F., The JAK kinases: Not just another kinases drug target, *Semin. Cell. Dev. Biol.* 19, 319–328, 2008.
7. Decker, T., and Müller, M., The continuing fascination with Jaksand Stats: An introduction, in *Jak-Stat Signaling: From Basics and Disease*, ed. T. Decker and M. Müller, pp. 1–4, Springer Verlag, Vienna, Austria, 2012.

JASPAR

JASPAR is a database for transcription factor binding.[1–3]

1. Khan, A., Fornes, O., Stigliani, A., et al., JASPAR 2018: Update of the open-access database of transcription factor binding profiles and its web framework, *Nucleic Acids Res.* 46(DI), D1284, 2018.
2. Garbelini, J.M.C., Kashiwabara, A.Y., and Sanches, D.S., Sequence motif finder using memetic algorithm, *BMC Bioinformatics* 19(1), 4, 2018.
3. Sugiaman-Trapman, D., Vitezic, M., Jouhilahti, E.M., et al., Characterization of the human RFX transcription factor family by regulatory and target gene analysis, *BMC Genomics* 19(1), 181, 2018.

JOHNSTON-OGSTON EFFECT

The Johnson-Ogston effect describes the effect of two or more components on sedimentation behavior in analytical ultracentrifugation.[1] The observation is that in a mixtures of two components with different sedimentation coefficients, there is an apparent increase in the amount of the smaller (less rapidly sedimenting) component with an apparent decrease in the amount of the larger (more rapidly sedimenting). The effect increases with increasing concentration of the analytes and is negligible or absent at low concentration. The effect presumably represents a concentration-dependent frictional interaction between the components. Understanding of the Johnston-Ogston effect is of value in the interpretation of analytical ultracentrifugation.[2–5] While analytical ultracentrifugation is not of high academic interest at the current time, the technique is of great importance in the biopharmaceutical industry.[6]

1. Johnston, J.P., and Ogston, A.G., A boundary anomaly found in the ultracentrifugation sedimentation of mixtures, *Trans. Faraday Soc.* 42, 789–799, 1946.
2. Speakman, P.T., Johnston-Ogston effect in the ultracentrifugation of solutions of denatured collagen, *Biochim. Biophys. Acta* 69, 480–484, 1963.
3. Janado, M., Nichol, L.W., and Dunstone, J.R., The Johnston-Ogston effect in sedimenting proteoglycan mixtures, *J. Biochem.* 71, 257–263, 1972.
4. Correia, J.J., Johnson, M.L., Weiss, G.H., and Yphantis, D.A., Numerical study of the Johnston-Ogston effect in two-component systems, *Biophys. Chem.* 5, 255–264, 1976.
5. Schumaker, V.N., Calcott, M.A., Spiegelberg, H.L., and Müller-Eberhard, H.J., Ultracentrifuge studies of the binding of IgG of different subclasses to the C1q subunit of the first component of complement, *Biochemistry* 15, 5175–5181, 1976.
6. Liu, J., Yadav, S., Andya, J., Demeule, B., and Shirt, S.J., Analytical ultracentrifugation and its role in development and research of therapeutical proteins, *Methods Enzymol.* 562, 441–476, 2015.

KARYOLOGY

Karyology is the study of the nucleus of the cell, specifically the chromosomes.[1,2] Karyology has used in the characterization of master cell banks and working cell banks for recombinant DNA products[3] and in cell therapy.[4]

1. Chiarelli, A.B., and Koen, A.L., *Comparative Karyology of Primates*, Moulton, The Hague, the Netherlands, 1979.
2. Macgregor, H.C., *An Introduction to Animal Cytogenetics*, Chapman & Hall, London, UK, 1993.

3. Petricciani, J.C., and Horaud, F.N., Karyology and tumorigenicity testing requirements: Past, present, and future, *Dev. Biol. Stand.* 93, 5–13, 1998.
4. Thépot, A., Morel, A.P., Justein, V., et al., Evaluation of tumorigenic risk of tissue-engineered oral mucosal epithelial cells by using combinatorial examinations, *Cell Transplant.* 19, 999–1006, 2010.

KATAL

Katal is an international standard (SI; Systems International d'Unites) unit for enzyme activity. A katal (kat) is defined as 1 mol/s. A unit for enzyme activity is defined by the IUBMB as 1 μmoL/min; then one unit of enzyme activity is equal to 16.67×10^{-9} kat or 16.67 nkat. This term is used more in clinical chemistry than basic biomedical investigation.[1–8]

1. Dybkær, R., Problems of quantities and units in enzymology, *Enzyme* 20, 46–64, 1975.
2. Lehmann, H.P., Metrication of clinical laboratory data in SI units, *Am. J. Clin. Pathol.* 65, 2–18, 1976.
3. Lehman, H.P., SI units, *CRC Crit. Rev. Clin. Lab. Sci.* 10, 147–170, 1979.
4. Bowers, G.N., Jr., and McComb, R.B., A unifying reference system for clinical enzymology: Aspartate aminotransferase and the International Clinical Enzyme Scale, *Clin. Chem.* 39, 1128–1136, 1984.
5. Powsner, E.R., SI quantities and units for American Medicine, *JAMA* 252, 1737–1741, 1984.
6. van Assendelft, O.W., The international system of units (SI) in historical perspective, *Am. J. Public Health* 77, 1400–1403, 1987.
7. Dybkær, R., and Storring, P.L., Application of IUPAC-IFCC recommendations on quantities and units to WHO biological reference materials for diagnostic use. International Union of Pure and Applied Chemistry (IUPAC) and International Federation of Clinical Chemistry (IFCC), *Eur. J. Clin. Chem. Clin. Biochem.* 33, 623–625, 1995.
8. Dybkær, R., The tortuous road to the adoption of katal for the expression of catalytic activity by the general conference on weights and measures, *Clin. Chem.* 48, 586–590, 2002.

KERATIN

Keratins are a large family of fibrous proteins which form intermediate filaments[1,2] around trichocytes and epithelial cells. The term keratin is derived from the Greek word for horn as some keratins form hard tissues. There are five types of proteins which form intermediate filaments in various cells: Type I and Type II are keratins. Type I keratins are acidic proteins

(Ip = 4.5–5.5) with a molecular weight of 40–64 kDa) and type II keratins are neutral/acidic proteins (Ip = 6.5–7.5) with a molecular weight of 52–62 kDa). There are further subdivisions of keratin where type Ia and type IIa form "hard" keratins in trichocytes while Ib and IIb form soft keratins in epithelial cells.[3] The hard keratins are characterized by a high content of cysteine.[4,5] As should be clear from the above, it is apparent that there is classification keratins as of "soft" and "hard" keratins, low-sulfur and high-sulfur keratins as well as other designations.[6,7] Type I keratins and type II keratins are classifications where there are 26 type I keratins and 26 type II keratins; type I keratins bind with type II keratins to form intermediate filaments[8] which show tissue-specific and cell-specific expression.[9] The reduction of disulfide bonds in keratin in hair is the basis of the permanent wave treatment in cosmetology.[10]

1. Lazarides, E., Intermediate filaments as mechanical integrators of cellular space, *Nature* 283, 249–256, 1980.
2. Fuchs, E., and Weber, K., Intermediate filaments: Structure, dynamics, function, and disease, *Annu. Rev. Biochem.* 63, 345–382, 1994.
3. Parry, D.A.D., and Smith, T.A., Keratin intermediate filaments: Similarities and differences with other members of the IF family, in *Fibrous Proteins*, ed. T. Scheibel, Chapter 6, pp. 77–91, Landes Bioscience, Austin, TX, 2008.
4. Jones, L.M., Simon, M., Watts, N.R., et al., Intermediate filament structure: Hard α-keratin, *Biophys. Chem.* 68, 82–93, 1997.
5. Parry, D.A.D., and North, A.C.T., Hard α-keratin intermediate filament chains: Substructure of the N- and C-terminal domains and the predicted structure and function of the C-terminal domains of type I and type II chains, *J. Struct. Biol.* 122, 67–75, 1998.
6. Fraser, R.D.B., MacRae, T.P., and Rogers, G.E., *Keratins Their Composition Structure and Biosynthesis*, Charles C. Thomas, Springfield, IL, 1972.
7. Bowden, P.E., Keratins and other epidermal proteins, in *Molecular Aspects of Dermatology*, Chapter 2, pp. 19–54, John Wiley & Sons, Chichester, UK, 1993.
8. Jacob, J.T., Coulombe, P.A., Kwan, R., and Omary, M.B., Type I and II keratin intermediate filaments, *Cold Spring Harb. Perspect. Biol.* 10(4), a018275, 2018.
9. Bowden, P.E., Keratins and other epidermal proteins, in *Molecular Aspects of Dermatology*, Chapter 2, pp. 19–54, John Wiley & Sons, Chichester, UK, 1993.
10. Suzuta, K., Ogawa, S., Takeda, Y., Kaneyama, K., and Arai, K., Intermediate disulfide cross-linked structural change induced by permanent wave treatment of human hair with thioglycolic acid, *J. Costmetic Sci.* 63, 177–196, 2012.

KINOME

The kinome is the sum of the various protein kinases in the genome of an organism.[1–6] Kinomics is the term that describes the study of the kinome in the genome of a given organism.[7–11]

1. Jacoby, E., Tresadern, G., Bembenek, S., et al., Extending kinome coverage by analysis of kinase inhibitor broad profiling data, *Drug Discov. Today* 20, 652–658, 2015.
2. Zulawski, M., and Schulze, W.X., The plant kinome, *Methods Mol. Biol.* 1306, 1–23, 2015.
3. Fleuren, E.D., Zhang, L., Wu, J., and Daly, R.J., The kinome "at large" in Cancer, *Nat. Rev. Cancer* 16, 83–98, 2016.
4. Baharani, A., Trost, B., Kisalik, A., and Napper, S., Technological advances for interrogating the human kinome, *Biochem. Soc. Trans* 45, 65–77, 2017.
5. Radu, M., and Chernoff, J., Recent advances in methods to assess the activity of the kinome, *F1000Res.* 6, 1004, 2017.
6. Wilson, L.J., Linley, A., Hammond, D.E., et al., New perspectives, opportunities, and challenging in exploring the human protein kinome, *Cancer Res.* 78, 15–29, 2018.
7. Vieth, M., Sutherland, J.J., Robertson, D.H., and Campbell, R.M., Kinomics: Characterizing the therapeutically validated kinase space, *Drug Discov. Today* 10, 839–846, 2005.
8. Johnson, S.A., and Hunter, T., Kinomics: Methods for deciphering the kinome, *Nat. Methods* 2, 17–25, 2005.
9. Gomase, V.S., and Tagore, S., Kinomics, *Curr. Drug. Metab.* 9, 255–258, 2008.
10. Kim, D.H., and Sim, T., Chemical kinomics: A powerful strategy for target deconvolution, *BMB Rep.* 43, 711–719, 2010.
11. Kindrachuk, J., Falcinelli, S., Wadda, J., et al., Systems kinomics for characterizing host responses to high-consequence pathogens at the NIH/NIAID integrated research facility—Frederick, *Pathol. Dis.* 71, 190–198, 2014.

KNOCKDOWN

Knockdown is a term used to describe the suppression/inhibition of the transcription of a specific protein by interfering with function of the mRNA encoding the protein in question. A knockdown may be accomplish with an antisense oligonucleotide or by RNA interference.[1] Antisense technology is based on Watson-Crick base pairing of an oligonucleotide to mRNA conceptually based on the interaction of tRNA with mRNA.[2–4] Antisense oligonucleotides act either by blocking the process of transcription[5] or by forming a duplex with the mRNA which is then sensitive to cleavage by RNAse H.[6,7] Small interfering RNA (siRNA) also act by base pairing with mRNA resulting in mRNA degradation.[8–11] Gene knockdown with siRNA dates to early work on

Caenorhabditis elegans.[12–14] The action of siRNA is complex involving the RNA-induced silencing complex (RISC) which involves the initial processing of an RNA duplex by nuclease culminating with guidance of a specific nuclease, argonaute, which cleaves the target mRNA.[15,16]

1. Allison, L.A., *Fundamental Molecular Biology*, pp. 258–264, Blackwell Publishing, Malden, MA, 2007.
2. Goodchild, J., Agrawal, S., Civeira, M.P., et al., Inhibition of human immunodeficiency virus replication by antisense oligodeoxynucleotides, *Proc. Natl. Acad. USA* 85, 5507–5511, 1988.
3. Zamecnik, P., History of antisense oligonucleotides, in *Antisense Therapeutics*, ed. S. Agrawal, Chapter 1, pp. 1–11, Humana Press, Totowa, NJ, 1996.
4. Toulme, J.J., Historical aspects of antisense oligodeoxynucleotides, in *Antisense Oligonucleotides and Antisense RNA: New Pharmacological and Therapeutic Agents*, ed B. Weiss, Chapter 1, pp. 1–16, CRC Press, Boca Raton, FL, 1997.
5. Crooke, S.,T., Basic principles of antisense technology, in *Antisense Drug Development Principles, Strategies, and Applications*, ed. S.T. Crooke, Chapter 1, pp. 1–28, Marcel Dekker, New York, 2001.
6. Zamaratski, E., Pradeepkumar, P.I., and Chattopadhyaya, J., A critical survey of the structure-function of the antisense oligo/RNA heteroduplex as substrate for RNase H, *J. Biochem. Biophys. Methods* 48, 189–208, 2001.
7. Kieplpinski, L.J., Hagedorn, P.H., Lindow, M., and Vinther, J., RNase H sequence preferences influence antisense oligonucleotide efficiency, *Nucleic Acids Res.* 45, 12932–12944, 2017.
8. Shan, G., RNA interference as a gene knockdown technique, *Int. J. Biochem. Cell Biol.* 42, 1243–1251, 2010.
9. Kelly, A., and Hurlstone, A.F., The use of RNAai technologies for gene knockdown in zebrafish, *Brief Funct. Genomics* 10, 189–196, 2011.
10. Lieberman, J., Manipulating the *in vivo* immune response by targeted gene knockdown, *Curr. Opin. Immunol.* 35, 63–72, 2015.
11. Leber, N., Kaps, L., Aslam, M., et al., SiRNA-mediated *in vivo* gene knockdown by acid-degradable cationic nanohydrogel particles, *J. Control. Release* 248, 10–23, 2017.
12. Lee, R.C., Feinbaum, R.L., and Ambros, V., The *C. elegans* heterochronicgene lin-4 encodes small RNAs with antisense complementarity to lin-14, *Cell* 75, 843–854, 1993.
13. Fire, A., Xu, S., Montgomery, M.K., et al., Potent and specific genetic interference by double-stranded RNA in *Caenorhabditis elegans*, *Nature* 391, 806–811, 1998.
14. Lee, R., Feinbaum, R., and Ambrox, V., A short history of a short RNA, *Cell* 116(2 Suppl), S89–S92, 2004.
15. Wilson, R.C., and Doudna, J.A., Molecular mechanisms of RNA interference, *Annu. Rev. Biophys.* 42, 217–239, 2013.
16. Piatek, M.J., and Werner, A., Endogenous siRNAs: Regulators of internal affairs, *Biochem. Soc. Trans.* 42, 1174–1179, 2013.

KNOCKIN

The term knockin is used describe the result of a "gain-of-function" mutation where a gene is added to the genome of an organism resulting the expression of a new protein.[1] A knockin has been used to evaluate the efficacy and toxicity of an monoclonal antibody in a mouse model.[2] Adeno-associated virus (AAV) has been used to deliver CRISPR/Cas 9 for the knock-in of human α-1-antitrypsin resulting in stable expression the protein.[3]

1. Geng, Y., Whoriskey, W., Park, M.Y., et al., Rescue of cyclin D1 deficiency by knockin cyclin E, *Cell* 97, 767–777, 1999.
2. Costa, M.J., Kudaravalli, J., Liu, W.-H., et al., A mouse model for evaluation of efficacy and concomitant toxicity of anti-huma CXCR4 therapeutics, *PLoS One* 13(3), e0194688, 2018.
3. Stephens, C.J., Kashentseva, E., Everett, W., Kaliberova, L., and Curiel, D.L., Targeted in vivo knockin of human alpha-1-antitrypsin cDNA using adenoviral delivery of CRISPR/Cas9, *Gene Therapy* 25, 139–156, 2018.

KNOCKOUT

The term knockout is usually used to describe the process/result of the disruption of the function of a specific gene in a cell or organism. A knockout differs from a knockdown in that a knockout can be inherited while a knockdown is a transient modification. The term knockout is commonly associated with a knockout mouse.[1,2] The process for obtaining a gene knockout is similar to that for a knockin that the original work involved double strand breakage of DNA follow by recombination. In case of knockout, the presence of non-homologous end-joining which is more error-prone than homologous end joining resulting in a defective (mutant) sequence[3] leading a knockout transgenic. A knockout results in the change in the expression of the gene in all tissues with no dependence on time or environment. A conditional knockout[4] is a knockout which can be confined to a specific tissue[5] or can be spatially and time dependent.[6] As with knock-ins, knockouts may also be generated by zinc-finger nuclease[7] or CRISPR/Cas9 or TALEN.[8] It must be empathized that knockout methods are genome editing techniques and results may differ from other loss-of-function approaches such as knockdown.[9]

1. Crawley, J.N., *What's Wrong with My Mouse? Behavioral Phenotyping of Transgenic and Knockout Mice*, Wiley-Interscience, Hoboken, NJ, 2007.

2. *Mouse Genetics; Methods and Protocols*, ed. S.R. Singh and Coppola, Humana Press, New York, 2014.
3. van Gent, D.C., and van der Burg, M., Non-homologous end-joining: A sticky affair, *Oncogene* 26, 7731–7740, 2007.
4. Lewandoski, M., Conditional control of gene expression in the mouse, *Nature Rev. Genetics* 2, 743–755, 2001.
5. Miyasaka, Y., Uno, Y., Yoshimi, K., CLICK: One-step generation of conditional knockout mice, *BMC Genomics* 19, 318, 2018.
6. Lobe, C.G., and Nagy, A., Conditional genome alternation in mice, *BioEssays* 20, 200–208, 1998.
7. Hauschild-Quintern, J., Petersen, B., Cost, G.J., and Niemann, H., Gene knockout and knockin by zinc-finger nucleases: Current status and perspectives, *Cell. Mol. Life Sci.* 70, 2969–2983, 2013.
8. Auer, T.O., and Del Bene, F., CRISPR/Cas9 and TALEN-mediated knock-in approaches in zebrafish, *Methods* 69, 142–150, 2014.
9. Housden, B.E., Muhar, M., Gemberling, M., et al., Loss-of-function genetic tools for animal models: Cross-species and cross-platform differences, *Nat. Rev. Genet.* 18, 24–40, 2017.

KRÜPPEL-LIKE FACTOR

Krüppel-like factors are a family of zinc finger transcription factors.[1,2] The name is derived from the *Drosophila* Krüppel embryonic pattern regulator.[3] There a number of Krüppel-like factors (KLFs) such as KLF4,[4] KLF10,[5] and KLF15.[6]

1. Schuh, R., Aicher, W., Gaul, U., et al., A conserved family of nuclear proteins containing structural elements of the zinc finger protein encoded by Krüppel, a Drosophila segmentation gene, *Cell* 47, 1025–1032, 1986.
2. *The Biology of Krüppel-like factors*, ed. R. Nagai, S.L. Friedman, and M. Kasuga, Springer, Tokyo, Japan, 2009.
3. Gaul, U., Seifert, E., Schuh, R., and Jäckle, H., Analysis of *Krüppel* protein distribution during early Drosophila development reveals posttranslational regulation, *Cell* 50, 639–647, 1987.
4. Ghaleb, A.M., and Yang, V.W., Krüppel-like factor 4 (KLF4): What we currently know, *Gene* 611, 27–37, 2017.
5. Memon, A., and Lee, W.K., KLF10 as a tumor suppressor gene and its TGF-β signaling, *Cancers* 10(6), 161, 2018.
6. Patel, S.K., Ramchand, J., Crocitti, V., and Burrell, L.M., Krüppel-like factor 15 is critical for the development of left ventricular hypertrophy, *Int. J. Mol. Sci.* 19:1303, 2018.

LABILE ZINC

Zinc is an essential mineral for most organisms. It is suggested that zinc is the second most important signaling metal in intra- and inter-cellular communication.[1] Intracellular zinc is either labile or tightly bound to proteins. Labile zinc is defined as either free zinc or loosely bound and free to exchange. Much of the zinc in the cell is tightly bound to protein and has been referred to as the zinc proteome.[2,3] Various methods have been developed for the measurement of intracellular labile zinc.[4,5] The concentration of labile zinc in monocytes is estimated to be 0.17 nM and 0.35 nM in lymphocytes.[6] Lower values for labile zinc have been suggested.[7] Total cellular zinc concentration has been estimated at 200 µM again suggesting that most of the intracellular zinc is tightly bound to proteins.[8] It is of interest that zinc can weakly bind to some gel filtration (size exclusion) matrices.[9–12]

1. Moret, W., Zinc in cellular regulation: The nature and significance of "zinc signals," *Int. J. Mol. Sci.* 18, 2285, 2017.
2. Eide, D.J., Zinc transporters and the cellular trafficking of zinc, *Biochim. Biophys. Acta* 1763, 711–722, 2006.
3. Maret, W., Zinc and the zinc proteome, *Met. Ions Life Sci.* 12, 479–501, 2013.
4. Yan, X., Kim, J.J., Jeong, H.S., et al., Low-affinity zinc sensor showing fluorescence response with minimal artifact, *Inorg. Chem.* 56, 4332–4240, 2017.
5. Chabosseau, P., Woodier, J., Cheung, R., and Rutter, G.A., Sensors for measuring subcellular zinc pools, *Mettalomics* 10, 229–239, 2018.
6. Hasse, H., Hebel, S., Engelhardt, G., and L., Rink, Flow cytometry measurement of labile zinc in peripheral blood mononuclear cells, *Anal. Biochem.* 352, 222–230, 2006.
7. Colvin, R.A., Holmes, W.R., Fontaine, C.P., and Maret, W., Cytosolic zinc buffering and muffling: Their role in intracellular zinc homeostasis, *Metallomics* 2, 306–307, 2010.
8. Krezel, A., and Maret, W., The biological inorganic chemistry of zinc ions, *Arch. Biochem. Biophys.* 611, 3–19, 2016.
9. Dugger, D.L., Stanton, J.H., Irby, B.N., et al., The exchange of twenty metal ions with the weakly acidic silanol group of silica gel, *J. Phys. Chem.* 68, 757–760, 1966.
10. Evans, G.W., Johnson, P.E., Brushmiller, J.G., and Ames, R.W., Detection of labile zinc-binding ligands in biological fluids by modified gel filtration chromatography, *Anal. Chem.* 51, 839–843, 1979.
11. Johnson, P.E., and Evans, G.W., Binding of zinc and copper to some filtration media, *J. Chromatog.* 188, 405–407, 1980.
12. Martn, M.T., Metal-free chromatographic media, *Methods Enzymol.* 188, 15–21, 1988.

LACTOFERRIN

Lactoferrin is an iron binding protein of very high affinity originally found in milk[1–4] and subsequently in other secreted biological fluids such as saliva.[5–7] Lactoferrin is also found specific granules of neutrophils and is released on neutrophil activation.[8–11] Lactoferrin is considered to play an important role in the non-specific defense process by sequestering iron required for bacterial growth.[12,13] There is interest in lactoferrin as diagnostic[14,15] and therapeutic.[16–18]

1. Masson, P.L., and Heremans, J.F., Metal-combining properties of human lactoferrin (red milk protein). I. The involvement of bicarbonate in the reaction, *Eur. J. Biochem.* 6, 579–584, 1968.
2. Johansson, B.G., Isolation of crystalline lactoferrin from human milk, *Acta Chem. Scand.* 23, 683–684, 1969.
3. Giansanti, F., Panella, G., Leboffe, L., and Antonini, G., Lactoferrin from milk: Nutraceutical and pharmacological properties, *Pharmaceuticals* (Basal), 9(4), 61, 2016.
4. Villavicencio, A., Rueda, M.S., Turin, C.G., and Ochoa, T.J., Factors affecting lactoferrin concentration in human milk: How much do we know? *Biochem. Cell Biol.* 95, 12–21, 2017.
5. Goldman, A.S., and Smith, C.W., Host resistance factors in human milk, *J. Pediatr.* 82, 1082–1090, 1973.
6. Dipaolo, C and Mandel, I.D., Lactoferrin concentration in human parotid saliva as measure by an enzyme-linked immunosorbent assay (ELISA), *J. Dent. Res.* 59, 1463–1465, 1980.
7. Reitamo, S., Kottinen, Y.T., and Segerberg-Konttinine, M., Distribution of lactoferrin in human salivary glands, *Histochemistry* 66, 285–291, 1980.
8. Lehrer, R.I., and Ganz, T., Antimicrobial polypeptides of human neutrophils, *Blood* 76, 2169–2181, 1990.
9. Yang, D., de la Rosa, G., and Tewary, P., and Oppenheim, J.J., Alarmins link neutrophils and dendritic cells, *Trends Immunol.* 30, 531–537, 2009.
10. Fernández-Delgado, L., Vega-Rioja, A., Ventura, I., et al., Release of lactoferrin by neutrophils from asthmatic patients, *PLoS One* 10(10), 0141278, 2015.
11. Zhao, X., Ting, S.M., Sun, G., et al., Beneficial role of neutrophils through function of lactoferrin after intracerebral hemorrhage, *Stroke* 49, 1241–1247, 2018.
12. Bullen, J.J., Rogers, H.J., and Griffiths, E., Role of iron in bacterial infection, *Curr. Top. Microbiol. Immunol.* 80, 1–35, 1978.
13. Legrand, D., Elass, E., Pierce, A., and Mazurier, J., Lactoferrin and host defense: An overview of its immuno-modulating and anti-inflammatory properties, *Biometals* 17, 225–229, 2004.
14. Wang, Y., Pei, F., Wang, X., et al., Diagnostic accuracy of fecal lactoferrin for inflammatory bowel disease: A meta-analysis, *Int. J. Clin. Exp. Pathol.* 8, 12319–12332, 2015.
15. Farah, R., Haraty, H., Salame, Z., et al., Salivary biomarkers for the diagnosis and monitoring of neurological diseases, *Biomed. J.* 41, 63–87, 2018.
16. Ammons, M.C., and Copié, V., Lactoferrin: A bioinspired, anti-biofilm therapeutic, *Biofouling* 29, 443–455, 2013.
17. Pammi, M., and Suresh, G., Enteral lactoferrin supplementation for prevention of sepsis and necrotizing enterocolitis in preterm infants, *Cochrane Database Syst. Rev.* 6, CD007137, 2017.
18. Moreno-Expósito, L., Illescas-Montes, R., Melguizo-Rodríguez, L., et al., Multifunctional capacity and therapeutic potential of lactoferrin, *Life Sci.* 195, 61–64, 2018.

LATARCINS

Latarcins are a group of peptides found in the venom of *Lachesana tarabavaevi*.[1,2] The name is derived from the species of spider from which the peptides were isolated. Latarcins are short basic peptides which have antibacterial and cytolytic activity; cytolytic activity could be reduced by fusing a peptide derived from latarcin 1 with nuclear localization sequence.[3] The cell-penetrating activity of latarcins has been used to deliver cargo to the interior of the cell.[4] It is suggested that latarcins are disordered in solution but adopt an α-helical amphipathic conformation on binding to membranes.

1. Kozlov, S.A., Vassilevski, A.A., Feofanov, A.V., et al., Latarcins, antimicrobial and cytolytic peptides from the venom of the spider *Lachesana tarabaevi* (Zodariidae) that exemplify biomolecular diversity, *J. Biol. Chem.* 281, 20983–20992, 2006.
2. Dubovski, P.V., Vassilevski, A.A., Kozlov, S.A., et al., Latarcins: Versatile spider venom peptides, *Cell. Mol. Life Sci.* 72, 4501–4522, 2015.
3. Budagavi, D.P., and Chugh, A., Antibacterial properties of latarcin 1 derived cell-penetrating peptide, *Eur. J. Pharm. Sci.* 115, 43–49, 2015.
4. Pannappan, N., and Chugh, A., Cell-penetrating and cargo-delivery ability of a spider toxin-derived peptide in mammalian cells, *Eur. J. Pharm. Biopharm.* 114, 149–153, 2017.

LECTINS

Lectins are a group of proteins that bind specifically to monosaccharides, disaccharides, and oligosaccharides and are characterized by the ability to agglutinate cells, polymerized oligosaccharides or precipitate polysaccharides and glycoproteins.[1] The agglutination and precipitation reactions are based on the multivalency of the majority of lectins; there are monovalent lectins which will not support agglutination, polymerization, or precipitation.[2–4] Ricin from castor bean was the first lectin identified in 1888 by Hermann Stillmark but there was no substantial interest in these proteins until much later.[5] Lectins are found in a variety of organisms including plants[6,7] and fungi.[8] There a variety of animal lectins characterized by specificity, tissue localization, and function.[9,10] Animal lectins include galactins which bind to β-D-galactoside and are associated with inflammation,[11] C-lectins, so named because they require the presence of calcium ions for binding, include endocytic lectins which are membrane proteins which bind and participate in the endocytosis of certain glycoproteins,[12,13] collectins, which are characterized by the presence of collagenous domain[14] and are pattern recognition molecules,[15] and selectins which mediate the interaction of leukocytes with endothelial cells.[16] Mannose binding lectins which can be classified as collectins initiate the lectin complement activation pathway.[17,18] Mannose-binding lectin (MBL) are also pattern recognition molecule binds to repetitive microbial surface patterns resulting in the activation of the MAST (MBL-associated serine protease) pathway which in turn can activate either the classical pathway or alternate pathway.

1. Sharon, N., and Lis, H., *Lectins*, 2nd edn., Introduction, Chapter 1, pp. 1–4, Kluwer Academic, Dordrecht, the Netherlands, 2003.
2. Thomasson, D.L., and Doyle, R.J., Monovalent concanavalin A, *Biochem. Biophys. Res. Commun.* 67, 1545–1552, 1975.
3. Tanaka, I., Abe, Y., Hamada, T., Yonemitsu, O., and Ishii, S., Monovalent monomer derivative of concanavalin A produced by photochemically induced alkylation, *J. Biochem.* 89, 1643–1646, 1981.
4. Shahzad-ul-Hussan, S., Gustchina, E., Ghirlando, R., Clore, G.M., and Bewley, C.A., Solution structure of the monovalent lectin microvirin in complex with Manα(1–2) Man provides a basis for anti-HIV activity with low toxicity, *J. Biol. Chem.* 286, 20788–20796, 2011.
5. Sharon, N., and Lis, H., *Lectins*, 2nd edn., History, Chapter 2, pp. 5–32, Kluwer Academic, Dordrecht, the Netherlands, 2003.
6. Puztai, A., *Plant Lectins*, Cambridge University Press, Cambridge, UK, 1991.
7. *Plant Glycobiology: A Sweet Role of Lectins, Glycoproteins, Glycolipids, and Glycans*, ed. C.A. Albenne, E.J.M. van Damme, E.I. Janet, and N.I. Lannoo, Fronteirs Media, S.A., Lausanne, Cham, Switzerland, 2015.
8. Varrot, A., Basheer, S.M., and Imberty, A., Fungal lectins: Structure, function and potential applications, *Curr. Opin. Struct. Biol.* 23, 678–685, 2013.
9. *Lectins Biomedical Perspectives*, ed. A. Duszta and S. Bardocz, Taylor & Francis Group, London, UK, 1995.
10. *Animal Lectins* A Functional View, ed. G.R. Vaste and H. Ahmed, CRC Press, Boca Raton, FL, 2007.
11. Sundblad, V. Morosi, L.G., Geffner, J.R., and Rabinovich, G.A., Galactin-1: A jack-of-all-trades in the resolution of acute and chronic inflammation, *J. Immunol.* 199, 3721–3736, 2017.
12. McAbee, D.D., Jiang, X., and Walsh, K.B., Lactoferrin binding to the rat asialoglycoprotein receptor requires the receptor's lectin properties, *Biochem. J.* 348, 113–117, 2000.
13. Johannes, L., Wunder, C., and Shafaq-Zadah, M., Glycolipids and lectins in endocytic uptake processes, *J. Mol. Biol.* 428, 4792–4818, 2016.
14. Howard, M., Farrar, C.A., and Sacks, S.H., Structural and functional diversity of collectins and ficolins and their relationship to disease, *Semin. Immunopathol.* 40, 75–85, 2018.
15. Degn, S.E., and Thiel, S., Humoral pattern recognition and the complement system, *Scand. J. Immunol.* 78, 181–193, 2013.
16. McEver, R.P., Selectins: Initiators of leucocyte adhesion and signalling at the vascular wall, *Cardiovasc. Res.* 107, 331–339, 2015.
17. Speth, C., Prodinger, M., Würzner, R., Stoibert, H., and Dierich, M.P., Complement, in *Fundamental Immunology*, 6th edn., ed. W.E. Paul, Chapter 33, pp. 1047–1078, Lippincott, Williams & Wilkens/Wolters Kluwer, Philadelphia, PA, 2008.
18. Paréj, K., Dobó, J., Závodszkym, P., and Gál, P., The control of the complement lectin pathway activation revisited, *Mol. Immunol.* 54, 415–422, 2013.

LINKAGE GROUP

A linkage group is a group of genes located at different loci on a chromosome but are inherited as a un instead of undergoing independent assortment.[1–3]

1. Haig, D., A brief history of human autosomes, *Philos. Trans. R. Soc. Lond. B Biol. Sci.* 354, 1447–1470, 1999.
2. Wallis, G.P., Cameron-Christie, S.R., Kennedy, H.L., et al., Interspecific hydridization causes long-term phylogenetic discordance between nuclear and mitochondrial genomes in freshwater fishes, *Mol. Ecol.* 26, 3116–3127, 2017.
3. Matsubara, K., Iwasaki, Y., Nishiki, I., Nomura, K., and Fujiwara, A., Identification of genetic linkage group 1-linked sequences in Japanese eel (*Anguilla japonica*) by single chromosome sorting and sequencing, *PLoS One* 13(5), e0197040, 2018.

LIPOFECTION

Lipofection was originally described as cellular membrane translocation of DNA for gene therapy via the use of cationic lipids which form a **liposome** which then fuses with the cell membrane of the target cell.[1] The liposome and its cargo are referred to as a **lipoplex**.[2,3] There is still use of liposome technology for the delivery DNA for gene therapy[4,5] as well as use for the delivery of small RNA species.[6,7] Lipofection is usually compared with electroporation for transfection efficiency.[8–10]

1. Felgner, P.L., Gadek, T.R., Holm, M., et al., Lipofection: A highly efficient, lipid-mediated DNA-transfection procedure, *Proc. Natl. Acad. Sci.* 84, 7413–7417, 1987.
2. Zuhorn, I.S., Kalicharan, R., and Hoekstra, D., Lipoplex-mediated transfection of mammalian cells occurs through the cholesterol-dependent clathrin-mediated pathway of endocytosis, *J. Biol. Chem.* 277, 18021–18028, 2002.

3. Hart, S.L., Lipid carriers for gene therapy, *Curr. Drug. Deliv.* 2, 423–438, 2005.
4. Giselbrecht, J., Janich, C., Pinnapireddy, S.F., et al., Overcoming the polycation dilemma—Explorative studies to characterise the efficiency and biocompatibility of newly designed lipofection reagents, *Int. J. Pharm.* 541, 81–92, 2018.
5. Fondello, C., Agnetti, L., Glikin, G.C., and Finaocchiaro, L.M.E., Mechanisms enhancing the cytotoxic effects of bleomycin plus suicide or interferon-β lipofection in metastatic human melanoma cells, *Anticancer Agents Med. Chem.* 18, 1338–1348, 2018.
6. Enlund, E., Fischer, S., Handrick, R., et al., Establishment of lipofection for studying miRNA function in human adipocytes, *PLoS One* 9(5), e98023, 2014.
7. Ikeda, S., Sugimoto, M., and Kume, S., Lipofection of siRNA into bovine 8–16-cell stage embryos using zone removal and the well-of-the well culture system, *J. Reproc. Dev.* 64, 199–202, 2018.
8. Van Tendeoo, V.F., Ponsaerts, P., Lardon, F., et al., Highly efficient gene delivery by mRNA electroporation in human hematopoietic cells: Superiority to lipofection and passing pulsing of mRNA and to electroporation of plasmid cDNA for tumor antigen loading of dendritic cells, *Blood* 98, 49–56, 2001.
9. Liu, J., Yu, T. Zhou, J., et al., Optimal transfection methods and comparison of PK-15 and Dulac cells for rescue of chimeric porcine circovirus type 1–2, *J. Virol. Methods* 208, 90–95, 2014.
10. Mars, T., Strazisar, M., Mis, K., et al., Electrotransfection and lipofection show comparable efficiency for *in vitro* gene delivery of primary human myeloblasts, *J. Membr. Biol.* 248, 273–283, 2015.

LIPOPHILIC

The term lipophilic usually refers to the affinity or a compound, object, or matrix for similar materials including hydrophobic materials such as non-polar lipid or chromatographic matrices such as C_{18}-silica. Lipophilicity refers to the property of a compound to dissolve in a non-polar solvent such as benzene or toluene. The lipophilicity of compound is frequently measured by distribution or partitioning in an *n*-octanol-water system and can be assigned a value such as Log P.[1,2] Lipophilicity can also be measured by chromatographic methods.[3,4] Lipophilicity is an important characteristic of drugs.[5–7]

1. Klopman, G., and Zhu, H., Recent methodologies for the estimation of *n*-octanol/water partition coefficients and their use in the prediction of membrane transport properties of drugs, *Mini Rev. Med. Chem.* 5, 127–133, 2005.
2. Martel, S., Begnaud, F., Schuler, W., et al., Limits of rapid log P dermination methods for highly lipophilic and flexible compounds, *Anal. Chim. Acta* 915, 90–101, 2016.
3. Markuszewski, M.J., Wiczling, P., and Kaliszan, R., High-throughput evaluation of lipophilicity and acidity by new gradient HPLC methods, *Comb. Chem. High Throughput Screen.* 7, 281–289, 2004.
4. Xu, L., Li, L., Huang, J., et al., Determination of the lipophilicity (log P o/w) of organic compounds by microemulsion liquid chromatography, *J. Biomed. Anal.* 102, 409–416, 2015.
5. Mannhold, R., The impact of lipophilicity in drug research: A case report on beta-blockers, *Mini Rev. Med. Chem.* 5, 197–205, 2005.
6. Gocan, S., Cimpan, G., and Comer, J., Lipophilicity measurements by liquid chromatography, *Adv. Chromatog.* 44, 79–176, 2006.
7. Arnott, J.A., and Planey, S.L., The influence of lipophilicity in drug discovery and design, *Expert Opin. Drug Discov.* 7, 863–875, 2012.

LIPOSOMES

Liposomes are relatively large (nano to micro) micelles primarily composed of polar lipids (phospholipids) but other compositions are being developed.[1–4] There is considerable interest in liposomes for drug delivery[5–8] and in non-medical applications.[9]

1. Duman, G., Aslan, I., Özer, A.Y., Inanc, I., and Taralp, A., Liposome, gel and lipogelosome formulations containing sodium hyaluronate, *J. Liposome Res.* 24, 259–269, 2014.
2. Palac, Z., Hurler, J., Škalko-Basnet, N., Filipović-Grčić, J., and Vanić, Ž., Elastic liposomes-in-vehicle formulations destined for skin therapy: The synergy between type of liposomes and vehicle, *Drug Dev. Ind. Pharm.* 41, 1247–1253, 2015.
3. Philippot, J.R., *Liposomes as Tools in Basic Research and Industry* (1994), CRC Press, Boca Raton, FL, 2017.
4. Villegas, M.R., Barza, A., and Vallet-Regi, M., Nanotechnological strategies for protein delivery, *Molecules* 23, 1008, 2018.
5. Allen, T.M., and Cullis, P.R., Liposomal drug delivery systems: From concept to clinical applications, *Adv. Drug Deliv. Rev.* 65, 36–48, 2013.
6. Madni, A., Sarfraz, M., Rehman, M., et al., Liposomal drug delivery: A versatile platform of challenging clinical applications, *J. Pharm. Pharm. Sci.* 17, 401–426, 2014.
7. Florence, A.T., *Liposomes in Drug Delivery*, CRC Press, Boca Raton, FL, 2017.
8. Miyazaki, M., Yuba, E., Hayashi, H., Harada, A., and Kono, K., Hyaluronic acid-based pH-sensitive polymer-modified liposomes for cell-specific intracellular drug delivery systems, *Bioconjug. Chem.* 29, 44–55, 2018.
9. *Handbook of Nonmedical Applications of Liposomes*, ed. Y. Barenholz and D.D. Lasic, CRC Press/Taylor & Francis Group, Boca Raton, FL, 2018.

LOCALIZED SURFACE PLASMON RESONANCE

Localized surface plasmon resonance is a label-free analytical method based on the use of noble metal (Ag, Au) nanoparticles as sensors for macromolecular interactions.[1-3] Localized surface plasmon resonance is a form of surface plasmon resonance and is based on the spectral properties (excitation of active surface electrons) of nanoparticles (3–100 nm) which are smaller than the incident light as compared to the bulk metal.[4] Localized surface plasmon resonance has been used for the measurement of peptide nucleic acid-DNA hybridization,[5] detection of specific DNA sequence by hybridization to oligonucleotide probes,[6] the measurement of prolactin in human serum,[7] and cancer biomarkers in various biological fluids.[8] It has been suggested that localized surface plasmon resonance is a technology which can be applied to developing countries.[9]

1. Willets, K.A., and Van Duyne, R.P., Localized surface plasmon resonance spectroscopy and sensing, *Annu. Rev. Phys. Chem.* 58, 267–297, 2007.
2. Long, Y.-T., and Jing, C., *Localized Surface Plasmon Resonance and Correlative Devices*, SpringerBriefs, Heidelberg, Germany, 2014.
3. Unser, S., Bruzas, I., He, J., and Sagle, L., Localized surface plasmon resonance biosensing: Current challenges and approaches, *Sensors* 15, 15684–15716, 2015.
4. Long, Y.-T., and Jing, C., Brief introduction to localized surface plasmon resonance and correlative devices, in *Localized Surface Plasmon Resonance and Correlative Devices*, Chapter 1, pp. 1–9, SpringerBriefs, Heidelberg, Germany, 2014.
5. Endo, T., Kerman, K., Nagatani, N., Takamura, Y., and Tamiya, E., Label-free detection of peptide nucleic acid-DNA hybridization using localized surface plasmon resonance based optical biosensor, *Anal. Chem.* 77, 6976–6984, 2005.
6. Soares, L., Csáki, A., Jatschka, J., et al., Localized surface plasmon resonance (LSPR) biosensing using gold nanotriangles: Detection of DNA hybridization events at room temperature, *Analyst* 139, 4964–4973, 2014.
7. Faridli, Z., Mahani, M., Torkzadeh-Mahani, M., and Fasihi, J., Development of a localized surface plasmon resonance-based gold nanobiosensor for the determination of prolactin hormone in human serum, *Anal. Biochem.* 495, 32–36, 2016.
8. Ferhan, A.R., Jackman, J.A., Park, J.H., Cho, N.J., and Kim, D.H., Nanoplasmonic sensors for detecting circulating cancer biomarkers, *Adv. Drug Deliv. Rev.* 125, 48–77, 2018.
9. Hammond, J.L., Bhalla, N., Rafiee, S.D., and Estrela, P., Localized surface plasmon resonance as a biosensing platform for developing countries, *Biosensors* 4, 172–188, 2014.

LOCUS CONTROL REGION

A locus is the position of a gene on a chromosome. All alleles of a gene occupy the same position on a chromosome. A locus control region is a *cis*-acting region on a gene locus which controls the expression of linked transgenes.[1,2] The locus control region for β-globin has been an object of considerable study.[3]

1. Li, Q., Harju, S., and Peterson, K.R., Locus control regions: Coming of age at a decade plus, *Trends Genet.* 15, 403–408, 1999.
2. Dean, A., On a chromosome far, far away: LCRs and gene expression, *Trends Genet.* 22, 38–45, 2006.
3. Ellis, J., and Pannell, D., The human β-globin locus control region, *Eur. J. Biochem.* 269, 1589–1899, 2002.

LONGINS AND LONGIN DOMAIN

A longin is an R-SNARE (soluble *N*-ethylmaleimide-sensitive factor [NSF] attachment protein receptors) that is common to all eukaryotes and is characterized by an amino terminal segment referred to as a longin domain.[1] A longin domain is a sequence of 110–120 amino acids in a α-β-α structure.[2,3] An R-SNARE (arginine-contributing SNAREs) contains an arginine at a specific position while Q-SNARE (glutamine-contributing SNAREs) have a glutamine at that position. The term longin was suggested to differentiate such domains from "brevins" which are shorter *N*-terminal regions found in vesicle-associated membrane proteins.[4] The longin domain in R-SNARE protein is involved in membrane fusion[5] and membrane trafficking.[6,7] Longin domains (non-SNARE longins) have also been implicated in the interaction of small GTPases with guanine exchange factors.[8,9] Phytolongins are also a class of non-SNARE longins in intracellular regulation including secretory pathways.[10]

1. Rossi, V., Banfied, D.K., Vacca, M., et al., Longins and their longin domains: Regulated SNARES and multifunctional SNARE regulators, *Trends Biochem. Sci.* 29, 682–687, 2004.
2. Reardon, D., and Farber, G.K., The structure and evolution of α/β barrel proteins, *FASEB J.* 9, 497–503, 1995.
3. Orengo, C.A., and Thornton, J.M., Alpha plus beta folds revisited: Some favoured motifs, *Structure* 1, 105–120, 1993.
4. Filippini, F., Rossi, V., Galli, T., et al., Longins: A new evolutionary conserved VAMP family sharing a novel SNARE domain, *Trends Biochem. Sci.* 26, 407–409, 2001.
5. Dietrich, L.E.P., Boeddinghaus, C., LaGrassa, T.J., and Ungermann, C., Control of eukaryotic membrane fusion by N-terminal domain of SNARE proteins, *Biochim. Biophys. Acta* 1641, 111–119, 2003.

6. De Franceschi, N., Wild, K., Schlacht, A., et al., Longin and GAF domains: Structural evolution and adaptation to the subcellular trafficking machinery, *Traffic* 15, 104–121, 2014.

7. Daste, F., Galli, T., and Tareste, D., Structure and function of longin SNAREs, *J. Cell Sci.* 128, 4263–4372, 2015.

8. Levine, T.P., Daniels, R.D., Wong, L.H., et al., Discovery of new longin and roadblock domains that form platforms for small GTPases in Regulator and TRAPP-II, *Small GTPases* 4, 62–69, 2013.

9. Ishida, M., Oguci, M.E., and Fukuda, M., Multiple types of guanine exchange factors (GEFs) for Rab small GTPases, *Cell Structure Function* 41, 61–79, 2016.

10. de Marcos Lousa, C., Soubeyrand, E., Bolognese, P., et al., Subcellular localization and trafficking of phytolongins (non-SNARE longins) in the plant secretory pathway, *J. Expt. Bot.* 67, 2627–2639, 2016.

LUMINESCENCE

Luminescence (cold light) is the emission of energy in the form of light as a result of a chemical reaction (chemiluminescence) or a biological reaction (bioluminescence).[1] One of the best-known examples of bioluminescence is the light emitted by a firefly. This is results of the action of an enzyme, luciferase, on a substrate, luciferin, in the presence of ATP where the energy of ATP is converted to light.[2,3] The luciferase reaction is used as a signal in a variety of analytical methods.[4,5] Luminescence is related to but different from fluorescence is the emission of energy (light) in response to incident light, usually at lower wavelength. There are compounds which are both luminogenic and fluorescent such as 5(5-azoluciferinyl)-2,3-dihydro-1,4-phthalazinedione (ALPDO).[6] Luminescence is also related to **phosphorescence** where phosphorescence, as with fluorescence, is light emission after irradiation but unlike fluorescence, phosphorescence persists after the removal of the irradiation source. Compounds can be both fluorescent and phosphorescent.[7] Electrochemilumescence (electrogenerated chemiluminescence) differs from all of the above in that excited states are generated at the surface of an electrode.[8] Electroluminescence is the generation of luminescence in the presence of an electrical current.[9]

1. *Luminescence Biotechnology Instruments*, ed. K. Van Dyke, C. Van Dyke, and K. Woodfork, CRC Press, Boca Raton, FL, 2002.

2. Fraga, H., Firefly luminescence: A historical perspective and recent developments, *Photochem. Photobiol. Sci.* 7, 146–158, 2008.

3. Viera, J., Pinto da Silva, L., and Esteves da Silva, J.A., Advances in the knowledge of light emission by firefly luciferin and oxyluciferin, *J. Photochem. Photobiol. B* 117, 33–39, 2012.

4. Lundin, A., Optimization of the firefly luciferase reaction for analytical purposes, *Adv. Biochem. Eng. Biotechnol.* 145, 31–62, 2014.

5. Kiyama, M., Saito, R., Iwano, S., et al., Multicolor bioluminescence obtained using firefly luciferin, *Curr. Top. Med. Chem.* 16, 2648–2655, 2016.

6. Sudharharan, T., and Reddy, A.R., A bifunctional luminogenic substrate for two luminescent enzymes: Firefly luciferase and horseradish peroxidase, *Anal. Biochem.* 271, 159–167, 1999.

7. Prodius, D., Wilk-Kozubek, M., and Mudring, A.V., Synthesis, structural characterization and luminescence properties of 1-carboxymethyl-3-ethylimidazolium chloride, *Acta Chrystallogr. C Struct. Chem.* 74, 653–658, 2018.

8. Richter, M.M., Electrochemiluminescence, *Chem. Rev.* 104, 3003–3036, 2004; Muzyka, K., Current trends in the development of the electrochemiluminescent immunosensors, *Biosens. Bioeclectron.* 54, 393–407, 2014.

9. Cirio, M., De Liberato, S., Lambert, N., and Nori, F., Ground state electroluminescence, *Phys. Rev. Lett.* 116, 113601, 2016.

LYSOSOME

A lysosome is an intracellular organelle in a eukaryotic cell responsible for **controlled** intracellular digestion of proteins and other cellular constituents.[1,2] Lysosomes are involved in the catabolism/digestion of intracellular and extracellular cargo. Autophagy is a process for digestion of intracellular materials (cellular self-digestion) through the formation of autophagosomes which fuse with lysosomes.[3,4] Lysosomal protein degradation is also involved in MHC class II antigen presentation via the endosomal pathway.[5-7] The interior of the lysosome is unique in being acidic[8] reflecting the action of an energy-dependent proton pump.[9]

1. Appelmans, F., Wattlaux, R., and de Duve, C., Tissue fractionation studies 5. The association of acid phosphatase with a special class of cytoplasmic granules in rat liver, *Biochem. J.* 59, 438–445, 1955.

2. Novikoff, A.B., Beufay, H., and de Duve, C., Electron microscopy of lysosome-rich fractions from rat liver, *J. Biochem. Biophys. Cytology* 25(4 Suppl), 179–184, 1956.

3. Mizushima, N., Levine, B., Cuervo, A.M., and Kliosky, D.J., Autophagy fights disease through cellular self-digestion, *Nature* 451, 1069–1075, 2008.

4. Saha, S., Panigrahi, D.P., Patil, S., and Bhutia, S.K., Autophagy in health and disease: A comprehensive review, *Biomed. Pharmacother.* 104, 485–495, 2018.

5. Hsing, L.C., and Rudensky, A.Y., The lysosomal cysteine proteases in MHC class II antigen presentation, *Immunol. Rev.* 207, 229–241, 2005.

6. Mellman, T., Antigen processing and presentation by dendritic cells: Cell biological mechanisms, *Adv. Exp. Med. Biol.* 560, 63–67, 2005.

7. van Kasteren, S.I., and Overkleeft, H.S., Endo-lysosomal proteases in antigen presentation, *Curr. Opin. Chem. Biol.* 23, 8–15, 2014.
8. de Duve, C., Lysosomes revisited, *Eur. J. Biochem.* 137, 391–397, 1983.
9. Rudnick G., ATP-driven H+ pumping into intracellular organelles, *Annu. Rev. Physiol.* 48, 403–413, 1986.

MACROLIDES

Macrolide are naturally occurring antibiotics characterized by a large macrocyclic ring.[1–3] Macrolides were originally characterized as a macrocyclic lactone antibiotic (polyoxo antibiotic, e.g. magnamycin) but the classification has expanded to include polyene and ionophoric compounds.[4] The size of the macrocyclic monolactone ring can vary from 8-membered to 62-membered while other classes somewhat smaller, although most of the interest in is ring sizes from 12 to 16 members.[5] The action of macrolide antibiotics is based on the blockage of the nascent peptide exit tunnel as well as the inhibition of ribosomal peptidyl transferase activity.[6–9] Resistance to macrolide antibiotics is association with mutations in the 23S rRNA component of the ribosomal peptidyl transferase.[10] See **nascent peptide exit tunnel**.

1. Woodward, R.B., Struktur und Biogenese der Macrolide. Eine neue Klasse von Naturstoffen, *Angew. Chem.* 60, 50–59, 1957.
2. *Macrolides Chemistry, Pharmacology and Clinical Uses*, ed. A.J. Bryskier, J.-P. Butzler, H.C. Neu, and P.M., Tulkens, Arnette Blackwell Press, Paris, Francis, 1993.
3. *Macrolide Antibiotics Chemistry, Biology and Practice*, 2nd edn., ed. S. Ōmura, Academic/Elsevier, Amsterdam, the Netherlands, 2002.
4. Masamune, S., Bates, G.S., and Corcoran, J.W., Macrolides. Recent progress in chemistry and biochemistry, *Angew. Chem. Int. Ed. Engl.* 15, 585–607, 1977.
5. Shimoi, K., and Ōmura, S., Discovery of new macrolides, in *Macrolide Antibiotics Chemistry, Biology, and Practice*, ed. S. Ōmura, Chapter 1, pp. 1–56, Academic/Elsevier, Amersterdam, the Netherlands, 2002.
6. Brisson-Noël, A., Trieu-Cuot, P., and Courvalin, P., Mechanism of action of spiramycin and other macrolides, *J. Antimicrob. Chemother.* 22(supp B), 13–23, 1988.
7. Schlünzen, F., Zarivach, R., Harms, J., et al., Structural basis for the interaction of antibiotics with the peptidyl transferase centre in eubacteria, *Nature* 413, 814–821, 2001.
8. Tenson, T., Lovmar, M., and Ehrenberg, M., The mechanism of action of macrolide, lincosomide and streptogramin B reveals the nascent peptide exit path in the ribosome, *J. Mol. Biol.* 330, 1005–1014, 2003.
9. Lin, J., Zhou, D., Steitz, T.A., Polikanov, Y.S., and Gagnon, M.G., Ribosome-targeting antibiotics: Modes of action, mechanisms of resistance, and implications for drug design, *Annu. Rev. Biochem.* 87, 451–478, 2018.
10. Douthwaite, S.R., and Vester, B., Macrolide resistance conferred by alterations to the ribosome target site, in *The Ribosome Structure, Function, Antibiotics, and Cellular Function*, ed. R.A. Garrett, S.R. Douthwaite, A. Liljas, A.T. Matheson, P.B. Moore, and H.F. Noller, Chapter 35, pp. 431–439, ASM Press, Washington, DC, 2000.

MACROPHAGE

Macrophages are multifunctional cells and are considered part of the cellular immune system.[1–5] In the classical sense, a macrophage is an immune system cell that is derived from a monocyte after passage through the endothelium into the tissue spaces in response to inflammation.[6] More recent thinking suggests that macrophages are also intrinsic to tissues.[7] More recent thinking suggests that macrophages are also intrinsic to tissues.[8] In addition to this resident tissue population, monocytes are converted into macrophages during the inflammatory responses Monocytes are converted into a heterogeneous population of macrophages.[9] It is suggested that, in reflection of the heterogeneity, macrophages can be both pro-inflammatory and anti-inflammatory.[10] Macrophages are heterogeneous with multiple functions. A macrophage can be a phagocytic cell[11,12] and an antigen presenting cell.[13,14] The uptake of LDL into macrophages lead to the formation of foam cells which play an important role in the pathogenesis of atherosclerosis.[15–18] Lung interstitial macrophages are important in pulmonary homeostasis.[19]

1. Horst, M., *The Human Macrophage System: Activity and Functional Morphology*, Karger, Basel, 1988; *Macrophage Biology and Activation*, ed. S.W. Russell and S. Gordon, Springer-Verlag, Berlin, 1992.
2. *Macrophage-Pathogen Interactions*, ed. B.S. Zwilling and T.K. Eisenstein, M. Dekker, New York, 1992.
3. *The Macrophage*, ed. B. Bernard and C.E. Lewis, Oxford University Press, Oxford, UK, 2002.
4. *Macrophages: Biology and Role in the Pathology of Diseases*, ed. S.K. Biswas and A. Mantovani, Springer and Science + Business, New York, 2014.
5. *Macrophages Origin, Functions and Biointervention*, ed. M. Kloc, Springer International, Cham, Switzerland, 2017.
6. Lin, H.S., Gordon, S., Gordon, S., Chen, D.M., and Kurtz, M., Conversion of monocytes to cells capable of anchorage-independent growth in vitro, *J. Exp. Med.* 153, 488–493, 1981.
7. Kratofil, R.M., Kubes, P., and Deniset, J.F., Monocyte conversion during inflammation and injury, *Arterioscler. Thromb. Vasc. Biol.* 37, 35–42, 2017.

8. Epelman, S., Lavine, K.J., and Randolph, G.J., Origin and function of tissue macrophage, *Immunity* 41, 21–35, 2014.
9. Jakubzick, C.W., Randolph, G.J., and Henson, P.M., Monocyte differentiation and antigen-presenting functions, *Nat. Rev. Immunol.* 17, 349–362, 2017.
10. Shapouri-Mognhaddam, A., Mohammadian, S., Vazini, H., et al., Macrophage plasticity, polarization, and function in health and disease, *J. Cell Physiol.* 233, 6425–6440, 2018.
11. Nagelkerke, S.Q., Dekkers, G., Kustiawan, I., et al., Inhibition of FcγR-mediated phagocytosis by IVIg is independent of IgG-Fc sialylation and FcγRIIb in human macrophages, *Blood* 124, 3709–3718, 2014.
12. Alvey, C., and Discher, D.E., Engineering macrophages to eat cancer: From "marker of self" CD47 and phagocytosis to differentiation, *J. Leukoc. Biol.* 102, 31–40, 2017.
13. Guiiliams, M., Bruhns, P., Saeys, Y., Hammad, H., and Lambrecht, B.N., The function of Fcγ receptors in dendritic cells and macrophages, *Nat. Rev. Immunol.* 14, 94–108, 2014.
14. Kashem, S.W., Haniffa, M., and Kaplan, D.H., Antigen-presenting cells in the skin, *Annu. Rev. Immunol.* 35, 469–499, 2017.
15. Schwartz, C.J., Valente, A.J., Sprague, E.A., et al., The pathogenesis of atherosclerosis: An overview, *Clin. Cardiol.* 14(2 Suppl 1), I1–I16, 1991.
16. Shashkin, P., Dragulev, B., and Ley, K., Macrophage differentiation to foam cells, *Curr. Pharm. Des.* 11, 3061–3072, 2005.
17. McLaren, J.E., Michael, D.R., Ashlin, T.G., and Ramji, D.P., Cytokines, macrophage lipid metabolism and foam cells: Implications for cardiovascular disease therapy, *Prog. Lipid Res.* 50, 331–347, 2011.
18. Patel, K.M., Strong, A., Tohyama, J., et al., Macrophage sortilin promotes LDL uptake, foam cell formation, and atherosclerosis, *Circ. Res.* 116, 789–796, 2015.
19. Schyns, J., Bureau, F., and Marichal, T., Lung interstitial macrophages: Past, present, and future, *J. Immunol. Res.* 2018, 5160794, 2018.

MACROPINOCYTOSIS

Pinocytosis (derived from the ancient Greek to drink) is defined as a process by which droplets of liquid are taken into a cell, now known to be by means of small vesicles formed by the pinching off of an invagination of the cell membrane.[1] Pinocytosis can be distinguished from phagocytosis which is the process by which solid particles (generally other cells or bacteria) are taken into a cell. Macropinocytosis is one of the several types of clathrin-independent endocytosis.[2] While both micropinocytosis and phagocytosis are both actin-mediated processes, phagocytosis involves a cell membrane receptors interaction with cargo, macropinocytosis is independent of receptor.[3,4] The process of micropinocytosis

involving the "ruffling" of the membrane which close up to form intracellular vesicles known as micropinosomes.[5] Macropinocytosis is a constitutive process in dendritic cells providing an efficient method for MHC-class-II-restricted antigen presentation.[6-8] Macropinocytosis is an important mechanism in the uptake of LDL by macrophages leading to the formation of foam cells.[9-11] The process of micropinocytosis and formation of macropinosomes provides a mechanism for providing nutrients to cancer cells[12] and for the delivery of drugs to tumor cells.[13] An arginine-rich peptide was shown to induce active micropinocytosis providing a mechanism for targeted drug delivery to the intracellular space.[14,15]

1. *Oxford English Dictionary*, Oxford University Press, Oxford, UK, 2018.
2. Ferreira, A.P.A., and Boucrot, E., Mechanisms of carrier formation during clathrin-independent endocytosis, *Trends Cell. Biol.* 28, 188–200, 2018.
3. Araki, N., Johnson, M.T., and Swansom, J.A., A role for phosphoinositide 3-kinase in the completion of micropinocytosis and phagocytosis by macrophages, *J. Cell Biol.* 135, 1249–1260, 1996.
4. Cardelli, J., Phagocytosis and micropinocytosis in *Dictyoselium*: Phosphoinositide-based processes, biochemically distinct, *Traffic* 2, 331–320, 2001.
5. Swanson, J.A., and Watts, C., Macropinocytosis, *Trends Cell Biol.* 5, 424–428, 1995.
6. Sallusto, F., Cella, M., Danieli, C., and Lanzavecchia, A., Dendritic cells use micropinocytosis and the mannose receptor to concentrate macromolecules in the major histocompatibility complex class II compartment: Downregulation by cytokines and bacterial products, *J. Expt. Med.* 182, 389–400, 1995.
7. von Delwig, A., Hilkens, C.M., Altmann, D.M., et al., Inhibition of macropinocytosis blocks antigen presentation of type II collagen in vitro and in vivo in HLA-DR1 transgenic mice, *Arthritis Res. Ther.* 8, R93, 2006.
8. Liu, Z., and Roche, P.A., Macropinocytosis in phagocytes: Regulation of MHC class-II-restricted antigen presentation in dendritic cells, *Front. Physiol.* 6, 1, 2015.
9. Anzinger, J.J., Chang, J., Xu, Q., et al., Native low-density lipoprotein uptake by macrophage colony-stimulating factor-differentiated human macrophages is mediated by micropinocytosis and micropinocytosis, *Arterioscler. Thromb. Vasc. Biol.* 30, 2022–2031, 2010.
10. Michael, D.R., Ashlin, T.G., Davies, C.S., et al., Differential regulation of macropinocytsosis in macrophages by cytokines: Implications for foam cell formation and atherosclerosis, *Cytokine* 64, 357–361, 2013.
11. Chellan, B., Reardon, C.A., Getz, G.S., and Bowman, H., Enzymatically modified low-density lipoprotein promotes foam cell formation in smooth muscle cells

via micropinocytosis and enhances receptor-mediated uptake of oxidized low-density lipoprotein, *Arterioscler. Thromb. Vasc. Biol.* 36, 1101–1113, 2016.

12. Recouvreux, M.V., and Commisso, C., Macropinocytosis: A metabolic adaptation to nutrient stress in cancer, *Front. Endocrinol.* 8:261, 2017.

13. Ha, K.D., Bidlingmaier, S.M., and Liu, B., Macropinocytosis exploitation by cancers and cancer therapeutics, *Front. Physiol.* 7, 381, 2016.

14. Melikov, K., and Chernomordik, L.V., Arginine-rich cell penetrating peptides: From endosomal uptake to nuclear delivery, *Cell. Mol. Life Sci.* 62, 2739–2749, 2005.

15. Nakase, I., Noguchi, K., Aoki, A., et al., Arginine-rich cell-penetrating peptide-modified extracellular vesicles for active micropinocytosis induction and efficient intracellular delivery, *Sci. Rep.* 17, 1991, 2017.

MADIN-DARBY CANINE KIDNEY (MDCK)

Madin-Darby Canine Kidney (MDCK) is a term describing a mammalian cell line (MDCK cells) used as model system to represent polarized epithelial cells.[1-4] MDCK cells are used to study viruses[5,6] and for the production of viral vaccines.[7,8]

1. Hidalgo, I.J., Assessing the absorption of new pharmaceuticals, *Curr. Top. Med. Chem.* 1, 385–401, 2001.

2. Cohen, D., and Musch, A., Apical surface formation in MDCK cells: Regulation by the serine/threonine kinase EMK1, *Methods* 30, 69–276, 2003.

3. Sidorenko, Y., and Reichl, U., Structured model of influenza virus replication in MDCK cells, *Biotechnol. Bioeng.* 88, 1–14, 2004.

4. Urquhart, P., Pang, S., and Hooper, N.M., *N*-Glycans as apical targeting signals in polarized epithelial cells, *Biochem. Soc. Symp.* 72, 39–45, 2005.

5. Sidorenko, Y., and Reichl, U., Structured model of influenza virus replication in MDCK cells, *Biotechnol. Bioeng.* 88, 1–14, 2004.

6. Lakdawala, S.S., Fodor, E., and Subbaro, K., Moving on out: Transport and packaging of influenza viral RNA into virions, *Annu. Rev. Virol.* 3, 411–427, 2016.

7. Genzel, Y., Designing cell lines for viral vaccine production: Where do we stand? *Biotechnol. J.* 10, 728–740, 2015.

8. Manini, J., Domnich, A., Amicizia, D., et al., Flucelvax (Optaflu) for seasonal influenza, *Expert Rev. Vaccines* 14, 789–804, 2015.

MAILLARD REACTION

The Maillard reaction (named after Louis-Camille Maillard)[1,2] is a reaction between a protein amino group, usually the epsilon-amino group of lysine and a reducing sugar/aldose which can proceed to form a large number of derivative products.[3-5] The initial observation by Maillard was the formation of a yellow-brown color on heating an aqueous solution of an amine and sugar.[5] There is an initial condensation reaction to form a Schiff base, which undergoes rearrangement to form an Amadori product. The Amadori product can then form a variety of products and, in the case of lysine, form cross-links between protein chains as well as the formation of derivatives known as advanced glycation end products (AGE) or Maillard reaction products.[6] The initial reaction between amines and sugars is in essence a reaction between an aldehyde and a ketone with the initial formation of an *N*-substituted α-hydroxy derivative which forms a Schiff base (an imine) derivative by dehydration.[7] A Maillard-type reaction can also occur with the amino group of guanine in nucleic acid[8] generating novel taste products.[9] There is considerable interest in the Maillard reaction in food chemistry for taste, nutrition, and color.[10-15] Acrylamide is formed by a Maillard-type reaction in food in a reaction involving asparagine and a carbonyl compound.[16,17] The Maillard reaction is also involved in the tanning of animal skin.[18] In addition, the Maillard reaction in important in the action of self-tanning products.[19] Advanced glycation end products formed by Maillard-type reactions are also of considerable medical interest.[20-26] Finally, the reaction of sugars with proteins in the Maillard reaction is glycation as opposed to glycosylation which involves a different type of chemistry in the linking of sugars to proteins and is the result of an enzyme-catalyzed reaction. The broad interest in the Maillard reaction has resulted in the application of proteomic technology to study the various Maillard products.[27-29]

1. Nurston, H.E., *The Maillard Reaction: Chemistry, Biochemistry, and Implications*, Royal Society of Chemistry, Cambridge, UK, 2010.

2. Hellwig, M., and Henle, T., Baking, ageing, diabetes: A short history of the Maillard reaction, *Angew. Chem. Int. Ed. Engl.* 53, 10316–10329, 2014.

3. Hodge, J.E., Chemistry of the browning reactions in model systems, *J. Agric. Food Chem.* 1, 928–943, 1953.

4. Martins, S.I.F.S., Jongen, W.M.F., and van Boekel, M.A.J.S., A review of Maillard reaction in food and implications to kinetic modeling, *Trends Food Sci. Technol.* 11, 364–373, 2001.

5. Swanson, J.A., and Watts, C., Macropinocytosis, *Trends Cell Biol.* 5, 424–428, 1995.

6. Sell, D.R., Biemel, K.M., Reihl, O., Glucosepane is a major protein cross-link of the senescent human extracellular matrix. Relationship with diabetes, *J. Biol. Chem.* 280, 12310–12315, 2005.

7. Sprung, M.M., A summary of the reactions of aldehydes with amines, *Chem. Rev.* 26, 297–338, 1940.

8. Papoulis, A., al-Abed, Y., and Bucala, R., Identification of N^2-(1-carboxyethyl) guanine ICEG) as a guanine advanced glycosylation end product, *Biochemistry* 54, 648–655, 1995.

9. Suess, B., Brockhoff, A., Degenhardt, A., et al., Human taste and umami receptor responses to chemosensorica generated by Maillard-type N^2-alkyl- and N^2-arylthiomethylation of guanosine-5′-monophosphates, *J. Agrc. Food Chem.* 62, 11429–11440, 2014.

10. *The Maillard Reaction in Foods and Nutrition,* ed. G.R. Wallen and M.S. Feather, American Chemical Society, Washington, DC, 1987.

11. *The Maillard Reaction in Food and Medicine,* ed. J.O'Brien, H.E. Nurston, M.J.C., Crabbe and J.M. Ames, Royal Society of Chemistry, Cambridge, UK, 1998.

12. Losso, J.N., *The Maillard Reaction Reconsidered. Cooking and Eating for Health*, CRC Press, Boca Raton, FL, 2015.

13. Yin, Z., Sun, Q., Zhang, X., and Jing, H., Optimised formation of blue Maillard reaction products of xylose and glycine model systems and associated antioxidant activity, *J. Sci. Food. Agric.* 94, 1332–1339, 2014.

14. Liska, D.J., Cook, C.M., Wang, D.D., and Szpylka, J., Maillard reaction products and potatoes: Have the benefits been clearly assessed? *Food Sci. Nutr.* 4, 234–249, 2015.

15. Khan, M.I., Jo, C., and Tang, M.R., Meat flavor precursors and factors influencing flavor precursors—A systemic review, *Meat Sci.* 110, 278–284, 2015.

16. Mottram, D.S., Wedzicha, B.L., and Dodsoon, A.T., Acrylamide is formed in the Maillard reaction, *Nature* 419, 448–449, 2002.

17. Stadler, R.H., Blank, I., Varga, N., et al., *Nature* 419, 2002.

18. Zyzak, D.V., Sanders, R.A., Stajonovic, M., et al., Acrylamide formation mechanism in heated foods, *J. Agric. Food Chem.* 51, 4782–4787, 2003.

19. Jung, K., Seifert, M., Herrling, T., and Fuchs, J., UV-generated free radicals (FR) in skin: Their prevention by sun screens and their induction by self-tanning agents, *Spectrochim. Acta A Mol. Biomol. Spectrosc.* 69, 1423–1428, 2008.

20. Smith, M.A., Taned, S., Richey, P.L., Advanced Maillard reaction end products are associated with Alzheimer disease pathology, *Proc. Natl. Acad. Sci. USA* 91, 5710–5714, 1994.

21. Njoroge, F.G., and Monnier, V.M., The chemistry of the Maillard reaction under physiological conditions: A review, *Prog. Clin. Biol. Res.* 304, 85–107, 1989.

22. Marko, D., Habermeyer, M., Keméy, M., et al., Maillard reaction products modulating the growth of human tumor cells in vitro, *Chem. Res. Toxicol.* 16, 48–55, 2003.

23. Takeguchi, M., Yamagishi, S., Iwaki, M., et al., Advanced glycation end product (age) inhibitors and their therapeutic implications in diseases, *Int. J. Clin. Pharmacol. Res.* 24, 95–1010, 2004.

24. Jing, H., and Nakamura, S., Production and use of Maillard products as oxidative stress modulators, *J. Med. Food* 8, 291–298, 2005.

25. Vistoli, G., De Maddis, D., Cipak, A., et al., Advanced glycoxidation and lipoxidation end products (AGEs and ALEs): An overview of their mechanism of formation, *Free Radic. Res.* 47(Suppl 1) 3–27, 2013.

26. Ott, C., Jacobs, K., Haucke, E., et al., Role of advanced glycation end products in cellular signaling, *Redox. Biol.* 2, 411–429, 2014.

27. Ames, J.M., Application of semiquantiative proteomics techniques to the Maillard reaction, *Ann. N. Y. Acad. Sci.* 1043, 2250235, 2005.

28. Renzone, G., Arena, S., and Scaloni, A., Proteomic characterization of intermediate and advanced glycation end-products in commercial milk samples, *J. Proteomics* 117, 12–23, 2015.

29. Soboleva, A., Schmidt, R., Vikhnina, M., Grishina, T., and Frolov, A., Maillard proteomics: Opening new pages, *Int. J. Mol. Sci.* 18, 2677, 2017.

MAJOR GROOVE AND MINOR GROOVE—DNA STRUCTURE

The major grooves and minor grooves are the channels or grooves formed when two complementary strands of DNA hybridize with each other to form a double helix. The major groove is shallow and wide (~22 Å wide) while the minor groove is deep and narrow (~11 Å wide) with the base of the grooves formed by the edges of the planer bases.[1] While the phosphate and sugar moieties are relatively hydrophilic, the nucleobases are quite hydrophobic. The edges of the bases which form the base of the grooves contain nitrogen and oxygen which can interact with aqueous solvent. The sequence of base pairs can serve a code for binding specific proteins.[2] The major groove is responsible for the majority of binding of protein, primarily transcription factors) by interaction with an α-helical segment[3] of helix-turn-helix protein.[4] Proteins have specific binding sites in the major and minor grooves of DNA.[5,6] Protein binding to minor groove occurs through electrostatic interaction.[7] Actinomycin d binds to duplex DNA with specificity providing by binding of the pentapeptide rings to DNA sequence in the minor groove.[8]

1. Sharma, R.H., and Sharma, M.H., *DNA Double Helix and the Chemistry of Cancer*, Chapter 5, Structure of DNA, pp. 87–136, Adenine Press, Schenectedy, New York, 1988.

2. Allison, L.A., *Fundamental Molecular Biology*, p. 22, Blackwell, Malden, MA, 2007.

3. Allison, L.A., *Fundamental Molecular Biology*, p. 342, Blackwell, Malden, MA, 2007.

4. Alberts, B., Johnson, A., Lewis, J., Raffi, M., Roberts, K., and Walter, P., *Molecular Biology of the Cell*, 2nd edn., Garland Publishing, London, UK, 2002.

5. Lamoureux, J.S., and Glover, J.N., Principles of protein-DNA recognition revealed in the structural analysis of Ndt80-MSE DNA complexes, *Structure* 14, 555–565, 2006.

6. Amanzadeh, E., Mohadabatkar, H., and Biria, D., Classification of DNA minor and major groove binding proteins according to the NLSs by data analysis methods, *Appl. Biochem. Biotechnol.* 174, 437–451, 2014.

7. Chiu, T.P., Rao, S., Mann, R.S., Honig, B., and Rohs, R., Genome-wide prediction of minor-groove electrostatic potential enables biophysical modeling of protein-DNA binding, *Nucleic Acids Res.* 45, 12565–12576, 2017.

8. Cravens, S.L., Navapanich, A.C., Geierstanger, B.H., Tahmassebi, D.C., and Dwyer, T.J., NMR solution structure of a DNA-actinomycin D complex containing a non-hydrogen-bonding pair in the binding site, *J. Am. Chem. Soc.* 132, 17588–17598, 2010.

MAJOR HISTOCOMPATIBILITY COMPLEX (MHC)

The major histocompatibility complex (MHC) or locus is a cluster of genes on chromosome 6 (chromosome 17 in the mouse) which encodes a family of membrane glycoproteins referred to as MHC protein or molecules which function as receptors.[1–3] MHC membrane glycoproteins are found in antibody presenting cells (APCs; professional antigen presenting cells, dendritic cells, macrophages, and B-cells) and "present" antigens to effector CD-4 and CD-8 T-cells.[4] MHC membrane glycoproteins are divided into two groups, MHC class I and MHC class II, which present antigens to the cellular immune system.[5] Antigen presentation by MHC class I uses peptides generated from foreign proteins, aging intracellular proteins, and misfolded proteins. Peptides for MHC class I antigen presentation are processed by proteosomes and aminopeptidases and bind to transporter associated with antigen presentation (TAP), which places them onto MHC class I heterodimer. The peptide-MHC class I heterodimer transported from the endoplasmic reticulum via the Golgi to the plasma membrane for presentation to CD 8+ T-cells stimulating the formation of cytotoxic T-cells. Although the majority of peptides for MHC class I antigen presentation are intracellular in origin, some peptides are obtained from adjacent cells (cross-presentation) through gap junctions.[6] MHC class II antigen presentation involves peptide presentation to CD4+ T-cells which activate B-cells to form plasma cells that synthesize and secrete antibody. Peptides for MHC class II antigen presentation are derived from the action of lysosomal proteases on extracellular proteins in endosomes or macropinosomes.[7,8] Digestion of proteins occurs in late endosomes/lysosomes (MHC class II compartment) yielding peptides which then exchanges with CLIP (class II associated li peptide) peptide bound to MHC II class complex (α-chain and β-chain). The MHC class II molecule-peptide complex is transported to the plasma membrane where it binds to a T cell receptor (TCR) on a CD4+ cell. Cross-presentation can also occur with MHC class II and has been suggested as term to define autophagy-dependent MHC-class II presentation of intracellular antigens.[9] There are some non-membrane proteins such as HLA-DM[10] and HLA-DO[11] which are encoded by the MHC and function in the processing of peptides for delivery to the MHC membrane glycoproteins.[12,13]

1. Lyczak, J.B., The major histocompatibility complex, in *Immunology, Infection, and Immunity*, ed. G.B. Pier, J.B. Lyczak, and L.M. Wetzler, Chapter 11, pp. 261–282, ASM Press, Washington, DC, 2004.

2. Petersdorf, E.W., The major histocompatibility complex: A model for understanding graft-versus-host disease, *Blood* 122, 1863–1872, 2013.

3. Wiseman, R.W., Karl, J.A, Bohn, P.S., et al., Haplessly hoping: Macaque major histocompatibility complex made easy, *ILAR J.* 54, 196–210, 2013.

4. Birnbaum, M.E., Mendoza, J.L., Sethi, D.K., et al., Deconstructing the peptide-MHC specificity of T cell recognition, *Cell* 157, 107, 1073–1087, 2014.

5. Neefjes, J., Jongsma, M.L., Paul, P., and Bakke, O., Towards a systems understanding of MHC class I and MHC class II antigen presentation, *Nat. Rev. Immunol.* 11, 823–836, 2011.

6. Saccheri, F., Pozzi, C., Avogadri, F., et al., Bacteria-induced gap junctions in tumors favor antigen cross-presentation and antitumor immunity, *Sci. Transl. Med.* 2, 44ra57, 2010.

7. Krawczyk, M., and Reith, W., Regulation of MHC class II expression, a unique regulatory system identified by the study of a primary immunodeficiency disease, *Tissue Antigens* 67, 183–197, 2006.

8. Kohoutek, J., Jabrane-Ferrat, N., and Peterlin, B.M., Expression of MHC II genes, *Curr. Top. Microbiol. Immunol.* 290, 147–170, 2005.

9. Valečka, J., Almeida, C.R., Su, B., Pierre, P., and Gatti, E., Autophagy and MHC-restricted antigen presentation, *Mol. Immunol.* 99, 163–170, 2018.

10. Pos, W., Sethi, D.K., and Wucherpfennig, K.W., Mechanisms of peptide repertoire selection by HLA-DM, *Trends Immunol.* 34, 495–501, 2013.

11. Poluektov, Y.O., Kim, A., and Sadegh-Nasseri, S., HLA-DO and its role in MHC Class II antigen presentation, *Front. Immunol.* 4, 260, 2013.

12. Mellins, E.D., and Stern, L.J., HLA-DM and HLA-DO, key regulators of MHC-II processing and presentation, *Curr. Opin. Immunol.* 26, 115–122, 2014.
13. Alder, L.N., Jiang, W., Bhamidipati, K., et al., The other function: Class II-restricted antigen presentation by B cells, *Front. Immunol.* 8, 319, 2017.

MAST CELL

A mast cell is a type of leukocyte found in tissues[1,2] and contains large basophilic secretory granules containing histamine, arachidonic acid metabolites, platelet activating factor and other biologically active materials,[3] cytokines and growth factors,[4] proteases such as chymase and tryptase,[5] and acid hydrolases such as arylsulfatase[6] which are released on activation of the mast cells by immunologic (IgE) release.[7] Basophils are also activated by IgE and have similarities to mast cells.[8] The various materials secreted by the mast cell is referred to as the mast cell secretome.[9,10] Mast cell secretory granules also contain MHC class-II proteins are released on activation and migrate to the surface[11] which do participate in antigen presentation.[12] Mast cells have been considered primarily as effector cells in the allergic response[13] but recent work has demonstrated a wider scope of activities.[14–16]

1. Krishnaswamy, G., Ajitawi, O., and Chi, D.S., The human mast cell: An overview, *Methods Mol. Biol.* 315, 13–34, 2006.
2. Wolf, A.A., and Goodridge, H.S., Mast cells reveal their past selves, *Immunity* 48, 1065–1067, 2018.
3. Wasserman, S.I., The mast cell: Its diversity of chemical mediators, *Int. J. Dermatol.* 19, 7–17, 1980.
4. Mukai, K., Tsai, M., Saito, H., and Galli, S.J., Mast cells as sources of cytokines, chemokines, and growth factors, *Immunol. Rev.* 282, 121–150, 2018.
5. Schwartz, L.B., Lewis, R.A., Seldin, P., and Austen, K.F., Acid hydrolases and tryptase from secretory granules of dispersed human lung mast cells, *J. Immunol.* 126, 1290–1294, 1981.
6. Schwartz, L.B., and Austen, K.F., Enzymes of the mass cell granule, *J. Invest. Dermatol.* 74, 349–359, 1980.
7. Choi, H.W., and Abraham, S.N., *In Vitro* and *In Vivo* IgE/antigen-mediated mast cell activation, *Methods Mol. Biol.* 1799, 71–80, 2018.
8. Varricchi, G., Raap, U., Rivellese, F., Marone, G., and Gibbs, B.F., Human mast cells and basophils—How are they similar and how are they different? *Immunol. Rev.* 282, 8–34, 2018.
9. Vukman, K.V., Försönits, A., Oszvald, Å., Tóth, E.A., and Buzás, E.I., Mast cell secretome: Soluble and vesicular components, *Semin. Cell Dev. Biol.* 67, 65–73, 2017.
10. Atiakshin, D., Buchwalow, I., Samoilova, V., and Tiemann, M., Tryptase as a polyfunctional component of mast cells, *Histochem. Cell Biol.* 149, 461–467, 2018.
11. Vincent-Schneider, H., Théry, C., Mazzeo, D., et al., Secretory granules of mast cells accumulate mature and immature MHC class II molecules, *J. Cell Sci.* 114, 323–334, 2001.
12. Kambayashi, T., and Laufer, T.M., Atypical MHC class II-expressing antigen-presenting cells: Can anything replace a dendritic cell? *Nature Rev. Immnol.* 14, 719–730, 2014.
13. Puxeddu, H., Ribetti, D., Crivellato, E., and Levi-Schaffer, F., Mast cells and eosinophils: A novel link between inflammation and angiogenesis in allergic diseases, *J. Allergy Clin. Immunol.* 116, 531–536, 2005.
14. Galli, S.J., Kalesnikoff, J., Grimbaldeston, M.A., Piliponsky, A.M., Williams, C.M., and Tsai, M., Mast cells as "tunable" effector and Immunoregulatory cells: Recent advances, *Annu. Rev. Immunol.* 23, 749–786, 2005.
15. Saito, H., Role of mast cell proteases in tissue remodeling, *Chem. Immunol. Allergy* 87, 80–84, 2005.
16. Sibilano, R., Frossi, B., and Pucillo, C.E., Mast cell activation: A complex interplay of positive and negative signaling pathways, *Eur. J. Immunol.* 44, 2558–2566, 2014.

METABOLIPIDOMICS

Metabolipidomics is the study of the metabolism of lipids (metabolipidome) in a cell, tissue or organism.[1] Metabolipidomiics is distinguished from lipidomics in that metabolipidomics is the study of the metabolism of the lipids, while lipidomics is the study of the static concentrations of all lipids.[2] There has been limited but consistent use of the term metabolipidomics to describe research.[3,4]

1. Bleijerveld, O.B., Howeling, M., Thomas, M.J., and Cui, Z., Metabolipidomics: Profiling metabolism of glycerophospholipid species by stable isotopic precursors and tandem mass spectrometry, *Anal. Biochem.* 352, 1–14, 2006.
2. Balgoma, D., Montero, O., Balboa, M.A., and Balsinde, J., Lipidomic approaches to th study of phospholipase A_2-regulated phospholipid fatty acid incorporation and remodeling, *Biochimie* 92, 645–650, 2010.
3. Rombaldova, M., Janovska, P., Kopecky, J., and Kuda, O., Omega-3 fatty acids promote fatty utilization and production of pro-resolving lipid mediators in alternatively activated adipose tissue macrophages, *Biochem. Biophys. Res. Commun.* 490, 1080–1085, 2017.
4. Zhang, Q., Wang, X., Yan, G., et al., Anti-versus pro-inflammatory metabololipidome upon cupping treatment, *Cell Physiol. Biochem.* 45, 1377–1389, 2018.

METABOLITE/METABOLIC PROFILING

The canonical definition of a metabolite is the end product of a specific biochemical (metabolic) pathway such as glycolysis or fatty acid synthesis. An intermediate metabolite is an intermediate in a metabolic pathway[1] or in the degradation of drugs.[2] A metabolic (biochemical) pathway may be the pathway (anabolic pathway) in the synthesis of a specific product or products such as that for the synthesis of fatty acids[3] or degradation (catabolic pathway) as in the metabolism of nucleic acid components.[4] A metabolic inhibitor is a compound that inhibits a metabolic pathway.[5] The term metabolic profiling (metabolite profiling) was used to describe the study of metabolites in biological fluids such as urine[6] and for the study of the metabolism of drugs.[7–9] While metabolic profiling, in general, is concerned with the study of a specific metabolic pathway, while metabolomics[10] is a more global approach.[11] There is considerable overlap in the current literature. It can be suggested that metabolic profiling developed into metabolomics[12] much in the same way that classical protein chemistry developed into proteomics.[13]

1. Krebs, H.A., and Johnson, W.A., Acetopyruvic acid (αγ-diketovaleric acid) as an intermediate metabolite in animal tissues, *Biochem. J.* 31, 772–779, 1937.
2. Li, J., Fang, J., Zhong, F., et al., Development and validation of a liquid chromatography/tandem mass spectrometry assay for the simultaneous determination of dabigatran etexilate, intermediate metabolite, and dabigatran in 50 μL rat plasma and its application to pharmacokinetic study, *J. Chromatog. B. Analyt. Technol. Biomed. Life Sci.* 973C, 110–119, 2014.
3. Mashima, T., Seimya, H., and Tsuruo, T., *De novo* fatty-acid synthesis and related pathways as molecular targets for cancer therapy, *Brit. J. Cancer* 100, 1369–1372, 2009.
4. Rivas, M., Becerra, A., and Lazcano, A., On the early evolution of catabolic pathways: A comparative genomics approach. I. The cases of glucose, ribose, and the nucleobases catabolic routes, *J. Mol. Evol.* 86, 27–46, 2018.
5. Webb, J.L., *Enzyme and Metabolic Inhibitors*, Academic Press, New York, 1963.
6. Lefevere, M.F., Verhaeghe, B.J., Declerck, D.H., et al., Metabolic profiling or urinary organic acids by single and multicolumn capillary gas chromatography, *J. Chromatog. Sci.* 27, 23–29, 1989.
7. Okujava, V.M., Chankvetadze, B.G., Rukhadze, M.D., Rogava, M.M., and Tkesheliadze, N.B., Use of normal-phase microcolumn high-performance liquid chromatography for the study of hydrolytic stability, metabolic profiling and pharmacokinetics of an antiepileptic drug, benzonal, *J. Pharm. Biomed. Anal.* 9, 465–473, 1991.
8. Claus, S.P., Development of personalized functional foods needs metabolic profiling, *Curr. Opin. Clin. Nutr. Metab. Care* 17, 667–673, 2014.
9. Suhre, K., Metabolic profiling in diabetes, *J. Endocrinol.* 221, R75–F85, 2014.
10. Dunn, W.B., and Ellis, D.I., Metabolomics: Current analytical platforms and methodologies, *Trends Anal. Chem.* 24, 285–294, 2005
11. Larive, C.K., Barding, G.A., Jr., and Dinges, M.M., NMR spectroscopy for metabolomics and metabolic profiling, *Anal. Chem.* 87, 133–146, 2015.
12. Griffin, J.L., The Cinderella story of metabolic profiling: Does metabolomics get to go to the functional genomics ball? *Philos. Trans. R. Soc. Lond. B Biol. Sci.* 361, 147–161, 2006.
13. Lundblad, R.L., *The Evolution of Protein Chemistry to Proteomics*, CRC Press, Boca Raton, FL, 2006.

METABOLOME

The metabolome is the sum of the various metabolites produced in a cell, tissue, or organism.[1–7] There has been considerable interest in the relationship between the host metabolome and the microbiome.[8–12]

1. Tweeddale, H., Notley-McRobb, L., and Perenci, T., Effect of slow growth on metabolism of *Escherichia coli*, as revealed by global metabolite pool ("metabolome") analysis, *J. Bacteriol.* 180, 5109–5116, 1998.
2. Oliver, S.G., Winson, M.K., Kell, D.B., and Baganz, F., Systematic functional analysis of the yeast genome, *Trends Biotechnol.* 16, 373–383, 1998.
3. Scalert, A., Brennan, L., Manach, C., et al., The food metabolome: A window over dietary exposur, *Am. J. Clin. Nutr.* 99, 1289–1308, 2014.
4. Nikiforev, A., Kulikova, V., and Ziegler, M., The human NAD metabolome: Functions, metabolism and compartmentalization, *Crit. Rev. Biochem. Mol. Biol.* 50, 284–297, 2015.
5. Zamboni, N., Ssaghatelian, A., and Patti, G.J., Defining the metabolome: Size; flux, and regulation, *Mol. Cell.* 58, 699–706, 2015.
6. Kell, D.B., and Oliver, S.G., The metabolome 18 years on: A concept comes of age, *Metabolomics* 12, 148, 2016.
7. Zierer, J., Jackson, M.A., Mastenmüller, G., et al., The fecal metabolome as a functional readout of the gut microbiome, *Nat. Genet.* 50, 790–795, 2018.
8. Li, Y.V., and Holmes, E., Metabolomics for understanding gut microbiome and host metabolic interplay, in *Human Microbiota and Microbiome*, ed. J.R. Marchesi and M. Egert, Chapter 11, pp. 154–178, CABI, Wallingford, UK, 2014.
9. Lamichhane, S., Sen, P., Dickens, A.M., Orešič, M., and Bertram, H.C., Gut metabolome meets microbiome: A methodological perspective to understand the relationship between host and microbe, *Methods* 149, 3–12, 2018.
10. Ye, J.Z., Li, Y.T., Wu, W.R., et al., Dynamic alterations in the gut microbiota and metabolome during the development of methionine-choline-deficient diet-induced nonalcoholic steatohepatitis, *World J. Gastroenterol.* 24, 2468–2481, 2018.
11. Sanguinetti, E., Collado, M.C., Marrachelli, V.G., et al., Microbiome-metabolome signatures in mice genetically prone to develop dementia, fed a normal or fatty diet, *Sci. Rep.* 8, 4907, 2018.

12. Xin, Y., Diling, C., Jian, Y., et al., Effects of oligosaccharides from *Morinda officinalis* on gut microbiota and metabolome of APP/PS1 transgenic mice, *Front. Neurol.* 9, 412, 2018.

METABOLOMICS

Metabolomics is the study of the metabolome. Ideally, the metabolome would be ideally, the non-biased identification/quantification of all metabolites in a biological system such as an organelle, cell, tissue, or organism (including plants).[1–6]

1. *Plant Metabolomics*, ed. K. Saito, R.A. Dixon, and L. Wilmitzer, Springer, Berlin, Germany, 2006.
2. Nabil, S., *Computational Metabolomics*, Nova Science, New York, 2011.
3. *Concepts in Plant Metabolomics*, ed. B.J. Nikolau and E.S. Wurtele, Springer, Dordrecht, the Netherlands, 2007.
4. *Metabolomics: From Fundamental to Clinical Applications*, ed. A. Sussulini, Springer, Cham, Switzerland, 2017.
5. *Mass Spectrometry-based Metabolomics: A Practical Guide*, ed. E. Fukasaki and S.P. Putri, CRC/Taylor & Francis, Boca Raton, FL, 2015.
6. *Chromatographic Methods in Metabolomics*, ed. E. Hyötyläinen and S., Wiedmer, Royal Society of Chemistry, Cambridge, UK, 2013.

METAGENOMICS

Metagenomics[1–3] is the genomic analysis of a mixed microbial population such as that found in an environmental sample[4–7] or in a microbiome.[8–12]

1. Schloss, P.D., and Handelsman, J., Biotechnological prospects from metagenomics, *Curr. Opin. Biotechnol.* 14, 303–310, 2003.
2. Riesenfled, C.S., Schloss, P.D., and Handelsman, J., Metagenomics: Genomic analysis of microbial communities, *Annu. Rev. Genet.* 38, 525–552, 2004.
3. Steele, H.L., and Streit, W.R., Metagenomics: Advances in ecology and biotechnology, *FEMS Microbiol. Lett.* 247, 105–111, 2005.
4. Bouhajja, E., Agathos, S.N., and George, I.F., Metagenomics: Probling pollutant fate natural and engineered ecosystems, *Biotechnol. Adv.* 34, 1413–1426, 2016.
5. Purohit, H.J., Kapley, A., Khardenavis, A., Qureshi, A., and Defale, N.A., Insights in waste management bioprocesses using genomic tools, *Adv. Appl. Microbiol.* 97, 121–170, 2016.
6. Quince, C., Walker, A.W., Simpson, J.T., Loman, N.J., and Segata, N., Shotgum metagenomics, from sampling to analysis, *Nat. Biotechnol.* 35, 833–844, 2017.
7. Zolfo, M., Asnicar, F., Manghi, P., et al., Profiling microbial strains in urban environments using metagenomic sequencing data, *Biol. Direct.* 13(1), 9, 2018.
8. Walker, A.W., Duncan, S.H., Louis, P., and Flint, H.J., Phylogeny, culturing, and metagenomics of the human gut microbiota, *Trends Microbiol.* 22, 267–274, 2014.
9. Han, M., Yang, P., Zhou, H., Li, H., and Ning, K., Metagenomics and single-cell omics data analysis for human microbiome research, *Adv. Exp. Med. Biol.* 939, 117–137, 2016.
10. Wolfe, B.E., Using cultivated microbial communities to dissect microbiome assembly: Challenges, limitations, and the path ahead, *mSystems* 3(2), e00161–17, 2018.
11. Verma, D., Garg, P.K., and Dubey, A.K., Insights into the human oral microbiome, *Arch. Microbiol.* 200, 525–540, 2018.
12. Heintz-Buschart, A., and Wilmes, P., Human Gut microbiome; function matters, *Trends Microbiol.* 26, 563–574, 2018.

METAPROTEOMICS

Metaproteomics is the proteomic analysis of mixed microbial communities such as those found in environmental samples where individual contributions of a specific organism cannot be identified[1–4] or in the microbiome.[5–8]

1. Wilmes, P., and Bond, P.L., The application of two-dimensional polyacrylamide gel electrophoresis and downstream analyses to a mixed community of prokaryotic microorganisms, *Environ. Microbiol.* 6, 911–920, 2004.
2. Kan, J., Hanson, T.E., Ginter, J.M., Wnag, K., and Chen, F., Metaproteomic analysis of Chesapeake Bay microbial communities, *Saline Systems* 1, 7, 2005.
3. Wilmes, P., and Bond, P.L, Metaproteomics: Studying functional gene expression in microbial ecosystems, *Trends Microbiol.* 14, 92–97, 2006.
4. Valenzuela, L., Chi, A., Beard, S., et al., Genomics, metagenomics and proteomics in biomining microorganisms, *Biotechnol. Adv.* 24, 195–209, 2006.
5. Kolmeder, C.A., and de Vos, W.M., Metaproteomics of our microbiome—Developing insight in function and activity in man and model systems, *J. Proteomics* 97, 3–16, 2014.
6. Mao, L., and Franke, J., Symbiosis, dysbiosis, and rebiosis-the value of metaproteomics in human microbiome monitoring, *Proteomics* 15, 1142–1151, 2015.
7. Moon, C., Stupp, G.S., Su, A.I., and Wolan, D.W., Metaproteomics of colonic microbiota unveils discrete protein functions among colitic mice and control groups, *Proteomics* 18, 1700391, 2018.
8. Li, L., Zhang, X., Ning, Z., et al., Evaluating in vitro culture medium of gut microbiome with orthogonal experimental design a metaproteomics approach, *J. Proteome Res.* 17, 154–163, 2018.

METAZOAN/METAZOA

A metazoan is an organism with differentiated cells and tissues and usually a discrete digestive tract with specialized cells. In an older definition, the metazoa was an informal group defined as multicellular animal; redundant as an animal defined as multicellular.[1] A consideration of the available literature would define metazoa as multicellular organisms with varying degrees or organization.[2,3] The evolution of unicellular forms to metazoan via multicellular two-dimensional forms was dependent on the presence of sufficient oxygen[4] and to a higher level of organization through the development of the electron transport system.[5]

1. *The Penguin Dictionary of Biology*, 10th edn., ed. M. Thain and M. Hickman, Penguin Group, London, UK, 2000.
2. *Concise Encyclopedia Biology*, H.A. Scott (translate/revision), Walter de Gruyter, Berlin, Germany, 1996.
3. *A Dictionary of Biology*, 10th edn., ed. R. Hines and E. Martin, Oxford University Press, Oxford, UK, 2015.
4. Runnegar, B., Oxygen and the early evolution of the metazoan, in *Metazoan Life without Oxygen*, ed. C. Bryant, Chapter 4, pp. 45–67, Chapman & Hall, London, UK, 1991.
5. Behm, C.A., Fumerate reductase and the evolution of the electron transport system, in *Metazoan Life without Oxygen*, ed. C. Bryant, Chapter 5, pp. 81–108, Chapman & Hall, London, UK, 1991.

METHYLOME

The methylome is the genome-wide collection of the various methylation reactions. The methylome includes the DNA methylome,[1–3] the RNA methylome,[4,5] and the protein methylome with includes various methylation product derived from lysine and arginine.[6,7] The methylation reactions are catalyzed by various enzymes including DNA methyltransferases (DNMT),[8,9] RNA methyltransferases (RMT),[10] lysine methyltransferases (KMT),[11] and arginine methyltransferases (PRMT, protein arginine methyltransferase).[12] PRMTs are a target in cancer therapy.[13] The majority of protein methylation occurs on histones, although there are other protein targets.[14] It should be noted that there are a large number of methyltransferase (MTs) for DNA, DNMT1, DUMT2, DUMT3a, and DUMT3b together with a DNMT-related protein, DNMT3L.[15] S-Adenosyl-L-methionine (AdoMet) is the methyl donor for the majority of methylation reactions; there are rare instances where the methyl group is derived from folate.[16] Derivatives of AdoMet have been developed to identify sites of intracellular modification.[17]

1. Krueger, F., Kreck, B., Franke, A., and Andrews, S.R., DNA methylome analysis using short bisulfite sequencing data, *Nat. Methods* 9, 145–151, 2012.
2. Sánchez-Romero, M.A., Cota, I., and Casadesús, J., DNA methylation in bacteria from the methyl group to the methylome, *Curr. Opin. Microbiol.* 25, 9–16, 2015.
3. Sun, Z., Cunningham, J., Slager, S., and Kocher, J.P., Base resolution methylome profiling: Considerations in platform selection, data preprocessing and analysis, *Epigenomics* 7, 813–828, 2015.
4. Sibbritt, T., Patel, H.R., and Preiss, T., Mapping and significance of the mRNA methylome, *Wiley Interdiscip. Rev. RNA* 4, 297–422, 2013.
5. Dominissini, D., Nachtergaele, S., Moshitch-Moshkovitz, S., et al., The dynamic N^1-methyladenosine methylome in eukaryotic messenger RNA, *Nature* 530, 441–446, 2016.
6. Carlson, S.M., and Gonzani, O., Emerging technologies to map the protein methylome, *J. Mol. Biol.* 426, 3350–3362, 2014.
7. Plank, M., Fischer, R., Geoghegan, V., et al., Expanding the yeast protein arginine methylome, *Proteomics* 15, 3232–3243, 2015.
8. Cheng, X., Structure and function of DNA methyltransferases, *Annu. Rev. Biophys. Biomol. Struct.* 24, 293–318, 1995.
9. Lyko, F., The DNA methyltransferase family: A versatile toolkit for epigenetic regulation, *Nature Rev. Genetics* 19, 81–92, 2018.
10. Haag, S., Sloan, K.E., Höbartner, C., and Bohnsack, M.T., *In Vitro* RNA methyltransferase activity, *Methods Mol. Biol.* 1562, 259–268, 2017.
11. Faines, P.Ø., Jakobsson, M.E., Davydova, E., Ho, A., and Malecki, J., Protein lysine methylation by seven-β-strand methyltransferases, *Biochem. J.* 473, 1995–2009, 2016.
12. Wolf, S.S., The protein arginine methyltransferase family: An update about function, new perspectives and the physiological role in humans, *Cell. Mol. Life Sci.* 66, 2109–2121, 2009.
13. Wang, Y., Hu, W., and Yuan, Y., Protein arginine methyltransferase 5 (PRMT5) as an anticancer target and its inhibitor discovery, *J. Med. Chem.* 61, 9439–9441, 2018.
14. Wang, R., and Luo, M., A journey toward biorthogonal profiling of protein methylation inside living cells, *Curr. Opin. Chem. Biol.* 17, 729–737, 2013.
15. Tost, J., DNA methylation. Introduction to the biology and the disease associated changes as a biomarker, in *DNA Methylation Methods and Protocols*, 2nd edn., ed. J. Tost, Chapter 1, pp. 3–20, Humana/Springer, New York, 2009.
16. Hamdane, D., Grosjean, H., and Fontecave, M., Flavin-dependent methylation of RNAs: Complex chemistry for a simple modification, *J. Mol. Biol.* 428, 4867–4881, 2016.
17. Deen, J., Vranken, C., Leen, V., et al., Methyltransferase-directed labeling of biomolecules and its applications, *Angew. Chem. Int. Ed.* 36, 5182–5200, 2017.

MICELLES

Micelles are a heterogeneous group of small (nanoscale) particles composed of individual molecules which can be considered an aggregate. A formal definition of a micelle is An individual particle of the dispersed phase of a colloidal system; *spec.* a spherical array formed by certain amphipathic molecules (e.g. soaps), especially one formed in aqueous solution in which the hydrophobic region of the array is enclosed by a polar shell.[1] A micelle is similar to but distinguished from a liposome.[2] One definition of liposome is a natural globule of fat or lipid suspended in the cytoplasm of a cell[1] and there are early papers which use this definition.[3] However, the definition rapidly moved to A minute artificial globule consisting of one or more layers of phospholipid enclosing an aqueous core, used experimentally as a model for biological membranes.[1] Current use would define liposomes as synthetic analogues of natural membranes with unilamellar or multilamellar structure.[4] Liposomes are generally composed of lipids, although there is work on the modification of these structures for improved performance.[5–8] In biochemistry and molecular biology, the term micelle was used in reference to a simple structure composed of polar lipids in aqueous solution forming an amphipathic layer with the polar groups directed toward solvent and non-polar groups clustered toward the interior.[9,10] However, a micelle can be composed of proteins or other organic materials.[11] Micelles derived from casein polymers have been extensively studies because of their presence in milk.[12–14] The term critical micellar concentration (CMC) defines the concentration when and amphipathic substance such as a fatty acid would transition from solution phase to micelle.[15,16] Micelles are used for drug delivery.[17,18] Micelles of various compositions are used to remove pollutants from soil (soil-washing).[19] See also **liposomes, nanotechnology**.

1. *Oxford English Dictionary*, Oxford University Press, Oxford, UK, 2019.
2. Peer, D., Karp, J.M., Hong, S., et al., Nanocarriers as an emerging platform for cancer therapy, *Nat. Nanotechnol.* 2, 751–760, 2007.
3. Angel, A., Studies on the compartmentalization of lipid in adipose cells. I: Subcellular distribution, composition, and transport of newly synthesized lipid: Liposomes, *J. Lipid. Res.* 11, 420–432, 1970.
4. *Liposomes Methods and Protocols*, ed. S.C. Basu and M. Basu, Humana Press, Totowa, NJ, 2002.
5. Murata, M., Yonamine, T., Tanaka, S., et al., Surface modification of liposomes using polymer-wheat germ agglutinin conjugates to improve the absorption of peptide drugs by pulmonary administration, *J. Pharm. Sci.* 102, 1281–1289, 2013.
6. Johannssen, T., and Lependies, B., Glycan-based cell targeting to modulate immune responses, *Trends. Biotechnol.* 35, 334–346, 2017.
7. Hameed, S., Bhattarai, P., and Sai, Z., Cerasomes and bicelles: Hybrid bilayered nanostructures with silica-like surface in cancer theranostics, *Front. Chem.* 6, 127, 2018.
8. *Liposome Technology*, ed. G. Gregoriadis, CRC Press/Taylor & Francis Group, Boca Raton, FL, 2018.
9. Hartley, G.S., *Aqueous Solutions of Paraffin-Chain Salts: A Study in Micelle Formation*, Hermann and cie, Paris, 1936.
10. Mukerjee, P., *Critical Micelle Concentrations of Aqueous Surfactant Systems*, US National Bureau of Standards, US Government Printing Office, Washington, DC, 1971.
11. Wang, J., Li, S., Han, Y., et al., Poly(ethylene glycol)-polylactide micelles for cancer therapy, *Front. Pharmacol.* 9, 202, 2018.
12. Bloomfield, V.A., and Mead, R.J., Jr., Structure and stability of casein micelles, *J. Dairy Sci.* 58, 592–601, 1975.
13. Silva, N.F., Saint-Jalmes, A., de Carvalho, A.F., and Gaucheron, F., Development of casein microgels from cross-linking of casein micelles by genipen, *Langmuir* 30, 10167–10175, 2014.
14. Redwan, E.M., Xue, B., Almehdar, H.A., and Uversky, V.N., Disorder in milk proteins: Caseins, intrinsically disordered colloids, *Curr. Protein Pept. Sci.* 16, 228–242, 2015.
15. Klevens, H.B., The critical micelle concentration of anionic soap mixtures, *J. Chem. Phys.* 14, 742, 1946.
16. Corrin, M.L., and Harkins, W.D., Determination of the critical concentration for micelle formation in solutions of colloidal electrolytes by the spectral change of a dye, *J. Am. Chem. Soc.* 69, 679–683, 1947.
17. Aliabadi, H.M., and Lavasanifar, A., Polymeric micelles for drug delivery, *Expert Opin. Drug Deliv.* 3, 139–162, 2006.
18. Zhou, Q., Zhang, L., Yang, T., and Wu, H., Stimuli-responsive polymeric micelles for drug delivery and cancer therapy, *Int. J. Nanomedicine* 13, 2921–2942, 2018.
19. Shah, A., Shahzad, S., Munir, A., et al., Micelles as soil and water decontamination agents, *Chem. Rev.* 116, 6042–6074, 2016.

MICROARRAY

The term microarray refers to an analytical technology where probes of known (usually) composition are used to identify and quantify analytes (targets) in (usually) complex mixtures. The probe is usually attached by either covalent or noncovalent binding to a matrix. The matrix is frequently a modified glass slide with the probes printed onto the slide. A labeled sample then applied to the probe surface; frequently a fluorescent label is used for the signal from the sample bound to the probe.[1,2] The use of PCR to amplify the signal increases sensitivity.[3] The data from DNA microarrays (and other probes such as proteins) can be expressed in the form of a "heat map"[4] to show increased or decreased gene expression.[5] There is considerable interest in the use of microarray technology to develop the lab-on-a-chip.[6] There are systems where the target is placed on the microarray surface and analyzed with a labeled probe. This approach has seen most use with proteins as an approach is referred to as reverse-phase protein microarray.[7,8] Microarray assays are based on high density of probes on a surface. Microarrays have 200 spots or elements/cm^2 while a **macroarray** would have 20 spots or elements/cm^2.[9] A microarray spot may have diameter of 6 mm and, in the case of small molecule synthesis such as an aptamer, contains 50–100 nmol compound while a microarray spot has a diameter of 0.1 mm and contains 50–100 pmols compound.[10] Macroarrays have been used to establish conditions for reactions in microarrays.[11] As should be obvious from the above, the term microarray is used most often in DNA microarray. The technology is based on the complementarity of DNA strands (molecular hybridization) as, for example, shown in the double helix.[12,13] DNA microarrays can process a very large number of samples so while the assay technology is relatively straightforward, although requiring robotics,[14,15] experimental design, and data analysis is a continuing challenge.[16–22] Microarray technology has been useful in the analysis of proteins.[23] Antibody or antibody fragments have been used as probes for protein microarray analysis and purified proteins have been used to screen for antibodies as for example with hybridoma supernatant fractions.[24] Reverse Phase Protein Microarray (RPPM) is the term used to describe the use of proteins as probes for microarrays.[25,26] Aptamers have been used in the protein microarrays[27,28] with SELEX (systematic evolution of ligands by exponential enrichment) for probe synthesis[29] which is a form of combinatorial chemistry[30] Peptide microarrays can be used for the assay/identification of proteolytic enzymes[31] and for the identification of epitopes.[32] Microarray technology can also be applied to the study of multiple tissue specimens with tissue microarrays where small tissue samples (0.5 mm) can be placed on glass slide.[33–36] Carbohydrates can also serve as a probe for the analysis of complex mixtures.[37]

1. Ramsey, G., DNA chips: State-of-the-art, *Nat. Biotechnol.* 16, 40–44, 1998.
2. Wagenknecht, H.A., Fluorescent DNA base modifications and substitutes: Multiple fluorophore labeling and the DETEQ concept, *Ann. N. Y. Acad. Sci.* 1130, 122–130, 2008.
3. Pierik, A., Boamfa, M., van Zelst, M., et al., Real time quantitative amplification detection on a microarray: Toward high multiplex quantitative PCR, *Lab. Chip.* 12, 1897–1902, 2012.
4. Dresen, I.M., Hüsing, J., Kruse, E., Boes, T., and Jöckel, K.H., Software packages for quantitative microarray-based gene expression analysis, *Curr. Pharm. Biotechnol.* 4, 417–437, 2003.
5. Fridley, K.M., Nair, R., and McDevitt, T.C., Differential expression of extracellular matrix and growth factors by embryoid bodies in hydrodynamic and static cultures, *Tissue Eng. Part C Methods* 20, 931–940, 2014.
6. Marzancola, M.G., Sedighi, A., and Li, P.C., DNA microarray-based diagnostics, *Methods Mol. Biol.* 1368, 161–178, 2016.
7. Tibes, R., Qiu, Y., Lu, Y., et al., Reverse-phase protein array: Validation of a novel proteomic technology and utility for analysis of primary leukemia specimens and hematopoietic stem cells, *Mol. Cacner Ther.* 5, 2512–2521, 2006.
8. Masuda, M., and Yamada, T., Signaling pathway profiling by reverse-phase protein array for personalized cancer medicine, *Biochim. Biophys. Acta* 1854, 651–657, 2015.
9. Reimer, U., Reineke, U., and Schneiden-Mergener, J., Peptide arrays: From macro to micro, *Curr. Opin. Biotechnol.* 13, 315–329, 2002.
10. Blackwell, H.E., Hitting the SPOT: Small-molecule macroarrays advance combinatorial synthesis, *Curr. Opin. Chem. Biol.* 10, 203–212, 2006.
11. Stansfield, H.E., Kulczewski, B.P., Lyband, K.E., and Jamieson, E.R., Identifying protein interactions with metal-modified DNA using microarray technology, *J. Biol. Inorg. Chem.* 14, 193–199, 2009.
12. Southern, E.M., DNA microarrays History and Overview, in *DNA Assays Methods and Protocols*, ed. J.B. Rampal, Chapter 1, pp. 1–15, Humana Press, Totowa, NJ, 2001.
13. Pirrung, M.C., and Southern, E.M., The genesis of microarrays, *Biochem. Mol. Biol. Education* 42, 106–113, 2014.
14. Auburn, R.P., Kreil, D.P., Meadows, L.A., et al., Robotic spotting of cDNA and oligonucleotide microarrays, *Trends Biotechnol.* 23, 374–279, 2005.
15. Ahmad, H., Sutherland, A., Shin, Y.S., et al., A robotics platform for automated batch fabrication of high density, microfluidics-based DNA microarrays, with applications to single cell, multiplex assays of secreted proteins, *Rev. Sci. Instrum.* 82(9), 094301, 2011.
16. Brazma, A., Hingamp, P., Quackenbush, J., et al., Minimum information about a microarray experiment (MIAME)-towards standards for microarray data, *Nat. Genet.* 29, 365–371, 2001.
17. Hackett, J.L., and Lesko, L.J., Microarray data—The US FDA, industry and academia, *Nature* 21, 742–743, 2003.
18. Mehta, T., Tanik, M., and Allison, D.B., Towards some epistemological foundations of statistical methods for high-dimensional biology, *Nat. Genet.* 36, 943–947, 2004.
19. Gorreta, F., Barzaghi, D., Van Meter, A.J., Chandhoke, V., and Del Diacco, L., Development of a new standard for microarray experiments, *Biotechniques* 36, 1002–1009, 2004.

20. Knudsen, S., *Guide to Analysis of DNA Microarray Data*, Wiley-Liss, Hoboken, NJ, 2004.

21. Li, S., and Li, D., *DNA Microarray Technology and Data Analysis in Cancer Research*, World Scientific Publisher, Singapore, 2008.

22. Amaratunga, D., Carbrera, J., and Shkedy, Z., *Exploration and Analysis of DNA Microarray and Other High-Dimensional Data*, 2nd edn., Wiley, Hoboken, NJ, 2014.

23. Windren, C., Antibody-based proteomics, *Adv. Exp. Med. Biol.* 926, 163–179, 2016.

24. Stoevesandt, O., and Taussig, M.J., Affinity proteomics: The role of specific binding reagents in human proteome analysis, *Expert Rev. Proteomics* 9, 401–414, 2012.

25. Wulfkuhle, J.D., Aquino, J.A., Calvert, V.S., et al., Signal pathway profiling of ovarian cancer from human tissue specimens using revers-phase protein microarrays, *Proteomics* 3, 2085–2090, 2003.

26. Pawlak, M., and Carragher, N.O., Reverse phase protein arrays elucidate mechanisms-of-action and phenotypic response in 2D and 3D models, *Drug Discov. Today. Technol.* 23, 7–16, 2017.

27. Witt, M., Walter, J.G., and Stahl, F., Aptamer microarrays-Current status and future prospects, *Microarrays* (Basal) 4, 115–132, 2015.

28. Albaba, D., Soomro, S., and Mohan, C., Aptamer-based screens of human body fluidsfo biomarkers, *Microarrays* (Basel) 4, 424–431, 2015.

29. Liu, X., Li, H., Jia, W., Chen, Z., and Xu, D., Selection of aptamers based on a protein microarray integrated with a microfluidic chip, *Lab. Chip.* 17, 178–185, 2016.

30. Lam, K.S., and Renil, M., From combinatorial chemistry to chemical microarray, *Curr. Opin. Chem. Biol.* 6, 353–358, 2002.

31. Lei, Z., Chen, H., Zhang, H., et al., Evaluation of matrix metalloproteinase inhibition by peptide microarray-based fluorescence assay on polymer brush substrate and in vivo assessment, *ACS Appld. Mater. Interfaces* 9, 44241–44250, 2017.

32. Richer, J., Johnston, S.A., and Stafford, P., Epitope identification from fixed-complexity random-sequenecy peptide microarrays, *Mol. Cell. Proteomics* 14, 136–147, 2015.

33. Rimm, D.L., Camp, R.L, Charette, L.A., et al., Tissue microarray: A new technology for amplification of tissue resources, *Cancer J.* 7, 24–31, 2001.

34. Bubendorf, L., Nocito, A., Moch, K., and Sauter, G., Tissue microarray (TMA) technology: Miniaturized pathology archives for high-throughput in situ studies, *J. Pathol.* 195, 72–79, 2001.

35. Fedor, H.L., and De Marzo, A.M., Practical methods for tissue microarray construction, *Methods Mol. Biol.* 103, 89–101, 2005.

36. Dancau, A.-M., Simon, R., Mirlacher, M., and Sauter, G., Tissue microarrays, in *Methods Mol. Biol.* 1381 (*Cancer Gene Profiling. Methods and Protocols.* ed. R. Grützmann and C.P Ilarsky), Chapter 3, pp. 53–65, Springer Science-Business Media, New York, 2016.

37. Zone, C., Venot, A., Li, X., et al., Heparan sulfate microarray reveals that heparan sulfate-protein binding exhibits different ligand requirements, *J. Am. Chem. Soc.* 139, 9534–9543, 2017.

MICRODIALYSIS

The term microanalysis refers to two different applications both of which require the use of a semipermeable membrane. The oldest application is the dialysis of small (micro) volumes of material.[1,2] While there are still some novel applications of microdialysis to study proteins,[3] the majority of current application of microdialysis refers to a process for sampling low-molecular weight metabolites in the extracellular space of tissues. The technique was developed to measure metabolites in brain tissue.[4,5] This technique is used for the study of tissue metabolism and pharmacokinetic studies. Microdialysis is accomplished through the use of a probe constructed as a concentric tube is implanted into a tissue and a perfusion fluid (a physiological solution such as Hank's balanced salt solution) enters through an inner tube flowing toward the distal end and, entering the space between the inner tube and the outer dialysis membrane flow back toward the proximal end of the probe. Dialysis takes place during the passage of fluid toward the proximal end and the exiting fluid is sampled for the analyte in question. It is viewed a noninvasive method of evaluated tissue metabolism.[6–9] The major use of microdialysis is in the study of pharmaceuticals.[10–13]

1. Englander, S.W., and Crowe, D., Rapid microdialysis and hydrogen exchange, *Anal. Biochem.* 12, 579–584, 1965.

2. Brand, P.H., and Stansbury, R., Improved microdialysis technique, *Anal. Biochem.* 94, 109–111, 1979.

3. Sun, S., Long, C., Tao, C., Meng, S., and Deng, B., Ultrasonic microdialysis coupled with capillary electrophoresis electrochemiluminescence study the interaction between trimetazidine dihydrochloride and human serum albumin, *Anal. Chim. Acta* 851, 37–42, 2014.

4. Zetterström, T., Vernet, U., Ungerstedt, U., et al., Purine levels in the intact rat brain studies with an implanted perfused hollow fibre, *Neurosci. Lett.* 29, 111–115, 1982.

5. Tossman, U., Eriksson, S., Delin., A., et al., Brain amino acids measured by intracerebral dialysis in portacaval shunted rats, *J. Neurochem.* 41, 1046–1051, 1983.

6. Lonnroth, P., and Smith, U., Microdialysis—A novel technique for clinical investigations, *J. Intern. Med.* 227, 295–300, 1990.

7. Ungerstedt, U., Microdialysis—Principles and applications for studies in animals and man, *J. Intern. Med.* 230, 365–373, 1991.

8. Thorell, A., Nygren, J., and Ljungqvist, O., Microdialysis method for measuring human metabolism, *Curr. Opin. Clin. Nutr. Metab. Care* 7, 515–52, 2004.

9. Abrahamsson, P., and Winso, O., An assessment of calibration and performance of the microdialysis system, *J. Pharm. Biomed. Anal.* 39, 730–734, 2005.

10. Hocht, C., Opezzo, J.A., and Taira, C.A., Microdialysis in drug discovery, *Curr. Drug. Discov. Technol.* 1, 269– 285, 2004.

11. Rooyackeres, O., Cano-Cebriaqn, M.J., Zornoza, T., Polache, A., and Granero, L., Quantitative in vivo microdialysis in pharmacokinetic studies: Some reminders, *Curr. Drug. Metab.* 6, 83–90, 2005.

12. *Applications of Microdialysis in Pharmaceutical Science*, ed. T.-U. Tsai, Wiley, Hoboken, NJ, 2011.

13. *Microdialysis in Drug Development*, ed. M. Miller, Springer Science-Business, New York, 2013.

MICROSATELLITE

A microsatellite is a linear sequence of DNA, which contains a variable number of short (1–6 bp) oligonucleotide repeats (simple sequence).[1,2] A microsatellite is also sometimes referred to as a simple sequence repeat.[3] A simple sequence length refers to sequences within microsatellite which can show polymorphism.[4] Together with minisatellites, microsatellites are also referred to as variable number of tandem repeats (VNTR).[5] Microsatellites are used for genetic mapping and show variability in oncological disorders. These sites are used for genetic mapping.[6] Microsatellite instability is a biomarker in oncological disorders.[7] Changes are measured by simple sequence length polymorphisms.[8] PCR is used in the analysis of microsatellite instability.[9,10]

1. Tautz, D., and Schlotterer, C., Simple sequences, *Curr. Opin. Genet. Dev.* 4, 832–837, 1994; Adams, R.H., Blackmon, H., Reyes-Velasco, J., et al., Microsatellite landscape evolutionary dynamics across 450 million years of vertebrate genome evolution, *Genome* 59, 295–310, 2016.

2. Adams, R.H., Blackmon, H., Reyes-Velasco, J., et al., Microsatellite landscape evolutionary dynamics across 450 million years of vertebrate genome evolution, *Genome*. 59, 295–310, 2016.

3. Mishima, K., Hirao, T., Watanabe, A., and Takata, K., Isolation and characterization of microsatellite markers for *Thujopsis dolabrata* var. *hondai* (Cupressaceae), *Am. J. Bot.* 99, e317–e319, 2012.

4. Panaud, O., Chen, X., and McCouch, S.R., Development of microsatellite markers and characterization of simple sequence length polymorphism (SSLP) in rice (*Oryza sativa* L.), *Mol. Gen. Genet.* 252, 598–607, 1996.

5. Gemayel, R., Vinces, M.D., Legendre, M., and Verstrepen, K.J., Variable tandem repeats accelerate evolution of coding and regulatory sequences, *Annu. Rev. Genet.* 44, 445–477, 2010.

6. Grover, A., and Sharma, P.C., Development and use of molecular markers: Past and present, *Crit. Rev. Biotechnol.* 36, 290–302, 2016.

7. Dudley, J.C., Lin, M.T., Le, D.T., and Eschleman, J.R., Microsatellite instability as a biomarker for PD-1 blockade, *Clin. Cancer Res.* 22, 813–820, 2016.

8. Hosseinzdeh-Colagar, A., Haghighatnia, J.M., Amiri, Z., Mohadjerani, M., and Tafrihi, M., Microsatellite (SSR) amplification by PCR usually led to polymorphic bands: Evidence which shows replication slippage occurs in extend or nascent DNA strands, *Mol. Biol. Res. Commun.* 5, 167–174, 2016.

9. Elfimova, N., Amer, W., and Odenthal, M., Analysis of microsatellite instability by microfluidic-based electrophoresis, *Methods Mol. Biol.* 919, 287–296, 2013.

10. Dandelot, E., and Gourdon, G., The flash-small-pool PCR: How to transform blotting and numerous hybridization steps into a simple denatured PCR, *BioTechniques* 64, 262–265, 2018.

MINICOLLAGEN

Minicollagens are a family of small collagens (14–16 gly-x-y repeats flanked by amino-terminal and carboxyl-terminal stretches of proline residues with repeated cysteine residues) universally in the nematocysts in cnidarians, sp. *cnidaria*.[1] Nematocysts are unique "tubules" that are ejected with great force (approximately 40,000 g) from cnidarians as a defense mechanism.[2] Minicollagens have the characteristic triple-helical structure associated with most collagens. The monomer form of minicollagen ii *Hydra* contain internal disulfide bonds in the amino- and carboxyl-terminal regions which undergo an exchange reaction to form a disulfide-like triple helix.[3,4] Minicollagen in combination with a 90 kDa glycoprotein, NOWA (Nematocyst outer wall antigen)[5] form the matrix for the nematocyst.[6–8] It is of interest that nematocyst protein is not soluble in SDS but is soluble in dithiothreitol. The unique properties of minicollagens are of interest in biotechnology.[9,10]

1. Kurz, E.M., Holstein, T.W., Petri, B.M., Engel, J., and David, C.N., Mini-collagens in Hydra nematocysts, *J. Cell Biol.* 114, 1159–1169, 1991.

2. Holstein, T., and Tardent, P., An ultrahigh-speed analysis of exocytosis: Nematocyst discharge, *Science* 223, 830–833, 1984.

3. Engel, U., Pertz, O., Fauser, C., et al., A switch in disulfide linkage during minicollagen assembly in *Hydro* nematocysts, *EMBO J.* 20, 3063–3073, 2001.

4. Tursch, A., Mercadante, D., Tennigkeit, J., Gräter, F., and Özbek, S., Minicollagen cysteine-rich domains encode distinct of polymerization to form stable nematocyst capsules, *Sci. Rep.* 6, 25709, 2016.

5. Engel, U., Özbek, S., Streigtwolf-Engel, R., et al., Nowa, a novel protein with minicollagen Cys-rich domains, is involved in nematocyst formation in *Hydra*, *J. Cell Sci.* 115, 3923–3934, 2002.

6. Özbek, S., Pokidysheva, E., Schwager, M., et al., The glycoprotein NOWA and minicollagens are part of a disulfide-linked polymer that forms the cnidarian nematocyst wall, *J. Biol. Chem.* 279, 52016–52023, 2004.

7. David, C.N., Özbek, S., Adamczyk, P., et al., Evolution of complex structures: Minicollagens shape the cnidarians nematocyst, *Trends Genet.* 24, 431–438, 2008.

8. Özbek, S., The cnidarian nematocyst: A miniature extracellular matrix with a secretory vesicle, *Protoplasma* 248, 635–640, 2011.

9. Weiher, F., Schatz, M., Steinem, C., and Geyer, A., Silica precipitation by synthesis minicollagens, *Biomacromolecules* 14, 683–687, 2013.

10. Yang, Y.I., Jung, D., Yang, B., Hwang, B.H., and Cha, H.J., Aquatic proteins with repetitive motifs provide insights to bioengineering of novel biomaterials, *Biotechnol. J.* 9, 1493–1502, 2014.

MINIPROTEIN

A miniprotein can be defined as the smallest linear sequence of amino acids which can independently fold into a unique three-dimensional structure thus differing from a peptide[1] based on work when the binding domain of protein A was reduced to the smallest functional form.[2] The size of miniproteins is approximately 40 amino acid residues.[3] There are some plant proteins which are described as miniproteins.[4] The carboxypeptidase inhibitor isolated by the Yellow Bell Pepper has a molecular weight of approximately 4 kDa; proteases inhibitors from other plant sources such as the lima bean are larger (9 kDa) but still small.[5] While the bulk of the work on miniproteins has focused on studies on protein conformation and folding, there has been work on synthesizing small proteins with biological activity.[6–8]

1. DeGrado, W.F., and Sosnick, T.R., Protein minimization: Downsizing through mutation, *Proc. Natl. Acad. Sci. USA* 93, 5680–5681, 1996.

2. Braisted, A.C., and Wells, J.A., Minimizing a binding domain from protein A, *Proc. Natl. Acad. Sci. USA* 93, 5688–5692, 1996.

3. Baker, E.G., Bartlett, G.J., Goff, K.L.P., and Woolfson, D.N., Miniprotein design: Past, present, and prospects, *Accts. Chem. Res.* 50, 2085–2092, 2017.

4. Cotabarren, J., Tellechea, M.E., Avilés, F.X., and Rivera, J.L., Biochemical characterization of the YBPCI miniprotein, the first carboxypeptidase inhibitor isolated from yellow bell pepper (*Capsicum annuum* L.), a novel contribution to the knowledge of miniproteins stability, *Protein Expr. Purif.* 144, 55–61, 2018.

5. Birk, Y., Lima bean trypsin inhibitors, *Mehods Enzymol.* 45, 707–709, 1976.

6. Vita, C., Vizzavona, J., Drakopoulou, E., Zinn-Justin, S., Gilquin, B., and Ménez, A., Novel miniproteins engineered by the transfer of active sites to small nature scaffolds, *Biopolymers* 47, 93–100, 1998.

7. Shen, X., Bogers, W.M., Yales, N.L., et al., Cross-linking of a CD4-mimetic miniprotein with HIV-1 Env gp140 alters kinetids and specificities of antibody responses against HIIV-1 Env in maques, *J. Virol.* 91, e00401–e00417, 2017.

8. Molinos-Albert, L.M., Bilbao, E., Agulló, L., et al., Proteoliposomal formulations of an HIV-1 gp41-based miniprotein elicit a lipid-dependent immunodominant response overlapping the 2F5 binding motif, *Sci. Rep.* 7, 40800, 2017.

MODULUS OF ELASTICITY

Elasticity is defined as the ability of a solid material to change its size and shape under the action of applied force but returns to its original shape when force is removed. An elastic material can be defined as a substance which changes shape in response to force without loss of energy (i.e. without breakage). A common example is the rubber band. A modulus is a numerical constant representing some properties of a substance, and equal to the ratio of a (usually mechanical) cause to the magnitude of its effect on the substance.[1] The modulus elasticity is the stress required to produce unit strain causing a change in length (Young's modulus) or a twist or shear (shear modulus) or a change volume (bulk modulus). In the case of Young' modulus, it is the force (applied load) per unit area/increase per unit length and, as with viscosity, the unit is the Pascal. Young's modulus is used frequently in biochemistry and biomechanics. Example of use of Young's modulus in biomechanics include the measurement of bone quality.[2,3] Young's modulus is also measured in collagen.[4–6] Young's modulus is a metric measured with atomic force microscopy to evaluate macromolecular structures.[7,8] **Pseudoelasticity** is term which was advanced to describe the response of biological tissues such as arteries.[9,10] The concept of pseudoelasticity is based on earlier observations that elasticity of living tissues is non-linear and the derived Young's modulus varied over a large range.[11] It is noted that tissue is anisotropic and does not meet the definition of an elastic body. **Shape memory alloys** have been described as being pseudoelastic.[12]

1. *Oxford English Dictionary,* Oxford University Press, Oxford, UK, 2019.

2. Rho, J.Y., Ashman, R.B., and Turner, C.H., Young's modulus of trabecular and cortical bone material: Ultrasonic and microtensile measurements, *J. Biomechanics* 26, 111–119, 1993.

3. Zhang, G., Deng, X., Guan, F., et al., The effect of storage time in saline solution on the material properties of cortical bone tissue, *Clin. Biomech.* 57, 56–66, 2018.

4. Manssor, N.A., Radzi, Z., Yahya, N.A., et al., Characteristics and Young's modulus of collagen fibrils from expanded skin using anisotropic controlled rate self-inflating tissue expander, *Skin Pharmocol.* 29, 55–62, 2016.

5. Ghanaeian, A., and Soheilifard, R., Mechanical elasticity of proline-rich and hydroxyproline-rich collagen-like triple-helices studied using steered molecular dynamics, *J. Mech. Behav. Biomed. Mater.* 86, 115–123, 2018.

6. Tang, M., Li, T., Pickering, E., et al., Steered molecular dynamics characterization of the elastic modulus and defomation mechanisms of single natural tropocollagen molecules, *J. Mech. Behav. Biomed. Mater.* 86, 359–367, 2018.

7. Takeda, S., Sakurai, T., Hui, S.-P., Fuda, H., and Chiba, H., Effects of enzymes on elastic modulus of low-density lipoproteins were investigated using atomic force microscopy, *Biochem. Biophys. Res. Commun.* 501, 607–611, 2018.

8. Dumitru, A.C., Conrard, L., Giudice, C.L., et al., High-resolution mapping and recognition of lipid domains using AFM with toxin-derivatized probes, *Chem. Commun.* 54, 6903, 2018.

9. Fung, Y.C., Fronek, K., and Patitucci, P., Pseudoelasticity of arteries and the choice of its mathematic expression, *Am. J. Physiol.* 237, H620–H631, 1979.

10. Fung, Y.C., *Mechanical Properties of Livng Tissues*, 2nd edn., Springer-Verlag, New York, 1993.

11. Fung, Y.C.B., Elasticity of soft tissue in simple elongation, *Am. J. Physiol.* 213, 1532–1544, 1967.

12. Pittaccio, S., Garavaglia, L., Ceriotti, C., and Passaretti, F., Applications of shape memory alloys for neurology and neuromuscular rehabilitation, *J. Funct. Biomater.* 6, 328–344, 2015.

MOLECULAR BEACONS

A molecular beacon is a DNA probe which is a single chain loop and stem structure. A fluorophore at the 5′-terminus is in proximity to a fluorescence quencher at the 3′-terminus is moved as shown below on the binding of the probe to a specific DNA or RNA sequence with an resulting increase in fluorescence.[1,2] The concept of the molecular beacon is related to fluorescence resonance energy transfer (FRET) where the signal of a fluorophore is altered by a change in relationship to a quencher.[3] FRET probes, such as labeled aptamers, can be used to study nucleic acids.[4,5] There have been significant advances in the chemistry of the reporter groups[6] including the use of quantum dots.[7] There is an issue with getting the molecular probes into a cell because of the negative charge on the nucleic acid which can be solved by the presence of arginine oligopeptides on the quantum dot-based molecular beacon.

1. Tyagi, S., and Kramer, F.R., Molecular beacons: Probes that fluoresce upon hybridization, *Nat. Biotechnol.* 14, 303–308, 1998.

2. Piatek, A.S., Tyagi, S., Pol, A.C., et al., Molecular beacon sequence analysis for detecting drug resistance in *Mycobacterium tuberculosis*, *Nature Biotechnol.* 16, 359–363, 1998.

3. Okamoto, K., and Sako, Y., Recent advances in FRET for the study of protein interactions and dynamics, *Curr. Opin. Struct. Biol.* 46, 16–43, 2017.

4. Li, J., Cao, Z.C., Tang, Z., Wang, K., and Tan, W., Molecular beacons for protein-DNA interaction studies, *Methods Mol. Biol.* 429, 209–224, 2008.

5. Junager, N.P.L., Kongsted, J., and Astakhova, K. Revealing nucleic acid mutations using Förster resonance energy transfer-based probes, *Sensors* 16, 1173, 2016.

6. Huang, K., and Marti, A.A., Recent trends in molecular beacon design and applications, *Anal. Bioanal. Chem.* 402, 3091–3102, 2012.

7. Lee, J., Moon, S.U., Lee, Y.S., et al., Quantum dot-based molecular beacon to monitor intracellular microRNAs, *Sensors* 15, 12872–12883, 2015.

MOLECULAR CLOCK

A molecular clock is best known as a device for placing a timescale on evolutionary events using genetic data.[1–8] However, the term molecular clock is also used to describe the genes that drive circadian rhythm.[9]

1. Zuckerkandl, E., On the molecular evolutionary clock, *J. Mol. Evol.* 26, 34–46, 1987.

2. Easteal, S., A mammalian molecular clock, *Bioessays* 14, 415–419, 1992.

3. Seoighe, C., Turning the clock back on ancient genome duplication, *Curr. Opin. Genet. Dev.* 13, 636–643, 2003.

4. Freitas, C., Rodrigues, S., Saude, L., and Palmeirim, I., Running after the clock, *Int. J. Dev. Biol.* 49, 317–324, 2005.

5. Renner, S.S., Relaxed molecular clocks for dating historical plant dispersal events, *Trends Plant Sci.* 10, 550–558, 2005.

6. Ho, S.Y.W., and Larson, G., Molecular clocks: When times are a-changing, *Trends Genet.* 22, 79–83, 2006.

7. Ho, S.Y., Duchêne, S., Molecular-clock methods for estimating evolutionary rates and timescales, *Mol. Ecol.* 23, 5947–5965, 2014.

8. Harfmann, B.D., Schroder, E.A., and Esser, K.A., Circadian rhythms, the molecular clock, and skeletal muscle, *J. Biol. Rhythms* 30, 84–94, 2015.

9. Sunar, I.K., Yao, H., Sellix, M.T., and Rahman, I., Circadian molecular clock in lung pathophysiology, *Am. J. Physiol. Lung Cell. Mol. Physiol.* 309, L1056–L1075, 2015.

MONOCOT (MONOCOTYLEDON)

Monocots (Monocotyledonae) are a taxon of angiospermae, flowering plants which have embryos with only one cotyledon (one seed leaf)[1,2] and represent approximately one-quarter of the plant kingdom with diverse members of major interest in biotechnology. Many monocots are of great economic interest either as food or materials. Bamboo has great use as a structural material in many societies.[3] Early work showed that it was possible engineer monocots such as rice and maize to obtain transgenic plants with improved crop performance.[4] More recently gene editing technologies such as CRISPR/CAS9 have been used to obtain plants with improved performance but not containing foreign DNA.[5,6]

1. Dahlgren, R., Clifford, H.T., and Yeo, P.F., *The Families of the Monocotyledons Structure, Evolution, and Toxonomy*, Springer-Verlag, Berlin, Germany, 1985.
2. *Monocots Systematic and Evolution,* ed. K.L. Wilson and D.A. Morrison, CSIRO Publishing, Collingwood, Victoria, Australia, 2000.
3. Lewis, M.W., and Hake, S., Keep on growing: Building and patterning leaves in the grasses, *Curr. Opin. Plant. Biol.* 29, 80–86, 2016.
4. Shimamoto, K., Gene expression in transgenic monocots, *Curr. Opin. Biotechnol.* 5, 158–162, 1994.
5. Gerasimova, S.V., Khlestkina, E.K., Kocheto, A.V., and Shumny, V.K., Genome editing system CRISPR/CAS9 and peculiarties of its application in monocots, *Russian J. Plant Physiol.* 64, 141–165, 2017.
6. Van Eck, J., Genome editing and plant transformation of solanaceous food crops, *Curr. Opin. Biotechnol.* 49, 35–41, 2018.

MONOCYTE

Monocytes (Mo) are a heterogeneous population of white blood cells (leukocytes)[1] which are the canonical precursors to tissue macrophages (Mø)[2-4] and dendritic cells (DC).[5,6] Monocytes circulate in the blood and migrate to the tissues where they become macrophages.[7] The transition of monocyte to macrophage can affected by recombinant human macrophage colony-stimulating factor.[8] Monocytes and macrophages may also be derived from human pluripotent stem cells.[9] Monocytes may also differentiate into osteoclasts.[9,10] There are studies suggesting that monocytes can transform into stem cells.[11,12] There is also evidence showing that monocytes can be transformed into endothelial cells.[13] Monocytes are considered to be peripheral blood mononuclear cells (PBMCs) together with B cell, NK (natural killer) cells, T cells, and plasmacytoid dendritic cells.[14] PBMCs have been shown enhance wound healing.[15-17]

1. Terry, R.L., and Miller, S.D., Molecular control of monocyte development, *Cell. Immunol.* 291, 16–21, 2014.
2. Bobryshev, Y.V., Monocyte recruitment and foam cell formation in atherosclerosis, *Micron* 37, 208–222, 2006.
3. Cathelin, S., Rébe, C., Haddaoui, L., et al., Identification of proteins cleaved downstream of caspases activation in monocytes undergoing macrophage differentiation, *J. Biol. Chem.* 281, 17779–17788, 2006.
4. Gordan, S., Macrophages and phagocytosis, in *Fundamental Immunology*, 6th edn., ed. W. Paul, Chapter 18, pp. 547–569, Wolters Kluwer Health/ Lippincott Williams & Wilkins, Philadelphia, PA, 2008.
5. Geissmann, F., Auffray, C., Palframan, R., et al., Blood monocytes: Distinct subsets, how they relate to dendritic cells, and their possible roles in the regulation of T-cell responses, *Immunol. Cell Biol.* 86, 398–408, 2008.
6. Geissman, F., Manz, M.G., Jung, S., et al., Development of monocytes, macrophages, and dendritic cells, *Science* 327, 656–661, 2010.
7. Bain, C.C., and Mowat, A.M., The monocyte-macrophage axis in the intestine, *Cell. Immunol.* 291, 41–48, 2014.
8. Wallner, S., Grandi, M., Konovalova, T., et al., Monocyte to macrophage differentiation goes along with modulation of the plasmalogen pattern through transcriptional regulation, *PLoS One* 9(4), e94102, 2014.
9. van Wilgenburg, B., Browne, C., Vowles, J., and Cowley, S.A., Efficient, long term production of monocyte-derived macrophages from human pluripotent stem cells under partially defined and fully-defined conditions, *PLoS One* 8(8), e71098, 2013.
10. Zhou, Y., Deng, H.W., and Shen, H., Circulating monocytes: An appropriate model for bone-related study, *Osteoporos Int.* 26, 2561–2572, 2015.
11. Zhao, Y., Glesne, D., and Huberman, E., A human peripheral blood monocyte-derived subset acts a pluripotenti stem cells, *Proc. Natl. Acad. Sci. USA* 100, 2426–2431, 2003.
12. Ungelfroren, H., Hyder, A., Schulze, M., et al., Peripheral blood monocytes as adult stem cells: Molecular characterization and improvements in culture conditions to enhance stem cell features and proliferative potential, *Stem Cells Int.* 2016, 7132751, 2016.
13. Arderiu, G., Espinosa, S., Peña, E., et al., Tissue factor variants induced monocyte transformation and trans-differentiation into endothelial-like cells, *J. Thromb. Haemost.* 15, 1689–1703, 2017.
14. Hornung, V., Rothenfusser, S., Britsch, S., et al., Quantitative expression of toll-like receptor 1–10 mRNA in cellular subsets of human peripheral blood mononuclear cells and sensitivity to CpG oligodeoxynucleotides, *J. Immunol.* 168, 4531–4537, 2002.
15. Hopper, N., Wardale, J., Brooks, R., et al., Peripheral blood mononuclear cells enhance cartilage repair in *in vivo* osteochondral defect model, *PLoS One* 10(8), e0133997, 2015.
16. Beer, L., Mildner, M., Gyongyöi, M., and Ankersmit, H.J., Peripheral blood mononuclear cell secretome for tissue repair, *Apoptosis* 21, 1336–1351, 2016.

17. Orlandi, C., Bondioli, E., Verturi, E., and Melandri, D., Preliminary observations of a new approach to tissue repair: Peripheral blood mononuclear cells in platelet-rich plasma injected into skin graft area, *Exp. Dermatol.* 27, 795–797, 2018.

MORPHOPROTEOMICS

Morphoproteomics employs the use of immunohisto-chemical techniques to study the various proteins in a tumor. Emphasis is placed on posttranslational modification and translocation of proteins which could be therapeutic targets.[1,2] There has been limited use of this term.

1. Brown, R.E., Morphoproteomic portrait of the mTOR pathway in mesenchymal chondrosarcoma, *Ann. Clin. Lab. Sci.* 34, 397–399, 2004.
2. Quesada, A.E., Nguyen, N.D., Rios, A., and Brown, R.E., Morphoproteomics identifies constitutive activation of the mTORC2/Akt and NF-κB pathways and expressions of IGF-R, Sir1, COX-2, and FASN in peripheral T-cell lymphomas: Pathogenetic implications and therapeutic options, *Int. J. Clin. Exp. Pathol.* 7, 8732–8739, 2014.

MUCUS/MUCINS

Mucus is a viscous biological fluid secretion containing water, ions, and proteins. Mucus is secreted by goblet cells,[1] specialized cells in the epithelia of the mucosal surfaces of intestinal tract, specialized cells in the epithelia of the mucosal surfaces of intestinal tract,[2,3] lungs,[4] cervix,[5] and other areas including the nasal passage. Mucus plays a protective role for the underlying mucosal surfaces.[6] Secretion of abnormal mucins has a role in the pathogenesis of cystic fibrosis.[7,8] The term mucin is used to describe a protein(s) which give the viscous properties of mucus secretions. There are a number of mucin genes which are responsible for the synthesis of both secreted and cell-bound mucins. Mucins are large with observed $M_r \geq 1000$ kDa and approaching 10000 kDa.[9] Mucins are glycoproteins with 50%–80% carbohydrate with oligosaccharide chains attached to serine and threonine residues. There has been some controversy over the shape of the mucin molecule but seem reasonable that is a random coil with an axial ratio greater than 100.[10,11] The high molecular weight and extended conformation account for the high viscosity of mucin which can be enhanced by the presence of other proteins[12] and other materials such as calcium ions.[13] Submaxilary gland secretion in the oral cavity defined as a mucous secretion which contains large amounts of mucin.[14,15] Mucins are encoded by the MUC gene in humans. There are 20+ MUC genes in humans.[16] Mucin may be secreted in a form that will polymerase or a form which will not polymerize. There is also membrane bound mucin which possesses a trans-membrane segment. Both membrane-bound mucin and secreted mucin contain large amounts of bound carbohydrate (50%–80% of total mass) present in chains of 2–20 monomer monosaccharide units bound to a protein of 100–500 kDa.[17] The membrane-bound mucin is a component of the glycocalyx on mucosal surfaces.[18] Mucins are characterized by high viscosity, high molecular weight ($\geq 10^6$), and a rigid structure.[19,20] Mucin has been reported to have catalytic activity.[21,22]

1. Knoop, K.A., and Newberry, R.D., Goblet cells: Multifaceted players in immunity at mucosal surfaces, *Mucosal Immunol.* 11, 1551–1557, 2018.
2. Okumura, R., and Takeda. K., Maintenance of intestinal homeostasis by mucosal barriers, *Inflamm. Regen.* 38, 5, 2018.
3. Martens, E.C., Neurmann, M., and Desai, M.S., Interactions of commensal and pathogenic microorganisms with the intestinal mucosal barrier, *Nat. Rev. Microbiol.*, in press (doi:10.1038/s41579-018-0036-x), 2018.
4. Symmes, B.A., Stefanski, A.L., Magin, C.M., and Evans, C.M., Role of mucins in lung homeostasis: Regulated expression and biosynthesis in health and disease, *Biochem. Soc. Trans.* 46, 707–719, 2018.
5. Curlin, M., and Bursac, D., Cervical mucus: From biochemical structure to clinical implications, *Front. Biosci.* 5, 507–515, 2013.
6. Thorpe, D., Stringer, A., and Butlet, R., Chemotherapy-induced mucositis: The role of mucin secretion and regulation, and the enteric nervous system, *Neurotoxicology* 38, 101–105, 2013.
7. Venkatakrishnan, V., Packer, N.H., and Thaysen-Andersen, M., Host mucin glycosylation plays a role in bacterial adhesion in lungs of individuals with cystic fibrosis, *Expert Rev. Respir. Med.* 7, 553–576, 2013.
8. Roesch, E.A., Nichols, D.P., and Chmiel, J.F., Inflammation in cystic fibrosis: An update, *Pediatric Pulmonol.* 53(S3), S30–S50, 2018.
9. Gillis, R.B., Adams, G.G., Wolf, B., et al., Molecular weight distribution analysis by ultracentrifugation: Adaptation of a new approach for mucins, *Carbohyd. Polym.* 93, 178–183, 2013.
10. Forstner, J.F., Jabbal, I., and Forstner, G.G., Goblet cell mucin of rat small intestine. Chemical and physical characterization, *Canad. J. Biochem.* 51, 1154–1166, 1973.
11. Sheehan, J.K., and Carlsted, I., Hydrodynamic properties of human cervical-mucus glycoproteins in 6 M-guanidinium chloride, *Biochem. J.* 217, 93–101, 1984.
12. List, S.J., Findlay, B.P., Forstner, G.G., and Forstner, J.B., Enhancement of the viscosity of mucin by serum albumin, *Biochem. J.* 175, 565–571, 1978.

13. Raynal, B.D.E., Hardingham, T.E., Sheehan, J.K., and Thornton, D.J., Calcium-dependent protein interactions in MUC5B provide reversible cross-links in salivary mucus, *J. Biol. Chem.* 278, 28703–28710, 2003.

14. Veerman, E.C., van den Keybus, P.A., Valentijin-Benz, M., and Nieuw Amerongen, A.V., Isolation of different high-Mr mucin species of human whole saliva, *Biochem. J.* 283, 807–811, 1992.

15. Thornton, D.J., Khan, N., Mehrotra, B., et al., Salivary mucin MG1 is comprised almost entirely of different glycosylated forms of the MUC5B gene product, *Glycobiology* 9, 293–302, 1999.

16. Ma, J., Rubin, R.K., and Voyhow, J.A., Mucins, mucus and goblets cells, *Chest* 154, 169–176, 2018.

17. Basil, R., and Turner, B.S., The biology of mucin: Composition, synthesis and organization, *Adv. Drug. Deliv. Res.* 124, 3–15, 2018.

18. Corfield, A.P., Mucins: A biologically relevant glycan barrier in mucosal protection, *Biochim. Biophys. Acta* 1850, 236–252, 2015.

19. Bansil, R., Stanley, E., and LaMont, J.T., Mucin biophysics, *Annu. Rev. Physiol.* 57, 635–657, 1995.

20. Zappone, B., Patil, N.J., Madsen, J.B., Pakkanen, K.I., and Lee, S., Molecular structure and equilibrium forces of bovine submaxillary mucin adsorbed at a solid-liquid interface, *Langmuir* 31, 4524–4533, 2015.

21. Shraga, N., Belgorodsky, B., and Gozin, M., Organic reactions promoted by mucin glycoproteins, *J. Am. Chem. Soc.* 131, 12074–12075, 2009.

22. Fernandez-Hermida, Y., Grande, G., Menarguez, M., Astorri, A.L., and Azagra, R., Proteomic markers in cervical mucus, *Protein Pept. Lett.* 25, 463–471, 2018.

MÜLLERIAN INHIBITING SUBSTANCE (ANTI-MÜLLERNIAN HORMONE)

Müllerian Inhibiting Substance (MIS), better known today as anti-Müllernian hormone (AMH), is a 140 kDa homeodimeric peptide hormone[1] which is processed by limited proteolysis (cleavage between R427 and S428) to yield a 25 kDa fragment which is the biologically active form with homology to the TGF-β family.[2,3] AMH (Anti-Mullerian hormone is the preferred nomenclature) inhibits the development of uterus and fallopian tubes; the lack of AMH permits the development of these structures as well as other aspects of female reproductive system.[4] AMH has other functions during the female reproductive cycle in the adult.[5] Blood levels in males are high in males in childhood and decrease at puberty. AMH levels in females are low or absent at birth, variable until 4 years, then increasing until 8 years and remaining constant at levels similar to the male during the reproductive years decreasing after menopause.[6] AMH was observed to inhibit the growth of ovarian cancer cells.[7] There have efforts to use AMH as a therapeutic for ovarian cancer.[8–10] A MAB-based therapeutic directed against the AMH receptors is also be being evaluated.[11]

1. Lane, A.H., and Donahoe, P.K., New insights into Mullerian inhibiting substance and its mechanism of action, *J. Endocrinol.* 158, 1–6, 1998.

2. Cate, R.L., Mattallano, R.J., Hessions, C., et al., Isolation of the bovine and human genes for Müllerian inhibiting substance and expression of the human gene in animal cells, *Cell* 45, 685–698, 1986.

3. Pepinsky, R.B., Sinclair, L.K., Chow, E.P., et al., Proteolytic processing of Mullerian inhibiting substance produces a transforming growth factor-β-like fragment, *J. Biol. Chem.* 263, 18961–18964, 1988.

4. Shahrokhi, S.Z., Kazerouni, F., and Ghaffari, F., Anti-Müllerian hormone: Genetic and environmental effects, *Clin. Chim. Acta* 476, 123–129, 2018.

5. Dewailly, D., Andersen, C.Y., Balen, A., et al., The physiology and clinical utility of anti-Mullerian hormone in women, *Hum. Reprod. Update* 20, 370–385, 2014.

6. Wong, R.R.Y., Worley, M.J., Jr., Chung, T.K.H., and Wong, Y.F., An update on Müllerian-inhibiting substance: Its potential application against ovarian cancer, *Endocr. Relat. Cancer* 21, R227–R233, 2014.

7. Masiakos, P.T., MacLaughlin, D.T., Maheswaran, S., et al., Human ovarian cancer cell lines, and primary ascites cells express the human Mullerian inhibiting substance (MIS) type II receptor, bind, and are responsive to MIS, *Clin. Cancer Res.* 5, 3488–3499, 1999.

8. Kim, J.H., MacLaughlin, D.T., and Donahoe, P.K., Mullerian inhibitory substance/anti-Müllerian hormone: A novel treatment for gynecological tumors, *Obstet. Gynecol. Sci.* 57, 343–357, 2014.

9. Pépin, D., Sosulski, A., Zhang, L., et al., AAV9 delivering a modified human Mullerian inhibiting substance as a gene therapy in patient-derived xenografts of ovarian cancer, *Proc. Natl. Acad. Sci. USA* 112, E4418–E4427, 2015.

10. Kushnir, V.A., Seifer, D.B., Barad, D.H., Sen, A., and Gleicher, N., Potential therapeutic applications of human anti-Müllerian hormone (AMH) analogues in reproductive medicine, *J. Assist. Reprod. Genet.* 34, 1105–1113, 2017.

11. Bougherara, H., Némati, F., Nicolas, A., et al., The humanized anti-human AMHRII mAb 3C23K exerts an anti-tumor activity against human ovarian cancer through tumor-associated macrophages, *Oncotarget* 8, 99950–99965, 2017.

MYELOID PROGENITOR CELL (MYELOID STEM CELL)

There are a variety of cells in whole blood constituting 30%–50% of total volume with the major portion being erythrocytes (red blood cells) which are responsible for the transport of oxygen and carbon dioxide between the pulmonary system and the tissue beds. The remaining cells are comprised of platelets (derived from megakaryocytes) which participate in blood coagulation (hemostasis). Other cells include granulocytes, monocytes, T-cells, B-cells, and NK-cells.[1] There is a common progenitor cell in the bone marrow, the **hematopoietic cell**, gives rise to the **common lymphoid progenitor** and the **common myeloid progenitor** (myeloid progenitor cell). The lymphoid progenitor is the precursor of the T-cell, B-cell, and NK-cells. The myeloid progenitor cell is the precursor of granulocyte, macrophages, erythrocytes, megakaryocytes, and mast cells (myeloid/erythroid series) in a controlled process.[2–7] Granulocytes include neutrophils, eosinophils, and basophils.[8] Acute myelogenous leukemia is due to malignant transformation of the hematopoietic stem cell.[9] Ceramide accumulation has been shown to induce apoptosis in myeloid cells while a derivative from the hydrolysis of ceramide, sphingosine-1-phosphate, promotes survival in these cells[10] and other cells.[11] These observations have suggested the acid ceramidase as a therapeutic target in acute myeloid leukemia[12] and ulcerative colitis.[13]

1. Yoder, M.C., Overview of stem cell biology, in *Hematology Basic Principles and Practice*, 5th edn., ed. R. Hoffman, R.J. Benz, Jr., Shattil, S.J., Furie, B., Silberstein, L.E., McGlave, P., and Heslop, H., Churchill Livingstone/Elsevier, Philadelphia, PA, 2009.
2. Burgess, A.W., and Metcalf, D., The nature and action of granulocyte-macrophage colony stimulating factors, *Blood* 56, 947–958, 1980.
3. Islam, A., Haemopoietic stem cells: A new concept, *Leuk. Res.* 9, 1415–1432, 1985.
4. Cannistra, S.A., and Griffin, J.D., Regulation of the production and function of granulocytes and monocytes, *Semin. Hematol.* 25, 173–188, 1988.
5. McNiece, I.K., Langley, K.E., and Zsebo, K.M., Recombinant human stem cell factor synergises with GM-CSF, G-CSF, IL-3 and epo to stimulate human progenitor cells of the myeloid and erythroid lineages, *Exp. Hematol.* 19, 226–231, 1991.
6. Morstyn, G., Hematopiesis in 2010, in *Twenty Years of G-CSF Clinical and Non-Clinical Discoveries*, ed. G. Molineux, M. Foote, and T. Arvedson, pp. 1–12, Springer Basal AG, Cham, Switzerland, 2010.
7. Zhang, J., Li, L., Baldwin, A.S., Jr., Friedman, A.D., and Paz-Priel, I., Loss of IKKβ but not NF-κB p65 skews differentiation toward myeloid over erythroid commitment and increases myeloid progenitor self-renewal and functional long-term hematopoietic stem cells, *PLoS One* 10(6), e130441, 2015.
8. Edwards, S.L., *Biochemistry and Physiology of the Neutrophil*, Cambridge University Press, Cambridge, UK, 1994.
9. Estrov, Z., The leukemic stem cell, in *Acute Myelogenous Leukemia Genetics, Biology, and Therapy*, ed. L. Najarajan, pp. 1–17, Springer Science + Business, New York, 2010.
10. Jarvis, W.D., Fornari, F.A., Traylor, R.S., et al., Induction of apoptosis and potentiation of ceramide-mediated cytotoxicity by sphingoid bases in human myeloid leukemia cells, *J. Biol. Chem.* 271, 8275–8284, 1996.
11. Espaillat, M.P., Kew, R.R., and Obeid, L.M., Sphingolipids in neutrophil function and inflammatory responses: Mechanisms and implications for intestinal immunity and inflammation in ulcerative colitis, *Adv. Biol. Regul.* 63, 140–155, 2017.
12. Tam. S.-F., Pearson, J.M., Feith, D.J., and Loughran, T.P., Jr., The emergence of acid ceramidase as a therapeutic target for acute myeloid leukemia, *Expt. Opin. Therapeut. Targets* 21, 583–590, 2017.
13. Espaillat, M.P., Snider, A.J., Zui, Z., et al., Loss of acid ceramidase in myeloid cells suppresses intestinal neutrophil recruitment, *FASEB J.* 32, 2339–2353, 2018.

NANOFILTRATION

Nanofiltration is the filtration of small (nano) particles from solvent using a filter with extremely small pores (0.001 micron [μm]).[1] Nanofiltration is finer than ultrafiltration (0.01 μm) but not as fine as reverse osmosis (0.0001 micron [μm]).[2] Nanofiltration is used during the processing of protein biopharmaceuticals.[3–5] There is use of nanofiltration in the food industry.[6,7] The major use of nanofiltration is in the water processing industry.[8–12]

1. *Nanofiltration: Principles and applications*, ed. A.J. Shäfer, A.G. Fane, and T.D. Waite, Elsevier Advanced Technology, Oxford, UK, 2005.
2. Jye, L.W., and Ismail, A.F., *Nanofiltration Membranes. Synthesis, Characterization, and Applications*, CRC Press, Boca Raton, FL, 2016.
3. Burnouf, T., and Radosevich, M., Nanofiltration of plasma-derived biopharmaceutical products, *Haemophilia* 9, 24–37, 2003.
4. Brandstätter, H., Schulz, P., Polunic, I., et al., Purification and biochemical characterization of functional complement factor H from human plasma fractions, *Vox. Sang.* 103, 201–212, 2012.
5. Chou, M.L., Lin, L.T., Devos, D., and Burnouf, T., Nanofiltration to remove microparticles and decrease the thrombogenicity of plasma: In vitro feasibility assessment, *Transfusion* 55, 2433–2444, 2015.
6. Rossano, R., D'Elia, A., and Riccio, P., One-step separation from lactose: Recovery and purification of major cheese-whey proteins by hydroxyapatite—A flexible procedure suitable for small- and medium-scale preparations, *Protein Expr. Purif.* 21, 165–169, 2001.

7. Salehi, F., Current and future applications for nanofiltration technology in the food processing, *Food Bioproducts Processing* 92, 161–177, 2014.
8. Berg, P., Hagmeyer, G., and Gimbel, R., Removal of pesticides and other micropollutants by nanofiltration, *Desalinization* 113, 205–208, 1997.
9. Radjenovic, J., Petrovic, M., Ventura, F., and Barceló, D., Rejection of pharmaceuticals in nanofiltration and reverse osmosis membrane drinking water treatment, *Water Res.* 42, 3601–3610, 2008.
10. Mondal, S., Wickramasinghe, S.R., Produced water treatment by nanofiltration and reverse osmosis membranes, *J. Membrane Sci.* 322, 162–170, 2008.
11. Bergman, R., *Reverse Osmosis and Nanofiltration* (AWWA Manual M46), 2nd., edn., American Water Works Association, Denver, CO, 2010.
12. Cloete, T.E., *Nanotechnology in Water Treatment Applications*, Caister Academic, Norfolk, UK, 2010.

NANOG

Nanog is a homeodomain transcription factor which is found in undifferentiated embryonic stem cells and is considered important for the maintenance of pluripotency.[1-8] The name of the *NANOG* gene is derived from the Celtic term for the land of eternal youth, Tir-Na-Nog.[9] There are 11 *NANOG* pseudogenes (e.g. *NANOGP8*), ten retropseudogenes and one duplicate pseudogene.[10] The NANOG transcription factor is of importance in the development of tumor cells.[11-13] A CRISPR/Cas 9 knockout of NANOG and NANOGP8 decreased the malignant potential of prostate cancer cell lines.[14]

1. Mitsui, K., Tokuzawa, Y., Itoh, H., et al., The homeoprotein Nanog is required for maintenance of pluripotency in mouse epiblast and ES cells, *Cell* 113, 631–642, 2003.
2. Chambers, I., Colby, D., Robertson, M., et al., *Cell* 113, 643–655, 2003.
3. Oh, J.H., Do, H.J., Yang, H.M., et al., Identification of a putative transactivation domain in human Nanog, *Exp. Mol. Med.* 37, 250–254, 2005.
4. Yates, A., and Chambers, I., The homeodomain protein Nanog and pluripotency in mouse embryonic stem cells, *Biochem. Soc. Trans.* 33, 1518–1521, 2005.
5. Silva, J., Chambers, I., Pollard, S., and Smith, A., Nanog promotes transfer of pluripotency after cell fusion, *Nature* 441, 997–1001, 2006.
6. Saunders, A., Faiola, F., and Wang, J., Pursuing self-renewal and pluripotency with the stem cell factor Nanog, *Stem Cells* 31, 1227–1236, 2013.
7. Lopez Novo, C., and Rugg-Gunn, P., Crosstalk between pluripotency factors and higher-order chromatin organization, *Nucleus* 7, 447–452, 2016.
8. Blinka, S., and Rao, S., Nanog expression in embryonic stem cells—An ideal model system to dissect enhancer function, *Bioessays*, 39, 1700086, 2017.
9. Fairbanks, D.J., *Relics of Eden The Powerful Evidence of Evolution in DNA*, Prometheus Books, Amherst, New York, 2007.
10. Fairbanks, D.J., *Relics of Eden The Powerful Evidence of Evolution in DNA*, Appendix 1, The story of NANOG and its pseudogenes, pp. 177–188, Prometheus Books, Amherst, New York, 2007.
11. Iv Santaliz-Ruiz, L.E., Xie, X., Old, M., Teknos, T.N., and Pan, Q., Emerging role of nanog in tumorigenesis and cancer stem cells, *Int. J. Cancer* 135, 2741–2748, 2014.
12. Gawlik-Rzemieniewska, N., and Bednarek, I., The role of NANOG transcriptional factor in the development of malignant phenotype of cancer cells, *Cancer Biol. Ther.* 17, 1–10, 2016.
13. Wong, O.G.W., and Cheung, A.N.Y., Stem cell transcription factor NANOG in cancers—is eternal youth a curse? *Expt. Opin. Therapeut. Targets* 20, 407–417, 2016.
14. Kawamura, N., Nimura, K., Nagano, H., et al., CRISPR/Cas 9-mediated gene knockout of NANOG and NANOGP8 decreases the malignant potential of prostate cancer cells, *Oncotarget* 6, 22361–22374, 2015.

NAR PROMOTER

The Nar promoter is the promoter region of the *nar* operon which encodes nitrate reductase in *Escherichia coli*.[1] The promoter is generally only maximally induced under anaerobic conditions. It has been shown that the *nar* promoter in some strains of *Escherichia coli* can be induced under condition of very low oxygen tension in the presence of nitrate. This observation has been used to develop some useful processes for recombinant protein expression in *Escherichia coli*.[2-4] The *nar* promoter has been engineered to provide a unique oxygen sensor.[5]

1. Li, S.F., and DeMoss, J.A., Promoter region of the *nar* operon of *Escherichia coli*: Nucleotide sequence and transcription initiation signals, *J. Bacteriol.* 169, 4614–4620, 1987.
2. Han, S.J., Chang, H.N., and Lee, J., Characterization of an oxygen-dependent inducible promoter, the *nar* promoter of *Escherichia coli*, to utilize in metabolic engineering, *Biotechnol. Bioeng.* 72, 573–577, 2001.
3. Hwang, H.J., Kim, J.W., Ju, S.Y., Park, J.H., and Lee, P.C., Application of an oxygen-inducible *nar* promoter systems for production of biochemicals in *Escherichia coli*, *Biotechnol. Bioeng.* 114, 468–473, 2017.
4. Lalwani, M.A., Zhao, E.M., and Avelos, J.L., Current and future modalities of dynamic control in metabolic engineering, *Curr. Opin. Biotechnol.* 52, 56–65, 2018.
5. Garcia, J.R., Cha, H.J., Rao, G., Marten, M.R., and Bentley, W.E., Microbial *nar*-GFP cell sensors reveal oxygen limitations in highly aerated laboratory-scale fermenters, *Microb. Cell Fact.* 8, 6, 2009.

NANOTECHNOLOGY

Nanotechnology is the study of particles, devices, substances having physical dimensions of 1–100 nanometers (10^{-9} meter; 0.001–0.100 micrometers).[1–9] The goal is to take existing technologies which are used on the "macro" level to the "nano" level. For example, a conventional assay might use 50 μL; an assay in nanotechnology would use samples in nL (nanoliter) quantities.[10–12]

1. Wilson, M., *Nanotechnology: Basic Science and Emerging Technologies*, Chapman & Hall, Boca Raton, FL, 2002.
2. Poole, C.P., and Owens, F.J., *Introduction to Nanotechnology*, Wiley, Hoboken, NJ, 2003.
3. Di Ventra, M., and Evoy, S., *Introduction to Nanoscale Science and Technology*, Kluwer Academic, Boston, MA, 2004.
4. Bhushan, B., *Springer Handbook of Nanotechnology*, Springer, Berlin, 2004.
5. Tiwari, A., and Turner, A.P.F., ed., *Biosensors Nanotechnology*, John Wiley & Sons, Hoboken, NJ, 2014.
6. Wang, B., ed., *RNA Biotechnology*, CRC Press, Boca Raton, FL, 2014.
7. Khudyakov, Y.E., and Pumpens, P., ed., *Viral Nanotechnology*, CRC Press, Boca Raton, FL, 2016.
8. Stine, K.J., *Carbohydrate Nanotechnology*, John Wiley & Sons, Hoboken, NJ, 2016.
9. Fulekar, M.H., *Environmental Nanotechnology*, CRC Press, Boca Raton, FL, 2018.
10. Gielen, E., van Vliet, L., Koprowski, B.T., et al., A fully unsupervised compartment-on-demand platform for precise nanoliter assays of time-dependent steady-state enzyme kinetics and inhibition, *Anal. Chem.* 85, 4761–4769, 2013.
11. Avesar, J., Rosenfeld, D., Truman-Rosentsvit, M., et al., Rapid phenotypic antimicrobial susceptibility testing using nanoliter arrays, *Proc. Natl. Acad. Sci. USA* 114, E5787–E5795, 2017.
12. Duewer, D.L., Kline, M.C., Romsos, E.L., and Toman, B., Evaluating droplet digital PCR for the quantification of human genomic DNA: Converting copies per nanoliter to nanograms nuclear DNA per microliter, *Anal. Bioanal. Chem.* 410, 2879–2887, 2018.

NASCENT PEPTIDE EXIT TUNNEL

The nascent peptide exit tunnel is a "tunnel"/pore starting at the peptidyl transferase center on the ribosome and ending on the solvent side on the large ribosomal subunit.[1–7] The mode of action of macrolide antibiotics is based on the blockage of the nascent exit channel thus prevent the exit of some but not all proteins from the bacterial ribosome.[8,9] See also **macrolide**.

1. Gabashvili, I.S., Gregory, S.T., Valle, M., et al., The polypeptide tunnel system in the ribosome and its gating in erythromycin resistance mutants of L4 and L22, *Mol. Cell.* 8, 181–188, 2001.
2. Tenson, T., and Ehrenberg, M., Regulatory nascent peptides in the ribosomal tunnel, *Cell* 108, 591–594, 2002.
3. Jenni, S., and Ban, N., The chemistry of protein synthesis and voyage through the ribosomal tunnel, *Curr. Opin. Struct. Biol.* 13, 212–219, 2003.
4. Vimberg, V., Ziong, L., Bailey, M., Tenson, T., and Mankin, A., Peptide-mediated macrolide resistance reveals possible specific interactions in the nascent peptide exit tunnel, *Mol. Microbiol.* 54, 376–385, 2004.
5. Baram, D., and Yonath, A., From peptide-bond formation to cotranslational folding: Dynamic, regulatory and evolutionary aspects, *FEBS Lett.* 579, 948–94, 2005.
6. Egea, P.F., Stroud, R.M., and Walter, P., Targeting proteins to membranes: Structure of the signal recognition particle, *Curr. Opin. Struct. Biol.* 15, 213–220, 2005.
7. Markin, A.S., Nascent peptide in the "birth canal" of the ribosome, *Trends Biochem. Sci.* 31, 11–16, 2006.
8. Kannan, K., and Mankin, A.S., Macrolide antibiotics in the ribosome exit tunnel: Species-specific binding and action, *Ann. N. Y. Acad. Sci.* 12241, 33–47, 2011.
9. Vazquez-Laslop, N., and Mankin, A.S., How macrolide antibiotics work, *Trends Biochem. Sci.* 43, 668–684, 2018.

NEPHELOMETRY

Nephelometry is the measurement of electromagnetic wave scattering in a direction different from the direct path of the transmitted light; for example, electromagnetic energy scattered at a 90° angle from the incident radiation. The first nephelometer was developed in 1894[1] and the technique saw considerable subsequent use in analytical chemistry.[2] The term nephelometry is derived from the Greek word for cloud. Nephelometry is used for the measurement of protein complexes including immune complexes.[3–6] Nephelometry has had considerable use for the measurement of immune complexes in monoglobinopathies but is being supplanted by other technologies.[7,8] Nephelometry is the method of choice in the plasma fractionation industry to measure the concentration of specific immunoglobulin in intravenous immunoglobulin preparations.[9,10] Nephelometry is frequently compared with turbimetry.[11] While nephelometry measures reflected light (scattered light), turbimetry measure loss of light transmission through a sample.

1. Richards, T.W., A revision of the atomic weight of strontium first paper: The analysis of strontium bromide, *Proc. Amer. Acad. Arts Sciences* 30, 369–389, 1894.
2. Yoe, J.H., *Photometric Chemical Analysis (Colorimetry and Nephelometry)*, Volume II (Nephelometry), John Wiley & Sons, New York, 1929.
3. Deverilli, I., and Reeves, W.G., Light scattering and absorption—Developments in immunology, *J. Immunol. Methods* 38, 191–204, 1980.

4. Blackstock, R., In vitro methods for detection of circulating immune complexes and other solution protein-protein interactions, *Ann. Clin. Lab. Sci.* 11, 262–268, 1981.

5. Steinberg, K.K., Cooper, G.R., Graiser, S.R., and Rosseneu, M., Some considerations of methodology and standardization of apolipoprotein A-I immunoassays, *Clin. Chem.* 29, 415–426, 1983.

6. Price, C.P., Spencer, K., and Whicher, J., Light-scattering immunoassay of specific proteins: A review, *Ann. Clin. Biochem.* 20, 1–14, 1983.

7. Willrich, M.A., and Katzmann, J.A., Laboratory testing requirements for diagnosis and follow-up of multiple myeloma and related plasma cell dyscrasias, *Clin. Chem. Lab. Med.* 54, 907–919, 2016.

8. Keren, D.F., and Schroeder, L., Challenges of measuring monoclonal proteins in serum, *Clin. Chem. Lab. Med.* 54, 947–961, 2016.

9. Tuerlinckx, D., Florkin, B., Ferster, A., et al., Pneumococcal antibody levels in children with PID receiving immunoglobulin, *Pediatrics* 133, e154–e162, 2014.

10. Mieschner, S.M., Huber, T.M., Kühne, M., et al., In Vitro evaluation of cytomegalovirus-specific hyperimmune globulins vs. standard intravenous immunoglobins, *Vox Sang.* 109, 71–78, 2015.

11. Dominici, R., Luarachi, P., and Franzini, C., Measurement of C-reactive protein: Two high sensitivity methods compared, *J. Clin. Lab. Anal.* 18, 380–284, 2004.

NEXT-GENERATION SEQUENCING

Next-generation sequencing refers to nucleic acid (using DNA) sequencing methods[1–3] which do not use the original sequencing technologies based on work in the Sanger laboratory[4,5] or the Maxam-Gilbert method.[6] The next-generation technologies have the capability of massive parallel sequencing (referred to as deep sequencing) where the challenge is as much in data analysis as design and execution of the experiment.[7–11]

1. Hardwick, S.A., Deveson, I.W., and Mercer, T.R., Reference standards for next-generation sequencing, *Nature Reviews Genetics* 18, 473–484, 2017.

2. Slatko, B.E., Goodnea, A.F., and Ausubel, F.M., Overview of next generation sequencing technologies, *Curr. Prot. Mol. Biol* 122(1), e59, 2018.

3. Adamiak, J., Otelwska, A., Tafer, H., et al., First evaluation of the microbiome of built cultural heritage by using the Ion Torrent next generation sequencing platform, *Intl. Biodeterioration & Biodegradation* 131, 11–18, 2018.

4. Sanger, F., and Coulson, A.R., A rapid method for determining sequences in DNA by primed synthesis with DNA polymerase, *J. Mol. Biol.* 94, 441–448, 1975.

5. Sanger, F., Nicklen, S., and Coulson, A.R. DNA sequencing with chain-terminating inhibitors, *Proc. Natl. Acad. Sci. USA* 74, 5463–5467, 1977.

6. Maxam, A.M., and Gilbert, W., A new method for sequencing DNA, *Proc. Natl. Acad. Sci. USA* 74, 560–564, 1977.

7. Ping, K.-P., *Next-Generation Sequencing and Sequence Data Analysis*, Bentham Science, Sharjah, United Arab Emirates, 2015.

8. *Computational Methods for Next Generation Sequencing Data Analysis*, ed. I. Măndou and A. Zelikovsky, John Wiley & Sons, Hoboken, NJ, 2016.

9. *Applications for Next-Generation Sequencing Data: Techniques, Approaches, and Applications*, ed. M. Elloumi, Springer, Cham, Switzerland, 2017.

10. Wang, X., *Next-Generation Sequencing Data Analysis*, CRC Press/Taylor & Francis Group, Boca Raton, FL, 2016.

11. Sung, W.-K., Algorithms for Next-Generation Sequencing, CRC Press/Taylor & Francis Group, Boca Raton, FL, 2017.

NIOSOMES

Niosomes are vesicles (a vesicular system; an organogel) formulated from non-ionic surfactants such monoesters of sorbitan such as sorbitan monostearate (Span™ 60) and cholesterol[1,2] or Tween® 20[3] which is a more complex non-ionic surfactant. Cholesterol is included in the formulation to improve the stability of the noisome. Niosomes are similar to liposomes as both are (at minimum) a bilayer lipid and are developed as vehicles for drug delivery.[4–7] Niosomes differ from liposomes in having a hydrophilic head such sorbitan while liposomes have a polar head such as the phosphoglycerol moiety of phospholipids. See **liposomes**.

1. Myung, Y., Yeom, S., and Han, S., A niosomal bilayer of sorbitan monostearate in complex with flavones: A molecular dynamics simulation study, *J. Liposome Res.* 26, 336–344, 2016.

2. Moghassemi, S., Hadjizadeh, A., and Omidfar, K., Formulation and characterization of bovine serum albumin-loaded noisome, *AAPS PharmSciTech.* 18, 27–33, 2017.

3. Mandal, S., Banerjee, C., Ghosh, S., Kuchlyan, J., and Sarkar, N., Modulation of the photophysical properties of curcumin in nonionic surfactant (Tween 20) forming micelles and niosomes: A comparative study of different microenvironments, *J. Phys. Chem. B.* 117, 6957–6968, 2013.

4. Choi, M.J., and Maibach, H., Liposomes and niosomes as topical drug delivery systems, *Skin Pharmacol. Physiol.* 18, 209–219, 2005.

5. Azeem, A., Anwer, M.K., and Talegaonkar, S., Niosomes in sustained and targeted drug delivery: Some recent advances, *J. Drug. Target.* 17, 671–689, 2009.

6. Abdelkader, H., Alani, A.W., and Alany, R.G., Recent advances in non-ionic surfactant vesicles (niosomes): Self-assembly, fabrication, characterization, drug delivery applications and limitations, *Drug. Deliv.* 21, 87–100, 2014.

7. Marinecci, C., Di Marzio, L., Rinaldi, F., et al., Niosomes from 80s to present: The state of the art, *Adv. Colloid Interface Sci.* 205, 197–206, 2014.

NONIDET P-40™ (NO LONGER AVAILABLE)

Nonidet P-40™ was a popular nonionic (polyoxythelene glycol derivative) detergent used for membrane protein solubilization[1,2] as well as for other purposes.[3–5] However, Nonidet P-40™ is no longer available and substitutes for Nonidet P-40™ have been advanced.[6] It would seem that most substitutes for Nonidet P-40™ are based a p-alkylphenyethoxylate (e.g. Triton X-114).

1. Linke, D., Detergents: An overview, *Methods Enzymol.* 463, 603–617, 2009.
2. Peach, M., Marsh, N., Miskiewicz, E.T., and MacPhee, D.J., Solubilization of proteins: The importance of lysis buffer choice, *Methods Mol. Biol.* 1312, 49–60, 2015.
3. Sanchez-Ferrer, A., Bru, R., and Garcia-Carmona, F., Phase separation of biomolecules in polyoxyethylene glycol nonionic detergents, *Crit. Rev. Biochem. Mol. Biol.* 29, 275–313, 1994.
4. Muro, M.D., Fernandez, C., and Moneo, I., Renaturation of blotting allergens increases the sensitivity of specific IgE detection, *J. Investig. Allergol. Clin. Immunol.* 6, 166–171, 1996.
5. Ono, C., Hirano, J., Okamoto, T., and Matsuura, Y., Evaluation of viral contamination in a baculovirus expression system, *Microbiol. Immunol.* 62, 200–204, 2018.
6. Sinha, S., Field, J.J., and Miller, J.H., Use of substitute Nonidet P-40 nonionic detergents in intracellular tubulin polymerization assays for screening of microtubule targeting agents, *Biochem. Cell Biol.* 95, 379–384, 2017.

NORTHERN BLOT

Northern blot is similar to Southern blot except a specific RNA sequence is detected with a labeled cDNA probe. The RNA targets are separated by electrophoresis and transferred to a PVDF membrane for reaction with the cDNA probe.[1–4] Current use is directed toward the detection of small RNA species[5,6] and long noncoding (LNC) RNA.[7] I could not find the first use of the term Northern blot but I do recall the name arising from the suggestion that RNA was the opposite of DNA and, hence, north is opposite of south ignoring the fact the term Southern blot did not arise from the study of a compass. The first example of a Northern blot appeared in 1977 where RNA separated in an agarose gel were transferred to a diazobenzyloxymethyl paper and assessed with DNA probes[8] which was followed by improvements in the technology.[9,10]

1. Hayes, P.C., Wolf, C.R., and Hayes, J.D., Blotting techniques for the study of DNA, RNA, and proteins, *BMJ* 299, 965–968, 1989.
2. Dallman, M.J., Montgomery, R.A., Larsen, C.P., Wanders, A., and Wells, A.F., Cytokine gene expression: Analysis using northern blotting, polymerase chain reaction and in situ hybridization, *Immunol. Rev.* 119, 163–179, 1991.
3. Raval, P., Qualitative and quantitative determination of mRNA, *J. Pharmacol. Toxicol. Methods* 32, 125–127, 1994.
4. Durrant, I., Enhanced chemiluminescent detection of horseradish peroxidase labeled probes, *Methods Mol. Biol.* 31, 147–161, 1994.
5. Aravin, A., and Tuschi, T., Identification and characterization of small RNAs involved in RNA silencing, *FEBS Lett.* 579, 5830–5840, 2005.
6. Damm, K., Bach, S., Müller, K.M., et al., Improved Northern blot detection of small RNAs using EDC crosslinking and DNA/LNA probes, *Methods Mol. Biol.* 1296, 41–51, 2015.
7. HU, X., Feng, Y., HU, Z., et al., Detection of long noncoding RNA expression by nonradioactive Northern blots, in *Long Noncoding RNAs: Methods and Protocols* (Methods in Molecular Biology, vol. 1402), Chapter 14, pp. 177–189, Springer Science + Business, New York, 2016.
8. Alwine, J.C., Kemp, D.J., and Stark, G.R., Method for detection of specific RNAs in agarose gels by transfer to diazobenzyloxymethyl-paper and hybridization with DNA probes, *Proc. Natl. Acad. Sci. USA* 74, 5350–5354, 1977.
9. Thomas, P.S., Hybridization of denatured RNA and small DNA fragments transferred to nitrocellulose, *Proc. Natl. Acad. Sci. USA* 77, 5201–5205, 1977.
10. Hamelin, R., Northern blot mapping: A procedure for mapping mRNA immobilized on nitrocellulose by probing end-labeled DNA fragments, *Anal. Biochem.* 175, 500–506, 1988.

NORTHWESTERN BLOT

The northwestern blot is a blotting technique which identifies RNA-binding proteins. The protein mixture is separated by gel electrophoresis and subsequently transferred to a PVDF or nitrocellulose membrane. RNA-binding proteins are identified through the binding of radiolabeled or fluorophore-labeled RNA oligomers,[1–4] Northwestern blot technology is also used to evaluate aptamer-protein interactions.[5,6] Northern blot technology was used to identify dsRNA binding proteins.[7] The **southwestern** blot assay uses DNA probes to identify DNA binding proteins.[8,9] Some minor directional blotting technologies included the eastern, Far-Eastern blot, far-western, and north northwestern blot.

1. Chen, X., Sadlock, J., and Schon, E.A., RNA-binding patterns in total human tissue proteins: Analysis by northwestern blotting, *Biochem. Biophys. Res. Commun.* 191, 18–25, 1993.

2. Hiriart, E., Bardouillet, L., Manet, E., et al., A region of the Epstein–Barr virus (EBV) mRNA export factor EB2 containing an arginine-rich motif mediates direct binding to RNA, *J. Biol. Chem.* 278, 37790–37798, 2003.

3. Zhao, S., Xue, Y., Hao, J., and Liang, C., The RNA binding properties and domain of Rice stripe virus nucleocapsid protein, *Virus Genes* 51, 276–282, 2015.

4. Zang, S., and Lin, R.J., Northwestern blot analysis: Detecting RNA-protein interaction after gel separation of protein mixture, *Methods Mol. Biol.* 1421, 111–125, 2016.

5. Sekiya, S., Noda, K., Nishikawa, F., et al., Characterization and application of a novel RNA aptamer against the mouse prion protein, *J. Biochem.* 139, 383–390, 2006.

6. Yoshida, Y., Sakai, N., Masuda, H., et al., Rabbit antibody detection with RNA aptamers, *Anal. Biochem.* 375, 217–222, 2008.

7. Schiff, L.A., Nibert, M.L., Co, M.S., Brown, E.G., and Fields, B.N., Distinct binding sites for zinc and double-stranded RNA in the reovirus outer capsid protein sigma 3, *Mol. Cell. Biol.* 8, 273–283, 1988.

8. Bowen, B., Steinberg, J., Laemmli, U.K., and Weintraub, H., The detection of DNA-binding proteins by protein blotting, *Nucleic Acids Res.* 8, 1–20, 1980.

9. Jia, Y., Nagore, L., and Jarrett, H., Southwestern blotting assay, *Methods Mol. Biol.* 1334, 85–99, 2015.

NOTCH

The term notch describes a family of receptors important in growth and development.[1–3] There are four members of the notch family of receptors in humans. The term notch is derived the prototype which was identified in *Drosophila* in 1919 with a report that a partial loss of gene function resulted in notches or serrations in the wing.[4,5] The interaction of notch with its ligands, delta, serrate, Lag-2 (DSL) on an opposing cell surface results in a conformational change (activation) in notch following by two proteolytic cleavages. The first cleavage is accomplished with ADAM-10 and the second by γ-secretase which releases the notch intracellular domain (NICD).[6,7] Abnormal activation of notch is observed in cancer.[8,9] Notch signaling is an emerging therapeutic target.[10–12]

1. Bray, S.J., Notch signalling: A simple pathway becomes complex, *Nature Rev. Mol. Cell Biol.* 7, 676–689, 2006.

2. Kopan, R., and Ilagan, M.X.G., The canonical notch signaling pathway: Unfolding the activation mechanism, *Cell* 137, 216–233, 2009.

3. Kovall, R.A., Gebelein, B., Springer, K.D., and Kopan, R., The canonical notch signaling pathway: Structure and biochemical insights into shape, sugar, and force, *Dev. Cell* 41, 228–241, 2017.

4. Moohr, O.L., Character changes caused by mutation of an entire region of a chromosome in drosophila, *Genetics* 4, 275–282, 1919.

5. Artavanis-Tsakonas, S., Rand, M.D., and Lake, R.J., Notch-signaling: Cell-fate control and signal integration in development, *Science* 284, 770–776, 1999.

6. Farnie, G., and Clarke, R.B., Mammary stem cells and breast cancer-role of notch signalling, *Stem Cell Rev.* 3, 169–175, 2007.

7. Chillakuri, C.R., Sheppard, D., Lea, S.M., and Handford, P.A., Notch receptor-ligand binding and activation: Insights from molecular studies, *Sem. Cell Dev. Biol.* 23, 421–428, 2012.

8. Grabher, C., von Boehmer, H., and Look, A.T., Notch 1 activation in the molecular pathogenesis of T-cell acute lymphoblastic leukemia, *Nature Rev. Cancer* 6, 347–369, 2006.

9. Zou, B., Zhou, X.-L., Lai, S.-Q., and Liu, J.-C., Notch signaling and non-small cell lung cancer, *Oncology Letters* 15, 3415–3421, 2018.

10. Groth, C., and Fortini, M.E., Therapeutic approaches to modulating Notch signaling: Current challenges and future prospects, *Sem. Cell Dev. Biol.* 21, 465–472, 2012.

11. Mirtschink, P., and Chavakis, T., The missed notch to bring down diabetes, *Trends Endocrinol. Metab.* 29, 448–450, 2018.

12. Venkatesh, V., Nataraj, R., Thangaraj, G.S., et al., Targeting Notch signalling pathway of cancer stem cells, *Stem Cell Investig.* 5, 5, 2018.

NUCLEAR FACTOR KAPPA B (NF-κB)

Nuclear factor kappa B (NF-κB) is a transcription factor that was originally described in B cell as protein which bound to the kappa (κ) chain of immunoglobulin (nuclear factor regulating expression of the Ig κ chain in B cells).[1,2] NF-κB is homologous with the cactus-dorsal system in *Drosophila*[3,4] where the destruction of cactus releases dorsal to translocate to the nucleus. It was recognized that NF-κB was common to all cells as an inactive form which, upon activation, translocates to the nucleus where there is a specific binding to DNA. The NF-κB family consists of homo- and heterodimers formed from five subunits, p50, p52, p65(RelA), cRel, and RelB.[5] The five subunits share a conserved amino-terminal sequence of approximately 300 amino acids known as the Rel homology region.[6] While the term NF-κB usually refers to the combination of the various subunits to form homo- and heterodimers, the most common form is the combination of p50/p65(RelA).[7,8] NF-κB is found in an inactive form in the cytosol of the cell, bound to an inhibitor protein (IκB) which is "inactivated" by phosphorylation by a cytosolic kinase, IκB kinase (IKK). There are several inhibitor proteins and several kinases.[9] The activated

NF-κB translocates to nucleus activating a number genes of including proinflammatory genes.[10] NF-κB action also inhibits apoptosis (programmed cell death) and possible necrosis as well as autophagy.[11,12] There are multiple factors which regulated the specificity of NF-κB interaction with genes including the action of IKK,[13] various combinations of the several monomers to form the active homodimer or heterodimer, post-translational modification of the various monomer/dimer units,[14] nuclear factors,[15,16] and sequence elements in the target gene sequence.[17,18]

1. Sen, R., and Baltimore, D., Inducibility of κ immunoglobulin enhancer-binding protein Nf-κB by a posttranslational mechanism, *Cell* 47, 921–928, 1986.
2. Ruddon, R.W., *Cancer Biology*, Oncogenes, Chapters 7, pp. 277–317, Oxford University Press, New York, 1995.
3. Ghosh, S., Gifford, A.M., Riviere, L.R., et al., Cloning of the p50 DNA binding subunit of NF-κB: Homology to *rel* and *dorsal*, *Cell* 62, 1019–1029, 1990.
4. Pires, B.R.B., Silva, R.C.M.C., Ferreira, G.M., and Abdelhay, E., NF-kappaB: Two sides of the same coin, *Genes* 9(1), 24, 2018.
5. Huxford, T., and Ghosh, G., Structural analysis of NF-κB and IκB proteins, in *NF-κB/Rel Transcription Factor Family*, ed. H.-C. Liou, Chapter 1, pp. 1–11, Landes Bioscience/Eureka, Georgetown, Texas, 2008.
6. Rushlow, C., and Warrior, R., The rel family of protein, *Bioessays* 14, 89–95, 1992.
7. Liu, J., Sodeoka, M., Lane, W.S., and Verdine, G.L., Evidence for a non-helical DNA-binding motif in the Rel homology region, *Proc. Natl. Acad. Sci. USA* 91, 908–912, 1994.
8. Tomida, A., and Tsuno, T., Drug resistance pathways as targets, in *Anticancer Drug Development*, ed. B.C. Baguley and D.J. Kerr, Chapter 5, pp. 77–90, Academic Press, San Diego, CA, 2002.
9. Li, Z.-W., and Karin, M., NF-κB signal transduction by IKK complexes, in *NF-κB/Rel Transcription Factor Family,* ed. H.-C. Liou, Landes/Eureka, Georgetown, TX, 2006.
10. O'Neil, D., and Steidler, L., Cytokines, chemokines and growth factors in the pathogenesis and treatment of inflammatory bowel disease, *Adv. Exptl. Med. Biol.* 520, 250–258, 2003.
11. Fan, Y., Dutte, J., Gupta, N., Fan, G., and Gélinger, C., Regulation of cell death by NF-κB and its role in tumorigenesis and therapy, *Adv. Exptl. Med. Biol.* 615, 223–350, 2008.
12. Ricci, M.S., and El-Deiry, W.S., The extrinsic pathway of apoptosis, in *Apoptosis, Senescence, and Cancer*, 2nd edn., ed. D.A. Gewirtz, S.E. Holt, and S. Grant, Chapter 2, pp. 31–54, Humana Press, Totowa, NJ, 2007.
13. Vincendeau, M., Hadian, K., Messias, A.C., et al., Inhibition of canonical NF-κB signaling by a small molecule targeting NEMO-ubiquitin interaction, *Sci. Rep.* 6, 18934, 2016.
14. Perkin, N.D., Post-translational modifications regulating the activity and function of the nuclear factor kappa b pathway, *Oncogene* 25, 6716–6730, 2006.
15. Campbell, K.J., and Perkins, N.D., Regulation of NF-kappaB function, *Biochem. Soc. Symp.* 73, 165–180, 2006.
16. Wan, F., and Lenardo, M.J., The nuclear signaling of NF-κB: Current knowledge, new insights, and future perspectives, *Cell Res.* 20, 24–33, 2010.
17. Leung, T.H., Hoffmann, A., and Baltimore, D. One nucleotide in a κB site can determine cofactor specificity for NF-κB dimers, *Cell* 118, 453–464, 2004.
18. Wang, V.Y.-F., Huang, W., Asagiri, M., et al., The transcriptional specificity of NF-κB dimers is coded within the κB DNA response elements, *Cell Rep.* 2, 824–839, 2012.

NUCLEAR MAGNETIC RESONANCE (NMR)

Nuclear magnetic resonance (NMR) is a technique which detects nuclear-spin orientation of an atom in an applied magnetic field.[1–4] NMR can be considered to be a form of spectroscopy based on the absorption and emission of electromagnetic radiation by certain nuclei (which have a dipole magnetic moment) when placed in a magnetic field.[5,6] The position (measured as a chemical shift) of a signal depends on the external field and the magnetic field in close proximity to the target nuclei. Of particular value in NMR is the proximately of groups that influence the characteristics of the target nuclei which has been known for some time.[7] As a result, identical nuclei in different molecules appear at different frequencies or fields (chemical shift) in different molecules. The data is the detection of a nuclear magnetic moment, usually measured as the chemical shift[8] from that of a standard such as 2,2-dimetyl-2-silapentane-5-sulfonate.[9] Magnetic resonance imaging (MRI) is a valuable diagnostic technique based on characteristics of water protons in tomographic sections of tissues[10–12] and in tissue engineering.[13] NMR is proving useful in metabolomics.[14,15] The application of NMR to the study of protein structure has become more useful reflecting an improvement in the technology[16–18] including solid-state NMR.[19,20]

1. Harris, R.K., *Nuclear Magnetic Resonance A Physicochemical View*, Longman Scientific, Harlow, Essex, UK, 1986.
2. Lambert, J.B., and Mazzola, E.P., *Nuclear Magnetic Resonance Spectroscopy: An Introduction to Principles, Applications, and Experimental Methods*, Pearson/Prentice Hall, Upper Saddle River, NJ, 2004.
3. Mitchell, T.N., and Costisella, B., *NMR—From Spectra to Structures: An Experimental Approach*, Springer, Berlin, Germany, 2004.

4. Friebolin, H., *Basic One- and Two-Dimensional NMR Spectroscopy*, Wiley-VCH, Weinheim, Germany, 2005.

5. Field, L.D., Fundamental aspects of NMR spectroscopy, in *Analytical NMR*. ed. L.D. Field and S. Sternhill, Chapter 2, John Wiley & Sons, Chichester, UK, 1989.

6. Akitt, J.W., and Mann, B.E., *NMR and Chemistry*, 4th edn., CRC Press, London, UK, 2000.

7. Dailey, B.P., and Shoolery, J.N., The electron withdrawal power of substituent groups, *J. Am. Chem. Soc.* 77, 3977–3981, 1955.

8. Bovey, E.A., *Nuclear Magnetic Resonance Spectroscopy*, 2nd edn., Chapter 3, The chemical shift, pp. 87–146, Academic Press, San Diego, CA, 1988.

9. Wishart, D.S., Bigam, C.G., Yao, J., et al., ^{1}H, ^{13}C and ^{15}N chemical shift referencing in biomolecular NMR, *J. Biomol. NMR* 6, 135–140, 1995.

10. Foster, M.A., *Magnetic Resonance in Medicine and Biology*, Chapter 10, NMR proton imaging, Pegammamon Press, Oxford, UK, 1984.

11. *Magnetic Resonance Imaging*, ed. C.L. Partain, Saunders, Philadelphia, PA, 1988.

12. Smith, R.C., and Lange, R.C., *Understanding Magnetic Resonance Imaging*, CRC Press, Boca Raton, FL, 1998.

13. Glover, J., *Magnetic Resonance Imaging*, Carcanet Publishing, Manchester, UK, 2008.

14. de Graaf, R., *In vivo* NMR spectroscopy techniques: Direct detection, MRS, kinetics and labels; fluxes; concentrations, in *Metabolomics by in vivo NMR*, ed. R.G. Shulman and D.L. Rothman, Chapter 2, pp. 7–29, John Wiley and Sons, Hoboken, NJ, 2005.

15. Wermter, F.C., Mitschke, N., Bock, C., and Dreher, W., Temperature dependence of ^{1}H NMR chemical shifts and its influence on estimated metabolite concentration, *Magn. Reson. Mater. Phy.* 30, 579–590, 2017.

16. Wishart, D.S., Sykes, B.D., and Richards, F.M., Relationship between nuclear magnetic resonance chemical shift and protein secondary structure, *J. Mol. Biol.* 222, 311–333, 1991.

17. Jiang, Y., and Kalodimos, C.G., NMR studies of large proteins, *J. Mol. Biol.* 429, 2667–2676, 2017.

18. Berjanskii, M.V., and Wishart, D.S., Unraveling the meaning of chemical shifts in protein NMR, *BBA Proteins and Proteomics* 1865, 1564–1775, 2017.

19. Müller, H., Etzkom, M., and Heise, H., Solid-state NMR, *Curr. Top. Chem.* 335, 121–156, 2013 (*Modern NMR Methodology,* ed. H. Heise and S. Matthews, Springer-Verlag, Berlin, Germany, 2013).

20. Lacabanne, D., Fogeron, M.L., Wiegand, T., et al., Protein sample preparation for solid-state NMR investigations, *Prog. Nucl. Magn. Reson. Spectrosc.* 110, 20–33, 2019.

NUCLEAR PORE COMPLEX

The nucleus of a eukaryotic cell is complex with little internal structure.[1] The nucleus is separated from the cytoplasm by the nuclear envelope. The nuclear pore complex is a large protein complex which spans the nuclear envelope (distance between the cytoplasm and the interior of the nucleus).[2,3] While the size of the channel of the nuclear pore complex permits the passive diffusion of materials up to 40 kDa, selective mechanisms permit the passage of much larger materials such a ribonucleoprotein complexes and viral proteins in a specific process.[4–6] Enabling passage through the nuclear pore complex is of biopharmaceutical interest including gene therapy applications.[7–10]

1. Robson, M.I., Rizzotto, A., and Schirmer, E.C., Sparial organization of the nucleus compartmentalizes and regulates the genome, in *Nuclear Pore Complexes in Genomic Organization, Function, and Maintenance*, ed. M.D. D'Angelo, Chapter 1, pp. 1–34, Springer AG, Cham, Switzerland, 2018.

2. Löschberger, A., Franke, C., Krohne, G., van de Linde, S., and Sauer, M., Correlative super-resolution fluorescence and electron microscopy of the nuclear pore complex with molecular resolution, *J. Cell Sci.* 127, 4351–4355, 2014.

3. von Appen, A., Kosinski, J., Sparks, L., et al., *In situ* structural analysis of the human nuclear pore complex, *Nature* 526, 140–143, 2015.

4. Rout, M.P., Atchison, J.D., Suprapto, A., et al., The yeast nuclear pore complex: Composition, architecture, and transport mechanism, *J. Cell Biol.* 148, 635–651, 2000.

5. Panté, N., and Kann, M., Nuclear pore complex is able to transport macromolecules with diameters of ~39 nm, *Mol. Biol. Cell* 13, 425–434, 2002.

6. Shahin, V., Nuclear pore complexes: Fascinating nucleo-cytoplasmic checkpoints, in *Nuclear Pore Complexes in Genomic Organization, Function, and Maintenance*, ed. M.D. D'Angelo, Chapter 3, pp. 63–86, Springer AG, Cham, Switzerland, 2018.

7. Mastrobattista, E., Oosting, R.S., Hennink, W.E., Koning, G.A., and Commelin, D.J.A., The nuclear pore complex: The gateway to successful nonviral gene delivery, *Pharmaceut. Res.* 23, 447–459, 2006.

8. Nicolson, S.C., and Samulski, R.J., Recombinant adeno-associated virus utilizes host cell nuclear import machinery to enter the nucleus, *J. Virol.* 88, 4132–4144, 2014.

9. Bai, H., Lester, G.M.S., Petishnok, L.C., and Dean, D.A., Cytoplasmc transport and nuclear import of plasmid DNA, *Biosci. Rep.* 37(6), BSR20160616, 2017.

10. Li, X., Kang, P., Chen, Z., et al., Rock the nucleus: Significantly enhanced nuclear membrane permeability and gene transfection by plasmonic nanobubble induced nanomechanical transduction, *Chem. Commun.* 54, 2479–2482, 2018.

NUCLEIC ACID TESTING (NAT)

Nucleic acid testing (nucleic acid amplification testing; NAT) is the use of PCR technology to test for the presence of nucleic acid sequences in biological materials for the presence of viral pathogens.[1] NAT was developed for assessing the safety of blood for transfusion[2-6] and for plasma for fractionation.[7-9] The term nucleic acid testing is also used for clinical diagnostic procedures[10] and for screening solid organ donations,[11-13] and tissue transplantation.[14] NAT is also used for the detection of allergens in food.[15-17]

1. *Nucleic Acid Testing for Human Disease*, ed. A. Lorincz, CRC Pres/Taylor & Francis Group, Boca Raton, FL, 2006.
2. Cardoso, M.S., Koerner, K., and Kubanek, B., Minipool screening by nucleic acid testing for hepatitis B virus, hepatitis C virus, and HIV: Preliminary results, *Transfusion* 38, 905–907, 1998.
3. Chamberland, M.E, Surveillance for bloodborne infections, *Thromb. Haemost.* 82, 494–499, 1999.
4. Drosten, C., Weber, M., Seifried, E., and Roth W.K., Evaluation of a new PCR assay with competitive internal control sequence for blood donor screening, *Transfusion* 40, 718–724, 2000.
5. Roth, W.K. Buhr, S., Drosten, C., and Seifried, E., NAT and viral safety in blood transfusion, *Vox Sang.* 78(Suppl 2), 257–259, 2000.
6. Mauk, M.G., Liu, C., Sadik, M., and Bau, H.H., Microfluidic devices for nucleic acid (NA) isolation, isothermal NA amplification, and real-time detection, *Methods Mol. Biol* 1256, 15–40, 2015.
7. Flanagan, P., and Snape, T., Nucleic acid technology (NAT) testing and the transfusion service: A rationale for the implementation of minipool testing, *Transfus. Med.* 8, 9–13, 1998.
8. Farrugia, A., Plasma for fractionation: Safety and quality issues, *Haemophlia* 10, 334–340, 2004.
9. Nucleic acid testing (NAT) for human immunodeficiency virus type 1 (HIV-1) and hepatitis C virus (HCV): Testing, product disposition, and donor referral and reentry, https://www.fda.gov/downloads/BiologicsBloodVaccines/GuidanceComplianceRegulatoryInformation/Guidances/Blood/UCM210270.pdf.
10. Chang, M., Wong, A.J.S., Raugi, D.N., et al., Clinical validation of a novel diagnostic HIV-2 total nucleic acid quantitative assay using the Abbot m2000 platform: Implications for complementary HIV-2 nucleic acid testing for the CDC 4th generation HIV diagnostic testing algorithm, *J. Clin. Virol.* 86, 56–61, 2017.
11. Lai, J.C., Kahn, J.G., Tavakol, M., Peters, M.G., and Roberts, J.P., Reducing infection transmission in solid organ transplantation through donor nucleic acid testing; a cost effectiveness analysis, *Am. J. Transplantation* 13, 2611–2618, 2013.
12. Kiberd, B., Cost-effeciveness of routine nucleic acid testing in organ donors, *Am. J. Transplant.* 14, 979–980, 2014.
13. Lai, J.C., Kahn, J.G., and Roberts, J.P., Author response: Reducing infection transmission in solid organ transplantation though donor nucleic acid testing: A cost-effectiveness analysis, *Am. J. Transplant.* 14, 981, 2014.
14. Pruss, A., Caspari, G., Krüger, D.H., et al., Tissue donation and virus safety: More nucleic acid amplification testing is needed, *Tranpl. Infect. Dis.* 12, 375–386, 2010.
15. Prado, M., Ortea, I., Vial, S., et al., Advanced DNA- and protein-based methods for the detection and investigation of food allergens, *Crit. Rev. Food Sci. Nutri.* 56, 2511–2542, 2016.
16. Graziano, S., Gulli, M., and Marmiroli, N., Detection of allergen coding sequences of kiwi, peach, and apple in processed food by qPCR, *J. Sci. Food Agric.* 98, 3129–3129, 2018.
17. Eischeid, A.C., and Stadig, S.R., A group-specific, quantitative real-time PCR assay for detection of crab. A crustacean shellfish allergen, in complex food matrices. *Food Chem.* 244, 224–231, 2018.

NUCLEOSOME

The nucleosome is the subunit of mammalial chromatin.[1-3] A nucleosome is an octomer of histone proteins associated with an approximate 140 bp segment of DNA. The octomer is composed of two each of histone H2A, histone H2B, histone H3, and histone H4. Nucleosomes are dynamic entities being subject to chemical modification (e.g. acetylation) and conformation change.[4-10] Nucleosomes can undergo degradation in inflammatory disorders and as free histones or DNA-bound histones are passively released into the circulation where they can have a variety of functions such as a providing pattern-associated recognition pattern activation of the immune system in sepsis.[11,12] Released nucleosomes be microbicidal and prothrombotic.[13] The nucleosome does present a therapeutic target.[14,15] There is particular interest in targeting lysine demethylase.[16-18]

1. Lewin, B., The nucleosome: Subunit of mammalian chromatin, *Nature* 254, 651–653, 1975.
2. Marion, C., and Roux, B., Nucleosome arrangement in chromatin, *Nucleic Acids Res.* 5, 4431–4434, 1978.
3. Wu, J., and Grunstein, M., 25 years after the nucleosome model: Chromatin modifications, *TIBS* 25, 619–623, 2000.
4. Sivolob, A., and Prunell, A., Nucleosome conformational flexibility and implications for chromatin dynamics, *Philos. Transact. A Math. Phys. Eng. Sci.* 362, 1519–1547, 2004.
5. Lieb, J.D., and Clarke, N.D., Control of transcription through intragenic patterns of nucleosome composition, *Cell* 123, 1187–1190, 2005.
6. Stockdale, C., Bruno, M., Ferreira, H., et al., Nucleosome dynamics, *Biochem. Soc. Symp.* 73, 109–119, 2006.
7. Reinberg, D., and Sims, R.J., 3rd, de facto nucleosome dynamics, *J. Biol. Chem.* 281, 23297–23301, 2006.
8. Polo, S.E., and Almouzni, G., Chromatin assembly: A basic recipe with various flavours, *Curr. Opin. Genetics Develop.* 16, 104–111, 2006.

9. Swygert, S.G., and Peterson, C.L., Chromatin dynamics: Interplay between remodeling enzymes and histone modifications, *Biochim. Biophys. Acta* 1839, 728–736, 2014.

10. Bornelöv, S., Reynolds, N., Xenophontos, M., et al., The nucleosome remodeling and deacetylation complex modulates chromatin structure at sites of active transcription to fine-tune gene expression, *Molec. Cell* 71, 58–72, 2018.

11. Chen, R., Kang, R., Fan, X.B., and Tang, D., Release and activity of histone in disease, *Cell Death Dis.* 5, e1370, 2014.

12. Silk, E., Zhao, H., Weng, H., and Ma, D., The role of extracellular histone in organ injury, *Cell Death Dis.* 8, e2812, 2017.

13. Szatmary, P., Huang, W., Criddle, D., Tepikin, A., and Sutton, R., Biology, role and therapeutic potential of circulating histones in acute inflammatory disorders, *J. Cell. Mol. Med.* 22, 4617–4629, 2018.

14. de Silva, I.T., de Oliveira, P.S., and Santos, G.M., Featuring the nucleosome surface as a therapeutic target, *Trends Pharmacol. Sci.* 36, 263–269, 2015.

15. Cabral, W.F., Machado, A.H., and Santos, G., Exogenous nucleosome-binding molecules: A potential new class of therapeutic drugs, *Drug Discov. Today* 21, 707–711, 2016.

16. Niwa, H., and Umehara, T., Structural insight into inhibitors of flavin adenine dinucleotide-dependent lysine demethylases, *Epigenetics* 12, 340–352, 2017.

17. Benton, C.B., Fiskus, W., and Bhalla, K.N., Targeting histone acetylation: Readers and writers in leukemia and cancer, *Cancer. J.* 23, 286–291, 2017.

18. Magliulo, D., Bernardi, R., and Messina, S., Lysine-specific demethylase 1A as a promising target in acute myeloid leukemia, *Front. Oncol.* 8, 255, 2018.

NUTRIGENOMICS

The science of nutrigenomics seeks to provide a molecular understanding for how common dietary chemicals (i.e. nutrition) affect health by altering the expression of an individual's genetic makeup with emphasis on disease prevention/treatment (personalized medicine). Nutrigenomics can be considered the genomics of nutrition.[1–7] An example is the use of proteomics to evaluate cancer biomarkers in response to **dietary intervention**.[8] Another focus is the use of omics technology to drive **personized nutrition**.[9] Nutrigenomics is also used in **cosmetology/dermatology**[10] and potentially in the development of cosmeceuticals.[11,12] Nutrigenomics is related to the concept of functional foods.[13] It is noted that the concept of **foodomics** has been advanced in relation to nutrigenomics.[14,15]

1. van Ommen, B., and Stierum, R., Nutrigenomics: Exploiting system biology in the nutrition and health arena, *Curr. Opin. Biotechnol.* 13, 517–721, 2002.

2. Muller, M., and Kersten, S., Nutrigenomics: Goals and strategies, *Nat. Rev. Genet.* 4, 315–322, 2003.

3. Bauer, M., Hamm, A., and Pankratz, M.J., Linking nutrition to genomics, *Biol. Chem.* 385, 593–596, 2004.

4. *Nutrigenomics: Application to the Development of Nutraceuticals and Cosmeceuticals*, Nova Science, Happauge, New York, 2013.

5. Carlberg, C., Ulven, S.M., and Molnár, F., *Nutrigenomics*, Springer AG, Cham, Switzerland, 2016.

6. *Nutrigenomics and Proteomics in Health and Disease Towards a systems-level understanding of gene-diet interactions*, 2nd edn., ed. M. Kussman and P.J. Stover, John Wiley & Sons, Chichester, West Sussex, 2017.

7. *Nutrigenomics and Nutraceuticals: Clinical Relevance and Disease Prevention*, ed. Y. Pathak and A.M. Ardekani, CRC Press/Taylor & Francis Group, Boca Raton, FL, 2017.

8. Schroll, M.M., and Hummon, A.B., Employing proteomics to understand the effects of nutritional intervention in cancer treatment, *Anal. Bioanol. Chem.* 410, 6371–6386, 2018.

9. van Ommen, B., van den Broek, T., de Hoogh, I., et al., Systems biology of personalized nutrition, *Nutr. Rev.* 75, 579–599, 2017.

10. Melnik, B.C., Linking diest to acne metabolomics, inflammation, and comedogenesis: At update, *Clin. Cosmet. Investig. Dermatol.* 8, 371–388, 2015.

11. Gao, X.-H., Zhang, L., Wei, H., and Chen, H.-D., Efficacy and safety of innovative cosmeceuticals, *Clinics Dermatol.* 26, 367–379, 2008.

12. Alfano, A., Corsuto, L., Finamore, R., et al., Valorization of olive mill wastewater by membrane processes to recover natural antioxidant compounds for cosmeceutical and nutraceutical applications of functional foods, *Antioxidants* 7, 72, 2018.

13. Claus, S.P., Development of personalized functional foods needs metabolic profiling, *Curr. Opin. Clin. Nutr. Metab. Care* 17, 567–573, 2014.

14. Ibáñez, C., Simó, C., Garcia-Cañas, V., Acunha, T., and Cifuentes, A., The role of direct high-resolution mass spectrometry in foodomics, *Anal. Bioanol. Chem.* 407, 6275–6287, 2015.

15. Braconi, D., Berhnardini, G., Millucci, L., and Santucci, A., Foodomics for human health: Current status and perspectives, *Expert Rev. Proteomics* 15, 153–164, 2018.

OGSTON SIEVING (OGSTON EFFECT)

Ogston sieving is a term used to describe the behavior of large DNA or RNA molecules on gel electrophoresis where the pore size of the gel matrix is equal or less than the radius gyration of the analyte; in other words, the analyte is considered as undeformable sphere.[1] The migration of a DNA polymer will depend on the distribution of analyte between the mobile phase and the gel on the ability of the analyte based on radius of gyration of the analyte and the pore size distribution of the gel. The concept of Ogston sieving is based on early work of Ogston on fiber matrices.[2,3] Ogston sieving is also be applicable to the behavior of proteins.[4] Ogston sieving is frequently compared with the reptation model of electrophoresis. The reptation model applied with DNA (or other large linear molecules) where the radius of gyration is larger than the pore size of the matrix.[5] The reptation or biased reptation model treats the migrating solute as a flexible material which can "snake" through the polymer gel network.[6,7] The term reptation is derived from zoology where it refers to the action of creeping of crawling, as in the manner of a snake.[8]

1. Durney, B.C., Crihfield, C.L., and Holland, L.A., Capillary electrophoresis applied to DNA: Determining and harnessing sequence and structure to advance bioanalyses (2009–2014), *Anal. Bioanal. Chem.* 407, 6923–6928, 2015.
2. Ogston, A.G., The spaces in a uniform random suspension of fibres, *Trans. Faraday Soc.* 54, 1754–1757, 1958.
3. Viovy, J.L., and Duke, T., DNA electrophoresis in polymer solutions: Ogston sieving, repatation and constraint release, *Electrophoresis* 14, 322–329, 1993.
4. Gerstner, A., Csapo, Z., Sasvari-Szekely, M., and Guttman, A., Ultrathin-layer sodium dodecyl sulfate gel electrophoresis of proteins: Effects of gel composition and temperature on the separation of sodium dodecyl sulfate-protein complexes, *Electrophoresis* 21, 834–840, 2000.
5. Durney, B.C., Crichtfield, C.L., and Holland, L.A., Capillary electrophoresis applied to DNA: Determining and harnessing sequence and structure to advance bioanalyses (2009–2014), *Anal. Bioanal. Chem.* 407, 6923–6928, 2015.
6. Viovy, J.L., Reptation theories of electrophoresis, *Mol. Biotechnol.* 6, 31–46, 1996.
7. Slater, G.W., DNA gel electrophoresis: The reputation model(s), *Electrophoresis* 30(Suppl 1), S181–S187, 2009.
8. *Oxford English Dictionary*, Oxford University Press, Oxford, UK, 2019.

OKAZAKI FRAGMENTS

Okazaki fragments are smaller fragments of DNA, complementary to the lagging DNA strand which are synthesized, which form short double-stranded segments and are then incorporated into the larger DNA molecule showing that replication can be a discontinuous process.[1–5]

1. Okazaki, R., Okazaki, T., Sakabe, K., Sugimoto, K., and Sugino, A., Mechanism of DNA chain growth. I. Possible discontinuity and unusual secondary structure of newly synthesized chains, *Proc. Natl. Acad. Sci. USA* 59, 598–605, 1968.
2. Alberts, B.M., Prokaryotic DNA replication mechanisms, *Philos. Trans. R. Soc. Lond. B Biol. Sci.* 317, 395–420, 1987.
3. Okazaki, T., Days weaving the lagging strand synthesis of DNA—A personal recollection of the discovery of Okazaki fragments and studies on discontinuous replication mechanism, *Proc. Jpn. Acad. Sci. Ser B Phys. Biol. Sci.* 93, 322–338, 2017.
4. Burgers, P.M.J., and Kunkel, T.A., Eukaryotic DNA replication fork, *Annu. Rev. Biochem.* 86, 417–438, 2017.
5. Stodola, J.L., and Burgers, P.M., Mechanism of lagging-strand DNA replication in eukaryotes, *Adv. Exp. Med. Biol.* 1042, 117–133, 2017.

OMP85 (OUTER MEMBRANE PROTEIN 85)

OMP85 (Outer Membrane Protein 85) is a family of proteins found (primarily) in gram-negative bacteria which participate in the formation of the outer membrane.[1–4] The canonical OMP85 proteins was described as a homologous group of 85 kDa outer membrane proteins cloned from *Neisseria gonorrhoeae* and *Neisseria meningitis*.[5] OMP85 proteins are also described in mitochondria[6–8] and chloroplasts.[9] There is a description of human homologs.[10]

1. Gentle, I.E., Burri, L., and Littigow, T., Molecular architecture and function of the Omp85 family of proteins, *Molecular Microbiol.* 58, 1216–1225, 2005.
2. Webb, C.T., Heinz, E., and Lithgow, T., Evolution of the β-barrel assembly machinery, *Trends Microbiol.* 20, 612–620, 2012.
3. Calmettes, C., Judd, A., and Moraes, T.F., Structural aspects of bacterial outer membrane protein assembly, *Adv. Exp. Med. Biol.* 883, 255–270, 2015.
4. Leyton, D.L., Belousoff, M.J., and Lithgow, T., The β-barrel assembly machinery complex, *Methods Mol. Biol.* 1329, 1–16, 2015.
5. Manning, D.S., Reschke, D.K., and Judd, R.C., Omp85 proteins of *Neisseria gonorrhoeae* and *Neisseria meningitidis* are similar to *Hemophilus* D-15-Ag and *Pasteurella multoida* OMP87, *Microb. Pathog.* 25, 11–21, 1998.
6. Ott, C., Utech, M., Goetz, M., Rudel, T., and Kozjak-Pvlovic, V., Requirements for the import of neiserrial Omp85 into the outer membrane of human mitochondria, *Biosci. Rep.* 33, e00028, 2013.
7. Simmerman, R.F., Dave, A.M., and Bruce, B.D., Structure and function of POTRA domains of Omp85/TPS superfamily, *Int. Rev. Cell Mol. Biol.* 308, 1–34, 2014.
8. Höhr, A.I.C., Lindau, C., Wirth, C., et al., Membrane protein insertion through a mitochondrial β-barrel gate, *Science* 359(6373), eaah6834, 2018.
9. Hsueh, Y.C., Nicolaisen, K., Fernie, A.R., et al., The outer membrane Omp85-like protein P39 influences metabolic homoeostasis in mature *Arabidopsis thaliana*, *Plant Biol.*(Stuttg) 20, 825–833, 2018.
10. Schleiff, E., Maier, E.G., and Becker, T., Omp85 in eukaryotic systems: One protein family with distinct functions, *Biol. Chem.* 392, 21–27, 2011.

ONCOGENE

The classic definition of the term oncogene is a gene that causes the transformation of normal cells into cancerous tumor cells, especially a viral gene that transforms a host cell into a tumor cell; a gene that encodes a protein product which will stimulate uncontrolled cellular proliferation. Onco as a combining form is derived from the Greek for "of or relating to swelling or tumors.[1] Oncogenes are derivatives of normal cellular genes.[2–13] The term **proto-oncogene** is defined as "originally: a normal cellular gene whose nucleotide sequence is similar to that of a viral oncogene." Later also: a cellular gene believed to have the capacity to become onogenic (e.g. by mutation or overactivity).[1] The are a number of proto-oncogenes identified as important in the development of cancer.[14–17]

1. *Oxford English Dictionary*, Oxford University Press, Oxford, UK, 2019.
2. Wiman, K.G., and Hayward, W.S., Rearrangement and activation of the *c-myc* gene in avian and human B-cell lymphomas, *Tumour Biol.* 5, 211–219, 1984.
3. Balmain, A., Transforming *ras* oncogenes and multistage carcinogenesis, *Br. J. Cancer* 51, 1–7, 1985.
4. Newbold, R.F., Malignant transformation of mammalian cells in culture: Delineation of stages and role of cellular oncogenes activation, *IARC Sci. Publ.* 67, 31–53, 1985.
5. Ratner, L., Josephs, S.F., and Wong-Staal, F., Oncogenes: Their role in neoplastic transformation, *Annu. Rev. Microbiol.* 39, 419–449, 1985.
6. *Genes, Oncogenes, and Hormones: Advances in Cellular and Molecular Biology of Breast Cancer*, ed. R.B. Dickson and M.E. Lipman. Kluwer Academic, Boston, MA, 1992.
7. *Oncogenes and Tumor Suppressor Genes in Human Malignancies*, ed. C.C. Benz and E.T. Liu, Kluwer Academic, Boston, MA, 1993.
8. Heskeh, R., *The Oncogene Handbook*, Academic Press, London, UK, 1994.
9. Cooper, G.M., *Oncogenes* 2nd edn., Jones and Bartlett, Boston, MA, 1995.
10. Ross, D.W., *Introduction to Oncogenes and Molecular Cancer Medicine*, Springer, New York, 1998.
11. Rak, J., *Oncogene-Directed Therapies*, Humana Press, Totowa, NJ, 2003.
12. Giehl, K., Oncogenic Ras in tumour progression and metastasis, *Biol. Chem.* 386, 193–205, 2005.
13. Kashyap, A. *Bioinformatics of Non Small Cell Lung Cancer and the Ras Proto-Oncogene*, Springer-Verlag, Heidelberg, Germany, 2015.
14. Nandi, D., Cheema, P.S., Jaiswal, N., and Nag, A., Foxm1: Repurposing an oncogene as a biomarker, *Semin. Cancer Biol.* 52, 74–84, 2018.
15. Fernandez, D., Sanchez-Arevalo, V.J., and de Alboran, I.M., The role of the proto-oncogene *c-myc* in B lymphocyte differentiation, *Crit. Rev. Immunol.* 32, 321–334, 2012.
16. Parinot, C., and Nandrot, E.F., A compressive review of mutations in the MERTK proto-oncogene, *Adv. Exp. Med. Biol.* 854, 259–265, 2016.
17. Romei, C., Ciampi, R., and Elisei, R., A comprehensive overview of the role of the RET proto-oncogene in thyroid carcinoma, *Nat. Rev. Endocrinol.* 12, 192–202, 2016.

ONCOGENOMICS

Oncogenomics is the genomics of cancer (cancer genomics). It involves the study of oncogenes by the use of such tools as microarrays to evaluate expression and mutation with such tools as DNA microarray, RFLP, and RNA seq to study the oncology process.[1–5] Precision oncogenoomics/personalized oncogenomics using circulating tumor-derived DNA is of increasing interest.[6–10]

1. Rosell, R., Monzo, M. O'Brate, A., and Taron, M., Translational oncogenomics: Toward rational therapeutic decision-making, *Curr. Opin. Oncol.* 14, 171–179, 2002.
2. Strausberg, R.L., Simpson, A.J., Old, L.J., and Riggins, G.J., Oncogenomics and the development of new cancer therapies, *Nature* 429, 469–474, 2004.
3. Jain, K.K., Role of oncoproteomics in the personalized management of cancer, *Expert Rev. Proteomics* 1, 49–55, 2004.
4. Lam, S.H., and Gong, Z., Modeling liver cancer using zebrafish: A comparative Oncogenomics approach, *Cell Cycle* 5, 573–577, 2006.
5. Carroll, S.L., The challenge of cancer genomics in rare nervous system neoplasms: Malignant peripheral nerve sheath tumors as a paradigm for cross-species comparative oncogenomics, *Am. J. Pathol.* 186, 464–477, 2016.
6. Marquardt, J.U., and Andersen, J.B., Liver cancer oncogenomics: Opportunities and dilemmas for clinical applications, *Hepat. Oncol.* 2, 79–93, 2015.
7. Sheffield, B.S., Tessier-Cloutier, B., Li-Chang, H., et al., Personalized oncogenomics in the management of gastrointestinal carcinomas-early experiences from a pilot study, *Curr. Oncol.* 23, e571–e575, 2016.
8. Wartman, L.D., The future of cancer treatment using precision oncogenomics, *Cold Spring Harb. Mol. Case Stud.* 4, a002824, 2018.
9. Campbell, C., and Greenfield, J.P., Precision oncogenomics in pediatrics: A personal reflection, *Cold Spring Harb. Mol. Case Stud.* 4, a002865, 2018.
10. Carpten, J.C., and Mardis, E.R., The era of precision oncogenomics, *Cold Spring Harb. Mol. Case Stud.* 4, a002915, 2018.

ONCONASE® (RANPIRNASE)

Onconase® (ranpirnase) is a ribonuclease isolated from amphibia.[1] Ranpirnase is homologous to pancreatic ribonuclease but has low activity in the hydrolysis of RNA but substantial cytolytic activity.[2,3] Ranpirnase was originally described as P-30 protein (Pannon) isolated from various verebrates.[4,5] Onconase® is being developed for clinical use in oncology.[6] Antibody-drug conjugate technology has been used to improve the specificity of Onconase® as an antibody-RNase conjugate (immunoRNase).[7–9] Onconase® (rampirnase) has also been suggested to inactivate Ebola virus.[10]

1. Ardelt, W., Mikulski, S.M., and Shogen, K., Amino acid sequence of an anti-tumor protein from *Rana Pipiens* oocytes and early embryos. Homology to pancreatic ribonuclease, *J. Biol. Chem.* 266, 245–251, 1991.
2. Wu, Y., Mikulski, S.M., Ardelt, W., et al., A cytotoxic ribonuclease. Study of the mechanism of onconase cytotoxicity, *J. Biol. Chem.* 268, 10686–10693, 1993.
3. Kim, B.M., Kim, H., Raines, R.T., et al., Glycosylation of onconase increases its conformational stability and toxicity for cancer cells, *Biochem. Biophys. Res. Commun.* 315, 976–983, 2004.
4. Darzynkiewicz, Z., Carter, S.P., Mikulski, S.M., Ardelt, W.J., and Shogen, K., Cytostatic and cytotoxic effects of Pannon (P-30 protein), a novel anticancer agent, *Cell Tissue Kinet.* 21, 169–182, 1988.
5. Mikulski, S.M., Ardelt, W., Shogen, K., Bernstein, E.H., and Menduke, H., Striking increase of survival of mice bearing M109 Madison carcinoma treated with a novel protein from amphibian embryos, *J. Natl. Cancer Inst.* 82, 151–153, 1990.
6. Smolewski, P., Witkowska, M., Zolinska, M., et al., Cytotoxic activity of the amphibian ribonucleases onconase and r-amphinase on tumor cells from B cell lymphoproliferative disorders, *Int. J. Oncol.* 45, 419–425, 2014.
7. Weber, T., Mavratzas, A., Kiesgen, S., et al., A humanized anti-CD22-onconase antibody drug conjugate mediates highly potent destruction of targeted tumor cells, *J. Immunol. Res.* 2015, 561814, 2015.
8. Jordaan, S., Akinrinamade, O.A., Nachreiner, T., et al., Updates in the development of immunoRNase for the selective killing of tumor cells, *Biomedicines* 6(1), E28, 2018.
9. Sun, M., Sun, L., Sun, D., et al., Targeted delivery of immune-RNase may improve cancer therapy, *Cancer Cell Int.* 18, 58, 2018.
10. Hodge, T., Draper, K., Brasel, T., et al., Antiviral effect of ranpirnase against Ebola virus, *Antiviral Res.* 132, 210–218, 2016.

OPERON

An operon can be defined as a unit of coordinated gene activity which regulates protein synthesis in prokaryotes, consisting of a linear sequence of structural genes with one or more regulatory regions.[1] The term was advanced by Jacob and Monod in 1960 as a genetic unit of coordinate expression.[2–4] While the concept of the operon is considered to be a universal mechanism, it has been studied most extensively in bacterial systems. The original study stemmed from work on the metabolism of sugars in *Escherichia coli* and was of such monumental significance that an entire book was dedicated to the *lac* operon.[5] The *nar* operon in *E. coli* is one or the more highly studied and interesting operon. The *nar* operon encodes nitrate reductase, the first enzyme in the process of using nitrate as terminal electron acceptor in a number of bacteria.[6–8] This system is described as the respiratory nitrate reductase system and enables these bacteria to be facultative anaerobes. The promoter region of the *nar* operon is generally only maximally induced under anaerobic conditions. It has been shown that the *nar* promoter in some strains of *E. coli* can be induced under condition of very low oxygen tension in the presence of nitrate. This observation has been used to develop some useful processes for recombinant protein expression in *E. coli*.[9–12]

1. *Oxford English Dictionary*, Oxford University Press, Oxford, UK, 2019.
2. Jacob, F., Perrin, D., Sanchez, C., and Monod, J., Operon: A group of genes with the expression coordinated by an operator. *C. R.Hebd. Seances Acad. Sci.* 250, 1727–1729, 1960.
3. Jacob, F., and Monod, J., Genetic regulatory mechanisms in the synthesis of proteins, *J. Mol. Biol.* 3, 318–356, 1961.
4. Jacob, F., The birth of the operon, *Science* 332, 767, 1961.
5. Muller-Hill, B., *The lac Operon: A Short History of a Genetic Paradigm*, Walter de Gruyter, Berlin, Germany, 1996.
6. Blasco, F., Pommier, J., Augier, V., Chippaux, M., and Giordano, G., Involvement of the narJ or narW gene product in the formation of active nitrate reductase in *Escherichia coli*, *Mol. Microbiol.* 6, 221–230, 1992.
7. Dubourdieu, M., and DeMoss, J.A, The narJ gene product is required for biogenesis of respiratory nitrate reductase in *Escherichia coli*, *J. Bacteriol.* 174, 867–872, 1992.
8. Hoffmann, T., Troup, B., Szabo, A., Hungerer, C., and Jahn, D., The anaerobic life of *Bacillus subtitlis*; cloning of the genes encoding the respiratory nitrate reductase system, *FEMS Microbiol. Lett.* 131, 219–225, 1995.
9. Han, S.J., Chang, H.N., and Lee, J., Characterization of an oxygen-dependent inducible promoter, the *nar* promoter of *Escherichia coli*, to utilize in metabolic engineering, *Biotechnol. Bioeng.* 72, 573–577, 2001.
10. Kim, N.J., Choi, J.H., Kim, Y.C., et al., Development of anaerobically inducible *nar* promoter expression vectors for the expression of recombinant proteins in *Escherichia coli*, *J. Biotechnol.* 151, 102–107, 2011.

11. Hwang, H.J., Kim, J.W., Ju, S.Y., Park, J.H., and Lee, P.C., Application of an oxygen-inducible *nar* promoter system in metabolic engineering for production of biochemicals in *Escherichia coli*, *Biotechnol. Bioengineer.* 114, 468–473, 2017.
12. Hwang, H.J., Lee, S.Y., Lee, P.C., Engineering and application of synthetic *nar* promoter for fine-tuning the expression of metabolic pathway genes in *Escherichia coli*, *Biotechnol. Biofuels.* 11, 103, 2018.

OPEN READING FRAME (ORF)

The canonical definition of an open reading frame (ORF) is a DNA sequence divisible by 3 which starts with an initiation codon (transcription start site), the AUG coding for methionine, and ending with a stop codon which encodes a protein.[1] There are other possibilities such as a sequence of triplet bases between two stop codons or a third involving splicing bordered by a donor and acceptor splice site.[2]

1. Brown, A., Shao, S., Murray, J., Hegde, R.S., and Ramakrishnan, Structural basis for stop codon recognition in eukaryotes, *Nature* 524, 493–496, 2015.
2. Sieber, P., Platzer, M., and Schuster, S., The definition of open reading frame revisited, *Trends Genet.* 34, 162–170, 2018.

OPSONIZATION

Opsonization is the process by which a foreign body, usually a bacterial cell, is coated with an antibody (an opsonin) and then destroyed by the subsequent process of phagocytosis by an immune cell, frequently a macrophage.[1,2] The canonical process of opsonization involves the reaction of an IgG protein with an antigen via the CDR in the amino-terminal portion of the antibody yielding an antigen-antibody complex. There is a conformational change in the C-terminal region of the molecule (the Fc domain) allowing binding to a specific receptor on the immune cell.[3] Neutrophils also participate in antibody-dependent opsonization.[4]

1. Lu, J., Marjon, K.D., Mold, C., Du Clos, T.W., and Sun, T.W., Pentraxins and Fc receptors, *Immunol. Rev.* 250, 230–238, 2012.
2. Sosale, N.G., Spinler, K.R., Alvey, C., and Discher, D.E., Macrophage engulfment of a call or nanoparticle is regulated by unavoidable opsonization, a species-specific 'marker of self' CD47, and target physiological properties, *Curr. Opin. Immunol.* 35, 107–112, 2015.
3. Joller, N., Weber, S.S., and Oxenius, A., Antibody-Fc receptor interactions in protection against intracellular pathogens, *Eur. J. Immunol.* 41, 899–897, 2011.
4. Thomsen, K., Christophersen, L., Jenson, P.Ø., et al., Anti-*Pseudomonas aeruginosa* IgY antibodies promote bacterial opsonization and augment the phagocytic activity of polymorphonuclear neutrophils, *Hum. Vaccin. Immunother.* 12, 1690–1699, 2016.

OPTICAL ACTIVITY

The canonical definition of optical activity is the ability of chemical compounds to rotate the plane of polarization of polarized light; compounds may be dextrorotatory (*d*)(+) or levorotatory (*l*)(−); (±) is used to indicate racemic mixtures. These signs are arbitrary as rotation can change with the wavelength of light. Optical activity is associated with asymmetric compounds.[1] Such compounds are defined as optically active or having chiral properties and characterized by polarimetry. The optical activity of a chemical compound is a chemical property and an index of stereochemical purity. Optical activity and the measurement of optical activity has a long history.[2,3] Optical Rotatory Dispersion (ORD) and Circular Dichroism are more complex measurements of optical activity used for study of polymer conformation. ORD is the change in the optical rotation of a sample with a change in the wavelength of the light.[4] Circular dichroism is a change in the velocity of light- and right-circularly polarized light as it passes through a sample (the differential absorption of left- and right-handed light).[5] It is suggested that CD is more useful than ORD, although advances in instrumentation has increased the use of ORD.[4] Interpretation of ORD can be challenging.[5] Raman optical activity (chiroptical Raman activity where the difference in Raman scattering intensity of left and right circularly polarized light is measured) is useful for the study of protein structure.[6–9]

1. Sharp, D.W.A., *Penguin Dictionary of Chemistry*, 2nd edn., Penguin Books, London, UK, 1990.
2. Charney, E., *The Molecular Basis of Optical Activity Optical Rotatory Dispersion and Circular Dichroism,* Chapter 1, Discovery, Development and Nomenclature, pp. 1–17. John Wiley & Sons, New York, 1979.
3. Lightner, D.A., and Gorst, J.E., *Organic Conformation Analysis and Stereocemistry,* Chapter 2, Optical activity, pp. 37–61, Wiley-VCH, New York, 2000.
4. Castiglioni, E., Abbate, S., and Longhi, G., Experimental methods for measuring optical rotatory dispersion: Survey and outlook, *Chirality* 23, 711–716, 2011.
5. Cowman, M.K., and Matsuoka, S., Experimental approaches to hyaluronan structure, *Carbohydr. Res.* 340, 791–809, 2005.
6. Barron, L.D., Magnetic vibrational optical activity in the resonance Raman spectrum of ferrocytochrome c, *Nature* 257, 372–374, 1975.

7. Weymuth, T., and Reiher, M., Characteristic Raman optical activity signatures of protein β-sheets, *J. Phys. Chem. B* 117, 11943–11953, 2013.
8. Martial, B., Lefèvre, T., and Auger, M., Understanding amyloid fibril formation using protein fragments: Structural investigations via vibrational spectroscopy and solid-state NMR, *Biophys. Rev.* 10, 1133–1149, 2018.
9. Haraguchi, S., Shingae, T., Fujisawa, T., et al., Spectroscopic ruler for measuring active-site distortions based on Raman optical activity of a hydrogen out-of-plane vibration, *Proc. Natl. Acad. Sci. USA* 115, 8671–8675, 2018.

OPTICAL ROTATORY DISPERSION (ORD)

Optical rotatory dispersion (ORD) is the measurement of the differential change in the velocity of light- and right-circularly polarized light as it passes through a sample. ORD has been used to study protein folding using time-resolved spectroscopy.[1,2] There was considerable early enthusiasm about the application of ORD to the study of protein conformation, it has been supplanted by other techniques such as NMR. ORD still has use in organic chemistry in combination with other techniques such as vibrational circular dichroism.[3–6]

1. Kliger, D.S., Chen, E., and Goldbeck, R.A., Probing kinetic mechanisms of protein function and folding with time-resolved natural and magnetic chiroptical spectroscopies, *Int. J. Mol. Sci.* 13, 683–697, 2012.
2. Chen, E., and Kliger, D.S., Deconstructing time-resolved optical rotatory dispersion kinetic measurements of cytochrome c folding: From molten globule to the native state, *Methods Mol. Biol.* 895, 405–419, 2012.
3. Mazzeo, G., Cimmino, A., Masi, M., et al., Importance and difficulties in the use of chiroptical methods to assign the absolute configuration of natural products: The case of phytotoxic pyrones and furanones produced by *Diplodia corticola, J. Nat. Prod.* 80, 2406–2415, 2017.
4. Covington, C.L., Raghavan, V., Smuts, J.P., Armstrong, D.W., and Polavarapu, P.L., Absolute configuration of an axially chiral sulfonate determined from its optical rotatory dispersion, electronic circular dichroism, and vibrational circular dichroism spectra, *Chirality* 29, 670–676, 2017.
5. Lesnichaya, M.V., Sukhov, G.B., Aleksandrova, G.P., et al., Chiroplasmonic magnetic gold nanocomposites produced by one-step aqueous method using κ-carrageenan, *Carbohydr. Polym.* 175, 18–26, 2017.
6. Vergura, S., Santoro, E., Masi, M., et al., Absolute configuration assignment to anticancer Amaryllidaceae alkaloid jonquailine, *Fitoerapia* 129, 78–84, 2018.

OPTICAL SWITCHES

On description of an optical switch in telecommunications is a switch that enables signals in optical fibers or integrated optical circuits (IOCs) to be selectively switched from one circuit to another.[1] An optical switch is formally described as a device that can be made to deflect, interrupt, or modify an incident beam of light when required, as by varying the optical transmission properties of a material by means of an applied electric or magnetic field.[2] An optical switch in chemistry can be a molecule that changes optical properties in response to light (electromagnetic radiation). The azobenzene linkage is of considerable interest in photochemistry because of facile photoisomerization.[3,4] The conversion of spiropyranes to merocyanine by UV absorbance at 365 nm is another optical switch where the merocyanine has absorbance at 500 nm while the spiropyrane lacks significant UV absorbance.[5] The merocyanine derivative can be converted to the spirolactone form by visible light (approximately 400–700 nm). It also noted that the conversion of a dinitro-derivative of the chromene ring permit the conversion of the spiropyran to a merocyanine can be accomplished with a thiol.[6]

1. Maier, M., *Optical Switching Networks*, Cambridge University Press, Cambridge, UK, 2018.
2. *Oxford English Dictionary*, Oxford University Press, Oxford, UK, 2019.
3. Yager, K.D., and Barrett, C.J., Novel photo-switching using azobenzene functional materials, *J. Photochem. Photobiol. A Chemistry* 182, 250–261, 2006.
4. Wie, Z., He, H., Chi, Z., Ran, X., and Guo, L., Two-photon isomerization triggers two-photon-excited fluorescence of an azobenzene derivative, *Spectrochim. Acta Pt. A Mol. Bimol. Spectroscopy* 206, 120–125, 2019.
5. Sakata, T., Yan, Y., and Marriott, G., Family of site-selective molecular optical switches, *J. Org. Chem.* 70, 2009–2013, 2005.
6. Tantges, B., Or, V., Carcia, J., Shaw, J.T., and Louis, A.Y., Preparation of a conjugation-ready thiol responsive molecular switch, *Tetrahedron Lett.* 56, 6569–6573, 2015.

ORFeome

The ORFeome is the number of protein-coding open reading frames (ORFs) in an organism. Determining the number of ORFs in an organism is a formidable task. One approach is to use algorithms to search DNA databases.[1,2] A human ORF-clone resource has been established in the Gateway vector format.[3,4] There is also a Harvard ORF database.[5] There are small ORFs (defined as a series of in-frame codons following a start codon and terminated with a stop codon) which should be considered as the encode functional peptides.[6,7] An ORF database (Xenbase) is available for *Xenopus laevis/Xenopus tropicalis*.[8]

1. Brent, M.R., Genome annotation past, present, and future. How to define an ORF at each locus, *Genome Res.* 8:399, 2007.

2. Woodcroft, B.J., Boyd, J.A., and Tyson, G.W., OrfM: A fast open reading reading frame predictor from metagenomic data, *Bioinformatics* 32, 2702–2703, 2016.

3. Bechtel, S., Rosenfelder, H., Duda, A., et al., The full-ORF clone resource of the German cDNA consortium, *BMC Genomics* 8, 399, 2007.

4. Wiemann, S., Pennacchio, C., Hu, Y., et al., The ORFeome collaboration: A genome-scale human ORF-clone resource, *Nature Methods* 13, 191–192, 2016.

5. http://horfdb.dfci.harvard.edu/.

6. Pueyo, J.I., Magny, E.G., and Couso, J.P., New peptides under the s(ORF)ace of the genome, *Trends Biochem. Sci.* 41, 665–678, 2016.

7. Couso, J.P., and Patraquim, P., Classification and function of small open reading frames, *Nat. Rev. Mol. Cell Biol.* 18, 575–589, 2017.

8. Karimi, K., Fortriede, J.D., Lotay, V.S., et al., Xenbase: A genomic, epigenomic and transcriptomic model organism database, *Nucleic Acids Res.* 46, D861–D868, 2018.

ORGANELLE PROTEOMICS

Organelle proteomics is the analysis of subcellular organelles such as mitochondria, nucleus, the endocytotic apparatus by proteomic techniques.[1-6] There has been some success in the study of "unusual" organelles such as cilia.[7] It would appear that the most significant applications in organelle proteomics have been with plants in the study of chloroplasts.[8-16]

1. Huber, L.A., Pfaller, K., ad Vistor, I., Organelle proteomics: Implications for subcellular fractionation in proteomics, *Circ. Res.* 92, 962–968, 2003.

2. Taylor, S.W., Fahy, E., and Ghosh, S.S., Global organellar proteomics, *Trends Biotechnol.* 21, 82–88, 2003.

3. Huber, L.A., Pfaller, K., ad Vistor, I., Organelle proteomics: Implications for subcellular fractionation in proteomics, *Circ. Res.* 92, 962–968, 2003.

4. Warnock, D.E., Fahy, E., and Taylor, S.W., Identification of protein associations in organelles, using mass spectrometry-based proteomics, *Mass Spectrom. Rev.* 23, 259–280, 2004.

5. Yates, J.R., 3rd, Gilchrist, A., Howell, K.E., and Bergeron, J.J., Proteomics of organelles and large cellular structures, *Nat. Rev. Mol. Cell Biol.* 6, 702–714, 2005.

6. Duclos, S., and Desjardins, M., Organelle proteomics, *Methods Mol. Biol.* 753, 117–128, 2011.

7. Boldt, K., van Reeuwijk, J., Lu, Q., et al., An organelle-specific protein landscape identifies novel diseases and molecular mechanisms, *Nat. Commun.* 7, 11491, 2016.

8. Jan van Wijk, K., Proteomics or the chloroplast: Experimentation and prediction, *Trends Plant Sci.* 5, 420–425, 2000.

9. Jarvis, P., Organeller proteomics: Chloroplasts in the spotlight, *Curr. Biol.* 14, R317–R319, 2004.

10. van Wijk, K.J., Plastid proteomics, *Plant Physiol. Biochem.* 42, 963–977, 2004.

11. Rutschow, H., Ytterberg, A.J., Frisco, G., Nilsson, R., and van Wijk, K.J., Quantitative proteomics of a chloroplast SRP54 soring mutant and its genetic interactions with CLPC1 in *Arabidopsis*, *Plant Physiol.* 148, 156–175, 2008.

12. van Wijk, K.J., and Baginsky, S., Plastid proteomics in higher plants: Current state and future goals, *Plant Physiol.* 155, 1578–1588, 2011.

13. Agrawal, G.K., Bourguignon, J., Rolland, N., et al., Plant organelle proteomics: Colleaborating for optimal cell function, *Mass Spectrom. Rev.* 30, 772–853, 2011.

14. Hossain, Z., Nouri, M.Z., and Komatsu, S., Plant cell organelle proteomics in response to abiotic stress, *J. Proteome Res.* 11, 37–48, 2012.

15. Carraretto, L., Teardo, E., Checchetto, V., et al., Ion channels in plant bioenergetic organelles, chloroplasts and mitochondria: From molecular identification to function, *Mol. Plant* 9, 371–395, 2016.

16. Pocsfalvi, G., Turiák, L., Ambrosone, A., et al., Protein biocargo of citrus fruit-derived vesicles reveals heterogeneous transport and extracellular vesicel populations, *J. Plant Physiol.* 229, 111–121, 2018.

ORTHOGONAL

In mathematics, the term orthogonal describes two lines intersecting at right angles (mathematics). In Euclidean space, two vectors are orthogonal if make an angle of $90°$ or if the angle of one vector is $0°$. The term is derived from the Greek *orthos* meaning straight, upright, vertical. The term orthogonal has been used to describe a variety of activities in biochemistry and molecular biology including protein purification and analysis. The term orthogonal was used in the process developed for the incorporation of unusual/novel amino acids into proteins. The process involved the identification of a suppressor tRNA and a compatible tRNA synthetase which can incorporate a novel amino acid into a position specified by an amber mutant codon.[1-3] *Escherichia coli* was the host organism for these early studies. The term orthogonal was used to indicate that neither tRNA or tRNA synthetase would function with the native transcription components in *E. coli*. The term orthogonal was not used in the original concept paper.[4] The orthogonal technique has been extended to mammalian cells.[5] The biorthogonal has been advanced to describe a chemical reaction which can occurs within a cell or organism without affecting the organism.[6–8] The work on orthogonal modification by engineering tRNA interaction provided unique amino acid residues for modification of protein by novel chemical reaction providing the basis for other biorthogonal modification in cells.[9–11] The term **orthogonal** also refers to purification, in particular, the purification of proteins, where two different techniques (multi-dimensional) relying on different properties of the proteins.[12,13] **Orthogonal analytical techniques** are also used for the characterization of biopharmaceutical proteins.[14–17]

1. Liu, D.R., Magliery, T.J., Pastrnak, M., and Schultz, P.G., Engineering a tRNA and aminoacyl-tRNA synthetase for the site-specific incorporation of unnatural amino acids into protein *in vivo*, *Proc. Natl. Acad. Sci. USA* 94, 10092–10097, 1997.
2. Wang, L., and Schultz, P.G., A general approach for the generation of orthogonal tRNAs, *Chem. Biol.* 8, 883–890, 2001.
3. Wang, L., Brock A., Heberich, B., and Schultz, P.G., Expanding the genetic code of *Escherichia coli*, *Science* 292, 498–500, 2001.
4. Noren, C.J., Anthony-Cahill, S.J., Griffith, M.C., and Schultz, P.G., A general method for site-specific incorporation of unnatural amino acids into proteins, *Science* 244, 182–188, 1989.
5. Köhrer, C., Sullivan, E.L., and RajBhandary, U.L., Complete set of orthogonal 21st aminoacyl-tRNA synthetase-amber, ochre and opal suppressor tRNA pairs: Concomitant suppression of three different termination codons in an mRNA in mammalian cells, *Nucl. Acids Res.* 21, 6200–6211, 2004.
6. Hang, H.C., Yu, C., Kato, D.L., and Bertozzi, C.R., A metabolic labeling approach toward proteomic analysis of mucin-type O-linked glycosylation, *Proc. Natl. Acad. Sci. USA* 100, 14846–14851, 2003.
7. van Swieten, P.F., Leeuwenburgh, M.A., Kessler, B.M., and Overkleeft, H.S., Bioorthogonal organic chemistry in living cells: Novel strategies for labeling biomolecules, *Org. Biomol. Chem.* 3, 20–27, 2005.
8. Sen Gupta, S., Kuzelka, J., Singh, P., Accelerated biorthogonal: A practical method for the ligation of diverse functional molecules to a polyvalent virus scaffold, *Bioconjug. Chem.* 16, 1572–1579, 2005.
9. Luo, X., Zambaldo, C., Liu, T., et al., Recombinant thiopeptides containing noncanonical amino acids, *Proc. Natl. Acad. Sci. USA* 113, 3615–3620, 2016.
10. Lee, T.C., Kang, M., Kim, C.H., et al., Dual unnatural amino acid incorporation and click-chemistry labeling to enable single-molecule FRET studies of p97 folding, *Chembiochem* 17, 981–984, 2016.
11. Yang, A.C., du Bois, H., Olsson, N., et al., Multiple click-selective tRNA synthetases expand mammalian cell-specific proteomics, *J. Am. Chem. Soc.* 140, 7046–7051, 2018.
12. Evans, C.R., and Jorgenson, J.W., Multidimensional LC-LC and LC-CE for high resolution separations of biologicals, *Anal. Bioanal. Chem.* 378, 1952–1961, 2004.
13. Cap, S., Pollasrtini, J., and Jiang, Y., Separation and characterization of protein aggregates and particles by field flow fractionation, *Curr. Pharm. Biotechnol.* 10, 382–390, 2009.
14. Righetti, P.G., Bioanalysis: Its past, present, and future, *Electrophoresis* 25, 2111–2127, 2004.
15. Carpenter, J.F., Randolph, T.W., Jiskoot, W., et al., Potential inaccurate quantitation and sizing of protein aggregates by size exclusion chromatography; essential need to use orthogonal methods to assure the quality of therapeutic protein products, *J. Pharm. Sci.* 99, 2200–2209, 2010.
16. Berkowitz, S.A., Engen, J.R., Mazzeo, J.R., and Jones, G.B., Analytical toos for characterizing biopharmaceuticals and the implications for biosimilars, *Nature Rev. Drug. Discov.* 11, 527–540, 2012.
17. Fekete, S., Veuthey, J.L., Beck, A., and Guillarme, D., Hydrophobic interaction chromatography for the characterization of monoclonal antibodies and related products, *J. Pharm. Biopharm. Anal.* 130, 3–18, 2016.

ORTHOLOGS

In genetics, the canonical definition of the term orthologs refers to genes in different organisms which have similar function (gene pairs which have arisen from speciation).[1–4] There are a number of examples of orthologs[5–10] which are contrasted with **paralogs** which are also homologs but result from gene duplication.[11–14]

1. Li., L., Stoeckert, C.J., Jr., and Roos, D.S., OrthoMCL: Identification of ortholog groups for eukaryotic genomes, *Genome Res.* 13, 2178–2189, 2003.
2. Sjölander, K., Datta, R.S., Shen, Y., and Shoffner, G.M., Ortholog identification in the presence of domain architecture rearrangement, *Brief Bioinform.* 12, 413–422, 2011.
3. Altenhoff, A.M., Boeckmann, B., Capella-Gutierrez, S., et al., Standardized benchmarking in the quest for orthologs, *Nat. Methods* 13, 425–430, 2016.
4. Miller, J.B., Pickett, B.D., and Ridge, P.G., Just Orthologs: A fast, accurate, and user-friendly ortholog identification algorithm, *Bioinformatics* 35, 546–552, 2018.
5. Hudson, B.D., Murdoch, H., and Milligan, G., Minireview: The effects of species ortholog and SNP variation on receptors for free fatty acids, *Mol. Endocrinol.* 27, 1177–1187, 2013.
6. Igaki, T., and Miura, M., The Drosophila TNF ortholog Eiger: Emerging physiological roles and evolution of the TNF system, *Semin. Immunol.* 26, 267–274, 2014.

7. Sun, M., Feng, X., Liu, Z., et al., An Orc1/Cdc6 ortholog functions as a key regulator in the DNA damage response in *Archaea*, *Nucleic Acids Res.* 46, 6697–6711, 2018.

8. Pertusa, M., Rivera, B., González, A., Ugarte, G., and Madrid, R., Critical role of the pore domain in the cold response to TRPM8 channels identified by ortholog functional comparison, *J. Biol. Chem.* 293, 12454–12471, 2018.

9. Baeza Garcia, A., Siu, E., Sun, T., et al., Neutralization of the *Plasmodium*-encoded MIF ortholog confers protective immunity against malaria infection, *Nat. Commun.* 9, 2714, 2018.

10. Dahal, G.P., and Viola, R.E., Structural insights into inhibitor binding to a fungal ortholog of aspartate semialdehyde dehydrogenase, *Biochem. Biophys. Res. Commun.* 503, 2848–2854, 2018.

11. Hlouchová, K., Navrátil, V., Tykvart, J., Sácha, P., and Konvalinka, J., GCPII variants, paralogs and orthologs, *Curr. Med. Chem.* 19, 1316–1322, 2012.

12. Desideri, E., Cavallo, A.L., and Baccarini, M., Alike, but different: RAF paralogs and their signaling outputs, *Cell* 161, 967–970, 2015.

13. Chung, K.P., Zeng, Y., and Jiang, L., COPII paralogs in plans: Functional redundancy or diversity? *Trends Plant. Sci.* 21, 758–769, 2016.

14. Widemam, J.G., Balacco, D.L., Fieblinger, T., and Richards, T.A., PDZ8 is not the "functional ortholog" of Mmm1, it is a paralog, *F1000Res.* 7, 1088, 2018.

OSMOSENSOR

An osmosensor is a cell surface receptor which measures the osmolality of the medium external to a cell. The cell or organisms will respond to the information provided by the osmosensor to adapt to the osmolality of the environment around the cell. Bacteria respond to changes in external osmotic changes by either accumulating or exporting solutes (osmolytes, inorganic ions); changes in internal solute concentration will result in changes in water concentration inside the cell.[1] Bacteria have specific membrane transporters which respond to osmotic stress (osmostress).[2] Yeast use the high osmolarity glycerol (HOG) pathway to adapt to high external osmolality.[3,4] The membrane receptor Sho1 is "activated" by high external osmolarity leading to the activation of the Hog1 map (mitogen-activated protein) kinase initiating the intracellular synthesis of glycerol is a process which can be described as osmodaptation.[5,6] The osmosensor and related pathways become far more complicated in metazoan organisms.[7–9] There is particular interest in transient receptor potential (TRP) channels as an osmosensor[10–12] recognizing that TRPV4 is pleiotropic.[13] There is a suggestion that cytoplasm can act as an osmosensor at the level or the mammalian cell.[14]

1. Wood, J.M., Bacterial responses to osmotic challenges, *J. Gen. Physiol.* 145, 381–388, 2014.

2. Poolman, B., Spitzer, J.J., and Wood, J.M., Bacterial osmosensing: Roles of membrane structure and electrostatics in lipid-protein and protein-protein interactions, *Biochim. Biophys. Acta* 1666, 88–104, 2004.

3. Van Wuytswinkel, O., Reiser, V., Siderius, M., et al., Response of *Saccharomyces cerevisiae* to severe osmotic stress: Evidence for a novel activation mechanism of the HOG MAP kinase pathway, *Mol. Microbiol.* 37, 382–397, 2000.

4. Tatebayashi, K., Yamamoto, K., Nagoya, A., et al., Osmosensing and scaffolding functions of the oligomeric four-transmembrane domain osmosensor Sho1, *Nature Commun.* 6, 6995, 2015.

5. McLaggan, D., Logan, T.M., Lynn, D.G., and Epstein, W., Involvement of γ-glutamyl peptides in osmoadaptation of *Escherichia coli*, *J. Bacteriol.* 172, 3631–3636, 1990.

6. Welsh, D.T., Reed, R.H., and Herbert, R.A., The role of trehalose in the osmoadaptation of *Escherichia coli* NCIB 9484, *J. Gen. Microbiol.* 137, 745–750, 1991.

7. Woudenberg-Vrenken, T.E., Bindels, R.J., and Hoenderop, J.G., The role of transient receptor potential channels in kidney disease, *Nat. Rev. Nephrol.* 5, 441–449, 2009.

8. Noda, M., and Sakuta, H., Central regulation of body-fluid homeostasis, *Trends Neurosci.* 36, 661–673, 2013.

9. Agnati, L.F., Marcoli, M., Leo, G., Maura, G., and Guidolin, D., Homeostasis and the concept of "interstitial fluids hierarchy": Relevance of cerebrospinal fluid sodium concentrations and brain temperature control, *Int. J. Mol. Med.* 39, 487–497, 2017.

10. Liedtke, W., TRPV4 as osmosensor: A transgenic approach, *Pflugers Arch.* 451, 176–180, 2005.

11. Shibasaki, K., TRPV4 ion channel as important ion sensors, *J. Anesth.* 30, 1014–1019, 2016.

12. Kumar, H., Lee, S.H., Kim, K.T., Zeng, X., and Han, I., TRPV4: A sensor for homeostasis and pathological events in the CNS, *Mol. Neurobiol.*, 55, 8695–8708, 2018.

13. Kanju, P., and Liedtke, W., Pleiotropic function of TRPV4 ion channels in the central nervous system, *Exp. Physiol.* 101, 1472–1476, 2016.

14. Fels, J., Orlov, S.N., and Grygovczyk, R., The hydrogel nature of mammalian cytoplasm contributes to osmosensing and extracellular pH sensing, *Biophys. J.* 96, 4276–4285, 2009.

OSTEOBLAST

Osteoblasts are bone-forming cells which secrete matrix proteins and mineral. Osteoblasts comprise 4%–6% of the cells in bone and are critical to the maintenance of bone mass.[1] **Osteocalcin** (originally described as bone gla protein) is a small protein or large peptide (ca. 5.5 kDa) which may contain γ-carboxyglutamic acid (GLA) and bind calcium ions.[2,3] Osteocalcin synthesized and secreted by osteoblasts during the process of bone formation as an approximately 10 kDa precursor.[4] The expression of osteocalcin can be enhanced by Vitamin D[5] but there are species differences in this effect.[6] Osteocalcin exists in two forms, a form containing 2–3 residues of GLA, which is incorporated into developing bone and an "undercarboxylated" form which is secreted and has been suggested to have an endocrine function in the regulation of glucose metabolism.[7,8] The carboxylated form of osteocalcin is suggested to have a role in the regulation of mineralization.[9] There interest in the therapeutic use of osteocalcin.[10,11] It has been reported that an increase in the undercarboxylated form of osteocalcin is associated with an increase in bone fractures.[12]

1. Capulli, M., Paone, R., and Rucci, N., Osteoblast and osteocyte: Games without frontiers, *Arch. Biochem. Biophys.* 561, 3–12, 2014.
2. Hauschka, P.V., Lian, J.B., Cole, D.E. c., and Gundberg, C.M., Osteocalcin and matrix Gla-protein: Vitamin K-dependent proteins in bone, *Physiol. Rev.* 69, 990–1047, 1989.
3. Zoch, M.L., Clemens, T.L., and Riddle, R.C., New insights into the biology of osteocalcin, *Bone* 82, 42–49, 2016.
4. Celeste, A.J., Rosen, V., Bruecker, J.L., et al., Isolation of the human gene for bone gla protein utilizing mouse and rat cDNA clones, *EMBO J.* 5, 1885–1890, 1986.
5. Lian, J., Stewart, C., Puchacz, E., et al., Structure of the rat osteocalcin gene and regulation of vitamin D-dependent expression, *Proc. Natl. Acad. Sci.* 86, 1143–1147, 1989.
6. van de Peppel, J., and van Leeuwen, J.P.T.M., Vitamin D and gene networks in human osteoblasts, *Front. Physiol.* 5, 137, 2014.
7. Gundberg, C.M., Lian, J.B., and Booth, S.L., Vitamin K-dependent carboxylation of osteocalcin: Friend or foe? *Adv. Nutrition* 3, 149–157, 2012.
8. Mirokami, A., Kawakubo-Yasukochi, T., and Hirata, M., Osteocalcin and its endocrine function, *Biochem. Pharmacol.* 132, 1–8, 2017.
9. Hasegawa, T., Ultrastructure and biological function of matrix vesicles in bone mineralization, *Histochem. Cell Biol.* 149, 389–304, 2018.
10. Ferron, M., McKee, M.D., Levine, R.L., Ducy, P., and Karsenty, G., Intermittent injections osteocalcin improve glucose metabolism and prevent type 2 diabetes in mice, *Bone* 50, 568–575, 2012.
11. Gupte, A.A., Sabek, O.M., Fraga, D., et al., Osteocalcin protects against nonalcoholic steatohepatitis in a mouse model of metabolic syndrome, *Endocrinology* 155, 4696–4705, 2014.
12. Hirakawa, H., Gatanaga, H., Ochi, H., et al., Antiretroviral therapy containing HIV protease inhibitors enhances fracture risk by impairing osteoblast differentiation and bone quality, *J. Infect. Dis.* 215, 1893–1897, 2017.

OSTEOCLAST

Osteoclasts are bone-degrading cells which have a limited life time and have an opposite function to osteoblasts.[1] Osteoclasts are formed (osteoclastogeneisis) from blood-derived monocytes in a process which involves the binding of receptor-activated NF-κB ligand (RANKL)[2] to the receptor-activated NF-κB (RANK) receptor.[3–5] A simplistic view of the process of osteoblast function is the dissolution of hard tissue (**osteolysis**). However, osteolysis is a sequential process[6,7] where the osteoclast attaches to the bard surface matrix establishing a microenvironment with the secretion of acid to dissolve the mineral component[8,9] followed by the degradation of the collagen I matrix by cathepsin K, a lysosomal cysteine protease.[10,11] Osteoprotegerin is glycoprotein showing sequence homology to the TNF superfamily which block the activation of osteoclasts.[12] There is significant interest in pharmacological modulation of osteoclast activity reflecting its role in the development of osteoporosis. Approaches have included the development of inhibitors of RANKL binding to RANK[13] and the development of inhibitors to cathepsin K.[14]

1. D'Amico, L., and Roato, H., Osteoclasts: The major actors in bone resorption, in *Osteoclasts: Morphology, Function, and Clinical Implications*, ed. A.J. Brown and J.S. Walker, Chapter 5, pp. 95–112, Nova Science Publishers, New York, 2012.
2. Willard, D., Chen, W.J., Barrett, G., Expression, purification, and characterization of the human receptor activator of NF-κB ligand (RANKL) extracellular domain, *Protein Expr. Purif.* 20, 48–57, 2000.
3. Nanke, Y., Kobashigawa, T., Yago, T., et al., RANK expression and osteoclastogenesis in human monocytes in peripheral blood from rheumatoid arthritis patients, *Biomed. Res. Intern.* 2016, 4874195, 2016.
4. Tsukasaki, M., Hamada, K., Okamoto, K., et al., LOX fails to substitute for RANKL in osteoclastogenesis, *J. Bone Mineral Res.* 32, 434–439, 2017.
5. Ono, T., and Nakashima, T., Recent advances in osteoclast biology, *Histochem. Cell Biol.* 149, 325–31, 2018.
6. Teitelbaum, S.L., Tondravi, M.M., and Ross, R.P., Osteoclasts, macrophages, and the molecular mechanisms of bone resorption, *J. Leukocyte Biol.* 61, 381–388, 1997.
7. Mbalaviele, G., Novack, D.V., Schett, G., and Teitelbaum, S.L., Inflammatory osteolysis: A conspiracy against bone, *J. Clin. Invest.* 127, 2030–2039, 2017.
8. Teitelbaum, S.L. Bone resorption by osteoclasts, *Science* 289, 1504–1508, 2000.
9. Teitelbaum, S.L., and Zou, W., The osteoclast cytoskeleton: How does it work? *IBMS BoneKEy* 8, 74–83, 2011.
10. Bossard, M.J., Tomaszek, T.A., Thompson, S.K., et al., Proteolytic activity of human osteoclast cathepsin K. Expression, activation, and substrate identification, *J. Biol. Chem.* 271, 12517–12524, 1996.

11. Garnero, P., Borel, O., Byrjalsen, I., et al., The collageno-lytic activity of cathepsin K is unique among mammalian proteinases, *J. Biol. Chem.* 273, 32347–32352, 1998.
12. Simonet, W.S., Lacey, D.L., Dunstan, C.R., et al., Osprotegerin: A novel secreted protein involved in the regulation of bone density, *Cell* 89, 309–319, 1997.
13. Lacey, D.L., Boyle, W.J., Simonet, W.S., et al., Bench to bedside: Elucidation of the OPG-RANK-RANKL pathway and the development of denosumab, *Nature Rev. Drug Discov.* 11, 401–419, 2012.
14. Drake, M.T., Clarke, B.L., Oursler, M.J., and Khosla, S., Cathepsin K inhibitors for osteoporosis: Biology, potential clinical utility, and lessons learned, *Endocr. Rev.* 38, 325–350, 2017.

OSTEOCYTE

The osteocyte is a considered to be a terminally differentiated osteoblast responsible for the control of osteoblast and osteoclast function.[1,2]

1. Prideaux, M., Findlay, D.M., and Atkins, G.J., Osteocytes: The master cells in bone remodeling, *Curr. Opin. Pharmacol.* 28, 24–30, 2016.
2. Joeng, K.S., Lee, Y.C., Lim, J., et al., Osteocyte-specific WNT1 regulates osteoblast function during bone homeostasis, *J. Clin. Invest.* 127, 2678–2688, 2017.

OSTEOPROTEGERIN (OPG)

Osteoprotegerin (OPG) is a secreted protein (401 amino acids) which is a paracrine factor in bone metabolism.[1] The primary structure deduced from the cDNA suggests that osteoprotegerin is a glycoprotein.[2] OPG is a member of the TGF superfamily without a transmembrane domain and inhibits the production of osteoclast by binding to RANKL[3] and hence inhibits the process of bone resorption. The OPG/RANKL/RANK system has importance in systems other than hard tissues (pleiotropic effect).[4–7] Heparin binds to osteoprotegerin and can enhance osteoclastic activity by inhibiting osteoprotegerin function.[8,9]

1. Hofbauer, L.C., Khosla, S., Dunstan, C.R., et al., The roles of osteoprotegerin and osteoprotegerin ligand in the paracrine regulation of bone resorption, *J. Bone Miner. Res.* 15, 2–12, 2000.
2. Simonet, W.S., Lacey, D.L., Dunstan, C.R., et al., Osteoprotegerin: A novel secreted protein involved in the regulation of bone density, *Cell* 309–319, 1997.
3. Boyce, B.F., and Xing, L., Biology of RANK, RANKL, and osteoprotegerin, *Arthritis Res.* 9(Suppl 1), S1, 2007.
4. Kong, Y.Y., Boyle, W.J., and Penninger, J.M., Osteoprotegerin ligand: A regulator of immune responses and bone physiology, *Immunol. Today* 21, 495–502, 2000.
5. Omland, T., Ueland, T., Jansson, A.M., et al., Circulating osteoprotegerin levels and long-term prognosis in patients with acute coronary syndromes, *J. Am. Coll. Cardiol.* 51, 627–633, 2008.
6. Liu, W., and Zhang, X., Receptor activator of nuclear factor-κB ligand (RANKL)/RANK/osteoprotegerin system in bone and other tissues, *Mol. Med.* 11, 3212–3218, 2015.
7. Weichhaus, M., Chung, S.T., and Connelly, L., Osteoprotegerin in breast cancer: Beyond bond remodeling, *Mol. Cancer* 14, 117, 2015.
8. Irie, A., Takami, M., Kubo, H., et al., Heparin enhances osteoclastic bone resorption by inhibiting osteoprotegerin activity, *Bone* 41, 165–174, 2007.
9. LI, B., Lu, D., Chen, Y., Zhao, M., and Zuo, L., Unfractionated heparin promotes osteoclast formation in vitro by inhibiting osteoprotegerin activity, *Int. J. Mol. Sci.* 17(4), E613, 2016.

OUT-OF-FRAME

The term out-of-frame refers to a change in the triplet reading sequence DNA or RNA resulting from a mutation which results in an alternative translation. Examples of mutation include the deletion of a base which in one case results in the switch of a tumor suppressor to an oncogene.[1] Another out-of-frame mutation resulting from base deletion resulted in a strange gain-of-function mutation where the base deletion in *EPO* interrupted translation of the primary *EPO* mRNA but resulted in excess EPO production from a normally noncoding sequence in another exon.[2] Alternative splicing of sequence elements of the pre-mRNA (can be introns, exons, or parts of an exon) can result in a shift of the reading frame when compared to an alternative mature mRNA processed from the same pre-mRNA resulting in a different product.[3]

1. He, S., and Liang, C., Frameshift ion of UVRAG: Switching a tumor suppressor to an oncogene in colorectal cancer, *Autophagy* 11, 1939–1940, 2015.
2. Zmajkovic, J., Lundberg, P., Nienhold, R., et al., A gain-of-function mutation in EPO in familial erythrocytosis, *New Engl. J. Med.* 378, 924–930, 2018.
3. Asselta, R., Rimoldi, V., Guenna, I., et al., Molecular characterization of in-frame and out-of-frame alternative splicing in coagulation factor XI pre-mRNA, *Blood* 115, 2065–2072, 2010.

OXYANION HOLE

The oxyanion hole is a feature of the active sites of hydrolytic enzymes such as lipases or chymotrypsin where the oxyanion of the transition state is stabilized by hydrogen bonding to amide nitrogen(s) on the enzyme.[1–5] In one case, a substrate (cocaine) is suggested to contribute to stabilization of the oxyanion intermediate in its hydrolysis by human carboxylesterase-1.[6] A novel receptor that uses an oxyanion hole to bind carboxylic acids as has been synthesized.[7]

1. Menard, R., and Storer, A.C., Oxyanion hole interactions in serine cysteine proteases, *Biol. Chem. Hoppe Seyler* 373, 393–400, 1992.
2. Whiting, A.K., and Peticolas, W.L., Details of the acyl-enzyme intermediate and the oxyanion hole in serine protease catalysis, *Biochemistry* 33, 552–561, 1994.
3. Johal, S.S., Cui, J., Marankan, F., Fu, W., et al., An oxyanion-hole selective serine protease inhibitor in complex with trypsin, *Bioorg. Med. Chem.* 10, 41–46, 2002.
4. Lee, L.C., Lee, Y.L., Leu, R.J., and Shaw, J.F., Functional role of catalytic triad and oxyanion hole-forming residues on enzyme activity of *Escherichia coli* thioesterase I/protease I/Phospholipase L1, *Biochem. J.* 397, 69–76, 2006.
5. Zhang, W., Sulea, T., Tao, L., et al., Contribution of active site residues to substrate hydrolysis by USP2: Insights into catalysis by ubiquitin specific proteases. *Biochemistry* 50, 4775–4785, 2011.
6. Yao, J., Chen, X., Zheng, F., and Zhan, C.G., Catalytic reaction mechanism for drug metabolism in human carboxylesterase-1: Cocaine hydrolysis pathway, *Mol. Pharm.* 15, 3871–3880, 2018.
7. Rubio, O.H., Mazo, S.D., Monleón, L.M., et al., A cleft type receptor which combines an oxyanion hole with electrostatic interactions, *Org. Biomol. Chem.* 15, 4571–4578, 2017.

OXYGEN ACTIVATION

Oxygen activation refers to the process converting dioxygen (O_2) to a reactive form such as superoxide.[1] Superoxide is formed by the one-electron reduction of dioxygen.[2,3] The formation of peroxide is another example of oxygen activation.[4]

1. Cue, L., Jr., Dioxygen activating enzymes, in *Inorganic Chemistry: Structure and Reactivity*, University Science Books, Sausalito, CA, 2007.
2. Mason, R.P., and Holtzman, J.L., The role of catalytic superoxide formation in the O_2 inhibition of nitroreductase, *Biochem. Biophys. Res. Commun.* 67, 1267–1274, 1975.
3. Wong, H.S., Dighe, P.A., Mezera, V., Monternier, P.A., and Brand, M.D., Production of superoxide and hydrogen peroxide from specific mitochondrial sites under different bioenergetic conditions, *J. Biol. Chem.* 292, 16804–16809, 2017.
4. Kovaleva, E.G., and Lipscomb, J.D., Versatility of biological non-heme Fe(II) centers in oxygen activation reactions, *Nature Chem. Biol.* 4, 186–193, 2008.

PALINDROME

The term palindrome refers to an oligonucleotide sequence which reads the same forwards and backwards. Palindromic sequences are frequently present at the sites of restriction class II enzyme cleavages where opposing strands read the same; that is the $3'{\rightarrow}5'$ sequence in one strand is the same as the $5'{\rightarrow}3'$ sequence in the opposing strand.[1,2] A large palindrome may be initiate by a short inverted repeat[3] resulting in genetic instability.[4]

1. Fuglsang, A., Distribution of potential type II restriction sites (palindromes) in prokaryotes, *Biochem. Biophys. Res. Commun.* 310, 280–285, 2003.
2. Tóth, E., Huszár, K., Bencsura, P., et al., Restriction enzymes body doubles and PCR cloning: On the general use of type IIs restriction enzymes for cloning, *PLoS One* 9(3), e90896, 2014.
3. Tanaka, H., Tapscott, S.J., Trask, B.J., and Yao, M.-C., Short inverted repeats initiate gene amplification through the formation of a large DNA palindrome in mammalian cells, *Proc. Natl. Acad. Sci. USA* 99, 8772–8777, 2002.
4. Leach, D.R., Long DNA palindromes, cruciform structures, genetic instability and secondary structure repair, *Bioassays* 16, 893–900, 1994.

PARACRINE

Paracrine is a term used in reference to a hormone or other biological effector such as a peptide growth factor or cytokine which has an effect on the cell or tissue immediately surrounding the cell or tissue responsible for the synthesis of the given compound.[1,2] The concept of a paracrine gland was introduced by Feyrter in 1952[3] and gained acceptance.[4,5] The concept is now well established.[6–8] Understanding and use of paracrine secretion have gained importance in regenerative medicine.[9,10] See **autocrine, endocrine**.

1. Franchimont, P., *Paracrine Control*, Saunders, Philadelphia, PA, 1986.
2. Piva, F., *Cell to Cell Communication in Endocrinology*, Raven Press, New York, 1988.
3. Feyrter, F., Über die These von den peripherin endokrinen (parakrinen) Drüsen, *Acta Neurovegetative* 4, 409–424, 1952.
4. Feyrter, F., Zur Lehre von den peripheren endokrinen (parakrinen) Drüsen des Menschen Neue Erkenntulisse, *Wien. Med. Wochenschr.* 106, 515–516, 1956.
5. Razenhofer, M., von den peripheren endokrinen (parakrinen) Drüsen, *Wien. Klin. Wochenshr.* 83, 22–31, 1971.
6. Morhayim, J., Rudjito, R., van Leeuwen, J.P., and van Driel, M., Paracrine signaling by extracellular vesicles via osteoclasts, *Curr. Mol. Biol. Rep.* 2, 48–55, 2016.

7. Nava, E., and Llorens, S., The paracrine control of vascular motion. A historical perspective, *Pharmacol. Res.* 113, 125–145, 2016.

8. Ibrahim, A., Neinast, M., and Arany, Z.P., Myobolites: Muscle-derived metabolites wth paracrine and systemic effects, *Curr. Opin. Pharmacol.* 34, 15–20, 2017.

9. Rafatian, G., and Davis, D.R., Heart-derived cell therapy 2.0: Paracrine strategies to increase therapeutic repair of injured myocardium, *Stem Cells* 36, 1794–1803, 2018.

10. Mytsyk, M., Isu, G., Cerino, G., et al., Paracrine potential of adipose stromal vascular fraction cells to recover hypoxia-induced loss of cardiomyocyte function, *Biotechnol. Bioeng.* 116, 132–142, 2018.

PARALOGS

Paralogs are genes within the same genome that have evolved by gene duplication.[1–8] Contrasted with orthologs which are also homologs but have arisen via speciation.[9,10]

1. Ohno, S., The one-to-four rule and paralogues of sex-determining genes, *Cell. Mol. Life Sci.* 55, 824–830, 1999.

2. Forterre, P., Displacement of cellular proteins by functional analogues from plasmids or viruses could explain puzzling phylogenies of many DNA informational proteins, *Mol. Microbiol.* 33, 457–465, 1999.

3. Gilbert, J.M., The evolution of engrailed genes after duplication and speciation events, *Dev. Gene. Evol.* 212, 307–318, 2002.

4. Ferrier, D.E., Hox genes: Did the vertebrate ancestor have a Hox14? *Curr. Biol.* 14, R210–R211, 2004.

5. Tsuru, T., Kawai, M., Mizutani-Ui, Y., Uchiyama, I., and Kobayashi, I., Evolution of paralogous genes: Reconstruction of genome rearrangements through comparison of multiple genomes with *Staphylococcus aureus*, *Mol. Biol. Evol.* 23, 1269–1285, 2006.

6. Hlouchová, K., Navrátil, V., Tykvart, J., Sácha, P., and Konvalinka, J., GCPII variants, paralogs and orthologs, *Curr. Med. Chem.* 19, 1316–1322, 2012.

7. Desideri, E., Cavallo, A.L., and Baccarini, M., Alike, but different: RAF paralogs and their signaling outputs, *Cell* 161, 967–970, 2015.

8. Chung, K.P., Zeng, Y., and Jiang, L., COPII paralogs in plans: Functional redundancy or diversity? *Trends Plant. Sci.* 21, 758–769, 2016.

9. Gupta, K., Selinsky, B.S., Bacterial and algal orthologs of prostaglandin H_2 synthase: Novel insights into the evolution of an integral membrane protein, *Biochim. Biophys. Acta* 1848, 83–94, 2015.

10. Tekaia, F., Inferring orthologs: Open questions and perspectives, *Genomics Insights* 9, 17–28, 2016.

PARTIAL MOLAR VOLUME

The partial molar volume of a solute is that volume of the solute in a solution when the concentration of the solute approaches zero (infinite dilution).[1,2] There is some early literature which uses the term partial specific volume for amino acids.[3,4] However, current literature reserves the use of partial specific volume for proteins[5,6] and other polymers.[7] The partial molar volume is calculated from experimental data (apparent molar volume).[8,9]

1. Kyte, J., *Structure in Protein Chemistry*, 2nd edn., Noncovalent Forces, Chapter 5, pp. 189–249, Garland Science, New York, 2007.

2. Zhao, H., Viscosity *B*-coefficients and standard partial molar volumes of amino acids, and their roles in interpreting the protein (stabilization), *Biophys. Chem.* 122, 157–183, 2006.

3. Bull, H.B., and Breese, K., Surface tension of amino acid solutions: A hydrophobicity scale of the amino acid residues, *Arch. Biochem. Biophys.* 161, 665–670, 1974.

4. Arakawa, T., and Timasheff, S.N., Preferential interactions of proteins with solvent components in aqueous amino acid solutions, *Arch. Biochem. Biophys.* 224, 19–177, 1983.

5. Hammes, G.G., *Physical Chemistry for the Biological Sciences*, Wiley-Interscience, Hoboken, NJ, 2007.

6. Miranda-Hernández, M.P., Valle-González, E.R., Ferreira-Gómez, D., et al., Theoretical approximations and experimental extinction coefficients of biopharmaceuticals, *Anal. Bioanal. Chem.* 408, 1523–1530, 2016.

7. Gohon, Y., Paylov, G., Timmins, P., et al., Partial specific volume and solvent interactions of amphipol A8–35, *Anal. Biochem.* 334, 318–334, 2004.

8. Singh, V., Sharma, G., and Gardas, R.L., Thermodynamic and ultrasonic properties of ascorbic acid in aqueous protic ionic liquid solutions, *PLoS One* 10(5), e012609, 2015.

9. Rodríguez, D.M., and Romero, C.M., Effect of temperature on the partial molar volumes and the partial molar compressibilities of α-amino acids in water and in aqueous solutions of strong electrolytes, *J. Mol. Liquids* 233, 487–498, 2017.

PARTIAL SPECIFIC VOLUME

The partial specific volume is closely related to the partial molal volume. Formally, it is the volume of a solute in a solution extrapolated to zero concentration.[1] There is some early literature which uses the term partial specific volume for amino acids.[2,3] However, a consideration of the current literature suggests that the term partial specific volume is reserved for use with polymers including proteins,[4] nucleic acids,[5,6] and other polymers.[7] The partial specific volume is sensitive to solvent composition and temperature.[8] Knowledge of the partial specific volumes of proteins is necessary for the determination of molecular weight by analytical ultracentrifugation.[9]

1. Hammes, G.G., *Physical Chemistry for the Biological Sciences*, Chapter 14, Hydrodynamics of Macromolecules, pp. 295–316, Wiley-Interscience, Hoboken, NJ, 2007.

2. Bull, H.B., and Breese, K., Surface tension of amino acid solutions: A hydrophobicity scale of the amino acid residues, *Arch. Biochem. Biophys.* 161, 665–670, 1974.

3. Arakawa, T., and Timasheff, S.N., Preferential interactions of proteins with solvent components in aqueous amino acid solutions, *Arch. Biochem. Biophys.* 224, 19–177, 1983.

4. Rogge, R.A., and Hansen, J.C., Sedimentation velocity analysis of large oligomeric chromatin complexes using interference detection, *Methods Enzymol.* 562, 349–362, 2015.

5. Hellman, L.M., Rodgers, D.W., and Fried, M.G., Phenomenological partial-specific volumes for G-quadruplex DNAs, *Eur. Biophys. J.* 39, 389–396, 2013.

6. Chaires, J.B., Dean, W.L., Le, H.T., and Trant, O., Hydrodynamic models of G-quadruplex structures, *Methods Enzymol.* 562, 287–304, 2015.

7. Wagner, M., Peitsch, C., Tauhardt, L., Schallon, A., and Schubert, U.S., Characterization of cationic polymers by asymmetric flow field-flow fractionation and multi-angle light scattering: A comparison with traditional techniques, *J. Chromgatog. A* 1325, 195–203, 2014.

8. Suzuki, M., Imao, A., Mogami, G., et al., Strong dependence of hydration state of F-actin on the bound Mg^{2+}/Ca^{2+} ions, *J. Phys. Chem. B* 120, 6917–6928, 2016.

9. Edelstein, S.J., and Schachman, H.K., The simultaneous determination of partial specific volumes and molecular weights with microgram quantities, *J. Biol. Chem.* 242, 206–311, 1967.

PEGylation

PEGylation is the process of the conjugation of a polyethylene glycol (PEG) chain to a different molecule, most often a protein. PEGylation was developed at Rutgers University in 1977.[1,2] PEGylation has been used to obtain derivatives of biopharmaceutical products with increased efficacy.[3,4] There are a variety of approaches to conjugation of PEG to proteins.[5] While the majority of PEGylation applications have been to peptides and proteins, PEG has been used to prepared derivatives of aptamers.[6,7] PEGylation is pleiotropic in improving the properties of a biopharmaceutical with a major effect on renal clearance.[8,9] PEGylation can reduce the immunogenicity of proteins[10,11] by a mechanism which has been described as immunocamouflage.[12]

1. Abuchowski, A., van Es, T., Palczuk, N.C., and Daves, F.F., Alteration of immunological properties of bovine serum albumin by covalent attachment of polyethylene glycol, *J. Biol. Chem.* 252, 3578–3581, 1977.

2. Abuchowski, A., McCoy, J.R., Palczuk, N.C., van Es, T., and Davis, F.F., Effect of covalent attachment of polyethylene glycol on immunogenicity and circulating life of bovine liver catalase, *J. Biol. Chem.* 252, 3582–3586, 1977.

3. Knop, K., Hoogenboom, R., Fischer, D., and Schubert, U.S., Poly(ethylene glycol) in drug delivery: Pros and cons as well as potential alternatives, *Angew. Chem. Int. Ed.* 49, 6288–6308, 2010.

4. *PEGylated Protein Drugs: Basic Science and Clinical Application*, ed. F.M. Veronese, Birkhäuser, Basel, Switzerland, 2009.

5. Pasur, G., and Veronese, F.M., Start of the art in PEGylation: The great versatility achieved after forty years of research, *J. Control. Rel.* 161, 461–472, 2012.

6. Da Pieve, C., Blackshaw, E., Missailidis, S., and Perkins, A.C., PEGylation and biodistribution of an anti-MUC1 aptamer in MCF-7 tumor bearing mice, *Bioconjug. Chem.* 23, 1377–1381, 2012.

7. Haruta, K., Otaki, N., Nagamine, M., et al., A novel PEGylation method for improving the pharmacokinetic properties of anti-interleukin-17A RNA aptamers, *Nucleic Acid Res.* 27, 36–44, 2017.

8. Knauf, M.J., Bell, D.P., Hirtzen, P., et al., Relationship of effective molecular size to systemic clearance in rate of recombinant interleukin-2 chemically modified with water-soluble polymers, *J. Biol. Chem.* 263, 15064–15070, 1988.

9. Clark, R., Olson, K., Fuh, G., et al., Long-acting growth hormones produced by conjugation with polyethylene glycol, *J. Biol. Chem.* 271, 21969–21977, 1996.

10. Katre, N.V., Immunogenicity of recombinant IL-2 modified by covalent attachment of polyethylene glycol, *J. Immunol.* 144, 209–213, 1990.

11. Lee, P.W., Isarov, S.A., Wallat, J.D., et al., Polymer structure and conformation alter the antigenicity of virus-like particle-polymer conjugates, *J. Am. Chem. Soc.* 139, 3312–3315, 2017.

12. Kyluik-Price, D.L., and Scott, M.D., Effects of methoxypoly(ethylene glycol) mediated immunocamouflage on leukocyte surface maker detection, cell conjugation, activation and alloproliferation, *Biomaterials* 24, 167–177, 2016.

PDZ-DOMAINS

A PDZ-domain characterizes a family of proteins involved in protein-protein interactions with a preference for binding to C-terminal regions of target proteins and are recognized as biological scaffolds supporting signaling complexes.[1-6] The PDZ acronym is derived from the combination of PDZ (**P**SD-95/Discs-large/**Z**O1;PSD-95, the *Drosophila* **D**iscs-Large septate junction protein and the epithelial junction protein **Z**O-1).[7] PDZ domains are important in G-coupled protein receptors.[8]

1. Fanning, A.S., and Anderson, J.M., Protein-protein interactions: PDZ domain networks, *Curr. Biol.* 6, 1385–1388, 1996.

2. Saras, J., and Heldin, C.H., PDZ domains bind carboxyl-terminal sequences of target proteins, *Trends Biochem. Sci.* 21, 455–458, 1996.

3. Harrison, S.C., Peptide-surface association: The case of PDZ and PTB domains, *Cell* 86, 341–343, 1996.
4. Ponting, C.P., Phillips C., Davies, K.E., and Blake, D.J., PDZ domains: Targeting signalling molecules to sub-membranous sites, *Bioessays* 19, 469–479, 1997.
5. Lasky, L.A., Skelton, N.J., and Sidhu, S.S., PDZ domains: Intracellular mediators of carboxyl-terminal protein recognition and scaffolding, in *Modular Protein Domains*, ed. G. Cesareni, M. Gimona, M. Sudol, and M. Yaffe, Chapter 13, pp. 257–278, Wiley-VCH, Weinheim, Germany, 2005.
6. Ernst, A., Appleton, B.A., Ivarsson, Y., et al., A structural portrait of the PDZ domain family, *J. Mol. Biol.* 426, 3509–3519, 2014.
7. Kennedy, M.B., Origin of PDZ (DHR, GLGF) domains, *Trends Biochem. Sci.* 20, 350, 1995.
8. Dunn, H.A., and Ferguson, S.S. PDZ protein regulation of G protein-coupled receptor trafficking and signaling pathways, *Mol. Pharmacol.* 88, 624–639, 2015.

PEPDUCINS

Pepducins are lipidated (*N*-terminal palmitoyl) *C*-terminal amidated peptides with the ability to penetrate cells. The oligopeptide structure of the pepducin is derived from the primary structure of the internal loops of the G-protein coupled receptor (GPCR).[1] It was reasoned that pepducins should act as allosteric effectors of GPCR interaction with G-protein.[2] The first application of this concept showed that the pepducin based on the third intracellular loop of the PAR-1 receptor inhibited activation of platelets by thrombin.[3,4] A pepducin was subsequently shown to inhibit the neutrophil inflammatory response.[5] Work has continued to develop pepducins, which will modulate GPCR function as therapeutic agents.[6–8] See also **cell penetrating peptide, G-protein coupled receptor**.

1. Carr, R., III and Benovik, J.L., From biased signalling to polypharmacology: Unlocking unique intracellular signalling using pepducins, *Biochem. Soc. Trans.* 44, 555–561, 2016.
2. Covic, L., Gresser, A.L., Talavera, J., Swift, S., and Kuliopulos, A., Activation and inhibition of G protein-coupled receptors by cell-penetrating membrane-tethered peptides, *Proc. Natl. Acad. Sci. USA* 99, 643–438, 2002.
3. Covic, L., Misra, M., Badar, J., Singh, C., and Kuliopulos, A., Pepducin-based intervention of thrombin-receptor signaling and systemic platelet activation, *Nat. Med.* 8, 1161–1165, 2002.
4. Kuliopulos, A and Covic, L., Blocking receptors on the inside: Pepducin-based intervention of PAR signaling and thrombosis, *Life Sci.* 74, 255–262, 2003.
5. Lomas-Neira, J., and Ayala, A., Pepducins: An effective means to inhibit GPCR signaling by neutrophils, *Trends Immunol.* 26, 619–621, 2005.
6. Carr, R., 3rd, Du, Y., Quoyer, J., et al., Development and characterization of pepducins as Gs-biased allosteric agonists, *J. Biol. Chem.* 289, 35669–35684, 2014.
7. Zhang, P., Covic, L., and Kuliopulos, A., Pepducins an other lapidated peptides as mechanistic probes and therapeutics, *Methods Mol. Biol.* 1324, 191–203, 2015.
8. Chaturvedi, M., Schilling, J., Beautrait, A., et al., Emerging paradigm of intracellular targeting of G protein-coupled receptors, *Trendsd Biochem. Sci.* 43, 533–546, 2018.

PEPTERGENTS (LIPID-LIKE PEPTIDES)

Peptergents, also known as lipid-like peptides, are small, self-assembling peptides with detergent properties which are quite useful for the study of membrane proteins.[1–3]

1. Yeh, J.I., Du, S., Tortajada, A., Paulo, J., and Zhang, S., Peptergents: Peptide detergents that improve stability and functionality of a membrane protein, Glycerol-3-phosphate dehydrogenase, *Biochemistry* 44, 16912–16919, 2005.
2. Kiley, P., Zhao, X., Vaughn, M., et al., Self-assembling peptide detergents stabilize isolated photosystem I on a dry surface for an extended time, *PLoS Biol.* 3, e230, 2005.
3. Veith, K., Martinez Molledo, M., et al., Lipid-like peptides and stabilize integral membrane proteins for biophysical and structural studies, *ChemBioChem.* 18, 1735–1742, 2017.

PEPTIDE APTAMERS

Aptamers are a class of chemical compounds that are designed to bind specifically to nucleic acids and proteins. Peptide aptamers are developed with SEXEX technology and are generally encoded in a "scaffold protein" to preserve conformation.[1–6]

1. Baines, I.C., and Colas, P., Peptide aptamers as guides for small-molecule drug discovery, *Drug. Discov. Today.* 11, 334–341, 2006
2. Li, J., Tap, S., Chen, X., Zhang, C.Y., and Zhang, Y., Peptide aptamers with biological and therapeutic applications, *Curr. Med. Chem.* 18, 4215–4222, 2011.
3. Gilbert, B., Simon, S., Dimitrova, V., Diaz-Latoud, C., and Arrigo, A.P., Peptide aptamers: Tools to negatively or positively module HSPB1(27) function, *Philos. Trans. R. Soc. Lond. B Biol. Sci.* 368, 1082–1101, 2013.
4. Leśniewska, K., Warbrick, E., and Ohkura, H., Peptide aptamers define distinct EB1- and EB3-binding motifs and interfere with microtubule dynamics, *Mol. Biol. Cell* 25, 1025–1036, 2014.
5. Reverdatto, S., Burz, D.S., and Xhekhtman, A., Peptide aptamers: Development and applications, *Curr. Top. Med. Chem.* 15, 1082–1101, 2015.

6. Goto, S., Tsukakoshi, K., and Ikebukuro, K., Development of aptamers against unpurified proteins, *Biotechnol. Bioeng.* 114, 2706–2716, 2017.

PEPTIDE NUCLEIC ACIDS

Peptide nucleic acids (PNAs) consist of a peptide backbone (aminoethylglycine) with nucleic acid base substituents.[1,2] Conventional peptide synthesis technology can be used for the preparation of peptide nucleic acids.[3] PNAs are stable in serum and bacterial extracts.[4] There is continued interest in the use of PNAs.[5–8] There is continued development of cell-penetrating derivatives of PNAs.[9–11] The synthesis of PNAs with analog bases has been reported.[12,13]

1. Nielsen, P.E., Egholm, M., Berg, R.H., and Burchardt, O., Sequence-selective recognition of DNA by strand displacement with a thymine-substituted polyamide, *Science* 254, 1497–1500, 1991.
2. Nielsen, P.E., Antisense peptide nucleic acids, *Curr. Opin. Mol. Ther.* 2, 282–287, 2000.
3. Zambaldo, C., Barluenga, S., and Winssinger, N., PNA-encoded chemical libraries, *Curr. Opin. Chem. Biol.* 26, 8–15, 2015.
4. Demidov, V.V., Frank-Kamenetsii, M.D., et al., Stability of peptide nucleic acids in human serum and cellular extracts, *Biochem. Pharmacol.* 48, 1310–1313, 1994.
5. Wu, J.C., Meng, Q.C., Ren, H.M., et al., Recent advances in peptide nucleic acid for cancer bionanotechnology, *Acta Pharmacol. Sin.* 38, 798–805, 2017.
6. Gahtory, D., Murtola, M., Smulders, M.M.J., et al., Facile functionalization of peptide nucleic acids (PNAs) for antisense and single nucleotide polymorphism detection, *Org. Biomol. Chem.* 15, 6710–6714, 2017.
7. Narenji, H., Gholizadeh, P., Aghazadeh, M., et al., Peptide nucleic acids (PNAs): Currently potential bactericidal agents, *Biomed. Pharmacother.* 93, 580–588, 2017.
8. Gupta, A., Mishra, A., and Puri, N., Peptide nucleic acids: Advanced tools for biomedical applications, *J. Biotechnol.* 259, 148–159, 2017.
9. Cordier, C., Boutimah, F., Bourdeloux, M., et al., Delivery of antisense peptide nucleic acids to cells by conjugation with small arginine-rich cell-penetrating peptide (R/W)9, *PLoS One* 9(8), e104999, 2014.
10. Kauffman, W.B., Fuselier, T., He., J., and Wimley, W.C., Mechanism matters: A taxonomy of cell penetrating peptide, *Trends Biochem. Sci.* 40, 749–764, 2015.
11. Readman, J.B., Dickson, G., and Coldham N.G., Tetrahdal DNA nanoparticle vector for intracellular delivery of targeted peptide nucleic acid antisense agents to restore antibiotic sensitivity in cefotaxime-resistant Escherichia coli, *Nucleic Acid Ther.* 27, 176–182, 2017.
12. Nielsen, P.E., PNA technology, in *Peptide Nucleic Acids Methods and Protocols*, ed. P.E. Nielsen, Humana, Totowa, NJ, 2002.
13. Tomori, T., Miyataka, Y., Sao, Y., et al., Synthesis of peptide nucleic acids containing pyridazine derivatives as cytosine and thymine analogs, and their duplexes with complementary oligodeoxnucleotides, *Org. Lett.* 17, 1609–1612, 2015.

PEPTIDOME

It is the peptide complement of a genome. Peptidomics is the study of the peptidome. The definition of a peptide in most studies is arbitrary based on size as determined by ultrafiltration[1–4] or size-exclusion chromatography.[5–7] While I don't know of a specific reference, it would seem that the upper limit of a peptide is 50 amino acids but there is no consensus such as document from a learned society or regulatory group. I recall several heated discussions on whether pancreatic RNAse was a small protein or a large peptide with biological activity while I was a research associate in the laboratory of Stanford Moore and William Stein at the Rockefeller University. See **miniprotein, osteoclast** (for osteocalcin).

1. Zheng, X., Baker, H., and Hancock, W.S., Analysis of the low molecular weight serum peptidome using ultrafiltration and a hybrid ion trap-Fourier transform mass spectrometry, *J. Chromatog. A.*, 1120, 173–184, 2006.
2. Wu, L., Li., H., Li., X., et al., Peptidomic analysis of cultured cardiomyocytes exposed to acute ischemic-hypoxia, *Cell Physiol. Biochem.* 41, 358–368, 2017.
3. Greening, D.W., and Simpson, R.J., Characterization of the low-molecular-weight human plasma peptidome, *Methods Mol. Biol.* 1619, 63–79, 2017.
4. Di Meo, A., Batruch, I., Yousef, A.G., et al., An integrated proteomic and peptidomic assessment of the normal human urinoma, *Clin. Chem. Lab. Med.* 55, 237–247, 2017.
5. Ueda, K., Saichi, N., Takami, S., et al., A comprehensive peptidome profiling technology for the identification of early detection biomarkers for lung carcinoma, *PLoS One* 6(4), e18567, 2011.
6. Gallego, M., Mora, L., and Toldrá, F., Peptidomics as a tool for quality control in dry-cured ham processing, *J. Proteomics* 147, 98–107, 2016.
7. Fesenko, I., Khazigaleeva, R., Govorun, V., and Invanov, B., Analysis of endogenous peptide pools of *Physomitrella patens* Moss, *Methods Mol. Biol.* 1719, 395–405, 2018.

PERFORIN

Perforin is a protein located in the granules of CD8 T-cells (cytotoxic T cells) and natural killer cells. Upon degranulation of these cells, perforin is released and inserts into the target cell's plasma membrane, forming a pore resulting in lysis of the target cell.[1–9]

1. Catalfamo, M., and Henkart, P.A., Perforin and the granule exocytosis cytotoxicity pathway, *Curr. Opin. Immunol.* 15, 522–527, 2003.
2. Ashton-Rickardt, P.G., The granule pathway of programmed cell death, *Crit. Rev. Immunol.* 25, 161–182, 2005.
3. Zhou, F., Perform: More than just a pore-forming protein, *Int. Rev. Immunol.* 29, 56–76, 2010.
4. Pipkin, M.E., Rao, A., and Lichtenheld, M.G., The transcriptional control of the perforin locus, *Immunol. Rev.* 235, 55–72, 2010.
5. Thiery, J., and Lieberman, J., Perforin: A key pore-forming protein for immune control of viruses and cancer, *Subcell. Biochem.* 80, 197–220, 2014.
6. Voskoboinik, I., Whisstock, J.C., and Trapani, J.A., Perforin and granzymes: Function, dysfunction and human pathology, *Nat. Rev. Immunol.* 15, 388–400, 2015.
7. Spicer, B.A., Conroy, P.J., Law, R.H.P., Voskoboinik, I., and Whisstock, J.C., Perforin-a key(shaped) weapon in the immunological arsenal, *Semin. Cell Dev. Biol.* 72, 117–123, 2017.
8. Goldstein, P., and Griffiths, G.M., An early history of T cell-mediated cytotoxicity, *Nat. Rev. Immunol.* 18, 527–535, 2018.
9. Behr, F.M., Chuwonpad, A., Stark, R., and van Gisbergen, K.P.J.M., Armed and ready: Transcriptional regulation of tissue-resident memory CD8 T cells, *Front. Immunol.* 9, 1770, 2018.

PEROXIREDOXINS

Peroxiredoxins are a group of antioxidant thioredoxin-dependent enzymes with a catalytic function in the detoxification of cellular-toxic peroxides.[1,2] The 2-cysteine peroxiredoxin (Prxs) is one member of a family of proteins with similar function.[3] The 2 cys peroxiredoxin is a homodimer with a cysteine on each dimer having a specific function. The catalytic activity of mammalian Prxs is dependent on a cysteine residue at the active site in the thiolate form. The reduction of the peroxide is associated with the conversion of the thiolate to a sufenic acid. The sulfenic acid is converted back the cysteine form via formation of a disulfide with a cysteine on the other homodimer which is reduced to regenerate the active site cysteine.[4] The sulfenic acid can be oxidized to sulfinic acid with excess peroxide in conditions of oxidative stress; Regeneration of the sulfenic acids requires an enzyme, cysteine sulfenic acid reductase (sulfiredoxin, Srx).[5,6]

1. Rhee, S.G., and Kil, I.S., Multiple functions and regulation of mammalian peroxiredoxins, *Annu. Rev. Biochem.* 86, 749–775, 2017.
2. Karplus, P.A., A primer on peroxiredoxin biochemistry, *Free Rad. Biol. Med.* 80, 183–190, 2015.
3. Perkins, A., Nelson, K.J., Parsonage, D., Poole, L.B., and Karplus, P.A., Peroxiredoxins: Guardians against oxidative stress and modulators of peroxide signaling, *Trends Biochem. Sci.* 40, 435–445, 2015.
4. Karplus *op cit.,* Veal, E.A., Underwood, Z.E., Tomalin, L.E., Morgan, B.A., and Pillay, C.S., Hyperoxidation of peroxiredoxin: Gain or loss of function? *Antioxid. Redox. Signal.* 28, 574–590, 2018.
5. Jönsson, T.J., and Lowther, W.T., The peroxiredoxin repair proteins, *Subcell. Biochem.* 44, 115–141, 2007.
6. Akter, S., Fu, I., Jung, Y., et al., Chemical proteomics reveals new targets of cysteine sulfenic acid reductase, *Nat. Chem. Biol.* 14, 995–1004, 2018.

PEROXYNITRITE

Peroxynitrite is an oxidizing/nitrating agent derived from the reaction of nitric oxide and superoxide which reacts with proteins, lipids, and nucleic acids. The reactions are complex, and in addition to oxidation reactions such as carbonyl formation and disulfide formation, there are reactions such as nitrosylation of cysteine and the nitration of tyrosine.[1–7] The reaction of tyrosine with peroxynitrite is sensitive to solvent environment with nitration favored in a hydrophobic environment as opposed to oxidation.[8]

1. Pryor, W.A., and Squadrito, G.L., The chemistry of peroxynitrite: A product from the reaction of nitric oxide with superoxide, *Am. J. Physiol.* 268, L699–L722, 1995.
2. Beckman, J.S., and Koppenol, W.H., Nitric oxide, superoxide, and peroxynitrite: The good, the bad, and ugly, *Am. J. Physiol.* 271, C1424–C1437, 1996.
3. Radi, R., Denicola, A., and Freeman, B.A., Peroxynitrite reactions with carbon dioxide-bicarbonate, *Methods Enzymol.* 301, 353–357, 1999.
4. Halliwell, B., Zhao, K., and Whiteman, M., Nitric oxide and peroxynitrite. The ugly, the uglier and the not so good: A personal view of the recent controversies, *Free Radic. Res.* 31, 651–669, 1999.
5. Ohmori, H., and Kanayama, N., Immunogenicity of an inflammation-associated product, tyrosine nitrated self-proteins, *Autoimmun. Rev.* 4, 224–229, 2005.
6. Hurd, T.R., Filipovska, A., Costa, N.J., et al., Disulphide formation on mitochondrial protein thiols, *Biochem. Soc. Trans.* 44, 1390–1393, 2005.
7. Niles, J.C., Wishnok, J.S., and Tannenbaum, S.R., Peroxynitrite-induced oxidation and nitration products of guanine and 8-oxoguanine: Structures and mechanisms of product formation, *Nitric Oxide* 14, 109–121, 2006.
8. Zhang, H., Joseph, J., Feix, J., et al., Nitration and oxidation of a hydrophobic tyrosine probe by peroxynitrite in membranes: Comparison with nitration and oxidation of tyrosine by peroxynitrite in aqueous solution, *Biochemistry* 40, 7675–7686, 2001.

PESCADILLO

The gene for pescadillo (*Pes*) was identified in zebrafish with the potential of encoding a protein with 562 amino acids. The gene appeared to be expressed across a broad range of species including humans.[1] Studies in zebrafish showed high level of expression in early development. Subsequent work in a murine cell culture system showed that pescadillo contained discrete structural motifs.[2] A pattern of expression in neural tissue was observed and it was suggested that it may be necessary for oncogenic transformation.[3,4] Pescadillo has been shown to be important for the formation of ribosomes in mammalian cells[5] and plant cells.[6,7] There is continued interest in the role of *Pes* in tumor development.[8-10]

1. Allende, M.L., Amsterdam, A., Becker, T., et al., Insertional mutagenesis in zebrafish identifies two novel genes, pescadillo and dead eye, essential for embryonic development, *Genes Dev.* 10, 3141–3155, 1996.
2. Haque, J., Boger, S., Li, J., and Duncan, D.A., The murine Pes1 gene encodes a nuclear protein containing a BRCT domain, *Genomics* 70, 201–210, 2000.
3. Kinoshita, Y., Jarell, A.D., Flaman, J.M., et al., Pescadillo, a novel cell cycle regulatory protein abnormally expressed in malignant cells, *J. Biol. Chem.* 276, 6656–6665, 2001.
4. Maiorana, A., Tu, X., Cheng, G., and Baserga, R., Role of pescadillo in the transformation and immortalization of mammalian cells, *Oncogene* 23, 7116–7124, 2004.
5. Kellner, M., Rohrmoser, M., Forné, I., et al., DEAD-box helicase DDX27 regulates 3′ end formation of ribosomal 47S RNA and stably associates with the PeBoW-complex, *Exp. Cell Res.* 334, 146–159, 2015.
6. Zografidis, A., Kopolas, G., Podia, V., et al., Transcriptional regulation and functional involvement of the *Arabidopsis* pescadillo ortholog AtPES in root development, *Plant Sci.* 229, 53–65, 2014.
7. Ahn, C.S., Cho, H.K., Lee, D.H., et al., Functional characterization of the ribosome biogenesis factors PES, BOP1, and WDR12 (PeBoW) and mechanisms of defective cell growth and proliferation by PeBoW deficiency in *Abribdopsis*, *J. Exp. Bot.* 67, 5217–5232, 2016.
8. Li, J., Zhuang, Q., Lan, X., et al., PES1 differentially regulates the expression of ERα and ERβ in ovarian cancer, *IUBMB Life* 65, 1017–1025, 2013.
9. Lázaro-Ibáñez, E., Lunavat, T.R., Jang, S.C., et al., Distinct prostate cancer-related mRNA cargo in extracellular vesicle subsets from prostate cell lines, *BMC Cancer* 17, 92, 2017.
10. Fan, P., Wang, B., Meng, Z., Zhao, J., and Jin, Z., PES1 is transcriptionally regulated by BRD4 and promotes cell proliferation and glycolysis in hepatocellular carcinoma, *Int. J. Biochem. Cell Biol.* 29, 104, 1–8, 2018.

PFAM

Pfam is a database used to organize protein sequence data to form protein families. The Pfam database was developed in 1997[1] and is based on the use of hidden Markov model (HHM, a hidden Markov model has a underlying or unobserved state process that follows a Markov chain)[2] profiles to identify proteins into families based on domain homology[3] (rather than short sequence) to a seed domain to comprise part A; part B consisted of protein sequence without homology match. Several hundred families were identified in this effort. Work over the past 20 years has expanded this database[4-6] where the most recent publications describe some 15,000 protein families.[7,8] See **domain**.

1. Sonnhammer, E.L.L., Eddy, S.R., and Durbin, R., Pfam: A comprehensive database of protein domain families based on seed alignments, *Proteins: Structure, Function Genetics* 28, 405–420, 1997.
2. Parida, L., *Pattern Discovery in Bioinformatics Theory and Algorithm*, Chapman & Hall/CRC, New York, 2008.
3. Williams, R.W., Xue, B., Uverskky, V.N., and Dunker, A.K., Distribution and cluster analysis of predicted intrinsically disordered protein Pfam domains, *Intrinsically Disord. Proteins* 1, e25724, 2013.
4. Bateman, A., Birney, E., Durbin, R., et al., The Pfam protein families database, *Nucleic Acids Res.* 28, 263–266, 2000.
5. Birney, E., Cerruti, L., et al., The Pfam protein families data base, *Nucl. Acids Res.* 30, 276–280, 2002.
6. Finn, R.D., Bateman, A., Clements, J., et al., Pfam: The protein families database, *Nucleic Acids Res.* 42, D222–D230, 2014.
7. Finn, R.D., Coggill, P., Eberhardt, R.Y., et al., The Pfam protein families database: Towards a more sustainable future, *Nucleic Acids Res.* 44, D279–D285, 2016.
8. Ovehinnikov, S., Park, H., Varghese, N., et al., Protein structure determination using metagenome sequence data, *Science* 355, 294–298, 2017.

PHARMACEUTICAL EQUIVALENTS

The FDA considers drug products to be pharmaceutical equivalents if they meet these three criteria: (1) they contain the same active ingredient(s), (2) they are of the same dosage form and route of administration, and (3) they are identical in strength or concentration.[1] Pharmaceutically equivalent drug products may differ in characteristics such as shape, release mechanism, labeling (to some extent), scoring, excipients (including colors, flavors, preservatives). Pharmaceutical equivalence is of importance in the development of generic drugs. The approval of a generic drug is dependent on showing equivalence to the innovator drug. Pharmaceutical equivalence may be equivalent to therapeutic equivalence in drugs but this may always be the case with conflicting studies on the relation of pharmaceutical equivalence and therapeutic equivalence.[2–5] The issue of pharmaceutical equivalence and therapeutic equivalence is a larger problem with biologics.[6,7]

1. https://www.fda.gov/Drugs/InformationOnDrugs/ucm079436.htm#P.
2. Vesga, O., Agudelo, M., Salazar, B.E., Rodriguez, C.A., and Zulanga, A.F., Generic vancomycin products fail *in vivo* despite being pharmaceutical equivalents of the innovator, *Antimicrob. Agents Chemother.* 54, 3271–3279, 2010.
3. Diaz, J.A., Silva, E., Arias, M.J., and Garzón, M., Comparative *in vitro* study of the antimicrobial activities of different commercial antibiotic products of vancomycin, *BMC Clin. Pharmacol.* 11, 9, 2011.
4. Gonzalez, J.M., Rodriguez, C.A., Zuluaga, A.F., Agudelo, M., and Vesga, O., Demonstration of therapeutic equivalence of fluconazole generic products in the neutropenic mouse model of disseminated candidiasis, *PLoS One* 10(11), e0141872, 2015.
5. Rodriguez, C.A, Adudelo, M., Aguilar, Y.A., Zuluaga, A.F., and Vesga, O., Impact on bacterial resistance of therapeutically nonequivalent gererics: The case of Piperacillin-Tazobactam, *PLoS One* 11(5), e0155806, 2016.
6. Subramanyam, M., Clinical development of biosimilars: An evolving landscape, *Bioanalysis* 5, 575–586, 2013.
7. Crommelin, D.J., Shah, V.P., Klebovich, I., et al., The similarity question for biologicals and non-biological complex drugs, *Eut. J. Pharm. Sci.* 76, 10–17, 2015.

PHARMACOGENOMICS

Pharmacogenomics (PGx) is the use of genomics to study the development and utilization of drugs; more specifically the effect of patient genetic variation on the pharmacokinetics/therapeutic response of drugs.[1] Pharmacogenomics is essential for the application of personalized medicine/precision medicine in medical practice.[2–4] One of the first examples of the application of pharmacogenomics was in the pharmacokinetics of warfarin.[5] A review in 2015 noted that variability in approximately 20 genes affected the pharmacokinetics of 80 drugs.[6,7]

1. Mooney, S.D., Progress towards the integration of pharmacogenomics in practice, *Hum. Genet.* 134, 459–465, 2015.
2. *Pharmacogenomics of Alcohol and Drugs of Abuse*, ed. A. Dasgupta and L. Langman, CRC Press, Boca Raton, FL, 2012.
3. *Pharmacogenomics: Challenges and Opportunities in Therapeutic Implementation*, ed. F.W.Y. Lam and L.H. Cavalleri, Academic Press, Oxford, UK, 2013.

4. *Immunopharmacogenomics*, ed. Y. Nakamura, Springer, Tokyo, Japan, 2015.
5. *Applying Pharmcogenomics in Therapeutics*, ed. Y. Feng and H.-G. XIa, CRC Press, Boca Raton, FL, 2016.
6. Drozda, K., Pacanowski, M.A., Grimstein, C., and Zineh, I., Pharmacogenetic labeling of FDA-approved drugs: A regulatory retrospective, *JACC Basic Transl. Sci.* 3, 545–549, 2018.
7. Relling, M.V., and Evans, W.E., Pharmacogenomics in the clinic, *Nature* 526, 343–350, 2015.

PHARMACOPHORE

The term pharmacophore refers to the totality of structural features of a compound (drug) (e.g. functional groups, stereochemistry) which provide for the pharmacological properties of said compound.[1] The knowledge of a pharmacophore (pharmacophore modeling) is used in drug design.[2–5]

1. Güner, O.F., and Bowen, J.P., Setting the record straight: The origin of the pharmacophore concept, *J. Chem. Inf. Model* 54, 1269–1283, 2014.
2. Güner, O.F, The impact of pharmacophore modeling in drug design, *IDrugs* 9, 567–572, 2005.
3. Güner, O., Clent, O., Kurogi, Y., Pharmacophore modeling and three dimensional database searching for drug design using catalyst: Recent advances, *Curr. Med. Chem.* 11, 2991–3005, 2004.
4. Pautasso, C., Troia, R., Genuardi, M., and Palumbo, A., Pharmacophore modeling technique applied for the discovery of proteasome inhibitors, *Expert Opin. Drug Discov.* 9, 931–943, 2014.
5. Lu, X., Yang, H., Chen, Y., et al., Development of pharmacophore modeling: Generation and recent applications in drug discovery, *Curr. Pharm. Des.* 24, 3424–3439, 2018.

PHARMACOPROTEOMICS

Pharmacoproteomics is the use of proteomics to elucidate mechanism of action of drugs.[1–6] It can also refer to the use of proteomics for drug discovery and development[7] and personalized medicine.[8]

1. Butler, G.S., Dean, R.A., Tam, E.M., and Overall, C.M., Pharmacoproteomics of a metalloproteinase hydroxamate inhibitor in breast cancer cells: Dynamics of membrane type 1 matrix metalloproteinase-mediated membrane protein shedding, *Mol. Cell. Biol.* 28, 4896–4914, 2008.
2. Saminathan, R., Bai, J., Sadrolodabaee, L., Karthik, G.M., et al., VKORC1 pharmacogenetics and pharmacoproteomics in patients on warfarin anticoagulant therapy: Thransthyretin precursor as a potential biomarker, *PLoS One* 5(12), e15064, 2010.

3. Dos Santos, S.C., Mira, N.P., Moreira, A.S., and Sá-Correia, I., Quantiative—and phosphor-proteomic analysis of the yeast response to the tyrosine kinase inhibitor imatinib to pharmacoproteomics-guided drug line extension, *OMICS* 16, 527–551, 2012.

4. Huang, Z.X., Tan, J.H., Li, T.W., et al., Influence of sinomenine on protein profiles on peripheral blood mononuclear cells from ankylosing spondylitis patients: A pharmacoproteomic study, *Chin. Med. J.* (Eng.) 126, 3645–3650, 2013.

5. Uchida, Y., Ohtsuki, S., and Terasaki, T., Pharmacoproteomics-based reconstruction of *in vivo* P-glycoprotein function at blood-brain barrier and brain distribution of substrate verapamil in pentylenetetrazole-kindled epilepsy, spontaneous epilepsy, and phenytoin treatment models, *Drug Metab. Dispos.* 12, 1719–1726, 2014.

6. Zohaib, M., Ansari, S.H., Shamsi, T.S., Zubarev, R.A., and Zarina, S., Pharmacoproteomics profiling of plasma from β-thalassemia patients in response to hydroxyurea treatment, *J. Clin. Pharmacol.* 59, 98–106, 2019.

7. Jain, K.K., Role of pharmacoproteomics in the development of personalized medicine, *Pharmacogenomics J.* 5, 331–336, 2004.

8. Witzmann, F.A., and Grant, R.A., Pharmacoproteomics in drug development, *Pharmacogenomics J.* 3, 69–76, 2003.

PHASE DIAGRAM

A phase diagram is a graph showing the relationship between the physical phases of a substance (e.g. solid, gas, liquid) over a range of conditions (usually temperature and pressure). A phase is generally defined as a homogeneous part of a heterogeneous system that is clearly separated from other phases of the substance, by a boundary. Phase diagrams are of value in a number of disciplines including geology, biology, physical chemistry, and separation science. Phase diagrams for water have been of particular interest where, in simple terms, the separation between ice and water as an example of a boundary between phases; however, the behavior of water is far more complex than two simple phases.[1–3] Regardless, it is easy to conceptualize an ice cube in a glass of water. Phase diagrams are of value in designing systems for the crystallization of proteins[4,5] and the distribution of lipids in model membranes.[6–10] Phase diagrams have been used to develop two-phase polymer systems for the separation of proteins and nucleic acids[11,12] It has been suggested that such partitioning can occur in the cytoplasm of a cell[13] forming "membraneless organelles."[14] The term phase diagram has been used to describe the distribution of a macromolecule between different states depending on ligand binding and the mechanism of ligand binding.[15–17]

A different approach to the use of the concept of phase diagram is presented in control of the mechanism of apoptosis, where the use of the term separatrix (a term from mathematics implying a boundary) to define phases representing concentrations pro-caspase 3 and XIAP (x-linked inhibitor of apoptosis).[18]

1. Dill, K.A., Truskett, T.M., Vlachy, V., and Hribar-Lee, B., Modeling water, the hydrophobic effect, and ion salvation, *Annu. Rev. Biochem. Biomol. Struct.* 34, 173–199, 2005.

2. Koga, K., and Tanaka, H., Phase diagram of water between hydrophobic surfaces, *J. Chem. Phys.* 122(10), 104711, 2005.

3. Conde, M.M., Vega, C., Tribello, G.A., and Slater, B., The phase diagram of water at negative pressures: Virtual ices, *J. Chem. Phys.* 131(3), 034510, 2009.

4. Asherie, N., Protein crystallization and phase diagrams, *Methods* 34, 266–272, 2004.

5. Baumgartner, K., Galm, L., Nötzold, J., et al., Determination of protein phase diagrams by microbatch experiments: Explaining the influence of precipitants and pH, *Int. J. Pharmaceutics* 479, 28–40, 2015.

6. Dorfler, H.D., Mixing behavior of binary insoluble phospholipid monolayers. Analysis of the mixing properties of binary lecithin and cephalin systems by application of several surface and spreading techniques, *Adv. Colloid Interface Sci.* 31, 1–110, 1990.

7. Mason, J.T., Investigation of phase transitions in bilayer monolayers, *Methods Enzymol.* 295, 468–494, 1998.

8. Crowe, J.H., Tablin, F., Tsvetkova, N., et al., Are lipid phase transitions responsible for chilling damage in human platelets? *Cryobiology* 38, 180–191, 1999.

9. Goñi, F.M., Alonso, A., Bagatelli, L.A., et al., Phase diagrams of lipid mixtures relevant to the study membrane rafts, *Biochim. Biophys. Acta* 1781, 665–684, 2008.

10. Shimokawa, N., Himeno, H., Hamada, T., et al., Phase diagrams and ordering in charged membranes, *J. Phys. Chem. B.* 128, 6358–6367, 2016.

11. Diamond, A.D., and Hsu, J.T., Aqueous two-phase systems for biomolecule separation, *Adv. Biochem. Eng. Biotechnol.* 47, 89–135, 1992.

12. Johansson, H.O., Matos, T., Luz, J.S., et al., Plasmid DNA partitioning and separation using poly(ethylene glycol)/poly(acrylate)/salt aqueous two-phase systems, *J. Chromatog. A* 1233, 30–35, 2012.

13. Tlostoguzov, V., Compositions and phase diagrams for aqueous systems based on proteins and polysaccharides, *Int. Rev. Cytol.* 132, 3–31, 2000.

14. Brady, J.P., Farber, P.J., Sekhar, A., et al., Structural and hydrodynamic properties of an intrinsically disordered region of a germ cell-specific protein on phase separation, *Proc. Natl. Acad. Sci. USA* 114, E8194–E8203, 2017.

15. Rösgen, J., and Hinz, H.-J., Phase diagrams: A graphical representation of linkage relations, *J. Mol. Biol.* 328, 255–271, 2003.

16. Ferreon, A.C., Ferreon, J.C., Bolen, D., and Rösgen, J., Protein phase diagrams II: Nonideal behavior o biochemical reactions in the presence of osmolytes, *Biophys. J.* 92, 245–256, 2007.

17. Ferreon, A.C., Ferreon, J.C., Wright, P.E., and Dennis, A.A., Modulation of allostery by protein intrinsic disorder, *Nature* 498, 390–394, 2013.

18. Aldridge, B.B., Gaudet, S., Lauffenburger, D.A., and Sorger, P.K., Lyapunov exponents and phase diagrams reveal multi-factorial control over TRAIL-induced apoptosis, *Mol. Syst. Biol.* 7, 553, 2011.

PHENOTYPE

The term phenotype refers to the physical manifestation of the genes of an organism, the collection of structure and function expressed by the genotype of an organism.[1–8] Phenotypic expression in an organism can be modified by "background effects" which are poorly understood but may reflect genetic interaction networks.[9]

1. Padykula, H.A., *Control Mechanisms in the Expression of Cellular Phenotypes*, Academic Press, New York, 1970.

2. Levine, A.J., *The Transformed Phenotype*, Cold Spring Harbor Laboratory Press, Cold Spring Harbor, NY, 1984.

3. Papaioannou, V.E., and Behringer, R.I., *Mouse Phenotypes: A Handbook of Mutation Analysis*, Cold Spring Harbor Laboratory Press, Cold Spring Harbor, NY, 2005.

4. *Immunology, phenotype first: How Mutations have established New Principles and Pathways in Immunology*, ed. Beutler, B.I., Springer, Berlin, Germany, 2008.

5. *Epigenetics: Linking Genotype and Phenotype in Development and Evolution*, ed. B.I. Hallgrimsson, B.I., and Hall, B.K., University of California Press, Berkeley, CA, 2011.

6. *Engineering Complex Phenotypes in Industrial Strains,* ed. R. Parnaik, Wiley, Hoboken, NJ, 2013.

7. Frommlet, F., Nakgorzata, B., and Ramsey, D.M., *Phenotypes and Genotypes: The Search for Influential Genes,* Springer, London, UK, 2016.

8. Akessadro, M., *Plant Evolutionary Developmental Biology: The Evolvability of the Phenotype*, Cambridge University Press, Cambridge, UK, 2018.

9. Hou, J., van Leeuwen, J., Andrews, B.J., and Boone, C., Genetic network complexity shapes background-dependent phenotypic expression, *Trends Genet.* 34, 576–586, 2018.

PHOSPHOLIPASE C

Phosholipase C is a term used to refer to a family of intracellular enzymes (isozymes)[1,2] central to many signal transduction pathways via effects on the mobilization of Ca^{2+} and protein kinase C.[3,4] Phospholipase C is best known for the conversion of phosphoinositol 4,5-bisphosphate to yield 1,4,5-inositol triphosphate which mobilizes calcium ions,[5–7] and diacylglycerol which activate protein kinase C.[8,9] Phospholipase C is involved in a variety of processes including the macrophage inflammatory response.[10]

1. Gresset, A., Sondek, J., and Harden, T.K., The phospholipase C isozymes and their regulation, *Subcell. Biochem.* 58, 61–94, 2012.

2. Lyon, A.M., and Tesmer, J.J., Structural insights into phospholipase C-β function, *Mol. Pharmacol.* 84, 488–500, 2013.

3. Kadamur, G., and Ross, E.M., Mammalian phospholipase C, *Annu. Rev. Physiol.* 75, 127–154, 2013.

4. Nakamura, Y., and Fukami, K., Regulation and physiological functions of mammalian phospholipase C, *J. Biochem.* 161, 315–321, 2017.

5. Litosch, I., and Fain, J.N., Regulation of phosphoinositide breakdown by guanine nucleotides, *Life Sci.* 39, 187–194, 1986.

6. Putney, J.W., Jr., Formation and actions of calcium-mobilizing messenger, inositol 1,4,5-trisphosphate, *Am. J. Physiol.* 252, G149–G157, 1987.

7. Bird, G.S., DeHaven, W.I., Smyth, J.T., and Putney, J.W., Jr., Methods for studying store-operated calcium entry, *Methods* 46, 204–212, 2008.

8. Shigeto, M., Cha, C.Y., Rorsman, P., and Kaku, K., A role of PLC/PKC-dependent pathway in GLP-1-stimulated insulin secretion, *J. Mol. Med.* 95, 361–368, 2017.

9. Trexler, A.J., and Tarasaka, J.W., Regulation of insulin exocytosis by calcium-dependent protein kinase C in beta cells, *Cell Calcium* 67, 1–10, 2017.

10. Zhu, L., Jones, C., and Zhang, G., The role of phospholipase C signaling in macrophage-mediated inflammatory response, *J. Immunol. Res.* 2018, 5201759, 2018.

Cis-PHOSPHORYLATION OR *Cis*-AUTOPHOSPHORYLATION

Cis-Phosphorylation or *cis*-autophosphorylation refers to a phosphorylation event where the kinase catalyzes the phosphorylation of itself as opposed to phosphorylation by another molecule of the same kinase (*trans*-phosphorylation).[1] The *cis*- and *trans*-reactions are not necessarily exclusive can occur on the kinase molecule.[2,3]

1. Cann, A.D., and Kohanski, R.A., *Cis*-autophosphorylation of juxtamembrane tyrosines in the insulin receptor kinase domain, *Biochemistry* 36, 7681–7689, 1997.

2. Greenswag, A.R., Muok, A., Li, X., and Crane, B.R. Conformational transitions that enable histidine kinase autophosphorylation and receptor array integration, *J. Mol. Biol.* 427, 3890–3907, 2015.

3. Zheng, W., Cai, X., Li, S., and Li, Z., Autophosphorylation mechanism of the ser/thr kinase stkl from *Staphylococcus aureus*, *Front. Microbiol.* 9, 758, 2018.

TRANS-PHOSPHORYLATION OR TRANS-AUTOPHOSPHORYLATION

Trans-phosphorylation or *Trans*-autophosphorylation is an autophosphorylation event where the kinase catalyzes the phosphorylation of another molecule of the same kinase as opposed to *cis*-phosphorylation where the kinase phosphorylates itself.[1-3] Frequently both *cis*- and *trans*-phosphorylation occur on the same molecule but it possible to assign the mechanism of the reaction.[4]

1. Kelly, J.D., Haldeman, B.A., Grant, F.J., et al., Platelet-derived growth factor (PDGF) stimulates PDGF subunit dimerization and inter-subunit *trans*-phosphorylation, *J. Biol. Chem.* 266, 8987–8992, 1991.
2. Chen, H., Xu, C.F., Ma, J., et al., A crystallographic snapshot of tyrosine *trans*-phosphorylation in action, *Proc. Natl. Acad. Sci. USA* 105, 19660–19665, 2008.
3. Hubbard, S.R., Mechanistic insights into regulation of JAK2 tyrosine kinase, *Front. Endocrinol.* 8, 361, 2018.
4. Frattali, A.L., Treadway, J.L., and Pessin, J.E., Transmembrane signaling by the human insulin receptor kinase. Relationship between intramolecular beta subunit *trans*- and *cis*-autophorylation and substrate kinase activation, *J. Biol. Chem.* 267, 195210–19528, 1992.

PHYTOREMEDIATION

Phytoremediation is the use of plants for removal (remediation) of toxic metals, most often from soil.[1-3] Soil bacteria, diazotrophs such as rhizobia, which are associated with nitrogen fixation, are important in the removal of metal ions from soil by plants.[4-6] It is noted that the term bioremediation is used to describe the process by which bacteria remove pollutants from soil and water while the term phytoremediation is used to describe the plant process recognizing the term phytoremediation is used to describe the process where organic compounds are jointly remediated by plants and bacteria.[7-9] Plants are also used to remove organic pollutants from soil,[10,11] although there are challenges with respect to the physical availability of organic compounds in soil.[12]

1. Arthur, E.L., Rice, P.J., Rice, P.J., et al., Phytoremediation—An overview, *Crit. Rev. Plant Sci.* 24, 109–122, 2005.
2. Ali, H., Khan, E., and Sajad, M.A., Phytoremediation of heavy metals—concepts and applications, *Chemosphere* 91, 869–881, 2013.
3. Bang, J., Kamala-Kannan, S., Lee, K.J., et al., Phytoremediation of heavy metals in contaminated water and soil using *Miscanthus* sp. Goedae-Uksaei 1, *Int. J. Phytoremediation* 17, 515–520, 2015.
4. Hao, X., Taghavi, S., Xie, P., et al., Photoremediation of heavy and transition metals aided by legume-rhizobia symbiosis, *Int. J. Phytoremediation* 16, 179–202, 2014.
5. Ullah, A., Mushtag, H., Ali, H., et al., Diazotrophs-assisted phytoremediation of heavy metals: A novel approach, *Environ. Sci. Pollut. Res. Int.* 22, 2505–2514, 2015.
6. El Aafi, N., Saidi, N., Maltouf, A.F., et al., Prospecting metal-tolerant rhizobia for phytoremediation of mining soils from Morocco using *Anthyllis vulneraria* L., *Environ. Sci. Pollut. Res. Int.* 22, 4500–4512, 2015.
7. Khan S., Afzal, M., Iqbal, S., and Khan, Q.M., Plant-bacteria partnerships for the remediation of hydrocarbon contaminated soils, *Chemosphere* 90, 1317–1332, 2013.
8. Bell, T.H., Joly, S., Pitre, FE., and Yergeau, E., Increasing phytoremediation efficiency and reliability using novel omics approaches, *Trends Biotechnol.* 32, 271–280, 2014.
9. Hussain, I., Aleti, G., Najdu, R., et al., Microbe and plant assisted-remediation of organic xenobiotics and its enhancement by genetically modified organisms and recombinant technology, *Sci. Total Environ.* 628–629, 1582–1599, 2018.
10. Olsen, P.E., Castro, A., Joern, M., et al., Comparison of plant families in a greenhouse phytoremediation study on an aged polycyclic aromatic hydrocarbon-contaminated soil, *J. Environ. Qual.* 36, 1461–1469, 2007.
11. Chandranshive, V.V., Kadam, S.K., Khandare, R.V., et al., *In situ* phytoremediation of dyes from textile wastewater using garden ornamental plants, effect on soil quality and plant growth, *Chemosphere* 210, 968–976, 2018.
12. Ouvrard, S., Leglize, P., and Morel, J.L., PAH phytoremediation: Rhizodegradation or rhizoattenuation? *Int. J. Phytoremediation* 16, 46–61, 2014.

PINOCYTOSIS

Pinocytosis is the process of transport of material (transcytosis) of substances from the extracellular space to the intracellular space, most frequently in a vesicle which is then internalized.[1] It is process that is separate from endocytosis and phagocytosis[2] in that it occurs in all cells and has been extensively studied in amoeba.[3-5] Pinocytosis is considered to an important mechanism in the uptake of LCL by aortic macrophages in the development of atherosclerosis.[6,7] See **macrophage, micropinocytosis**.

1. Holter, H., Pinocytosis, *Int. Rev. Cytology* 8, 481–504, 1959.
2. Boihdanowicz, M., and Grinstein, S., Role of phospholipids in endocytosis, phagocytosis, and macropinocytosis, *Physiol. Rev.* 93, 69–106, 2013.
3. Klein, G., and Satre, M., Kinetics of fluid-phase pinocytolsis in *Dictyostellum discoideum* amoeba, *Biochem. Biophys. Res. Commun. Res. Commun.* 138, 1146–1152, 1986.
4. Josefsson, J.O., Arvidson, G., and Cobbold, P., Possible regulation of cation-induced pinocytosis in *Amoeba proteus* by phospholipase A, *Eur. J. Cell Biol.* 46, 200–206, 1988.

5. Prusch, R.D., and Roscoe, J.C., A possible signal-coupling role for cyclic AMP during endocytosis in *Amoeba proteus*, *Tissue Cell* 25, 141–149, 1993.

6. Kluth, H.S., Fluid-phase pinocytosis of LDL by macrophages: A novel target to reduce macrophage cholesterol accumulation in atherosclerotic lesions, *Curre. Pharm. Des.* 19, 5865–5872, 2013.

7. Anzinger, J.J., Jin, X., Palmer, C.S., et al., Measurement of aortic cell fluid-phase pinocytosis in vivo by flow cytometry, *J. Vasc. Res.* 54, 195–199, 2017.

PIPETTE (PIPET)

First, unknown to me, there has been a serious issue with the term pipette. The question is, is it pipette or pipet? Fortunately this issue has been addressed and while the result in not binding, it would appear that the preferred term is pipette.[1] A pipette is defined as "A slender tube of small calibre used for obtaining a known small volume of a liquid," especially in laboratory work, and often incorporating a swollen central reservoir; pipette is also a verb defined as "To draw (*off*) by means of a pipette; to transfer (*into*) by means of a pipettes."[2] Regardless of the volume delivered, the major quality attribute for pipetting, whether 10 mL or 10 μL is accuracy.[3–9] There is a need for consistent periodic calibration of pipettes and training of operators.[10,11] Specific operator technique is also important.[12,13] There has been a series of studies on the effect of laboratory conditions (ambient temperature, barometric pressure) which can be significant sources of error.[14] While accuracy is important, contamination during transfer can be a problem with clinical samples.[15]

While I recognize that instrumentation and technology have markedly improved over the past 20 years, there was an assay issue that took me from Los Angeles to Switzerland to solve an assay problem involving a classic 96-well microplate. There was a major discrepancy in potency of an expensive biologic between laboratories. The problem was solved when was determined that the angle of the pipette tip to wall of the microplate well was critical for adequate mixing. Pipette tips from mircopipettes are used for solid-phase extraction in sample preparation.[16–20] The term pipette is also used to describe the patch-clamp pipette which is used in electrophysiology.[21–23] Instrumentation continues to advance.[24]

1. Gold, M., Pipette vs. pipet-which one is correct? https://www.artel-usa.com/pipette-vs-pipet/.

2. *Oxford English Dictionary*, Oxford University Press, Oxford, UK, 2019.

3. Greendyke, R.M., Wormer, J.L., and Banzhaf, J.C., Quality assurance in the blood bank. Studies of technologist performance, *Am. J. Clin. Pathol.* 71, 287–290, 1979.

4. Pecci, J., Ryan, C., and Kahn, T., Source of errors on using a positive-displacement pipette in hepatitis B testing, *Clin. Chem.* 25, 335–336, 1979.

5. Hedges, A.J., Estimating the precision of serial dilutions and viable bacterial counts, *Int. J. Food Microbiol.* 76, 207–214, 2002.

6. Bertermann, R., Pipet quality control: A microliter of prevention, *Amer. Biotechnol. Lab.* 18–24, 2004.

7. Curtis, R., Minimizing liquid delivery risk: Pipets as sources of errors, *Amer. Lab.* March, 8–9, 2007.

8. Rakhankulova, M., Stavrou, S.W., Yuen, A.P., et al., Micropipette tips—The unsung heroes of mass spectrometry, *Rapid Commun. Mass Spectrom.* 22, 2349–2354, 2008.

9. Ghasemzadeh, N., Wilhemsen, T.W., Nyberg, F., and Hjerten, S., Precautions to improve the accuracy of quantitative determinations of biomarkers in clinical diagnostics, *Electrophoresis* 31, 2722–2729, 2010.

10. Curtis, R.H., and Rodriguez, G., Pipet performance verification: An important part of method validation, *Amer. Lab.* 12–17, 2004.

11. Carle, A.B., Rodriguez, G.W., and Curtis, R.H., Transferability of pipet Calibrations and proficiency of operators: Prerequisites for method validation and method transfers, *Amer. Biotechnol. Lab.* 10–13, 2009.

12. Vaccaco, W., Minimizing liquid delivery: Operators as sources of error, *Amer. Lab.* September, 16–18, 2007.

13. Carle, A.B., Rodriguez, G.W., and Curtis, R.H., Transferability of pipet. Calibrations and proficiency of operators: Prerequisites for method validation and method tansfers, *Amer. Biotechnol. Lab.* 10–13, 2009.

14. https://www.aweimagazine.com/article/extreme-pipetting-313.

15. Hopkins, H., Oyibo, W., Luchavez, J., et al., Blood transfer devices for malaria rapid diagnostic tests: Evaluation of accuracy, safety and ease of use, *Malar. J.* 10, 30, 2011.

16. Wang, H. So, P.K., Ng, T.T., and Yao, Z.P., Rapid analysis of raw solution samples by C18 pipette-tip electrospray ionization mass spectrometry, *Anal. Chim. Acta* 844, 1–7, 2014.

17. Zhang, Y. Zhao, Y.G., Chen, W.S., et al., Three-dimensional ionic liquid-ferrite functionalized graphene oxide for pipette-tip solid phase extraction of 16 polycyclic aromatic hydrocarbons in human blood sample, *J. Chromatog A* 1552, 1–9, 2018.

18. Fresco-Cala, B., and Cárdenas, S., Potential of nanoparticle-based hybrid monoliths as sorbents in microextraction techniques, *Anal. Chim. Acta* 1031, 15–27, 2018.

19. Simões, N.S., de Oliveira, H.L., da Silva, R.C.S., Hollow mesoporous structured molecularly imprinted polymer as adsorbent in pipette-tip solid-phase extraction for the determination of antiretrovirals from plasma of HIV-infected patients, *Electrophoresis*, 39, 2581–2589, 2018.

20. Mastrianni, K.R., Kemnitzer, and W.E., Miller, K.W.P., A novel, automated dispersive pipette extraction technology greatly simplifies catecholamine sample preparation for downstream LC-MS/MS analysis, *SLAS Technol.* 24, 117–123, 2019.

21. Stuart, G., and Spruston, N., Probing dendritic function with patch pipettes, *Curr. Opin. Neurobiol.* 5, 389–394, 1995.

22. Danker, T., Braun, F., Silbernagl, N., and Guenther, E., Catch and patch: A pipette-based approach for automating patch clamp that enable cell selection and fast compound application, *Assay Drug Dev. Technol.* 14, 144–155, 2016.

23. Stockslager, M.A., Capocasale, C.M., Holst, G.L., et al., Optical method for automated measurement of glass micropipette tip geometry, *Precis. Eng.* 46, 88–95, 2016.

24. Beroz, J., and Hart, A.J., Universal handheld micropipette, *Rev. Sci. Instrum.* 87, 115112, 2016.

PIRANHA SOLUTION

Piranha solution is a mixture of concentrated sulfuric acid and hydrogen peroxide (as an example, a 7:3(v/v) ratio of 98% H_2SO_4 [concentrated sulfuric acid] and 30%(w/v) H_2O_2) which is used for the cleaning of glass and other surfaces.[1–7] A slightly different ratio of reagents (6/4,v/v) has been used.[8] A basic piranha solution composed of ammonium hydroxide and hydrogen peroxide (again in 70/30 ratio) has been described[9,10] which provided somewhat different results with a titanium surface.

1. Guo, W., and Ruckenstein, E., Crosslinked glass fiber affinity membrane chromatography and its application to fibronectin separation, *J. Chromatog. B Technol. Biomed. Life Sci.* 795, 61–72, 2003.

2. Ziegler, K.J., Gu, Z., Peng, H., et al., Controlled oxidative cutting of single-walled carbon nanotubes, *J. Amer. Chem. Soc.* 127, 1541–1547, 2005.

3. Wang, M., Liechti, K.M., Wang, Q., and White, J.M., Self-assembled monolayers: Fabrication with nanoscale uniformity, *Langmuir* 21, 1848–1857, 2005.

4. Szuneritz, S., and Boukherroub, R., Preparation and characterization of thin films of SiO(x) on gold substrates for surface plasmon resonance studies, *Langmuir* 22, 1660–1663, 2006.

5. Petrovykh, D.Y., Kimura-Suda, H., Opdahl, A., et al., Alkanethiols on platinum: Multicomponent self-assembled monolayers, *Langmuir* 14, 2578–2587, 2006.

6. Hoshiya, N., Shimoda, M., Yoshikawa, H., et al., Sulfur modification of Au via treatment with Piranha solution provides low-Pd releasing and recyclable Pd material, SAPd, *J. Am. Chem. Soc.* 132, 7270–7272, 2010.

7. de Vos, W.M., Cattoz, B., Avery, M.P., Cosgrove, T., and Prescott, S.W., Adsorpion and surfactant-mediated desorption of poly(vinylpyrrolidone) on plasma- and piranha-cleaned silica surfaces, *Langmuir* 30, 8425–8431, 2014.

8. Maji, D., Lahiri, S.K., and Das, S., Study of the hydrophilicity and stability of chemically modified PDMS surface using piranha and KOH solution. *Surface Interface Analysis* 44, 62–69, 2012.

9. Nazarov, D.V., Zemtsova, E.G., Vallev, R.Z., and Smirnov, V.M. Formation of micro- and nanostructures on the nanotitanium surface by chemical etching and deposition of titania films by atomic layer deposition (ALD), *Materials* (Basal) 8, 8366–8377, 2015.

10. Nazarov, D.V., Zemtsova, E.G., Solokhin, A.Y., Valiev, R.Z., and Smirnov, V.M., Modification of the surface topography and composition of ultrafine and coarse grained titanium by chemical etching, *Nanomaterials* (Basel) 7, E15, 2017.

PLASTID

The canonical definition of plastid is "an organelle in the cytoplasm of a plant cell bound by a double membrane and usually containing pigment or food substance."[1] Plastids are suggested to the evolutionary result of the process of endosymbiosis[2,3] where a bacteria (Cyanobacter) was taken into a eukaryotic "host" by phagocytosis eventually resulting in a plastid (as an endosymbiont).[3,4] Plastids develop into different organelles such as chromoplasts and chloroplasts during the development of the plant.[5–7] Following maturation the organelles degenerate eventually forming a plastid in dry seeds. Endosymbiosis is also suggested to be responsible for the presence of mitochondria in eukaryotic cells.[8,9]

1. *Oxford English Dictionary*, Oxford, UK, 2019.

2. Zimorski, V., Ku, C., Martin, W.F., and Gould, S.B., Endosymbiotic theory for organelle origins, *Curr. Opin. Microbiol.* 22, 38–46, 2014.

3. Cavalier-Smith, T., Membrane heredity and early chloroplast evolution, *Trends Plant. Sci.* 5, 175–182, 2000.

4. Dorrell, R.G., and Howe, C.J., Integration of plastids with their hosts: Lessons learned from dinoflagellates, *Proc. Natl. Acad. Sci. USA* 112, 10247–10254, 2015.

5. Lopez-Juez, E., and Pyke, K.A., Plastids unleashed: Their development and their integration in plant development, *Int. J. Dev. Biol.* 49, 557–577, 2005.

6. Toyoshima, Onda, Y., Shiina, T., and Nakahira, Y., Plastid transcription in higher plants, *Crit. Rev. Plant Sci.* 24, 59–81, 2005.

7. Allorent, G., Courtois, F., Chevalier, F., and Lerbs-Mache, S., Plastic gene expression during chloroplast differentiation and dedifferentiation into non-photosynthetic plastids during seed formation, *Plant Mol. Biol.* 82, 59–70, 2013.

8. Archibald, J.M., Endosymbiosis and eukaryotic cell evolution, *Curr. Biol. Rev.* 25, R911–R921, 2015.

9. Allen, J.F., Why chloroplasts and mitochondria retain their own genomes and genetic systems: Colocation for redox regulation of gene expression, *Proc. Natl. Acad. Sci. USA* 112, 10231–10238, 2015

PLATE NUMBER

Plate number is one of several properties of a chromatographic column term used to estimate performance. A plate is a separation instance or moment that a solute encounters during passage through a chromatographic column. The higher the number of plates, the more possibility for high resolution but such resolution depends on the individual behavior of solutes (see resolution). Plates may be theoretical or effective plates. The efficiency of a column is measured in the number of plates referred to as plate number (N) (also referred to as column efficiency).[1] A plate number may be theoretical or more often determined from experimental data. One equation for plate number (N). $N = 5.54(t_r/W_{1/2})^2$ where t_r is band retention time and $W_{1/2}$ is peak width at peak half-height. There are other algorithms but this is the most common formula. Plate number is as important in gas chromatography as it is liquid chromatography.[2–4] Plate number is an objective measure which can be used to compare chromatographic systems.[5–10]

1. Seidel-Morgenstern, A., Schulte, M., and Epping, A., Fundamental and general terminology, in *Preparative Chromatography*, 2nd edn., H. Schmidt-Traub, M. Schulte, and A. Seidel-Morgenstern, Chapter 2, pp. 7–46. Wiley-VCH Verlag GmbH, Weinheim, Germany, 2013.
2. Moretti, P., Vezzani, S., and Castello, G., Prediction of theoretical plate number in isothermal gas chromatographic analysis on capillary columns, *J. Chromatog. A* 1133, 305–314, 2006.
3. Yan, X., Yang, J., Wang, Q., and Liu, Y., Theoretical tools for predicting optimal cross-sectional shapes in microgas chromatography, *J. Sep. Sci.* 36, 1537–1544, 2013.
4. Kurganov, A.A., Korolev, A.A., Shiryaeva, V.E., Popova, T.P., and Kanateva, A.Y., Kinetic efficiency of polar monolithic capillary columns in high-pressure gas chromatography, *J. Chromatog.* 1315, 162–166, 2013.
5. Mahesan, B., and Lai, W., Optimization of selected chromatographic responses using a designed experiment at the fine-tuning stage in reversed-phase high-performance liquid chromatographic method development, *Drug Dev. Ind. Pharm.* 27, 585–590, 2001.
6. Chester, T.L., and Teremmi, S.O., A virtual-modeling and multivariate-optimization examination of HPLC parameter interactions and opportunities for saving analysis time, *J. Chromatog. A.* 1096, 16–27, 2005.
7. Lohrmann, M., Schulte, M., and Strube, J., Generic method for systematic phase selection and method development of biochromatographic processes. Part I. Selection of a suitable cation-exchanger for the purification of a pharmaceutical protein, *J. Chromatog. A* 1092, 89–100, 2005.
8. Nishi, H., and Nagamatsu, K., New trend in the LC separation analysis of pharmaceuticals—High performance separation by ultra high-performance liquid chromatography (UHPLC) with core-shell particle C18 columns, *Anal. Sci* 30, 205–211, 2014.
9. Sultan, Y., Magan, N., and Medina, A., Comparison of five different C18 HPLC analytical columns for the analysis of ochratoxin A in different matrices, *J. Chromatog. B Analyt. Technol. Biomed. Life Sci.* 971, 89–93, 2014.
10. Ito, M., Shimizu, K., and Nakatani, K., Three-dimensional representation method using pressure, time, and number of theoretical plates to analyze separation conditions in HPLC columns, *Anal. Sci.* 34, 137–142, 2018.

PLECKSTRIN HOMOLOGY-LIKE DOMAIN (PHLD)

The Pleckstrin homology-like domain (PHLD) is a protein domain consisting of 100–120 amino acids, which binds phosphoinositide and other activators such as heterotrimeric G proteins and participates in the process of signal transduction.[1,2] The term Pleckstrin was advanced in 1989 to describe a 47 kDa protein (P47) which had been shown to be substrate for protein kinase C during platelet activation.[3] The name was derived from the platelet protein Pleckstrin (platelet and leukocyte C kinase substrate and KFARKSTRRSIR) as most likely phosphorylation site identified as a substrate for protein kinase C.[4,5] There are a large number of proteins that contains the PH Domain[6,7] and it has been suggested there is a role for the PH domain in interactions with the cytoskeleton. The Pleckstrin homology-like domain superfamily (PH-like superfamily, accession number d17171)[8] contains a large number of members in several families. The Pleckstrin homology-like domain family A (PHLDA) has been the subject of most study with three members.[9] PHLDA1 is identical with TDAG651 (T-cell death associated gene 51).[10–12] PHLDA1 was recognized early a factor in T-cell death as well as negative regulator of cell growth and the prevention of apoptosis in tumor cells.[13] Subsequent work has shown that PHLDA1 inhibits Erb receptors (e.g. EGFR) by preventing receptor dimerization and, as a result, downstream activation of Akt.[9,14] Several studies suggest that downregulation of PHLDA1 promotes tumor development as well as tumor cell migration.[15] PHLDA2 has been identified as an inhibitor of Akt signally by inhibiting translocation repressing tumor development.[16] Inhibition of Akt is based on the ability of PHLDA2 to bind membrane lipid (phosphatidylinositol). PHLDA2 is also a maternally imprinted gene[17] important in fetal development.[18,19] PHLDA2 has been proposed as a cancer biomarker[20] as has PHLDA1.[21] PHLDA3 is unique in that it is a small protein (144 amino acids) consisting mostly of a single PH domain[22] which functions as an inhibitor of Akt. It is noted that

Akt has a PH domain.[23] Other examples of PH domains include dynamin[24] and p210 BCR-ABL.[25]

1. Musacchio, A., Gibson, T., Rice, P., Thompson, J., and Saraste, M., The PH domain: A common piece in the structural patchwork of signalling proteins, *Trends Biochem. Sci.* 18, 343–348, 1993.
2. Gilson, T.J., Hyvönen, M., Musacchio, A., Saraste, M., and Birney, E., PH domain: The first anniversary, *Trends Biochem. Sci.* 19, 349–353, 1994.
3. Haslam, R.J., Lynham, J.A., and Fox, J.E., Effects of collagen, ionophore A23187 and prostaglandin E1 on the phosphorylation of specific proteins in blood platelets, *Biochem. J.* 178, 397–406, 1979.
4. Tyers, M., Rachubinski, R.A., Stewart, M.I., et al., Molecular cloning and expression of the major protein kinase C substrate of platelets, *Nature* 333, 470–473, 1988.
5. Tyers, M., Haslam, R.J., Rachubinski, R.A, and Harley, C.B., Molecular analysis of pleckstrin: The major protein kinase C substrate of platelets, *J. Cell. Biochem.* 40, 133–145, 1989.
6. Musacchio, A., Gibson, T., Rice, P., Thompson, J., and Saraste, M., The PH domain: A common piece in the structural patchwork of signalling proteins, *Trends Biochem. Sci.* 18, 343–348, 1993.
7. Lemmon, M.A., Ferguson, K.M., and Abrams, C.S., Pleckstrin homology domains and the cytoskeleton, *FEBS Lett.* 513, 71–76, 2002.
8. https://www.ncbi.nlm.nih.gov/Structure/cdd/cddsrv.cgi?uid=327399.
9. Chen, Y., Takikawa, M., Tsutumi, S., et al., PHLDA1, another PHLDA family member that inhibits Akt, *Cancer Sci.* 109, 3532–3542, 2018.
10. Kuske, M.D.A., and Johnson, J.P., Assignment of the human PHLDA1 gene to chromosome 12q15 by radiation hybrid mapping, *Cytogenetics Cell Genetics* 89, 1, 2000.
11. Sellheyer, K., and Nelson, P., Follicular stem cell marker PHLDA1 (TDAG51) is superior to cytokeratin-20 In differentiating between trichoepithelioma and basal cell carcinoma in small biopsy specimens, *J. Cutaneous Pathol.* 38, 542–550, 2011.
12. Coleman, S.K., Cao, A.W., Rebalka, I.A., et al., The Pleckstrin homology like domain family member TDAG51, is temporally regulated during skeletal muscle regeneration, *Biochem. Biophys. Res. Commun.* 495, 499–505, 2018.
13. Kuske, M.D.A., and Johnson, J.P., Assignment of the human PHLDA1 gene to chromosome 12q15 by radiation hybrid mapping, *Cytogenetics Cell Genetics.* 89, 1, 2000.
14. Magi, S., Iwamoto, K., Yumoto, N., et al., Transcriptionally inducible Plecstrin homology-like domain, family A, member 1, attenuates ErB receptor oligomerization, *J. Biol. Chem.* 293, 2206–2218, 2018.
15. Bonatto, N., Carlini, M.J., de Bessa Garcia, A., and Nagai, M.A., PHLDA1 (Pleckstrin homology-like domain, family A, member 1) knockdown promotes migration and invasion of MCF1OA breast epithelial cells, *Cell Adhesion Migration* 12, 37–46, 2018.
16. Wang, X., Li, G., Koul, S., et al., PHLDA2 is a key oncogene-induced negative feedback inhibitor of EGFR/ErbB2 signaling via interference with AKT signaling, *Oncotarget* 9, 24914–24926, 2018.
17. Moore, G.E., Ishida, M., Demetriou, C., et al., The role and interaction of imprinted genes in human fetal growth, *Phil. Trans. R. Soc. B* 370, 20140074, 2015.
18. Salas, M., John, R., Saxema, A., et al., Placental growth retardation due to loss of imprinting of *Phlda2*, Mech. Devel. 121, 1199–1210, 2004.
19. Tunster, S.J., Creeth, H.D.J., and John, R.M., The imprinted *Phlda2* gene modulates a major endocrine compartment of the placenta to regulate placental demands for maternal resources, *Dev. Biol.* 409, 251–260, 2016.
20. Quanz, M., Bender, E., Kopitz, C., et al., Preclinical efficacy of the noval monocarboxylate 1 inhibitor BAY-8002 and associated markers of resistance, *Mol. Cancer Ther.* 17, 2285–2296, 2018.
21. Sellheyer, K., and Nelson, P., Follicular stem cell marker PHLDA1 (TDAG51) is superior to cytokeratin-20 In differentiating between trichoepithelioma and basal cell carcinoma in small biopsy specimens, *J. Cutaneous Pathol.* 38, 542–550, 2011.
22. Kwase, T., Ohki, R., Shibata, T., et al., PH domain-only protein PHLDA3 is a p53 regulated repressor of Akt, *Cell* 136, 535–550, 2009.
23. Agamasu, C., Ghanam, R.J., Xu, F., et al., The interplay between calmodulin and membrane interactions with the Pleckstrin homology domain of Akt, *J. Biol. Chem.* 292, 251–263, 2017.
24. Dar, S., and Pucadyll, T.J., The Pleckstrin-homology domain of dynamin is dispensible for membrane constriction and fission, *Mol. Biol. Cell.* 28, 152–160, 2017.
25. Shimasaki, K., Watanabe-Takahashi, M., Umeda, M., et al., Pleckstrin homology domain of p210 BCR-ABL interacts with cardiolipin to regulate its mitochondrial translocation and subsequent mitophagy, *Genes Cells* 23, 22–34, 2018.

PLEIOTROPIC

Pleiotropic is described as the condition of pleiotropy where pleiotropy is defined as the production by a single gene of two of more apparently unrelated phenotypic effects.[1-3] The definition has been extended to describe other biochemical events such as an effector molecule associated with more than a single effect such as insulin[4,5] or insulin-like growth factor.[6-8] Pleiotropic activity has been referred to as "moonlighting" with one example being glyceraldehyde-3-phosphate dehydrogenase where the protein has different activities dependent on subcellular localization.[9] The pleiotropic effects of statins has been the subject of considerable study.[10-12]

1. *Oxford English Dictionary*, Oxford University Press, Oxford, UK, 2019.
2. Leroi, A.M., Bartke, A., De Benedictis, G., et al., What evidence is there for the existence of individual genes with antagonistic pleiotropic effects? *Mech, Ageing Dev.* 126, 421–429, 2005.
3. Carbone, M.A., Jordan, K.W., Lyman, R.F., et al., Phenotypic variation and natural selection at catsup, a pleiotropic quantitative trait gene in *Drophila*, *Curr. Biol.* 16, 912–919, 2006.
4. Smith, R.M., Harada, S., and Jarett, L., Insulin internalization and other signaling pathways in the pleiotropic effects of insulin, *Int. Rev. Cytol.* 173, 243–280, 1997.
5. Cariou, B., Pleiotropic effects of insulin and GLP-1 receptor agonists: Potential benefits of the association, *Diabetes Metab.* 41(6 Suppl 1), 6S28–6S35, 2015.
6. Salminen, A., and Kaarniranta, K., Insulin/IGF-1 paradox of aging: Regulation via AKT/IKK/NF-κB signaling, *Cell Signal.* 22, 573–577, 2010.
7. Ashpole, N.M., Logan, S., Yabluchanskiy, A., et al., IGF-1 has sexually dimorphic, pleiotropic, and time-dependent effects on healthspan, pathology, and lifespan, *Geroscience* 39, 129–145, 2017.
8. Arroba, A.T., Campos-Caro, A., Aguilar-Diosdado, M., and Valverde, A.M., IGF-1, inflammation and retinal degeneration: A close network, *Front. Aging Neurosci.* 10, 203, 2018.
9. Sirover, M.A., Pleiotropic effects of moonlighting glyceraldehyde-3-phosphate dehydrogenase (GAPDH) in cancer progression, invasiveness, and metastases, *Cancer Metastasis Rev.* 37, 665–676, 2018.
10. Marfarlane, S.I., Muniyappa, R., Francisco, R., and Sowers, J.R., Pleiotropic effects of statins: Lipid reduction and beyond, *J. Clin. Endocrinol. Metabol.* 87, 1451–1458, 2002.
11. Davies, J.T., Delfino, S.F., Feinberg, C.E., et al., Current and emerging uses of statins in clinical therapeutics: A review, *Lipid Insights* 9, 13–29, 2016.
12. Bharami, A., Parsamanesh, N., Atkin, S.L., et al., Effect of statins on toll-like receptors: A new insight to pleioptropic effects, *Pharmacol. Res.* 135, 230–238, 2018.

POISSON DISTRIBUTION

The Poisson distribution is a probability density function that is an approximation to the biomodal distribution and is characterized by its mean being equal to its variance. A more formal definition is a frequency distribution which gives the probability of a number of discrete events occurring in a certain time interval, or of a particular number of successes out of a given number of trials.[1] The practical result is the familiar bell-shaped curve for a theoretical distribution.[2] The Poisson distribution is based on the concept that each event/measurement/data point is independent of any other event/measurement/data point.[3] There are a number of texts discussing the role of the Poisson Distribution in statistical analysis.[4–8]

1. *Oxford English Dictionary*, Oxford University Press, Oxford, UK, 2019.
2. Koyama, K., Hokunan, H., Hasegawa, M., Kawamura, S., and Koseki, S., Do bacterial numbers follow a theoretical Poisson distribution? Comparison of experimentally obtained numbers of single cells with random number generation via computer simulation, *Food Microbiol.* 60, 49–53, 2016.
3. Hayat, M.J., and Higgins, M., Understanding Poisson registration, *J. Nurs. Educ.* 53, 207–215, 2014.
4. Consul, P.C., *Generalized Poisson Distribution: Properties ond Appications*, Marcel Dekker, New York, 1989.
5. Mezei, L.M., *Practical Spreadsheet Statistics and Curve Fitting for Scientists and Engineers*, Prentice Hall, Englewood Cliffs, NJ, 1990.
6. Heldt, J.J., *Quality Sampling and Reliability: New Uses for the Poisson Distribution*, St. Lucie Press/CRC Press, Boca Raton, FL, 1999.
7. Dowdy, S.M., and Wearden, S., *Statistics for Research*, Wiley, New York, 1991.
8. Balakrishnan, N., and Nevzorov, V.B., *A Primer on Statistical Distributions*, Wiley, Hoboken, NJ, 2003; Shui, F., *The Poisson-Dirichlet Distribution and Related Topics: Models and Asymptotic Behaviors*, Springer-Verlag, Berlin, Germany, 2010.

POLYADENYLATION

The term polyadenylation refers to the attachment of approximately 200 adenyl residues to the 3′-end of Pre-messenger RNA during the process of transcription. Polyadenylation is one of three events which occur during the processing of transcription. The other two events are 5′-capping with a guanosine derivative[1,2] and RNA splicing by spliceosomes to remove introns.[3] Termination of transcription by 3′-cleavage is followed by polyadenylation. The sequence 5′-AAUAAA-3′ is one of the upstream signals for polyadenylation.[4] Polyadenylation was the first pre-mRNA modification to be observed when an increase in the content of polyadenylic acid in sea urchin embryos was observed following fertilization.[5] Subsequent work showed that the increase in polyadenylic acid was due to the polyadenylation of mRNA and was association with the translocation of the polyadenylated mRNA to the ribosomal fraction for translation.[6,7] Polyadenylation is a signal, together 5′-capping that the mRNA is ready to be exported to the ribosomes in the cytoplasm by the nuclear pore complex.[8,9]

1. Jurado, A.R., Tan, D., Jiao, X., and Kiledjian, M., Structure and function of pre-RNA capping quality control and 3′-end processing, *Biochemistry* 53, 1882–1898, 2014.
2. Martinez-Rucobo, F.W., Kohler, R., van de Waerbeemd, M., et al., Molecular basis of transcription-coupled pre-mRNA capping, *Molec. Cell* 58, 1079–1089, 2015.
3. Jurica, M.S., and Moore, M.J., Pre-mRNA splicing: Awash in a sea of proteins, *Molec. Cell* 12, 5–14, 2003.
4. Fitzgerald, M., and Shenk, T., The sequence 5′-AAUAAA3′ forms part of the recognition site for polyadenylation of late SV40 mRNAs, *Cell* 24, 251–260, 1981.
5. Slater, D.W., Slater, I., and Gillespie, D., Post-fertilization synthesis of polyadenylic acid in sea urchin embryos, *Nature* 240, 333–337, 1972.
6. Slater, I., Gillespie, D., and Slater, D.W., Cytoplasmic adenylation and processing of material RNA, *Proc. Natl. Acad. Sci. USA* 70, 406–411, 1973.
7. Wilt, F.H., Polyadenylation of maternal RNA of sea urchin eggs after fertilization, *Proc. Natl. Acad. Sci. USA* 70, 2345–2349, 1973.
8. Darnell, J.E., Jr., Reflections on the history of pre-mRNA processing and highlights of current knowledge: A unified picture, *RNA* 19, 443–460, 2013.
9. Alberts, B., Johnson, A., Lewis, J., Morgan, D., and Raft, M., *Molecular Biology of the Cell*, 5th edn., Chapter 6, How cells read the genome from DNA to RNA, pp. 299–368, Garland Science/CRC Press, Abington, UK, 2015.

POLYMERASE CHAIN REACTION (PCR)

The polymerase chain reaction (PCR)[1] was developed by Kerry Mullis in 1983 and is a mainstay of molecular biology. The history of the development of the PCR has been described[2] as well as its importance for biotechnology.[3] PCR is a method for amplification of DNA or RNA for analysis or used in recombinant DNA technology.[4–7] There are a number of version of the PCR reaction which are shown in Table PCR 1. There some variations of the PCR reaction such the panhandle PCR[8,9] and vectoretter PCR[10–12] used for genomic sequencing which are not shown. While the bulk of PCR is used for genomic diagnostics and recombinant DNA work, there is use of PCR for the amplification of barcodes in DNA chemical libraries.[13,14] Primed *in situ* labeling (PRINS) is a technical approach related to PCR where a DNA probe is used to bind to denatured cellular DNA and serve a primer

for a PCR reaction where the product can be visualized with a label such a biotin or digotoxigen (both as dUTP derivatives).[15–17]

1. Mullis, K.B., and Faloona, F.A., Specific synthesis of DNA in vitro via a polymerase-catalyzed chain reaction, *Methods Enzymol.* 155, 335–350, 1987.
2. Mullis, K.B., The usual origin of the polymerase chain reaction, *Sci. Am.* 262, 56–61, 1990.
3. Robinson, P., *Making PCR: A story of biotechnology,* University of Chicago Press, Chicago, IL, 1996.
4. McPherson, M., and Møller, S., *PCR*, 2nd edn., Garland Science/Taylor & Francis Group, New York, 2006.
5. *Real-Time PCR*, ed. M.J. Dorek, Taylor & Francis Group, Abington, UK, 2006.
6. *PCR Technology: Current Innovations,* 3rd edn., ed. T. Nolan and S.A. Bustin, CRC Press, Boca Raton, FL, 2013.
7. *Quantitative Real-Time PCR Methods and Protocols*, ed. R. Biasoni and A. Rosi, Humana/Springer, Clifton, NJ, 2014.
8. *PCR Primer Design*, ed. C. Basu, Humana/Springer, Clifton, NJ, 2015.
9. Jones, D.H., and Winistorfer, S.C., Sequence specific generation of a DNA panhandle permits PCR amplification of unknown flanking DNA, *Nucleic Acids Res.* 20, 595–600, 1992.
10. Megonigal, M.D., Rappaport, E.F., Wilson, R.B., et al., Panhandle PCR for cDNA: A rapid method for isolation of *MLL* fusion transcripts involving unknown partner genes, *Proc. Natl. Acad. Sci. USA* 97, 9597–9602, 2000.
11. Arnold, C., and Hodgson, I.J., Vectorette PCR: A novel approach to genomic walking, *Genome Res.* 1, 39–42, 1991.
12. Proffitt, J., Fenton, J., Pratt, G., Yates, Z., and Morgan, G., Isolation and characterization of recombinant events involving immunoglobulin heavy chain switch regions in multiple myeloma using long distance vectorette PCR (LDV-PCR), *Leukemia* 13, 1100–1107, 1999.
13. Hilario, E., Fraser, L.G., and McNeilage, M., Trinucleotide repeats as bait for vectorette PCR: A tool for developing genetic mapping markers, *Mol. Biotechnol.* 42, 320–326, 2009.
14. Franzini, R.M., and Randolph, C., Chemical space of DNA-encoded libraries, *J. Med. Chem.* 59, 6629–6644, 2016.
15. Zimmermann, G., and Neri, D., DNA-encoded chemical libraries: Foundations and applications in lead discovery, *Drug Discov. Today.* 21(11), 1828–1834, 2016.
16. Koch, J., Primed *in situ* labeling as a fast and sensitive method for the detection of specific DNA sequences in chromosomes and nuclei, *Methods* 9, 122–128, 1996.
17. Speel, E.J., Ramaekers, F.C., and Hopman, A.H., Primed *in situ* nucleic acid labeling combined with immunocytochemistry to simultaneously localize DNA and proteins in cells and chromosomes, *Methods Mol. Biol.* 226, 453–464, 2003.

Description of Various Technologies for Nucleic Acid Amplification Based on the Polymerase Chain Reaction (PCR)

PCR Technique	Description	References
PCR[a]	The original technique uses a DNA polymerase to extend two opposed primers flanking a segment of DNA designated as the target region. Early work designated the target region as the amplicon[1,2] and this terminology is still used.[3] The fundamental process involves the initial separation of double-stranded DNA sample by heat denaturation. After cooling, primer, enzyme, Mg^{2+} and the mixture of deoxynucleotide triphosphates in buffer (e.g. Tris) are added. This process is repeated and the original amplicon continues to be copied at a linear rate, the transcripts are transcribed at an exponential rate.[4,5] The original technique used a Klenow fragment of DNA polymerase[6] which lacked the intrinsic exonuclease activity seen with DNA polymerases. The thermal lability of the Klenow fragment required the addition of fresh enzyme after each thermal denaturation cycle.[7,8] The use of a thermostable DNA polymerase such as Taq polymerase[9] allowed the reaction to proceed without the addition of fresh enzyme at each cycle. Given the exponential nature of the PCR reaction, it is possible to obtain a ten million-fold amplification of an amplicon.[4,7,b]	1–9
Nested PCR	Nested PCR is a variation of PCR where a second set of primers internal on the amplicon relative to the original primers is used to focus on a shorter DNA sequence. Nested PCR is used to increase the sensitivity and fidelity of the PCR reaction.[10–12]	10–12
Inverse PCR	Inverse PCR is a technique which permits the determination of DNA sequence flanking the target region.[13–16] This approach is dependent on the presence of one restriction site inside the target region and a different restriction site in the flanking regions. A segment of DNA containing the target sequence and flanking regions is obtained by one restriction enzyme or by reverse transcriptase. A second strand of DNA is obtained to yield a double-stranded DNA which is then circularized by DNA ligase. A linear DNA is obtained by restriction enzyme cleavage in the target region and a PCR product is obtained by primers directed "out" from opposing ends of the target region. Inverse PCR has proved useful for chromosome walking.[17]	13–17
RT-PCR	RT-PCR is the PCR using RNA as the source of the amplicon. A polydT primer is frequently used for preparation of the first cDNA copy reflecting the presence of a polyA tail on mRNA. A single primer is then used to make the second DNA chain which is then amplified with normal PCR process.[18] RT-PCR is used for measurement of gene expression in tissues[19,20] and single cells.[20–22]	18–22
Real Time PCR	Real Time PCR uses a fluorescent signal to measure the progress of strand duplication. This is accomplished the use of oligonucleotide probes containing a fluorophore[23,24] which hybridizes with the PCR product or with the use of a dye such as ethidium bromide or cyanine dyes,[25] which intercalate into double-stranded DNA sequence with a change in spectral characteristics.[23,26] The use of fluorescent probes to measure PCR product has permitted the development of instrumentation to measure the progress of PCR in "real-time" [27] rather than by electrophoretic analysis following amplification. Real-time RT-PCR is a method to measure mRNA levels.[28] In this context, the technique is referred to as quantitative real-time RT-PCR.[29]	23–29
qPCR	Current qPCR uses the measurement technologies of real-time PCR to measure the concentration of a specific DNA species.[30] Real-time PCR coupled with RT-PCR permits the accurate quantitative determination of messenger RNA concentrations.[31] There are many considerations in the application of this technique to the measurement of mRNA levels.[31–34]	30–33
dPCR	dPCR is a variation of PCR where a complex DNA sample is diluted to an extent that a single drop contains on a single DNA species.[35–38] This is intended to improve the specificity of the PCR reaction with complex mixtures such as present in the preparation of DNA libraries.[39–41] This technique is also described as digital droplet PCR.[42] dPCR has been adapted for use with microfluidic systems[43] permitting analysis of single cells.[44]	35–44b
Emulsion PCR	Emulsion PCR is an extension of dPCR where the components of a PCR reaction are separated into oil droplet.[45–48] Solid-phase reaction technology with beads has been used in emulsion PCR.[49,50] Emulsion PCR has been used for amplification of single DNA molecules.[46,51,a]	45–51
Multiplex PCR	A process where multiple primers are used to obtain products from multiple target sequences in genomic DNA.[52] Multiplex PCR was originally used to define genomics deletions Duchenne muscular dystrophy.[53] Multiplex PCR continues to be used for diagnosis of genomic rearrangements[54] and identification of pathogens.[55]	52–55
Anchored PCR Ligation PCR		

[a] Abbreviations are PCR, polymerase chain reaction; RT-PCR, reverse transcriptase-PCR; qPCR, quantitative PCR; dPCR, digital PCR

[b] For example, 25 cycles with 70% amplification efficiency would produce 1 μg of PCR product from 1 pg of target sequence. (From Table 1.1 in Newton, C.R., and G.A. Graham, *PCR*, 2nd edn., Bios Science, Oxford, UK, 1997.)

REFERENCES

1. Baran, N., Lapidot, A., and Manor, H., Unusual sequence element found at the end of an amplicon, *Mol. Cell. Biol.* 7, 2636–2640, 1987.

2. Chang, F., and Li, M.M., Clinical application of amplicon-based next-generation sequencing in cancer, *Cancer Genet.* 206, 413–419, 2013.

3. Pabinger, S., Ernst, K., Pulverer, W.S., et al., Analysis and visualization tool for targeted amplicon bisulfite sequencing on Ion Torrent sequencers, *PLoS One* 11(7), e0160227, 2016.

4. Newton, C.R., and Graham, A., *PCR*, 2nd edn., Bios/Springer, Oxford, UK, 1997.

5. McPherson, M.J., and Møller, S, G, *PCR*, Bios/Springer, Oxford, UK, 2000.

6. Mullis, K.B., and Faloona, F.A., Specific synthesis of DNA *in vitro* via polymerase-catalyzed chain reaction, *Methods Enzymol.* 155, 335–350, 1987.

7. Salik, R.K., Gelfand, D.H., Stoffel, S., et al., Primer-directed enzymatic amplification of DNA with a thermostable DNA polymerase, *Science* 239, 487–491, 1988.

8. Syvänen, A.C., Bengtatröm, M., Tenhunen, J., and Söderlund, H., Quantification of polymerase chain reaction products by affinity-based hybrid collection, *Nucleic Acids Res.* 16, 11327–11338, 1988.

9. Liu, C.C., and LiCata, V.J., The stability of Taq DNA polymerase results from a reduced entropic folding penalty; identification of other thermophilic proteins with similar folding thermodynamics, *Proteins* 82, 785–793, 2014.

10. Porter-Jordan, K., Rosenberg, E.I., Keiser, J.F., et al., Nested polymerase chain reaction assay for the detection of cytomegalovirus overcomes false positives caused by contamination with fragmented DNA, *J. Med. Virol.* 30, 85–91, 1990.

11. Borchers, K., and Slater, J., A nested PCR for the detection and differentiation of EHV-1 and EHV-4, *J. Virol. Methods* 45, 331–336, 1993.

12. Mijatovic-Rustempasic, S., Esona, M.D., Williams, A.L., and Bowen, M.D., Sensitive and specific nested PCR assay for detection of rotovirus A in samples with a low viral load, *J. Virol. Methods* 236, 41–46, 2016.

13. Ochman, H., Gerber, A.S., and Hard, D.L., Genetic applications of an inverse polymerase reaction, *Genetics* 120, 621–623, 1988.

14. Zilberberg, N., and Gurevitz, M., Rapid isolation of full length cDNA clones by "inverse PCR": Purification of a scorpion cDNA family encoding α-neurotoxins, *Analyt. Biochem.* 209, 203–205, 1993.

15. Huang, S-H., Inverse polymerase chain reaction: An efficient approach to cloning cDNA ends, *Molec. Biotechnol.* 2, 15–22, 1994.

16. Pavlopoulos, A., Identification of DNA sequences that flank a known region by inverse PCR, *Methods Mol. Biol.* (*Molecular Methods for Evolutionary Genetics*) 772, 267–275, 2011.

17. Trinh, Q., Zhu, P., Shi, H., et al., A-T linker adapter polymerase chain reaction for determining flanking sequences by rescuing inverse PCR or thermal asymmetric interlaced PCR products, *Anal. Biochem.* 466, 24–26, 2014.

18. Ohan, N.W., and Jeikkila, J.J., Reverse transcription-polymerase chain reaction: An overview of the technique and its applications, *Biotechnol. Advances* 11, 13–29, 1993.

19. Salonga, D.S., Danenburg, K.D., Grem, J., et al., Relative gene expression in normal and tumor tissue by quantitative RT-PCR, *Methods in Molecular Biology* 191, 83–98, 2002.

20. Hashimoto, A., Matsui, T., Tanaka, S., et al., Laser-mediated microdissection for analysis of gene expression in synovial tissue, *Modern Rheumatol,* 17, 185–190, 2007.

21. Dixon, A.K., Richardson, P.J., Pinnock, R.D., and Lee, K., Gene expression analysis at the single-cell level, *Trends Pharm. Sci.* 21, 65–70, 2000.

22. Phiilips, J.K., and Lipski, J., Single-cell RT-PCR as a tool to study gene expression in central and peripheral autonomic neurons, *Autonomic Neurosci.* 86, 1–13, 2000.

23. Chminggi, M., Monereau, S., Pernet, P., et al., Specific real-time PCR vs. fluorescent dyes for serum free DNA quantification, *Clin. Chem. Lab. Med.* 45, 993–995, 2007.

24. Faltin, B., Zengele, R., and von Stetten, F., Current methods for fluorescence-based universal sequence-dependent detection of nucleic acids in homogenous assay and clinical applications, *Clin. Chem.* 59, 1567–1582, 2013.

25. Bruijns, B.B., Tiggelaar, R.M., and Gardeniers, J.G., Fluorescent cyanine dyes for the quantification of low amounts of dsDNA, *Anal. Biochem.* 511, 74–79, 2016.

26. McCarthy, M.T., and O'Callaghan, C.A., Solid-phase-reader quantification of specific PCR products by measurement of band-specific ethidium bromide fluorescence, *Anal. Biochem.* 447, 30–32, 2014.

27. Oste, C.C., PCR Instrumentation: Where do we stand? in *The Polymerase Chain Reaction*, ed. K.B. Mullis, F. Ferré, and R.A. Gibbs, pp. 165–173, Birkhäuser, Boston, MA, 1994.

28. Blashke, V., Reich, K., Blaschke, S., Zipprich, S., and Neumann, C., Rapid quantitation of proinflammatory and chemoattractant cytokine expression in small tissue samples and monocyte-derived dendritic cells: Validation of a new real-time RT-PCR technology, *J. Immunol. Methods* 246, 79–90, 2000.

29. Winer, J., Jung, C.K.S., Shackel, I., and Williams, W.P., Development and validation of real-time quantitative reverse transcriptase-polymerase chain reaction for monitoring gene expression in cardiac monocytes in vitro, *Anal. Biochem.* 270, 41–49, 1999.

30. Dymond, J.S., Explanatory chapter: Quantitative PCR, *Methods Enzymol.* 529, 279–289, 2013.

31. Bustin, S.A., Benes, V., Garson, J.A., et al., The MIQE guidelines: Minimum information for publication of quantitative real-time PCR experiments, *Clin. Chem.* 55, 611–622, 2009.

32. Bustin, S.A., Why the need for qPCR publication guidelines? The case for MIQE, *Methods* 50, 217–226, 2010.

33. Lanoix, D., Lacasse, A.A., St-Pierre, J., et al., Quantitative PCR pitfalls: The case of the human placenta, *Mol. Biotechnol.* 52, 234–243, 2012.

34. Sanders, R., Mason, D.J, Foy, C.A., and Hugget, J.F., Considerations for accurate gene expression measurements by reverse transcription quantitative PCR when analyzing clinical samples, *Anal. Bioanal. Chem.* 406, 6471–6483, 2014.

35. Sykes, P.J., Neoh, S.H., Brisco, M.J., et al., Quantitation of targets for PCR by use of limiting dilution, *Biotechniques* 13, 444–449, 1992.

36. Vogelstein, B., and Kinzler, K.W., Digital PCR, *Proc. Natl. Acad. Sci. USA* 96, 9236–9241, 1999.

37. Bizouarn, F., Introduction to Digital PCR, in *Methods Mol. Biol. (Quantitative Real-Time PCR. Method and Protocols)* 1160, 27–40, 2014.

38. Huggett, J.F., Cowen, S., and Foy, C.A., Considerations for digital PCR as an accurate molecular diagnostic tool, *Clin. Chem.* 61, 79–88, 2015.

39. Persson, M.A., Combinatorial libraries, *Int. Rev. Immunol.* 10, 53–63, 1993.

40. Pollock, S., Thomas, D.Y., and Jansen, G., PCR-based unidirectional deletion method for creation of comprehensive cDNA libraries, *Biochim. Biophys. Acta* 1723, 265–269, 2005.

41. Aigrain, L., Gu, Y., and Quail, M.A., Quantification of next generation sequencing library preparation protocol efficiencies using droplet digital PCR assays—A systematic comparison of DNA library preparation kits for Illumina sequencing, *BMC Genomics* 17, 458, 2016.

42. Zonta, E., Garlan, F., Pécuchet, N., et al., Multiplex detection of rare mutations by picoliter droplet based digital PCR: Sensitivity and specificity, *PLoS One* 11(7), e0159094, 2016.

43. Zhang, Y., and Jiang, H-R., A review on continuous-flow microfluidic PCR in droplets: Advances, challenges and future, *Anal. Chim. Acta* 914, 7–16, 2016.

44. Ma, S., Loufakis, D.N., Cao, Z., et al., Diffusion-based microfluidic PCR for "one-pot" analysis of cells, *Lab Chip* 124, 2905–2909, 2014.

45. Tawfik, D.S., and Griffiths, A.D., Man-made cell-like compartments for molecular evolution, *Nature Biotechnol.* 16, 652–656, 1998.

46. Nakano, M., Komatsu, J., Matsuura, S-I., et al., Single-molecule PCR using water-in-oil emulsion, *J. Biotechnol.* 102, 117–124, 2003.

47. Williams, R., Peisajovich, S.G., Miller, O.J., et al., Amplification of complex gene libraries by emulsion PCR, *Nature Methods* 3, 545–550, 2006.

48. Schültze, T., Rubelt, F., Repkow, J., et al., A streamlined protocol for emulsion polymerase chain reaction and subsequent purification, *Anal. Biochem.* 410, 155–157, 2011.

49. Takaaki, K., Takei, Y., Ohtsuka, M., et al., PCR amplification from single DNA molecules on magnetic beads in emulsion: Application for high-throughput screening for transcription factor targets, *Nucleic Acids Res.* 33, e150/1–e150/9, 2005.

50. Hueninger, T., Wessels, H., Fischer, C., Paschke-Kratzin, A., and Fischer, M., Just in time selection: A rapid semi-automated SELEX of DNA aptamers using magnetic separation and beads, emulsion, amplification, and magnetics, *Anal. Chem.* 86, 10940–10947, 2014.

51. Orkunoglu-Suer, F., Harralson, A.F., Frankfurter, D., Gindoff, P., and O'Brien, T.J., Targeted single molecule sequencing methodology for ovarian hyperstimulation syndrome, *BMC Genomics* 16, 264, 2015.

52. Edwards, M.C., and Gibbs, R.A., Multiplex PCR: Advantages, development, and applications, *Genomic Res.* 3(4), S65–S75, 1994.

53. Chamberlain, J.S., Gibbs, R.A., Ranier, J.E., Nguyen, P.N., and Caskey, C.T., Deletion screening of the Duchenne muscular dystrophy locus via multiplex DNA amplification, *Nucleic Acids Res.* 16, 11141–11156, 1988.

54. De Lellis, L., Curia, M.C., Veschi, S., et al., Methods for routine diagnosis of genomic rearrangements: Multiplex PCR-based methods and future perspectives, *Exp. Rev. Mol. Diagn.* 8, 41–52, 2008.

55. Chang, S.S., Hseih, W.H, Liu, T.S., et al., Multiplex PCR system for rapid detection of pathogens in patients with presumed sepsis—A systemic review and meta-analysis, *PLoS One* 8(5), e62323, 2013.

POLYVINYLPYRROLIDONE (PVP)

Polyvinylpyrrolidone (PVP) is a polymer similar to poly(ethylene)glycol (PEG) is that it is readily soluble in water. PVP is synthesized by the free-radical polymerization of *N*-vinylpyrrolidinone (1-vinyl-2-pyrrolidinone). The final size of the polymer is controlled by choice of experimental conditions. PVP has been useful in a limited number of applications in biotechnology. There was early work suggesting that PVP at low concentrations (< 1% w/v) prevented aggregation of a monoclonal antibody.[1] More recent work has used PVP as mimic for intracellular polymers in the study of protein crowding.[2,3] PVP protected lactate dehydrogenase from inactivation during lyophilization by prevent dissociation (molecular crowding/preferential exclusion) and protecting from the decrease in pH (phosphate buffers[4] during freezing.[5] PVP has some direct therapeutic use as a carrier for drugs[6–8] and as a carrier for iodine (povidone-iodine) as a disinfectant.[9–12]

1. Gombotz, W.R., Pankey, S.C., Phan, D., et al., The stabilization of a human IgM monoclonal antibody with poly(vinylpyrrolidone), *Pharm. Res.* 11, 624–632, 1994.

2. Charlton, L.M., Barnes, C.O., Li, C., et al., Residue-level interrogation of macromolecular crowding effects on protein stability, *J. Am. Chem. Soc.* 130, 6826–6830, 2008.

3. Smith, A.E., Zhang, Z., Pielak, G.J., and Li, C., NMR studies of protein folding and binding in cells and cell-like environments, *Curr. Opin. Struct. Biol.* 30, 7–16, 2015.

4. van den Berg, L., and Rose, D., Effect of freezing on the pH and composition of sodium and potassium phosphate solutions: The reciprocal system—KH_2PO_4-Na_2HPO_4-H_2O, *Arch. Biochem. Biophys.* 81, 319–329, 1959.

5. Anchordoquy, T.J., and Carpenter, J.F., Polymers protect lactate dehydrogenase during freeze-drying by inhibiting dissociation in the frozen state, *Arch. Biochem. Biophys.* 332, 231–238, 1996.

6. Kaneda, Y., Tsutsumi, Y., Yoshioka, Y., et al., The use of PVP as a polymeric carrier to improve the plasma half-life of drugs, *Biomaterials* 25, 3259–3266, 2004.

7. Yang, M., Xie, S., Li, Q., et al., Effects of polyvinyl-pyrrolidone both as a binder and pore-former on the release of sparingly water-soluble topiramate from ethylcellulose coated pellets, *Int. J. Pharm.* 465, 187–196, 2014.

8. Van Duong, T., and Van den Mooter, G., The role of the carrier in the formulation of pharmaceutical solid dispersions. Part II: Amorphous carriers, *Expert Opin. Drug Deliv.* 13, 1681–1694, 2016.

9. Art, G., Combination povidone-iodine and alcohol formulations more effective, more convenient versus formulations containing either iodine or alcohol alone: A review of the literature, *J. Infus. Nurs.* 28, 314–320, 2005.

10. Bigliardi, P.L., Alsagoff, S.A.L., El-Kafrawi, H.Y., et al., Povidone iodine in wound healing: A review of current concepts and practices, *Int. J. Surg.* 44, 260–268, 2017.

11. Grzybowski, A., Karclaerz, P., and Myers, W.G., The use of povidone-iodine in ophthalmology, *Curr. Opin. Ophthalmol* 29, 19–32, 2018.

12. López-Cano, M., Kraft, M., Curell, A., et al., A meta-analysis of prophylaxis of surgical site infections with topical application of povidone iodine before primary closure, *World J. Surg.* 43, 374–384, 2018.

1. *Post-Translational Modifications in Plants*, ed. N. Battey, H.G. Dickinson, and A.M. Hetheringto, Cambridge University Press, Cambridge, UK, 1993.

2. Grave, D.J., *Co- and Post-Translational Modification of Proteins: Chemical Principles and Biological Effects*, Oxford University Press, New York, 1994.

3. Walsh, C., *Posttranslational Modification of Proteins: Expanding Nature's Inventory*, Robers and Company, Englewood, CO, 2006.

4. Walsh, G., *Post-Translational Modification of Protein Biopharmaceuticals*, Wiley-VCH, Weinhem, Germany, 2009.

5. *Analysis of Protein Post-Translational Modifications by Mass Spectrometry*, ed. J.R. Griffin and R.D. Unwin, John Wiley & Sons, Hoboken, NJ, 2016.

6. Wold, F., *In vivo* chemical modification of proteins (post-translational modification), *Annu. Rev. Biochem.* 50, 783–814, 1981.

7. Yan, S.C., Grinnell, B.W., and Wold, F., Post-translational modification of proteins: Some problems left to solve, *Trends Biochem. Sci.* 14, 264–268, 1989.

8. Krishna, R.G., and Wold, F. Post-translational modification of proteins, *Adv. Enzymol. Relat. Areas Mol. Biol.* 67, 265–298, 1993.

9. Berkner, K.L., Vitamin K-dependent carboxylation, *Vitam. Horm.* 78, 131–156, 2008.

10. Bartesaghi, S., and Radl, R., Fundamentals on the biochemistry and peroxynitrite and protein tyrosine nitration, *Redpx. Biol.* 14, 618–625, 2018.

11. Sales Gil, R., de Castro, I.J., Berihun, J., et al., Protein phosphatases at the nuclear envelope, *Biochem. Soc. Trans.* 46, 173–182, 2018.

12. *Reversible Protein Acetylation* (Novartis Foundation Symposium 259), ed. G. Bock and J. Goodie, John Wiley & Sons, Chichester, UK, 2004.

13. Walsh, C.T., Garneau-Tsodikova, S., and Gatto, G.J., Jr., Protein posttranslational modifications: The chemistry of proteome diversification, *Ange, Chem. Int. Ed.* 44, 7342–7372, 2005.

POST-TRANSLATIONAL MODIFICATION

A post-translational modification is a covalent modification of a protein, which may be reversible, following translation of the RNA to form the nascent polypeptide chain.[1–5] There are several excellent reviews[6–8] of the early work in this area which are quite useful. At that time, while there was information on the chemical nature of the modification, the function of the modifications was largely unknown.[7] A post-translational modification may be enzyme catalyzed as in the case of γ-carboxylation[9] or chemical as in the case of nitration by peroxynitrite;[10] the modification may be reversible as the in case of phosphorylation[11] and acetylation[12] or irreversible in the case of γ-carboxylation[9] and nitration by peroxynitrite.[10] There are a large number of post-translation modifications involving diverse amino acids.[13]

PRE-INITIATION COMPLEX

The pre-initiation complex is a complex of general transcription factors (GTFs) that are formed at each replication start point/origin at the start of S phase and is required for the action of RNA polymerase II.[1–5] The process of formation of the preinitiation complex starts with the loading of the Mcm2-7 (minichromosome maintenance 2-7) helicase complex onto chromatin during the G1 phase[4,6] in a process facilitated by origin recognition complex[7–9] in a process referred to as licensing.[10–12] This prereplication complex serves as the matrix for the formation of the preinitiation complex as the cell moves into S phase. While most of the work has been performed with the Pol II system, a preinitiation complex participates in the Pol III system.[13]

1. Roeder, R.G., The complexities of eukaryotic transcription initiation: Regulation of preinitiation complex assembly, *Trends Biochem. Sci.* 16, 402–408, 1991.
2. Parker, M.W., Botchan, M.R., and Berger, J.M., Mechanisms of DNA replication initiation in eukaryote, *Crit. Rev. Biochem. Mol. Biol.* 52, 107–144, 2017.
3. Kelly, T., Historical perspectives of eukaryotic DNA replication, *Adv. Exp. Med. Biol.* 1042, 41, 2017.
4. Schilbach, S., Hartsche, M., Tegunov, D., et al., Structures of transcription pre-initiation complex with TFIIH and mediator, *Nature* 551, 204–209, 2017.
5. Nozawa, K., Schneider, T.R., and Cramer, P., Core mediator structure at 3.4 Å extends model of transcription initiation complex, *Nature* 545, 248–251, 2017.
6. Powell, S.K., MacAlpine, H.K., Prinz, J.A., et al., Dynamic loading of and redistribution of the Mcm2-Y helicase complex through the cell cycle, *Embo J.* 34, 531–543, 2015.
7. Hua, X.H., and Newport, J., Identification of a preinitiation step in DNA replication that is independent of origin recognition complex and cdc6, but dependent on cdk2, *J. Cell Biol.* 140, 271–281, 1998.
8. Li, H., and Stillman, B., The origin recognition complex: A biochemical and structural view, *Subcell. Biochem.* 62, 37–58, 2012.
9. MacAlpine, D.M., Orchestrating the human DNA replication program, *Proc. Natl. Acad. Sci. USA* 113, 9136–9138, 2016.
10. Cyetic, C.A., and Walter, J.C., Getting a grip on licensing; mechanism of stable Mcm2–7 loading onto replication origins, *Mol. Cell* 21, 143–144, 2006.
11. Gros, J., Kumar, C., Lynch, G., et al., Post-licensing specification of eukaryotic replication origins by facilitated Mcm2–7 sliding along DNA, *Mol. Cell* 60, 797–807, 2015.
12. Sugimoto, N., and Fujita, M., Molecular mechanism for chromatin regulation during MCM loading in mammalian cells, *Adv. Exp. Med. Biol.* 1042, 61–78, 2017.
13. Male, G., von Appen, A., Glatt, S., et al., Architecture of TFIIIC and its role in RNA polymerase III preinitiation complex assembly, *Nat. Commun.* 6, 7387, 2015.

PRIMASE (DNA PRIMASE)

Primase is a RNA polymerase that catalyzes polymerization of ribonucleoside 5′-triphosphates to form RNA primers in as a sequence which is directed by DNA template (primer) during the process of single-strand DNA replication.[1–5] DNA polymerase α-primase complex synthesizes a short (8–10 nucleotide) RNA which is then extended with dNTPs to create a primer for further DNA synthesis by Pol δ on the lagging stand[6,7] and Pol ε on the leading strand.[7] The primase is a component of the replisome responsible for DNA replication.[8]

1. Foiani, M., Lucchini, G., and Plevani, P., The DNA polymerase alpha-primase complex couples DNA replication, cell-cycle progression and DNA-damage response, *Trends Biochem. Sci.* 22, 424–427, 1997.
2. Arezi, B., and Kuchta, R.D., Eurkaryotic DNA primase, *Trends Biochem. Sci.* 25, 572–576, 2000.
3. Frick, D.N., and Richardson, C.C., DNA primases, *Annu. Rev. Biochem.* 70, 39–80, 2001.
4. Benkovic, S.J., Valentine, A.M., and Salinas, F., Replisome-mediated DNA replication, *Annu. Rev. Biochem.* 70, 181–208, 2001.
5. MacNeil, S.A., DNA replication: Partners in the Okazaki two-step, *Curr. Biol.* 11, F842–F844, 2001.
6. Stodola, J.L., and Burgers, P.M., Mechanism of lagging-strand DNA replication in eukaryotes, *Adv. Exp. Med. Biol.* 1042, 117–133, 2017.
7. Pellegrini, L., The Pol α-primase complex, in *The Eukaryotic Replisome: A Guide to Protein Structure and Function*, ed. S. MacNeill, Chapter 6, pp. 157–169, Springer Science + Business, Dordrecht, the Netherlands, 2012.
8. MacNeill, S., Composition and dynamics of the eukaryotic replisome: A brief overview, in *The Eukaryotic Replisome: A Guide to Protein Structure and Function*, ed. S. MacNeill, Chapter 1, pp. 1–17, Springer Science + Business, Dordrecht, the Netherlands, 2012.

PROFESSIONAL PHAGOCYTES/ PROFESSIONAL ANTIGEN PRESENTING CELLS

Polymorphonuclear granulocytes, monocytes, and macrophages have been described as professional phagocytes responsible for the majority of phagocytosis.[1–3] Dendritic cells are also considered professional phagocytes.[3,4] Nonprofessional phagocytes include fibroblasts and epithelial cells with cross-talk with professional phagocytes.[5] Professional antigen presentation cells (pAPCs) include B-cells (B-lymphocytes), macrophages (Møs), and dendritic cells.[6] Most cells have MHC (major histocompatibility complex) I locus for presenting peptide from intracellular proteins such as derived from viruses. A number of cells have MHC II locus for capturing exogenous antigens. However, possession of an MHC II locus does not necessarily licence a cell as a pAPC. pAPCs have been suggested to have several characteristics; the ability to present and MHC II—peptide complex to a CD4+ T cell, the presence of costimulatory agents to stimulate the T cell and the ability to secrete supportive cytokines.[7,8] Dendritic cells have been described as the most active professional APC.[8–10] There are other cells (atypical MHC class II cells[8]) such as γδ T-cells,[7,11] mast cells,[12] and neutrophils.[13] It has been suggested[14] that pAPC capability can be transferred from dendritic cells to non-APC cells providing "MHC-dressed cells" by a process called trogocytosis.[15] This process of the transfer of exosomes (extracellular vesicles)[16] has been suggested to be useful for cancer therapy.[17]

1. Rabinovitch, M., Professional and non-profession phagocytes: An introduction, *Trends Cell Biol.* 5, 85–87, 1995.
2. Arandjelovic, S., and Ravichandran, K.S., Phagocytosis of apoptotic cells in homeostasis, *Nat. Immunol.* 16, 907–917, 2015.
3. Boe, D.M., Curris, B.J., Chen, M.M., Ippolito, J.A., and Kovacs, E.J., Extracellular traps and macrophages: New roles for the versatile phagocyte, *J. Leukoc. Biol.* 97, 1023–1035, 2015.
4. Savina, A., and Amigorena, S., Phagocytosis and antigen presentation in dendritic cells, *Immunol. Rev.* 219, 143–156, 2007.
5. Han, C.Z., Juncadella, I.J., Kinchen, J.M., Macrophages redirect phagocytosis by non-professional phagocytes and influence inflammation, *Nature.* 529, 570–574, 2016.
6. Blander, M.J., The many ways tissue phagocytes respond to dying cells, *Immunol.* Rev. 277, 158–173, 2017.
7. Brandes, M., Willimann, K., and Moser, B., Professional antigen-presentation function by human γδ T cells, *Science* 309, 264–268, 2005.
8. Kambayashi, T., and Laufer, T.M., Atypical MHC class II-expressing antigen-presenting cells: Can anything replace a dendritic cell? *Nat. Rev. Immunol.* 14, 719–730, 2014.
9. Delamarre, L., and Mellman, I., Cell biology of antigen processing and presentation, in *Fundamental Immunology*, 6th edn., ed. W.E. Paul, Chapter 20, pp. 614–630, Wolters Klower/Lippincott Williams & Wilkins, Philadelphia, PA, 2008.
10. Mellman, I., Turley, S.J., and Steinman, R.M., Antigen processing for amateurs and professionals, *Trends Cell Biol.* 8, 231–237, 1998.
11. Himoudi, N., Morgenstern, D.A., Yan, M., et al., Human γδ lymphocytes are licensed for professional antigen presentation by interaction with opsonized target cells, *J. Immunol.* 188, 1708–1715, 2012.
12. Galli, S.J., and Gaudenzio, N., Human mast cells as antigen-presenting cells: When is this role important *in vivo*? *J. Allergy Clin. Immunol.* 141, 92–93, 2018.
13. Vono, M., Lin, A., Norrby-Teglund, A., et al., Neutrophils acquire the capacity for antigen presentation to memory CD4+ T cells in vitro and ex vivo, *Blood* 129, 1991–2001, 2017.
14. Nakayama, M., Antigen presentation by MHC-dressed cells, *Front. Immunol.*5, 672, 2015.
15. LeMaoult, J., Caumartin, J., and Carosella, E.D., Exchanges of membrane patches (trogocytosis) split theoretical and actual functions of immune cells, *Hum. Immunol.* 68, 240–243, 2007.
16. Lindenbregh, M.F.S., and Stoorvogel, W., Antigen presentation by extracellular vesicles from professional antigen presenting cells, *Annu. Rev. Immunol.* 36, 435–459, 2018.
17. Pitt, J.M., Andre, F., Amigorena, S., et al., Dendritic cell-derived exosomes for cancer therapy, *J. Clin. Invest.* 126, 1224–1232, 2016.

PROMOTER ELEMENT

A promoter element is a segment of DNA sequence where RNA polymerase binds and initiates transcription.[1,2] The bacterial system for transcription is simple; RNA polymerase in the presence of sigma factor binds tightly to the DNA sequence at the promoter site and proceeds with the synthesis of RNA until termination with the release of sigma factor and mature RNA.[1] A single gene has a single promoter element. The process of transcription is more complex in eukaryotes where there are multiple general transcription factors which bind to RNA polymerase II (the most common polymerase, known as Pol II) at the promoter site within the gene control region. The TATA box in the promoter regions is located 25 bases upstream from the transcription start site and serves to bind one of the general transcription factor (TFIID).[1] The term promoter has also been used to describe the effect of chemicals such as benzyl acetate on carcinogenesis.[3]

1. Alberts, B., Johnson, A., Lewis, J., Morgan, D., and Raff, M., *Molecular Biology of the Cell*. 6th edition, Chapter 6, pp. 299–368, Garland Science/Taylor & Francis Group, New York, 2018.
2. King, R.C., Stanfield, W.D., and Mulligan, P.K. A Dictionary of Genetics, 7th edn., Oxford University Press, Oxford, UK, 2006.
3. Longnecker, D.S., Roebuck, B.D., Curphey, T.J., and MacMillan, D.L., Evaluation of promotion of pancreatic carcinogenesis in rats by benzyl acetate, *Food Chem. Toxicol.* 28, 665–668, 1990.

PROTAMINE

Protamine is a basic protein characterized by a high content of arginine (50%–70%), smaller than histones and replace histones during spermatogenesis.[1–4] In the process of replacing histones in chromatin, the chromatin condenses protecting DNA from damage.[4] Protamines have a long history dating 1874.[5] Protamines are relatively small proteins with molecular weight ranging from 5 kDa to 10 kDa.[6] Examples of small protamines include that isolated from the dog fish (designated Z3); molecular weight of approximately 4200 (determined by density gradient centrifugation; gel filtration did yield accurate results).[7] This protamine also contained only five amino acids; arginine (20), glycine (6), serine (3), alanine (1), and tyrosine (1). Another protamine (Z2) isolated from the dog-fish was quite different, larger and more varied amino acid content), with a high content of cysteine (4), lysine (6), and arginine (17) as well as amount of other amino acids.[8] The change in protein composition during spermatogenesis in the dog fish first involves the replacement of histones by two proteins, S1 and S2, which are rich in arginine and lysine with cysteine absent and are thought to be intermediate between histones in protamines.[9] Most mammals have a single protamine designated P1; mouse and human have another protamine, P2, in addition to P1.[10-15] Protamines have had considerable use as a therapeutic product. Protamine has been used to neutralize heparin anticoagulant activity.[16-20] The combination of protamine with insulin was observed to extend circulatory half-life in product known as insulin-Hagedorn.[21-25] Protamine or protamine derivatives (low molecular weight protamine) have been used for non-viral delivery of DNA into cells for gene therapy,[26] the delivery of RNA therapeutics,[27] and a Cas9 ribonucleoprotein complex.[28] Low molecular weight fragments of protamine have been prepared by enzymatic hydrolysis which may have improved therapeutic properties.[29-31]

1. Ando, T., Yamasaki, M., and Suzuki, K., *Protamines Isolation Characterization Structure and Function*, Springer-Verlag, New York, 1973.
2. Meistrich, M.L., Mohapatra, B., Shirley, C.R., and Zhao, M., Roles of transition nuclear proteins in spermiogenesis, *Chromasoma* 111, 483–488, 2003.
3. Aoki, V.W., and Carrell, D.T., Human protamines and the developing spermatid: Their structure, function, expression and relationship with male infertility, *Asian J., And rol.* 5, 315–324, 2003.
4. Steger, K., and Balhorn, R., Sperm nuclear protamines. A checkpoint to control sperm chromatin quality, *Anat. Histol. Embryol.* 47, 273–279, 2018.
5. Miescher, F., Das Protamin, eine neue organische Base aud den Samenfäden, des Rheinlachses, *Berichte* 7, 376–379, 1874.
6. Carroll, W.R., Callanan, M.J., and Saroff, H.A., Physical and chemical properties of protamine from the sperm of salmon (*Oncorhynchus tschawytscha*). II. Anion binding characteristics, *J. Biol. Chem.* 234, 2314–2316, 1959.
7. Sautiére, P., Briand, G., Gusse, M., and Chevaillier, P., Primary structure of a protamine isolated from the sperm nuclei of the dog-fish *Scyllirhinus canicullus*, *Biochim. Biophys. Acta* 119, 251–255, 1981.
8. Martinage, A., Gusse, M., Bélaiche, D., Sautiére, P., and Chevaillier, P., Amino acid sequence of a cysteine-rich, arginine-rich sperm protamine of the dog-fish (*Scylliorhinus caniculus*), *Biochim. Biophys. Acta* 831, 172–178, 1985.
9. Cheuviere, M., Laine, B., Sautiere, P., and Chevaillier, P., Purification and characterization of two basic spermatid-specific proteins isolatedfrom the dog fish *Scylliorhinus caniculus*, *FEBS Letters* 153, 231–235, 1983.
10. McKay, D.J., Renaux, B.S., and Dixon, G.H., Human sperm protamines. Amino-acid sequence of two forms of protamine P2, *Eur. J. Biochem.* 156, 5–8, 1986.
11. Bellue, A.R., McKay, D.J., Renaux, B.S., and Dixon, G.H., Purification and characterization of mouse protamines P1 and P2. Amino acid sequence of P2, *Biochemistry* 27, 2890–2897, 1988.
12. Wouters-Tyrou, D., Martinage, A., Chevaillier, P., and Sautiére, P., Nuclear basic proteins in spermiogenesis, *Biochimie* 80, 117–128, 1998.
13. Balhorn, R., The protamine family of sperm nuclear proteins, *Genome Biology* 8, 227, 2007.
14. Soler-Ventura, A., Castillo, J. de la Iglesia, A., et al., A step-by-step detailed protocol and brief review of protamine alterations *Protein Pept. Lett.* 25, 424–437, 2018.
15. Balhorn, R., Steger, K., Bergmann, M., et al., New monoclonal antibodies specific for mammalian protamines P1 and P2, *Syst. Biol. Reprod. Med.* 31, 1–24, 2018.
16. Cowley, L.L., and Lam, C.R., The neutralization of heparin by protamine, *Surgery* 24, 97–99, 1948.
17. Parkin, T.W., and Kvale, W.F., Neutralization of the anticoagulant effects of heparin with protamine (salmine), *Am. Heart J.* 37, 333–342, 1949.
18. Gordon, L.A., Perkins, H.A., and Richards, V., Studies in regional heparinization. I. The use of simultaneous neutralization with protamine; preliminary studies, *N.Engl. J. Med.* 255, 1025–1029, 1956.
19. Boer, C., Meesters, M.I., Veerhack, P., and Vonk A.B.A., Anticoagulant and side-effects of protamine in cardiac surgery, *Br. J. Anaesth.* 126, 914–927, 2018.
20. Glauser, B.R., Santos, G.R.C., Silvan, J.D., et al., Chemical and pharmacological aspects of neutralization of heparins form different animal sources by protamine, *J. Thromb. Haemost.* 16, 1789–1799, 2018.
21. Hagedorn, H.C., Jensen, B.N., Krarup, N.B., and Wodstrup, I., Protamine insulinate, *J. Am. Med. Assoc.* 106, 177–180, 1936.
22. Khowaja, A., Alkhaddo, J.B., Rana, Z., and Fish, L., Glycermic control in hospitalized patients with diabetes receiving corticosteroids using a neutral protamine Hagedorn insulin protocol: A randomized clinical trial, *Diabetes Ther.* 9, 1647–1655, 2018.
23. Alemayehu, B., Speiser, J., Bloudek, L., and Sarnes, E., Cost associated with long-acting insulin analogues in patients with diabetes, *Am. J. Manag. Care* 24(8 Spec. No.), SP265–SP272, 2018.
24. Lipska, K.J., Parker, M.M., Moffet, H.H., Huang, E.S., and Karter, A.J., Association of initiation of basal insulin analogues vs. neutral protamine Hagedorn insulin with hypoglycemia-related emergency department of visits of hospital admissions and with glycemic control in patients with type 2 diabetes, *JAMA* 320, 53–62, 2018.
25. Gotham, D., Barber, M.J., and Hill, A., Production costs and potential prices for biosimilars of human insulin and insulin analogues, *BMJ Glob. Health* 3(5), e000850, 2018.
26. El-Aneed, A., An overview of current delivery systems in cancer gene therapy, *J. Control Release* 94, 1–14, 2004.
27. Kauffman, K.J., Webber, M.J., and Anderson, D.G., Materials for non-viral intracellular delivery of messenger RNA therapeutics, *J. Control Release* 240, 227–240, 2016.
28. Kim, S.M., Shin, S.C., Kim, E.E., et al., Simple in vivo gene editing via direct self-assembly of Cas9 ribonucleoprotein complexes for cancer treatment, *ACS Nano* 12, 7750–7760, 2018.

29. Chang, L.-C., Lee, H.-F, Yang, Z., and Yang, V.C., Low molecular weight Pergamon (LMWP) as nontoxic heparin/low molecular weight heparin antidote(I): Preparation and characterization, *AAPS Pharmsci* 3(2), 17, 2001.

30. Kharidia, R., Friedman, K.A., and Liang, J.F., Improved gene expression using low molecular weight peptides produced from protamine sulfate, *Biochemistry* (Moscow) 73, 1162–1168, 2008.

31. Zhang, L., Shi, Y., Song, Y., et al., The use of low molecular weight protamine to enhance oral absorption of exenatide, *Int. J. Pharmaceutics* 547, 265–273, 2018.

PROTEASE/PROTEOLYTIC ENZYME/PEPTIDASE

A protease/proteolytic enzyme catalyzes the hydrolysis of a peptide bond in a protein; the hydrolysis of the peptide bond can be described as the action of a peptidase.[1] There a large number of proteases; 477 in *Drosophila melanogaster*, 405 in *Escherichia coli* and 600 in *Homo sapiens*.[2] A simple classification of proteases can divides these enzymes into two functional categories and four chemical categories. The functional categories are regulatory[3–6] and digestive.[7–9] Examples of regulatory proteolysis is proprotein processing by furin and the processes of blood coagulation while digestive enzyme include enzyme like pepsin, trypsin, and chymotrypsin found in mammalian digestive systems. There are digestive enzymes of considerable therapeutic interest found in blood-sucking nematodes[10] which are of interest as therapeutic targets.[11] Chemical categories describe the functional groups at enzyme active site and include serine proteases such as trypsin or chymotrypsin, cysteine proteases such as papain and the caspases, aspartic acid proteases such as pepsin, and metalloproteinases such as ADAM proteases and matrix metalloproteinase (MMP). There has been some discussion of the various approaches for the classification of the proteases.[12–15] MEROPS, the current classification system for peptidases[16–18] evolved from earlier work.[19,20] which organized peptidases into types. families and clans. There is extensive compilation of information on peptidases based on MEROPS classification.[21,22]

1. Rawlings, N.D., Protease families, evolution and mechanism of action, in *Proteases, Structure and Function*, ed. K. Brix and W. Stocker, Chapter 1, pp. 1–36, Springer Verlag, Wien, Austria, 2013.

2. Rawlings, N.D., Waller, M., Barrett, A.J., and Bateman, A., *MEROPS*; the database of proteolytic enzymes, their substrates and inhibitors, *Nucl. Acids Res.* 42, D503–D509, 2014.

3. *Proteases and Biological Control*, ed. E.I. Reich, D.B. Rifkin, and E. Shaw, Cold Spring Harbor Laboratory Press, Cold Spring Harbor, NY, 1975.

4. *Regulatory Proteolytic Enzymes and Their Inhibitors*, ed. S. Magnusson, Pergamon, Press, Oxford, UK, 1978.

5. Neurath, H., Proteolytic enzymes, past and present, *Fed. Proc.* 44, 2907–2913, 1983.

6. *Proteases and the Regulation of Biological Processes*, ed. J. Saklatvala and H. Nagase, Portland Press, London, UK, 2003.

7. *Molecular and Cellular Basis of Digestion*, ed. P. Desnuelle, E. Norén, O., and Sjöström, H., Elsevier, Amsterdam, the Netherlands, 1986.

8. Janiak, M.C., Digestive enzymes of human and nonhuman primates, *Evol. Anthropol.* 25, 253–266, 2016.

9. Caffrey, C.R., Goupil, L., Rebello, K.M., Dalton, J.P., and Smith, D., Cysteine proteases as digestive enzymes in parasitic helminths, *PLoS Negl. Trop. Dis.* 12, 0005840, 2018.

10. Williamson, A.L., Brindley, P.J., Knox, D.P., Hotez, P.J., and Loukas, A., Digestive proteases of blood-feeding nematodes, *Trends Parasitol.* 19, 417–423, 2003.

11. Pearson, M.S., Ranjit, N., and Loukas, A., Blunting the knife: Development of vaccines targeting digestive proteases of blood-feed helminth parasites, *Biol. Chem.* 391, 901–911, 2010.

12. Bergman, M., A classification of proteolytic enzymes, *Adv. Enzymol.* 2, 49–68, 1942.

13. Hartley, B.S., Proteolytic enzymes, *Annu. Rev. Biochem.* 29, 45–72, 1960.

14. Friedrich, P., and Bozóky, Z., Digestive versus regulatory proteases: On calpain action *in vivo*, *Biol. Chem.* 386, 609–612, 2005.

15. López, C., and Bond, J.S., Proteases: Multifunctional enzymes in life and disease, *J. Biol. Chem.* 283, 30433–30437, 2008.

16. Rawlings, N.D., and Barrett, A.J., MEROPS: The peptidases database, *Nucleic Acids Res.* 27, 325–331, 1999.

17. Rawlings, N.D., Barrett, A.J., and Bateman, A., MERPOS: The database of proteolytic enzymes, their substrates and inhibitors, *Nucleic Acids Res.* 40, D343–D350, 2012.

18. Rawlings, N.D., Waller, M., Barrett, A.J., and Bateman, A., MEROPS: The database of proteolytic enzymes, their substrates and inhibitors, *Nucleic Acids Res.* 42, D503–D509, 2014.

19. Rawlings, N.D., Barrett, A.J., Thomas, P.D., et al., The MEROPS database of proteolytic enzymes, their substrates and inhibitors in 2017 and a comparison with peptidases in the PANTHER database, *Nucleic Acids Res.* 46, D624–D632, 2017.

20. Rawllings, N.D., and Barrett, A.J., Evolutionary families of peptidases, *Biochem. J.* 290, 205–218, 1993.

21. Barrett, A.J., and Rawlings, N.D., Families and clans of serine peptidases, *Arch. Biochem. Biophys.* 318, 247–250, 1995.

22. *Handbook of Proteolytic Enzymes*, 3rd edn., ed. N.D. Rawlings and G. Salvesen, *Academic Press*, Boston, MA, 2013.

PROTEASE-ACTIVATED RECEPTOR (PAR)

Protease-activated receptors (PARs) are a family of 4 G-protein coupled receptors in which the ligand (tethered ligand) is intrinsic to the receptor protein and exposed by proteolysis in the *N*-terminal external region.[1–6] PARs may also be activated by peptides homologous to the tethered ligand exposed by proteolysis (thrombin receptor activation peptide, TRAP).[7–10] The protease-activated receptor was first described in platelets by Coughlin and colleagues[11–14] and by another group in France[15] using fibroblasts. Since the original work, four PARs have been described on a wide variety of cell types. It should be noted that there are proteases which inactivate PARs such as plasmin and neutrophil elastase which inactivate PAR1.[16] Below is a partial listing of the characteristics of PAR obtained from various sources.[1,4,16]

Protease Activated Receptors

Receptor Designation	Cell	Activating Enzyme
PAR1	Platelets	Thrombin
	Leukocytes	Activated protein C
	Fibroblasts	Cathepsin G
	Neurons	Matrix
	Keratinocytes	metalloproteinase-1
	Smooth muscle cells	Trypsin
		Granzyme
PAR2	Endothelial cells	Tissue factor/factor VIIa
	Leukocytes	Factor Xa
	Vascular smooth	Tryptase
	muscle cells	Kallikrein-related
	Epithelial cells	peptidase-5
		Trypsin
PAR3	Vascular smooth	Thrombin
	muscle cells	
	Platelets	
	Astrocytoma cells	
PAR4	Megakaryocytes	Thrombin
	Skeletal muscle cells	MASP-1
	Vascular endothelial	Plasmin
	cells	Trypsin
	Human islets	Gingipain

1. Ossovskaya, V.S., and Bunnett, N.W., Protease-activated receptors: Contribution to physiology and disease *Physiol. Rev.* 84, 579–621, 2004.
2. Soh, U.J., Dores, M.R., Chen, B., and Trejo, J., Signal transduction by protease-activated receptors, *Br. J. Pharmacol.* 160, 191–203, 2010.
3. Alberelli, M.A., and De Candia, E., Functional role of protease activated receptors in vascular biology, *Vascul. Pharmacol.* 62, 72–81, 2014.
4. Guenther, F., and Melzig, M.F., Protease-activated receptors and their biological role—Focused on skin inflammation, *J. Pharm. Pharmacol.* 67, 1623–1633, 2015.
5. Nieman, M.T., Protease-activated receptors in hemostasis, *Blood* 128, 169–177, 2016.
6. Hamilton, J.R., and Trejo, J., Challenges and opportunities in protease-activated receptor drug development, *Annu. Rev. Pharmacol. Toxicol.* 57, 349–373, 2017.
7. Levine, L., α-Thrombin and trypsin use different receptors to stimulate arachidonic acid metabolism, *Prostaglandins* 47, 437–449, 1994.
8. Debeir, T., Benavides, J., and Vigé, X., Dual effects of thrombin and a 14-amino acid peptide agonist of the thrombin receptor on septal cholinergic neurons, *Brain Res.* 708, 159–166, 1996.
9. Ceruso, M.A., McComsey, D.F., Leo, G.C., et al., Thrombin receptor-activating peptides (TRAPs): Investigation of bioactive conformations via structure-activity, spectroscopic, and computational studies, *Biooorg. Med. Chem.* 7, 2353–2371, 1999.
10. Hollenberg, M.D., Mihara, K., Polley, D., et al., Biased siginalling and proteinase-activated receptors (PARs): Targeting inflammatory disease, *Br. J. Pharmacol.* 171, 1180–1194, 2014.
11. Vu, T.K., Hung, D.T., Wheaton, V.I., and Coughlin, S.R., Molecular cloning of a functional thrombin receptor reveals a novel proteolytic mechanism of receptor activation, *Cell* 64, 1057–1068, 1991.
12. Coughlin, S.R., Vu, T.K., Hung, D.T., and Wheaton, V.I., Expression cloning and characterization of a functional thrombin receptor reveals a novel proteolytic mechanism of receptor activation, *Semin. Thromb. Hemost.* 18, 161–166, 1992.
13. Coughlin, S.R., Thrombin signalling and protease-activated receptors, *Nature* 407, 258–264, 2000.
14. Coughlin, S.R., Protease-activated receptors in hemostasis, thrombosis and vascular biology, *J. Thromb. Haemost.* 3, 1800–1814, 2005.
15. Rasmussen, U.B., Vouret-Cravieri, V., Jallet, S., et al., cDNA cloning and expression of a hamster alpha-thrombin receptor coupled to Ca²⁺ mobilization, *FEBS Lett.* 288, 123–128, 1991.
16. Hollenberg, M.D, Hansen, K.K., Mihara, K., and Ramachandran, R., Proteolytic enzymes and cell signaling: Pharmacological lessons, in *Proteases and Their Receptors in Inflammation*, ed. N. Vergnolle and M. Chignard, pp. 1–25, Springer Basal, Basal, Switzerland, 2011.

PROTEASE INHIBITOR COCKTAIL

A protease inhibition cocktail is a mixture of protease inhibitors that is used to preserve protein integrity by preventing proteolysis during the processing of samples for subsequent analysis. The term cocktail refers to a mixture of components which may distilled spirits such as Manhattan, food as in lobster cocktail, or chemicals.[1] A protease inhibitor cocktail is composed of a broad spectrum of protease inhibitors intends to inhibit the diverse proteolytic enzymes found in tissue extracts and biological fluids. A protease inhibitor cocktail became available as more proteases were identified. Many inhibitors were developed in the course of the of the mechanism of catalysis by these newly identified enzymes. Early work used a single inhibitor such as benzamidine as an inhibitor,[2] but it was recognized that multiple inhibitors were needed.[3-5] The term protease inhibitor cocktail was introduced in the early 1990s.[6,7] Protease inhibitor cocktails are available from a variety of commercial sources. There are other ways to prevent unwanted proteolysis in the preparation of samples for electrophoresis.[8] The term protease cocktail is also used to refer to the combination of therapeutic protease inhibitors used in AIDS therapy.[9-12]

1. *Oxford English Dictionary,* Oxford University Press, Oxford, UK, 2018.
2. Radcliffe, R., and Nemerson, Y., Activation and control of factor VII by activated factor X and thrombin. Isolation and characterization of a single chain form of factor VII, *J. Biol. Chem.* 250, 388–395, 1975.
3. Johnson, R.A., Jakobs, K.H., and Schultz, G., Extraction of the adenylate cyclase-activating factor of bovine sperm and its identification as a trypsin-like protease, *J. Biol. Chem.* 260, 114–121, 1985.
4. Nanoff, C., Jacobson, K.A., and Stiles, G.L., The A_2 adenosine receptor: Guanine nucleotide modulation of agonist binding is enhanced by proteolysis, *Mol.Pharmacol.* 39, 130–135, 1991.
5. Palmer, T.M., Jacobson, K.A., and Stiles, G.L., Immunological identification of A_2 adenosine receptors by two antipeptide antibody preparations, *Mol. Pharmacol.* 43, 391–397, 1992.
6. Takei, Y., Marzi, I., Kauffman, F.C., et al., Increase in survival time of liver transplants by protease inhibitors and a calcium channel blocker nisoldipine, *Transplantation* 50, 14–20, 1990.
7. Ledwith, B.J., Cahill, M.K., Losse, L.S., et al., Measurement of plasma angiotensin II: Purification by cation-exchange chromatography, *Anal. Biochem.* 213, 349–355, 1993.
8. Castellanos-Serra, L., and Paz-Lago, D., Inhibition of unwanted proteolysis during sample preparation: Evaluation of its efficacy in challenge experiments, *Electrophoresis* 23, 1745–1753, 2002.
9. Tamamura, H., and Fujii, N., Two orthogonal approaches to overcome multi-drug resistant HIV-1s: Development of protease inhibitors and entry inhibitors based on CXCR4 antagonists, *Curr. Drug Targets Infect. Disord.* 3, 103–110, 2004.
10. Wicovsky, A., Siegmund, D., and Wajant, H., Interferons induce proteolytic degradation of TRAILR4, *Biochem. Biophys. Res. Commun.* 337, 184–190, 2005.
11. Liu, L., Mugundu, G.M., Kirby, B.J., et al., Quantification of human hepatocytes cytochrome P450 enzymes and transporters induced by HIV protease inhibitors using new validated LC-MS/MS cocktail assays and RT-PCR, *Biopharm. Drug. Dispos.* 33, 207–217, 2012.
12. Su, C.T., Ling, W.L., Lua, W.H., Haw, Y.X., and Gan, S.K., Structural analyses of 2015-updated drug-resistant mutations in HIV-1 protease: An implication of protease inhibitor cross-resistance, *BMC Bioinformatics* 17(Suppl 19), 500, 2016.

PROTEASOME

Proteostasis refers to the maintenance of the intracellular proteome.[1] The proteome is product of synthesis and degradation. Inside the cell, protein degradation occurs either via the proteasome or via autophagy with the lysosomes.[2] The proteasome is responsible for 80% of the degradation of intracellular protein; maintenance or enhancement of proteasome function has been suggested to positively affect the aging process.[3,4] The proteasome is a multi-subunit complex that functions in the degradation of intracellular proteins in eukaryotic cell.[5-8] There is a not a single proteasome but a variety[7] based on structure, function as in immunoproteasomes, and tissue location[9] such as the thymoproteasome, which is found in cortical thymic epithelial cells.[10] Regardless of source, the proteasome is composed of a 20S particle referred to the core particle or catalytic subunit,[8,11] which is combined with one or two 19S regulatory particles in eukaryotes subunits to form the canonical 26S proteasome.[11] It has been noted[11] that while the 26S designation is commonly used, it has been determined that 26S complex (which contains two 19S particles) can be a 30.3S complex[12] (S is an abbreviation for the Svedberg which is a unit of time for the movement of a particle in centrifugal field, 10–13 seconds). As work progresses, it clear that there is more heterogeneity in the eukaryotic proteasome.[7] The immunoproteasome has an 11S regulatory particle which enables ATP-independent process of proteins to yield peptides for presentation to MHC class 1 complex.[13,14] The 20S standard proteasome accepts proteins presented by the regulatory particles. The proteins enter the interior of the 20S and are hydrolyzed to peptides catalyzed by N-terminal threonine residues on three of the several β chains.[11] Each of the three chains has different specificity: caspase-like, trypsin-like and chymotrypsin-like. The hydroxyl group of the N-terminal threonine provides the nucleophilic attack on the carboxy group of the sisscle peptide bond (in analogy to serine hydroxyl group of a serine protease) with the amino group of the *N*-terminal threonine providing the base catalysis (in analogy to the histidine residue of serine proteases). The isolated β chains lack this catalytic capability. Proteins designated for hydrolysis by proteasomes are usually marked by polyubiquitinylation, although there is evidence that markedly unfolded proteins may also be recognized by proteasomes in the absence of polyubiquitinylation. An example is the degradation of oxidized proteins.[15] The process of protein presentation by the regulatory particle requires ATP.[8,16] Elucidation of this requirement provided as explanation for the earlier observations of a requirement for ATP for hydrolysis of proteins by cellular extracts.[17] The proteasome is a therapeutic target in cancer.[18-20] The immunoproteasome was suggested a variant of the standard proteasome inducible by IFN-γ in 1993.[21] There was more work in this area but debate about the immunoproteasome continued to 2001.[22] The immunoproteasome is accepted today as structurally different from the standard immunoproteasome with the replacement of the three catalytic β chains.[23] There is interest in the immunoproteasome as a therapeutic target.[24]

1. Klaips, C.L., Jayaraj, G.C., and Hartl, F.U., Pathways of cellular proteostasis in aging and disease, *J. Cell Biol.* 217, 51–63, 2018.
2. Sands, W.A., Page, M.M., and Selman, C., Proteostasis and ageing: Insights from long-lived mutant mice, *J. Physiol.* 595, 6283–6390, 2017.
3. Kruegel, U., Robison, B., Dange, T., et al., Elevated proteasome capacity extends replicative lifespan in *Saccharomyces cerevisiae*, *PLoS Genet.* 7(9), e1002253, 2011.
4. Chondrogianni, N., Georgila, K., Kourtis, N., Tavernarakis, N., and Gonos, E.S., 20S proteasome activation promotes life span extension and resistance to proteotoxicity in *Caenorhabditis elegans*, *FASEB J.* 29, 611–622, 2015.
5. Arrigo, A.P., Tanaka, K., Goldberg, A.L., and Welch, W.J., Identity of the 19S "prosome" particle with the large multifunctional protease complex of mammalian cells (the proteasome), *Nature* 331, 192–194, 1988.
6. Enenkel, C., Yeast proteasome structure and biogenesis, in *The Proeasome in Neurodegeneration*, ed. L. Stefanis and J.N. Keller, Chapter 1, pp. 1–16, Springer Science + Business, New York, 2006.
7. Dahlmann, B., Mammalian proteasome subtypes: Their diversity in structure and function, *Arch. Biochem. Biophys.* 591, 132–140, 2016.
8. Collins, G.A., and Goldberg, A.L., The logic of the 26S proteasome, *Cell* 169, 792–806, 2017.
9. Kniepert, A., and Groettrup, M., The unique functions of tissue-specific proteasomes, *Trends Biochem. Sci.* 39, 17–24, 2013.
10. Murata, S., Takahama, Y., and Tanaka, K., Thymoproteasome: Probable role in generating positively selecting peptides, *Curr. Opin. Immunol.* 20, 192–196, 2008.
11. Marques, A.J., Palanimurugan, R., Maias, A.C., Ramos, P.C., and Dohman, R.J., Catalytic mechanism and assembly of the proteasome, *Chem. Rev.* 109, 1509–1536, 2009.
12. Yoshimura, T., Kameyama, K., Takagi, T., et al., Molecular characterization of the "26S" proteasome complex from rat liver, *J. Struct. Biol.* 111, 200–211, 1993.
13. Kaur, G., and Batra, S., Emerging role of immunoproteasomes in pathophysiology. *Immunol. Cell Biol.* 94, 812–820, 2016.
14. Eskandari, S.K., Seelen, M.A.J., Lin, G., and Azzi, J.R., The immunoproteasome: An old player with a novel and emerging role in alloimmunity, *Am. J. Transplant.* 17, 3033–3039, 2017.
15. Jung, T., Höhn, A., and Grune, T., The proteasome and the degradation of oxidized proteins: Part II—protein oxidation and proteasomal degradation, *Redox Biol.* 2, 99–104, 2014.
16. Wehmer, M., Rudeck, T., Beck, G., et al., Structural insights into the functional ATPase module of the 26S proteome, *Proc. Natl. Acad. Sci. USA* 114, 1305–1310, 2017.
17. McGuire, M.J., Croall, D.E., and DeMartino, G.N., ATP-stimulated proteolysis in soluble extracts of BHK21/C13 cells. Evidence for multiple pathways and a role for an enzyme related to the high-molecular weight protease, micropain, *Arch. Biochem. Biophys.* 262, 273–285, 1988.
18. Manasanch, E.E., and Orlowski, R.Z., Proteasome inhibitors in cancer therapy, *Nat. Rev. Clin. Oncol.* 14, 417–433, 2017.
19. Vandross, A., Proteasome inhibitor based therapy for treatment of newly diagnosed multiple myeloma, *Semin. Clin. Oncol.* 44, 381–384, 2017.
20. Yong, K., Gonzalez-McQuire, S., Szabo, Z., Schoen, P., and Hajek, R. The start of a new wave: Developments in proteasome inhibition in multiple myeloma, *Eur. J. Haematol.* 101, 220–236, 2018.
21. Gaczumska, M., Rock, K.I., and Goldberg, A.L., Role of proteasomes in antigen presentation, *Enzyme & Protein* 47, 354–369, 1993.
22. Van den Eynde, B.J., and Morel, S., Differential processing of class-1-restricted epitopes by the standard proteome and the immunoproteasome, *Curr. Opin. Immunol.* 13, 147–159, 2001.
23. Besler, M., Kirk, C.J., and Groettrup, M., The immunoproteasome in antigen process and other immunological functions, *Curr. Opin. Immunol.* 26, 74–80, 2013.
24. Miller, Z., Ao, L., Kim, K.B., and Lee, W., Inhibitors of the immunoproteasome: Current status and future directions, *Curr. Pharm. Res.* 19, 4140–4151, 2013.

PROTEIN DISULFIDE ISOMERASE

The protein disulfide isomerase (PDI) family is composed on number of enzymes with varied function.[1] The cananonical function of these enzymes is the oxidative folding of enzymes in the intracellular secretory pathway.[2–4] Protein disulfide isomerase activity was discovered in the early 1960s.[5,6] It should be noted that this observation was part of a body of work for which Anfinsen received the Nobel Prize in Chemistry in 1972; the other winners were Stanford Moore and William Stein. While the initial focus on the PDI family focused on their role in catalyzing the formation of disulfide bonds in proteins, these enzymes are oxidoreductases[7–9] which can catalyze the oxidation of cysteine residues in proteins during folding as well as the reduction of disulfide bonds. Protein disulfide isomerase has also gained importance in biopharmaceutical manufacturing using bacterial systems such as *Escherichia coli* (*E. coli*).[10] Bacterial expression systems such *E. coli* are useful in that there is high level of products but present problems in the lack of glycosylation and the production of proteins in inclusion bodies. The proteins in inclusion bodies needs to be reduced in the presence of chaotropic agents such as guanidine. The reduced proteins need then to be oxidized with the correct formation of disulfide bonds. PDI has been useful in improving the process of the refolding of proteins in the manufacture of biopharmaceutical proteins in bacterial expression systems.[11–16]

Some PDIs (ERp57 and ERp5) are secreted by endothelial cells and platelets and localized to the surfaces of these cells[17] where they can contribute to thrombus formation by catalyzing the allosteric disulfide exchange reaction in proteins such as tissue factor.[18–20] Other work suggest a more complex role for PDIs in thrombosis.[21]

1. Benham A.M., The protein disulfide isomerase family: Key players in health and disease, *Antioxid. Redox. Signal.* 16, 781–789, 2012.
2. Servier, C.S., and Kaiser, C.A., Conservation and diversity of the cellular disulfide bond formation pathways, *Antioxid. Redox Signal.* 8, 797–811, 2006.
3. Bulleid, N.J., and Ellgaard, L., Multiple ways to make disulfides, *Trends Biochem. Sci.* 36, 485–492, 2011.
4. Bechtel, T.J., and Weerapana, E., From structure to redox: The diverse functional roles of disulfides and implications in disease, *Proteomics* 17, 1600391, 2017.
5. Goldberger, R.F., Epstein, C.J., and Anfinsen, C.B., Acceleration of reactivation of reduced bovine pancreatic ribonuclease by a microsomal system from rat liver, *J. Biol. Chem.* 238, 628–635, 1963.
6. Venetianer, P., and Straub, F.B., The enzymic reactivation of reduced ribonuclease, *Biochim. Biophys. Acta* 67, 166–168, 1963.
7. Wang, L., Wang, X., and Wang, C.C., Protein disulfide-isomerase, a foldling catalyst and a redox-regulated chaperone, *Free Radic. Biol. Med.* 83, 305–313, 2015.
8. Trevelin, S.C., and Lopes, L.R., Protein disulfide isomerase and Nox: New partners in redox signaling, *Curr. Pharm. Dex.* 21, 59, 5951–5963, 2015.
9. Soares Moretti, A.I., Martins Laurindo, F.R., Protein disulfide isomerase: Redox connections in and out of the endoplasmic reticulum, *Arch. Biochem. Biophys.* 617, 106–119, 2017.
10. Berlec, A., and Strukelj, B., Current state and recent advances in *Escherichia coli*, yeasts and mammalian cells, *J. Ind. Microbiol. Biotechnol.* 40, 257–274, 2013.
11. Noiva, R., Enzymic catalysis of disulfide formation, *Protein Expr. Purif.* 5, 1–13, 1994.
12. Kang, S.H., Kim, D.M., Kim, H.J., et al., Cell-free production of aggregation-prone proteins in soluble and active forms, *Biotechnol. Prog.* 21, 1412–1419, 2005.
13. Groff, D., Armstrong, S., Rivers, P.J., et al., Engineering toward a bacterial "endoplasmic reticulum" for the rapid expression of immunoglobulin proteins, *MAbs* 6, 671–678, 2014.
14. Mamipour, M., Yousefi, M., and Hasanzadeh, M., An overview on molecular chaperones enhancing solubility of expressed recombinant proteins with correct folding, *Int. J. Biol. Macromol.* 102, 367–375, 2017.
15. Rodriguez, C., Nam, D.H., Kruchowy, E., and Ge, X., Efficient antibody assembly in *E. coli* periplasm by disulfide bond folding factor co-expression and culture optimization, *Appl. Biochem. Biotechnol.* 183, 520–529, 2017.
16. Roth, R., van Zyl, P., Tsekoa, T., et al., Co-expression of sulphydryl oxidase and protein disulfide isomerase in *Escherichia coli* allows for production of soluble CRM$_{197}$, *J. Appl. Microbiol.* 122, 1402–1411, 2017.
17. Flaumenhaft, R., and Furie, B., Vascular thiol isomerases, *Blood* 128, 893–901, 2016.
18. Versteeg, H.H., and Ruf, W., Tissue factor coagulant function is enhanced by protein-disulfide isomerase independent of oxidoreductase activity, *J. Biol. Chem.* 282, 25416–25424, 2007.
19. Chen, V.M., Tissue factor de-encryption, thrombus formation, and thiol-disulfide exchange, *Semin. Thromb, Hemost.* 39, 40–47, 2013,
20. Zelaya, H., Rothmeier, A.S., and Ruf, W., Tissue factor at the crossroad of coagulation and cell signaling, *J. Thromb. Haemost.* 16, 1941–1952, 2018.
21. Essex, D.W., and Wu, Y., Multiple protein disulfide isomerases support thrombosis, *Curr. Opin. Haematol.* 25, 395–402, 2018.

PROTEIN TYROSINE PHOSPHATASES

Protein tyrosine phosphatases (PTPs) are members of a family of hydrolytic enzymes that catalyze the dephosphorylation of protein-bound *O*-tyrosine phosphate.[1,2] The phosphorylation of proteins is one of the most common post-translational modification with reversible medication occurring primarily at serine, threonine, and tyrosine with modification also occurring at histidine and aspartic acid[3] as well as phosphoarginine.[4] The importance of PTPs in the regulation of biological activity has been well documented.[5–12] The PTP family is a diverse group with an 107 genes in *Homo sapiens*.[13] PTPs are subject to redox regulation[14-16] by modification of a cysteine residue at the enzyme active site which is characterized by a low pKa (~5).[17,18] Oxidation of the active site cysteine to cysteine sulfenic acid by hydrogen peroxide results in inactivation which can be reversed by biological thiols providing a basis for redox regulation.[19] However, further oxidation the sulfenic acid or sulfonic acid derivative is essentially irreversible. There is a unique mechanism for preventing further oxidation of is provided by the formation of a sulfenyl-amide at the enzyme active site,[20,21] which is reversed by sulfhydryl compounds. Oxidation can also result in the formation of an internal disulfide bond providing protection.[22] Reflecting their complex role in regulation,[23-25] PTPs are a drug target.[26,27]

1. Pils, B., and Schultz, J., Evolution of the multifunctional protein tyrosine phosphatase family, *Mol. Biol. Evol.* 21, 625–631, 2004.

2. Tonks, N.K., Protein tyrosine phosphatases—from housekeeping enzymes to master regulators of signal transduction, *FEBS J.* 280, 346–278, 2013.

3. Walsh, C.T., Garneau-Tsodikova, S., and Gatto, G.J.,Jr., Protein posttranslational modifications: The chemistry of proteome diversifications, *Angew. Chem. Int. Ed.* 44, 7242–7272, 2005.

4. Ouyang, H., Fu, C., Fu, S., et al., Development of a stable phosphoarginine analogy for producing phosphoarginine antibodies, *Org. Biomol. Chem.* 14, 1925–1929, 2016.

5. Fischer, E.H., Tonks, N.K., Charbonneau, H., et al., Protein tyrosine phosphatases: A novel family of enzymes involved in transmembrane signaling, *Adv. Second Messenger Phosphoprotein Res.* 24, 272–279, 1990.

6. Calya, X., Goris, J., Hermann, J., et al., Phosphotyrosyl phosphatase activity of the polycation-stimulated protein phosphatases and involvement of dephosphorylation in cell cycle regulation, *Adv. Enzyme Reg.* 39, 265–285, 1990.

7. Burridge, K., Sastry, S.K., and Salfee, J.L., Regulation of cell adhesion by protein-tyrosine phosphatases. I. Cell-matrix adhesion, *J. Biol. Chem.* 281, 15593–15596, 2006.

8. Sallee, J.L., Wittchen, E.S., and Burridge, K., Regulation of cell adhesion by protein-tyrosine phosphatases. II. Cell-cell adhesion, *J. Biol. Chem.* 281, 16189–16192, 2006.

9. Fousteri, G., Liossis, S.N., and Battaglia, M., Roles of the protein tyrosine phosphatase PTPN22 in immunity and autoimmunity, *Clin. Immunol.* 149, 556–565, 2013.

10. Dubreuil, V., Sap, J., and Harroch, S., Protein tyrosine phosphatase regulation of stem and progenitor cell biology, *Semin. Cell Dev. Biol.* 37, 82–89, 2015.

11. Ohtake, Y., Saito, A., and LI, S., Diverse functions of protein tyrosine phosphatase in the nervous and immune systems, *Exp. Neurol.* 302, 196–204, 2018.

12. Tonks., N.K., Time to shine the spotlight on the protein tyrosine phosphatase family of signal transducing enzymes, in *Protein Tyrosine Phosphatases in Cancer*, ed. B.G. Neel and N. Tonks, pp. 1–12, Springer Science + Business Media, New York, 2016.

13. Boivin, B., and Tonks, N.K., Analysis of the redox regulation of protein tyrosine phosphatase superfamily members utilizing a cysteine-labeling assay, *Methods Enzymol.* 474, 35–50, 2010.

14. Xu, Y., and Neel, B.G., Redox regulation of PTPs in metabolism: Focus on assays, in *Protein Tyrosine Phosphatases: Control of Metabolism*, ed. K.K. Bence, Chapter 1, pp. 1–26, Springer Science + Business Media, New York, 2013.

15. Griffiths, H.R. Gao, D., Pararasa, C., Redox regulation in metabolic programming and inflammation, *Redox. Biol.* 12, 50–57, 2017.

16. Zhang, Z.Y., and Dixon, J.E., Active site labeling of the *Yersinia* protein tyrosine phosphatase: The determination of the *pKa* of the active site cysteine and the function of the conserved histidine 402, *Biochemistry* 32, 9340–9345, 1993.

17. Pregel, M.M., and Store, A.C., Active site titration of the tyrosine phosphatases SHP-1 and PTP1B using aromatic disulfides. Reaction with the essential cysteine residue in the active site, *J. Biol. Chem.* 272, 23552–23558, 1997.

18. Bhattacharya, S., LaButti, J.N., Seiner, D.R., and Gates, K.S., Oxidative inactivation of protein tyrosine phosphatase 1B by organic hydroperoxides, *Bioorg. Med. Chem. Lett.* 18, 5856–5659, 2008.

19. van Montfort, R.L., Congreve, M., Tisi, D., Carr, R., and Jhoti, H., Oxidation state of the active-site cysteine in protein tyrosine phosphatase 1B, *Nature* 423, 773–777, 2003.

20. Shetty, V., and Neubert, T.A., Characterization of novel oxidation products of cysteine in an active site motif peptide for PTB1B, *J. Am. Soc. Mass Spectrom.* 20, 1540–1548, 2009.

21. Parsons, Z.D., and Gates, K.S., Thiol-dependent recovery of catalytic activity from oxidized protein tyrosine phosphatases, *Biochemistry* 52, 6412–6423, 2013.

22. Mustelin, T., and Taskén, K., Positive and negative regulation of T-cell activation through kinases and phosphatases, *Biochem. J.* 371, 15–27, 2003.

23. Roskoski, R.,Jr., Src kinase regulation by phosphorylation and dephosphorylation, *Biochem. Biophys. Res. Commun.* 331, 1–14, 2005.

24. Tonks, N.K., Time to shine the spotlight on the protein tyrosine phosphatase family of signal transducing enzymes, in *Protein Tyrosine Phosphatases in Cancer*, pp. 1–12, Springer Science + Business Media, New York, 2016.

25. Vidović, D., and Schürer, S.C., Knowledge-based characterization of similarity relationships in the human protein-tyrosine phosphatase family for rational inhibitor design, *J. Med. Chem.* 52, 6649–6659, 2009.
26. Popov, D., Novel protein tyrosine phosphatase 1B inhibitors: Interaction requirements for improved intracellular efficacy in type 2 diabetes mellitus and obesity control, *Biochem. Biophys. Res. Commun.* 410, 377–381, 2011.
27. Stanford, S.M., and Bottini, N., Targeting tyrosine phosphatases: Time to end the stigma, *Trends Pharmacol. Sci.* 38, 524–540, 2017.

PROTEOME

The proteome can be defined as "the entire complement of proteins that is (or can be) expressed by a cell, tissue, or organism."[1] Another way is the total expressed protein content of a genome. The term proteome was advanced in 1995 to describe work on the expressed protein content of *Mycoplasma*.[2] The concept was rapidly adopted[3–9] and while there has been made great progress, challenges remain.[10] The majority of current work focuses on the definition of the proteome of organelles such as mitochondria[11–13] or biological fluids.[14–16] RNA-seq is used to complement canonical proteomic analysis to more fully define genome expression[17] but may overestimate the number of expressed proteins.[18]

1. *Oxford English Dictionary*, Oxford University Press, Oxford, UK, 2018.
2. Wasinger, V.C., Cordwell, S.J., Cerpa-Poljak, A., et al., Progress with gene-product mapping of the Mollicutes: *Mycoplasma genitalium*, *Electrophoresis* 16, 1090–1094, 1995.
3. Kahn, P., From genome to proteome: Looking at a cell's proteins, *Science* 270, 369–370, 1995.
4. Wilkens, M.R., Sanchez, J.C., Gooley, A.A., et al., Progress with proteome projects: Why all proteins expressed by a genome should be identified and how to do it, *Biotechnol. Genet. Eng. Rev.* 13, 19–50, 1996.
5. Figeys, D., Gygi, S.P., Zhang, Y., et al., Electrophoresis combined with novel mass spectrometry techniques: Powerful tools for the analysis of proteins and proteomics, *Electrophoresis* 19, 1811–1818, 1998.
6. Blackstock, W.P., and Weir, M.P., Proteomics: Quantitative and physical mapping of cellular proteins, *Trends Biotechnol.* 17, 121–127, 1999.
7. Bradshaw, R.A., Proteomics—Boom or bust? *Mol. Cell. Proteomics* 1, 177–178, 2002.
8. Bradshaw, R.A., and Burlingame, A.L., From proteins to proteomics, *IUBMB Life* 57, 267–272, 2005.
9. Domon, B., and Aebersold, R., Mass spectrometry and protein analysis, *Science* 312, 212–217, 2006.
10. Segura, V., Garin-Muga, A., Gurueaga, E., and Corrales, F.J., Progress and pitfalls in finding the "missing proteins" from the human proteome map, *Expert Rev. Proteomics* 14, 9–14, 2017.
11. Czarna, M., Kolodziejczak, M., and Janska, H., Mitochondrial proteome studies in seeds during germination, *Proteomics* 4(2), E19, 2016.
12. Wang, Y., Zhand, J., Li, B., and He, Q.Y., Proteomic analysis of mitochondria: Biological and clinical progresses in cancer, *Expert Rev. Proteomics* 14, 891–903, 2017,
13. Go, Y.M., Fernandes, J., Hu, X., Uppal, K., and Jones, D.P., Mitochondrial network responses in oxidative physiology and disease, *Free Radic. Biol. Med.* 166, 31–40, 2018.
14. Kwasnik, A., Tonry, C., Ardle, A.M., et al., Proteomes, their compositions and their sources, *Adv. Exp. Med. Biol.* 919, 3–21, 2016.
15. Csösz, É., Kalló, C., Márkus, B., et al., Quantitative body fluid proteomics in medicine—A focus on minimal invasiveness, *J. Proteomics* 153, 30–43, 2017.
16. Jimenez-Luna, C., Torres, C., Ortiz, R., et al., Proteomics biomarkers in body fluids associated with pancreatic cancer, *Oncotaget* 9, 16573–16587, 2018.
17. Zhao, W., Fitzgibbon, M., Bergan, L., et al., Identifying abundant immunotherapy and other targets in solid tumors; Integrating RNA-seq and mass spectrometry proteomics data sets, *Cancer J.* 23, 108–114, 2017.
18. Tress, M.L., Abascal, F., and Valencia, A., Alternative splicing may not be the key to proteome complexity, *Trends Biochem. Sci.* 42, 98–100, 2017.

PROTEOMETABOLISM

Proteometabolism is the metabolism of the proteome. The term is used only infrequently[1–3] and appears to be equivalent to protein metabolism,[4] although I could not find a statement to that effect.

1. He, M., Zhu, C., Dong, K., et al., Comparative proteome analysis of embryo and endosperm reveals central differential expression proteins involved in wheat seed germination, *BMC Plant Biol.* 15, 97, 2015.
2. Dan, W., Liu. Y.-L., Li, G.-Y., et al., Integrated hepatic transcriptional and serum metabolic studies on circulating nutrient metabolism in diurnal laying hens, *Oncotarget* 8, 113885–113894, 2017.
3. Zhang, D.D., Liu, J.L., Jiang, T.M., et al., Influence of *Kluyveromyces marxianus* on proteins, peptides, and amino acid in *Lactobacillus*-fermented milk, *Food Sci. Biotechnol.* 26, 739–748, 2017.
4. Ren, X.X., Xue, J.Q., Wang, S.L., et al., Proteomic analysis of tree peony (*Paeonia ostii* "Feng Dan") seed germination affected by low temperature, *J. Plant Physiol.* 224–225, 56–67, 2018.

PROTEOMICS

Proteomics is the study of the proteome which is not technology limited. It is the qualitative and quantitative study of the proteome under various conditions, including protein expression, modification, localization, and function, and protein–protein interactions, as a means of understanding biological processes. Proteomics replaced protein chemistry as a term to study proteins.[1]

1. Lundblad, R.L., The Evolution of Protein Chemistry to Proteomics: Basic Science to Clinical Application, CRC Press, Boca Raton, FL, 2006.

PROTO-ONCOGENE (PROTOONCOGENE)

A proto-oncogene is a normal cellular gene, usually associated with regulation, whose activation or modification to an oncogene is linked to malignant transformation (gain of function mutation).[1-4] A protooncogene can also be defined as a progenitor of an oncogene. A proto-oncogene can become an oncogene either by transformation by a virus (retrovirus)[3,5] or by "disturbance" such as chromosomal translocation,[6,7] or point mutation at their location in a chromosome. *c-Myc,* which encodes a transcription factor is one of the most studied of the proto-oncogenes.[7-11]

1. Bishop, J.M., Oncogenes and proto-oncogenes, *J. Cell. Physiol. Suppl.* 4, 1–5, 1986.
2. Bishop, J.M., and Hannfusa, W., Proto-oncogenes in normal and neoplastic cells, in *Scientific American Molecular Oncology,* ed. J.M. Bishop and R.A. Weinberg, Scientific American, New York, Chapter 4, pp. 61–83, 1996.
3. Perantoni, A.O., Cancer-associated genes, in *The Biological Basis of Cancer,* 2nd edn., ed. R.G. MacKinnell, R.E. Parchmont, A.O. Perantoni, S. Damganov, and G.B. Pierce, Chapter 5, pp. 145–154 Cambridge University Press, New York, 2006.
4. Alberts, B., Johnson, A., Lewis, J., Morgan, D., and Raff, M., *Molecular Biology of the Cell,* Chapter 20, Cancer, pp. 1091–1144, Garland Science/Taylor & Francis Group, New York, 2014.
5. Poletti, V., and Mavilio, F., Interactions between retroviruses and the host cell genome, *Mol. Ther. Methods Clin. Dev.* 8, 31–41, 2017.
6. Cory, S., Activation of cellular oncogenes in hemopoietic cells by chromosome translocation, *Adv. Cancer Res.* 47, 189–243, 1986.
7. Timakhov, R.A., Tan, Y., Rao, M., et al., Recurrent chromosomal rearrangements implicate oncogenes contributing to T-cell lymphomagenesis in Lck-MyrAkt2 transgenic mice, *Genes Chromosomes Cancer* 48, 786–794, 2009.
8. Dejure, F.R., and Eilers, M., MYC and tumor metabolism: Chicken and egg, *EMBO J.* 36, 3409–3420, 2017.
9. Schick, M., Harbringer, S., Nilsson, J.A., and Keller, U., Pathogenesis and therapeutic targeting of aberrant MYC expression in haematological cancers, *Br. J. Haematol.* 179, 724–738, 2017.
10. Trop-Steinberg, S., and Azar, Y. Is Myc an important biomarkers? Myc expression in immune disorders and cancer, *Am. J. Med. Sci.* 355, 67–85, 2018.
11. Casey, S.C., Baylot, V., and Felsher, D.W., The MYC oncogenei is a global regulator of the immune response, *Blood* 131, 2007–2015, 2018.

ProtParam

ProtParam is a program which allows the calculation of a number of physical, chemical, and functional properties for a protein from the known amino acid sequence.[1-13]

1. http://www.expasy.ch/tools/protparam.html.
2. Kutty, R.K., Kutty, G., Kambardur, R., et al., Molecular characterization and developmental expression of a retinoid- and fatty acid-binding glycoprotein from *Drosophila.* A putative lipophorin, *J. Biol. Chem.* 271, 20641–20649, 1996.
3. Menhart, N., Mitchell, T., Lusitani, D., Topouzian, N., and Fung, L.W.-M., *J. Biol. Chem.* 271, 30410–30416, 1996.
4. Wallach, T.M., and Segal, A.W., Stoichiometry of the subunits of flavocytochrome b_{558} of the NADPH oxidase of phagocytes, *Biochem. J.* 320, 33–38, 1996.
5. Fontes, W., Sousa, M.V., Aragã, J.B., and Morhy, L., Determination of the amino acid sequence of the plant cytolysin enterolobin, *Arch. Biochem. Biophys.* 347, 201–207, 1997.
6. Rotticci, D., Norin, T., Hult, K., and Martinelle, M., An active-site titration method for lipases, *Biochim. Biophys. Acta* 1483, 132–140, 2000.
7. Bickmore, W.A., and Sutherland, H.G.E., Addressing protein localization within the nucleus, *EMBO J.* 21, 1248–1254, 2002.
8. Bendtsen, J.D., Jensen, L.J., Blom, N., von Heijne, G., and Brunak, S., Feature-based prediction of non-classical and leaderless protein secretion, *Protein. Eng. Des. Select.* 17, 349–256, 2004.
9. Seddigh, S., Comprehensive comparison of two protein family of P-ATPase (13A1 and 13A3) in insects, *Comput. Biol. Chem.* 68, 266–281, 2017.
10. Szerszunowicz, T., Nalecz, D., and Dziuba, M., Selected bioinformatic tools and MS (MALDI-TOF, PMF) techniques used in the strategy for the identification of oat proteins after 2-DE, *Methods Mol. Biol.* 1536, 253–270, 2017.
11. Davishi, F., Zarei, A., and Madzak, C., In silico and in vivo analysis of signal peptides effect on recombinant glucose oxidase production in nonconventional yeast *Yarrowia lipolytica,* *World J. Microbiol. Biotechnol.* 34(9), 128, 2018.

12. Paramanik, V., Krishnan, H., and Kumar Thakur, M., Estrogen receptor α- and β-interacting proteins contain consensus secondary structures: An in silico study, *Ann. Neurosci.* 25, 1–10, 2018.
13. Tu, M., Wang, C., Chen, C., et al., Identification of a novel ACE-inhibitory peptide from casein and evaluation of the inhibitory mechanisms, *Food Chem.* 256, 98–104, 2018.

PROXIMAL PROMOTER REGION

The proximal promoter region is a region located 30–1900 bp upstream from the transcription start site (promoter) and usually contains multiple transcription factor binding sites (*cis*-regulatory elements).[1–7] Proximal promoter regions are also important in the regulation of transcription to yield long, noncoding RNA (lncRNA).[8] There is evidence that transcription also occurs in the proximal promoter regions yielded small interfering RNAs (siRNAs) which can modulate downstream transcription.[9,10]

1. van de Klundert, F.A., Jansen, H.J., and Bloemendal, H., A proximal promoter element in the hamster desmin upstream regulatory region is responsible for activation by myogenic determination factors, *J. Biol. Chem.* 269, 220–225, 1994.
2. Petrovic, N., Black, T.A., Fabian, J.R., et al., Role of proximal promoter elements in regulation of rennin gene transcription, *J. Biol. Chem.* 271, 22499–22505, 1996.
3. Mori, A., Kaminuma, Ogama, K., Okudaira, H., and Akiyama, K., Transcriptional regulation of IL-5 gene by nontransformed human T cells through the proximal promoter element, *Intern. Med.* 39, 618–625, 2000.
4. Ghosh-Choudhury, N., Choudhury, G.G., Harris, M.A., et al., Autoregulation of mouse BMP-2 gene transcription is directed by the proximal promoter element, *Biochem. Biophys. Res. Commun.* 286, 101–108, 2001.
5. Rentsendorj, O., Nagy, A., Sinko, I., et al., Highly conserved proximal promoter element harbouring paired Sox9-binding sites contributes to the tissue- and developmental stage-specific activity of the matrilin-1 gene, *Biochem. J.* 389, 705–716, 2005.
6. Levine, M., Paused RNA polymerase II as a developmental checkpoint, *Cell* 145, 502–511, 2011.
7. Huminiecki, K., and Horbańczuk, J., Can we predict gene expression by understanding proximal promoter architecture? *Trends. Biotechnol.* 35, 530–546, 2017.
8. Alam, T., Medvedeva, Y.A., Jia, H., et al., Promoter analysis reveals globally differential regulation of human long noncoding RNA and protein-coding genes, *PLoS One* 9(10), e109443, 2011.
9. Cinghu, S., Yang, P., Kosak, J.P., et al., Intragenic enhancers attenuate host gene expression, *Mol. Cell* 58, 104–117, 2017.
10. Pande, A., Brosius, J., Makalowska, I., Makalowski, W., and Raabe, C.A., Transcription interference by small transcripts in proximal promoter regions, *Nucleic Acids Res.* 46, 1069–1088, 2018.

PSEUDOGENES

The concept of pseudogene was advanced in 1977 to explain the finding of a defective 5S DNA which could not be transcribed.[1] It was suggested that the most reasonable explanation was gene duplication followed by mutation (unprocessed pseudogenes); however, the possibility of production of a pseudogene by reverse transcription of mRNA (processed pseudogenes) was also mentioned. Several years later, a review discussed processed pseudogenes arising from the reverse transcription of mRNA.[2] Current thinking[3] estimates that there are approximately 14,000 human pseudogenes with approximately 10,500 processed pseudogenes, 3000 unprocessed pseudogenes,[4,5] and 160 unitary pseudogenes.[6]

1. Jacq, C., Miller, J.R., and Brownlee, G.G., A pseudogene structure in 5S DNA of *Xenopus laevis, Cell* 12, 109–120, 1977.
2. Vanin, E.F., Processed pseudogenes: Characteristics and evolution, *Annu. Rev. Genet.* 19, 253–272, 1985.
3. Grandier, D., and Johnsson, P., Pseudogene-expressed RNAs: Emerging roles in gene regulation and disease, *Curr. Topics Microbiol. Immunol.* 394, 111–126, 2016.
4. Mancuso, D.J., Tuley, E.A., Westfield, L.A., et al., Human von Willebrand factor gene and pseudogene: Structural analysis and differentiation by polymerase chain reactins, *Biochemistry* 30, 253–269, 1991.
5. Park, C.S., Lee, H.S., Lee, H.Y., and Krishna, G., An unprocessed pseudogene of inducible nitric oxide synthetase gene in human, *Nitric Oxide* 1, 294–300, 1997.
6. Zhang, Z.D., Frankish, A., Hunt, T., Harrow, J., and Gerstein, M., Identification and analysis of unitary pseudogene: Historic and contemporary gene losses in human and other primates, *Genome Biol.* 11(3), R26, 2010.

PSYCHOGENOMICS

The process of applying the tools of genomics, transcriptomics, and proteomics to understand the molecular basis of behavioral abnormalities.[1–3] There is limited use of the descriptor.

1. Nestler, E.J., Psychogenomics: Opportunities for understanding addiction, *J. Neurosci.* 21, 8324–8327, 2001.
2. Bufe, B., Bresln, P.A.S., Kuhn, C., et al., The molecular basis of individual differences in phenylthiocarbamide and propylthiouracil bitterness perception, *Curr. Biol.* 15, 322–327, 2005.
3. Levy, F., Applications of pharmacogenetics in children with attention-deficit/hyperactivity disorder, *Pharmacogenomics and Personalized Medicine* 7, 349–356, 2014.

PSYCHROPHILIC

Psychrophilic is a term used to describe microorganisms (psychrophiles)[1–13] and describing enzymes which function at less than 20°C. A formal definition is "Of an organism, esp. a bacterium: Capable of growing at temperatures close to freezing; having an optimum growth temperature of less than 20°C."[14]

1. Bolter, M., Ecophysiology of psychrophilic and psychro-tolerant microorganisms, *Cell. Mol. Biol.* 50, 563–573, 2004.
2. Cavicchioli, R., Cold-adapted archaea, *Nat. Rev. Microbiol.* 4, 331–343, 2006.
3. Margesin, R., and Miteva, V., Diversity and ecology of psychrophilic microorganisms, *Res. Microbiol.* 162, 346–361, 2011.
4. Buzzini, P., Branda, E., Goretti, M., and Turchetti, B., Psychrophilic yeasts from worldwide glacial habitats: Diversity, adaptation strategies and biotechnological potential, *FEMS Microbiol. Ecol.* 82, 217–241, 2012.
5. De Maayer, P., Anderson, D., Cary, C., and Cowan, D.A., Some like it cold: Understanding the survival strategies of psychophiles, *EMBO Rep.* 15, 508–517, 2014.
6. Alcaino, J., Cifuentes, V., and Baeza, M., Physiological adaptations of yeasts living in cold environments and their potential applications, *World J. Microbiol. Biotechnol.* 31, 1467–1473, 2015.
7. Feller, G., and Gerday, C., Psychrophilic enzymes: Hot topics in cold adaptation, *Nat. Rev. Microbiol.* 1, 200–208, 2003.
8. Zecchinon, L., Oriol, A., Netzel, U., et al., Stability domains, substrate-induced conformational changes and hinge-bending motions in a psychrophilic phosphoglyc-erate kinase. A microcalorimetric study, *J. Biol. Chem.* 280, 41307–41314, 2005.
9. Feller, G., Protein stability and enzyme activity at extreme biological temperatures, *J. Phys. Condens. Matter* 22, 323101, 2010.
10. Cavicchioli, R., Charlton, T., Ertan, H., et al., Biotechnological uses of enzymes from psychrophiles, *Microbiol. Biotechnol.* 4, 449–460, 2011.
11. Maiangwa, J. Ali, M.S., Salleh, A.B., et al., Adaptational properties and applications of cold-active lipases from psychrophilic bacteria, *Extremophiles* 19, 235–247, 2015.
12. Sarmiento, F., Peralta, R., and Blamey, J.M., Cold and hot extremozymes: Industrial relevance and current trends, *Front. Bioeng. Biotechnol.* 3, 148, 2015.
13. Feller, G., Protein folding at extreme temperature: Current issues, *Semin. Cell Dev. Biol.* 84, 129–137, 2017.
14. *Oxford English Dictionary*, Oxford University Press, Oxford, UK, 2019.

PULL DOWN

Pull down (also pull-down or pulldown) is a term used to describe the process of the capture of a protein, a protein complex, or other macromolecule by binding to an immobilized capture reagent such as an antibody. This process enable the capture of a specific entity as well as the mild isolation of nucleosome components such as chromatin[1–5] including methyl lysine readers (chromatin readers).[6,7] Pull down methodology has also been used to study the interaction of RNA with proteins[8–10] as well as the identification of protein binding small molecules in drug development.[11–14]

1. Kloet, S.L., Baymaz, H.I., Makowski, M., et al., Towards elucidating the stability, dynamics and architecture of the nucleosome remodeling and deacetylase complex by using quantitative interaction proteomics, *FEBS J.* 282, 1774–1785, 2015.
2. Massie, C.E., Methods to identify chromatin-bound protein complexes: From Genome-wide to locus-specific approaches, *Methods Mol. Biol.* 1443, 139–150, 2016.
3. Hermans, N., Huisman, J.J., Brower, T.B., et al., Toehold-enhanced LNA probes for selective pull down and single-molecule analysis of native chromatin, *Sci. Rep.* 7(1), 16721, 2017.
4. Matysiak, J., Lesbats, P., Mauro, E., et al., Modulation of chromatin structure by the FACT histone chaperone complex regulates HIV-1 integration, *Retrovirology* 14(1), 39, 2017.
5. Isogawa, A., Fuchs, R.P., and Fujii, S., Versatile and efficient chromatin pull-down methodology based on DNA triple helix formation, *Sci. Report.* 8(1), 5925, 2018.
6. Vermeulen, M., Identifying chromatin readers using a SILAC-based histone peptide pull-down approach, *Methods Enzymol.* 512, 137–160, 2012.
7. Musselman, C.A., and Kutateladze, T.G., Preparation, biochemical analysis, and structure determination of methyllysine readers, *Methods Enzymol.* 573, 345–362, 2016.
8. Barra, J., and Leucci, E., Probing long noncoding RNA-protein interactions, *Front. Mol. Biosci.* 4, 45, 2017.
9. Bierhoff, H., Analysis of lncRNA-protein interactions by RNA-protein pull-down assays and RNA immunoprecipitation (RIP), *Methods Mol. Biol.* 1686, 241–250, 2018.
10. Cipriano, A., and Ballarino, M., The ever-evolving concept of the gene: The use of RNA/protein experimental techniques to understand genome functions, *Front. Mol. Biosci.* 5, 20, 2018.
11. Lee, H., and Lee, J.W., Target identification for biologically active small molecules using chemical biology approaches, *Arch. Pharm. Res.* 39, 1193–1201, 2016.
12. Yoon, S., and Rossi, J.J., Emerging cancer-specific therapeutic aptamers, *Curr. Opin. Oncol.* 29, 366–374, 2017.
13. Zhu, D., Guo, H., Chang, Y., et al., Cell- and tissue-based proteome profiling and dual imaging of apoptosis markers with probes derived Venetoclax and Idasanutlin, *Angew. Chem. Int. Ed. Engl.* 57, 9284–9289, 2018.
14. Webster, L.A., Thomas, M., Urbaniak, M., et al., Development of chemical proteomics for the foltatome and analysis of the kinetoplastid folateome, *ACS Infect. Dis.* 4, 1475–1483, 2018.

PULSED-FIELD GEL ELECTROPHORESIS

A gel electrophoretic technique for the analysis of very large DNA molecules. It usually uses an agarose gel matrix with alternating current in that the direction of the electric field is changed (or pulsed) periodically for separation.[1–5] The technique continues to see use in diagnostics for the identification of microorganisms.[6–11]

1. Schwartz, D.C., and Cantor, C.R., Separation of yeast chromosome-size DNAs by pulsed field gradient gel electrophoresis, *Cell* 37, 67–75, 1984.
2. Cantor, C.R., Smith, C.L., and Mathew, M.K., Pulsed-field gel electrophoresis of very large DNA molecules, *Ann. Rev. Biophys. Biophys. Chem.* 17, 287–304, 1988.
3. Lat, E., Birren, B.W., Clark, S.M., Simon, M.I., and Hood, L., Pulsed field gel electrophoresis, *Biotechniques* 7, 34–42, 1989.
4. Olson, M.V., Separation of large DNA molecules by pulsed-field gel electrophoresis. A review of the basic phenomenology, *J. Chromatog.* 470, 377–383, 1989.
5. Dukhin, A.S., and Dukhin, S.S., A periodic capillary electrophoresis method using an alternating current electric field for separation of macromolecules, *Electrophoresis* 26, 2149–213, 2005.
6. Miao, J., Chen, L., Wang, J., et al., Current methodologies on genotyping for noscocomial pathogen methicillin-resistant *Staphylococcus aureus* (MSRA), *Microb. Pathog.* 107, 17–28, 2017.
7. Valsdottir, F., Elfarsdottir, J.A., Gudlaugsson, O., and Himarsdottir, I., Long-lasting outbreak due to CTS-M-15-producing *Klebsiella pneumoniae* ST336 in a rehabilitation ward: Report and literature review, *J. Hosp. Infect.* 97, 42–51, 2017.
8. Lee, F., Diagnostics and laboratory role in outbreaks, *Curr. Opin. Infect. Dis.* 30, 419–424, 2017.
9. Abbasi, M., BaseriSalehi, M., Bahador, N., and Taherikalani, M., Antibiotic resistance patterns and virulence determinants of different SCCmec and pulsotypes of *Staphylococcus aureus* isolated from a major hospital in Ilam, Iran, *Open Microbiol. J* 11, 221–223, 2017.
10. Kaushik, A., and Kest, H., Pediatric methicillin-resistant *Staphylococcus aureus* osteoarticular infections, *Microorganisms* 6(2), E40, 2018.
11. Nutman, A., and Marchaim, D., "How to do it"–a molecular investigation of a hospital outbreak, *Clin. Microbiol. Infect.*, in press (doi:10.1016/j.cmi.2018.09.017), 2018.

PULSE RADIOLYSIS

Pulse radiolysis[1,2] uses very short (nanosecond) intense pulses of ionizing radiation to generate transient high concentrations of reactive species such as the hydrated electron, the radical water cation, and hydroxyl radical.[3,4] Pulse radiolysis of water provides hydroxy radicals and hydrated electrons which are useful for modification of proteins,[4–9] nucleic acids,[10–13] and carbohydrates.[14–16]

1. Salmon, G.A., and Sykes, A.G., Pulse radiolysis, *Methods Enzymol.* 227, 522–534, 1993.
2. *Radiation Applications*, ed. H. Kudo, Springer Nature, Singapore, 2018.
3. Ma, J., Wang, F., and Mostafavi, M., Ultrafast chemistry of water radical cation, $H_2O^{•+}$, in aqueous solutions, *Molecules* 23, E244, 2018.
4. Maleknia, S.D., Kieselar, J.G., and Downard, K.M., Hydroxyl radical probe of the surface of lysozyme by synchrotron radiolysis and mass spectrometry, *Rapid Commun. Mass Spectrom.* 16, 53–61, 2002.
5. Bataille, C., Baldacchino, G., Cosson, R.P., et al., Effect of pressure on pulse radiolysis reduction of proteins, *Biochim. Biophys. Acta* 1724, 432–439, 2005.
6. Nakuna, B.N., Sun, G., and Anderson, V.E., Hydroxyl radical oxidation of cytochrome c by aerobic radiolysis, *Free Radic. Biol. Med.* 37, 1203–1213, 2004.
7. Takamoto, K., and Chance, M.R., Radiolytic protein footprinting with mass spectrometry to probe the structure of macromolecular complexes, *Annu. Rev. Biophys. Biomol. Struct.* 35, 151–276, 2006.
8. Houée-Levin, C., and Bobrowski, K., The use of the methods of radiolysis to explore the mechanisms of free radical modifications in proteins, *J. Proteomics* 92, 51–62, 2013.
9. Carroll, L., Pattison, D.I., Davies, J.B., et al., Formation and detection of oxidant-generated tryptophan dimers in peptides and proteins, *Free Radic. Biol. Med.* 113, 132–142, 2017.
10. Kobayashi, K., Evidence of formation of adenine dimer cation radical in DNA: The importance of adenine base stacking, *J. Phys. Chem.* 114, 5600–5604, 2010.
11. Chatgilialoglu, D., D'Angelantonio, M., Kciuk, G., and Bobrowski, K., New insights into the reaction paths of hydroxyl radicals with 2'-deoxyguanosine, *Chem. Res. Toxicol.* 24, 2200–2206, 2011.
12. Hata, K., Urushibara, A., Yamashita, S., et al., Chemical repair activity of free radical scavenger edaravone: Reduction reactions with dGMP hydroxyl radical adducts and suppression of base lesions and AP sites on irradiated plasmid DNA, *J. Radiat. Res.* 56, 59–66, 2015.
13. Ma, J., Marignier, J.L., Pernot, P., et al., Direct observation of the oxidation of DNA bases by phosphate radicals formed under radiation: A model of the backbone-to-base hole transfer, *Phys. Chem. Chem. Phys.* 20, 14927–14937, 2018.
14. Edimecheva, I.P., Kisel, R.M., Shadyro, O.I., et al., Homolytic cleavage of the *O*-glycoside bond in carbohydrates: A steady-state radiolysis study, *J. Radiat. Res.* 46, 319–324, 2005.
15. Ponomarev, A.V., and Ershov, B.G., Radiation-induced high-temperature conversion of cellulose, *Molecules* 19, 16877–16908, 2014.
16. Yamashita, S. Ma, J., Marigneir, J.L., et al., Radiation-induced chemical reactions in hydrogel of hydroxypropyl cellulose (HPC): A pulse radiolysis study, *Radiat. Res.* 186, 650–658, 2016.

QUANTUM DOTS

Quantum dots are fluorescent semiconducting (usually CdSe surrounded by a passivation shell) nanocrystals[1-3] used in the imaging of cells and subcellular particles where quantum dots are considered to have considerable advantage over other fluorescent imaging approaches.[4-6] Quantum dots have also been used in homogeneous immunoassays.[7]

1. *Quantum Dots*, ed. E. Borovitskaya and M.S. Shur, World Publishing, Singapore, 2002.
2. *Nanocrystal Quantum Dots*, ed. V.L. Klimur, CRC Press/Taylor & Francis Group, Boca Raton, FL, 2010.
3. *Self-Assembled Quantum Dots*, ed. Z.M. Wang, Springer, New York, 2018.
4. Lidke, D.S., and Arndt-Jovin, D.J., Imaging takes a quantum leap, *Physiology* 19, 322–325, 2004.
5. Arya, H., Kaul, Z., Wadhwa, R., Taira, K., Hirano, T., and Kaul, S.C., Quantum dots in bio-imaging: Revolution by the small, *Biochem. Biophys. Res. Commun.* 378, 1173–1177, 2005.
6. Bentzen, E.L., Tomlinson, I.D., Mason, J., et al., Surface modification to reduce nonspecific binding of quantum dots in live cell assays, *Bioconjugate Chem.* 16, 1488–1494, 2005.
7. Takkinen, K., and Žvirbliene, A., Recent advances in homogeneous immunoassays based on resonance energy transfer, *Curr. Opin. Biotechnol.* 55, 16–22, 2019.

QUANTUM YIELD

Quantum yield is a measure of the efficiency of fluorescence or similar technique such as phosphorescence. In most applications, quantum yield is the percentage of incident energy emitted after absorption.[1] The higher the quantum yield, the greater the intensity of the fluorescence, luminescence, or phosphorescence. Quantum yield is a metric which has is used to express the effect of quenching on fluorescence[2] with application to the study of protein structure.[3,4] Quantum yield is also used to express the effect of quenching on tryptophan phosphorescence in proteins.[5-7] Quantum yield is also used to characterize the state of chlorophyll in plants.[8]

1. Persico, M., and Granucci, G., *Photochemistry A Modern Theoretical Perspective*, Chapter 1, Introduction to Photochemistry, Springer International Publishing AG, Cham, Switzerland, 2018.
2. Anger, P., Bharadwaj, P., and Novotny, L., Enhancement and quenching of single-molecule fluorescence, *Phys. Rev. Lett.* 96, 113002, 2006.
3. Lehrer, S.S., Solute perturbation of protein fluorescence. The quenching of the tryptophyl fluorescence of model compounds and of lysozyme by iodide ions, *Biochemistry* 10, 3254–3263, 1971.
4. Zelent, B., Bialas, C., Gryczynski, I., et al., Tryptophan fluorescence yields and lifetimes as a probe of conformational changes in human glucokinase, *J. Fluoresc.* 27, 1621–1631, 2017.
5. Berger, J.W., and Vanderkooi, J.M., Characterization of lens α-crystalline tryptophan microenvironments by room temperature phosphorescence spectroscopy, *Biochemistry* 28, 5501–5508, 1989.
6. Eftink, M.R., Ramsay, G.D., Burns, L., et al., Luminescence studies with trp repressor and its single-tryptophan mutants, *Biochemistry* 32, 9189–9198, 1993.
7. Kerwin, B.A., Aoki, K.H., Gonelli, M., and Strambini, G.B., Differentiation of the local structure around tryptophan 51 and 64 in recombinant human erythropoietin by tryptophan phosphorescence, *Photochem. Photobiol.* 84, 1172–1181, 2008.
8. Krasnosky, A.A., and Kovalev, Y.V., Spectral and kinetic parameters of phosphorescence of triple chlorophyll *a* in the photosynthetic apparatus in plants, *Biochemistry* (Moscow) 79, 349–361, 2014.

RAMAN SPECTROSCOPY (ALSO CALLED RAMAN SCATTERING)

Raman spectroscopy is a form of spectroscopy discovered in 1928[1] which measures vibrational modes in molecules. In that sense Raman spectroscopy is similar to infrared spectroscopy which is also based on measurement of vibrational modes in the wavelength range of $\sim 10^6$–10^4 cm^{-1}).[2-4] The emitted signal is weak and has been referred to as feeble fluorescence. A stronger signal is obtained by surface-enhanced Raman spectroscopy (SERS), which uses selected nanostructures to amplify the signal obtained from an analyte adsorbed to a matrix.[4,5] Raman spectroscopy has a distinct advantage over infrared spectroscopy is that Raman spectroscopy can be used for aqueous solutions and can be used for the study of biological macromolecules[6-9] including proteins,[10-15] carbohydrates,[16-18] and nucleic acids.[19-21] The ability to work with analytes in aqueous environments enables the application of Raman spectroscopy to the manufacture and characterization of biopharmaceutics.[22-27] Raman spectroscopy is also used for the analysis of biological tissues and biological fluids.[28-38]

1. Raman, C.V., and Krishnan, K.S., A new type of secondary radiation, *Nature* 121, 501–502, 1928
2. Ferraro, J.R., Nakamoto, K., and Brown, C.W., *Introductory Raman Spectroscopy*, 2nd edn., Academic Press/Elsevier, San Diego, CA, 2003.
3. Vandenabeele, P., *Practical Raman Spectroscopy: An Introduction*, John Wiley & Sons, Chichester, UK, 2013.

4. Prochazka, M., *Surface-Enhanced Raman Spectroscopy Bioanalytical Biomolecular and Medical Applications,* Springer International Publishing AG, Cham, Switzerland, 2016.

5. Stiles, P.L., Dieringer, J.A., Shah, N.C., and Van Duyne, P.V., Surface-enhanced Raman spectroscopy, *Annu. Rev. Anal. Chem.* 1, 601–626, 2008.

6. Warshel, A., Interpretation of resonance Raman spectra of biological molecules, *Annu. Rev. Biophys. Bioeng.* 6, 273–300, 1977.

7. Barron, L.D., Hecht, L., Blanch, E.W., and Bell, A.F., Solution structure and dynamics of biomolecules from Raman optical activity, *Prog. Biophys. Mol. Biol.* 73, 1–49, 2000.

8. Blanch, E.W., Hecht, L., and Barron, L.D., Vibrational Raman optical activity of proteins, nucleic acids, and viruses, *Methods* 29, 196–209, 2003.

9. Harrington, M.J., Wasko, S.S., Masic, C., et al., Pseudoelastic behavior of a natural material is achieved via reversible changes in protein backbone conformation, *J. R. Soc. Interface* 9, 2911–2922, 2012.

10. Kitagawa, T., Investigation of higher order structures of proteins by ultraviolet resonance Raman spectroscopy, *Prog. Biophy. Mol. Biol.* 58, 1–18, 1992.

11. Loehr, T.M., and Sanders-Loehr, J., Techniques for obtaining resonance Raman spectra of metalloproteins, *Methods Enzymol.* 226, 431–470, 1993.

12. Spiro, T.G., and Wasbotten, I.H., CD as a vibrational probe of heme protein active sites, *J. Inorgan. Biochem.* 99, 34–44, 2005.

13. Budhavaram, N.K., and Barone, J.R., Quantifying amino acid and protein substitution by Raman spectroscopy, *J. Raman Spectrosc.* 42, 355–362, 2011.

14. Kurowuski, D., Van Duyne, R.P., and Lednev, I.K., Exploring the structure and formation mechanism of amyloid fibrils by Raman spectroscopy: A review, *Analyst* 140, 4967–4980, 2015.

15. Khan, E., Mishra, S.K., and Kumar, A., Emerging methods for structural analysis of protein aggregation, *Protein Pept. Lett.* 24, 331–339, 2017.

16. Mathlouthi, M., and Koenig, J.L., Vibrational spectra of carbohydrates, *Adv. Carbohydr. Chem. Biochem.* 44, 7–89, 1986.

17. Wiercigroch, E., Szafraniec, E., Czamara, K., et al., Raman and infrared spectroscopy of carbohydrates: A review, *Spectrochim. Acta A Mol. Biomol. Spectrosc.*185, 317–335, 2017.

18. Venuti, V., Rossi, B., Mele, A., et al., Tuning structural parameters for the optimization of drug delivery performance of cyclodextrin-based nanosponges, *Expert Opin. Drug Deliv.* 14, 311–340, 2017.

19. Ghomi, M., Letellier, R., Liquier, J., and Taillandier, E., Interpretation of DNA vibrational spectra by normal coordinate analysis, *Int. J. Biochem.* 22, 691–699, 1990.

20. Benevides, J.M., Overman, S.A., and Thomas, G.J., Jr., Raman, polarized Raman and ultraviolet resonance Raman spectroscopy of nucleic acids and their complexes, *J. Raman Spectrosc.* 36, 279–299, 2005.

21. Garcia-Rico, E., Alvarez-Puebla, R.A., and Guerrini, L., Direct surface-enhanced Raman scattering (SERS) spectroscopy of nucleic acids: From fundamental studies to real-life applications, *Chem. Soc. Rev.* 47, 49009–4923, 2018.

22. De Beer, T.R.M., Allesø, M., Goethals, F., et al., Implementation of a process analytical technology system in a freeze-drying process using Raman spectroscopy for in-line process monitoring, *Anal. Chem.* 79, 7992–8003, 2007.

23. Wen, Z.-Q., Raman spectroscopy of protein pharmaceuticals, *J. Pharmaceut. Sci.* 96, 2861–2878, 2007.

24. McGoverin, C.M., Rades, T., and Gordon, K.C., Recent pharmaceutical applications of Raman and terahertz spectroscopies, *J. Pharmaceut. Sci.* 97, 4598–4621, 2008.

25. Jamieson, L.E., Asiala, S.M., Gracie, K., Faulds, K., and Graham, D., Bioanalytical measurements enabled by Surface-Enhanced Raman Scattering (SERS) probes, *Annu. Rev. Anal. Chem.* 10, 415–537, 2017.

26. Buckley, K., and Ryder, A.G., Applications of Raman spectroscopy manufacturing: A short review, *Appl. Spectrosc.* 71, 1085–1116, 2017.

27. Matthews, T.E., Smelko, J.P., Berry, B., et al., Glucose monitoring and adaptive feeding of mammalian cell culture in the presence of strong autofluorescence by near infrared Raman spectroscopy, *Biotechnol. Prog.* 34, 1574–1580, 2018.

28. Evans, J.W., Zawadzki, R.J., Liu, R., et al., Optical coherence tomography and Raman spectroscopy of the *ex-vivo* retina, *J. Biophotonics* 2, 398–406, 2009.

29. Matousek, P., and Stone, N., Emerging concepts in deep Raman spectroscopy of biological tissue, *Analyst* 134, 1058–1066, 2009.

30. Chan, K.L.A., Zhang, G., Tomic-Canic, M., et al., A coordinated approach to cutaneous wound healing: Vibrational microscopy and molecular biology, *J. Cell Mol. Med.* 12, 2145–2145, 2008.

31. Crane, N.J., Brown, T.S., Evans, K.N., et al., Monitoring the healing of combat wounds using Raman spectroscopic mapping, *Wound Repair Regener.* 18, 409–416, 2010.

32. Flach, C.R., and Moore, D.J., Infrared and Raman imaging of ex vivo skin, *Int. J. Cosmetic Sci.* 35, 125–135, 2013.

33. Mohammed, D., Crowther, J.M., Matts, P.J., Hadgraft, J., and Lane, M.E., Influence of niacinamide containing formulations on the molecular and biophysical properties of the stratum corneum, *Int. J. Pharm.* 441, 192–201, 2013.

34. Bocklitz, T., Bräutigam, K., Urbanek, A., et al., Novel workflow for combining Raman spectroscopy and MALDI-MSI for tissue based studies, *Anal. Bioanal. Chem.* 407, 7865–7873, 2015.

35. Musto, P., Calarco, A., Pannico, M., et al., Hyperspectral Raman imaging of human prostatic cells: An attempt to differentiate normal and malignant cell lines by univariate and multivariate data analysis, *Spectrochim. Acta Part A Mol. Biomol. Spectrosc.* 173, 476–483, 2017.

36. Pielesz, A., Biniaś, D., Sarna, E., et al., Active antioxidants in *ex-vivo* examination of burn wound healing by
means of IR and Raman spectroscopies-Preliminary
comparative research, *Spectrochim. Acta Part A Mol.
Biomol. Spectrosc.* 173, 924–930, 2017.

37. Agarwal, S., Lloyd, W.R., Loder, S.J., et al., Combined
reflectance and Raman spectroscopy to assess degree of
in vivo angiogenesis after tissue injury, *J. Surg. Res.* 209,
174–177, 2017.

38. Bunaciu, A.A., Fleschin, S., Hoang, V.D., and Aboul-
Enein, H.Y., Vibrational spectroscopy in body fluids
analysis, *Crit. Rev. Anal. Chem.* 47, 67–75, 2017.

RANDOMIZATION

An unbiased process by which individual sample or
process units are assigned to an experimental group.
Randomization is used extensively in assigning subjects
in clinical trials.[1–6] Random numbers may also be used
to identify lot numbers in manufacturing. It is difficult
for an individual or group to assignment random numbers. There are internet sites available to generate random numbers and random assignments.[7,8] Mendelian
randomization is a method of statistical analysis that uses
generic variants to make casual inferences about modifi-
able risk factors.[9–11] Mendelian randomization is based on
the Mendel's second law (law of independent association;
law of independent assortment).

1. Katz, M.H., *Study Design and Statistical Analysis
A Practical Guide for Clinicians*, Cambridge University
Press, New York, 2008.

2. Lachin, J.M., Statistical properties of randomization in
clinical trials, *Control. Clin. Trials* 9, 289–311, 1988.

3. Abel, U., and Koch, A., The role of randomization in
clinical trials: Myths and beliefs, *J. Clin. Epidemiol.* 52,
487–497, 1999.

4. Rosenberger, W.F., and Lachin, J.M., *Randomization in
Clinical Trials*, 2nd edn., John Wiley & Sons, Hoboken,
NJ, 2016.

5. Manco-Johnson, M.J., Kempton, C.L., Reding, M.T.,
et al., Randomized, controlled parallel-group trial of routine prophylaxis vs. on-demand treatment with sucrose-
formulated recombinant factor VIII in adults with severe
hemophilia A (SPINART), *J. Thromb. Haemost.* 11,
1119–1127, 2013.

6. Kim, J., and Shin, W., How to do random allocation (randomization), *Clin. Orthop. Surg.* 6, 103–109, 2014.

7. https://www.randomizer.org/.

8. https://www.random.org/lists/.

9. Lawlor, D.A., Harbord, R.M., Sterne, J.A.C., Timpson,
N., and Smith, G.D., Mendelian randomization: Using
genes as instruments for making causal inferences
in epidemiology, *Statistics Medicine* 27, 1133–1163,
2008.

10. Nitsch, D., Molokhia, M., Smeeth, L., et al., Limits to
causal inference based on Mendelian randomization:
A comparison with randomized controlled trials, *Am. J.
Epidemiol.* 163, 397–403, 2006.

11. Zoccali, C., Testa, A., Spoto, B., et al., Mendelian randomization: A new approach to studying epidemiology
in ESRD, *Am. J. Kidney Dis.* 47, 332–341, 2006.

REAL-TIME PCR; REAL-TIME RT-PCR

Real time PCR permits the assay of the rate of amplicon formation during replication in the PCR reaction.[1]
Conventional PCR amplicons are measured either by
size analysis or sequence analysis and while there is
a relation of amplicon number to target number in the
early phases, such a quantitative relationship is lost at
high levels of amplification. Real-time PCR use FRET
with a donor/acceptor pair.[1–11] The use of fluorescence
to measure the synthesis of amplicons permits the measurement of amplification in real time with the use of
appropriate instrumentations. Real-time RT-PCR is an
approach to quantitative use of the reverse transcriptase-
polymerase chain reaction (RT-PCR) to measure messenger RNA and viral pathogen RNA.[12–18] This is an
adaptation of techniques which were based on the use
of fluorescent tags to measure PCR amplicons in real
time and has proved useful for the study of gene expression where real-time RT-PCR is used to "validate" other
approaches to gene expression analysis such as the use of
DNA microarrays.[12–20]

1. Lee, L.G., Connell, C.R., and Bloch, W., Allelic discrimination by nick-translation PCR with fluorogenic probes,
Nucleic Acids Res. 21, 3761–3766, 1993.

2. Mullah, B., Livak, K., Andrus, A., and Kenney, P.,
Efficient synthesis of double dye-label oligodeoxyribo-
nucleotide probes and their application in a real-time
PCR, *Nucleic Acids Res.* 26, 1026–1031, 1998.

3. Edwards, K.J., and Saunders, K.A., Real-time PCR used
to measure stress-induced changes in the expression of
the genes of the aliginate pathway of *Pseudomonas aeruginosa*, *J. Appl. Microbiol.* 91, 29–37, 2001.

4. Brechtbuehl, K., Whalley, S.H., Dusheiko, G.M., and
Saunders, N.A., A rapid real-time quantitative poly-
merase chain reaction for hepatitis B virus, *J. Virol.
Methods* 93, 105–113, 2001.

5. Edwards, K.J., and Saunders, K.A., Real-time PCR used
to measure stress-induced changes in the expression of
the genes of the aliginate pathway of *Pseudomonas aeruginosa*, *J. Appl. Microbiol.* 91, 29–37, 2001.

6. Brechtbuehl, K., Whalley, S.H., Dusheiko, G.M., and
Saunders, N.A., A rapid real-time quantitative poly-
merase chain reaction for hepatitis B virus, *J. Virol.
Methods* 93, 105–113, 2001.

7. Giulietti, A., Overbergh, L., Valckx, D., et al., An overview of real-time quantitative PCR: Applications to quantify cytokine gene expression, *Methods* 25, 386–401, 2001.
8. Mackay, I.M., Arden, K.E., and Nitsche, A., Real-time PCR in virology, *Nucleic Acids Res.* 30, 1292–1305, 2002.
9. Klein, D., Quantification using real-time PCR technology: Applications and limitations, *Trends Mol. Med.* 8, 257–260, 2002.
10. *Real Time PCR. An Essential Guide*, ed. K. Edwards, J. Logan, and N. Saunders, *Horizon Biosciences*, Wymandham, Norfolk, UK, 2004.
11. Bustin, S.A., Benes, V., Nolan, T., and Pfaffi, M.W., Quantitative real-time RT-PCR—A perspective, *J. Mol. Endocrinol.* 34, 597–601, 2005.
12. Bustin, S.A., and Mueller, R., Real-time reverse transcription PRC (qRT-PCR) and its potential use in clinical diagnosis, *Clin. Sci.* 109, 365–379, 2005.
13. Delenda, C., and Gaillard, C., Real-time quantitative PCR for the design of lentiviral vector analytical assays, *Gene Ther.* 12(Suppl 1), S36–S50, 2005.
14. Kubista, M., Andrade, J.M., Bengtsson, M., et al., The real-time polymerase chain reaction, *Mol. Aspects Med.* 27, 95–125, 2006.
15. Kuypers, J., Wright, N., Ferrenberg, J., et al., Comparison of real-time PCR assays with fluorescent-antibody assays for diagnosis of respiratory virus infections in children, *J. Clin. Microbiol.* 44, 2382–2388, 2006.
16. Kozera, B., and Rapacz, M., Reference genes in real-time PCR, *J. Appl. Genet.* 54, 391–406, 2013.
17. Navarro, R., Serano-Heras, G., Castaño, M.J., and Solera, J., Real-time PCR detection chemistry, *Clin. Chim. Acta* 439, 231–250, 2015.
18. Wittwer, C.T., Democratizing the real-time PCR, *Clin. Chem.* 63, 924–925, 2017.
19. Kralik, P., and Ricchi, M., A basic guide to real time PCR in microbial diagnostics: Definitions, parameters, and everything, *Front. Microbiol.* 8, 108, 2017.
20. Wang, Y., Glenn, J.S., Winters, M.A., et al., A new dual-targeting real-time RT-PCR assay for hepatitis D virus RNA detection, *Diagn. Microbiol. Infect. Dis.* 92, 112–117, 2018.

RECEPTOR ACTIVITY MODIFYING PROTEINS (RAMPs)

Receptor activity modifying proteins (RAMPs) are accessory proteins to the function (ligand binding and signaling of G-protein coupled receptors (GPCRs).[1] Receptor activity modifying proteins/peptides (RAMPs) were identified in work to elucidate the functions of a specific GPCR, the calcitonin-receptor-like receptor (CRLR), where RAMP1 was necessary to transport CRLR to the cell surface as a receptor for calcitonin-gene-related peptide.[2] Subsequent work has shown that the CRLR functions as a heterodimer of the class B GPCR calcitonin receptor-like receptor (CLR) and RAMP1[3,4] with RAMP1 modifying the function of CLR by allosteric interaction.[4] While much work has been focused on the receptor for the calcitonin gene-related peptide (CGRP) and other class B GPCRs, there is interest in other GPCRs.[5–17]

1. Routledge, S.J., Ladds, G., and Poyner, D.R., The effects of RAMPs upon cell signalling, *Mol. Cell. Endocrinol.* 449, 12–20, 2017.
2. McLatchie, L.M., Fraser, M.J., Main, M.J., et al., RAMPs regulate the transport and ligand specificity of the calcitonin-receptor-like receptors, *Nature* 393, 333–339, 1998.
3. Simms, J., Uddin, R., Sakmar, T.P., et al., Photoaffinity cross-linking and unnatural amino acid mutagenesis reveal insights into calcitonin gene-related peptide binding to the calcitonin receptor-like receptor/receptor activity-modifying protein 1 (CLR/RAMP1) complex, *Biochemistry* 57, 4915–4922, 2018.
4. Liang, Y.-L., Khoshouer, M., Deganutti, G., et al., Cryo-EM structure of the active, G_s-protein complexed, human CGRP receptor, *Nature* 561, 492–497, 2018.
5. Foord, S.M., and Marshall, F.H., RAMPs: Accessory proteins for seven transmembrane domain receptors, *Trends Pharmacol. Sci.* 20, 184–187, 1999.
6. Sexton, P.M., Abiston, A., Morfis, M., et al., Receptor activity modifying proteins, *Cell Signal.* 13, 73–82, 2001.
7. Fischer, J.A., Muff, R., and Born, W., Functional relevance of G-protein-coupled-receptor-associated proteins, exemplified by receptor-activity-modifying proteins (RAMPs), *Biochem. Soc. Trans.* 30, 455–460, 2002.
8. Morfis, M., Christopolous, A., and Sexton, P.M., RAMPs: 5 years on. Where to now? *Trends Pharmacol. Sci.* 34, 596–601, 2003.
9. Udawela, M., Hay, D.L., and Sexton, P.M., The receptor activity modifying protein family of G protein coupled receptor accessory proteins, *Sem. Cell Dev. Biol.* 15, 299–308, 2004.
10. Young, A., Receptor pharmacology, *Adv. Pharmacol.* 52, 47–65, 2005.
11. Archbold, J.K., Flanagan, J.U., Watkins, H.A., Gingell, J.J., and Hay, D.L., Structural insights into RAMP modification of secretin family G protein-coupled receptors: Implications for drug development, *Trends Pharmacol.* 32, 591–600, 2011.
12. Sexton, P.M., Poyner, D.R, Simms, J., Christopoulos, A., and Hay, D.L., RAMPs as drug targets, *Adv. Exp. Med. Biol.* 744, 61–74, 2012.
13. Bomberger, J.M., Parameswaran, N., and Spielman, W.S., Regulation of GPCR trafficking by RAMPs, *Adv. Exp. Med. Biol.* 744, 25–37, 2012.
14. Klein, K.R., Matson, B.C., and Caron, K.M., The expanding repertoire of receptor activity modifying protein (RAMP) function, *Crit. Rev. Biochem. Mol. Biol.* 51, 65–71, 2016.

15. Hay, D.L., Walker, C.S., Gingell, J.J., et al., Receptor activity-modifying proteins: Multifunctional G protein-coupled receptor accessory proteins, *Biochem. Soc. Trans.* 44, 568–573, 2016.

16. Gingell, J., Simms, J., Barwell, J., et al., An allosteric role for receptor activity-modifying proteins in defining GPCR pharmacology, *Cell Discov.* 2, 16012, 2016.

17. Barbash, G., Lorenzen, E., Persson, T., Huber, T., and Sakmar, T.P., GPCRs globally coevolved with receptor activity-modifying proteins, RAMPs, *Proc. Natl. Acad. Sci. USA* 114, 12015–12020, 2017.

RECEPTOR TYROSINE PROTEIN KINASES

The phosphorylation and dephosphorylation of proteins has evolved into a critical control mechanism in biology has been known for some time since the work of Krebs and Fischer.[1–4] The early work identified serine and threonine as sites of phosphorylation; phosphotyrosine was identified as a site of post-translation modification in 1980.[5] A receptor protein tyrosine kinase was found to be associated with the EGF receptor in 1980[6] and with the insulin receptor in 1983.[7] Subsequent work has shown that there a large number of receptor protein tyrosine kinases classified by the nature of the ligand (e.g. EGF, insulin, PDGF, VEGF).[8,9] There are a number of cytoplasmic protein tyrosine kinases referred to as non-receptor protein tyrosine kinases[10,11] including JAK kinases.[12]

1. Fischer, E.H., and Krebs, E.G., Conversion of phosphorylase b to phosphorylase a in muscle extracts, *J. Biol. Chem.* 216, 121–132, 1955.

2. Fischer, E.H., and Krebs, E.G., Relationship of structure to function of muscle phosphorylase, *Fed. Proc.* 25, 1511–1520, 1966.

3. Fischer, E.H., Cellular regulation by protein phosphorylation, *Biochem. Biophys. Res. Commun.* 430, 865–867, 2013.

4. Thorner, J., Hunter, T., Cantley, L.C., and Sever, R., Signal transduction: From the atomic age to the post-genomic era, *Cold Spring Harb. Perspect. Biol.* 6(12), a022913, 2014.

5. Hunter, T., and Sefton, B.M., Transforming gene product of Rous sarcoma virus phosphorylates tyrosine, *Proc. Natl. Acad. Sci. USA* 77, 1131–1315, 1980.

6. Ushiro, H., and Cohen, S., Identification of phosphotyrosine as a product of epidermal growth factor-activated protein kinase in A-431 cell membranes, *J. Biol. Chem.* 255, 8363–8365, 1980.

7. Kasuga, M., Fujita-Yamaguchi, Y., Blithe, D.L., and Kahn, C.R., Tyrosine-specific protein kinase activity is associated with the purified insulin receptor, *Proc. Natl. Acad. Sci. USA* 80, 2137–2141, 1983.

8. *Receptor Tyrosine Kinases: Family and Subfamilies*, ed. D.L. Wheeler and Y. Yarden, Humana/Springer International Publishing AG, Cham, Switzerland, 2015.

9. Alberts, B., Johnson, A., Lewis, J., Morgan, D., and Raff. Roberts, P., and Walter, P., *Molecular Biology of the Cell.*, Garland Science/Taylor & Francis Group, New York, 2015.

10. Tsygankov, A.Y., Non-receptor protein kinases, *Front. Biosci.* 8, s595–s635, 2003.

11. Gocek, E., Non-receptor protein tyrosine kinases signaling pathways in normal and cancer cells, *Crit. Rev. Clin. Lab. Sci.* 51, 125–137, 2014.

12. Hubbard, S.R., Mechanistic insights into regulation of JAK2 tyrosine kinase, *Front. Endocrinol.* 8, 361, 2018.

RECEPTOR-ACTIVATOR OF NF-κB (RANK) AND RECEPTOR-ACTIVATOR OF NF-κB LIGAND (RANKL)

Receptor-activator of NF-κB (RANK) and receptor-activator of NF-κB ligand (RANKL)[1] are both membrane proteins which were described as members of the TNF family factors critical for osteoclast differentiation (osteoclastogenesis).[2,3] RANK is a trimeric membrane protein which associates with TNF-associated factor (TRAF) on binding of RANKL resulting in activation of Nf-κB and certain MAP kinases. RANKL (OPGL, osteoprotegerin ligand; TRANCE, TNF-related activation-induced cytokine) is found as membrane protein on a number of cells and function either as membrane-bound or is a soluble form released by proteolysis (matrix membrane proteases).[1] Osteoprotegerin (OPG) functions to regulate the RANK/RANKL system by competing with RANKL for binding to RANK and thus inhibiting of osteoclastogenesis.[4–6] RANKL is a therapeutic target for a monoclonal antibody, denusomab in the treatment of osteoporosis[7] and in multiple myeloma.[8] Although most interest in RANK/RANKL has focused on bone, this system is of importance in the immune system[8–11] and the female reproductive system.[12]

1. Nakashima, T., and Takayanagi, H., RANK and RANKL family members, in *Encyclopedia of signaling methods,* ed. S. Choi, Springer Science and Business, New York, 2012.

2. Suda, T., Takahashi, N., Udagawa, N., et al., Modulation of osteoclast differentiation and function by new members of the tumor necrosis factor, *Endocrine Rev.* 20, 345–357, 1999.

3. Takahashi, N., Udagawa, N., and Suda, T., A new member of the tumor necrosis family, OPG/OPGL/TRANCE/RANKL regulates osteoclast differentiation and function, *Biochem. Biophys. Res. Commun* 256, 449–455, 1999.

4. Yasuda, H., Shima, H., Nakagawa, N., et al., Identity of osteoclastognesis inhibitory factor (OCIF) and osteoprotegerin (OPG): A mechanism by which OPG/OCIF inhibits osteoclastogenesis *in vitro*, Endocrinology 139, 1329–1237, 1998.

5. Khosla, S., The OPG/RANKL/RANK system, *Endocrinology* 142, 5050–5055, 2001.

6. Theoleyre, S., Wittrant, Y., Tat, S.K., et al., The molecular triad OPG/RANK/RANKL: Involvement in the orchestration of pathophysiological bone remodeling, *Cytokine & Growth Factor Rev.* 15, 457–475, 2004.

7. Deeks, E.D., Denosumab: A review in postmenopausal osteoporosis, *Drugs Aging* 35, 163–173, 2018.

8. Raje, N.S., Bhatta, S., and Terpos, E., Role of the RANK/RANKL pathway in multiple myeloma, *Clin. Cancer Res.* 25, 12–20, 2019.

9. Weitzmann, M.N., Bone and the immune system, *Toxicol. Pathol.* 45, 911–934, 2017.

10. Totsuka, T., Kanai, T., Nemoto, Y., et al., RANK/RANKL signalling pathways182m 65 is critically involved in the function of CD4+CD25+ regulatory T cells in chronic colitis, *I. Immunol.* 182, 6079–6087, 2009.

11. Ahem, E., Smyth, M.J., Dougall, W.C., and Terry, M.W.L., Role of the RANKL-RANK axis is antitumor immunity—Implications for therapy, *Nat. Rev. Clin. Oncol.* 15, 676–693, 2018.

12. Meng, Y.H., Zhou, W.J., Jin, L.P., et al., RANKL-mediated harmonious dialogue between fetus and mother guarantees smooth gestation by inducing decidual M2 macrophage polarization, *Cell Death Dis.* 8(10), e3105, 2017.

RECEPTORS FOR ADVANCED GLYCATION END PRODUCTS (AGE) (RAGE)

RAGE are cell-surface receptors for advanced glycation end products (AGEs) as well as other ligands.[1,2] RAGE are members of the immunoglobulin superfamily of receptors[3,4] and are considered to be pattern-recognition receptors.[5–7] Most work on RAGE has focused on its role in inflammation.[8–12] The presence of AGE in processed animal feed is thought to be responsible for increased inflammation in the gut with a negative effect on the immune response necessitating the use of antibiotics.[13] The importance of RAGE in the inflammatory response is important for a variety of pathologies including diabetes[14–16] and Alzheimer's disease and other neurological disorders.[17–19] RAGE receptors are described as multi-ligand receptors[20,21] which can be activated by other ligands such polyphosphate[22] and S100 proteins.[23–25]

1. Schmidt, A.M., and Stern, D.M., Receptor for AGE (RAGE) is a gene within the major histocompatibility class III region: Implications for host response mechanisms in homeostasis and chronic disease, *Front. Biosci.* 6, D1151–D1160, 2001.

2. Bucciarelli, L.G., Wendt, T., Rong, L., et al., RAGE is a multiligand receptor of the immunoglobulin superfamily: Implications for homeostasis and chronic disease, *Cell. Mol. Life. Sci.* 59, 1117–1128, 2002.

3. Williams, A.F., and Barclay, A.N., The immunoglobulin superfamily-domains for cell surface recognition, *Annu. Rev. Immunol.* 6, 381–405, 1988.

4. Schmidt, A.M., Hori, O., Cao, R., et al., A novel cellular receptor for advanced glycation end products, *Diabetes* 45(Suppl 3), S77–S80, 1996.

5. Xie, J., Reverdatto, S., Frolov, A., et al., Structural basis for pattern recognition by the receptor for advanced glycation end products (RAGE), *J. Biol. Chem.* 283, 27255–27268, 2008.

6. Kawai, T., and Akira, S., The role of pattern-recognition receptors in innate immunity: Update on Toll-like receptors, *Nat. Immunol.* 11, 373–384, 2010.

7. Kato, J., Agalave, N.M., and Svensson, C.I., Pattern recognition receptors in chronic pain: Mechanisms and therapeutic implications, *Eur. J. Pharmacol.* 788, 261–273, 2016.

8. Yan, S.F., Ramasamy, R., Naka, Y., and Schmidt, A.M., Glycation, inflammation, and RAGE. A scaffold for the macrovascular complications of diabetes and beyond, *Circ. Res.* 93, 1159–1169, 2003.

9. Ramasamy, R., Vannucci, S.J., Yan, S.S., Herold, K., San, S.F., and Schmidt, A.M., Advanced glycation end products and RAGE: A common thread in aging, diabetes, neurodegeneration, and inflammation, *Glycobiology* 15, 16R–28R, 2005.

10. Kierdorf, K., and Frit, G., RAGE regulation and signaling in inflammation and beyond, *J. Leukoc. Biol.* 94, 55–68, 2013.

11. Byun, K., Yoo, Y., Son, M., et al., Advanced glycation end-products produced systemically and by macrophages: A common contributor to inflammation and degenerative diseases, *Pharmacol. Ther.* 177, 44–55, 2017.

12. Palanissami, G., and Paul, S.F.D., RAGE and its ligands: Molecular interplay between glycation, inflammation, and hallmarks of cancer—a review, *Horm. Cancer* 9, 295–325, 2018.

13. Teodorowicz, M., Hendriks, W.H., Wichers, H.J., and Savelkoul, H.F.J., Immunomodulation by processed animal feed: The role of Maillard reaction products and advanced glycation end-products (AGEs), *Front. Immunol.* 9, 2088, 2018.

14. Bierhaus, A., Humpert, P.M., Stern, D.M., Arnold, B., and Nawroth, P.P., Advanced glycation end product receptor-mediated cellular dysfunction, *Ann. N.Y. Acad. Sci.* 1043, 676–680, 2005.

15. Jensen, L.J., Ostergaard, J., and Flyvbjerg, A., AGE-RAGE and AGE cross-link interaction: Important players in the pathogenesis of diabetic kidney disease, *Horm. Metab. Res.* 37(Suppl. 1), 26–34, 2005.

16. Chiu, C.J., Rabbani, N., Rowan, S., et al., Studies of advanced glycation end products and oxidation biomarkers for type 2 diabetes, *Biofactors* 44, 281–288, 2018.

17. Cai, Z., Liu, N., Wang, C., et al., Role of RAGE in Alzheimer's disease, *Cell. Mol. Neurobiol.* 36, 483–495, 2016.

18. Ramasamy, R., Shekhtman, A., and Schmdt, A.M., The multiple faces RAGE—opportunities for therapeutic intervention in aging and chronic disease, *Expert Opin. Ther. Targets* 20, 431–446, 2016.

19. Ray, R., Juranek, J.K., and Rai, V., RAGE axis in neuroinflammation, neurodegeneration and its emerging role in the pathogenesis of amyotrophic lateral sclerosis, *Neurosci. Biobehav. Rev.* 62, 48–55, 2016.

20. Koch., M., Chitayat, S., Dattilo, B.M., et al., Structural basis for ligand recognition and activation of RAGE, *Structure* 18, 1342–1352, 2010.

21. Fritz, G., RAGE: A single receptor fits multiple ligands, *Trends. Biochem. Sci.* 36, 625–632, 2011.

22. Hassanian, S.M., Avan, A., and Ardesshirylajimi, A., Inorganic polyphosphoate: A key modulator of inflammation, *J. Thromb. Haemost.* 15, 213–218, 2017.

23. Leclerc, E., Fritz, G., Vetter, S.W., and Heizmann, C.W., Binding of S100 proteins to RAGE: An update, *Biochim. Biophys. Acta* 1793, 993–1007, 2009.

24. Pruenster, M., Vogl, T., Roth, J., and Sperandio, M., S100A8/A9: From basic science to clinical application, *Pharmacol. Ther.* 167, 120–131, 2016.

25. Ma, L., Sun, P., Zhang, J.C., Zhang, Q., and Yao, S.L., Proinflammatory effects of S100A8/A9 via TLR3 and RAGE signaling pathways in BV-2 microglial cells, *Int. J. Mol. Med.* 40, 31–38, 2017.

RECEPTOROME

That portion of the proteome that function via ligand recognition at the cell surface (receptors).[1-3] There is particular interest in the G-protein-coupled receptor receptorome (GPCRome).[1,4-8]

1. Kroeze, W.K., Sheffler, D.J., and Roth, B.L., G-protein-coupled receptors at a glance, *J. Cell Sci.* 115, 4868–4869, 2003.

2. Armbruster, B.N., and Roth, B.L., Mining the receptorome, *J. Biol. Chem.* 280, 5129–5132, 2005.

3. Roth, B.L., Receptor systems: Will mining the receptorome yield novel targets for pharmacotherapy, *Pharmacol. Ther.* 108, 59–64, 2005.

4. Amisten, S., Salehi, A., Rorsman, P., Jones, P.M., and Persaud, S.J., An atlas and functional analysis of G-protein coupled receptors in human islets of Langerhans, *Pharmcol. Ther.* 139, 359–391, 2013.

5. Amisten, S., Neville, M., Hawkes, R., et al., An atlas of G-protein coupled receptor expression and function in human subcutaneous adipose tissues, *Pharmacol. Ther.* 146, 61–93, 2015.

6. Amisten, S., Quantification of the mRNA expression of G protein-coupled receptors in human adipose tissue, *Methods Cell Biol.* 132, 73–105, 2016.

7. Kroeze, W.K., Sassano, M.F., Huang, X.P., et al., PRESTO-Tango as an open-source resource for interrogation of the druggable human GPCRome, *Nat. Struct. Mol. Biol.* 22, 362–369, 2015.

8. Hahnel, S., Wheeler, N., Lu, Z., et al., Tissue-specific transcriptome analyses provide new insights into GPCR signalling in adult *Schistosoma mansoni*, *PLoS Pathog.* 14(1), e1006718, 2018.

RECEPTOSOME

The receptosome is a cytoplasmic organelle resulting from the endocytosis of receptor-ligand complexes.[1-4] The term receptosome is not extensively used and there appears to be an overlap in the use of the terms receptosome, phagosome, and endosome. However, the use of the term receptosome seems to imply the occurrence of processing events in the recepotosome after internationalization.[5,6]

1. Willingham, M.C., and Pastan, I., The receptosome: An intermediate organelle of receptor-mediated endocytosis in cultured fibroblasts, *Cell* 21, 67–77, 1980.

2. Pastan, I.L., and Willingham, M.C., Journal of the center of the cell: Role of the receptosome, *Science* 214, 504–509, 1981.

3. Chitambar, C.R., and Zivkovic-Gilgenbach, Z., Role of the acidic receptosome in the uptake and retention of 67 Ga by human leukemic HL60 cells, *Cancer Res.* 50, 1484–1487, 1990.

4. Navarte, I., Schwend, T., and Gustafson, J.-A., Proteomics analysis of the estrogen receptor α receptosome, *Mol. Cell. Proteomics* 9, 1411–1422, 2010.

5. Fritsch, J., Zingler, P., Särchen, V., et al., Role of ubiquitination and proteolysis in the regulation of prp- and anti-apoptotic TNF-R1 siginaling, *Biochim. Biophys. Acta Mol. Cell Res.* 1864, 2139–2146, 2017.

6. Stephan, M., Edelmann, B., Winoto-Morbach, S., et al., Role of caspases in CD95-induced biphasic activation of acid sphingomyelinase, *Oncotarget* 8, 20067–20085, 2017.

REFRACTIVE INDEX (INDEX OF REFRACTION)

The refractive index can also be defined as "the ratio of the velocity of light (or other electromagnetic radiation) in a standard medium (usually air or a vacuum) to its velocity in a specified medium, or (equivalently), the ratio between the sines of the angles of incidence and refraction of a ray of light passing from a standard medium into the specified medium."[1] The refractive index of a solution is dependent on temperature, wavelength of the incident light, and concentration of solute. Refractive index measurements are also of value in the characterization of solids.[2] The refractive index measurement has a long history of use in the determination of protein concentration.[3,4] Protein conformation influences refractive index measurements.[5,6] The refractive index of a solution of lysozyme was observed to increase on proteolysis by pepsin.[7] There is extensive use of refractometry to measure protein concentration in veterinary medicine reflecting the availability of portable instrumentation.[8,9] Changes in the refractive index of solutions have been used to measure solute concentration in techniques such as analytical ultracentrifugation[10] and the chromatography of carbohydrates.[11] Techniques based on refractive index have been used to study cells and tissues.[12–15] The principle of refractive index measurements provides the basis for surface plasmon resonance.[16–18] More recently, refractive index has provided the based for measurement of macromolecules on surfaces.

1. *Oxford English Dictionary*, Oxford University Press, Oxford, UK, 2018.
2. Batsanov, S.S., Ruchkin, E.D., and Poroshina, I.A., *Refractive indices of solids*, Springer Nature, Singapore, 2016.
3. Barer, R., and Tkaczyk, S., Refractive index of concentrated protein solutions, *Nature* 173, 821–822, 1954.
4. Anderle, H., and Weber, A., Rediscovery and revival of analytical refractometry for protein determination: Recombining simplicity with accuracy in the digital era, *J. Pharm. Sci.* 105, 1097–1103, 2016.
5. Bornhop, D.J., Kammer, M.N., Kussrow, A., Flowers, R.A., 2nd, and Meiler, J., Origin and prediction of free-solution interaction studies performed label-free, *Proc. Natl. Acad. Sci. USA* 113, E1595–E1604, 2016.
6. Khago, D., Bierma, J.C., Roskamp, K.W., Kozyuk, N., and Martin, R.W., Protein refractive index increment is determined by conformation as well as composition, *J. Phys. Condens. Matter* 30(43), 435101, 2018.
7. Sarimov, R.M., Matveyeva, T.A., and Binhi, V.N., Laser interferometry of the hydrolytic changes in protein solutions: The refractive index and hydration shells, *J. Biol. Phys.* 44, 345–360, 2018.
8. Gupta, S., and Stockham, S.L., Refractometric total protein concentration in icteric serum from dogs, *J. Am. Vet. Med. Assoc.* 244, 63–67, 2014.
9. Buczinski, S., and Vandeweerd, J.M., Diagnostic accuracy of refractometry for assessing bovine colostrum quality: A systematic review and meta-analysis, *J. Dairy Sci.* 99, 7381–7394, 2016.
10. Brautigam, C.A., Padrick, S.B., and Sohuck, P., Multi-signal sedimentation velocity analysis with mass conservation for determining the stoichiometry of protein complexes, *PLoS One* 8(5), e62694, 2013.
11. Cheong, K.L., Wu, D.T., Zhao, J., and Li, S.P., A rapid and accurate method for the quantitative estimation of natural polysaccharides and their fractions using high-performance size exclusion chromatography coupled with multi-angle laser light scattering and refractive index detector, *J. Chromatog. A* 1400, 98–106, 2015.
12. Tearney, G.J., Brezinski, M.E., Southern, J.F., et al., Determination of the refractive index of highly scattering human tissue by optical coherence tomography, *Optics Letters* 20, 2258–2260, 1995.
13. Tainaka, K., Kuno, A., Kubota, S.I., Murakami, T., and Ueda, H.R., Chemical principles in tissue clearing and staining protocols for whole-body cell profiling, *Annu. Rev. Cell Dev. Biol.* 32, 713–741, 2016.
14. Goth, W., Lesicko, J., Sacks, M.S., and Tunnell, J.W., Optical-based analysis of soft tissue structures, *Annu. Rev. Biomed. Eng.* 18, 357–385, 2016.
15. Boothe, T., Hilbert, L., Heide, M., et al., A tunable refractive index matching medium for live imaging cells, tissues and model organisms, *Elife* 6, e27240, 2017.
16. Stenberg, E., Persson, B., Roos, H., and Urbaniczky, C., Quantitative determination of surface concentration of protein with surface plasmon resonance using radiolabeled proteins, *J. Colloid Interface Sci.* 143, 513–526, 1991.
17. Patching, S.G., Surface plasmon resonance spectroscopy for characterization of membrane protein-ligand interactions and its potential for drug discovery, *Biochim. Biophys. Acta* 1838, 43–55, 2015.
18. *Handbook of Surface Plasmon Resonance*, ed. R.B.M. Schasfoort, Royal Society of Chemistry, Cambridge, UK, 2017.

REGULATORS OF G PROTEIN SIGNALING (RGS)

The binding of ligand to G protein coupled receptors (GPCRs) results in the activation of G proteins. The activation of a G protein which is a trimer involves the replacement of GDP with GRP in the Gα subunit with the concomitant dissociation of the G$\beta\gamma$ heterodimer. Both the α subunit with bound GTP and the $\beta\gamma$ heterodimer are active and will remain active as long as the GTP is bound to the Gα subunit. Hydrolysis of the bound GTP in the Gα subunit results in loss of activity and reformation of the G protein trimer. While the Gα subunit has intrinsic GTPase activity, such activity is not sufficient and require RGS proteins to enhance the rate of hydrolysis of GTP acting as a GTPase-activating protein (GAP).[1–3] Thus, RGS proteins are considered to be inhibitors of GPCR signaling. It also becoming apparent that RGS proteins have other functions than negative regulation of GPCR signaling.[3,4] The RGS proteins are characterized by the presence of a sequence (RGS sequence) responsible for binding to the Gα subunit.[5] A similar regulatory system exists in plants with some significant differences.[6,7]

1. Woodard, G.E., Jardin, I., Berna-Erro, A., Salido, G.M., and Rosado, J.A., Regulators of G-protein-signaling proteins: Negative modulators of G-protein coupled receptor signaling, *Int. Rev. Cell Mol. Biol.* 317, 97–183, 2015.
2. Jules, J., Yang, S., Chen, W., and Li, Y.-P., Role of regulators of G protein signaling proteins in bone physiology and pathophysiology, *Prog. Mol. Biol. Transl. Sci.* 133, 47–75, 2015.
3. Sjögren, B., The evolution of regulators of G protein signalling proteins as drug targets—20 years in the making: IUPHAR review 21, *Brit. J. Pharmacol.* 174, 427–437, 2017.

4. Sethakorn, N., Yau, D.M., and Dulin, N.O., Non-canonical functions of RGS proteins, *Cell Signal.* 22, 1274–1281, 2010.

5. Tesmer, J.J., Structure and function of regulator of G protein signaling homology domains, *Prog. Mol. Biol. Transl. Sci.* 86, 75–113, 2009.

6. Pandey, S., Heterotrimeric G-protein regulatory circuits in plants: Conserved and novel mechanisms, *Plant Signal. Behavior* 12, e1325983, 2017.

7. Hackenberg, D., McKain, M.R, Lee, S.G., et al., Gα and regulator of G-protein signaling (RGS) protein pairs maintain functional compatibility and conserved interaction interfaces throughout evolution despite frequent loss of RGS proteins in plants, *New Phytol.* 216, 562–575, 2017.

REGULATORY TRANSCRIPTION FACTOR (TRANSCRIPTIONAL REGULATORS)

A regulatory transcription factor (transcriptional regulator) is a protein or protein complex, which interacts with a *cis*-regulatory region (*cis*-regulatory sequence) on a gene (usually in the major groove of the DNA) to enhance or suppress the rate of transcription. A regulatory transcription factor is not considered a part of the basal transcription apparatus as is a general transcription factor such as TFIID (TFII, transcription factor for polymerase II, the assignment of letter D is arbitrary).[1] A regulatory transcription factor is specific for a gene product and is usually defined as directly related to that gene product as is in inferno regulatory factor-1 (IRF-1).[2,3] The are now nine members of the interferon regulatory family influencing various tissues.[4] The Myc family of transcriptional factors are likely the most important regulatory transcription factors best known as product of *Myc* oncogenes. Myc regulatory transcriptional factors are important in normal function[5–8] but are best known as the product of the *c-Myc* protooncogene and its role in oncognesis.[5–11] c-Myc has molecular weight of 48 kDa and functions as a heterodimer with MAX.[12]

1. Bieniossek, C., Papai, G., Schaffitzel, G., et al., The architecture of human general transcription factor TFIID core complex, *Nature* 493, 699–702, 2013.

2. Miyamoto, M., Fujita, T., Kimura, Y., et al., Regulated expression of a gene encoding a nuclear factor, IRF-1, that specifically binds to IFN-β gene regulatory elements, *Cell* 54, 903–913, 1988.

3. Fujita, T., Kimura, Y., Miyamoto, N., Barsoumian, E.L., and Taniguchi, T., Induction of endogenous IFN-α and IFN-β genes by a regulatory transcription factor, IRF-1, *Nature* 337, 270–272, 1989.

4. Tamura, T., Yanai, H., Savitsky, D., and Taniguchi, T., The IRF family Transcription factors in immunity and oncogenesis, *Annu. Rev. Immunol.* 26, 535–584, 2008.

5. Trumpp, A., Rrefaeli, Y., Oskarsson, T., et al., c-Myc regulates mammalian body size by controlling cell number but not cell size, *Nature* 414, 768–773, 2001.

6. Khattar, E., and Tergaonkar, V., Transcriptional regulation of telomerase reverse transcriptase (TERT) by MYC, *Front. Cell Devel. Biol.* 5, 1, 2017.

7. Casey, S.C., Baylot, V., and Felsher, D.W., MYC: Master regulator of immune privilege, *Trends Immunol.* 38, 298–305, 2017.

8. Casey, S.C., Baylot, V., and Felsher, S.W., The MYC oncogene is a global regulator of the immune response, *Blood* 131, 2007–2015, 2018.

9. Dang, C.V., MYC on the path to cancer, *Cell* 149, 22–35, 2012.

10. Dejure, F.R., and Eilers, M., MYC and tumor metabolism: Chicken and egg, *EMBO J.* 36, 3409–3420, 2017.

11. Kalkat, M., De Melo, J., Hickman, K.A., et al., MYC deregulation in primary human cancers, *Genes* (Basel) 8(6), E151, 2017.

12. Wechsler, D.S., and Dang, C.V., Opposite orientation of DNA bending by c-Myc and Max, *Proc. Natl. Acad. Sci. USA* 89, 7635–7639, 1992.

RESURRECTION PLANTS

Resurrection plants usually found in arid regions which adopt a compact shape during water deprivation and changes shape upon rehydration.[1–7] Resurrection plants are described as desiccation-resistant plants which can survive cellular water content below 10% while drought-resistant plants can survive unless water content drops below 60%.[7] **Trehalose**, an unusual disaccharide, accumulates in resurrection plants and is thought to be association with desiccation resistance as an osmoprotectant.[8,9] Octulose is also seen in resurrection plants; however, it is not clear that octulose has a function such as described for trehalose.[10] Trehalose has received considerable interest as a protective excipient in the processing of biopharmaceutical products.[11–14] There is also interest in using trehalose as a therapeutic.[15]

1. Kranner, I., Beckett, R.P., Wornik, S., Zorn, M., Preifhofer, H.W., Revival of a resurrection plant correlates with its antioxidant status, *Plant J.* 31, 13–24, 2002.

2. Schluepmann, H., Pellny, T., van Dijken, A., Smeeken, S., and Paul, M., Trehalose 6-phosphate is indispensable for carbohydrate utilization and growth in *Arabidopsis thaliana*, *Proc. Natl. Acad. Sci. USA* 100, 6849–6854, 2003.

3. Jones, L., and McQueen-Mason, S., *FEBS Lett.* 559, 61–65, 2004.

4. Helseth, L.E., and Fischer, T.M., Physical mechanisms of rehydration in *Polypodium polypodioides*, a resurrection plant, *Phys. Rev. E. Stat. Nonlin. Soft Matter. Phys.* 71(6 Pt 1):061903, epub, 2005.

5. Challabathula, D., Puthur, J.T., and Bartels, D., Surviving metabolic arrest: Photosynthesis during desiccation and rehydration in resurrection plants, *Ann. N.Y. Acad. Sci.* 365, 89–99, 2016.

6. Bechtold, U., Plant life in extreme environments: How do you improve drought tolerance? *Front. Plant Sci.* 9, 543, 2018.

7. Callabathula, D., Zhang, Q., and Bartels, D., Protection of photosynthesis in desiccation-tolerant resurrection plants, *J. Plant Physiol.* 227, 84–92, 2018.

8. Avonce, N., Leyman, B., Thevelein, J., and Iturriaga, G., Trehalose metabolism and glucose sensing in plants, *Biochem. Soc. Trans.* 33, 276–279, 2005.

9. Williams, B., Njaci, I., Mogaddam, L., et al., Trehalose accumulation triggers autophagy during plant desiccation, *PLoS Genet.* 11(12), 310005705, 2015.

10. Zhang, Q., and Bartels, D., Octulose: A forgotten metabolite? *J. Exp. Bot.* 68, 5689–5694, 2017.

11. Bragg, J.T., D'Ambrosio, H.K., Smith, T.J., et al., Esterified trehalose analogues protect mammalian cells from heat shock, *ChemBioChem* 18, 1863–1870, 2017.

12. Kanojia, G., Ten Have, R., Brugmans, D., et al., The effect of formulation on spray dried Sabin inactivated polio vaccine, *Eur. J. Pharm. Biopharm.* 129, 21–29, 2018.

13. Yang, X., Hui, Q., Yu, B., et al., Design and evaluation of lyophilized fibroblast growth factor 21 and its protection against ischemia cerebral injury, *Bioconjug. Chem.* 29, 287–295, 2018.

14. Zhang, X., Yu, X., Wang, Y.A., and Zhao, J., Dose reduction of bone morphogenetic protein-2 for bone regeneration using a delivery system based on lyophilization with trehalose, *Int. J. Nanomedicine* 13, 403–414, 2018.

15. Portbury, S.D., Hare, D.J., Finkelstein, D.I., and Adlard, P.A., Trehalose improves traumatic brain injury-induced cognitive impairment, *PLoS One* 12(8), e0183683, 2017.

RETROMER/RETROMER COMPLEX

The retromer complex is a multi-protein device that mediates endosomal protein sorting in guiding transport back to the membrane surface as in receptor recycling or in transport to the *trans*-Golgi network.[1–7] Retriever is another mechanism for cargo recycling.[8]

1. Pfeffer, S.R., Membrane transport: Retromer to the rescue, *Curr. Biol.* 11, R109–R111, 2001.

2. Seaman, M.N.J., Recycle your receptors with retromer, *Trends Cell Biol.* 15, 68–75, 2005.

3. Griffin, C.T., Trejo, J., and Magnuson, T., Genetic evidence for a mammalian retromer complex containing sorting nexins 1 and 2, *Proc. Natl. Acad. Sci. USA* 102, 15173–15177, 2005.

4. Gullapalli, A., Wolfe, B.L., Griffin, C.T., Magnuson, T., and Trejo, J., An essential role of SNX1 in lysosomal sorting of protease-activated receptor-1: Evidence for retromer-, Hrs-, and Tsg101-independent functions of sorting nexins, *Mol. Biol. Cell* 17, 1228–1238, 2006.

5. Lucas, M., and Hierro, A., Retromer, *Curr. Biol.* 27, R687–R689, 2017.

6. Purushothaman, L.K., and Ungermann, C., Cargo induces retromer-mediated membrane remodeling on membranes, *Mol. Biol. Cell* 29, 2709–2719, 2018.

7. Kovtun, O., Leneva, N., Bykov, Y.S., et al., Structure of the membrane-assembled retromer coat determined by cryo-electron tomography, *Nature* 561, 561–564, 2018.

8. McNally, K.E., Faulkner, R., Steinberg, F., et al., Retriever is a multiprotein complex for retromer-independent endosomal cargo recycling, *Nat. Cell Biol.* 19, 1214–1225, 2017.

RETRO-TRANSLOCATION (RETROTRANSLOCATION)

Retrotranslocation and retro-translocation appear to refer to the same process so the term retrotranslocation will be used reflecting a slightly greater number of PubMed entries. Retrotranslocation is a process by which misfolded proteins or other incorrect translation products are transported from the lumen of the endoplasmic reticulum to the cytoplasm for subsequent degradation (endoplasmic reticulum-associated degradation; ERAD).[1–6] Retrotranslocation is also a process for mitochondrial proteins.[7,8]

1. Johnson, A.E., and Haigh, N.G., The ER translocon and retrotranslocation: Is the shift into reverse manual or automatic? *Cell* 102, 709–712, 2000.

2. Svedine, S., Wang, T., Halaban, R., and Herbert, D.N., Carbohydrates act as sorting determinants in ER-associated degradation of tyrosinase, *J. Cell. Sci.* 117, 2937–2949, 2004.

3. Schulze, A., Sandera, S., Buerger, E., et al., The ubiquitin-domain protein HERP forms a complex with components of the endoplasmic reticulum associated degradation pathway, *J. Mol. Biol.* 354, 1021–1027, 2005.

4. Nakatsukasa, K., and Brodsky, J.L., The recognition and retrotranslocation of misfolded proteins from the endoplasmic reticulum, *Traffic* 9, 861–870, 2008.

5. Hampton, R.Y., and Sommer, T., Finding the will and the way of ERAD substrate retrotranslocation, *Curr. Opin. Cell Biol.* 24, 460–466, 2012.

6. Guerriero, C.J., Reutter, K.R., Augustine, A.A., et al., Transmembrane helix hydrophobicity is an energetic barrier during the retrotranslocation of integral membrane ERAD substrates, *Mol. Cell Biol.* 28, 2076–2090, 2017.

7. Todt, F., Cakir, Z., Reichenbach, F., et al., Differential retrotranslocation of mitochondrial Bax and Bak, *EMBO J.* 34, 67–80, 2015.

8. Bragoszewski, P., Wasilewski, M., Sakowska, P., et al., Retro-translocation of mitochondrial intermediate space proteins, *Proc. Natl. Acad. Sci.* 112, 7713–7718, 2015.

REVERSE IMMUNOLOGY

Reverse immunology is the elucidation of the structure of minor histocompatibility antigens (miHA) found on tumor cells and grafts (stem cells, tissues such as liver) used in allogeneic blood and organ transplantation.[1]

The approach is based on the identification of peptides which arise from antigens (miHA) processed by proteasomes, which would react with activated T cells.(CTLs).[2,3] Initial work was based on the identification of tumor specific antigens, peptides based on the sequence of the selected antigens predicted *in silico*, and the reactivity of the peptides with activated T cell determined first by binding to MHC and subsequently by reactivity with activated T-cells.[4] The *in silico* approach has not been as successful as hoped; a more recent approach involved the characterization of the HLA peptidome.[5] Reverse immunology is an approach in contrast to **forward immunology** which can involve the culture of autologous peripheral blood monocytes with tumor cells followed by identification of the antigens responsible for the T cell response.[1,6] There are other approaches to identifying the antigen(s) responsible for T cell activation using forward immunology.[6,7]

1. Zilberberg, J., Feinman, R., and Korngold, R., Strategies for the identification of T cell-recognized tumor antigens in hematological malignancies for improved graft-versus-tumor responses after allogeneic blood and marrow transplantation, *Biol. Blood Marrow Transplant.* 21, 1000–1007, 2015.
2. Boon, T., and van der Bruggen, P., Human tumor antigens recognized by T lymphocytes, *J. Exp. Med.* 183, 725–729, 1996.
3. Tanzarella, S., Fleischhauer, K., van Endert, P., Bordignon, C., and Traversari, C., Characterization of antigenic peptide epitopes by reverse immunology: Induction of cytotoxic T lymphocytes specific for exogenous peptide only, *Int. J. Cancer* 72, 912–915, 1997.
4. Viatte, S., Alves, P.M., and Romero, P., Reverse immunology approach for the identification of CD8 T-cell-defined antigens: Advantages and hurdles, *Immnol. Cell Biol.* 84, 318–330, 2006.
5. Hornbrink, P., Hassan C., Kester, M.G.D., et al., Discovery of T cell epitopes implementing HLA-peptidomics into a reverse immunology approach, *J. Immunol.* 190, 3869–3877, 2013.
6. Kimura, S., Kozakai, Y., Kawaguchi, S., et al., Clonal T-cell response against autologous pleomorphic malignant fibrous histiocytoma antigen presented by retrieved HLA-A*0206, *J. Orthopaedic Res.* 26, 271–278, 2008.
7. Oostrvogels, R., Minnema, M.C., van Elk, M., et al., Towards effective and safe immunotherapy after allogeneic stem cell transplantation: Identification of hematopoietic-specific minor histocompatibility antigen UTA2–1, *Leukemia* 27, 642–649, 2013.

REVERSE MICELLE

A reverse micelle or inverted micelle is a stable assembly of a surfactant around an aqueous core where the lipophilic part of the surfactant is directed toward the exterior which is a non-polar solvent and the charged portion is directed toward the aqueous core. Reverse micelles have been used for the stabilization of proteins and study of enzymes in organic solvents[1–6] including studies on molecular crowding,[7–10] for protein purification[11–17] and for drug delivery.[18–20]

1. Grandi, C., Smith, R.E., and Luisi, P.L., Micellar solubilization of biopolymers in organic solvents. Activity and conformation of lysozyme in isooctane reverse micelles, *J. Biol. Chem.* 256, 837–843, 1981.
2. Nicot, C., and Waks, M., Proteins as invited guests of reverse micelles: Conformational effects, significance, applications, *Biotechnol. Genet. Eng. Rev.* 13, 267–314, 1996.
3. Tuena de Gomez-Puyou, M., and Gomez-Puyou, A., Enzymes in low-water systems, *CRC Rev. Biochem. Mol. Biol.* 33, 53–89, 1998.
4. Orlich, B., and Schomäcker, R., Enzyme catalysis in reverse micelles, *Adv. Biochem. Eng. Biotechnol.* 75, 185–208, 2002.
5. Marhuenda-Egea, F.C., and Bonete, M.J., Extreme halophilic enzymes in organic solvents, *Curr. Opin. Biotechnol.* 13, 385–389, 2002.
6. Eskici, G., and Axelsen, P.H., Amyloid beta peptide folding in reveres micelles, *J. Am. Chem. Soc.* 139, 9566–9575, 2017.
7. Hilaire, M.R., Abaskharon, R.M., and Gai, F., Biomolecular crowding arising from small molecules, molecular constraints, surface packing, and nano-confinement, *J. Chem. Lett.* 6, 2546–2553, 2015.
8. Honeggar, P., and Steinhauser, O., Revival of collective water structure and dynamics in reverse micelles brought about by protein encapsulation, *Phys. Chem. Chem. Phys.* 20, 22932–22945, 2018.
9. Ganguly, A., Paul, B.K., and Das, S., Modulation of probe-genomic DNA interaction within the confined interior of a reverse micelle: Is the bulk-like properties of water truly achieved in large reverse micelles? *Int. J. Biol. Macromol.* 118, 1203–1210, 2018.
10. Cheng, K., Wu, Q., Zhang, Z., et al., Crowding and confinement can oppositely affect protein stability, *ChemPhysChem* 19, 3350–3355, 2018.
11. Bernert, J.T., Jr., and Sprecher, H., Solubilization and partial purification of an enzyme involved in rat liver microsomal fatty acid chain elongation: Beta-hydroxyacyl-CoA dehydrase, *J. Biol. Chem.* 254, 11584–11590, 1979.
12. Leser, M.E., Wei, G., Luisi, P., and Maestro, M., Application of reverse micelles for the extraction of proteins, *Biochem. Biophys. Res. Commun.* 135, 629–635, 1986.
13. Luisi, P.L., and Magid, L.J., Solubilization of enzymes and nucleic acids in hydrocarbon micellar solutions, *CRC Crit. Rev. Biochem.* 20, 409–474, 1986.
14. Krishna, S.H., Srinivas, N.D., Ragnavarao, K.S., and Karanth, N.G., Reverse micellar extraction for downstream processing of proteins/enzymes, *Adv. Biochem. Eng. Biotechnol.* 75, 1190183, 2002.

15. Wan, J., Guo, J., Miao, Z., and Guo, X., Reverse micellar extraction of bromolain from pineapple peel—Effect of surfactant structure, *Food Chem.* 197, 450–456, 2016.
16. Yin, T., Lin, M., Wan, J., and Cao, X., Molecular interaction mechanisms in reverse micellar extraction of microbial transglutaminase, *J. Chromatog. A.* 1511, 25–36, 2017.
17. Zhao, X., Liu, H., Zhang, X., and Zhu, H., Comparison of structures of walnut protein fractions obtained through reverse micelles and alkaline extraction with isoelectric purification, *Int. J. Biol. Macromol.* 125, 1214–1220, 2019.
18. Muller-Goymann, C.C., Physicochemical characterization of colloidal drugery systems such as reverse micelles, vesicles, liquid crystals, and nanoparticles for topical administration, *Eur. J. Pharm. Biopharm.* 58, 343–356, 2004.
19. Nguyen, T.B.T., Li, S., and Deratanti, A., Reverse micelles prepared from amphiphilic polylactide-b-poly(ethylene glycol) block copolymers for controlled release of hydrophilic drugs, *Int. J. Pharm.* 495, 154–161, 2015.
20. Chen, Y., Liu, Y., Yao, Y., Zhang, S., and Gu, Z., Reverse micelle-based water-soluble nanoparticles for simultaneous bioimaging and drug delivery, *Org. Biomol. Chem.* 15, 3232–3238, 2017.

REVERSE-PHASE PROTEIN ARRAY

Reverse-phase protein array (RPPA) is microarray technology where dilutions of a heterogeneous sample such as a cell lysate is applied to matrix and probed with antibodies to determine the presence of specific analytes. The term reverse is used to indicate that, contrary to a conventional proteins microarray where the probes are on the matrix, it is the sample that is applied to the matrix.[1] There are mechanisms for the normalization of RPPA data.[2] RPPA is being used extensively to study disease processes with emphasis on oncology[3–7] as well as for drug development.[8–12]

1. Yuan, Y., Hong, K., Lin, Z.T., et al., Protein arrays III: Reverse-phase protein arrays, *Methods Mol. Biol.* 1654, 279–289, 2017.
2. Chiechi, A., Normalization of reverse phase protein microarray data: Choosing the best normalization analyte, *Methods Mol. Biol.* 132, 77–89, 2016.
3. Paweletz, C.P., Charboneau, L., Bichsel, V.E., et al., Reverse phase protein microarrays which capture disease progression show activation of pro-survival pathways at the cancer invasion front, *Oncogene* 20 1981–1989, 2001.
4. Masuda, M., and Yamada, T., Signaling pathway profiling using reverse-phase protein array and its clinical applications, *Expert Rev. Proteomics* 14, 607–615, 2017.
5. Patil, V., and Mahalingam, K., A four-protein expression prognostic signature predicts clinical outcome of lower-grade glioma, *Gene* 679, 57–64, 2018.
6. Du, D., Ma, W., Yates, M.S., et al., Predicting high-risk endometrioic carcinomas using proteins, *Oncotarget* 9, 19704–19715, 2018.
7. Kornblau, S.M., Ruvolo, P.P., Wang, R.Y., et al., Distinct protein signatures of acute myeloid leukemia bone-marrow derived stromal cells are prognostic for patient survival, *Haematologica* 103, 810–821, 2018.
8. Lu, Y., Ling, S., Hedge, A.M., et al., Using reverse-phase protein arrays as pharmacodynamic assays for functional proteomics, biomarker discovery, and drug development in cancer, *Semin. Oncol.* 43, 576–483, 2016.
9. Li, J., Zhao, W., Akbani, G., et al., Characterization of human cancer cell lines by reverse-phase protein arrays, *Cancer Cell* 31, 225–239, 2017.
10. Pawlak, M., and Carragher, N.O., Reverse phase protein arrays elucidate mechanisms-of-action and phenotypic response in 2D and 3D models, *Drug Discov. Today Technol.* 23, 7–16, 2017.
11. Huang, X., Cao, M., Wu, X., et al., Anti-leukemia activity of NSC-743380 in SULT1A2-expressing acute myeloid leukemia cells is associated with inhibitions of cFLIP expression and P13K/AKT/mTOR activities, *Oncotarget* 8, 102150–102160, 2017.
12. Aslan, O., Cremona, M., Morgan, C., et al., Preclinical evaluation and reverse phase protein array-based profiling of P13K and MEK inhibitors in endometrial carcinoma in vitro, *BMC Cancer* 18:168, 2018.

REVERSE TRANSCRIPTASE

A reverse transcriptase is an enzyme which catalyzes the formation of DNA from an RNA template.[1–4] Reverse transcriptase are critical for the replication of RNA viruses such as HIV and is major drug targets for AIDS and other RNA viral diseases such as hepatitis B.[5–9] Reverse transcriptase activity is a critical part of telomerase function.[10–13]

1. O'Conner, T.E., Reverse transcriptase- progress, problems and prospects, *Bibl. Haematol.* 39, 1265–1181, 1973.
2. Wu, A.M., and Gallo, R.C., Reverse transcriptase, *CRC Crit. Rev. Biochem.* 3, 289–347, 1975.
3. Verma, I.M., The reverse transcriptase, *Biochim. Biophys. Acta* 473, 1–38, 1977.
4. Gerard, G.F., Reverse transcriptase, in *Enzymes of Nucleic Acid Synthesis and Modification*, Vol 1, DNA enzymes, ed. S.T. Jacob, Chapter 1, pp. 1–38, CRC Press, Boca Raton, FL, 2018.
5. *Reverse Transcriptase Inhibitors in HIV/AIDS Therapy*, ed. G. Skowron and R.D. Ogdon, Humana Press, Totowa, NJ, 2006.
6. *Human Immunodeficiency Virus Rescriptase: A Bench-to-Beside Success*, ed. M. Götte and S. LeGrice, Springer, New York, 2013.
7. Chan, A.H., Lee, W.G., Spâsov, K.A., et al., Covalent inhibitors for eradication of drug-resistant HIV-1 reverse transcriptase: From design to protein crystallography, *Proc. Natl. Acad. Sci. USA* 114, 9725–9730, 2017.

8. Elmessaoudi-Idrissi, M., Blondel, A., Ketani, A., et al., Virtual screening in hepatitis B virus drug discovery: Current state-of-the-art and future perspectives, *Curr. Med. Chem.* 25, 2709–2721, 2018.

9. Rai, M.A., Pannek, S., and Fichtenbaum, C.J., Emerging reverse transcriptase inhibitors for HIV-1 infection, *Expert Opin. Emerg. Drugs* 23, 149–157, 2018.

10. Teichroeb, J.H., Kim, J., and Betts, D.H., The role of telomeres and telomerase reverse transcriptase isoforms in pluripotency induction and maintenance, *RNA Biol.* 13, 707–719, 2016.

11. Webb, C.J., and Zakian, V.A., Telomerase RNA is more than a DNA template, *RNA Biol.* 13, 683–689, 2016.

12. Dey, A., and Chakrabarti, K., Current perspectives of telomerase structure and function in eukaryotes with emerging views on telomerase in human parasites, *Int. J. Mol. Sci.* 19, E3333, 2018.

13. Wang, Y., and Feigon, J., Structural biology of telomerase and its interaction at telomeres, *Curr. Opin. Struct Biol.* 42, 77–87, 2017.

REVERSE TRANSCRIPTASE—POLYMERASE CHAIN REACTION (RT-PCR)

A variation of the PCR technique in which cDNA is made from RNA via reverse transcription. The cDNA is then amplified using standard PCR protocols.[1–10] RT-PCR was used to measure transcriptomes and can be used in combination with RNA-seq.[11,12]

1. Mocharla, H., Mocharla, R., and Hodes, M.E., Coupled reverse transcription-polymerase chain reaction (RT-PCR) as a sensitive and rapid method for isozyme genotyping, *Gene* 93, 271–275, 1990.

2. Weis, J.H., Tan, S.S., Martin, B.K., and Willwer, C.T., Detection of rare mRNAs via quantitative RT-PCR, *Trends Genet.* 8, 263–264, 1992.

3. Akoury, D.A., Seo, J.J., James, C.D., and Zaki, S.R., RT-PCR detection of mRNA recovered from archival glass slide smears, *Mol. Pathol.* 6, 195–200, 1993.

4. Silver, J., Maudru, T., Fujita, K., and Repaske, R., An RT-PCR assay for the enzyme activity of reverse transcriptase capable of detecting single virions, *Nucleic Acids Res.* 21, 3593–3594, 1993.

5. Taniguchi, A., Kohsaka, H., and Carson, D.A., Competitive RT-PCR ELISA: A rapid, sensitive and non-radioactive method to quantitate cytokine mRNA, *J. Immunol. Methods* 169, 101–109, 1994.

6. Prediger, E.A., Quantitating mRNAs with relative and competitive RT-PCR, *Methods Mol. Biol.* 160, 49–63, 2001.

7. Joyce, C., Quantitative RT-PCR. A review of current methodologies, *Methods Mol. Biol.* 193, 83–92, 2002.

8. Ransick, A., Detection of mRNA by in situ hybridization and RT-PCR, *Methods Mol. Biol.* 74, 601–620, 2004.

9. Bachman, J., Reverse-transcription PCR (RT-PCR), *Methods Enzymol.* 530, 67–74, 2013.

10. Khan-Malek, R., and Wang, Y., Statistical analysis of quantitative RT-PCR results, *Methods Mol. Biol.* 1641, 281–296, 2017.

11. Costa, C., Giménez-Capitán, A., Karachaliou, N., and Rosell, R., Comprehensive molecular screening: From the RT-PCR to the RNA-seq, *Trans. Lung Cancer Res.* 2, 87–91, 2013.

12. Menyhárt, O., Harami-Papp, H., Sukumar, S., et al., Guidelines for the selection of functional assays to evaluate the hallmarks of cancer, *Biochim. Biophys. Acta* 1866, 300–319, 2016.

RHO FACTOR (RHO PROTEIN)

A ring-shaped homohexameric bacterial protein encoded by the *rho* gene which regulates RNA polymerase activity by terminating the process of transcription.[1–3] Rho factor is possibly more properly described as transcription termination factor Rho.[4,5]

1. Richardson, J.P., Rho-dependent termination and ATPases in transcript termination, *Biochim. Biophys. Acta* 1577, 251–260, 2002.

2. Banerjee, S., Chalissery, J., Bandey, I., and Sen, R., Rho-dependent transcription termination: More questions than answers, *J. Microbiol.* 44, 11–22, 2006.

3. Mitra, P., Ghosh, G., Hiafeezunnisa, M., and Sen, R., Rho protein: Roles and mechanisms, *Annu. Rev. Microbiol.* 71, 687–709, 2017.

4. Grylak-Mielnicka, A., Bidnenko, V., Bardowski, J., and Bidnenkom E., Transcription termination factor Rho: A hub linking diverse physiological processes in bacteria, *Microbiology* 162, 433–447, 2016.

5. Kriner, M.A., Sevostyanova, A., and Groisman, E.A., Leaning from the leaders: Gene regulation by the transcription termination factor Rho, *Trends Biochem. Sci.* 41, 690–699, 2016.

RHOMBOID

Rhomboid is a term describing a family of transmembrane proteins which can be intramembrane serine proteases widely distributed in prokaryotes[1,2] and eukaryotes,[3] which can function as secretases.[4] There are inactive (noncatalytic) forms of rhomboid in mammals which have been described as rhomboid pseudoproteases.[5] Rhomboid proteases have an active site serine as a nucleophile for catalysis but are classical serine proteases in that the active site has a his-ser dyad while classical serine proteases (chymotrypsin-like proteases) have a his-ser-asp triad.[4,6] Rhomboid proteases are monomeric proteins[7] which required lipid for function.[8] It has been possible to isolate rhomboid proteases from membranes and stabilize them in lipid nanodisks.[9] PARL is a mitochondrial rhomboid protease.[10] There is interest in the development of inhibitors of rhomboid proteases for therapeutic use.[11] Rhomboid (*rho* gene) was found during mutagenesis studies in *Drosophila*.[12,13] Rhomboid was subsequently shown to function in the ectopic activation of EGF-receptors in *Drosophila* implying release of membrane bound EGF.[14] It should be noted that *rho* (gene) should not be confused with transcription termination factor Rho.

1. Sampathkumar, P., Mak, M.W., Fischer-Witholt, S.J., et al., Oligomeric state study of prokaryote rhomboid proteases, *Biochim. Biophys. Acta* 1818, 3090–3097, 2012.
2. Panigraphi, R., and Lemieux, M.J., Functional implications of domain organization within prokaryotic rhomboid proteases, *Adv. Exp. Med. Biol.* 883, 107–117, 2015.
3. Urban, S., A guide to the rhomboid protein superfamily in development and disease, *Sem. Cell Dev. Biol.* 60, 1–4, 2016.
4. Lastum, V.L., Grieve, A.G., and Freeman, M., Substrates and physiological functions of secretase rhomboid proteases, *Sem. Cell Dev. Biol.* 60, 10–18, 2016.
5. Lemberg, M.K., and Adrain, C., Inactive rhomboid proteins: New mechanisms with implications in health and disease, *Sem. Cell Dev. Biol.* 60, 29–37, 2016.
6. Shokhen, M., and Albeck, A., How does the exosite of rhomboid protease affect substrate processing and inhibition, *Protein Science* 26, 2355–2366, 2017.
7. Kreutzbeger, A.J.B., and Urban, S., Single-molecule analyses reveal rhomboid proteins are strict and functional monomers in the membrane, *Biophys. J.* 115, 1755–1761, 2018.
8. Paschkowsky, S., Oestereich, F., and Munter, L.M., Embedded in the membrane: How lipids confer activity and specificity to intramembrane proteins, *J. Membrane Biol.* 251, 369–378, 2018.
9. Barniol-Xicota, M., and Verhelst, S.H.L., Stable and functional rhomboid proteases in lipid nanodisc by using diisobutylene/maleic acid copolymers, *J. Am. Chem. Soc.* 140, 14557–14567, 2018.
10. Spinazzi, M., and De Strooper, B., PARL: The mitochondrial rhomboid protease, *Sem. Cell Devel. Biol.* 60, 19–28, 2016.
11. Strisovsky, K., Rhomboid protease inhibitors: Emerging tools and future therapeutics, *Sem. Cell Devel. Biol.* 60, 52–62, 2016.
12. Jürgens, G., Wieschaus, E., Nüsslein-Volhard, C., and Kluding, H., Mutations affecting the pattern of the larval cuticle in *Drosophila melanogaster*. II. Zygotic loci on the third chromosome, *Rous's Arch. Dev. Biol.* 193, 283–295, 1984.
13. Bier, E., Jan, L.Y., and Jan, Y.N., *Rhomboid*, a gene required for dorsoventral axis establishment and peripheral nervous system development in *Drosophila melanogaster*, *Genes & Devel.* 4, 190–203, 1990.
14. Noll, R., Sturtevant, M.A., Gollapudi, R.R., and Bier, E., New functions of the *Drosophila* rhomboid gene during embryonic and adult development are revealed by a novel genetic method, enhancer piracy, *Development* 120, 2329–2338, 1994.

RIBOSWITCH

A riboswitch is a mechanism to regulate mRNA expression in prokaryotes.[1,2] Certain metabolites (e.g. riboflavin, thiamine pyrophosphate, some amides such as serine, flavin mononucleotide) can bind to a specific region (riboswitch) on a messenger RNA causing a conformational change in the mRNA regulating expression. Riboswitches were earlier described as the *RFN* (riboflavin) element.[3,4] A riboswitch is usually located in the 5′-untranslated region (leader sequence) upstream from the initiator codon and consists of an aptamer which binds the ligand (sensory domain and regulatory domain).[5,6] Riboswitches are potential therapeutic targets in bacterial infection[7,8] and as control of transgene cytotoxicity in AAV transfection.[9]

1. Romby, P., and Springer, M., Translational control in prokaryotes, in *Translational Control in Biology and Medicine*, ed. M.B. Matthews, N. Sonnenberg, and J.W.B. Hershy, Chapter 26, pp. 803–827, Cold Spring Harbor Laboratory Press, Cold Spring Harbor, NY, 2007.
2. McCown, P.J., Corbino, K.A., Stav, S., Sherlock, M.E., and Breaker, R.R., Riboswitch diversity and distribution, *RNA* 23, 995–1011, 2017.
3. Gelfand, M.A., Mironov, A.A., Jomantas, J., et al., A conserved RNA structure element involved in the regulation of bacterial riboflavin synthesis genes, *Trends Genet.* 15, 439–442, 1999.
4. Serganov, A., Huang, L., and Patel, D.J., Coenzyme recognition and gene regulation by a flavin mononucleotide riboswitch, *Nature* 458, 233–237, 2009.
5. Kazanov, M.D., Vitreschak, A.G., and Gelfand, M.S., Abundance and functional diversity of riboswitches in microbial communities, *BMC Genomics* 8, 347, 2007.
6. Mehdizadeh, A.E., Hejazi, M.S., and Barzegar, A., Riboswitches: From living biosensors to novel targets of antibiotics, *Gene* 592, 244–259, 2016.
7. Deigan, K.E., and Ferré-D'Amaré, A.R., Riboswitches: Discovery of drugs that target bacterial gene-regulatory RNAs, *Acc. Chem. Res.* 44, 1329–1338, 2011.

8. Wang, H., Mann, P.A., Ziao, L., et al., Dual-targeting small-molecule inhibitors of the *Staphylococcus aureus* FMN riboswitch disrupt riboflavin homeostasis in an infectious setting, *Cell. Biol.* 24, 576–588, 2017.

9. Strobel, B., Klauser, B., Hartig, J.S., et al., Riboswitch-mediated attenuation of transgene cytotoxicity increases Adeno-associated virus vector yields in HEK-293 cells, *Mol. Ther.* 23, 1582–1591, 2015.

RING-FINGER PROTEINS/ RING-FINGER DOMAINS

The term RING (Really Interesting New Gene)-finger[1–3] which is a concept related to zinc finger,[4,5] describes a domain defined by a unique zinc-binding motif. This motif was first described in RING1 gene[2] and RING1 protein was subsequently shown to act as a repressor of transcription.[6] Following work has shown that the RING motif occurs in a wide variety of proteins including enzymes (ligases) involved in ubiquitination[7–12] including the Cbl (casitas B-linage lymphoma) ubiquitin ligases[13–15] and muscle-specific RING finger proteins (MuRFs).[12,16–19]

1. Saurin, A.J., Borden, K.L., Boddy, M.N., and Freemont, P.S., Does this have a familiar RING? *Trends Biochem. Sci.* 21, 208–214, 1996.

2. Lovering, R., Hanson, I.M., Borden, K.L., et al., Identification and preliminary characterization of a protein motif related to the zinc finger, *Proc. Natl. Acad. Sci. USA* 90, 2112–2116, 1993.

3. Eisenhaber, B., Chumak, N., Eisenhaber, F., and Hauser, M.T., The ring between the ring fingers (RBR) protein family, *Genome Biol.* 8(3), 209, 2007.

4. Freemont, P.S., Hanson, I.M., and Trowsdale, J., A novel cysteine-rich sequence motif, *Cell* 64, 483–484, 1991.

5. Borden, K.L.B., and Freemont, P.S., The RING finger domain: A recent example of a sequence-structure family, *Curr. Opin. Struct. Biol.* 6, 395–401, 1996.

6. Satijn, D.P.E., Gunster, M.J., van der Vlag, J., et al., RING1 is associated with the polycomb group protein complex and acts as a transcriptional repressor, *Mol. Cell. Biol.* 17, 4105–4113, 1997.

7. Jackson, P.K., Eldridge, A.G., Freed, E., et al., The lore of the RINGs: Substrate recognition and catalysis by ubiquitin ligases, *Trends Cell Biol.* 10, 429–439, 2000.

8. Guzmán, P., The prolific family of RING-H2 ubiquitin ligases, *Plant Signal. Behav.* 7, 1014–1921, 2012.

9. Tomar, D., and Singh, R., TRIM family proteins; emerging class of RING E3 ligases as regulator of the NF-κB pathway, *Biol. Cell* 107, 22–40, 2015.

10. Zheng, N., and Shabek, N., Ubiquitin ligases: Structure, function, and regulation, *Annu. Rev. Biochem.* 86, 129–157, 2017.

11. Kumar, B., Roy, A., Veettil, M.V., and Chandra, B., Insight into the roles of E3 Ubiquitin ligase c-Cbl, ESCRT machinery and host cell signaling in Kaposi's sarcoma-associated herpesvirus entry and trafficking, *J. Virol.* 92(4), 01376–17, 2018.

12. Borlepawar, A., Frey, N., and Rangrez, A.Y., A systematic view on E3 ligase Ring TRIMmers with a focus on cardiac function and disease, *Trends Cardiovasc. Med.* 29, 1–8, 2019.

13. Smit, L., and Borst, J., The Cbl family of signal transduction molecules, *Crit. Rev. Oncol.* 8, 359–379, 1997.

14. Liu, Q., Zhou, H., Langdon, W.Y., and Zhang, J., E3 ubiquitin ligase Cbl-b in innate and adaptive immunity, *Cell Cycle* 13, 1875–1884, 2014.

15. Li, M., Kales, S.C., Ma, K., et al., Balancing protein stability and activity in cancer: A new approach for identifying driver mutations affecting CBL ubiquitin ligase activation, *Cancer Res.* 76, 561–571, 2016.

16. Gregorio, C.C., Perry, C.N., and McElhinny, A.S., Functional properties of the titin/connectin-associated proteins, the muscle-specific RING finger proteins (MURFs), in striated muscle, *J. Muscle Res. Cell Motil.* 26, 389–400, 2005.

17. Gregorio, C.C., Perry, C.N., and McElhinny, A.S., Functional properties of the titin/connectin-associated proteins, the muscle-specific RING finger proteins (MURFs), in striated muscle, *J. Muscle Res. Cell Motil.* 14, 1–12, 2006.

18. Tacchi, L., Bickerdike, R., Secombes, C.J., and Martin, S.A., Muscle-specific RING finger (MuRF) cDNAs in Atlantic salmon (*Salmo salar*) and their role as regulators of muscle protein degradation, *Mar. Biotechnnol.* 14, 35–45, 2012.

19. Mayans, O., and Labeit, S., MuRFs, specialized members of the TRIM/RBCC family with roles in the regulation of the trophic state of muscle and its metabolism, *Adv. Exp. Med. Biol.* 700, 119–129, 2012.

RNA CAPPING

RNA capping is the capping mRNA synthesized by RNA Pol II. This process is critical for gene expression in eukaryotes and viruses but is absent in bacterial and archaeal systems.[1–3] RNA capping refers to the addition of a N^7-methylguanosine to the 5′-end of the messenger RNA after 20–30 nucleotides have been added by RNA polymerase. This modification requires three enzymes to convert the final triphophosphate linkage to the methylguanine base. The first step is the removal of the terminal phosphoryl residues from the 5′-nucleotide triphosphate in the growing mRNA chain. The second step is the transfer of guanidine monophosphate from guanidine triphosphate to the 5′-diphosphate nucleotide in the growing oligonucleotide chain followed by methylation of the 5′-terminal guanidine nucleotide. The N^7-methyl-guanidine residue serves to identify an RNA synthesized in the nuclease intended for synthesis of protein translation, designates the start of transcription as well contributing to the stability of the mRNA by preventing degradation.[4] The presence of an unusual methylated guanosine at the 5-terminal of messenger RNA was described in 1974.[5,6] Subsequent work showed that the placement of the 5′-terminal cap was a multistep synthetic process[7,8] resulting in the currently accepted three step process.[9]

1. Bentley, D.L, Coupling mRNA processing with transcription in time and space, *Nat. Rev. Genet.* 15, 163–175, 2014.
2. Ramanathan, A., Robb, G.B., and Chan, S.H., mRNA capping: Biological functions and applications, *Nucleic Acids Res.* 44, 7511–7526, 2016.
3. Aregger, M., and Cowing, V.H., Regulation of mRNA capping the cell cycle, *RNA Biol.* 14, 11–14, 2017.
4. Shatkin, A.J., Capping of eukaryotic RNA, *Cell* 9, 645–653, 1976.
5. Reddy, R., Ro-Choi, T.S., Henning, D., and Busch, H., Primary sequence of U-1 nuclear ribonucleic acid of Novikoff hepatoma ascites cells, *J. Biol. Chem.* 249, 6486–6494, 1974.
6. Rottman, F., Shatkin, A.J., and Perry, R.P., Sequences containing methylated nucleotides at the 5′ termini of messenger RNAs: Possible implications for processing, *Cell* 3, 197–199, 1974.
7. Winicov, I., and Perry, R.P., Synthesis methylation, and capping of nuclear RNA by a subcellular system, *Biochemistry* 15, 5039–5046, 1976.
8. Groner, Y., Gilboa, E., and Aviv, H., Methylation and capping of RNA polymerase II primary transcripts by HeLa nuclear homogenates, *Biochemistry* 17, 977–982, 1978.
9. Shatkin, A.J., and Manley, J.L., The ends of the affair: Capping and polyadenylation, *Nat. Struct. Biol.* 7, 838–842, 2000.

3. Filipowicz, W., RNAi: The nuts and bolts of the RISC machine, *Cell* 122, 17–20, 2005.
4. Hutvagner, G., Small RNA asymmetry in RNAi: Function in RISC assemble and gene regulation, *FEBS Lett.* 579, 5850–5857, 2005.
5. Hammond, S.M., Dicing and slicing: The core machinery of the RNA interference pathway, *FEBS Lett.* 579, 5822–5829, 2005.
6. Gilmore, I.R., Fox, S.P., Hollins, A.J., and Akhtar, S., Delivery strategies for siRNA-mediated gene silencing, *Curr. Drug Deliv.* 3, 147–155, 2006.
7. Azlan, A., Dzaki, N., and Azzam, G., The executor of small RNA function, *J. Genet. Geomics* 43, 481–494, 2016.
8. Zhu, L., Jiang, H., Sheong, F.K., et al., Understanding the core of RNA interference: The dynamic aspects of the Argonaute-mediated processes, *Prog. Biophy. Mol. Biol.* 128, 39–46, 2017.
9. Sheu-Gruttadaruia, J., and MacRae, I.J., Structural foundations of RNA silencing by Argonaute, *J. Mol. Biol.* 429, 2619–2639, 2017.
10. Olina, A.V., Kulbachinsky, A.V., Aravin, A.A., and Esyuina, D.M., Argonaute proteins and mechanisms of RNA interference in eukaryotes and prokaryotes, *Biochemistry* (Moscow) 83, 483–497, 2018.
11. Zhang, R., Jing, Y., Zhang, H., et al., Comprehensive evolutionary analysis of the major RNA-induced silencing complex members, *Sci. Rep.* 8(1), 14189, 2018.
12. Michlewski, G., and Caceres, J.F., Post-translational control of miRNA biogenesis, *RNA*, in press (doi:10.1261/rna/o68692.118), 2018.
13. Ponnusamy, M., Yan, K.-W., Liu, C.-Y., Li, P.-F., and Wang, K., PIWI family emerging as a decisive factor of cell fate: An overview, *Eur. J. Cell Biol.* 96, 746–757, 2017.
14. Sturm, Á., Perczel, A., Ivics, Z., and Vellai, T., The Piwi-piRNA pathway: Road to immortality, *Aging Cell* 16, 906–911, 2017.

RNA-INDUCED SILENCING COMPLEX (RISC)

The RNA-induced silencing complex (RISC) is a complex formed from the interaction of interfering RNA (RNA interference, RNAi) from small interfering RNAs (siRNA) or microRNAs (miRNAs) with mRNA-protein (Argonaut protein). RISC formation results in post-transcriptional gene silencing as a result of mRNA cleavage.[1–12] A related function is provided by PIWI (P-element induced wimpy testis) which in combination with piRNA silences transposons among other suggested functions[13] and has been related to the process of aging.[14]

1. Sontheimer, E.J., Assembly and function of RNA silencing complexes, *Nat. Rev. Mol. Cell Biol.* 6, 127–138, 2005.
2. Tang, G., siRNA and miRNA: An insight into RISCs, *Trends Biochem. Sci.* 30, 106–114, 2005.

RNA INTERFERENCE (RNAi)

RNA interference (RNAi) refers to the inhibition of gene transcription mediated through the production of small interfering RNA fragments (siRNA) from longer double-stranded RNA[1,2] or microRNA (miRNA).[3,4] siRNA can be delivered inside the cell, for example, by a lentiviral-mediated process,[5] a liposome-mediated process,[6] or electroporation.[7] MicroRNA (miRNA) is generated *in vivo* from the cleavage of short hairpin RNA (shRNA).[8] These fragments, in combination with a protein (Argonaute), binds to messenger RNA result in destruction of the mRNA. RNA interference is also referred to as RNA silencing.[8,9] The laboratory application of RNA silencing is known as knock-down[10] as there is, in principle, a transient block in gene expression. The concept of knockdown is in contrast to knockout where the gene (DNA) can be inactivated.[11] There are approaches such as Cas9 which can be used to either activate or inactivate genes.[12]

1. Fire, A., Xu, S., Montgomery, M.K., et al., Potent and specific genetic interference by double-stranded RNA in *Caenorhabditis elegans*, *Nature* 391, 806–811, 1998.
2. Elbashir, S.M., Harborth, J., Lendeckel, W., et al., Duplexes of 21-nucleotide RNAs mediate RNA interference in cultured mammalian cells, *Nature* 411, 494–498, 2001.
3. Filipowicz, W., RNAi: The nuts and the bolts of the RISC machine, *Cell* 122, 17–20, 2005.
4. Herkenhoff, M.E., Oliveira, A.C., Nachtgall, P.G., et al., Fishing into the microRNA transcriptome, *Front. Genet.* 9, 88, 2018.
5. Qin, X.-F., An, D.S., Chen, I.S.Y., and Baltmore, D., Inhibiting HIV-1 infection in human T cells by lentiviral-mediated delivery of small interfering RNA against CCR5, *Proc. Natl. Acad. Sci. USA* 100, 183–188, 2003.
6. Landen, C.N.,Jr., Chavez-Reves, A., Bucana, C., et al., Therapeutic *EphA2* gene targeting *in vivo* using neutral liposomal small interfering RNA delivery, *Cancer Res.* 65, 6910–6918, 2005.
7. Golzio, M., and Teissie, J., siRNA delivery via electropulsation: A review of the basic processes, *Methods Mol. Biol.* 1121, 81–98, 2014.
8. Fellmann, C., and Lowe, S.W., Stable RNA interference rules for silencing, *Nature Cell Biol.* 16, 10–18, 2014.
9. Saito, K., Miyoshi, K., Siomi, M.C., and Siomi, H., The key features of RNA silencing, in *RNA Technologies and Their Applications*, ed. V.A. Erdmann and J. Barciszewski, pp. 1–28, Springer Verlag, Berlin, Germany, 2010.
10. Shan, G., RNA interference as a gene knockdown technique, *Int. J. Biochem. Cell Biol.* 42, 1243–1251, 2010.
11. Lillis, A.P., Van Duyn, L.B., Murphy-Ullrich, J.E., and Strickland, D.K., LDL receptor-related protein 1: Unique tissue-specific functions revealed by selective gene knockout studies, *Physiol. Rev.* 88, 887–913, 2008.
12. Dahlman, J.E., Abudayyeh, O.O., Joung, J., et al., Orthogonal gene knockout and activation with a catalytically active Cas9 nuclease, *Nat. Biotechnol.* 33, 1159–1161, 2015.

RNA POLYMERASES

RNA polymerases are enzymes responsible for the biosynthesis of DNA-directed RNA synthesis. RNA polymerase is a nucleotide transferase that synthesizes RNA from ribonucleotides. In bacteria there is only one RNA polymerase.[1,2] Archaea also have a single RNA polymerase.[3–5] Eukaryotic cells have three RNA polymerases.[6] RNA polymerase I (polI) catalyzes the synthesis of ribosomal RNA species in the form of a precursor pre-rRNA (45S) which is processed into other species such as 5.8 S, 28 S and 18S RNA.[6–8]

RNA polymerase II[9–12] is responsible for the synthesis of mRNA,[13–15] snoRNA (small nuclear RNA),[16] miRNA (microRNA),[17,18] and other RNA species.[6] RNA polymerase III (polIII) synthesizes various noncoding RNAs including tRNA (transfer RNAs) and other smaller RNA species.[6,19]

1. Lathe, R., RNA polymerase of *Escherichia coli*, *Curr. Top. Microbiol. Immunol.* 83, 37–91, 1978.
2. Darst, S.A., Bacterial RNA polymerase, *Curr. Opin. Struct. Biol.* 11, 155–162, 2001.
3. Geiduschek, E.P., and Ouhammouch, M., Archaeal transcription and its regulators, *Mol. Microl.* 56, 1397–1407, 2005.
4. Hirata, A., Klein, B.J., and Murakami, K.S., The x-ray crystal structure of RNA polymerase from Archaea, *Nature* 451, 851–857, 2008.
5. Hirata, A., and Murakami, K.S., Archaeal RNA polymerase, *Curr. Opin. Struct. Biol.* 19, 724–731, 2009.
6. Alberts, B., Hunt, T., Johnson, A., et al., *Molecular Biology of the Cell*, Chapter 6, How cells read the genome: From DNA to protein, Chapter 6, pp. 299–369, Garland Science, New York, 2015.
7. Tsang, C.K., Bertram, P.G., Ai, W., Drenan, R., and Zheng, X.F.S., Chromatin-mediated regulation of nucleolar structure and RNA Pol I localization by TOR, *The EMBO J.* 22, 6045–6056, 2003.
8. Sadian,Y., Tafur, L., Kosinski,J., et al., Structural insights into transcription initiation by yeast RNA polymerase I, *Embo J.* 36, 2698–2709, 2017,
9. Young, R.A., RNA polymerase II, *Annu. Rev. Biochem.* 60, 689–715, 1991.
10. Cramer, P., Bushnell, D.A., and Kornberg, R.D., Structural basis of transcription: RNA polymerase II at 2.8 Ångstrom resolution, *Science* 292, 1863–1876, 2001.
11. Hahn, S., Structure and mechanism of the RNA polymerase II transcription machinery, *Nature Struct. Mol. Biol.* 11, 394–403, 2004.
12. Chen F.X., Smith, E.R., and Shilatiford, A., Born to run: Control of transcription elongation by RNA polymerase II, *Nat. Rev. Mol. Cell Biol.* 19, 464–478, 2018.
13. Adhya, S.L., *RNA Polymerase and Associated Factors*, Academic Press, San Diego, CA, 1996.
14. *Eukaryotic Gene Transcription*, ed. S. Goodbourn, IRL Press at Oxford University Press, Oxford, UK, 1996.
15. Richter, J.D., *mRNA Formation and Function*, Academic Press, San Diego, CA, 1997.
16. Bachellerie,J.P.,Cavaillé,J.,andHüttenhofer,A.,The expanding snoRNA world, *Biochemie* 84, 775–790, 2002.
17. Lee, Y., Kim, M., Han, J., et al., MicroRNA genes are transcribed by RNA polymerase II, *EMBO J.* 23, 4051–5080, 2004.
18. Ross, J.S., Carlson, J.A., and Brock, G., miRNA: The new gene silencer, *Am. J. Clin. Pathol.* 128, 830–836, 2007.
19. Abascal-Palacios, G., Ramsay, E.P., Beuron, F., Morris, E., and Vannini, A., Structural basis of RNA polymerase III transcription initiation, *Nature* 552, 301–306, 2018.

RNA-seq

RNA-seq is the term used for RNA-sequence analysis as applied to the determination of the transcriptome including noncoding RNA.[1-4] While there are variations on the technique, RNA-seq involves the isolation of RNA from a cell or tissue, the preparation of cDNA from the RNA or fragments thereof, determination of the cDNA sequence by next generation sequencing, and reading the RNA sequences from the cDNA sequence. RNA-seq does require sophisticated data analysis.[5-7] While there are other methods such as DNA microarray analysis for study of gene expression,[8] RNA-seq is emerging as the preferred method.[9-11]

1. Mortazavi, A., Williams, B.A., McCue, K., Schaeffer, L., and Wold, B., Mapping and quantifying mammalian transcriptomes by RNA-seq, *Nature Methods* 5, 621–628, 2008.
2. Marioni, J.C., Mason, C.E., Mane, S.M., Stephens, M., and Gilad, Y., RNA-seq: An assessment of technical reproducibility and comparison with other gene expression arrays, *Genome Res.* 18, 1509–1517, 2008.
3. Wang, Z., Gerstein, M., and Snyder, M., RNA-seq: A revolutionary tool for transcriptomics, *Nat. Rev. Genet.* 10, 57–63, 2009.
4. Croucher, N.J., and Thomson, N.R., Studying bacterial transcriptomes using RNA-seq, *Curr. Opin. Micobiol.* 13, 619–624, 2010.
5. Monger, C., Kelly, P.S., Gallagher, C., et al., Towards next generation CHO cell biology: Bioinformatics methods for RNA-Seq based expression profiling, *Biotechnol. J.* 10, 950–966, 2015.
6. Conesa, A., Madrigal, P., Tarazona, S., A survey of best practices for RNA-seq data analysis, *Genome Biol.* 17, 13, 2016.
7. Poplawski, A., Marini, F., Hess, M., et al., Systematically evaluating interfaces for RNA-seq analysis from a life scientist perspective, *Brief Bioinform.* 17, 213–223, 2016.
8. Lee, J.Y., Tokumoto, M., Fujiwara, Y., and Satoh, M., Gene expression analysis using DNA microarray in HK-2 human proximal tubular cells treated with cadmium, *J. Toxicol. Sci.* 38, 959–962, 2013.
9. Creecy, J.P., and Conway, T., Quantitative bacterial transcriptomics with RNA-seq, *Curr. Opin. Microbiol.* 23, 133–140, 2015.
10. Zhang, W., Yu, Y., Hertwig, F., et al., Comparison of RNA-seq and microarray-based models for clinical endpoint prediction, *Genome Biol.* 16, 133, 2015.
11. Sumitomo, S., Nagafuchi, Y., Tsuchida, Y., et al., Transcriptome analysis of peripheral blood from patients with rheumatoid arthritis: A systematic review, *Inflamm. Regen.* 38, 21, 2018.

RNA SPLICING

RNA splicing is a form of RNA editing which involves the removal of introns from the sequence of a pre-mRNA following Pol II transcription of DNA to form an uninterrupted coding sequence (mature RNA transcript).[1-3] RNA splicing is not a static process and alternative splicing[4,5] yield multiple messages from a single pre-mRNA transcript. Alternative splicing is of importance in oncology.[6,7] A **spliceosome**, a complex of proteins and nucleic acids, responsible for the process of splicing.[8-11] Backsplicing of exons or lariat introns[12] is responsible for the formation of circular RNA species which are thought to have a regulatory function.[13-15]

1. Sharp, P.A., The discovery of split genes and RNA splicing, *Trends Biochem. Sci.* 30, 279–281, 2005.
2. Matlin, A., Clark, F., and Smith, C.W., Understanding alternative splicing: Toward a cellular code, *Nat. Rev. Mol. Cell. Biol.* 6, 386–398, 2005.
3. Stetefeld, J., and Ruegg, M.A., Structural and functional diversity generated by alternative mRNA splicing, *Trends Biochem. Sci.* 30, 510–521, 2005.
4. Baralle, F.E., and Giudice, J., Alternative splicing as a regulator of development and tissue identity, *Nat. Rev. Mol. Cell Biol.* 18, 437–451, 2017.
5. Bush, S.J., Chen, L., Tovar-Corona, J.M., and Urrutia, A.O., Alternative splicing and the evolution of phenotypic novelty, *Philos. Trans. R. Soc. Lond. B Biol. Sci.* 372(1713), 201504474, 2017.
6. El Marabti, E., and Younis, I., The cancer spliceosome: Reprogramming of alternative spicing in cancer, *Front. Mol. Biosci.* 5, 80, 2018.
7. Paschalis, A., Sharp, A., Welti, J.C., et al., Alternative splicing in prostate cancer, *Nat. Rev. Clin. Oncol.* 15, 663–675, 2018.
8. Plaschka, C. Lin., P.C., and Nagai, K., Structure of a pre-catalytic spliceosome, *Nature* 546, 617–621, 2017.
9. Wilkinson, M.E., Fica, S.M., Galej, W.P., et al., Postcatalytic spliceosome structure reveals mechanism of 3'-splice site selection, *Science* 358, 1283–1288, 2017.
10. Shi, Y., Mechanistic insights into precursor messenger RNA splicing by the spliceosome, *Nat. Rev. Mol. Cell Biol.* 18, 655–670, 2017.
11. Bohnsack, M.T., and Sloan, K.E., Modifications in small nuclear RNAs and their roles in spliceosome assembly and function, *Biol. Chem.* 399, 1265–1276, 2018.
12. Wan, R., Yan, C., Bai, R., Lei, J., and Shi, Y., Structure of an intron lariat spliceosome from *Saccharomyces cerevisiae*, *Cell* 171, 120–132, 2017.
13. Salzman, J., Circular RNA expression: Its potential regulation and function, *Trends Genet.* 32, 309–316, 2016.
14. Ebbesen, K.K., Hansen, T.B., and Kjems, J., Insights into circular RNA biology, *RNA Biol.* 14, 1035–1045, 2017.
15. Holdt, L.M., Kohlmaier, A., and Teupser, D., Circular RNAs as therapeutics agents and targets, *Front. Physiol.* 9, 1262, 2018.

RIBONUCLEASE III (RNase III)

RNase III was identified as a enzyme involved in degradation in bacteria.[1] Subsequent work showed the RNase III was involved in the metabolism of double-stranded RNA (dsRNA)[2] and in the generation of biological dsRNA species involved in RNA silencing.[3] RNase III constitutes a family of enzymes involved in the processing of dsRNA and gene regulation.[4] Examples include DICER[5–7] and Drosha.[8–10]

1. Nicholson, A.W., Function, mechanism and regulation for bacterial ribonuclease, *FEMS Microbiol. Rev.* 23, 371–390, 1999.
2. Lamontagne, B., Larose, S., Boulanger, J., and Elela, S.A., The RNase III family: A conserved structure and expanding functions in eukaryotic dsRNA metabolism, *Curr. Issues Mol. Biol.* 3, 71–78, 2001.
3. Conrad, C., and Rauhut, R., Ribonuclease III: New sense from nuisance, *Int. J. Biochem.* 34, 116–129, 2002.
4. Court, D.L., Gan, J., Liang, Y.H., et al., RNase III: Genetics and function: Structure and mechanism, *Annu. Rev. Genet.* 47, 405–431, 2013.
5. Tijsterman, M., and Plasterk, R.H., Dicers at RISC; the mechanism of RNAi, *Cell* 117,1–3, 2004.
6. Svobodova, E., Kubikova, J., and Svoboda, P., Production of small RNAs by mammalian Dicer, *Pflugers Arch.* 468, 1089–1102, 2016.
7. Song, M.S., and Rossi, J.J., Molecular mechanism of Dicer: Endonuclease and enzymatic activity, *Biochem. J.* 474, 1603–1618, 2017.
8. Carnell, M.A., and Hannon, G.J., RNase III enzymes and the initiation of gene silencing, *Nat. Struct. Mol. Biol.* 11, 214–218, 2004.
9. Lee, Y., Ahn, C., Han, J., et al., The nuclear RNase III Drosha initiates microRNA processing, *Nature* 425, 415–419, 2003.
10. Kim, B., Jeong, K., and Kim, V.N., Genome-wide mapping of DROSHA cleavage sites on primary microRNAs and noncanonical substrates, *Mol. Cell* 66, 258–269, 2017.

ROLLING

Rolling is a term used to describe the initial interaction between a neutrophil and the luminal wall of a blood vessel (endothelium)[1,2] in process involving interaction between proteins expressed by neutrophils and endothelial cells wall proteins.[3–5] Rolling is preceded by margination of the neutrophils[6,7] and is prior to transit to diapedesis transit to interstitial space through the endothelium).[8,9]

1. Sundd, P., Pospieszalska, M.K., Cheung, L.S., Konstantopoulos, K., and Ley, K., Biomechanics of leukocyte rolling, *Biorheology* 48, 1–35, 2011.
2. Sundd, P., and Pospieszalska, M.K., and Ley, K., Neutrophil rolling at high shear: Flattening, catch bond behavior, tethers and slings, *Mol. Immunol.* 55, 59–69, 2013.
3. von Andrian, U.H., Chambers, J.D., Berg, E.L., et al., L-selectin mediates neutrophil rolling in inflamed venules through sialyl LewisX-dependent and -independent recognition pathways, *Blood* 82, 182–191, 1993.
4. McEver, R.P., Selectins: Initiators of leucocyte adhesion and signalling at the vascular wall, *Cardiovasc. Res.* 107, 331–339, 2015.
5. Zuchtriegel, G., Uhl, B., Hessenauer, M.E.T., et al., Spatiotemporal expression dynamics of selectins govern the sequential extravasation of neutrophils and monocytes in the acute inflammatory response, *Arteriosler. Thromb. Vasc. Biol.* 35, 899–910, 2015.
6. Ley, K., Molecular mechanisms of leucocyte recruitment in the inflammatory process, *Cardiovasc. Res.* 32, 733–742, 1996.
7. Pearson, M.J., and Lipowsky, H.H., Effect of fibrinogen on leukocyte margination and adhesion in postcapillary venules, *Microcirculation* 11, 295–306, 2004.
8. Marki, A., Esko, J.D., Pries, A.R., and Ley, K., Role of the endothelial surface layer in neutrophil recruitment, *J. Leukoc. Biol.* 98, 503–515, 2015.
9. Filippi, M.D., Mechanism of diapedesis: Importance of the transcellular route, *Adv. Immunol.* 129, 25–53, 2016.

RTX (REPEATS IN TOXINS) TOXINS

RTX (Repeats in Toxins) toxins are a family of toxins produced by gram-negative bacteria.[1,2] Canonical RTX toxins can be divided into two categories. Cytolysins are pore-forming proteins such a hemolysins which attack erythrocytes and other eukaryotic cells.[3] The leukotoxins are more specific with specificity toward leukocytes such as macrophages and are important in the process of inflammation,[4,5] However, the RTX toxin family of proteins is quite heterogeneous ranging in size from 40 kDa to 600 kDa[6]; the designation of toxin is contained within the name but the family also contained proteases and other enzymes.[6] The various members of the RTX toxin family the presence of a variable number nonapeptide repeats of glycine and aspartic acid which bind calcium ions. The members of the RTX toxin family also share a common secretory pathway. There are some RTX toxins which are quite different from the canonical cytolysins described above such as the adenyl cyclase toxin from *Bordetella*[7] and the MARTX toxins.[8] Enzymes in the RTX toxin family include a serralysin protease from *Serrratia marcescens*[9] and lipases.[10]

1. Coote, J.G., Structural and functional relationship among the RTX toxin determinants of Gram-negative bacteria, *FEMS Microbiol. Rev.* 8, 137–161, 1992.
2. Lally, E.T., Hill, R.B., Kleba, I.R., and Korostoff, J., The interaction between RTX toxins and target cells, *Trends Microbiol.* 7, 356–361, 1995.

3. Benz, R., Channel formation by RTX-toxins of pathogenic bacteria: Basis of their biological activity, *Biochim. Biophys. Acta* 1858, 526–537, 2016.

4. Johansson, A., *Aggregatibacter actinomycetemcomitans* leukotoxin: A powerful tool with capacity to cause imbalance in the host inflammatory response, *Toxins* 3, 242–259, 2011.

5. Malachowa, N., Kobayashi, S.D., Braughton, K.R., et al., *Staphylococcus aureus* leukotoxin GH promotes inflammation, *J. Infect. Dis.* 206, 1185–1193, 2012.

6. Linhartová, I., Bumba, L., Mašín, J., et al., RTX proteins: A highly diverse family secreted by a common mechanism, *FEMS Microbiol. Rev.* 34, 1076–1112, 2010.

7. Novak, J., Cerny, O., Osickova, A., et al., Structure-function relationships underlying the capacity of *Bordetella* adenylate cyclase toxin to disarm host phagocytes, *Toxins* 9, 300, 2017.

8. Satchell, K.J.F., Structure and function of MARTX toxins and other large repetitive RTX proteins, *Annu. Rev. Microbiol.* 65, 71–90, 2011.

9. Zhang, L., Morrison, A.J., and Thibodeau, P.H., Interdomain contacts and the stability of serralysin protease from *Serratia marcescens*, *PLoS One* 10(9), 0138419, 2015.

10. Ali, M.S., Ganasen, M., Rahman, R.N., et al., Cold-adapted RTX lipase from antartic *Pseudomonas* sp. strain AMS8: Isolation, molecular modeling and heterologous expression, *Protein J.* 32, 317–325, 2013.

S+/L−

The term S+/L− refers to an indicator cell line containing murine sarcoma virus (S+) but does not contain murine leukemia virus (L−) (sarcoma+/leukemia−) which is used to detect replication competent retroviruses such as murine leukemia retroviruses which may be present in producer cell lines or retroviral vectors. The S+/L− assay is common in the manufacturing of various biopharmaceutical products including gene therapy products.[1–6]

1. Adamson, S.R., Experiences of virus, retrovirus and retrovirus-like particles in Chinese hamster ovary (CHO) and hybridoma cells used for production of protein therapeutics, *Dev. Biol. Stand.* 93, 89–96, 1998.

2. Forestell, S.P., Dando, J.S., Böhnlein, E., and Rigg, R.J., Improved detection of replication-competent retrovirus, *J. Virol. Methods* 60, 171–178, 1996.

3. Chen, J., Reeves, L., Sanburn, N., et al., Packaging cell lines DNA contamination of vector supernatants: Implication for laboratory and clinical research, *Virology* 262, 187–197, 2001.

4. Reeves, L., Duffy, L., Koop, S., Fyffe, J., and Cornetta, K., Detection of ecotropic replication-competent retroviruses: Comparison of S+/L− assays, *Human Gene Therapy* 13, 1783–1790, 2002.

5. Duffy, L., Koop, S., Fyffe, J., and Cornetta, K., Extended S+/L− assay for detecting replication-competent retroviruses pseudotype 3d with the RD114 viral envelope, *Preclinica*, 53–59, 2003.

6. Hashimoto-Gotoh, A., Yoshikawa, R., and Miyazawa, T., Comparison between S+L− assay and LacZ marker rescue assay for detecting replication-competent gamma-retroviruses, *Biologicals* 43, 363–368, 2015.

S100 PROTEINS

S100 proteins are a multifunctional family of proteins with intracellular and extracellular function[1–4] The seminal member of the family, S100, was described as an acidic protein found in nervous issues and was distinguished by solubility in saturated ammonium sulfate (100% saturation).[5] S100 proteins are known for their ability to bind calcium ions.[6,7]

1. Passey, R.J., Xu, K., Hume, D.A., and Geczy, C.L., S100A8: Emerging functions and regulations, *J. Leukocyte Biol.* 66, 549–556, 1999.

2. Heizmann, C.W., The multifunctional S100 protein family, *Methods Mol. Biol.* 172, 69–80, 2002.

3. Emberley, E.D., Murphy, L.C., and Watson, P.H., S100 proteins and their influence on pro-survival pathways in cancer, *Biochem. Cell Biol.* 82, 508–515, 2004.

4. Donato, R., Cannon, B.R., Sorci, G., et al., Functions of S100 proteins, *Curr. Mol. Med.* 13, 24–57, 2013.

5. Moore, B.W., A soluble protein characteristic of the nervous system, *Biochem. Biophys. Res. Commun.* 19, 739–744, 1965.

6. Lin, H., Andersen, G.R., and Yatime, L., Crystal structure of human S100A8 in complex with zinc and calcium, *BMC Struct. Biol.* 16(1), 8, 2016.

7. Melville, Z., Aligholizadeh, E., McKnight, L.E., X-ray crystal structure of human calcium-bound S100A1, *Acta Crystallogr. F Struct. Biol. Commun.* 73, 215–221, 2017.

SACTIPEPTIDES

Sactipeptides are a unique group of peptides characterized by a thioether crosslink between cysteine and the α-carbon of another amino acid.[1,2] Sactipeptides are among a number of unusual peptides synthesized by bacteria with antibiotic activity.[3] Sactipeptides are synthesized on ribosomes with the thioether bond formed by the action of sactisynthase, a radical SAM enzyme.[4,5]

1. Kawulka, K., Sprules, T., McKay, R.T., Structure of subtilosin A, an antimicrobial peptide from *Bacillus subtills* with unusual posttranslational modification linking cysteine sulfur α-carbons of phenylalanine and threonine, *J. Am. Chem. Soc.* 125, 4726–4727, 2003.

2. Lohans, C.T., and Vederas, J.C., Structural characterization of thioether bridged bacteriocins, *J. Antibiotics* 67, 23–30, 2015.

3. Arnison, P.G., Bibb, M.J., Bierbaum, G., et al., Ribosomally synthesized and post-translationally modified peptide natural products: Overview and recommendations for a universal nomenclature, *Nat. Prod. Rep.* 30, 108–160, 2013.

4. Flühe, L., and Marahiel, M.A., Radical *S*-adenosylmethionine enzyme catalyzed thioether bond formation in sactipeptide biosynthesis, *Curr. Opin. Chem. Biol.* 17, 605–612, 2013.

5. Grell, T.A.J., Kincannon, W.M., Bruender, N.A., et al., Structural and spectroscopic analyses of the sporulation killing factor biosynthetic enzyme SkfB, a bacterial AdoMet radical sactisynthase, *J. Biol. Chem.* 293, 17349–17361, 2018.

SAPONINS

Saponins are a group of bioactive glycosides found in a variety of plants. Saponins consist of a to terpene component known as an aglycone or sapogenins coupled with a carbodrate[1] Saponins are important as pharmaceutical product, cosmetics, and foods.[2,3] Tubeimosides (terpene saponins) are suggested to be of importance in oncology.[4] It is of interest that gut microbiota metabolized saponins to bioactive forms.[5] It has been reported that saponins can act as adjuvants in the activation of T-cell and antigen presenting cells.[6]

1. Moses, T., Papadopoulos, K.K., and Osbourn, A., Metabolic and functional diversity of saponins, biosynthetic intermediates and semi-synthetic derivatives, *Crit. Rev. Biochem. Mol. Biol.* 49, 439–462, 2014.

2. Murthy, H.N., Dandin, V.S., Park, S.-Y., and Park, K.-Y., Quality, safety and efficacy profiling ginseng adventitious roots produced in vitro, *Appl. Microbiol. Biotechnol.* 102, 7309–7317, 2018.

3. Singh, B., Singh, J.P., Singh, N., and Kaur, A., Saponins in pulses and their health promoting activities: A review, *Food Chem.* 233, 540–549, 2017.

4. Islam, M.S., Wang, C., Zheng, J., et al., The potential role of tubeimosides in cancer prevention and treatment, *Eur. J. Med. Chem.* 162, 109–121, 2019.

5. Kim, D.-H., Gut microbiota-mediated pharmacokinetics of ginseng saponins, *J. Ginseng Res.* 42, 255–263, 2018.

6. Marciani, D.J., Elucidating the mechanisms of action of saponin-derived adjuvants, *Trends Pharmacol. Sci.* 39, 573–585, 2018.

SAPOSINS

Saposin is a term that was given[1-3] to describe small proteins which act as cofactors (e.g. sphingolipid activator protein, coglucosidase) in the hydrolysis of sphingolipids.[4-7] There are four saposins, A, B, C, and D, which are generated from a common precursor, prosaposin.[8] Saposins are suggested to act as detergents in solubilizing sphingolipids. Saposins have been suggested to function in the transfer of phospholipids[9] and in the load of lipids onto CD1 in the process of the presentation of lipid antigens.[10]

1. Morimoto, S., Martin, B.M., Kishimoto, Y., and O'Brien, J.S., Saposin D: A sphingomylinase activator, *Biochem. Biophys. Res. Commun.* 156, 403–410, 1988.

2. Morimoto, S., Martin, B.M., Yamamoto, Y., et al., Saposin A: Second cerebrosidase activator protein, *Proc. Natl. Acad. Sci. USA* 86, 3389–3393, 1989.

3. O'Brien, J.S., and Kishimoto, Y., Saposin proteins: Structure, function, and role in human lysosomal storage disorders, *FASEB J.* 5, 301–308, 1991.

4. Berent, B.L., and Radin, N.S., β-Glucosidase activator protein from bovine spleen ("coglucosidase"), *Arch. Biochem. Biophys.* 208, 248–260, 1981.

5. Li, Y.T., and Li, S.C., Activator proteins for the catabolism of glycosphingolipids, *Adv. Exp. Med. Biol.* 174, 213–226, 1984.

6. Inui, K., and Wenger, D.A., Biochemical, immunological, and structural studies on a sphingolipid activator proteins (SAP-1), *Arch. Biochem. Biophys.* 233, 556–564, 1984.

7. Conzelmann, E., and Sandhoff, K., Activator proteins for lysosomal glycolipid hydrolysis, *Methods Enzymol.* 138, 792–815, 1987.

8. Vaccaro, A.M., Salivioli, R., Tatti, and Ciaffoni, F., Saposins and their interactions with lipids, *Neurochemical Res.* 24, 307–314, 1999.

9. Ciaffoni, F., Tatti, M., Boe, A., et al., Saposin B binds and transfers phospholipids, *J. Lipid Res.* 47, 1045–1053, 2006.

10. Garrido-Arandia, M., Cuevas-Zuviria, B., Diaz-Perales, A., and Pacios, L.E., A comparative study of human saposins, *Molecules* 23(2), E422, 2018.

SCAFFOLD

The term scaffold has several terms of importance in biochemistry and molecular biology. In combinatorial chemistry or parallel synthetic strategy, a scaffold is the common platform which serves the core for synthesis of individual chemical species.[1-6] The term scaffold is also used for matrices for dimensional cell culture[7-11] with emphasis on tissue engineering.[12-20]

1. Barry, J.F., Davis, A.P., and Pérez-Payan, M., A trifunctional steroid-based scaffold for combinatorial chemistry, *Tetrahedron Letters* 40, 2849–2852, 1999.

2. Batra, S., Rastogi, S.K., Kundu, B., Patra, A., and Bhaduri, A.P., A novel isoxazole-based scaffold for combinatorial chemistry, *Tetrahedron Letters* 41, 5971–5974, 2000.

3. Lee, M.-L., and Schneider, G., Scaffold architecture and pharmacophoric properties of natural products and trade drugs: Application in the design of natural product-based combinatorial libraries, *J. Comb. Chem.* 3, 284–289, 2001.

4. Batra, S., Srinivasan, T., Rastogi, S.K., et al., Combinatorial synthesis and biological evaluation of isoxazole-based libraries as antithrombotic agents, *Bioorg. Med. Chem. Lett.* 12, 1905–1908, 2002.

5. Ortholand, J.Y., and Ganesan, A., Natural products and combinatorial chemistry: Back to the future, *Curr. Opin. Chem. Biol.* 8, 271–280, 2004.

6. Janssen, G.V., van den Heuvel, J.A.C., Megens, R.P., Benninghof, J.C.I., and Ovaa, H., Microwave-assisted diastereoselective two-step three-component synthesis for rapid access to drug-like libraries of substituted for rapid access to drug-like libraries of substituted 3-amino-β-lactams, *Bioorg. Med. Chem.* 26, 41–49, 2018.

7. Dutta, R.C., and Dutta, A.K., Cell-interactive 3D-scaffold: Advances and applications, *Biotechnol. Adv.* 27, 334–339, 2009.

8. Hollister, S.J., Scaffold engineering: A bridge to where? *Biofabrication* 1(1), 012001, 2009.

9. Rossi, F., and van Griensven, M., Polymer functionalization as a powerful tool to improve scaffold performance, *Tissue Eng. Part A* 20, 2043–2041, 2014.

10. Nair, A., and Tang, L., Influence of scaffold design on host immune and stem cell responses, *Semin. Immunol.* 29, 62–71, 2017.

11. Yuan, H., Xing, K., and Hsu, H.Y., Trinity of three-dimensional (3D) scaffold, vibration and 3D printing on cell culture application: A systematic review and indicating future direction, *Bioengineering* (Basel) 5(3), E57, 2018.

12. Hammond, J.S., Beckingham, I.J., and Shakesheff, K.M., Scaffolds for liver tissue engineering, *Expert Rev. Med. Devices* 3, 21–27, 2006.

13. Hollister, S.J., Porous scaffold design for tissue engineering, *Nat. Mater.* 4, 518–524, 2005.

14. Li, C., Vepari, C., Jin, H.J., Kim, H.J., and Kaplan, D.L., Electrospun silk-BMP-2 scaffolds for bone tissue engineering, *Biomaterials*, 27(16), 3115–3124, 2006.

15. van Lieshout, M.I., Vaz, C.M., Rutten, M.C., Peters, G.W., and Baaijens, F.P., Electrospinning versus knitting: Two scaffolds for tissue engineering of the aortic valve, *J. Biomater. Sci. Polym. Ed.* 17, 77–89, 2006.

16. Rai, V., Dilisio, M.F., Dietz, N.E., and Agrawal, D.K., Recent strategies in cartilage repair: A systematic review of the scaffold development and tissue engineering, *Biomed. Mater. Res. A.* 105, 2343–2354, 2017.

17. Ning, L., and Chen, X., A brief review of extrusion-based tissue scaffold bio-printing, *Biotechnol. J.* 12(8), 1600671, 2017.

18. Ovsianikov, A., Khademhosseini, A., and Mironov, V., The synergy of scaffold-based and scaffold-free tissue engineering strategies, *Trends Biotechnol.* 36, 348–357, 2018.

19. Zhou, Y., Chyu, J., and Zumwalt, M., Recent progress of fabrication of cell scaffold by electrospinning technique for articular cartilage tissue engineering, *Int. J. Biomater.* 2018, 1953636, 2018.

20. Chen, X., Fan, H., Deng, X., et al., Scaffold structural microenvironmental cues to guide tissue regeneration in bone tissue applications, *Nanomaterials* (Basel) 8(11), E960, 2018.

SCRAMBLED PEPTIDE

A scrambled peptide is a random sequence generated from the same amino acids in a test peptide. This approach is used to determine specificity of the biological activity of a peptide.[1-8] In other words, the use of a scrambled peptide established the importance of sequence as opposed to composition.

1. Ohki, K., Kumagai, K., Mitsuda, S., Takano, T., Kimura, T., and Ikuta, K., Characterization of a unique scrambled peptide derived from the CD4 CDR3-related region which shows substantial activity for blocking HIV-1 infection, *Vaccine* 11, 682–686, 1993.

2. Gordon, Y.J., Huang, L.C., Romanowski, E.G., et al., Human cathelicidin (LL-37), a multifunctional peptide, is expressed by ocular surface epithelia and has potent antibacterial and antiviral activity, *Curr. Eye. Res.* 30, 385–394, 2005.

3. Loiarro, M., Sette, C., Gallo, G., et al., Peptide-mediated interference of TIR domain dimerization in MyD88 inhibits interleukin-1-dependent activation of NF-κB, *J. Biol. Chem.* 280, 15809–15814, 2005.

4. Arumugam, T.V., Chan S.L., Jo, D.-G., et al., Gamma secretase-mediated Notch signaling worsens brain damage and functional outcome in ischemic stroke, *Nature Med.* 12, 621–623, 2006.

5. Yoshida, Y., Kurokawa, T., Nishikawa, Y., et al., Laminin-1-derived scrambled peptide AG73T disaggregates laminin-1-induced ovarian cancer cell spheroids and improves the efficacy of cisplatin, *Int. J. Oncol.* 32, 673–681, 2008.

6. Jordan, R.E., Fernandez, J., Brezski, R.J., et al., A peptide immunization approach to counteract a *Staphylococcus aureus* protease defense against host immunity, *Immunol. Lett.* 172, 29–39, 2016.

7. Mao, Y., Nguyen, T., Tonkin, R.S., et al., Characterisation of Peptide 5 systemic administration for treating traumatic spinal cord injured rats, *Exp. Brain Res.* 235, 3033–3048, 2017.

8. Zeng, B., Devadoss, D., Wang, S., et al., Inhibition of pressure-activated cancer cell adhesion by FAK-derived peptides, *Oncotarget* 8, 98051–98067, 2017.

Sec-DEPENDENT

The term Sec-dependent refers the general secretory pathway which in bacteria refers to the translocation of proteins across the cytoplasmic membrane into the periplasm in bacteria or the translocation of proteins across the endoplasmic reticulum in eukaryotes.[1,2] The Sec pathways involve the participation of specific proteins[3] such as PpiD.[4]

1. Stephenson, K., Sec-dependent protein translocation across biological membranes: Evolutionary conservation of an essential protein transport pathway, *Mol. Memb. Biol.* 22, 17–28, 2005.

2. Beckwith, J., The Sec-dependent pathway, *Res. Microbiol.* 164, 497–504, 2013.

3. Rusch, S.L., and Kendall, D.A., Interactions that drive Sec-dependent bacterial protein transport, *Biochemistry* 46, 9665–9673, 2007.

4. Fürst, M., Zhou, Y., Merfort, J., and Müller, M., Involvement of PprD in Sec-dependent protein translocation, *Biochim. Biophys. Actg Mol. Cell. Res.* 1865, 273–280, 2018.

SECRETASE

The term secretase is used to describe those proteolytic activities involved in the processing of amyloid precursor protein (APP) to yield the soluble circulating amyloid protein. There are three described secretases involved in amyloid processing that are defined by the site of cleavage in APP; α-Secretase also known as ADAM10,[1,2] β-secretase also known as BACE1 (β-site APP cleaving enzyme 1),[3,4] and γ-secretase which contains presenilin as the catalytic component.[5–7] Secretases have been involved in activity other than cleavage of amyloid proteins.[8–14]

1. Vincent, B., Regulation of the α-secretase ADAM10 at transcriptional, translational and post-translational levels, *Brain Res. Bull.* 126, 154–169, 2016.

2. Peron, R., Vatanabe, I.P., Manzine, P.R., Camis, A., and Cominetti, M.R., Alpha-secretaase ADAM10 regulation: Insights into Alzheimer's disease treatment, *Pharmaceuticals* (Basel) 11(1), E12, 2018.

3. Araki, W., Post-translational regulation of the β-secretase BACE1, *Brain Res. Bull.* 126, 170–177, 2016.

4. Moussa, C.E., Beta-secretase inhibitors in phase I and phase II clinical trials for Alzheimer's disease, *Expert. Opin. Investig. Drugs* 26, 1131–1136, 2017.

5. Tomita, T., Molecular mechanism of intramembrane proteolysis by γ-secretase, *J. Biochem.* 156, 195–201, 2014.

6. Stiller, I., Lizák, B., and Bánhegyi, G., Physiological functions of presenilins: Beyond γ-secretase, *Curr. Pharm. Biotechnol.* 15, 1019–1025, 2014.

7. Aguayo-Ortiz, R., and Dominguez, L., Simulating the γ-secretase enzyme: Recent advances and future directions, *Biochemie* 147, 130–135, 2018.

8. Hoooper, N.M., Karran, E.H., and Turner, A.J., Membrane protein secretases, *Biochem. J.* 321, 265–279, 1997.

9. Mezyk, R., Browska, M., and Bereta, J., Structure and functions of tumor necrosis factor-alpha converting enzyme, *Acta Biochim. Pol.* 50, 625–645, 2003.

10. Wolfe, M.S., and Kopan, R., Intramembrane proteolysis, *Science* 305, 1119–1123, 2004; The term secretase has been used to describe the activity responsible for the release of TNF from membranes.

11. Lee, S.M., Jeong, Y.H., Kim, H.M., et al., Presenilin enhancer-2 (PSENEN), a component of the gamma-secretase complex, is involved in adipocyte differentiation, *Domest. Anim. Endocrinol.* 37, 170–180, 2009.

12. Han, J., and Shen, Q., Targeting γ-secretase in breast cancer, *Breast Cancer* 4, 83–90, 2012.

13. Inoue, T., Zhang, P., Zhang, W., et al., γ-secretase promotes membrane insertion of the human papillomavirus L2 capsid protein during virus infection, *J. Cell. Biol.* 217, 3545–3559, 2018.

14. Merilahti, J.A.M., and Elenius, K., Gamma-secretase-dependent signaling of receptor tyrosine kinases, *Oncogene*, in press (doi:10.1038/s41388-018-045-z), 2018.

SELECTIVITY FACTOR

In one definition, the selectivity factor is the kinetics discrimination shown by a compound in reacting with two or more position on the same compound such as benzene or toluene (e.g. *meta* vs *para*)[1] or in the kinetic discrimination of racemic mixtures.[2,3] It is quantitatively expressed by ratios of rate constants of the competing reactions, or by the decadic logarithms of such ratios.[1–3] It also refers to the differential affinity of compounds to a chromatographic matrix. Chromatographic selectivity is a determining factor in resolution between various components of a mixture and can be expressed as the ratio of the retention time of two components of a mixture.[4–9] In this context, the selectivity factor may be referred to as separation factor or just selectivity. The term selectivity factor also describes a transcription factor (SL-1) for RNA polymerase I (Pol I).[10–15]

1. Brown, H.C., and Smoot, C.R., Isomer distribution and partial rate factors in the gallium bromide catalyzed alkylation of benzene and toluene. The selectivity factor, S_f in electrophilic substitution, *J. Am. Chem. Soc.* 78, 6255–6259, 1956.

2. Ferreira, E.M., and Strolz, B.M., The palladium-catalyzed oxidative kinetic resolution of secondary alcohols with molecular oxygen, *J. Am. Chem. Soc.* 123, 7725–7726, 2001.

3. Das, S., Majumdar, N., De, C.K., et al., Asymmetric catalysis of the carbonyl-amine condensation: Kinetic resolution of primary amines, *J. Am. Chem. Soc.* 139, 1357–1359, 2017.

4. Glajch, J.L., Kirkland, J.J., and Squire, K.M., Optimization of solvent strength and selectivity for reversed-phase liquid chromatography using an interactive mixture-design statistical technique, *J. Chromatog.* 199, 57–79, 1980.

5. Sellergren, B., Ekberg, B., and Mosbach, K., Molecular imprinting of amino acid derivatives in microporous polymers. Demonstration of substrate- and enantioselectivity by chromatographic resolution of racemic mixtures of amino acid derivatives, *J. Chromatog.* 347, 1–10, 1985.

6. Sander, L.C., and Wise, S.A., Effect of phase length on column selectivity for the separation of polycyclic aromatic hydrocarbons by reversed-phase liquid chromatography, *Anal. Chem.* 59, 2309–2313, 1987.

7. Rathnasekara, R., and El Rassi, Z., Polar silica-based stationary phases. Part II- Neutral silica stationary phases with surface bound maltose and sorbitol for hydrophilic interaction liquid chromatography, *J. Chromatog. A.* 1508, 24–32, 2017.

8. Gritti, F., Besner, S., Cormier, S., and Gilar, M., Applications of high-resolution recycling liquid chromatography: From small to large molecules, *J. Chromatog. A* 1524, 108–120, 2017.

9. De Boevre, M., Van Poucke, C., and Ediage E.N., Ultra-high-performance supercritical fluid chromatography as a separation tool for *Fusarium* mycotoxins and their modified forms, *J. AOAC Intn.*101, 627–632, 2018.

10. Learned, R.M., Cordes, S., and Tjian, R., Purification and characterization of a transcription factor that confers promoter specificity to human RNA polymerase I, *Mol. Cell. Biol.* 5, 1358–1369, 1985.

11. Comai, L., Tanese, N., and Tjian R., The TATA-binding protein and associated factors are integral components of the RNA polymerase I transcription factor, SL1, *Cell* 68, 965–976, 1992.

12. Rudloff, U., Eberhard, D., and Grummt, I., The conserved core domain of the human TATA binding protein is sufficient to assemble the multisubunit RNA polymerase I-specific transcription factor SL1, *Proc. Natl. Acad. Sci. USA* 91, 8229–8233, 1994.

13. Comai, L., Song, Y., Tan, C., and Bui, T., Inhibition of RNA polymerase I transcription in differentiated myeloid leukemia cells by inactivation of selectivity factor 1, *Cell Growth Differ.* 11, 63–70, 2000.

14. Xu, S., and Hori, R.T., Identification of a domain within human TAF(I)48, a subunit of selectivity factor I, that interacts with helix 2 of TBP, *Gene* 338, 177–186, 2004.

15. Russell, J., and Zomerdijk, J.C., The RNA polymerase I transcription machinery, *Biochem. Soc. Symp.* (73), 203–216, 2006.

SELEX

SELEX is an acronym for systematic evolution of nucleic acid ligands by exponential enrichment. This is an iterative process based on combinatorial chemistry product short single-stranded oligonucleotides with specific binding properties for a specific target.[1-6] The initial work on SELEX focuses on the development of aptamers specific for individual proteins. More recent work has extended SELEX for the development of aptamers specific for cells.[7-12]

1. Tuerk, C., and Gold, L., Systematic evolution of ligands by exponential enrichment: RNA ligands to bacteriophage T4 DNA polymerase, *Science* 249, 505–510, 1990.

2. Klug, S.J., and Famulok, M., All you wanted to know about SELEX, *Mol. Biol. Rep.* 20, 97–107, 1994.

3. Joyce, G.J., In vitro evolution of nucleic acids, *Curr. Opin. Struct. Biol.* 4, 331–336, 1994.

4. Stoltenburg, R., Reinemann, C., and Strehlitz, B., FluMag-SELEX as an advantageous method for DNA aptamer selection, *Anal. Bioanal. Chem.* 383, 83–91, 2005.

5. Gopinath, S.C.B., Methods developed for SELEX, *Anal. Bioanal. Chem.* 387, 171–182, 2007.

6. Darmostuk, M., Rimpelova, S., Ghelcova, H., and Ruml, T., Current approaches in SELEX: An update to aptamer selection technology, *Biotechnol. Adv.* 33, 1141–1161, 2015.

7. Phillips, J.A., Lopez-Colon, D., Zhu, A., Xu, Y., and Tan, W., Applications in cancer cell biology, *Anal. Chim. Acta* 621, 101–108, 2008.

8. Fang, X., and Tan, W., Aptamers generated from cell-SELEX for molecular medicine: A chemical biology approach, *Accts. Chem. Res.* 43, 48–57, 2010.

9. Fafinska, J., Czech, A., Sitz, T., Ignatova, Z., and Hahn, U., DNA aptamers for the malignant transformation marker CD24, *Nucleic Acid Ther.* 28, 326–334, 2018.

10. Li, W.M., Zhou, L.L., Zheng, M., and Fang, J., Selection of metastatic breast cancer cell-specific aptamers for the capture of CTCs with a metastatic phenotype by cell-SELEX, *Mol. Ther. Nucleic Acids* 12, 707–717, 2018.

11. Haghighi, M., Knanahmad, H., and Palizban, A., A selection and characterization of single-stranded DNA aptamers binding human B-cell surface protein CD20 by cell-SELEX, *Molecules* 23(4), E715, 2018.

12. Kaur, H., Recent developments in cell-SELEX technology for aptamer selection, *Biochim. Biophys. Acta Gen. Subj,* 1862, 2323–2329, 2018.

SEPARASE

Separase is a large (Mr≈220 kDa)[1] cysteine protease which dissolves cohesion in the metaphase t0 anaphase transition in mitotic procession.[2-6] This is highly regulated process involving inhibition by the chaperone securin and cyclin B1 prior to anaphase.[7-9] Separase is activated by the ubiquitin-dependent proteolytic degradation of securing.[10,11]

1. Viadiu, H., Stemmann, O., Kirschner, M.W., and Walz, T., Domain structure of separase and its binding to securing as determined by EM, *Nature Struc. Mol. Biol.* 12, 552–553, 2005.

2. Uhlmann, F., Secured cutting: Controlling separase at the metaphase to anaphase transition, *EMBO Rep.* 2, 487–492, 2001.

3. Hearing, C.H., and Nasmyth, K., Building and breaking bridges between sister chromatids, *Bioessays* 25, 1178–1191, 2003.

4. Uhlmann F., The mechanism of sister chromatid cohesion, *Exp. Cell Res.* 296, 80–85, 2004.

5. Ross, K.E., and Cohen-Fix, O., Separase: A conserved protease separating more than just sisters. *Trends Cell Biol.* 12(1), 1–3, 2002.

6. Hirano, T., Chromosome dynamics during mitosis, *Cold Spring Harb. Perspect. Biol.* 7(6), a015792, 2015.

7. Yanagida, M., Cell cycle mechanisms of sister chromatid separation: Roles of Cut1/separin and Cut2/securin. *Genes Cells* 5, 1–8, 2000.
8. Shindo, N., Kumada, K., and Hirota, T., Separase sensor reveals dual roles for separase coordinating cohesion cleavage and Cdk1 inhibition, *Develop. Cell.* 23, 112–123, 2012.
9. Luo, S., and Tong, L., Structural biology of the separase-securin complex with crucial roles in chromosome segregation, *Curr. Opin. Struct. Biol.* 49, 114–122, 2018.
10. Farr, K.A., and Cohen-Fix, O., The metaphase to anaphase transition: A case of productive destruction, *Eur. J. Biochem.* 263, 14–19, 1999.
11. Wei, R., Li, B., Guo, J., et al., Smurf1 targets securing for ubiquitin-dependent degradation and regulates the metaphase-to-anaphase transition, *Cell Signal.* 38, 60–66, 2017.

SEPARATION FACTOR

Separation factor (also known as selectivity factor) is designated by the term α and refers to the relative affinity of two components for a chromatographic matrix and related to the resolution. By definition the separation factor is larger than 1 and could be described by the following expression; $\alpha = t_2/t_1$ where t_2 is the elution time for the apex of the more slowly moving solute and t_1 is the elution time for the apex of the more rapidly moving solute.[1-5] The term separation factor is used in separation science, mainly in chromatography[6] but also in other techniques such as capillary electrophoresis.[7] In this sense, separation factor differs from selectivity factor which is used in contexts outside of separation science. See **selectivity factor**.

1. Chen, Y., Kele, M., Quinones, I., Sellergren, B., and Guiochon, G., Influence of the pH on the behavior of an imprinted polymeric stationary phase—Supporting evidence for a binding site model, *J. Chromatog. A* 927, 1–17, 2001.
2. Avramescu, M.E., Borneman, Z., and Wessling, M., Mixed-matrix membrane adsorbers for protein separation, *J. Chromatog. A* 1006, 2003.
3. Ziomek, G., Kaspereit, M., Jezowski, J., Seidel-Morgenstern, A., and Antos, D., Effect of mobile phase composition on the SMB processes efficiency. Stochastic optimization of isocratic and gradient operation, *J. Chromatog. A* 1070, 111–124, 2005.
4. Lesellier, E., and Tchapla, A., A simple subcritical chromatographic test for an extended ODS high performance liquid chromatography column classification, *J. Chromatog. A.* 1100, 45–59, 2005.
5. Lapointe, J.F., Gauthier, S.F., Pouliot, Y., and Bouchard, C., Selective separation of cationic peptides from a tryptic hydrolyzate of beta-lactoglobulin by electrofiltration, *Biotechnol. Bioeng.* 94, 223–233, 2006.
6. Khatiashvili, T., Kakava, R., Matarashvili, I., et al., Separation of enantiomers of selected chiral sulfoxides with cellulose tris(4-chloro-3-methylphenylcarbamate)-based chiral columns in high-performance liquid chromatography with very high separation factor, *J. Chromatog. A* 1545, 59–66, 2018.
7. Bowser, M.T., Bebault, G.M., Peng, X., and Chen, D.D., Redefining the separation factor: A potential pathway to a unified separation science, *Electrophoresis* 18, 2928–2934, 1997.

SERCA

Sarcoplasmic reticulum Ca^{2+} ATPase, responsible for calcium ion transport.[1,2]

1. Martonosi, A.N., and Pikula, S., The structure of the Ca^{2+}-ATPase of sarcoplasmic reticulum, *Acta Biochim. Pol.* 50, 337–365, 2003.
2. Strehler, E.E., and Treiman, M., Calcium pumps of plasma membrane and cell interior, *Curr. Mol. Med.* 4, 323–335, 2004.

SEREX

Serological identification of antigens by recombinant expression cloning.[1-4]

1. Sahin, U., et al., Human neoplasms elicit multiple specific immune responses in the autologous host, *Proc. Natl. Acad. Sci. USA* 92, 11810–11813, 1995.
2. Chen, Y.-T., et al., A testicular antigen aberrantly expressed in human cancers detected by autologous antibody screening, *Proc. Natl. Acad. Sci. USA*, 94, 1914–1918, 1997.
3. Fernandez, M.F., et al., Improved approach to identify cancer-associated autoantigens, *Autoimmun. Rev.* 4, 230–235, 2005.
4. www.licr.org/SEREX.html; www2.licr.org/Cancer ImmunomeDB/.

SERIAL LECTIN AFFINITY CHROMATOGRAPHY

The use of a series of two or more lectin affinity chromatography columns of known specificity for the fractionation of oligosaccharides, glycoproteins, or glycopeptides into structurally distinct groups.[1-7]

1. Cummings, R.D., and Kornfeld, S., Fractionation of asparagine-linked oligosaccharides by serial lectin-agarose affinity chromatography. A rapid, sensitive, and specific technique, *J. Biol. Chem.* 257, 11235–11240, 1982.
2. Qiu, R., and Regnier, F.E., Comparative glycoproteomics of N-linked complex-type glycoforms containing sialic acid in human serum, *Anal. Chem.* 77, 7725–7231, 2005.

3. Durham, M., and Regnier, F.E., Targeted glycoproteomics: Serial lectin affinity chromatography in the selection of *O*-glycosylation sites on proteins form the human blood proteome, *J. Chromatog. A* 1132, 165–173, 2006.
4. Yamashita, K., and Ohkura, T., Determination of glycan motifs using serial lectin affinity chromatography, *Methods Mol. Biol.* 1200, 79–92, 2014.
5. Zhu, F., Clemmer, D.E., and Trinidad, J.C., Characterization of lectin binding affinities *via* direct LC-MS profiling: Implications for glycopeptide enrichment and separation strategies, *Analyst* 142, 65, 2017.
6. Lehoux, S., and Ju, T., Separation of two distinct *O*-glycoforms of human IgA by serial lectin chromatography follow by mass spectrometry *O*-glycan analysis, *Method Enzymol.* 585, 67–75, 2017.
7. Zhang, C., Rodriguez, E., Bi, C., et al., High performance affinity chromatography and related separation methods for the analysis of biological and pharmaceutical agents, *Analyst* 143, 374, 2018.

SERPIN

Serpin developed into a term in own right. The term serpin was developed as an acronym for serine protease inhibitor[1] but is now considered to be a structurally homologous superfamily of proteins having masses in the range of 40 kDa to 100 kDa.[2–7] Serpins are considered to be metastable proteins such the transition to a stable form is associated with the inactivation of the cognate protease(s).[8–14] The ability of a serpin to be able to fold to a "stable" metastable state is an interesting problem.[15]

1. Carroll, R.W., and Travis, J., *α*-1-antitrypsin and the serpins: Variation and countervariation, *Trends Biochem. Sci.* 10, 20–24, 1985.
2. Hunt, L.T., and Dayhoff, M.O., A surprisingly new protein superfamily containing ovalbumin, antithrombin III, and alpha-1-proteinase inhibitor, *Biochem. Biophys. Res. Commun.* 95, 864–871, 1980.
3. Potempa, J., Korzus, E., and Travis, J., The serpin superfamily of proteinase inhibitors: Structure, function, and regulation, *J. Biol. Chem.* 269, 15957–15960, 1994.
4. Gettins, P.G., Patston, P.A., and Olson, S.T., *Serpins: Structure, Function and Biology*, R.G. Landes, Austin, Texas, 1995.
5. *Chemistry and Biology of Serpins* (*Advances in Experimental Medicine and Biology*, volume 415), ed. F.C. Church, Plenum Press, New York, 1997.
6. *Serpins and Protein Kinase Inhibitors: Novel Functions, Structural Features and Molecular Mechanisms*, ed. B. Georgiev and S. Markovski, Nova Scientific Publishers, New York, 2010.
7. *The Serpin Family: Proteins with Multiple Functions in Health and Disease*, Springer International Publishing, Cham, Switzerland, 2015.
8. Gettins, P., Patson, P.A., and Schapira, M., The role of conformational change in serpin structure and function, *Bioessays* 15, 461–467, 1993.
9. Schulze, A.J., Huber, R., Bode, W., and Engh, R.A., Structural aspects of serpin inhibition, *FEBS Lett.* 344, 117–124, 1994.
10. Lawrence, D.A., The role of reactive-center loop mobility in the serpin inhibitory mechanism, *Adv. Exp. Med. Biol.* 425, 99–108, 1997.
11. Whisstock, J., Skinner, R., and Lesk, A.M., An atlas of serpin conformations, *Trends Biochem. Sci.* 23, 63–67, 1998.
12. Gettins, P.G., Serpin structure, mechanism, and function, *Chem. Rev.* 102, 4751–4804, 2002.
13. Huntington, J.A., Shape-shifting serpins—Advantages of a mobile mechanism, *Trends Biochem. Sci.* 31, 427–435, 2006.
14. Whisstock, J.C., and Bottomley, S.P., Molecular gymnastics: Serpin structure, folding and misfolding, *Curr. Opin. Struct. Biol.* 16, 761–768, 2006.
15. Rao, V.V.H.G., and Gosavi, S., On the folding of a structurally complex protein to its metastable active state, *Proc. Natl. Acad. Sci. USA* 115, 1998–2003, 2018.

SHOTGUN PROTEOMICS

Shotgun proteomics (also known as bottom up proteomics) is method for the identification of proteins in complex mixtures based on mass spectrometric analysis of peptides obtained by the enzymatic or chemical digestion of the entire proteome. A naturally occurring protein mixture such as cell extract, blood plasma or other biological fluid is reduced, alkylated, and subjected to tryptic hydrolysis. The tryptic hydrolysis is fractionated by liquid chromatography and analyzed by mass spectrophotometry.[1–7]

1. Yao, X., Freas, A., Ramirez, J., Demirev, P.A., and Feselau, C., Proteolytic [18]O labeling for comparative proteomics: Model studies with two serotypes of adenovirus, *Anal. Chem.* 73, 2836–2842, 2001.
2. Wolters, D.A., Washburn, M.P., and Yates, J.R., III, An automated multidimensional protein identification technology for shotgun proteomics, *Anal. Chem.* 73, 5683–5690, 2001.
3. Liu, H., Sadygov, R.G., and Yates, J.R., III, A model for random sampling and estimation of relative protein abundance in shotgun proteomics, *Anal. Chem.* 76, 4193–4201, 2004.
4. Rauniyar, N., and Yates, J.R., Isobaric labeling-based relative quantification in shotgun proteomics, *J. Proteome Res.* 13, 5393–5309, 2014.
5. Lereim, R.R., Oveland, E., Beryen, F.S., Vaudel, M., and Barsnes, H., Visualization, inspection and interpretation of shotgut proteomics identification results, *Adv. Exp. Med. Biol.* 919, 227–235, 2016.

6. The, M., and Käll, L., Integrated identification and quantification error probabilities for shotgun proteomics, *Mol. Cell Proteomics* 18, 561–570, 2019.

7. HaileMariam, M., Equez, R.V., Singh, H., et al., S-Trap, an ultrafast sample-preparation approach for shotgun proteomics, *J. Proteome Res.* 17, 2917–2924, 2018.

SHUGOSHIN

The term shugoshin (Japanese word for guardian spirit) describes protein family having a role in the centromeric protection of cohesion; protects the centromeric cohesion at meiosis I by inhibiting the action of separase on cohesion.[1–10] Shugoshin may consist of a single protein, Sgo1 in *Saccharomyces cerevisiae* MEI-S332 in *Drosophila,* or two proteins SGO1 and SGO2 in humans.[11]

1. Kitajima, T.S., Kawashima, S.A., and Watanabe, Y., The conserved kinetochore protein shugoshin protects centromeric cohesion during meiosis, *Nature* 427, 510–517, 2005.

2. Salic, A., Waters, J.C., and Mitchison, T.J., Vertebrate shugoshin links sister centromere cohesion and kinetochore microtubule stability in mitosis, *Cell* 118, 567–578, 2004; Goulding, S.E., and Earnshaw, W.C., Shugoshin: A centromeric guardian senses tension, *Bioessays* 27, 588–591, 2005.

3. Watanabe, Y., Shugoshin: Guardian spirit at the centromere, *Curr. Opin. Cell. Biol.* 17, 590–595, 2005.

4. Stemmann, O., Boos, D., and Gorr, I.H., Rephrasing anaphase: Separase FEARs shugoshin, *Chromosoma* 113, 409–417, 2005.

5. Mcgee, P., Molecular biology: Chromosome guardian on duty, *Nature* 441, 35–37, 2006.

6. Gregan, J., Spirek, M., and Rumpf, C., Solving the shugoshin puzzle, *Trends Genet.* 24, 205–207, 2008.

7. Macy, B., Wang, M., and Yu, H.G., The many faces of shugoshin, the "guardian sprit," in chromosome segregation, *Cell Cycle* 8, 35–37, 2009.

8. Clift, D., and Marston, A.L., The role of shugoshin in meiotic chromosome segregation, *Cytogenet. Genome Res.* 133, 234–242, 2011.

9. Gutiérrez-Caballero, C., Cebollaro, L.R., and Pendás, A.M., Shugoshins: From protectors of cohesion to versatile adaptors at the centromere, *Trends Genet.* 28, 351–360, 2012.

10. Buehl, C.J., and Kuo, M.H., Critical role of Shugoshin and histones as tension sensors during mitosis, *Curr. Genet.* 64, 1215–1219, 2018.

11. Watanabe, Y., Sister chromatid cohesion along arms and at centromeres, *Trends Genet.* 21, 405–412, 2005.

SIGMA FACTOR

Sigma factor is a general transcription factor for bacterial RNA polymerase which is essential for the start of transcription and dissociates from bacterial RNA polymerase as the end of transcription.[1–5]

1. Mooney, R.A., Darst, S.A., and Landick, R., Sigma and RNA polymerase: An on-again, off-again relationship? *Mol. Cell.* 20, 335–345, 2005.

2. Wigneshwerraj, S.R., Burrows, P.C., Bordes, P., et al., The second paradigm for activation of transcription, *Prog. Nucl. Acid Res. Mol. Biol.* 79, 339–369, 2005.

3. Alberts, B., Johnson, A., Lewis, J., et al., *Molecular Biology of the Cell,* 6th edn., Chapter 6, How cells read the genome: From DNA to protein, pp. 299–368, Garland Science/Taylor & Francis Group, New York, 2014.

4. Marchetti, M., Malinowska, A., Heller, I., and Wuite, G.J.L., How to switch the motor on: RNA polymerase initiation steps at the single molecules level, *Protein Sci.* 26, 1303–1313, 2017.

5. Davis, M.C., Kesthely, C.A., Franklin, E.A., and MacLellan, S.R., The essential activities of the bacterial sigma factor, *Canad. J. Microbiol.* 63, 89–99, 2017.

SIGNALOSOME

A signalosome is a large intracellular protein complex ($M_r \approx 400$ kDa) which can have a variety of functions depending on composition.[1–5] Some signalosomes (e.g. COP9, JabI)[3] have been considered to be zomes.[6] I could not find a specific definition for zomes, but an internet search suggests that the term can refer to a building of irregular construction. The first signalosome was identified as a macromolecular complex in *Arabidopsis* which regulates constitutive photomorphogenesis).[7,8] It was subsequently shown that there was homology between COP9 and the regulatory subunit of the 26S proteasome.[9–11] The nature of the signalosome has extended beyond these initial observations.[4–6,12–16] A relationship of the signalosome to the endosome has been suggested.[17]

1. Dubiel, D., Rockel, B., Naumann, M., and Dubiel, W., Diversity of COP9 signalosome structures and functional consequences, *FEBS Lett.* 589, 2507–2513, 2015.

2. Meister, C., Gulko, M.K., Köhler, A.M., and Braus, G.H., The devil is in the details: Comparison between COP9 signalosome (CSN) and the LID of the 26S proteasome, *Curr. Gener.* 62, 129–136, 2016.

3. LI, P., Xie, L., Gu, Y., Li, J., and Xie, J., Roles of multifunctional COP9 signalosome complex in cell fate and implications for drug discovery, *J. Cell. Physiol.* 232, 1246–1253, 2017.

4. DeBruine, Z.J., Xu, H.E., and Melcher, K., Assembly and architecture of the Wnt/β-catenin signalosome at the membrane, *Brit. J. Pharmacol.* 174, 4564–4574, 2017.

5. Kumar, S., and Jain, S., Immune signaling by supramolecular assemblies, *Immunology* 155, 435–445, 2018.

6. Chang, E.C., and Schwechheimer, C., ZOMES III: The interface between signalling and proteolysis, *EMBO Reports* 5, 1041–1045, 2004.

7. Wei, N., Chamovitz, D.A., and Deng, X.-W., Arabidopsis COP9 is a component of A novel signaling complex mediating light control of development, *Cell* 79, 117–124, 1994.

8. Chamovitz, D.A., Wei, N., Osterlund, M.T., et al., The COP9 complex: A novel multisubunit nuclear regulator involved in light control of a plant developmental switch, *Cell* 86, 115–121, 1996.

9. Glickman, M.H., Ruben, D.M., Coux, O., et al., A subcomplex of the proteasome regulatory particle is required for ubiquitin-conjugate degradation and related to the COP-singnalosome and eIF3, *Cell* 94, 615–623, 1998.

10. Seeger, M., Kraft, R., Ferrell, K., et al., A novel protein complex involved in signal transduction possessing similarities to 26S proteasome subunits, *FASEB J.* 12, 469–478, 1998.

11. Wei, N., Tsuge, T., Serino, G., et al., The COP9 complex is conserved between plants and mammals and is related to the 26S proteasome regulatory complex, *Current Biol.* 8, 919–922, 1998.

12. Jane-wit, D., Surovtseva, Y.V., Qin, L., Complement membrane attack complexes activate noncanonical NF-κB by forming an Akt+ NIK+ signalosome on Rab5+ endosomes, *Proc. Natl. Acad. Sci. USA* 112, 9686–9691, 2015.

13. Harrison, B.J., Venkat, G., Lamb, J.L., et al., The adaptor protein CD2AP is a coordinator of neurotrophin signaling-mediated axon arber plasticity, *J. Neurosci.* 36, 4259–4275, 2016.

14. Venuti, A., Pastori, C., Siracursano, G., et al., The abrogation of phosphorylation plays a relevant role in the CCR5 signalosome formation with natural antibodies to CCR5, *Viruses* 10(1), E9, 2017.

15. Galgano, D., Onnis, A., Pappaloardo, E., et al., The T-cell IFT20 interactome reveals new players in immune synapse assembly, *J. Cell. Sci.* 130, 1110–1121, 2017.

16. Gorby, C., Martinez-Fabregas, J., Wilmes, S., and Morago, I., Mapping determinnants of cytokine signaling via protein engineering, *Front. Immunol.* 9, 2143, 2018.

17. Perret, E., Lakkaraju, A., Deborde, S., et al., Evolving endosomes: How many varieties and why? *Curr. Opin. Cell Biol.* 17, 423–434, 2005.

SIGNAL RECOGNITION PARTICLE

A signal recognition particle is a targeting chaperone involved in the transmembrane transport of proteins.[1–5] The action of the signal recognition particle involves the recognition of the signal peptide.

1. Pool, M.R., Signal recognition particles in chloroplasts, bacteria, yeast, and mammals, *Molec. Membrane Biol.* 22, 3–15, 2004.

2. Akopian, D., Shen, K., Zhang, X., and Shan, S.O., Signal recognition particle: An essential protein-targeting machine, *Annu. Rev. Biochem.* 82, 693–721, 2013.

3. Zhang, X., and Shan, S.O., Fidelity of cotranslational protein targeting by the signal recognition particle, *Annu. Rev. Biophys.* 43, 381–408, 2014.

4. Gupta, S., Roy, M., and Ghosh, A., The archaeal signal recognition particle: Present understanding and future perspective, *Curr. Microbiol.* 74, 284–297, 2017.

5. Mercier, E., Holtkamp, W., Rodnina, M.V., and Wintermeyer, W., Signal recognition particle binding to translating ribosomes before emergence of a signal anchor sequence, *Nucleic Acids Res.* 45, 11858–11866, 2017.

SIGNATURE DOMAIN

The signature domain is an amino acid sequence that is closely conserved within a group of proteins and is considered unique to that group of proteins which is also called a protein family. The sequences may or may not have homologous function.[1] In this sense, the use of the term signature is related to historical use of this term to describe a physical property or feature of a plant or other natural object as an indication of pharmacological impact because of relation of such feature to the body part.[2,3] One of the most studied example is the C1q domain.[4–8] The term signature domain has broad use.[9–14]

1. Bakker, F.T., and Dunwell, J.M., Phylogeny, function, and evolution of the cupins, a structurally conserved, functionally diverse superfamily of proteins, *Mol. Biol. Evolution* 18, 593–605, 2001.

2. *Oxford English Dictionary*, Oxford University Press, Oxford, UK, 1989.

3. Webster's Third International Dictionary, Unabridged *Dictionary* 1996.

4. Bérubé, N.G., Swanson, X.H., Bertram, M.J., et al., Cloning and characterization of CRF, a novel C1q-related factor, expressed in areas of the brain involved in motor function, *Mol. Brain Res.* 63, 233–240, 1999.

5. Kishore, U., Gaboriaud, C., Waters, P., et al., C1q and tumor necrosis factor superfamily: Modularity and versatility, *Trends Immunol.* 25, 551–561, 2004.

6. Ghai, R., Waters, P., Roumenina, L.T., et al., C1q and its growing family, *Immunobiology* 212, 253–266, 2007.

7. Liu, F., Tan, A., Yang, A., et al., C1q11/Ctrp14 and C1q14/Ctrp11 promote angiogenesis of endothelial cells through activation of ERK1/2 signal pathway, *Mol. Cell. Biochem.* 424, 57–67, 2017.

8. Ghebrehiwet, B., Kandov, E., Kishore, U., and Peerschke, E.I.B., Is the A-chain the engine that drives the diversity of C1q functions? Revisiting its unique structure, *Front. Immunol.* 9, 162, 2018.

9. Tousidou, E., Nanopoulos, A., and Manolopoulos, Y., Improved methods for signature-tree construction, *The Computer Journal* 43, 301–314, 2000.

10. Ye, Y., and Godzik, A., Comparative analysis of protein domain organization, *Genome Res.* 14, 343–353, 2004.

11. Carlson, C.B., Bernstein, D.A., Annis, D.S., et al., *Nat. Struct. Mol. Biol.* 12, 910–914, 2005.

12. Tan, K., Duquette, M., Joachimiak, A., and Lawler, J., The crystal structure of the signature domain of cartilage oligomeric matrix protein: Implications for collagen, glycosaminoglycan and integrin binding, *FASEB J.* 23, 2490–2501, 2009.

13. Liem, R.K., Cytoskeletal integrators: The spectrin superfamlly, *Cold Sprint Harb. Perspect. Biol.* 8(10), a1081259, 2016.

14. Gupta, A., Agarwal, R., Singh, A., and Bhatnagar, S., Calcium-induced conformational changes of thrombospondin-1 signature domain: Implications for vascular disease, *J. Recept. Signal. Transduct. Res.* 37, 239–251, 2017.

SINGLE-CHAIN Fv FRAGMENT (scFv)

scFv is a synthetic (usually recombinant) peptide/protein composed of the V_L and V_H domains of an antibody linked by a peptide.[1–8] scFv are usually developed using phage display technology and, as relatively small (30 kDa) protein, can be obtained via expression in a variety of systems.[9–18] The scFv fragment can be expressed a fusion protein to enable targeting of a therapeutic component.[11,15,18–23] scFv fragments is a component of many bispecific antibodies.[24–33] It is possible to express the scFv inside the cell (intracellular expression) as intrabodies for analytical and therapeutic purposes.[34–40]

1. Leath, C.A., 3rd., Douglas, J.T., Curiel, D.T., and Alvarez, R.D., Single-chain antibodies: A therapeutic modality for cancer gene therapy, *Int. J. Oncol.* 24, 765–771, 2004.

2. Holliger, P., and Hudson, P.J., Engineered antibody fragments and the rise of single domains, *Nat. Biotechnol.* 23, 1126–1136, 2005.

3. Röthlisberger, D., Honengger, A., and Plückthun, A., Domain interactions in the Fab fragment: A comparative evaluation of the single-chain Fv and Fab format engineered with variable domains of different stability, *J. Mol. Biol.* 347, 773–789, 2005.

4. Ahmad, Z.A., Yeap, S.K., Ali, A.M., et al., scFc antibody: Principles and clinical application, *Clin. Dev. Immunol.* 2012, 980250, 2012.

5. Crivianu-Gaita, V., and Thompson, M., Aptamers, antibody scFv, and antibody Fab' fragments: An overview and comparison of three of the most versatile biosensor recognition elements, *Biosens. Bioelectron.* 85, 32–45, 2016.

6. Keller, T., Kalt, R., Raab, I., et al., Selection of scFv antibody fragments binding to human blood versus lymphatic endothelial surface antigens by direct cell phage display, *PLoS One* 10(5), e0127169, 2015.

7. Li, K., Zettlitz, K.A., Lipianskaya, J., et al., A fully human scFv phage display library for rapid antibody fragment reformatting, *Protein Eng. Design Selection* 28, 307–315, 2015.

8. Gaciarz, A., and Ruddock, L.W., Complementarity determining regions and frameworks contribute to the disulfide bond independent folding of intrinsically stable scFv, *PLoS One* 12(12), e0189964, 2017.

9. Chadd, H.E., and Chamow, S.M., Therapeutic antibody expression technology, *Curr. Opin. Biotechnol.* 12, 188–194, 2001.

10. de Graaf, M., van der Meulen-Mulleman, I.H., Pinedo, H.M., and Haisma, H.J., Expression of scFvs and scFv fusion proteins in eukaryotic cells, *Methods Mol. Biol.* 178, 379–387, 2002.

11. Kim, S.-E., Expression and purification of recombinant immunotoxin—A fusion protein stabilizes a single-chain Fv (scFv) in denaturing condition, *Prot. Express. Purif.* 27, 85–89, 2003.

12. Xavier, S., Gopi Mohan, C., Nair, S., Menon, K.N., and Vijayachandran, L.S., Generation of humanized single-chain fragment variable immunotherapeutic against EGFR variant III using baculovirus expression system and *in vitro* validation, *Int. J. Biol. Macromol.* 124, 17–24, 2018.

13. Wang, Y., Shan, Y., Gao, X., et al., Screening and expressing HIV-1 specific antibody fragments in *Saccharomyces cerevisiae*, *Mol. Immunol.* 103, 279–285, 2018.

14. Xiong, C., Mao, Y., Wu, T., et al., Optimized expression and characterization of a novel fully human bispecific single-chain diabody targeting vascular endothelial growth factor 165 and programmed death-1 in *Pichia pastoris* and evaluation of antitumor activity in vivo, *Int J Mol. Sci.* 19(10), E2900, 2018.

15. Lonoce, C., Marusic, C., Morrocchi, E., et al., Enhancing the secretion of a glyco-engineered Anti-CD20 scFv-Fc antibody in hairy root cultures, *Biotechnol. J.* 14, 1800081, 2019.

16. Vermeulen, J.G., Burt, F., van Heerden, E., et al., Evaluation of *in vitro* refolding vs cold shock expression: Production of a low yielding single chain variable fragment, *Protein Expr. Purif.* 151, 62–71, 2019.

17. Osaki, T., Nakanishi, T., Aoki, M., et al., Expression in *Escherichia coli* of a single-domain antibody-tumor necrosis factor α fusion protein specific for epidermal growth factor receptor, *Monoclon. Antib. Immunodiagn. Immunother.* 37, 20–25, 2018.

18. Bochichhio, A., Jordaan, S., Losasso, V., et al., Designing the sniper: Improving targeted human cytolytic fusion proteins for anti-cancer therapy via molecular simulation, *Biomedicine* 5(1), E9, 2017.

19. Fercher, C., Keshvari, S., McGluckin, M.A., and Barnard, R.T., Evolution of the magic bullet: Single chain antibody fragments for the targeted delivery of immunomodulatory proteins, *Exp. Biol. Med.* (Maywood) 243, 166–183, 2018.

20. Angelini, A., Miyabe, Y., Newsted, D., et al., Directed evolution of broadly crossreactive chemokine blocking antibodies efficacious arthritis, *Nat. Commun.* 9(1), 1461, 2018.

21. Kim, S., Kim, H., Jo, D.H., et al., Bispecific anti-mPDGFRβ x continue scFv-C(κ)-scFv fusion protein and continine-duocarmycin can form antibody-drug conjugate-like complexes that exert cytotoxicity against pPDGFRβ expressing cells, *Methods* 154, 125–135, 2019.

22. Zou, Y., Luo, W., Guo, J., et al., NK cell-mediated anti-leukemia cytotoxicity is enhanced using a NKG2D ligand MICA and anti-CD20 scfv chimeric protein, *Eur. J. Immunol.* 48, 1750–1763, 2018.

23. Fu, W., Sun, H., Zhao, Y., et al., Targeting delivery of CD44s-siRNA by scFv overcomes de novo resistance to cetuximab in triple negative breast cancer, *Mol. Immunol.* 99, 124–133, 2018.

24. Pluckthun, A., and Pack, P., New protein engineering approaches to multivalent and bispecific antibody fragments, *Immuntechnology* 3, 93–105, 1997.

25. Hudson, P.J., and Kortt, A.A., High avidity scFv multimers; diabodies and triabodies, *J. Immunol. Methods* 231, 177–189, 1999.

26. Lunde, E., Lauvrak, V., Rasmussen, I.B., et al., Troybodies and pepbodies, *Biochem. Soc. Trans.* 30, 500–506, 2002.

27. Cao, Y., and Suresh, M.R., Bispecific antibodies as novel bioconjugates, *Bioconjug. Chem.* 9, 635–640, 1998.

28. Schirrmann, T., Al-Halabi, L., Dübe, S., and Hust, M., Production systems for antibodies, *Front. Biosci.* 13, 4576–4594, 2008.

29. Ahmad, Z.A., Yeap, S.K., Ali, A.M., et al., scFv antibody: Principles and clinical application, *Clin. Dev. Immunol.* 2012, 980250, 2012.

30. Byrne, H., Conroy, P.J., Whisstock, J.C., and Kennedy, R.J., A tale of two specificities: Bispecific antibodies for therapeutic and diagnostic applications, *Trends Biotechnol.* 31, 621–632, 2013.

31. Yu, S., Li, A., Liu, Q., et al., Recent advances of bispecific antibodies in solid tumors, *J. Hematol. Oncol.* 10, 155, 2017.

32. Li, Y., A brief introduction of IgG-like bispecific antibody purification: Methods for removing product-related impurities, *Protein Express. Purif.* 155, 112–119, 2019.

33. Dimasi, N., Fleming, R., Wu, H., and Gao, C., Molecular engineering strategies and methods for the expression and purification of IgG-based bispecific bivalent antibodies, *Methods* 154, 77–86, 2019.

34. Visintin, M., Meli, G.A., Cannistraci, I., and Cattnaeo, A., Intracellular antibodies for proteomics, *J. Immunol. Methods* 290, 135–153, 2004.

35. Lobato, M.N., and Rabbitts, T.H., Intracellular antibodies as specific reagents for function ablation: Future therapeutic molecules, *Curr. Mol. Med.* 4, 519–528, 2004.

36. Marschall, A.L., Dübel, S., and Böldicke, T., Recent advances with ER targeted intrabodies, *Adv. Exp. Med. Biol.* 917, 77–93, 2016.

37. Renaud, E., Martinaeu, P., and Guglielmi, L., Solubility characterization and imaging of intrabodies using GFP-fusions, *Methods Mol. Biol.* 1575, 165–174, 2017.

38. Che Omar, M.T, Expression of functional anti-p24 scFv 183-H12–5C in HEK293T and Jurkat T cells, *Adv. Pharm. Bull.* 7, 299–312, 2017.

39. Nguyen, T.D., Nagamune, T., and Kawahara, M., A suicide switch directly eliminates intracellular scFv oligomers in the cytoplasm of mammalian cells, *Biotechnol. J.* 14, 1800350l, 2019.

40. Caucheteur, D., Robin, G., Parez, V., and Martineau, P., Construction of a synthetic antibody gene library for the selection of intrabodies and antibodies, *Methods Mol. Biol.* 1701, 239–253, 2018.

SITE-SPECIFIC PEGylation

Site-Specific PEGylation is a method which permits the conjugation of a poly(ethylene)glycol chain at a specific site in a protein. Site-specific pegylation can involve conjugation at glycan chain by glycopegylation with is an enzyme-catalyzed process[1–3] or by coupling of a hydrazide derivative of poly(ethylene)glycol to a periodate oxidized glycan chain.[4–6] Another approach uses the insertion of a cysteine residue by site-directed mutagenesis into the amino acid sequence of a protein which can be selectively modified by a maleimide derivative of PEG.[7–9] A related approach used the incorporation of a non-canonical amino acid, *p*-azidophenylalanine, and coupling of PEG via the Staudinger ligation.[10] Another approach is based on the selective modification of the *N*-terminal amino acid which (usually) has a lower pKa than the ε-amino groups of lysine.[11–14] Site-specific coupling of PEG to the carboxyl terminal residue has been reported.[15]

1. DeFrees, S., Wang, Z.G., Xing, R., et al., GlycoPEGylation of recombinant therapeutic proteins produced in *Escherichia Coli*, *Glycobiology* 16, 833–843, 2006.

2. Pasut, G., and Veronese, F.M., State of the art in PEGylation: The great versatility achieved after forty years of research, *J. Control. Release* 161, 461–472, 2012.

3. Giorgi, M.E., Agusti, R., and Lederkremer, R.M., Carbohydrate PEGylation, an approach to improve pharmaceutical potency, *Beilstein J. Org. Chem.* 10, 1433–1444, 2014.

4. Zalipsky, S., Functionalized poly(ethylene glycol) for preparation of biological relevant conjugates, *Bioconjug. Chem.* 6, 150–165, 1995.

5. Roberts, M.J., Bentley, M.D., and Harris, J.M., Chemistry for peptide and protein PEGylation, *Adv. Drug Deliv. Rev.* 64, 116–127, 2012.

6. Ritter, D.W., Roberts, J.R., and McShane, M.J., Glycosylation site-targeted PEGylation of glucose oxidase retains native enzyme activity, *Enzyme Microb. Technol.* 52, 279–285, 2013.

7. Goodson, R.J., and Katre, N.V., Site-directed pegylation of recombinant interleukin-2 at its glycosylation site, *Bio/Technology* 8, 343–345, 1990.

8. Xiong, C.Y., Natarajan, A., Shi, X.B., Denardo, G.L., and Denardo, S.J., Development of tumor targeting anti-MUC-1 multimer: Effects of di-scFv unpaired cysteine location on PEGylation and tumor binding, *Protein Eng. Des. Sel.* 19, 359–367, 2006.

9. Pan, L.Q., Wang, H.B., Lai, J., et al., Site-specific PEGylation of a mutated-cysteine residue and its effect on tumor necrosis factor (TNF)-related apoptosis-inducing ligand (TRAIL), *Biomaterials* 34, 9115–9123, 2013.

10. Hoffman, E., Streichert, K., Nischan, N., et al., Stabilization of bacterially expressed erythropoietin by single site-specific introduction of short branched PEG chains at naturally occurring glycosylation sites, *Mol. Biosyst.* 12, 1750–1755, 2016.

11. Gaertner, H.E., and Offord, R.E., Site-specific attachment of functionalized poly(ethylene glycol) to the amino terminus of proteins, *Bioconjug. Chem.* 7, 38–44, 1996.

12. Narimatsu, S., Yoshioka, Y., Watanabe, H., et al., Lysine-deficient lymphotoxin-α mutant for site-specific PEGylation, *Cytokine* 56, 589–493, 2011.

13. Zhou, Z., Zhang, J., Sun, L., Ma, G., and Su, Z., Comparison of site-specific PEGylation of the N-terminus of interferon beta-1b: Selectivity, efficiency, and in vivo/in vitro activity, *Bioconjug. Chem.* 25, 138–146, 2014.

14. Sung, I.T., Lee, M., Lee, H., et al., PEGylation and HAylation via catechol: α-amine-specific reaction at N-terminus of peptides and proteins, *Acta Biomater.* 43, 50–60, 2016.

15. Falciani, C., Lozzi, L., Scali, S., et al., Site-specific pegylation of an antimicrobial peptide increases resistance to *Pseudomonas aeruginosa* elastase, *Amino Acids* 46, 1403–1407, 2014.

SMALL INTERFERING RNA (siRNA)

A short-length double-stranded RNA (21–27 nucleotides in length) derived from intracellular double-stranded RNA by the action of specific endonucleases such as RNAse III (see **Dicer, Drosha**). The siRNA stimulates the cellular machinery to cut up messenger RNA thus inhibiting the process of transcription; this is process called knockdown.[1–4] There is substantial interest in the therapeutic use of siRNA.[5–8]

See **RNA-induced silencing complex (RISC), RNA interference.**

1. Kim, V.N., Small RNAs: Classification, biogenesis, and function, *Molecules and Cells* 19, 1–15, 2005.

2. Myers, J.W., and Ferrell, J.E., Jr., Silencing gene expression with Dicer-generated siRNA pools, in RNA Silencing. Methods and Protocols, ed. G.G. Carmichael, Humana Press, Totowa, NJ, Chapter 8, pp. 93–196, 2005.

3. Aravin, A., and Tuschi, T., Identification and characterization of small RNAs involved in RNA silencing, *FEBS Lett.* 579, 5830–5840, 2005.

4. Bass, B.L., Double-stranded RNA as a template for gene silencing, *Cell* 101, 235–238, 2000.

5. Liu, Y., Chen, J., Tang, Y., et al., Synthesis and characterization of quaternized poly(β-amino ester) for highly efficient delivery of small interfering RNA, *Mol. Pharm.* 15, 4558–4567, 2018.

6. Aljuffali, I.A., Lin, Y.K., and Fang, J.Y., Noninvasive approach for enhancing small interfering RNA delivery percutaneously, *Expert Opin. Drug. Deliv.* 13, 265–280, 2016.

7. Wu, D., Han, H., Xing, X., et al., Ideal and reality: Barricade in the delivery of small interfering RNA for cancer therapy, *Curr. Pharm. Biotechnol.* 17, 237–247, 2016.

8. Ruigrok, M.J.R., Frijlink, H.W., and Hinrichs, W.L.J., Pulmonary administration of small interfering RNA: The route to go? *J. Control. Release* 235, 14–23, 2016.

SMALL TEMPORAL RNA (stRNA)

Small temporal RNAs were identified as small antisense RNAs in *Caenorhabditis elegans* which are expressed only a specific stage in development and encode proteins involved in specific developmental timing events.[1–3] There is a limited literature for sTRNA as such as stRNAs are considered to be microRNAs (miRNAs).[3,4]

1. Pasquinelli, A.E., Reinhart, B.J., Slack, R., et al., Conservation of the sequence and temporal expression of *let-7* heterochronic regulatory RNA, *Nature* 408, 86–89, 2000.

2. Moss, E.G., RNA interference: It's a small RNA world, *Current Biology* 11, R772–R775, 2001.

3. Lee, R.C., and Ambros, V., An extensive class of small RNAs in *Caenorhabditis elegans*, *Science* 294, 862–864, 2001.

4. Bashirullah, A., Pasquinelli, A.E., Kiger, A.A., et al., Coordinate regulation of small temporal RNAs at the onset of *Drosophila* metamorphosis, *Devel. Biol.* 259, 1–8, 2003.

SMALL NUCLEAR RIBONUCLEOPROTEIN PARTICLE (snRNP)

Small nuclear ribonucleoprotein particles (snRNPs) (U1, U2, U4, U5, U6) are components of the spliceosome which are important in the recognition of the introns and splice site definition.[1–4] The individual snRNPs consist of a small uridine-rich nuclear RNA and a number of proteins.[5] The RNA components are characterized by the presence of a modified nucleotides such as 2,2,7-trimethylguanosine as a 5'cap. The cryoelectron microscopic structures of pre-catalytic spliceosome and associated snRNPs have been reported.[6,7] While there were earlier reports of ribonucleoprotein complexes,[8–10] the first isolation of small nuclear ribonucleoprotein particles was reported in 1975.[11] It was subsequently shown that a snRNP (U1) was required for the splicing of adenoviral RNA.[12]

1. Newman, A.J., The role of snRNP in pre-mRNA splicing, *The EMBO J.* 16, 5797–5800, 1997.
2. Graveley, B.R., Sorting out the complexity of SR protein functions, *RNA* 6, 1197–1211, 2000.
3. Will, C.L., and Luhrmann, R., Spliceosomal UsnRNP biogenesis, structure and function, *Curr. Opin. Cell. Biol.* 13, 290–301, 2001.
4. Turner, I.A., Norman, C.R., Churcher, M.J., and Newman, A.J., Roles of the U5 snRNP in spliceosome dynamics and catalysis, *Biochem. Soc. Trans.* 32, 928–931, 2004.
5. Patel, S., and Bellini, M., The assembly of a spiceosomal small nuclear ribonucleoprotein particle, *Nucleic Acids Res.* 36, 6482–6491, 2008.
6. Plaschka, C., Lin, P.C., and Nagai, S.K., Structure of a pre-catalytic spliceosome, *Nature* 546, 617–621, 2017.
7. Zhan, X., Yan, C., Zhang, X., Lei, J., and Shi, Y., Structures of the human pre-catalytic spliceosome and its precursor spliceosome, *Cell Res.* 28, 1129–1140, 2018.
8. Rorem, E.S., and Machlis, L., The ribonucleoprotein nature of large particles in the meiosporagia of Allomyces, *J. Biophys. Biochem. Cytol.* 3, 879–888, 1957.
9. Lovett, J.S., Chemical and physical characterization of "nuclear caps" isolated from *Blastocladiella* zoospores, *J. Bacteriol.* 85, 1235–1246, 1963.
10. Spirin, A.S., Informosomes, *Europ. J. Biochem.* 10, 20–35, 1969.
11. Raj, N.B.K., Ro-Cho, T.S., and Busch, H., Nuclear ribonucleoprotein complexes containing U1 and U2 RNA, *Biochemistry* 14, 4380–4385, 1975.
12. Yang, V.W., Lerner, M.R., Steitz, J.A., and Flint, S.J., A small nuclear ribonucleoprotein is required for splicing of adenoviral early RNA sequences, *Proc. Natl. Acad. Sci. USA* 78, 1371–1375, 1975.

SMART PROBES

A smart probe is a molecular entity probe which emits a signal only when bound to a specific target inside of a cell.[1,2] A smart nucleic acid probe is different from a molecular beacon as a smart nucleic acid probe relies on interaction with a guanine nucleotide in the oligonucleotide component (a hairpin). When the oligonucleotide component binds to a specific sequence in the target (complementary target sequence), there is a conformational change in the oligonucleotide component relieving the quenching of the fluorescent moiety. This approach is different from FRET (Förster Resonance Energy Transfer/Fluorescence Resonance Energy Transfer) but there are examples of the use of FRET reagents as smart probes.[3–6] There has been some use of biorthogonal technology in smart probes.[7,8]

1. Knemeyer, J.-P., Marmé, N., and Sauer, M., Probes for detection of specific DNA sequences at the single-molecule level, *Anal. Chem.* 72, 3717–3724, 2000.
2. Stöhr, K., Häfner, B., Nolte. O., Wolfrum, J., Sauer, M., and Herten, D.-P., Species-specific identification of Mycobacterial 16S rRNA PCR amplicons using smart probes, *Anal. Chem.* 77, 7195–7203, 2005.
3. Chang, E., Miller, J.S., Sun, J., et al., Protease-activated quantum dot probes, *Biochem. Biophys. Res. Commun.* 334, 1317–1321, 2005.
4. Fernandez, A., and Vendrell, M., Smart fluorescent probes for imaging macrophage activity, *Chem. Soc. Rev.* 45, 1182–1196, 2016.
5. Li, J., Zhang, Y., and Cheng, Z., FRET imaging of enzymatic activities using smart probes, *Methods Mol. Biol.* 1444, 37–44, 2016.
6. Saito, Y., Bag, S.S., Kusakabe, Y., et al., Dual-labeled oligonucleotide probe for sensing adenosine *via* FRET: A dual alternative to SNPs genotyping, *ChemComm* 2007, 2133–2135, 2007.
7. Shieh, P., and Bertozzi, C.R., Design strategies for biorthogonal smart probes, *Org. Biomol. Chem.* 12, 9307–9320, 2014.
8. Ji, X., Ji, K., Chittavong, V., et al., Click and fluoresce: A bioorthogonally activated smart probe for wash-free fluorescent labeling of biomolecules, *J. Org. Chem.* 82, 1471–1476, 2017.

SNARE PROTEINS

SNARE (soluble NSF [*N*-ethylmaleimide sensitive factor] attachment protein [SNAP] receptors) proteins participate in eukaryotic membrane fusion.[1–8] It is suggested that vesicle SNARE proteins fuse with target SNAP proteins during processes such as exocytosis.[9,10] A vesicular SNARE (v-SNARE) can fuse with a target SNARE to form a transmembrane complex (SNAREpin) resulting in membrane fusion.[11,12] At the completion of membrane fusion, the *trans* SNARE complex is designated as *cis*-SNARE complex. The SNARE components are dissociated by NSF (*N*-ethylmaleimide sensitive factor), an ATPase, in combination with a cofactor, SNAP (soluble NSF attachment protein), into v-SNARE and t-SNARE components which participate into another round membrane fusion.[13]

1. Ferro-Novick, S., and Jahn, R., Vesicle fusion from yeast to man, *Nature* 370, 191–193, 1994.
2. Rothman, J.E., and Warren, G., Implications of the SNARE hypothesis for intracellular membrane topology and dynamics, *Curr. Biol.* 4, 220–233, 1994.
3. Morgan, A., Exocytosis, *Essays Biochem.* 30, 77–95, 1995.
4. Pelham, H.R., SNAREs and the secretory pathway-lessons from yeast, *Exp. Cell Res.* 247, 1–8, 1997.
5. Hay, J.C., SNARE complex structure and function, *Exp. Cell Res.* 271, 10–21, 2001.

6. Dietrich, L.E.P., Boedinghaus, C., LaGrassa, J.T., and Ungermann, C., Control of eukaryotic membrane fusion by N-terminal domains of SNARE proteins, *Biochim. Biophys. Acta* 1641, 111–119, 2003.

7. Hong, W., SNAREs and traffic, *Biochim. Biophys. Acta* 1744, 493–517, 2005.

8. Montecucco, C., Schiavo, G., and Pantano, S., SNARE complexes and neuroexocytosis: How many, how close? *Trends Biochem. Sci.* 30, 367–372, 2005.

9. Sotirakis, E., and Galli, T., Exocytosis: Lessons from SNARE mutants, in *Molecular Mechanism of Exocytosis*, ed. R. Regazzi, Chapter 1, pp. 1–9, Landes Bioscience, Austin, TX, and Springer Business Media, New York, 2007.

10. Moore, D.J., and Mollenhauer, H.H., *The Golgi Apparatus*, Function, Chapter 8, pp. 155–185, Springer Business and Science, New York, 2009.

11. Hong, W., and Lev, S., Tethering the assembly of SNARE complexes, *Trends Cell Biol.* 24, 35–43, 2014.

12. Bombardier, J.P., and Munson, M., Three steps forward, two steps back: Mechanistic insights into the assembly and disassembly of the SNARE complex, *Curr. Opin. Chem. Biol.* 29, 66–71, 2015.

13. Ryu, J.-K., Jahn, R., and Yoon, T.-Y., Progresses in understanding N-ethylmaleimide sensitive factor (NSF) mediated disassembly of SNARE complexes, *Biopolymers* 105, 518–531, 2016.

SOAP

A soap is a substance formed by the combination of certain oils and fats with alkaline bases and used for washing/cleansing purposes. by the combination of certain oils and fats with alkaline bases and used for washing or cleansing purposes. Soap is prepared from natural oils and fats and is precipitated by the ions (notably calcium) present in hard water.[1] Soaps were prepared by the treatment of animal fats with natural bases such lye in a process today described as saponification.[2] Bile acids have been described as intestinal soaps[3,4] but are more complex than that.[5] The concept of bile acids as soaps is based on the ability of bile acids to solubilize lipids.[6] Soaps are usually compared with detergents. Detergents have some properties similar to soaps[8] and can be ionic detergents[7] or non-ionic detergents.[9,10] See **detergent**.

1. *Oxford English Dictionary*, Oxford University Press, Oxford, UK, 2018.

2. Preston, W.C., The Modern Soap Industry, Part I, *J. Chem. Educ.* 2, 1035–1044, 1925.

3. Hofmann, A.F., and Roda, A., Physicochemical properties of bile acids and their relationship to biological properties; an overview of the problem, *J. Lipid Res.* 25, 1477–1489, 1984.

4. Hoffman, A.F., The continuing importance of bile acids in liver and intestinal disease, *Annals Int. Med.* 159, 2647–2658, 1999.

5. Kuipers, F., Bloks, V.W., and Groen, A.K., Beyond intestinal soap—Bile acids in metabolic control, *Nat. Rev. Endocrinol.* 10, 488–498, 2014.

6. Carey, M.C., and Small, D.M., The characteristics of mixed micellar solutions with particular reference to bile, *Amer. J. Med.* 49, 590–608, 1970.

7. Helenius, A., McCaslin, D.R., Fries, E., and Tanford, D., Properties of detergents, *Methods in Enzymol.* 56, 734–749, 1979.

8. Friedman, M., and Wolf, R., Chemistry of soaps and detergents: Various types of commercial products and their ingredients, *Clinic Dermatology* 14, 7–13, 1996.

9. Khamlichi, S., Loirat, M.J., Blanchard, D., et al., Influence of the size of the polar head of non-ionic detergents on membrane proteins immunoaffinity purification, *J. Biochem. Biophys. Methods* 29, 123–134, 1994.

10. Lichtenberg, D., Ahyayauch, H., Alonso, A., and Goñi, F.M., Detergent solubilization of lipid bilayers: A balance of driving forces, *Trends Biochem. Sci.* 38, 85–93, 2013.

SOFT IONIZATION

The term soft ionization describes ionization techniques such as fast atom bombardment (FAD), electrospray ionization (ESI), or matrix-assisted laser desorption/ionization (MALDI) that result in the desorption and ionization of analyst without fragmentation while hard ionization techniques such as electron ionization result in fragmentation of the analytes.[1–4]

1. Casy, A.F., Mass spectrometry as an aid to the identification of ergots and dihydroergots: Comparison of hard and soft ionization techniques, *J. Pharmaceut. Biomed. Anal.* 12, 41–46, 1994.

2. Hejazi, L., Guilhaus, M., Hibbert, D.B., and Ebrahimi, D., Gas chromatography with parallel hard and soft ionization mass spectrometry, *Rapid Commun. Mass Spectrom.* 29, 91–99, 2014.

3. Tranchida, P.Q., Aloisi, I., Giocastro, B., and Mondello, L., Current state of comprehensive two-dimensional gas chromatography-mass spectrometry with focus on processes of ionization, *Trends. Anal. Chem.* 105, 360–366, 2018.

4. Wang, Y., Sun, J., Qiao, J., Ouyang, J., and Na, N., A "soft" and "hard" ionization method for comprehensive studies of molecules, *Anal. Chem.*, 90, 14095–14099, 2018.

SOMATIC HYPERMUTATION

The term somatic hypermutation describes the increased rate of mutation in the variable region of immunoglobulin genes which allows for diversity of immune recognition.[1–21]

1. Steele, E.J., Rothenfluh, H.S., and Both, G.W., Defining the nucleic acid substrate for somatic hypermutation, *Immuno. Cell Biol.* 70, 129–144, 1992.
2. George, J., and Clafin, L., Selection of B cell clones and memory B cells, *Semin. Immunol.* 4, 11–17, 1992.
3. Neuberger, M.S., and Milstein, C.S., Somatic hypermutation, *Curr. Opin. Immunol.* 7, 24–254, 1995.
4. Hengstschlager, M., Maizels, N., and Leung, H., Targeting and regulation of immunoglobulin gene somatic hypermutation and isotype switch recombination, *Prog. Nucleic Acid Res. Mol. Biol.* 50, 67–99, 1995.
5. Steele, E.J., Rothenflug, H.S., and Blanden, R.V., Mechanism of antigen-driven somatic hypermutation of rearranged immunoglobulin V(D)J genes in the mouse, *Immuno. Cell Biol.* 75, 82–95, 1997.
6. Rajewsky, K., Clonal selection and learning in the antibody system, *Nature* 381, 751–758, 1996.
7. Storb, U., Peters, A., Klotz, E., et al., *Cis*-acting sequences that affect somatic hypermutation of Ig genes, *Immunol. Rev.* 162, 153–160, 1998.
8. Neuberger, M.S., Ehrenstein, M.R., Klix, N., et al., Monitoring and interpreting the intrinsic features of somatic hypermutation, *Immunol. Rev.* 162, 107–116, 1998.
9. Kuppers, R., Goossens, T., and Klein, U., The role of somatic hypermutation in the generation of deletions and duplications in human Ig V region genes and chromosomal translocations, *Curr. Top. Microbiol. Immunol.* 246, 193–198, 1999.
10. Harris, R.S., Kong, Q., and Maizels, N., Somatic hypermutation and the three R's: Repair, replication and recombination, *Mutat. Res.* 436, 157–178, 1999.
11. Jacobs, H., and Bross, L., Towards an understanding of somatic hypermutation, *Curr. Opin. Immunol.* 13, 208–218, 2001.
12. Maul, R.W., and Gearhart, P.J., Controlling somatic hypermutation in immunoglobulin variable and switch regions, *Immunol. Res.* 47, 113–122, 2010.
13. Schroeder, H.W., Jr., and Cavacini, P.J., Controlling somatic hypermutation in immnoguln variable and switch regions, *J. Allergy Clin. Immunol.* 125(2 Suppl 2), S41–S52, 2010.
14. Sariasak, H., and Gearhart, P.J., Does DNA repair occur during somatic hypermutation? *Semin. Immunol.* 24, 287–292, 2012.
15. Detanico, T., St. Clair, J.B., Aviszus, K., et al., Somatic mutagenesis in autoimmunity, *Autoimmunity* 46, 102–114, 2013.
16. Robins, H., Immunosequencing: Applications of immune repertoire deep sequencing, *Curr. Opin. Immunol.* 25, 646–652, 2013.
17. King, D.J., Bowers, P.M., Kehry, M.R., and Horlick, R.A., Mammalian cell display and somatic hypermutation in vitro for human antibody discovery, *Curr. Drug. Discov. Technol.* 11, 56–64, 2014.
18. Steele, E.J., Somatic hypermutation in immunity and cancer. Critical analysis of strand-based and codon-context mutation signatures, *DNA Repair* (Amst) 45, 1–24, 2016.
19. Methot, S.P., and Di Noia, J.M., Molecular mechanisms of somatic hypermutation and class switch recombination, *Adv. Immunol.* 133, 37–87, 2017.
20. Chaudhary, N., and Wesemann, D.R., Analyzing immunoglobulin repertoires, *Front. Immunol.* 9, 462, 2018.
21. Schramm, C.A., and Douek, D.C., Beyond hot spots: Biases in antibody somatic hypermutation and implications for vaccine design, *Front. Imunnol.* 9, 1876, 2018.

SOUTHERN BLOTTING

Southern blotting describes a technique which uses a labeled (^{32}P or biotin) complementary oligonucleotide/polynucleotide to identify denatured DNA which has been transferred by absorption from an agarose gel to another matrix, such a nitrocellulose membrane. The term Southern refers to Edward M Southern who developed the technique.[1-4] There has been a consistent use of Southern blotting.[5-14] Other technologies are being advanced to supplement or replace the Southern blot.[15,16] There is variability in the capitalization of Southern as it is personal name as well as the name of a technique.[17,18] It is further noted that the use of Southern as a descriptor has spawned a variety of analytical technologies based on blotting having directional names (e.g. Northern, Western).[18]

1. Southern, E., Southern blotting, *Nature Protocols* 1, 518–525, 2006.
2. Southern, E.M., Detection of specific sequences among DNA fragments separated by gel electrophoresis, *J. Mol. Biol.* 98, 503–517, 1975.
3. Southern, E.M., Detection of specific sequences among DNA fragments separated by gel electrophoresis, 1975, *Biotechnology* 24, 122–139, 1992.
4. Southern, E.M., Blotting at 25, *Trends Biochem. Sci.* 25, 585–588, 2000.
5. *Protocols for Nucleic Acid Analysis by Nonradioactive Probes*, Humana, Totowa, NJ, 1994.
6. Kelly, K.F., Southern Blotting, *Proc. Nutr. Soc.* 55, 591–597, 1996.
7. Keichle, F.L., DNA technology in the clinical laboratory, *Arch. Pathol. Lab. Med.* 123, 1151–1153, 1999.
8. Porchet, N., and Aubert, J.P., Southern blot analysis of large DNA fragments, *Methods Mol. Biol.* 125, 313–321, 2000.
9. Voswinkel, J., and Gause, A., From immunoglobulin gene fingerprinting to motif-specific hybridization: Advances in the analysis of B lymphoid clonality in rheumatic diseases, *Arthritis Res.* 4, 1–4, 2002.
10. Wong, L.J., and Boles, R.G., Mitochondrial DNA analysis in clinical laboratory diagnostics, *Clin. Chim. Acta* 354, 1–20, 2005.
11. Rose, M.G., Degar, B.A., and Berliner, N., Molecular diagnostics of malignant disorders, *Clin. Adv. Hematol. Oncol.* 2, 650–660, 2004.

12. Mellars, G., and Gomez, K., Mutation detection by southern blotting, *Methods Mol. Biol.*688, 281–291, 2011.

13. Glenn, G., and Andreou, L.V., Analysis of DNA by southern blotting, *Methods Enzymol.*529, 47–63, 2013.

14. Tzeng, C.C., Tsai, L.P., Chang, Y.K., et al., A 15-year-long southern blotting analysis of FMR1 to detect female carriers and for prenatal diagnosis of fragile X syndrome in Taiwan, *Clin. Genet.* 92, 217–220, 2017.

15. Addis, M., Serrenti, M., Meloni, C., Cau, M., and Melis, M.A., Triplet-primed PCR is more sensitive than southern blotting-long PCR for the diagnosis of myotonic dystrophy type 1, *Genet. Test. Mol. Biomarkers* 16, 1428–1431, 2012.

16. Stefano, B., Patrizia, B., Matteo, C., and Massimo, G., Inverse PCR and quantitative PCR as alternative methods to southern blotting analysis to assess transgene copy number and characterize the integration site in transgenic woody plants, *Biochem. Genet.* 54, 291–305, 2016.

17. *The Chicago Manual of Style*, 15th edn., University of Chicago Press, Chicago, IL, 2003.

18. Klionsky, D.J., Blame it on southern, but it's a western blot, *Autophagy* 13, 1–2, 2017.

SOUTHWESTERN BLOTTING

Southwestern blotting describes an analytical procedure used to identify the specific binding of a DNA sequence to a protein which uses a technical approach similar to Southern blotting and western blotting.[1] A protein mixture is separated by electrophoresis and the resulting electrophoretogram is transferred to a PVDF membrane by electrophoresis. The proteins are renatured on the membrane and a ^{32}P-labeled oligodeoxyribonucleotide probe of defined sequence is used to identify proteins which bind to specific nucleotide sequence.[1] Other labels such as cyanine dyes or fluorescein can be used as a label for oligonucleotide probe.[2] The concept of using a labeled deoxyribonucleotide to identify proteins binding such specific sequence was developed in 1980[3] and has seen consistent use[1,2,4–15] Southwestern blotting is also used for histochemistry[16] and for ELISA.[17,18] I was unable to find the first use of the term "southwestern blot" but a paper published in 1989[19] suggested the used of the term "southwestern blot" to describe the combination of a protein blotting procedure and specific DNA interaction with a protein. **Northwestern blotting**[20–22] described a procedure similar to southwestern blotting but uses RNA instead of DNA.

1. Jia, Y., Nagore, L., and Jarrett, H., Southwestern blotting assay, *Methods Mol. Biol.* 1334, 85–99, 2015.

2. Franke, C., Gräfe, D., Bartsch, H., and Bachmann, M.P., Use of nonradioactive detection method for North- and South-Western Blot, *Methods Mol. Biol.* 1314, 63–71, 2015.

3. Bowen, B., Steinberg, J., Laemmli, U.K., and Weintraub, H., The detection of DNA binding proteins by protein binding, *Nucleic Acids Res.* 8, 1–20, 1980.

4. Miskimins, W.K., Roberts, M.P., McCelland, A., and Ruddle, F.H., Use of a protein-blotting procedure and a specific DNA probe to identify nuclear proteins that recognize the promoter region of the transferrin receptor gene, *Proc. Natl. Acad. Sci. USA* 82, 6741–6744, 1985.

5. Hübscher, U., Double replica southwestern, *Nucleic Acids Res.* 15, 5486, 1987.

6. Fuetterer, J., and Hohn, T., Involvement of nucleocapsids in reverse transcription: A general phenomena?. *Trends Biochem. Sci.* 12, 92–95, 1987.

7. Silva, C.M., Tully, D.B., Petch, L.A., Jewell, C.M., and Cidlowski, J.A., Application of a protein-blotting procedure to the study of human glucocorticoid receptor interactions with DNA, *Proc. Natl. Acad. Sci. USA* 84, 1744–1748, 1987.

8. Zhu, Q., Andrisani, O.M., Pot, D.A., and Dixon, J.E., Purification and characterization of a 43-kDa transcription factor required for rat somatostatin gene expression, *J. Biol. Chem.* 264, 6550–6556, 1989.

9. Burstein, K.L., Jewell, C.M., and Cidlowski, J.A., Human glucocorticoid receptor cDNA contains sequences sufficient for receptor down-regulation, *J. Biol. Chem.* 265, 7284–7291, 1990.

10. Won, K.-A., and Baumann, H., NF-AB, a liver-specific and cytokine inducible nuclear factor that interacts with the interleukin-1 response element of the rat α_1-acid glycoprotein gene, *Mol. Cell. Biol.* 11, 3001–3008, 1991.

11. Ogura, M., Takatori, T., and Tsuro, T., Purification and characterization of NF-R1 that regulates the expression of the human multidrug resistance (MDR1) gene, *Nucleic Acids Res.* 20, 5811–5817, 1992.

12. Kwast-Welfeld, J., de Belle, I., Walker, P.R., Whitfield, J.F., and Sikorska, M., Identification of a new cAMP response element-binding factor by southwestern blotting, *J. Biol. Chem.* 268, 19851–19585, 1993.

13. Liu, Z., and Jacob, S.T., Characterization of a protein that interacts with the rat ribosomal gene promoter and modulates RNA polymerase I transcription, *J. Biol. Chem.* 269, 16618–16625, 1994.

14. Handen, J.S., and Rosenberg, H.F., An improved method for Southwestern blotting, *Front. Biosci.* 2, c9–c11, 1997.

15. Coffman, J.A., and Yuh, C.H., Identification of sequence-specific DNA binding proteins, *Methods Cell Biol.* 74, 653–675, 2004.

16. Fedorov, A.V., Lukyanov, D.V., and Podgornaya, O.T., Identification of the proteins specifically binding to the rat LINE1 promoter, *Biochem. Biophys. Res. Commun.* 340, 553–559, 2006.

17. Jiang, D., Jia, Y., Zhou, Y., and Jarrett, H.W., Two-dimensional southwestern blotting and characterization of transcription factor on-blot, *J. Proteome Res.* 8, 3693–3701, 2008.

18. Hishikawa, Y., Damavandi, E., Izumi, S., and Koji, T., Molecular histochemical analysis of estrogen receptor alpha and beta expression in the mouse ovary: In situ hybridization and Southwestern histochemistry, *Med. Electron Microsc.* 36, 67–73, 2003.

19. Fukuda, I., Nishiumi, S., Yabushita, Y., et al., A new southwestern chemistry-based ELISA for detection of aryl hydrocarbon receptor transformation: Application to the screening of its receptor agonists and antagonists, *J. Immunol. Methods* 287, 187–201, 2004.

20. Lelong, J.-C., Prevost, G., Lee, K., and Crepin, M., South western blot mapping: A procedure for simultaneous characterization on DNA binding proteins and their specific genomic DNA target sites, *Anal. Biochem.* 179, 299–303, 1989.

21. Chen, X., Sadlock, J., and Schon, E.A., RNA-binding patterns in total human tissue, *Biochem. Biophys. Res. Commun.* 191, 18–25, 1993.

22. Zang, S., and Lin, R.J., Northwestern blot analysis: Detecting RNA-protein interaction after gel separation of protein mixture, *Methods Mol. Biol.* 1421, 111–125, 2016.

SPECIFIC HEAT

Specific heat is the amount of heat required to raise the temperature of one gram of a substance by 1°C; specific heat of water is one calorie (4.184 joule); **heat of fusion** is the amount of thermal energy to melt one mole of a substance at the melting point; also referred to as latent heat of fusion, kcal/mole or kJ/mole. **Heat of vaporization** is the amount of energy required to convert one mole of a substance to vapor at the boiling point; also referred to as the latent heat of vaporization, kcal/mole or kJ/mole.

SPECIFICITY

Specificity can have several definitions in biotechnology. In the process of assay validation, specificity is the ability of an assay to recognize a single analyte in a sample which might contain closely related species; for example, in DNA microarray assays, specificity would be the ability of a probe to bind to a unique target sequence and produce a signal proportional of the amount of that specific target sequence only. Also referred to as selectivity. The definition from the ICH[1] is "Specificity is the ability to assess unequivocally the analyte in the presence of components which may be expected to be present. Typically, these might include impurities, degradants, matrix, etc." Specificity in clinical diagnosis is the proportion (ratio) of negative tests on individuals to the number individuals without a given condition.[2] Specificity is contrasted with sensitivity which is the ratio of positive tests to the number of individuals with a clinically established condition. Specificity is also used to describe the performance of antibodies.[3]

1. Validation of Analytical Procedures: Text and Methodology Q2(R1), ICH (International Conference on the Harmonisation of Technical Requirements for Registration of Pharmaceuticals for Human Use) https://www.ich.org, 2005.

2. Geleijnse, M.L., Krenning, B.J., van Dalen, B.M., et al., Factors affecting sensitivity and specificity of diagnostic testing: Dobutamine stress echocardiography, *J. Am. Soc. Echocardiorgr* 22, 1199–1208, 2009.

3. Priest, J.W., Plucinski, M.M., Huber, C.S., et al., Specificity of the IgG antibody response to *Plasmodium falciparum, Plasmodium vivax, Plasmodium maleriae,* and *Plasmodium ovale* MSP1$_{19}$ subunit proteins in multiplexed serological assays, *Malaria J.* 17, 417, 2018.

SPECTROSCOPY/SPECTROMETRY

Spectroscopy describes the discipline which measures the interaction of electromagnetic radiation with materials including scattering, absorption, and emission. It does not necessarily include chemical effects such as bond formation or free radical formation. It does include some aspects of photochemistry which a specialized form of energy transduction. The term spectrometry has also been used to describe the interaction the interaction of electromagnetic radiation with matter; the first use was for the measurement of the index of refraction. The term spectrometry is currently used in mass spectrometry.

SPECTRUM/SPECTRA

An **emission spectrum** is a pattern of emissions from a particle following the application of energy. The emissions may be in form of electromagnetic waves such as observed in spectroscopy[1,2] or in the form of mass such as that observed in mass spectrometry. An **absorption spectrum** is the pattern of absorption of electromagnetic radiation by a particle as a function of wavelength.[3] Spectra can be considered to be the plural of spectrum.

1. Werts, M.H., Jukes, R.T.F., and Verhoeven, J.W., The emission spectrum and the radiative lifetime of Eu^{3+} in luminescent lanthanide complexes, *Phys. Chem. Chem. Phys.* 4, 1542–1548, 2002.

2. Pope, R.M., and Fry, E.S., Absorption spectrum (380–700 nm) of pure water. II. Integrating cavity measurements, *Applied Optics* 36, 8710–8723, 1997.

3. Eng, J.K., McCormack, A.L., and Yates, J.R.,III., An approach to correlate tandem mass spectral data of peptides with amino acid sequences in a protein database, *J. Am. Sco. Mass Spectrom.* 5, 976–989, 1994.

Sp1 TRANSCRIPTION FACTORS

Sp1 (specificity protein 1) transcription factors are a family of zinc finger transcription factors widely expressed in mammalian cells which binds to GC-rich promoter elements.[1-4]

1. Dynan, W.S., and Tjian, R., Isolation of transcription factors that discriminate between different promoters recognized by RNA polymerase II, *Cell* 32, 669–680, 1983.
2. Lomberk, G., and Urrutia, R., The family feud: Turning off Sp1 by Sp1-like KLF proteins, *Biochem. J.* 392, 1–11, 2005.
3. O'Connor, L., Gilmour, J., and Bonifer, C., The role of the ubiquitously expressed transcription factor Sp1 in tissue-specific transcriptional regulation and in disease, *Yale J. Biol. Med.* 89, 513–525, 2016.
4. Vizcaino, C., Mansilla, S., and Portugal, J., Sp1 transcription factor: A long-standing target in cancer chemotherapy, *Pharmacol. Ther.* 152, 111–124, 2015.

SPLICED-LEADER *TRANS*-SPLICING

Spliced-leader *trans*-splicing is process mediated by a spiceosome where a short RNA sequence derived from the 5′-end of a non-mRNA (SL-RNA, spliced-leader donor RNA) to an acceptor site (3′-spice acceptor site) on a pre-RNA molecule.[1-5] As a result, a diverse group of mRNA molecules in an organism acquire a common 5′-sequence.[4,5]

1. Murphey, W.J., Watkins, K.P., and Agabian, N., Identification of a novel Y branch structure as an intermediate in trypanosome mRNA processing: Evidence for trans splicing, *Cell* 47, 517–525, 1986.
2. Bruzik, J.P., Van Doren, K., Hirsh, D., and Steitz, J.A., Trans splicing involves a novel form of small nuclear ribonucleoprotein particles, *Nature* 335, 559–562, 1988.
3. Layden, R.E., and Eisen, H., Alternate trans-splicing in *Trypanosoma equiperdum*: Implication for splice site selection, *Mol. Cell. Biol.* 8, 1352–1360, 1988.
4. Hastings, K.E.M., SL trans-splicing: Easy come or easy go? *Trends Genet.* 21, 240–247, 2005.
5. Krchňáková, Z., Krajčovič, J., and Vesteg, M., On the possibility of an early evolutionary origin for the spliced leader *trans*-splicing, *J. Mol. Evol.* 85, 37–45, 2017.

SPLICEOSOME

The spliceosome is a complex of RNA and protein components which functions in the process of RNA splicing in ribosomes.[1-8] Prokaryote RNA mRNA is less complex than eukaryotic mRNA and are not subject to RNA splicing. Eukaryotic RNA species that participate in spliceosome function include U1, U2, U4, U5, and U6. These RNA species are rich in uridine which recognize species sequences at the 5′ and 3′ sites on the pre-mRNA. The regions between these specific sites is excised that the exons are joined together in the splicing process resulting in mature RNA.

1. Robash, M., and Seraphin, B., Who's on first? The U1 snRNP-5′ splice site interaction and splicing, *Trends in Biochem. Sci.* 16, 187–190, 1991.
2. Garcia-Blanco, M.A., Messenger RNA reprogramming by spliceosome-mediated RNA trans-splicing, *J. Clin. Invest.* 112, 474–480, 2003.
3. Kramer, A., Frefoglia, F., Huang, C.J., Malhaupt, F., Nesic, D., and Tanackovic, G., Structure-function analysis of the U2 snRNP-associated splicing factor SF3a, *Biochem. Soc. Trans.* 33, 439–442, 2005.
4. Herzel, L., Ottoz, D.S.M., Alpert, T., and Neugebauer, K.M., Splicing and transcription touch base: Co-transcriptional spliceosome assembly and function, *Nat. Rev. Mol. Cell. Biol.* 18, 637–650, 2017.
5. Fica, S.M., and Nagai, K., Cryo-electron microscopy snapshots of the spliceosome: Structural insights into a dynamic ribonucleoprotein machine, *Nat. Struct. Mol. Biol.* 24, 791–799, 2017.
6. Shi, Y., Mechanistic insights into precursor messenger RNA splicing by the spliceosome, *Nat. Rev. Mol. Cell. Biol.* 18, 655–670, 2017.
7. Vazquez-Arango, P., and O'Reilly, D., Variant snSNPs: New players within the spliceosome system, *RNA Biology* 15, 17–25, 2018.
8. Galej, W.P., Structural studies of the spliceosome: Past, present and future perspectives, *Biochem. Soc. Trans.* 46, 1407–1422, 2018.

SPLICING SILENCERS

Splicing silencers are weakly interacting *cis*- and *trans*-factors that repress constitutive and alternative splicing during mRNA processing.[1-4] There are exonic spicing silencers (ESS)[5-7] and intronic splicing silencers (ISS).[8,9] Splicing silencers are distinct from transcriptional silencing also known as transcriptional repression.

1. Staffa, A., and Cochrane, A., Identification of positive and negative splicing regulatory elements within the terminal tat-rev exon of human immunodeficiency virus type 1, *Mol. Cell. Biol.* 15, 4597–4605, 1995.
2. Puzzoli, U., and Sironi, M., Silencers regulate both constitutive and alternative splicing events in mammals, *Cell. Mol. Life Sci.* 62, 1579–1604, 2005.
3. Wang, Z., and Burge, C.B., Splicing regulation: From a parts lists of regulatory elements to an integrated splicing code, *RNA* 14, 802–813, 2008.
4. Lee, Y., and Rio, D.C., Mechanisms and regulation of alternative pre-mRNA splicing, *Annu. Rev. Biochem.* 84, 291–323, 2015.

5. Amendt, B.A., Si, Z.H., and Stoltzfus, C.M., Presence of exon splicing silencers with human immunodeficiency virus type 1 tat exon 2 and tat-rev exon 3: Evidence for inhibition mediated by cellular factors, *Mol. Cell. Biol.* 15, 4606–4615, 1995.

6. Chew, S.L., Baginsky, L., and Eperon, I.C., An exonic splicing silencer in the testes-specific DNA ligase III beta exon, *Nucleic Acids Res.* 28, 402–410, 2000.

7. Horan, L., Yasuhara, J.C., Kohlstaedt, L.A., and Rio, D.C., Biochemical identification of new splicing repression at the Drosophila P-element exonic splicing silencer, *Genes Dev.* 29, 2298–2311, 2015.

8. Jain, N., Morgan, C.E., Rife, B.D., Salemi, M., and Tolbert, B.S., Solution structure of the HIV-1 intron splicing silencer and its interactions with the UP domain of heterogeneous nuclear ribonucleoprotein (hnRNP) A1, *J. Biol. Chem.* 291, 2331–2344, 2016.

9. Park, S.K., Zhou, X., Pendleton, K.E., et al., A conserved splicing silencer dynamically regulates O-GlcNac transferase intron retention and O-GlcNac homeostasis, *Cell Rep.* 20, 1088–1099, 2017.

SR FAMILY OF PROTEINS

SR proteins (Serine and arginine rich proteins) is a family of phylogenetically conserved proteins, which are essential cofactors in the splicing which occurs during the maturation of messenger RNA.[1–8] SR proteins are characterized by the presence of an *N*-terminal RNA recognition motif or motifs and a C-terminal region characterized by repeated arginine/serine residues.[1,9] While the early work was focused on the role of SR proteins in splicing activities important for mRNA maturation, subsequent work has shown that SR proteins in mRNA export and translation.[10,11]

1. Zahler, A.M., Lane, W.S., Stolk, J.A., and Roth, M.R., SR proteins: A conserved family of pre-mRNA splicing factors, *Genes Dev.* 6, 837–847, 1992.

2. Birney, E., Kumar, S., and Krainer, A.R., Analysis of the RNA-recognition motif and RS and RBB domains: Conservation in metazoan pre-mRNA splicing factors, *Nuc. Acids Res.* 25, 503–5816, 1993.

3. Ramchatesingh, J., Zahler, A.M., Neugebauer, K.M., Roth, M.B., and Cooper, T.A., A subset of SR proteins activates splicing of the cardiac troponin T alternative exon by direct interactions with an exonic enhancer, *Mol. Cell. Biol.* 15, 4898–4907, 1995.

4. McNally, L.M., and McNally, M.T., SR protein splicing factors interact with the Rous sarcoma virus negative regulator of splicing elements, *J. Virol.* 70, 1163–1172, 1996.

5. Katsarou, M.E., Papakyriakou, A., Katsaros, N., and Scorilas, A., Expression of the C-terminal domain of novel human SR-A1 protein: Interaction with the CTD domain of RNA polymerase II, *Biochem. Biophys. Res. Commun.* 334, 61–68, 2005.

6. Zahler, A.M., Purification of SR protein splicing factors, *Methods. Mol. Biol.* 118, 419–432, 1999.

7. Sanford, J.R., Ellis, J., and Cáceres, J.F., Multiple roles of arginine/serine-rich splicing factors in RNA processing, *Biochem. Soc. Trans.* 33, 443–446, 2005.

8. Rasheva, V.I., Knight, D., Borko, P., Marsh, K., and Frolov, M.V., Specific role of the SR protein splicing factors B52 in cell cycle control in *Drosophila*, *Mol. Cell. Biol.* 26, 3468–3477, 2006.

9. Ma, X., and He, F., Advances in the study of SR protein family, *Genomics Proteomics Bioinformatics* 1, 2–8, 2003.

10. Hammarskold, M.-L., and Rekosh, D., SR proteins: To shuttle or not to shuttle, that is the question, *J. Cell Biol.* 216, 1875–1877, 2017.

11. Jeong, S., SR proteins: Binders, regulators, and connectors of RNA, *Mol. Cells* 40, 1–9, 2017.

STAINING

Staining is a process by which contrast is introduced into a sample such as a tissue section or an electrophoretogram. The process of staining uses an organic chemical referred to as a stain or dye.[1–3] In positive staining, the item of interest is "staining" (absorbs the stain); in negative staining, the item of interest is unreactive and the background absorbs the stain providing the necessary contrast.

1. Hayat, M.A., *Stains and Cytochemical Methods,* Plenum Press, New York, 1993.

2. Horobin, R.W., *Conn's Biological Stains: A Handbook of Dyes, Stains and Fluorochromes for Use in Biology and Medicine*, Bios Publishers, Oxford, UK, 2002.

3. Sabris, R.W., *Handbook of Biological Dyes and Stains: Synthesis and Industrial Applications*, Wiley-Blackwell, Hoboken, NJ, 2010.

STANDARD CONDITIONS (STANDARD STATE)

The standard state or standard conditions is used to define conditions

Pressure: 1 atm; Temperature: 25°C (298°K); all solutions are 1 molar.

STANDARD ELECTRODE POTENTIAL

The value ($E°$) for the standard electromotive force of a cell in which hydrogen under standard conditions is oxidized to hydronium ions (solvated protons) at the left-hand electrode. This value is used as a standard to measure electrode potentials.

STANDARD FREE ENERGY

A thermodynamic function designated G (after Walter Gibbs, frequently referred to as the Gibbs free energy). The change in G (ΔG) for a given reaction provides the information on the amount of energy derived from the reaction and is a product of the changes in enthalpy and entropy: $\Delta G = \Delta H - T\Delta S$. The standard free energy designated $\Delta G°$ indicates the values are those obtained for standard conditions. ΔG is negative for a thermodynamically favorable reaction. See **enthalpy** and **entropy**.

STARK EFFECT

The Stark effect is the effect of an electrical field on the absorption/emission of spectrum of a compound resulting in splitting. In the α–canonical example of the microwave spectrum of a gas, the splitting is proportional to the dipole moment and the magnitude of the dipole moment may be derived from the spectrum.[1] There are number of examples of the Stark effect in biochemistry including the effect of the electric field of an α-helix on spectrum of a covalently attached probe (4-[methylamino]benzoic acid),[2,3] the effect of an electric field on the spectrum of tryptophan providing insight into the fluorescence properties,[4] the effect of a local electric field on the fluorescence of a 3-hydroxyflavone dye coupled to a lysine residue,[5] the vibrational splitting of the spectrum carbon monoxide which measures the magnitude and direction of the internal electric effect in the Xe4 cavity of a myoglobin mutant,[6] providing the rationale for the spectral changes of red fluorescent proteins,[7] and the establishment of an electrostatic mechanism for the binding of Ras and Rap1a to the Ras binding domain of the RalGDS.[8] In this latter study,[8] cysteine residues were engineered into the RalGDS binding site for Ras, converted to cyanocysteine providing a thiocyanate (nitrile) functional group serving as spectral probe.

1. Silbey, R.J., Alberty, R.A., and Bawendi, M.G., *Physical Chemistry*, 4th edn., p. 474, John Wiley & Sons, Hoboken, NJ, 2005.
2. Lockhart, D.J., and Kim, P.S., Internal Stark effect measurement of the electric field at the amino terminus of an α-helix, *Science* 257, 947–951, 1992.
3. Sitkoff, D., Lockhart, D.J., Sharp, K.A., and Honig, B., Calculation of electrostatic effects at the amino terminal of an α helix, *Biophys. J.* 67, 2251–2260, 1994.
4. Pierce, D.W., and Boxer, S.A., Stark effect spectroscopy of tryptophan, *Biophysical J.* 68, 1583–1591, 1995.
5. Klymchenko, A.S., Avilov, S.V., and Demchenko, A.P., Resolution of Cys and Lys labeling of α-crystallin with site-sensitive fluorescent 3-hydroxyflavone dye, *Anal. Biochem.* 329, 43–57, 2004.
6. Lehle, H., Kriegl, J.M., Nienhaus, K., et al., Probing electric fields in protein cavities by using the vibrational Stark effect of carbon monoxide, *Biophys. J.* 88, 1978–1990, 2005.

7. Drobizher, M., Tillo, S., Makarov, N.S., Hughes, T.E., and Rebane, A., Color changes in red fluorescent proteins are due to internal quadratic Stark effect, *J. Phys. Chem. B Letters* 113, 12860–12864, 2009.
8. Stafford, A.J., Ensign, D.L., and Webb, L.J., Vibrational Stark effect spectroscopy at the interface of Ras and Rap1A bound to the Ras binding domain of RalGDS reveals an electrostatic mechanism of protein-protein interaction, *J. Phys. Chem.* 114, 15331–15544, 2010.

STATISTICAL POWER

Statistical power can be defined as the probability of obtaining a statistically significant result. A more formal definition is 1-probability of a type II error where a type II error is defined as the erroneous retention of a false null hypothesis.[1-3] There are varied applications of the principle of statistical power in biochemistry and molecular biology.[4-8] In general, the statistical power increases with the number of subjects/observations in a study. It is essential to consult with a statistician **before** not after starting a large study to determine the power required to obtain statistically valid results. Do not expect a statistician to solve problems of inadequate study design after the fact.

1. Gerstman, B.B., *Basic Biostatistics. Statistics for Public Health Practice*, Jones and Bartlett Publishers, Sudbury, MA, 2001.
2. Feinstein, A.R., *Principles of Medical Statistics*, Chapman and Hall/CRC Press, Boca Raton, FL, 2002.
3. *Encyclopaedic Companion to Medical Statistics*, ed. B.S. Everitt and C.R. Palmer, Hodden Arnold, London, UK, 2005.
4. Rose, J.E., Behm, F.M., Westman, E.C., and Johnson, M, Dissociating nicotine and nonnicotine components of cigarette smoking, *Pharmacol. Biochem. Behavior* 67, 71–81, 2000.
5. Faul, F., Erdfelder, E., Buchner, A., and Lang, A.-G., Statistical power analyses using G*Power 3.1: Tests for correlation and regression analyses, *Behavioral Res. Methods* 4, 1149–1160, 2005.
6. Bourgon, R., Gentleman, R., and Huber, W., Independent filtering increases detection power for high-throughput experiments, *Proc. Natl. Acad. Sci. USA* 107, 9546–9551, 2010.
7. Goodpaster, A.M., Romick-Rosedale, L.E., and Kennedy, M.A., Statistical significance analysis of nuclear magnetic resonance-based metabolomics data, *Anal. Biochem.* 401, 134–143, 2010.
8. Graham, E.B., Wieder, W.R., Leff, J.W., et al., Do we need to understand microbial communities to predict ecosystem function? A comparison of statistical models of nitrogen cycling processes, *Soil Biol. Biochem.* 68, 279–282, 2014.

STEROID HORMONE RECEPTOR (SHR)

Steroid hormone receptors are members of the nuclear receptor family.[1–4] The functional aspects of Steroid hormone receptors consist of an amino terminal domain (DBD) which contains two zinc fingers which bind DNA and a ligand-binding domain (LBD) in the C-terminal region of the molecule.[5,6] Steroid hormone receptors are ligand-activate transcription factors which influence protein synthesis by enhancing specific mRNA production. There is particular interest in the role of steroid receptors in oncology.[7–9]

1. Giguere, V., Ong, E.S., Segui, P., and Evans, R.M., Identification of a receptor for the morphogen retinoic acid, *Nature* 330, 624–629, 1987.
2. Petkovich, M., Brand, N.J., Krust, A., and Chambon, P., A human retinoic acid receptor which belongs to the family of nuclear receptor, *Nature* 330, 444–451, 1987.
3. Mangelsdorf, D.J., Thummel, C., Beato, M., et al., The nuclear receptor family: The second decade, *Cell* 83, 835–839, 1995.
4. Lazar, M.A., Maturing of the nuclear receptor family, *J. Clin. Invest.* 127, 1123–1125, 2017.
5. *Molecular Biology of Steroid and Nuclear Hormone Receptors*, ed. L.P., Freedman, Birkhäuser, Boston, MA, 1998.
6. Lavery, D.N., and McEwan, I.J., Structure and functions of steroid receptor AF1 transactivation domains: Induction of active conformations, *Biochem. J.* 391, 449–464, 2005.
7. Leehy, K.A., Regan Anderson, R.M., Danial, A.R., Lange, C.A., and Ostrander, J.H., Modifications to glucocorticoid and progesterone receptors alter cell fate in breast cancer, *J. Mol. Endocrinol.* 56, R99–R114, 2016.
8. D'Uva, G., and Lauriola, M., Towards the emerging crosstalk: ERBB family and steroid hormones, *Semin. Cell Dev. Biol.* 50, 143–152, 2016.
9. Truong, T.H., and Lange, C.A., Deciphering steroid receptor crosstalk in hormone-derived cancers, *Endocrinology* 159, 3897–3907, 2018.

STOCHASTIC

Referring to a random distribution of data or information. Stochastic is equivalent to random. Stochastic also has a meaning in music referring to composition where the basic sound structure is determined but where internal detail may be left to chance.[1] Systematic would be an antonym to stochastic.

1. *Oxford English Dictionary*, Oxford University Press, Oxford, UK, 2019.

STOCHASTIC/STOCHASTIC PROCESS

The term stochastic denotes involving or containing random errors. A stochastic process is a process consisting of a series of random variables (x_t), where t assumes values in a certain range of T.[1] The term stochastic process and random process are considered to be interchangeable. The concept of stochastic and stochastic process in of increasing importance in biochemistry with the advent of sophisticated analytical techniques and the ability to study single cells.[2,3] Stochastic is contrasted with coordinated[4] or deterministic[5] in describing a process.

1. *The Cambridge Dictionary of Statistics*, ed. B.S. Everitt, Cambridge University Press, Cambridge, UK, 1998.
2. Elowitz, M.B., Levine, A.J., Siggia, E.D., and Swain, P.S., Stochastic gene expression in a single cell, *Science* 297, 1183–1186, 2002.
3. Engl, C., Noise in bacterial gene expression, *Biochem. Soc. Trans.*, in press (doi:10.1042/BST20180500), 2019.
4. Lee, R.G., Rudler, D.L., Rackham, O., and Filipovska, A., Is mitochondrial gene expression coordinated or stochastic? *Biochem. Soc. Trans.* 46, 1239–1246, 2018.
5. Iioka, T., Takahashi, S., Yoshida, Y., et al., A kinetics study of ligard substitution reaction on dinuclear platinum complexes: Stochastic versus deterministic approach, *J. Comput. Chem.* 40, 279–285, 2019.

STRUCTURAL BIOLOGY

Structural biology is a discipline focuses on the study of the secondary, tertiary, and higher structures of proteins in the proteome and other macromolecules including macromolecular complexes.[1–18] Structural biology uses as variety of technologies most of which were developed for the characterization of proteins, nucleic acids, and polysaccharides including but limited to the use of crystallography,[19–21] mass spectrometry,[22,23] nuclear magnetic resonance,[24,25] and cryo-electron microscopy (cryo-EM).[26–30]

1. Smith, C.U.M., *Molecular Biology: A Structural Approach,* MIT Press, Cambridge, MA, 1968.
2. Devons, S., *Biology and the Physical Sciences*, Columbia University Press, New York, 1969.
3. Rhodes, D., and Schwabe, J.W., Structural biology. Complex behavior, *Nature* 352, 478–479, 1991.
4. Riddihough, G., Structural biology. Picture an enzyme at work, *Nature* 362, 793, 1993.
5. Diamond, R., *Molecular Structures in Biology*, Oxford University Press, Oxford, UK, 1993.
6. Waksman, G., and Caparon, M., *Structural Biology of Bacterial Pathogenesis*, ASM Press, Washington, DC, 2005.

7. Weiner, S., Sagi, I., and Addadi, L., Structural biology. Choosing the crystallization path less traveled, *Science* 309, 1027–1028, 2005.

8. Sundstrom, S., and Martin, N., *Structural Genomics and High Throughput Structural Biology*, Taylor & Francis, Boca Raton, FL, 2006.

9. Chiu, W., Baker, M.L., and Almo, S.C., Structural biology of cellular machines, *Trends Cell Biol.* 16, 144–150, 2006.

10. Aravind, L., Iyer, L.M., and Koonin, E.V., Comparative genomics and structural biology of the molecular innovations of eukaryotes, *Curr. Opin. Struct. Biol.* 16, 409–419, 2006.

11. Luckey, M., *Membrane Structural Biology: With Biochemical and Biophysical Foundations*, Cambridge University Press, Cambridge, UK, 2008.

12. Liljas, A., Liljas, L., Piskur, J., et al., *Textbook of Structural Biology*, World Scientific Publishers, Hackensack, NJ, 2009.

13. *Plant Structural Biology: Hormonal Regulations,* ed. T. Hakoshima and J. Hejátko, Springer Science and Business, Cham, Switzerland, 2018.

14. Wang, Y., and Feigon, J., Structural biology of telomerase and its interaction at telomeres, *Curr. Opin. Struct. Biol.* 47, 77–87, 2018.

15. Hasan, S.S., Sevvana, M. Kuhn, R.J., and Rossman, M.G., Structural biology of Zika virus and other flaviviruses, *Nat. Struct. Mol. Biol.* 25, 13–20, 2018.

16. Shi, R., Shen, X.X., Rokas, A., and Eichman, B.F., Structural biology of the HEAT-like repeat family of DNA glycosylases, *Bioessays* 40, e1800133, 2018.

17. Audet, M., and Stevens, R.C., Emerging structural biology of lipid G-protein coupled receptors, *Protein Sci.* 28, 292–304, 2019.

18. Reis, R., and Moraes, I., Structural biology and structure-function relationships of membrane proteins, *Biochem. Soc. Trans.* 47, 47–61, 2019.

19. Johansson, L.C., Stauch, B., Ishchenko, A., and Cherezov, V., A bright future for serial femtosecond crystallography with XFELs, *Trends Biochem. Sci.* 42, 749–762, 2017.

20. Mizohata, E., Nakane, T., Fukuda, Y., Nango, E., and Iwata, S., Serial femtosecond crystallography at the SACLA: Breakthrough to dynamic structural biology, *Biophys. Rev.* 10, 209–218, 2018.

21. Selikhanov, G.K., Fando, M.S., Dontsova, M.V., and Gabdukhakov, A.G., Investigations of photosensitive proteins by serial crystallography, *Biochemistry* (Mosc) 83(Suppl 1), S163–S175, 2018.

22. Calabrese, A.N., and Radford, S.E., Mass spectrometry-enabled structural biology of membrane proteins, *Methods* 147, 1870–205, 2018.

23. Chavez, J.D., and Bruce, J.E., Chemical cross-linking with mass spectrometry: A tool for systems structural biology, *Curr. Opin. Chem. Biol.* 48, 8–18, 2019.

24. Demers, J.P., Fricke, P., Shi, C., Chevelkov, V., and Lange, A., Structural determination of supra-molecular assemblies by solid-state NMR: Practical considerations, *Prog. Nucl. Magn. Reson. Spectrosc.* 109, 51–78, 2018.

25. Shimada, I., Ueda, T., Kofuku, Y., Eddy, M.T., and Wüthrich, K., GPCR drug discovery: Integrating solution NMR data with crystal and cryo-EM structures, *Nat. Rev. Drug Discov.*, in press (doi:10.1038/nrd.2018.180), 2019.

26. Henderson, R., From electron crystallography to single particle cryoEM (Nobel Lecture), *Angew. Chem. Int. Ed. Engl.* 57, 10804–10825, 2018.

27. Parent, K.N., Schrad, J.R., and Cingolani, G., Breaking symmetry in viral icosahedral capsids as seen through the lenses of X-ray crystallography and cyrp-electron microscopy, *Viruses* 10, E67, 2018.

28. Brown, A., and Shao, S., Ribosomes and cryo-EM: A duet, *Curr. Opin. Struct. Biol.* 52, 1–7, 2018.

29. Cheng, Y., Single-particle cryo-EM-How did it get here and where will it go, *Science* 361, 876–880, 2018.

30. Cheng, Y., Membrane protein structural biology in the era of single particle cryo-EM, *Curr. Opin. Struct. Biol.* 52, 58–63, 2018.

STRUCTURAL GENOMICS

Structural genomics is a discipline focusing on the determination of the three-dimensional structure of all gene products of the genome (physical aspects of the genome)[1-8] using a variety of techniques including x-ray crystallography, nuclear magnetic resonance, and cryo-electron microscopy. The key in differentiating structural genomics from related activities such as structural biology and structural proteomics is the emphasis on 3-dimensional structure and elucidation of protein folds. The current focus of structural genomics is directed toward drug discovery and other therapeutic approaches.[9-13]

1. Gaasterland, T., Structural genomics taking shape, *Trends Genet.* 14, 135, 1998.

2. Montellione, G.T., and Anderson, S., Structural genomics: Keystone for a human proteome project, *Nat. Struct. Biol.* 6, 11–12, 1999.

3. Zarembinski, T.I., Hung, L.W., Mueller-Dieckmann, H.J., et al., Structure-based assignment of the biochemical function of a hypothetical protein: A test case of structural genomics, *Proc. Natl. Acad. Sci. USA* 95, 15189–15193, 1998.

4. Elofsson, A., and Sonnhammer, E.L., A comparison of sequence and structure protein domain families as a basis for structural genomics, *Bioinformatics* 15, 480–500, 1999.

5. Skolnick, J., Fetrow, J.S., and Kolinski, A., Structural genomics and its importance for gene function analysis, *Nat. Biotechnol* 18, 283–287, 2000.

6. Burley, S.K., and Bonnano, J.B., Structural genomics of proteins from conserved biochemical pathways and processes, *Curr. Opin. Struct. Biol.* 12, 383–391, 2002.

7. Lundstrom, K., Structural genomics of GPCRs, *Trends Biotechnol.* 23, 103–108, 2005.

8. Grabowski, M., Niedzialkowska, E., Zimmerman, M.D., and Minor, W., The impact of structural genomics: The first quindecinnial, *J. Struct. Funct. Genomics* 17, 1–16, 2016.

9. Stacy, R., Anderson, W.F., and Myler, P.J., Structural genomics support for infectious disease drug design, *ACS Infect. Dis.* 1, 127–129, 2015.

10. Franklin, M.C., Cheung, J., Rudolph, M.J., et al., Structural genomics for drug design against the pathogen *Coxiella burnetil, Proteins* 83, 2124–2136, 2015.

11. Bradley, A.R., Echalier, A., Fairhead, M., et al., The SGC beyond structural genomics: Redefining the role of 3D structures by coupling genomic stratification with fragment-based discovery, *Essays Biochem.* 61, 495–503, 2017.

12. Waldmann, T.A., JAK/STAT pathway directed therapy of T-cell leukemia/lymphoma: Inspired by functional and structural genomics, *Mol. Cell. Endocrinol.* 451, 66–70, 2017.

13. Varga, J., Dobson, L., Reményi, I., and Tusnády, G.E., TSTMP: Target selection for structural genomics of human transmembrane proteins, *Nucleic Acids Res.* 45(D1), D325–D330, 2017.

STRUCTURAL PROTEOMICS

Structural proteomics is the study of the primary, secondary, and tertiary structure of the proteins in a proteome including functional predictions from primary structure.[1–17] Structural proteomics uses a number of techniques including x-ray crystallography and chemical modification. There is conceptional overlap between structural proteomic and other disciplines such as structural biology and structural genomics.

1. Jhoti, H., High-throughput structural proteomics using x-rays, *Trends Biotechnol.* 19 (10 Suppl), S67–S71, 2001.

2. Norin, M., and Sundstrom, M., Structural proteomics: Developments in structure-to-function, predictions, *Trends Biotechnol.* 20, 79–84, 2002.

3. Mylvagenam, S.E., Prahbakaran, M., Tudor, S.S., et al., Structural proteomics: Methods in deriving protein structural information and issues in data management, *Biotechniques* March Suppl., 42–46, 2002.

4. Sali, A., Glaseser, R., Earnest, T., and Baumeister, W., From words to literature in structural proteomics, *Nature* 422, 216–225, 2003.

5. Lefkovits, I., Functional and structural proteomics: A critical appraisal, *J. Chromatog. B. Anal. Technol. Biomed. Life. Sci.* 787, 1–10, 2003.

6. Jung, J.W., and Lee, W., Structure-based functional discovery of proteins: Structural proteomics, *J. Biochem. Mol. Biol.* 37, 28–34, 2004.

7. Yakunin, A.F., Yee, A.A., Savchenko, A., et al., Structural proteomics: A tool of genome annotation, *Curr. Opin. Chem. Biol.* 9, 42–48, 2004.

8. Liu, H.L., and Hsu, J.P., Recent developments in structural proteomics for protein structure determination, *Proteomics* 5, 2056–2068, 2005.

9. Vinarov, D.A., and Markley, J.L, High-throughput automated platform for nuclear magnetic resonance-based structural proteomics, *Expert Rev. Proteomics* 2, 49–55, 2005.

10. Banci, L., Bertini, I., Luchinat, C., and Mori, M., NMR in structural proteomics and beyond, *Prog. Nucl. Magn. Spectrosc.* 56, 247–266, 2010.

11. Petrotchenko, E.V., and Borchers, C.H., Crosslinking combined with mass spectrometry for structural proteomics, *Mass Spectrom. Rev.* 29, 862–876, 2010.

12. Donnarumma, D., Faleri, A., Costantino, P., Rappuoli, R., and Norais, N., The role of structural proteomics in vaccine development; recent advances and future prospects, *Expert Rev. Proteomics* 13, 55–68, 2016.

13. Leitner, A., Cross-linking and other structural proteomic techniques: How chemistry is enabling mass spectrometry applications in structural biology, *Chem. Sci.* 7, 4792–4803, 2016.

14. Kar, U.K., Simonian, M., and Whitelegge, J.P., Integral membrane proteins: Bottom-up, top-down and structural proteomics, *Expert. Rev. Proteomics* 14, 715–723, 2017.

15. Zhang, B., Cheng, M., Rempel, D., and Gross, M.L., Implementing fast photochemical oxidation of proteins (FPOP) as a footprinting approach to solve diverse problems in structural biology, *Methods* 144, 94–103, 2018.

16. Leitner, A., A review of the role of chemical modification methods in contemporary mass spectrometry-based proteomics research, *Anal. Chim. Acta* 1000, 2–19, 2018.

17. Hernychová, L., Rosůlek, M., Kádek, A., et al., The C-type lectin-like receptor NKrp1b: Structural proteomics reveals features affecting protein conformation and interactions, *J. Proteomics* 196, 162–172, 2016.

SUMOylation

SUMOylation is a term describing the modification of proteins with small ubiquitin-like modifier (SUMO).[1] There are 4 SUMO proteins which are members of ubiquitin-like protein family.[2–7] The majority of SUMO substrate proteins are located in the nucleus.[4,6] There are diverse functions of sumoylation.[8,9] The process of sumoyllation, like ubiquination, is a reversible, complex process.[8,10]

1. *Sumoylation: Molecular Biology and Biochemistry,* Horizon Biosciences, Wynmondham, UK, 2004.

2. Müller, S., Hoege, C., Pyrowolakis, G., and Jenisch, S., SUMO, ubiquitin's mysterious cousin, *Nat. Rev. Molec. Cell Biol.* 2, 202–210, 2001.

3. Watts, F.Z., SUMO modification of proteins other than transcription factors, *Semin. Cell Dev. Biol.* 15, 211–220, 2004.

4. Gill, G., SUMO and ubiquitin in the nucleus: Different functions, similar mechanisms? *Genes Dev.* 18, 2046–2059, 2004.

5. Navotchova, M., Budhiraja, R., Coupland, G., Eisenhaber, F., and Bachmair, A., SUMO conjugation in plants, *Planta* 220, 1–8, 2004.

6. Bossis, G., and Melchior, F., Regulation of SUMOylation by reversible oxidation and SUMO conjugating enzymes, *Mol. Cell.* 21, 349–357, 2006.

7. Adorisio, S., Fierabracci, A., Muscari, I., et al., SUMO proteins: Guardians of immune system, *J. Autoimmunity* 84, 21–28, 2017.

8. Creton, S., and Jentsch, S., Snapshot: The SUMO system, *Cell* 143, 848–848.el, 2010.

9. Jakobs, A., Koehnke, J., Hinstedt, F., et al., Ubc9 fusion-directed SUMOylation (UFDS): A method to analyze function of protein SUMOylation, *Nature Methods* 4, 245–250, 2007.

10. Ovaa, H., and Vertegaal, A.C.O., Probing ubiquitin and SUMO conjugation and deconjugation, *Biochem. Soc. Trans.* 46, 423–436, 2018.

SURFACE PLASMON RESONANCE

Surface plasmon resonance is a technique which uses affinity binding to measure the rate of interaction between biomolecules and amount of an analyte bound to a probe on gold surface.[1–12] Conceptually surface plasmon resonance is related to other binding assays such as ELISA assays. In surface plasmon resonance, binding is measured by the increase in mass on a target probe which is bound to a surface. Frequently gold is the surface. Incident light is refracted from the surface and measured as reflectance (surface plasmon resonance). See also **localized surface plasmon resonance**.

1. Englebienne, P., Van Hoonacker, AS., and Verhas, M., Surface plasmon resonance: Principles, methods and applications in biomedical sciences, *Spectroscopy* 17, 255–273, 2003.

2. Smith, E.A., and Corn, R.M., Surface plasmon resonance imaging as a tool to monitor biomolecular interactions in an array-based format, *Appl. Spectros.* 57, 320A–332A, 2003.

3. Lee, J.H., Yan, Y., Marriott, G., and Corn, R.M., Quantitative functional analysis of protein complexes on surfaces, *J. Physiol.* 563, 61–71, 2005.

4. Piehler, J., New methodologies for measuring protein interactions in vivo and in vitro, *Curr. Opin. Struct. Biol.* 15, 4–14, 2005.

5. Buijs, J., and Franklin, G.C., SPR-MS in functional proteomics, *Brief Funct. Genomic Proteomic* 4, 39–47, 2005.

6. Pattnaik, P., Surface plasmon resonance: Applications in understanding receptor-ligand interaction, *Appl. Biochem. Biotechnol.* 126, 76–92, 2005.

7. Homola, J., Vaisocherova, H., Dostalek, J., and Piliarik, M., Multi-analyte surface plasmon resonance biosensing, *Methods* 37, 26–36, 2005.

8. *Surface Plasmon Resonance Based Sensors*, ed. J. Dostálek, Springer, Berlin, Germany, 2006.

9. Oliveira, L.C., Lima, A.M.N., Thirstrup, C., and Neff, H.F., *Surface Plasmon Resonance Sensors: A Materials Guide to Design and Optimization,* Springer, Cham, Switzerland, 2015.

10. Olaru, A., Bala, C., Jaffrezic-Renault, N., and Aboul-Enein, H.Y., Surface plasmon resonance (SPR) biosensors in pharmaceutical analysis, *Crit. Res. Anal. Chem.* 45, 97–105, 2015.

11. *Handbook of Surface Plasmon Resonance*, ed. R.B.M. Schasfoort, Royal Society of Chemistry, Cambridge, UK, 2017.

12. Simon, L., and Gyurcsányi, R.E., Multiplexed assessment of the surface density of DNA probes on DNA microarrays by surface plasmon resonance imaging, *Anal. Chim. Acta* 1047, 131–138, 2019.

SURFACE TENSION

Surface tension (γ) is the force exerted by bulk solution on the surface molecules of a solution. Surface energy was defined by the potential energy per unit surface area,[1] but is now defined as the energy required for a unit change of surface (force/unit length; N/m^{-2}). In the case of water, surface tensions at 25°C is 71.97×10^{-3} N m^{-1} or 71.97 mN m^1 at 25°C.[2] While it is common to think as surface tension as a force preventing a molecule from leaving the fluid phase and going into the vapor phase, it is useful to consider surface tension as creating a thin, elastic sheet at the air–surface interface.[3,4] It is noted that while most attention is given to surface tension of liquids at air–liquid interfaces, solids also have surface tension.[4] Water molecule do strongly interact with each other providing a rationale for the value of 71.97 mN m^{-1} while that of acetone is 23.7 mN m^{-1} [2] results from a lesser self-association of acetone. The surface tension of water decreases with increasing temperature with a value of 58.8 nM m^{-1} at 100°C.[2,5] Some others values of interest are 485.56 mN m^{-1} for mercury (Hg), 954 mN m^{-1} for scandium (Sc), and 62.5 mN m^{-1} for ethylene glycol. A more complete listing of values for surface tension for various compounds and solutions are available elsewhere.[5] Pulmonary surfactant is a membrane-bound lipid/protein which reduces the surface tension of water in the lung permitting effective alveolar function.[6,7] See also **surfactants**.

1. Miller, F., Jr., *College Physics*, Harcourt, Brace & World, New York, 1959.

2. Silbey, R.J., Alberty, R.A., and Bawendi, M.G., *Physical Chemistry*, 4th edn., John Wiley & Sons, Hoboken, NJ, 2005.

3. Guyton, A.C., Moffatt, D.S., and Adair, T.H., Role of alveolar surface tension in transepithelial movement of fluid, in *Pulmonary Surfactant,* ed. B. Robertson, L.M.G. Van Golde, and J.J. Batenburg, Chapter 5, pp. 171–185, Elsevier, Amsterdam, the Netherlands, 1984.

4. Hill, B.A., *The Biology of Surfactant*, Cambridge University Press, Cambridge, UK, 1988.

5. *Handbook of Chemistry and Physics*, ed. D.R. Lide, CRC Press/Taylor & Francis Group, Boca Raton, FL, 2005–2006.

6. *Pulmonary Surfactant*, ed. B. Robertson, L.M.G. Van Holde, and J.J. Batenburg, Elsevier, Amsterdam, the Netherlands, 1984.

7. Bernhard, W., Lung surfactant: Function and composition in the context of development and respiratory physiology, *Ann. Anat.* 208, 146–150, 2016.

SURFACTANT

The term surfactant dates to the 1950s when it was developed as a shortened version of surface-active agent. A surfactant can be defined as a substance that reduces or otherwise affects the surface tension of water or other liquid; a surface-active agent.[1] A **pulmonary surfactant** is a mixture of surface-active agents (mainly lipoproteins) coating the alveoli of the lungs, which reduce alveolar surface tension and contribute to the elasticity of the lungs.[1] Surfactants are amphipathic/amphiphilic molecules which tend to migrate to surfaces or interfaces in solutions (at equilibrium, the concentration of a surfactant is higher at the interface than the concentration in bulk solution).[2–14] The term detergent is sometimes used interchangeably with surfactant; the purist might consider the term detergency to reflect on cleansing which is one of the several properties of surfactants. Surfactants can also be described as dispersing agents, emulsifiers, foaming agents, stabilizers, solubilizers or wetting agents depending on their performance activity and effect on final product. Surfactants can be divided into four broad chemical categories; anionic compounds such as soaps which are sodium salts of long-chain alkyl carboxylic acids (alkanoic acids); cationic compounds such as alkyl amine derivatives such as Triton™ RW; amphoteric derivatives; and nonionic surfactants such as alkylphenol ethoxylates (Igepal™) and anhydrosorbitol esters (Tween derivatives). Surfactants are used extensively in the solubilization of membrane proteins and phospholipids.[15–20] Surfactants have been advanced as alternatives to organic solvents in samples extraction.[21,22] Nonionic surfactants have an effect (drag reduction) on fluid flow at low concentrations.[23,24] Pulmonary surfactant is a unique combination of lipid and protein associated the membrane of the aveolus.[25–28]

1. *Oxford English Dictionary*, Oxford University Press, Oxford, UK, 2019.

2. *Kirk-Othmer Encyclopedia of Chemical Technology*, 3rd edn., Vol. 22, Wiley-Interscience, New York, 1983.

3. *Nonionic Surfactants*, ed. M.J. Schick, Marcel-Dekker, New York, 1966.

4. Attwood, D., and Florence, A.T., *Surfactant Systems: Their Chemistry, Pharmacy, and Biology*, Chapman and Hall, London, UK, 1983.

5. Cross, J., *Anionic Surfactants Analytical Chemistry*, Marcel Dekker, New York, 1998.

6. van Oss, N.M., *Nonionic Surfactants Organic Chemistry*, Marcel Dekker, New York, 1998.

7. Holmberg, K., *Novel Surfactants Preparation, Applications, and Biodegradability,* Marcel Dekker, New York, 1998.

8. Kwak, J.C.T., *Polymer-Surfactant Systems*, Marcel Dekker, New York, 1998.

9. Hus, J.-P., Interfacial Forces and Fields Theory and Applications, Marcel Dekker, New York, 1999.

10. Pefferkorn, E., *Interfacial Phenomena in Chromatography*, Marcel Dekker, New York, 1999.

11. Myers, D., *Surfaces, Interfaces, and Colloid: Principles and Applications*, Wiley-VCH, New York, 1999.

12. Broze, G., *Handbook of Detergents*, Marcel Dekker, New York, 1999.

13. *Physical Properties of Lipids*, ed. A.G. Marangani and S.S. Narine, Marcel-Dekker, New York, 2002.

14. Myers, D., *Surfactant Science and Technology*, 3rd edn. Chapter 1, An overview of surfactant science and technology, John Wiley & Sons, Hoboken, NJ, 2006.

15. Lichtenberg, D., Robson, R.J., and Dennis, E.A., Solubilization of phospholipid by detergents. Structural and kinetic aspects, *Biochim. Biophys. Acta* 737, 285–304, 1983.

16. Dennis, E.A., Micellization and solubilization of phospholipid by surfactants, *Adv. Colloid Interface Sci.* 26, 155–175, 1986.

17. Silvius, J.R., Solubilization and functional reconstitution of biomembrane components, *Annu. Rev. Biophys. Biomol. Struct.* 21, 323–348, 1992.

18. Henry, G.D., and Sykes, B.D., Methods to study membrane protein structure in solution, *Methods Enyzmol.* 239, 515–535, 1994.

19. Bowie, J.H., Stabilizing membrane proteins, *Curr. Opin. Struct. Biol.* 11, 397–402, 2001.

20. Seddon, A.M., Curow, P., and Booth, B.J., Membrane proteins, lipids and detergents: Not just a soap opera, *Biochim. Biophys. Acta* 1666, 105–117, 2004.

21. Moradi, M., and Yamini, Y., Surfactant roles in modern sample preparation techniques: A review, *J. Sep. Sci.* 35, 2319–2340, 2012.

22. Ma, F., Liu, F., Xu, W., and Li, L., Surfactant and chaotropic agent assisted sequential extraction/on-pellet digestion (SCAD) for enhanced proteomics, *J. Proteome Res.* 17, 2744–2754, 2018.

23. Jacobs, E.W., Anderson, G.W., Smith, C.A., et al., Drag reduction using high molecular weight fractions of poly-ethylene oxide, in *Drag Reduction in Fluid Flows. Techniques for Friction Control*, ed. R.H.J. Sellin and R.T. Moses, Ellis-Horwood, Chichester, NY, 1989.

24. Drappier, J., Divoux, T., Amarouchene, Y., et al., Turbulent drag reduction by surfactants, *Europhysics Lett.* 74, 362–368, 2006.

25. *Pulmonary Surfactant*, ed. B. Robertson, L.M.G. Van Holde, and J.J. Batenburg, Elsevier, Amsterdam, the Netherlands, 1984.

26. Hill, B.A., *The Biology of Surfactant*, Cambridge University Press, Cambridge, UK, 1988.

27. Bernhard, W., Lung surfactant: Function and composition in the context of development and respiratory physiology, *Ann. Anat.* 208, 146–150, 2016.

28. Knudsen, L., and Ochs, M., The micromechanics of lung alveoli: Structure and function of surfactant and tissue components, *Histochem. Cell Biol.* 150, 661–676, 2018.

SURROGATE BIOMARKER/ SURROGATE ENDPOINT

A surrogate biomarker is a biomarker which can be used in place of or in addition to a clinical observation for diagnosis or prognosis.[1–9] A surrogate endpoint has been defined as "A biomarker that is intended to substitute for a clinical endpoint. A surrogate endpoint is expected to provide clinical benefit (or harm or lack of benefit or harm) based on epidemiologic, therapeutic, pathophysiologic, or other scientific evidence."[10,11] There is extensive use of surrogate endpoints in clinical research.[12–20]

A surrogate biomarker can be a surrogate endpoint but a surrogate biomarker can be used in other applications of biomarkers.

1. Morrish, P.K., How valid is dopamine transporter imaging as a surrogate marker in research trials on Parkinson's disease? *Mov. Disord.* 18(Suppl 7), S63–S70, 2003.

2. Bowdish, M.E., Arcasoy, S.M., Wilt, J.S., et al., Surrogate markers and risk factors for chronic lung allograft dysfunction, *Am. J. Transplant.* 4, 1171–1178, 2004.

3. Kantarci, K., and Jack, C.R., Jr., Quantitative magnetic resonance techniques as surrogate markers of Alzheimer's disease, *NeuroRx* 1, 196–205, 2004.

4. Ebos, J.M, Lee, C.R., Bogdanovic, E., et al., Vascular endothelial growth factor-mediated decrease in plasma soluble vascular endothelial growth factor receptor-2 levesl a surrogate biomarker for tumor growth, *Cancer Res.* 68, 521–529, 2008.

5. Chen, S.C., and Kontoyiannis, D.P., New molecular and surrogate biomarker-based tests in the diagnosis of bacterial and fungal infection in febrile neutropenic patients, *Curr. Opin. Infect. Dis.* 23, 567–577, 2010.

6. Lasa, A., Garcia, A., Alonso, C., et al., Molecular detection of peripheral blood breast cancer mRNA transcripts as a surrogate biomarker for circulating tumor cells, *PloS One* 8(9), e74059, 2013.

7. Yagyu, S., Iehara, T., Tanaka, S., et al., Serum-based quantification of MYCN gene amplification in young patients with neuroblastoma: Potential utility as a surrogate biomarker for neuroblastoma, *PLoS One* 11(8), e0161039, 2016.

8. Larsen, M.A., Isaksen, V.T., Moen, O.S., et al., Leptin to adiponectin ratio—A surrogate biomarker for early detection of metabolic disturbances in obesity, *Nutr. Metab. Cardiovasc. Dis.* 28, 1114–1121, 2018.

9. Gu, Z., He., Y., Zhang, Y., et al., Postprandial increase in serum CA125 as a surrogate biomarker for early diagnosis of ovarian cancer, *J. Transl. Med.* 16, 114, 2018.

10. Biomarkers Definitions Working Group, Biomarkers and surrogate endpoints: Preferred definitions and conceptual framework, *Clin. Pharmacol. Therapeutics* 69, 89–95, 2001.

11. Johannsson, G., Bidlingmaier, M., Biller, B.M.K., et al., Growth Hormone Research Society perspective on biomarkers of GH action in children and adults, *Endocrine Connections* 7, R126–R134, 2018.

12. Hilsenbeck, S.G., and Clark, G.M., Surrogate endpoints in chemoprevention of breast cancer: Guidelines for evaluation of new biomarkers, *J. Cell. Biochem. Suppl.* 17G, 205–211, 1993.

13. Kluft, C., Principles of use of surrogate markers and endpoints, *Maturitas* 47, 293–298, 2004.

14. Lieberman, R., Evidence-based medical perspectives: The evolving role of PSA for early detection, monitoring of treatment response, and as a surrogate end point of efficacy for intervention in men with different clinical risk states for the prevention and progression of prostate cancer, *Am. J. Ther.* 11, 501–506, 2004.

15. Li, Z., Chines, A.A., and Meredith, M.P., Statistical validation of surrogate endpoints: Is bone density a valid surrogate for fracture? *J. Musculoskelet. Neuronal Interact.* 4, 64–74, 2004.

16. Wier, C.J., and Walley, R.J., Statistical evaluation of biomarkers as surrogate endpoints: A literature review, *Stat. Med.* 25, 183–203, 2006.

17. Patel, R.B., Vadganathan, M., Samman-Tahhan, A., et al., Trends in utilization of surrogate endpoints in contemporary cardiovascular clinical trials, *Am. J. Cardiol.* 117, 2845–1850, 2016.

18. Fiteni, F., Westeel, V., and Bonnetain, F., Surrogate endpoints for overall survival in lung cancer trials: A review, *Expert Rev. Anticancer Ther.* 17, 447–454, 2017.

19. Bikdeli, B., Punnathinont, N., Akram, Y., et al., Two decades of cardiovascular trials with primary surrogate endpoints: 1990–2011, *J. Am. Heart Assoc.* 6(3), e005285, 2017.

20. Wickström, K., and Moseley, J., Biomarkers and surrogate endpoints in drug development: A European regulatory view, *Invest. Ophthalmol. Vis. Sci.* 58, BIO27–BIO33, 2017.

SYSTEMS BIOLOGY

Systems biology is the integration of data at the genomic, transcriptomic, proteomic, and metabolomic levels including functional and structural data to formulate a mathematical expression(s) to explain biological function.[1–8] Systems biology has become more diffuse but the focus remain on the acquisition of data and integrative analysis with emphasis on global analysis as opposed to a reductionist approach.[9–12]

1. Ideker, T., Galitski, T., and Hood, L., A new approach to decoding life: Systems biology, *Annu. Rev. Genomics Hum. Genet.* 2, 343–372, 2001.
2. van der Greef, J., Stroobant, P., and van der Heijden, R., The role of analytical sciences in medical systems biology, *Curr. Opin. Chem. Biol.* 8, 559–565, 2004.
3. Levesque, M.P., and Benfey, P.N., Systems biology, *Curr. Biol.* 14, R179–R189, 2004.
4. Weston, A.D., and Hood, L.J., Systems biology, proteomics, and the future of health care: Toward predictive, preventative, and personalized medicine, *J. Proteome Res.* 3, 179–196, 2004.
5. Kirschner, M.W., The meaning of systems biology, *Cell* 121, 503–504, 2005.
6. *Systems Biology: Definitions and Perspectives*, ed. L. Alberghina and H.V. Westerhoff, Springer, Berlin, Germany, 2005.
7. Philippi, S., and Kohler, J., Addressing the problems with life-science databases for traditional uses and systems biology, *Nat. Rev. Genet.* 7, 482–488, 2006.
8. Palsson, B., *Systems Biology: Properties of Reconstructed Networks*, Cambridge University Press, Cambridge, UK, 2006.
9. *Systems Biology*, ed. R.A. Meyers, Wiley-Blackwell, Weinheim, Germany, 2012.
10. *Systems Biology*, ed. M.G. Katze, Springer, Berlin, Germany, 2013.
11. *Systems Biology*, ed. J. Nielsen and S. Hofmann, Wiley-VCH, Weinheim, Germany, 2017.
12. *Systems Biology*, ed. N. Rajewsky, J. Stefan, and J. Barciszewski, Springer, Cham, Switzerland, 2018.

TARGET OF RAPOMYCIN (TOR)

TOR (target of rapomycin) is a highly conserved serine/threonine protein kinase, which is a regulator of cell homeostasis and cell growth; the mammalian target of Rapomycin (mTOR).[1,2] Rapamycin, a macrolide, was identified in 1975 as product from *Streptomyces hygroscopicus* which was an antifungal antibiotic.[3,4] TOR as target for the action of rapamycin was suggested by studies in 1991 on cell cycle arrest in yeast,[5] although such was suggested by earlier studies.[6] Subsequent studies that the effect of rapamycin was directed against a protein kinase in mammals.[7–9] Subsequent work identified mTOR as the protein kinase[10–13] Current work shows that mTOR is a heterotrimer (approximately 298 kDa)[2,8,10] consisting of a catalytic subunit (mTOR), a regulatory-associated protein of target of rapamycin (RAPTOR), and a mammalian lethal with SEC13 protein 8 (mLSTR8).[2] mTOR has a major role in mediating the effect of nutrients and growth factors of cell growth and differentiation.[2,14]

1. Har, N., and Sonenberg, N., Upstream and downstream of mTOR, *Genes & Development* 18, 1926–1945, 2004.
2. Hindupur, S.K., González, A., and Hall, M.N., The opposing action of target of Rapomycin and AMP-activated protein kinase in cell growth, in *Size Control in Biology from Organelles to Organisms*, ed. R. Heald, I.K. Hariharan, and D.B. Wake, pp. 221–240, Cold Spring Harbor Press, Cold Spring Harbor, NY, 2015.
3. Vézena, C., Kudelski, A., and Sehgal, S.N., Rapamycin (AY-22,989), a new antifungal antibiotic. I. Taxonomy of the producing streptomycete and isolation of the active principle, *J. Antibiotic* 28, 721–726, 1975.
4. Sehgal, S.N., Baker, H., and Vézena, C., Rapamycin (AY-22,989), a new antifungal antibiotic. II Fermentation, isolation and characterization, *J. Antibiotics* 28, 727–732, 1975.
5. Heitman J., Movva, N.R., and Hall, M.N., Targets for cell cycle arrest by the immunosuppressant rapamycin in yeast, *Science* 253, 905–909, 1991.
6. Singh, K. Sun, S., and Vézina, C., Rapamycin (AY-22,989), a new antifungal antibiotic. IV Mechanism of action, *J. Antibiot.* 32, 630–645, 1979.
7. Alvers, M.W., Williams, R.T., Brown, E.J., et al., FKBP-rapamycin inhibits a cyclin-dependent kinase activity and cyclin D1-Cdk association in early G1 of an osteosarcoma cell line, *J. Biol. Chem.* 268, 22825–22829, 1993.
8. Sabatini, D.M., Erdjument-Bromage, H., Lui, M., et al., RAFT1: A mammalian protein that binds to FKBP12 in a rapamycin-dependent fashion and is homologous to yeast TORs, *Cell* 78, 35–42, 1994.
9. Chiu, M.I., Katz, H., and Berlin, V., RAPT1, a mammalian homolog of yeast Tor, interacts with the FCBP12/rapamycin complex, *Proc. Natl. Acad. Sci. USA* 91, 12574–12578, 1994.
10. Hara, K., Yonezawa, K., Kozlowski, M.T., et al., Regulation of eIF-4E BP1 phosphorylation by mTOR, *J. Biol. Chem.* 272, 26457–26463, 1997.
11. Nishiuma, T., Hara, K., Tsujishita, Y., et al., Characterization of the phosphoproteins and protein kinase activity in mTOR immunoprecipitates, *Biochem. Biophys. Res. Commun.* 252, 440–444, 1998.
12. Gingras, A.-C., Raught, B., and Sonenberg, N., Regulation of translation initiation by FRAP/mTOR, *Genes & Development* 15, 807–826, 2001.
13. Laplante, M., and Sabatini, D.M., mTOR signaling in growth control and disease, *Cell* 149, 274–293, 2012.
14. Livi, G.P., Halcyon dayas of TOR: Reflections on the multiple independent discovery of the yeast and mammalian TOR proteins, *Gene,* in press (doi:10.1016/j.gene.2018.12.046), 2019.

TARGETED PROTEOMICS

The original definition of targeted proteomics was the analysis of a defined portion of a proteome such as a glycoproteome, phosphoproteome, ribosomal proteins, or a specific tissue proteome.[1-5] The concept of target proteomics has now been modified to describe procedures which analyze a narrow range of product ions using techniques such as selected reaction monitoring/multiple reaction monitoring to measure a specific protein.[6-10]

1. Knepper, M.A., and Masilamani, S., Targeted proteomics in the kidney using ensembles of antibodies, *Acta Physiol. Scand.* 173, 11–21, 2001.
2. Warcheid, B., and Fenselau, C., A targeted proteomics approach to the rapid identification of bacterial cell mixtures by matrix-assisted laser desorption/ionization mass spectrometry, *Proteomics* 4, 2877–2892, 2004.
3. Mirzaei, H., and Regnier, F., Structure specific chromatographic selection in targeted proteomics, *J. Chromatog. B Analyt. Technol. Biomed. Life. Sci.* 817, 23–34, 2005.
4. Freije, J.F., and Bischoff, R., The use of affinity sorbents in targeted proteomics, *Drug. Discov. Today Technol.* 3, 5–11, 2006.
5. Portelius, E., Zetterberg, H., Gobom, J., Andreasson, U., and Blennow, K., Targeted proteomics in Alzheimer's disease: Focus on amyloid-β, *Expert Rev. Proteomics* 5, 225–237, 2008.
6. Bereman, M.S., MacLean, B., Tomazela, D.M., Liebler, D.C., and MacCoss, M.J., The development of selected reaction monitoring methods for targeted proteomics via empirical refinement, *Proteomics* 12, 1134–1141, 2012.
7. Ebhardt, H.A., Root, A., Sander, C., and Aebersold, R., Applications of targeted proteomics in systems biology and translational medicine, *Proteomics* 15, 3193–3208, 2015.
8. Shi, T., Song, E., Nie, S., et al., Advances in targeted proteomics and applications to biomedical research, *Proteomics* 16, 2160–2182, 2016.
9. Borràs, E., and Sabidó, E., What is targeted proteomics? A concise revision of targeted acquisition and targeted data analysis in mass spectrometry, *Proteomics* 17, 1700180, 2017.
10. Arsova, B., Watt, M., and Usadel, B., Monitoring of plant protein post-translational modifications using targeted proteomics, *Front. Plant Sci.* 9, 1168, 2018.

TELOMERASE

Telomerase is a ribonucleoprotein complex (a reverse transcriptase; human telomerase reverse transcriptase, hTERT)[1] which catalyzes the synthesis of DNA at the ends of chromosomes and confers replicative immortality to cells and considered to be important in the aging process.[1-10] Telomerase functions to extend the telomere which shortens during each cycle of cell division.[11] Under normal conditions in humans, the activity of telomerase is repressed resulting in senescence.[11,12] Telomerase activity is not inhibited in cancer cells; inhibition of telomerase is a therapeutic target.[13-19]

1. Sandin, S., and Rhodes, D., Telomerase structure, *Curr. Opin. Struct. Biol.* 25, 104–110, 2014.
2. Blackburn, E.H., Greider, C.W., Henderson, E., et al., Recognition and elongation of telomeres by telomerase, *Genome* 31, 553–560, 1989.
3. Lamond, A.I., Tetrahymena telomerase contains an internal RNA template, *Trends Biochem. Sci.* 14, 202–204, 1989.
4. Greider, C.W., Telomeres, telomerase and senescence, *Bioessays* 12, 363–369, 1990.
5. Greider, C.W., Telomerase and telomere-length regulation: Lessons from small eukaryotes to mammals, *Cold Spring Harb. Symp. Quant. Biol.* 58, 719–723, 1993.
6. Rhyu, M.S., Telomeres, telomerase, and immortality, *J. Natl. Cancer Inst.* 87, 884–894, 1995.
7. Buchkovich, K.J., Telomeres, telomerase, and the cell cycle, *Prog. Cell Cycle Res.* 2, 187–195, 1996.
8. Flores, I., Benetti, R., and Blasco, M.A., Telomerase regulation and stem cell behavior, *Curr. Opin. Cell Biol.* 18, 254–260, 2006.
9. Hahn, W.C., Telomere and telomerase dynamics in human cells, *Curr. Mol. Med.* 5, 227–231, 2005.
10. Blackburn, E.H., Telomeres and telomerase: Their mechanisms of action and the effects of altering their functions, *FEBS Lett.* 579, 859–862, 2005.
11. Smith, S., Telomerase can't handle the stress, *Genes Dev.* 32, 597–599, 2018.
12. Zvereva, M.I., Shcherabakova, D.M., and Dontsova, O.A., Telomerase: Structure, functions, and activity regulation, *Biochemistry* (Mosc.) 75, 1563–1583, 2010.
13. Harley, C.B., Kim, N.W., Prowse, K.R., et al., Telomerase, cell immortality, and cancer, *Cold Spring Harb. Symp. Quant. Biol.* 59, 307–315, 1994.
14. Ulmer, G.A., Telomere maintenance in clinical medicine, *Am. J. Med.* 117, 262–269, 2004.
15. Shin, J.S., Hong, A., Solomon, M.J., and Lee, C.S., The role of telomeres and telomerase in the pathology of human cancer and aging, *Pathology* 38, 103–113, 2006.
16. Chen, H., Li, Y., and Tollefsbol, T.O., Strategies targeting telomerase inhibition, *Mol. Biotechnol.* 41, 194–199, 2009.
17. Shawi, M., and Autexier, C., Telomerase, senescence and ageing, *Mech. Ageing Dev.* 129, 3–10, 2008.
18. Cassar, L., Nicholls, C., Pinto, A.R., et al., TGF-beta receptor mediated telomerase inhibition, telomere shortening and breast cancer cell senescence, *Protein Cell* 8, 39–54, 2017.
19. Hannen, R., and Bartsch, J.W., Essential roles of telomerase reverse transcriptase hTERT in cancer stemness and metastasis, *FEBS Lett.* 592, 2023–2031, 2017.

THERANOSTIC OR THERAGNOSTIC

Theranostic[1–5] or theragnostic[6–10] both refer the use of a diagnostic procedure which can also be a therapeutic agent. Theranostic appears to be the preferred term based on extent usage as per PubMed; as of January 2019, there were 4000+ references to theranostic while 200+ references to theragnostic. A cursory consideration of the literature suggests a greater use of the term theragnostic in radiation therapy/oncology.

1. Picard, F.J., and Bergeron, M.G., Rapid molecular theranostics in infectious disease, *Drug Discov. Today.* 7, 1092–1101, 2002.
2. Bavelaar, B.M., Lee, B.Q., Gill, M.R., Falzone, N., and Vallis, K.A, Subcellular targeting of theranostic radionuclides, *Front. Pharmacol.* 9, 996, 2018.
3. Ahmedova, A., Todorov, B., Burdzhiev, N., and Goze, C., Copper radiopharmaceuticals for theranostic applications, *Eur. J. Med. Chem.* 157, 1406–1425, 2018.
4. Werner, R.A., Welch, A., Kircher, M., et al., The theranostic promise for neuroendocrine tumors in the late 2010s—Where do we stand, where do we go? *Theranostics* 8, 6088–6100, 2018.
5. Khalid, U., Vi., C., Henri., J., et al., Radiolabelled aptamers for theranostic treatment of cancer, *Pharmaceuticals* (Basal) 12, E2, 2018.
6. Bentzen, S.M., Theragnostic imaging for radiation oncology: Dose-painting by numbers, *Lancer Oncol.* 6, 112–117, 2005.
7. Srivastava, S.C., Paving the way to personalized medicine: Production of some promising theragnostic radionuclides at Brookhaven National Laboratory, *Semin. Nucl. Med.* 42, 151–163, 2012.
8. Cho, J.-H., Ha, N-R., Koh, S.-H., and Yoon, M.-Y., Design of PKCδ-specific small peptide as a theragnostic agent for glioblastoma, *Anal. Biochem.* 495, 63–70, 2016.
9. Lee, H.J., Yoon, Y.I., and Bae, Y.J., Theragnostic ultrasound using microbubbles in the treatment of prostate cancer, *Ultraconography* 35, 3), 309–317, 2016.
10. Uthaman, S., Huh, K.M., and Park, I.K., Tumor microenvironment-responsive nanoparticles for cancer theragnostic applications, *Biomater. Res.* 11, 11, 2018.

THERAPEUTIC EQUIVALENCE (TE)

The US Food and Drug Administration (FDA) has the following information in its glossary.[1]

Drug products classified as therapeutically equivalent can be substituted with the full expectation that the substituted product will produce the same clinical effect and safety profile as the prescribed product. Drug products are considered to be therapeutically equivalent **only** if they meet these criteria:

- They are pharmaceutical equivalents (contain the same active ingredient(s); dosage form and route of administration; and strength).
- They are assigned by FDA the same therapeutic equivalence codes starting with the letter "A". To receive a letter "A", FDA
  - Designates a brand name drug or a generic drug to be the Reference Listed Drug (RLD).
  - Assigns therapeutic equivalence codes based on data that a drug sponsor submits in an ANDA to scientifically demonstrate that its product is bioequivalent (i.e. performs in the same manner as the Reference Listed Drug).

THERAPEUTIC EQUIVALENCE (TE) CODES

The coding system for therapeutic equivalence evaluations allows users to determine whether FDA has evaluated a particular approved product as therapeutically equivalent to other pharmaceutically equivalent products (first letter) and to provide additional information on the basis of FDA's evaluations (second letter). Sample TE codes: AA, AB, BC (More on TE Codes).

- FDA assigns therapeutic equivalence codes to pharmaceutically equivalent drug products. A drug product is deemed to be therapeutically equivalent ("A" rated) only if:
  - A drug company's approved application contains adequate scientific evidence establishing through *in vivo* and/or *in vitro* studies the bioequivalence of the product to a selected reference listed drug.
  - Those active ingredients or dosage forms for which no *in vivo* bioequivalence issue is known or suspected.
  - Some drug products have more than one TE Code.
  - Those products which the FDA does not seem to be therapeutically equivalent are "**B**" rated.

OVER-THE-COUNTER DRUGS ARE NOT ASSIGNED TE CODES

Bioequivalence is related concept with more application to the pharmacokinetics of drugs as opposed to biologics. The following is definition of bioequivalence from the US Food and Drug Administration.[2]

Bioequivalence. Bioequivalence is the absence of a significant difference in the rate and extent to which the active ingredient or active moiety in pharmaceutical equivalents or pharmaceutical alternatives becomes available at the site of drug action when administered at the same molar dose under similar conditions in an appropriately designed study. Section 505 (j)(8)(B) of the FD&C Act describes one set of conditions under which a test and reference listed drug (see Section 1.4) shall be considered bioequivalent:

- The rate and extent of absorption of the [test] drug do not show a significant difference from the rate and extent of absorption of the [reference] drug when administered at the same molar dose of the therapeutic ingredient under similar experimental conditions in either a single dose or multiple doses; or
- The extent of absorption of the [test] drug does not show a significant difference from the extent of absorption of the [reference] drug when administered at the same molar dose of the therapeutic ingredient under similar experimental conditions in either a single dose or multiple doses and the difference from the [reference] drug in the rate of absorption of the drug is intentional, is reflected in its proposed labeling, is not essential to the attainment of effective body drug concentrations on chronic use, and is considered medically insignificant for the drug.

Where these above methods are not applicable (e.g. for drug products that are not intended to be absorbed into the bloodstream), other scientifically valid *in vivo* or *in vitro* test methods to demonstrate bioequivalence may be appropriate.

For example, bioequivalence may sometimes be demonstrated using an *in vitro* bioequivalence standard, especially when such an *in vitro* test has been correlated with human *in vivo* bioavailability data. In other situations, bioequivalence may sometimes be demonstrated through comparative clinical trials or pharmacodynamic studies.

Drug products including biologics can be considered to be therapeutically equivalent if such products can be substituted for brand product/prescribed product/originator product with the full expectation that such substituted product will produce the same clinical effect and safety as the brand product/prescribed product/originator product. Therapeutic equivalence is a critical component in the development of biosimilar products.[3-6]

1. https://www.fda.gov/drugs/informationondrugs/ucm079436.htm.
2. https://www.fda.gov/drugs/developmentapprovalprocess/ucm079068.htm.
3. Papamichael, K., Van Stappen, Jairath, V., et al., Review article; pharmacological aspects of anti-TNF biosimilars in inflammatory bowel diseases, *Aliment. Pharmacol. Ther.* 42, 1158–1169, 2015.
4. Cohen, S.B., Alten, R., Kameda, H., et al., A randomized controlled trial comparing PF-06438179/GP1111 (an infliximab biosimilar) and infliximab reference product for the treatment of moderate to severe active rheumatoid arthritis despite methotrexate therapy, *Arthritis Res. Ther.* 20(1), 155, 2018.
5. Fleischmann, R.M., Alten, R., Pileckyte, M., et al., A comparative clinical study of PF-06410293, a candidate adalmumab biosimilar and adalimumab reference product (Humira®) in the treatment of active rheumatoid arthritis, *Arthritis Res. Ther.* 20(1), 178, 2018.
6. Frapaise, F.S., The end of phase 3 clinical trials in biosimiliars development? *Biodrugs* 32, 319–324, 2018.

THERMAL CONDUCTIVITY

Thermal conductivity can be defined as the rate of heat transfer by conduction through unit thickness, across unit area for unit difference of temperature. The SI unit is W/m K (watt/meter Kelvin).[1] Values for thermal conductivity of a variety of materials can be found in the *CRC Handbook of Chemistry and Physics*.[1] Thermal conductivity is an important characteristic of biological tissues[2-9] and biomaterials.[10-16] There are several good sources of information on thermal conductivity.[17,18]

1. *CRC Handbook of Chemistry and Physics*, 99th edn., ed. J.R. Rumble, CRC Press, Boca Raton, FL, 2018.
2. Harting, R., and Pfeiffenberger, U., Thermal conductivity of bovine and pig retina: An experimental study, *Grafes Arch. Clin. Exp. Ophthalmol.* 219, 290–291, 1982.
3. Miller, J.H., Wilson, W.E., Swenberg, C.E. et al., Stochastic model of free radical yields in oriented DNA exposed to densely ionizing radiation at 77K, *Int. J. Radiat. Biol. Relat. Stud. Phys. Chem. Med.* 53, 901–907, 1988.
4. Arkin, H., Holmes, K.R., and Chen, M.M., A technique for measuring the thermal conductivity and evaluating the "apparent conductivity" concept in biomaterials, *J. Biomech. Eng.* 111, 276–282, 1989.
5. Cheng, J., Shoffner, M.A., Bhattacharya, A., and Mahajan, R.L., Temperature dependence of thermal conductivity of biological tissues, *Physiol. Meas.* 24, 769–783, 2003.
6. Liang, X.M., Sekar, P.K., Zhao, G., et al., High accuracy thermal conductivity measurement of aqueous cryoprotective agents and semi-rigid biological tissues using a microfabricated thermal sensor, *Sci. Rep.* 5, 10377, 2015.
7. Jiang, Z.D., Zhao, G., and Lu, G.R., Measurement of thermal conductivity of porcine liver in the temperature range of cryotherapy and hyperthermia (250 ~ 315 k) by a thermal sensor made of micron-scale enameled copper wire, *Cryo Letters* 37, 427–431, 2016.

8. Walker, K.E., Baldini, T., and Lindeque, B.G., Thermal conductivity of human bone in cryoprobe freezing as related to density, *Orthopedics* 40, 90–94, 2017.

9. Fajardo, J.E., Carlevaro, C.M., Vericat, F., et al., Effect of the trabecular bone microstructure on measuring its thermal conductivity: A computer modeling-based study, *J. Therm. Biol.* 77, 131–136, 2018.

10. Bowman, H.F., Cravallo, E.G., and Woods, M., Theory, measurement, and application of thermal properties of biomaterials, *Annu. Rev. Biophys. Bioeng.* 4, 43–80, 1975.

11. Valvano, J.W., Cochran, J.R., and Diller, K.D., Thermal conductivity and diffusivity of biomaterials measured with self-heated thermistors, *Int. J. Thermophysics* 6, 301–311, 1985.

12. Rabin, Y., The effect of temperature-dependent thermal conductivity in heat transfer simulations of frozen biomaterials, *Cryo Letters* 21, 163–170, 2000.

13. Bhattacharya, S., Dhar, P., Das, S.K., et al., Colloidal graphite/graphene nanostructures using collagen showing enhanced thermal conductivity, *Int. J. Nanomedicine* 9, 1287–1298, 2014.

14. Mortazavi, B., Pötschke, M., and Cuniverti, G., Multiscale modeling of thermal conductivity of polycrystalline graphene sheets, *Nanoscale* 6, 3344–3352, 2014.

15. Zhang, Y.G., Zhu, Y.J., Chen, F., and Sun, T.W., Biocompatible, ultralight, strong hydroxyapatite networks based on hydroxyapatite microtubes with excellent permeability and ultralow thermal conductivity, *ACS Appl. Mater. Interfaces* 9, 7918–7928, 2017.

16. Vinothini, K., Rajendran, N.K., Ramu, A., et al., Folate receptor targeted delivery of paclitaxel to breast cancer cells via folic acid conjugated graphene oxide grafted methyl acrylated nanocarrier, *Biomed. Pharmacother.* 110, 906–917, 2019.

17. Berman, R., *Thermal Conduction in Solids*, Oxford University Press/Clarendon Press, Oxford, UK, 1976.

18. Fisher, T.S., *Thermal Energy at the Nanoscale*, World Scientific, Singapore, 2014.

THERMOPHILIC

Thermophilic is a term literally meaning "loving heat." A formal definition is "requiring a high temperature for development, as certain bacteria."[1] As suggested by the definition, the term is used most often to describe microorganisms which grow at elevated temperatures found, for example, in natural hot springs.[2–5] In molecular biology, the most famous thermophilic bacteria is *Themus aquaticus* which provide the TAQ polymerase responsible for the success of the polymerase chain reaction (PCR).[6–10] The thermal stability of the TAQ polymerase permits the thermal denaturation of duplex product of the reaction allowing for another cycle without the addition of new polymerase. Other thermostable enzymes are proving useful in a variety of applications.[11–21]

1. *Oxford English Dictionary*, Oxford University Press, Oxford, UK, 2019.

2. Amend, J.P., and Shock, E.L., Energetics of overall metabolic reactions of thermophilic and hyperthermophilic Archaea and bacteria, *FEMS Microbiol. Rev.* 25, 175–243, 2001.

3. Ubieta, M.S., Donati, E.F., Chann, K.G., et al., Thermophiles in the genomic era: Biodiversity, science, and applications, *Biotechnol. Adv.* 33, 633–647, 2015.

4. Nishihara, A., Matsuura, K., Tank, M., et al., Nitrogenase activity in thermophilic chemolithoautotrophic bacteria in the phylum Aquificae isolated under nitrogen-fixing conditions from Nakabusa hot springs, *Microbes Envion.* 33, 394–401, 2018.

5. Yasir, M., Qureshi, A.K., Khan, I., et al., Culturomics-based taxomic diversity of bacterial communities in the hot springs of Saudi Arabia, *OMICS* 23, 17–27, 2019.

6. Vosberg, H.P., The polymerase chain reaction: An improved method for the analysis of nucleic acids, *Human Genet.* 83, 1–15, 1989.

7. Chow, V.T., Tham, K.M., and Bernard, H.U., *Thermus aquaticus* DNA polymerase-catalyzed chain reaction for the detection of human papillomaviruses, *J. Virol. Methods* 27, 101–112, 1990.

8. Schaffer, A.L., Wojnar, W., and Nelson, W., Amplification, detection, and automated sequencing of gibbon interleukin-2 mRNA by *Thermus aquaticus* DNA polymerase reverse transcription and polymerase chain reaction, *Anal. Biochem.* 190, 292–296, 1990.

9. Spiess, A.N., Mueller, N., and Ivell, R., Trehalose is a potent PCR enhancer: Lowering of DNA melting temperature and thermal stabilization of taq polymerase by the disaccharide trehalose, *Clin. Chem.* 50, 1256–1259, 2004.

10. Rejali, N.A., Moric, E., and Wittwer, C.T., The effect of single mismatches on primer extension, *Clin. Chem.* 64, 801–809, 2018.

11. Lasa, I., and Berenguer, J., Thermophilic enzymes and their biotechnology potential, *Microbiologica* 9, 77–89, 1993.

12. Russell, R.J., and Taylor, G.L., Engineering thermostability: Lessons from the thermophilic proteins, *Curr. Opin. Biotechnol.* 6, 370–374, 1995.

13. Radianingtyas, H., and Wright, P.C., Alcohol dehydrogenases from thermophilic and hyperthermophilic archae and bacteria, *FEMS Microbiol. Rev.* 27, 593–616, 2003.

14. Egorova, K., and Antranikian, G., Industrial relevance of thermophilic Archaea, *Curr. Opin. Microbiol.* 8, 649–655, 2005.

15. Tu, T., Meng, K., Huang, H., et al., Molecular characterization of a thermophilic endo-polygalacturonase from *Thielavia arenaria* X27 with high catalytic efficiency and application potential in the food and feed industries, *J. Agric. Food Chem.* 62, 12686–12694, 2014.

16. Zerva, A., Christakopoulos, P., and Topakas, E., Characterization and application of a novel class II thermophilic peroxidase from *Myceliophthora thermophilia* in biosynthesis of polycatechol, *Enzyme Microb. Technol.* 75–76, 49–56, 2015.

17. Xia, W., Xu, X., Qian, L., et al., Engineering a highly active thermophilic β-glucosidase to enhance its pH stability and saccharification performance, *Biotechnol. Biofuels* 9, 147, 2016.

18. Dumorné, K., Córdova, D.C., Astorga-Eló, M., and Regnaneathan, P., Extremozymes: A potential source for industrial applications, *J. Microbiol. Biotechnol.* 27, 649–659, 2017.

19. Sun, Q., Chen, F., Geng, F., et al., A novel aspartic protease from *Rhizomucor michel* expressed in *Pichia pastoris* and its application on meat tenderization and preparation of turtle peptides, *Food Chem.* 245, 570–577, 2018.

20. Haq. I.U., Tahir, S.F., Aftab, M.N., et al., Purification and characterization of a thermostable cellobiohydrolase from *Thermotoga petrophilia, Protein Pept. Lett.* 25, 1003–1014, 2018.

21. Flores-Fernández, C.N., Cárdenas-Fernández, M., Drobirjevic, D., et al., Novel extremophilic proteases from *Pseudomonas aeruginosa* M211, and their application in the hydrolysis of dried distiller's grain with solubles, *Biotechnol. Prog.* 35, e2728, 2019.

THIOLASE/THIOLASE SUPERFAMILY

The term thiolase describes an enzyme activity which catalyzes the final step in β-oxidation of fatty acids[1–3] now known as 3-ketoacyl-CoA thiolase (3-oxoacyl-CoA thiolase).[4–9] The canonical reaction is the catalysis of the reaction between a 3-ketoacyl-CoA and CoA (coenzyme A) to yield an acyl-CoA two carbons shorter than the parent 3-ketoacyl-CoA and acetyl-CoA; the acetyl-CoA can be used for energy generation.[10] The process of β-oxidation starts with the dehydrogenation distal to the carbonyl group, the addition of water across the double bond followed by dehydrogenation resulting a 3-keto group. The majority of fatty acid catabolism occurs in peroxisomes and, to a lesser extent, mitochrondria.[11–14] It is important to recognize that members of the thiolase superfamily are important in biosynthetic reactions via the synthesis of acetoacetyl-CoA.[15,16] The degradative reaction of thiolase, the production of acyl-CoA and acetyl-CoA, is thermodynamically favored; an excess of CoA is thought to drive the biosynthetic reaction.[17]

1. Lynen, F., Wessely, L., Wieland, O., and Rueff, L., Zur β-Oxydation der Fettsäuren, *Angewandte Chem.* 64, 687, 1952.

2. Goldman, D.S., Studies on the fatty acid oxidizing system of animal tissues. VII. The β-ketoacyl coenzyme A cleavage enzyme, *J. Biol. Chem.* 208, 345–351, 1954.

3. Mazzei, Y., Negrel, R., and Ailhaud, G., Purification and some properties of thiolase from *Escherichia coli*, *Biochim. Biphys. Acta* 220, 129–131, 1970.

4. Miyazawa, S., Furuta, S., Osumi, T., Hashimoto, T., and Ui, N., Properties of peroxisomal 3-keto-coA thiolase from rat liver, *J. Biochem.* 90, 511–519, 1981.

5. Yamashita, H., Itsuki, A., Kimoto, M., Hiernori, M., and Tsuji, H., Acetate generation in rat liver mitochondria; acetyl-CoA hydrolase activity is demonstrated by 3-ketoacyl-CoA hydrolase is demonstrated by 3-ketoacyl-CoA thiolase, *Biochim. Biophys. Acta* 1761, 17–23, 2006.

6. Arnauld, S., Fidaleo, M., Clémencet, M.C., et al., Modulation of the hepatic fatty acid pool in peroxisomal 3-ketoacyl-CoA thiolase B-null mice exposed to the selective PPARalpha agonist Wy14,643, *Biochimie* 91, 1376–1386, 2009.

7. Kim, J., and Kim, K.J., Crystal structure and biochemical properties of REH16_A1887, the 3-ketoacyl-CoA thiolase from *Rastonia eutropha* H16, *Biochem. Biophys. Res. Commun.* 459, 547–552, 2015.

8. Kiema, T.R., Harijan, R.K., Strozyk, M., et al., The crystal structure of human mitochondrial 3-ketoacyl-CoA thiolase (T1): Insight into the reaction mechanism of its thiolase and thioesterase activities, *ActA Crystallogrr. D Biol. Crystallog.* 70, 3212–3225, 2014.

9. Kim, J., and Kim, K.J., Purification, crystallization and preliminary X-ray diffraction analysis of 3-ketoacyl-CoA thiolase A1887 from *Ralstonia eutopha* H16, *Acta Crystallogr. F. Struct. Biol. Commun.* 71, 758–762, 2016.

10. Matthews, C.K., van Holde, K.E., and Ahern, K.G., *Biochemistry*, 3th edn., p. 644, Addison, Wesley Longman, San Francisco, CA, 2000.

11. Igual, J.C, González-Bosch, C., Dopazo, J., and Pérez-Ortín, J.E., Pylogenetic analysis of the thiolase family. Implications for the evolutionary origin of peroxisomes, *J. Mol. Evolution* 35, 147–155, 1992.

12. Van Veldhaven, P.P., and Mannaerts, G.P., Role and organization of peroximsomal β-oxidation, *Adv. Exp. Med. Biol.* 466, 261–273, 2002.

13. Lautruffe, N., Nicolas-Frances, V., Clemencet, K.-L., et al., Gene regulation of peroxisomal enzymes by nutrients, hormones, and nuclear signaling factors in animal and human species, *Adv. Exp. Med. Biol.* 544, 225–236, 2003.

14. Wanders, R.J.A., Van Roermund, C.W.T., Visser, W.F., et al., Peroxisomal fatty acid alpha- and beta-oxidation in health and disease: New insights, *Adv. Exp. Med. Biol.* 544, 293–302, 2003.

15. Haapalainen, A.M., Meriläinen, G., and Wierenga, R.K., The thiolase superfamily: Condensing enzymes with diverse reaction specificities, *Trends Biochem. Sci.* 31, 64–71, 2006.

16. Torres-Salas, P., Bernal, V., López-Gallego, F., et al., Engineering Erg10 thiolase from *Saccharomyces cerevisiae* as a synthetic toolkit for the production of branched-chain alcohols, *Biochemistry* 57, 1338–1348, 2018.

17. Modis, Y., and Wierenga, R.K., A biosynthetic thiolase in complex with a reaction intermediate: The crystal structure provides new insights into the catalytic mechanism, *Structure* 7, 1279–1290, 1999.

THIOREDOXIN(S)

Thioredoxin is small protein functioning as an important reducing agent in biological systems and is considered to be a major regulator of redox reactions in the cell.[1-13] Thioredoxin is maintained in the reduced state by thioredoxin, a selenoprotein,[14] which is a target for chemotherapy.[15-17] Glutaredoxins are small enzymes which also function in redox control systems[18-21] Glutaredoxins are dependent on glutathione to catalyze disulfide exchange reactions.[22]

1. Holmgren, A., Thioredoxin, *Annu. Rev. Biochem.* 54, 237–271, 1985.
2. Martin, J.L., Thioredoxin-a fold for all reasons, *Structure* 3, 245–250, 1995.
3. Aslund, F., and Beckwith, J., The thioredoxin superfamily: Redundancy, specificity, and gray-area genomics, *J. Bacteriol.* 181, 1375–1379, 1999.
4. Arrigo, A.P., Gene expression and the thiol redox state, *Free Radic. Biol. Med.* 27, 936–944, 1999.
5. Holmgren, A., Antioxidant function of thioredoxin and glutaredoxin systems, *Antioxid. Redox Signal.* 2, 811–820, 2000.
6. Arner, E.S.J., and Holmgren, A., Physiological functions of thioredoxins and thioredoxin reductase, *Eur. J. Biochem.* 267, 6102–6109, 2000.
7. Burke-Gaffney, A., Callister, M.E., and Nakamura, H., Thioredoxin: Friend or foe in human disease? *Trends Pharmacol. Sci.* 26, 398–404, 2005.
8. Stefankova, P., Kollarova, M., and Barak, I., Thioredoxin—Structural and functional complexity, *Gen. Physiol. Biophys.* 24, 3–11, 2005.
9. Koc, A., Mathews, C.K., Wheeler, L.J., Gross, M.K., and Merrill, G.F., Thioredoxin is required for deoxyribonucleotide pool maintenance during S phase, *J. Biol. Chem.* 281, 15058–15063, 2006.
10. Sies, H., Berndt, C., and Jones, D.P., Oxidative stress, *Annu. Rev. Biochem.* 86, 715–748, 2017.
11. Meyer, Y., Belin, C., Delorme-Hinoux, V., Reichheld, J.P., and Riondet, C., Thioredoxin and glutaredoxin system in plants: Molecular mechanisms, crosstalks, and functional significance, *Antioxid. Redox. Signal.* 17, 1124–1160, 2012.
12. Sengupta, R., and Holmgren, A., Thioredoxin and thioredoxin reductase in relation to reversible *S*-nitrosylation, *Antioxid. Redox Signal.* 18, 259–269, 2013.
13. Lu, J., and Holmgren, A., The thioredoxin antioxidant system, *Free Radic. Biol. Med.* 66, 75–87, 2014.
14. Ren, X., Zou, L., Lu, J., and Holmgren, A., Selenocysteine in mammalian thioredoxin reductase and application of ebselen as a therapeutic, *Free Radic. Biol. Med.* 127, 238–247, 2018.
15. Zhang, J., Li, X., Han, X. Liu, R., and Fang, J., Targeting the thioredoxin systems for cancer therapy, *Trends Pharmacol. Sci.* 38, 794–808, 2017.
16. Scalcon, V., Bindoli, A., and Rigobello, M.P., Significance of the mitochondrial thioredoxin reductase in cancer cells: An update on role, targets and inhibitors, *Free Radic. Biol. Med.* 127, 62–79, 2018.
17. Yan, X., Zhang, X., Wang, L., et al., Inhibition of thioredoxin/thioredoxin reductase induces synthetic lethality in lung cancers with compromised glutathione homeostasis, *Cancer Res.* 79, 125–132, 2019.
18. Holmgren, A., Thioredoxin and glutathioredoxin systems, *J. Biol. Chem.* 264, 13963–13966, 1989.
19. Fernandes, A.P., and Holmgren, A., Glutaredoxins: Glutathione-dependent redox enzymes with functions far beyond a simple thioredoxin backup system, *Antioxid. Redox. Signal.* 6, 63–74, 2004.
20. Ströher, E and Millar, A.H., The biological role of glutaredoxins, *Biochem. J.* 446, 333–348, 2012.
21. Lillig, C.H., and Berndt, C., Glutaredoxins in thiol/disulfide exchange, *Antioxid. Redox. Signal.* 18, 1654–1665, 2013.
22. Xiao, X., La Fontaine, S., Bush, A.I., and Wedd, A.G., Molecular mechanisms of glutaredoxin enzymes: Versatile hubs for thiol-disulfide change between proteins and glutathione, *J. Mol. Biol.* 431, 158–177, 2019.

TIME-OF-FLIGHT

The term time-of-flight designates techniques and apparatus that depend on the time taken by particles to traverse a set distance, as, for example, the separation of ions according to their mass in mass spectrometry. Time-of-flight mass spectrometry (TOF-MS) measures flight time of ions; lighter ions travel a greater distance that heavier ions; mass proportional to time squared; converted to m/z by calibration with standards.[1-7] The term time-of-flight is also used in other applications such as measurement of blood flow[8-10] and flagella length.[11]

1. Cotter, R.J., Time-of-flight mass spectrometry: An increasing role in the life sciences, *Biomed. Environ. Mass Spectrom.* 18, 513–532, 1989.
2. Guilhaus, M., Selby, D., and Mlynski, V., Orthogonal acceleration time-of-flight mass spectrometry, *Mass Spectrom. Rev.* 19, 65–107, 2000.
3. Belu, A.M., Graham, D.J., and Castner, D.G., Time-of-flight secondary ion mass spectrometry: Techniques and applications for the characterization of biomaterial surfaces, *Biomaterials* 24, 3635–3653, 2003.
4. Seibert, V., Wiesner, A., Buschmann, T., and Meuer, J., Surface-enhanced laser desorption ionization time-of-flight mass spectrometry (SELDI TOF-MS) and ProteinChip technology in proteomics research, *Pathol. Res. Pract.* 200, 83–94, 2004.
5. Vestal, M.L., and Campbell, J.M., Tandem time-of-flight mass spectrometry, *Methods Enzymol.* 402, 79–108, 2005.
6. Boesl, U., Time-of-flight mass spectrometry: Introduction to the basics, *Mass Spectrom. Rev.* 36, 86–109, 2017.

7. Wolk, D.M., and Clark, A.E., Matrix-assisted laser desorption time-of-flight mass spectrometry, *Clin. Lab. Med.* 38, 471–486, 2018.

8. Kochar, R., Khandelwal, N., Singh, P., and Suri, S., Arterial contamination: A useful indirect sign of cerebral sino-venous thrombosis, *Acta Neurol. Scand.* 114, 139–142, 2006.

9. Han, S., Granwehr, J., Garcia, S., et al., Auxiliary probe design adaptable to existing probes for remote detection NMR, MRI, and time-of-flight tracing, *J. Magn. Reson.*, 182, 260–272, 2006.

10. Baghaie, A., Schnell, S., Bakhshinejad, A., et al., Curvelet transform-based volume fusion for correcting signal loss artifacts in time-of-flight magnetic resonance angiography data, *Comput. Biol. Med.* 99, 142–153, 2018.

11. Ishikawa, H., and Marshall, W.F., Testing the time-of-flight model for flagellar length sensing, *Mol. Biol. Cell* 28, 3447–3456, 2017.

TISSUE MICROARRAY

A microarray consisting of cores (0.6 mm in diameter for example) of tissue samples embedded in a paraffin block. Samples are taken from existing paraffin block sections This technology allows multiple samples to be processed at the same time under the same conditions.[1–16] This is an effective method which is cost-effective for processing large numbers of samples.[17,18] The development of tissue marcroarrays[19,20] is a method which uses larger specimens (0.8 × 1.0 cm) to obtain a larger field of coverage.

1. Moch, H., Schrami, P., Bubendorf, L., et al., High-throughput tissue microarray analysis to evaluated genes uncovered by cDNA microarray screening in renal cell carcinoma, *Am. J. Pathol.* 154, 981–986, 1999.

2. Kallioniemi, O.P., Wagner, U., Kononen, J., and Sauter, G., Tissue microarray technology for high-throughput molecular profiling of cancer, *Hum. Mol. Genet.* 10, 657–662, 2001.

3. Rao, J., Seligson, D., and Hemstreet, G.P., Protein expression analysis using quantitative fluorescence image analysis on tissue microarray slides, *BioTechniques* 32, 928–930, 2002.

4. Rubin, M.A., Dunn, R., Strawderman, M., and Pienta, K.J., Tissue microarray sampling strategy for prostate cancer biomarker analysis, *Am. J. Surg. Pathol.* 26, 312–219, 2002.

5. Hedvat, C.V., Hedge, A., Chaganti, R.S., et al., Application of tissue microarray technology to the study of non-Hodgkin's and Hodgkin's lymphoma, *Hum. Pathol.* 33, 968–974, 2002.

6. Kim, W.H., Rubin, M.A., and Dunn, R.L., High-density tissue microarray, *Am. J. Surg. Pathol.* 26, 1236–1238, 2002.

7. Parker, R.L., Huntsman, D.G., Lesack, D.W., et al., Assessment of interlaboratory variation in the immuno-histochemical determination of estrogen receptor status using a breast cancer tissue microarray, *Am. J. Clin. Pathol.* 117, 723–728, 2002.

8. Giltnane, J.M., and Rimm, D.L., Technology insight: Identification of biomarkers with tissue microarray technology, *Nat. Clin. Pract. Oncol.* 1, 104–111, 2004.

9. Zimpfer, A., Schonberg, S., Lugli, A., et al., Construction and validation of a bone marrow tissue microarray, *J. Clin. Pathol.*, 60, 57–61, 2006.

10. Avninder, S., Ylaya, K., and Hewitt, S.M., Tissue microarray: A simple technology that has revolutionized research in pathology, *J. Postgrad. Med.* 54, 158–162, 2008.

11. Camp, R.L., Neumeister, V., and Rimm, D.L., A decade of tissue microarrays: Progress in the discovery and validation of cancer biomarkers, *J. Clin. Oncol.* 26, 5630–5637, 2008.

12. Pallares, J., Santacana, M., Puente, S., et al., A review of the applications of tissue microarray technology in understanding the molecular features of endometrial carcinoma, *Anal. Quant. Cytol. Histol.* 31, 217–226, 2009.

13. Simon, R., Applications of tissue microarray technology, *Methods Mol. Biol.* 664, 1–16, 2010.

14. Franco, R., Caraglia, M., Facchini, G., Abbruzzese, A., and Botti, G., The role of tissue microarray in the era of target-based agents, *Expert Rev. Anticancer Ther.* 11, 859–869, 2011.

15. Barrette, K., van dea Oord, J.J., and Garmyn, M., Tissue microarray, *J. Invest. Dermatol.* 134, 1–4, 2014.

16. Albanghali, M., Green, A., Rakha, E., et al., Construction of tissue microarrays from core needle biopsies—A systematic literature review, *Histopathology* 68, 323–332, 2016.

17. Hsu, F.D., Nielsen, T.D., Alkushi, A., et al., Tissue microarrays are an effective and quality assurance tool for diagnostic immunohistochemistry, *Mod. Pathol.* 15, 1374–1380, 2002.

18. Shergill, I.S., Shergill, N.K., Arya, M., and Patel, H.R., Tissue microarrays: A current medical research tool, *Curr. Med. Res. Opin.* 20, 707–712, 2004.

19. Wang, L., Deavers, M.T., Malpica, A., Silva, E.G., and Liu, J., Tissue macroarray: A simple and cost-effective method for high-throughput studies, *Appl. Immunohistochem. Mol. Morphol.* 11, 174–176, 2003.

20. Dias, E.P., Picciani, B.L.S., Santos, V.C.B.C., and Cunha, K.S., A simple technique to contruct tissue macroarrays, *J. Clin. Pathol.* 71, 890–894, 2018.

TITIN

Titin is a very large protein (mass of approximately 3 million Daltons) which is the third-most abundant protein in vertebrate striated muscle and has a role in providing sarcomeric alignment and recoil. Titin is a single chain protein which extends from the M line to the Z line forming a thick filament.[1-12] **Connectin** was a term used to describe an elastic protein in myofibrils,[13,14] which was shown to be identical with titin.[15]

1. Fulton, A.B., and Isaacs, W.B., Titin, a huge, elastic sarcomeric protein with a probable role in morphogenesis, *Bioessays* 13, 157–161, 1991.
2. Trinick, J., Understanding the functions of titin and nebulin, *FEBS Lett.* 307, 44–48, 1992.
3. Kellermeyer, M.S., and Grama, L., Stretching and visualizing titin molecules: Combining structure, dynamics and mechanics, *J. Muscle Res. Cell Motil.* 23, 499–511, 2002.
4. Tskhovrebova, L., and Trinick, J., Titin: Properties and family relationships, *Nat. Rev. Mol. Cell Biol.* 4, 679–689, 2003.
5. Granzier, H.L., and Labeit, S., The giant protein titin: A major player in myocardial mechanics, signaling, and disease, *Circ. Res.* 94, 284–295, 2004.
6. Lange, S., Ehler, E., and Gautel, M., From A to Z and back? Multicompartment proteins in the sarcomere, *Trends Cell Biol.* 16, 11–18, 2006.
7. LeWinter, M.M., Wu, Y., Labeit, S., and Granzier, H., Cardiac titin: Structure, functions, and role in disease, *Clin. Chim. Acta* 375, 1–9, 2007.
8. Krüger, M., and Linke, W.A., The giant protein titin: A regulatory node that integrates myocyte signaling pathways, *J. Biol. Chem.* 286, 9905–9912, 2011.
9. LeWinter, M.M., and Granzier, H.L., Titin is a major human disease gene, *Circulation* 127, 938–944, 2013.
10. Dos Remedios, C., and Gilmour, D., An historical perspective of the discovery of titin filaments, *Biophys. Rev.* 9, 179–188, 2017.
11. Dos Remedios, C.G., An historical perspective of the discovery of titin filaments—Part 2, *Biophys. Rev.* 10, 1201–1203, 2017.
12. Herzog, W., The multiple roles of titin in muscle contraction and force production, *Biophys. Rev.* 10, 1187–1199, 2018.
13. Maruyama, K., Matsubara, S., Natori, R., Nonmura, Y., and Kimura, S., Connetin, an elastic protein of muscle. Characterization and function, *J. Biochem.* 82, 317–337, 1977.
14. Maruyama, K., Connectin, an elastic filamentous protein of striated muscle, *Int. Rev. Cytol.* 104, 81–114, 1986.
15. Maruyama, K., Kimura, S., Ohashi, K., and Kuwano, Y., Connectin, an elastic protein of muscle. Identification of "titin" with connectin, *J. Biochem.* 89, 701–709, 1981.

TOLL-LIKE RECEPTOR

The term toll-like receptors is derived from the relationship of these proteins to the membrane receptor encoded by the *toll* gene in *Drosophila*.[1-4] Toll-like receptors in mammals are immune cell receptors which recognize infectious agents and stimulate activation of the adaptive immune system.[5-16] Toll-like receptors are pathogen recognition receptors important in the non-specific (innate) immune response.[17-19]

1. Kuno, K., and Matsushima, K., The IL-1 receptor signaling pathway, *J. Leukoc. Biol.* 56, 542–547, 1994.
2. Meister, M., Lemaitre, B., and Hoffman, J.A., Antimicrobial peptide defense in *Drosophila*, *Bioessays* 19, 1019–1026, 1997.
3. Dushay, M.S., and Eldon, E.D., *Drosophila* immune responses as models for human immunity, *Am. J. Hum. Genet.* 62, 10–14, 1998.
4. O'Neill, L.A., and Greene, C., Signal transduction pathways activated by the IL-1 receptor family: Ancient signaling machinery in mammals, insects, and plants, *J. Leukoc. Biol.* 63, 650–657, 1998.
5. Aderem, A., and Ulevitch, R.J., Toll-like receptors in the induction of the innate immune response, *Nature* 406, 782–77, 2000.
6. Aderem, A., Role of the Toll-like receptors in inflammatory response in macrophages, *Crit. Care Med.* 29 (7 Suppl), S16–S18, 2001.
7. Beutler, B., and Rietschel, E.T., Innate immune sensing and its roots: The story of endotoxin, *Nat. Rev. Immunol.* 3, 169–176, 2003.
8. Philpott, D.J., and Girardin, S.E., The role of Toll-like receptors and Nod proteins in bacterial infection, *Mol. Immunol.* 41, 1099–1108, 2004.
9. Pasare, C., and Medzhitov, R., Toll-like receptors: Linking innate and adaptive immunity, *Adv. Exp. Med. Biol.* 560, 11–18, 2005.
10. O'Neill, L.A., How Toll-like receptors signal: What we know and what we don't know, *Curr. Opin. Immunol.* 18, 3–9, 2006.
11. Kreig, A.M., Therapeutic potential of Toll-like receptor 9 activation, *Nat. Rev. Drug Discov.* 5, 471–484, 2006.
12. Turvey, S.E., and Hawn, T.R., Towards subtlety: Understanding the role of Toll-like receptor signaling in susceptibility to human infections, *Clin. Immunol.* 120, 1–9, 2006.
13. *Toll-Like Receptors in Inflammation*, ed. L.A.J O'Neill and E. Brint, Birkhäuser Verlag, Basel, Switzerland, 2005.
14. *Toll-like Receptors (TLRs) and Innate Immunity*, ed. S. Bauer and G. Hartmann, Springer Verlag, Berlin, Germany, 2008.
15. *Toll-like Receptors; Roles in Infection and Neuropathology*, ed. T. Kiellan, Springer Verlag, Berlin, Germany, 2009.
16. *Toll-like Receptors: Practice and Methods*, ed. C.E. McCoy, Humana Press, New York, 2016.
17. Shimizu, T., Structural insights into ligand recognition and regulation of nucleic acid-sensing Toll-like receptors, *Curr. Opin. Struct. Biol.* 47, 52–59, 2017.

18. Marquest, M., Ferreira, A.R., and Ribeiro, D., The interplay between human cytomegalovirus and pathogen recognition receptors signaling, *Viruses* 10, E514, 2018.
19. Vijay, K., Toll-like receptors in immunity and inflammatory disease: Past, present, and future, *Int. Immunopharmacol.* 59, 391–412, 2018.

TonB

TonB is one component of a membrane receptor in gram-negative bacteria responsible for the transport of iron chelate (siderophores) as well as some other materials such as carbohydrates, Vitamin B_{12} and nickel complexes.[1–3] The transport process is energy-dependent and TonB is responsible for energy transduction.

1. Postle, K., TonB and the gram-negative dilemma, *Mol. Microbiol.* 4, 2019–2025, 1990.
2. Postle, K., and Kadner, R.S., Tough and go: Trying TonB to transport, *Mod. Microbiol.* 49, 869–882, 2003.
3. Noinaj, N., Guillier, M., Barnard, T.J., and Buchanan, S.K., TonB-dependent transporters: Regulation, structure, and function. *Annu. Rev. Microbiol.* 64, 43–60, 2010.

TONOPLAST

The tonoplast is the membrane surrounding a vacuole in a plant cell.[1–8] Tonoplast function is essential for the maintenance of turgor by the vacuole.[7,9–12]

1. Barbeir-Brygoo, H., Renaudin, J.P., and Guern, J., The vacuolar membrane of plant cells: A newcomer in the field of biological membranes, *Biochimie* 68, 417–425, 1986.
2. Bertl, A., and Slayman, C.L., Complex modulation of cation channels in the tonoplast and plasma membrane of *Saccharomyces cerevisiae*: Single-channel studies, *J. Exp. Biol.* 172, 271–287, 1992.
3. Neuhaus, J.M., and Rogers, J.C., Sorting of proteins to vacuoles in plant cells, *Plant Mol. Biol.* 38, 127–144, 1998.
4. Luttge, U., The tonoplast functioning as the master switch for circadian regulation of crassulacean acid metabolism, *Planta* 211, 761–769, 2000.
5. Gattolin, S., Sorieul, M., and Frigerio, L., Tonoplast intrinsic proteins and vacuolar identity, *Biochem. Soc. Trans.* 38, 769–773, 2010.
6. Rojas-Pierce, M., Targeting of tonoplast proteins to the vacuole, *Plant Sci.* 211, 132–136, 2013.
7. Neuhaus, H.E., and Trentmann, O., Regulation of transport processes across the tonoplast, *Front. Plant. Sci.* 5, 460, 2014.
8. Regon, P., Panda, P., Kshetrimayum, E., and Panda, S.K. Genome-wide comparative analysis of tonoplast intrinsic protein (TIP) genes in plants, *Funct. Integr. Genomics* 14, 617–629, 2014.
9. MacRobbie, E.A., Control of volume and turgor in stomatal guard cells, *J. Membr. Biol.* 210, 131–142, 2006.
10. Li, Z., Zhou, M., Hu, Q., et al., Manipulating expression of tonoplast transporters, *Methods Mol. Biol.* 913, 359–369, 2012.
11. Zhang, H., Zhao, F.G., Tang, R.J., et al., Two tonoplast MATE proteins function as turgor-regulating chloride channels in *Arabidopsis*, *Proc. Natl. Acad. Sci. USA* 114, E2036–E2045, 2017.
12. Krüger, F., and Schumacher, K., Pumping up the volume—Vacuole biogenesis in *Arabidopsis thaliana*, *Semin. Cell Dev. Biol.* 80, 106–112, 2018.

TOP-DOWN PROTEOMICS

Top-down proteomics is the mass spectrometric analysis of intact proteins as opposed to bottom-up-proteomics where mass spectrometry is used to analyze peptides derived from the proteolytic enzyme digests of proteins.[1–10]

1. Ge, Y., Lawhorn, G., ElNagger, E., et al., Top down characterization of larger proteins (45 kDa) by electron capture dissociation mass spectrometry, *J. Am. Chem. Soc.* 124, 672–678, 2002.
2. Nemeth-Cawley, J.F., Tangarone, B.S., and Rouse, J.C., "Top Down" characterization is a complementary technique to peptide sequencing for identifying protein species in complex mixtures, *J. Proteome Res.* 2, 495–505, 2003.
3. Williams, T.L., Monday, S.R., Edelson-Mammel, S., Buchanan, R., and Musser, S.M., A top-down proteomics approach for differentiating thermal resistant strains of *Enterobacter sakazakii*, *Proteomics* 5, 4161–4169, 2005.
4. Demirev, P.A., Feldman, A.B., Kowalski, P., and Lin, J.S., Top-down proteomics for rapid identification of intact microorganisms, *Anal. Chem.* 77, 7455–7461, 2005.
5. Du, Y., Parks, B.A., Sohn, S., Kwast, K.E., and Kelleher, N.L., Top-down approaches for measuring expression ratios of intact yeast proteins using Fourier transform mass spectrometry, *Anal. Chem.* 78, 686–694, 2006.
6. Tholey, A., and Becker, A., Top-down proteomics for the analysis of proteolytic events—Methods, applications and perspectives, *Biochim. Biophys. Acta Mol. Cell. Res.* 1864, 2191–2199, 2017.
7. Chen, B., Brown, K.A., Lin, Z., and Ge, Y., Top-down proteomics: Ready for prime time? *Anal. Chem.* 90, 110–127, 2018.
8. Schaffer, L.V., Rensvold, J.W., Shortreed, M.R., et al., Identification and quantification of murine mitochondrial proteoforms using an integrated top-down and intact-mass spectrometry, *J. Proteome Res.* 17, 3526–3536, 2018.
9. Toby, T.K., Fornelli, L., Srzentić, K., et al., A comprehensive pipeline for translational top-down proteomics from a single blood draw, *Nat. Protocols* 14, 119–152, 2019.
10. Lin, Z., Wei, L., Cai, W., et al., Simultaneous quantification of protein expression and modifications by top-down targeted proteomics: A case of sarcomeric subproteome, *Mol. Cell Proteomics* 18, 594–605, 2019.

TOPOISOMERASE

The term topoisomerase describes a family of enzymes which alter the topology of DNA by catalyzing relaxation and unknotting of the double-stranded DNA complex.[1] This action is required for DNA replication and the process of transcription.[2,3] This is accomplished through the alteration of the supercoiling of the DNA helix by transient strand breakage[1,4] where the topoisomerase is acting as a reversible nuclease.[3] Topoisomerase I cleaves one strand of DNA[5] while Topoisomerase II cleaves both strands of the DNA helix.[1,4,6] Topoisomerase activity is a target for cancer chemotherapy.[7–12]

1. Forterre, P., Introduction and historical perspectives, in *DNA Topoisomerases and Cancer. Cancer Drug Discovery and Development*, ed. Y. Pommier, Chapter 1, pp. 1–52, Humana/Springer Science Business, New York, 2012.
2. Pommier, Y., Sun, Y., Huang, S.N., and Nitiss, J.L., Roles of eukaryotic topoisomerases in transcription, replication and genomic stability, *Nat. Rev. Mol. Cell Biol.* 17, 703–721, 2016.
3. Alberts, B., Johnson, A., Lewis, J., et al., *Molecular Biology of the Cell*, 6th edn., pp. 252–254, Garland Science/Taylor & Francis Group, New York, 2012.
4. Osheroff, N., Biochemical basis for the interactions of type I and type II topoisomerases with DNA, *Pharmacol. Ther.* 41, 223–241, 1989.
5. Champoux, J.J., Human DNA topoisomerse I. Structure, enzymology and biology, in *DNA Topoisomerases and Cancer. Cancer Drug Discovery and Development*, ed. Y. Pommier, Chapter 2, pp. 53–69, Humana/Springer Science Business, New York, 2012.
6. Berger, J.M., and Osheroff N., Structure and mechanism of eukaryotic type IIA topoisomerase, in *DNA Topoisomerases and Cancer. Cancer Drug Discovery and Development*, ed. Y. Pommier, Chapter 4, pp. 87–101, Humana/Springer Science Business, New York, 2012.
7. Glisson, B.S., and Ross, W.E., DNA topoisomerase II: A primer on the enzyme and its unique role as a multidrug target in cancer chemotherapy, *Pharmacol. Ther.* 32, 89–106, 1987.
8. Giochard, S.M., and Danks, M.K., Topoisomerase enzymes as drug targets, *Curr. Opin. Oncol.* 11, 482–489, 1999.
9. Martincic, D., and Hande, K.R., Topoisomerase II inhibitors, *Cancer Chemother. Biol. Response Modif.* 22, 101–121, 2005.
10. de Almeida, S.M.V., Ribeiro, A.G., de Lima Silva, G.C., et al., DNA binding and topoiomserase inhibition: How can these mechanisms be explored to design more specific anticancer agents? *Biomed. Pharmcother.* 96, 1538–1556, 2017.
11. Mehta, A., Awah, C.U., and Sonabend, A.M., Topoisomerase II poisons for glioblastoma: Existing challenges and opportunities to personalize therapy, *Front. Neurol.* 9, 459, 2018.
12. Hevéner, K., Verstak, T.A., Lutat, K.E., Riggsbee, D.L., and Mooney, J.W., Recent developments in topoisomerase-targeted cancer chemotherapy, *Acta Pharm. Sci.* 8, 844–861, 2018.

TRANS-ACTIVATION

Trans-activation is the enhancement of transcription (transcriptional activation) by a transcription factor expressed by a gene at one locus binding to a different locus on DNA and influencing the activity of RNA polymerase.[1–6]

1. Roizman, B., Kristie, T., McKnight, J.L., et al., The trans-activation of herpes simplex virus gene expression: Comparison of two factors and their cis sites, *Biochimie* 70, 1031–1043, 1988.
2. Nevins, J.R., Mechanisms of viral-mediated trans-activation of transcription, *Adv. Virus Res.* 37, 35–83, 1989.
3. Green, N.M., Cellular and viral transcriptional activators, *Harvey Lect.* 88, 67–96, 1992–1993.
4. de Folter, S., and Angenent, G.C., Trans meets cis in MADS science, *Trends Plant Sci.* 11, 223–231, 2006.
5. Campbell, K.J., and Perkins, N.D., Regulation of NF-κB function, *Biochem. Soc. Symp.* 73, 165–180, 2006.
6. Belakvadi, M., and Fondell, J.D., Role of the mediator complex in nuclear hormone receptor signaling, *Rev. Physiol. Biochem. Pharmacol.* 156, 23–43, 2006.

TRANSCRIPTION

Transcription is the process by which genetic information is transferred from DNA to RNA.[1] Transcription is a complex process with a history of discovey.[2–19]

1. Alberts, B., Johnson, A., Lewis, J., et al., *Molecular Biology of the Cell*, 6th edn., Chapter 6, How cells read the genome: From DNA to protein, pp. 299–368, Garland Science/Taylor & Francis Group, New York, 2014.
2. Hames, B.D., and Glover, D.M., *Transcription and Splicing*, IRL Press, Oxford, UK, 1988.
3. Neidle, S., *DNA Structure and Recognition*, IRL Press, Oxford, UK, 1994.
4. Baumann, P., Qureshi, S.A., and Jackson, S.P., Transcription: New insights from studies on Archaea, *Trends Genet.* 11, 279–283, 1995.
5. Singer, M., and Berg, P., *Exploring Genetic Mechanisms*, University Science Books, Sausalito, CA, 1997.

6. Lewin, B., *Genes VII*, Oxford University Press, Oxford, UK, 2000.

7. Lodish, H.F., *Molecular Cell Biology*, W.H. Freeman, New York, 2000.

8. Brown, W.M., and Brown, P.M., *Transcription*, Taylor & Francis Group, London, UK, 2002.

9. Lee, D.K., Seol, W., and Kim, J.S., Custom DNA-binding proteins and artificial transcription factors, *Curr. Top. Med. Chem.* 3, 645–657, 2003.

10. Mondal, N., and Parvin, J.D., Transcription from the perspective of the DNA: Twists and bumps in the road, *Crit. Rev. Eukaryot. Gene Expr.* 13, 1–8, 2003.

11. Olson, M.O.J., *The Nucleolus*, Landes Bioscience, Georgetown, TX, 2004.

12. Sausville, EA., and Holbeck, S.L., Transcription profiling of gene expression in drug discovery and development: The NCI experience, *Eur. J. Cancer* 40, 2544–2549, 2004.

13. Uesugi, M., Synthetic molecules that modulate transcription and differentiation: Hints for future drug discovery, *Comb. Chem. High Throughput Screen.* 7, 653–659, 2004.

14. *DNA Conformation and Transcription*, ed. T. Ohyama, Landes Bioscience/Springer, Georgetown, Texas, 2005.

15. Beljanski, M., *The Regulation of DNA Replication and Transcription*, Demons Medical Publishing, New York, 2013.

16. Lavelle, C., Pack, unpack, bend, twist, pull, push: The physical side of gene expression, *Curr. Opin. Genet. Dev.* 25, 74–84, 2014.

17. Shapiro, J.A., Physiology of the read-write genome, *J. Physiol.* 592, 2319–2341, 2014.

18. Blombach, F., Smollett, K.L., Grohmann, D., and Werner, F., Molecular mechanism of transcription initiation-structure, function, and evolution of TFE/TFIIE-like transcription factors and open complex formation, *J. Mol. Biol.* 428, 2592–2606, 2016.

19. Jarroux, J., Morillon, A., and Pinskaya, M., History, discovery, and classification on lncRNAs, *Adv. Exp. Med. Biol.* 1008, 1–46, 2017.

TRANSCRIPTION FACTORS

Transcription factors are protein or protein complexes that bind to regions which are intrinsic to the DNA sequence of a regulated gene and control the process of transcription. Transcription factors can be general transcription factors that are required for the basal transcription apparatus or regulatory transcription factors which may bind upstream or downstream from the transcription initiation site and either enhance or suppress the rate of transcription.[1–14] See **NF-κB**, **promoter elements**, **RNA polymerase**, **general transcription factors**, and **regulatory transcription factors**.

1. *Transcriptional Regulation*, ed. S.L. McKnight and K.R. Yamamoto, Cold Spring Harbor Press, Cold Spring Harbor, NY, 1992.

2. Goodbourn, S., *Eukaryotic Gene Transcription,* IRL Press at Oxford, Oxford, UK, 1996.

3. *Transcription Factor Protocols*, ed. M.J. Tymms, Humana, Totowa, NJ, 2000.

4. *Transcription Factors*, ed. J. Locker, Academic Press(Bios), Oxford, UK, 2001.

5. Michalik, L., and Wahli, W., Involvement of PPAR nuclear receptors in tissue injury and wound repair, *J. Clin. Invest.* 116, 598–606, 2006.

6. Kikuchi, A., Kishida, S., and Yamamoto, H., Regulation of Wnt signaling by protein-protein interaction and post-translational modification, *Exp. Mol. Med.* 28, 1–10, 2006.

7. Sharrocks, A.D., PIAS proteins and transcriptional regulation—More than just SUMO E3 ligases? *Genes Dev.* 20, 754–758, 2006.

8. Campbell, K.J., and Perkins, N.D., Regulation of NF-kappaB function, *Biochem. Soc. Symp.* (73), 165–180, 2006.

9. Russell, J., and Zomerdijk, J.C., The RNA polymerase I transcription machinery, *Biochem. Soc. Sym.*(73), 203–216, 2006.

10. Gross, P., and Oelgeschlarger, T., Core promoter-selective RNA polymerase II transcription, *Biochem. Soc. Symp.*(73), 225–236, 2006.

11. *A Handbook of Transcription Factors*, ed. T.R. Hughes, Springer, Dordrecht, the Netherlands, 2010.

12. Thorsten, W., *Predicting Transcription Factor Complexes: A Novel Approach to Data Integration in Systems Biology*, Springer Spektrum, Wiesbaden, Germany, 2015.

13. *Transciptomics and Gene Regulation*, ed. J. Wu., Springer, Dorddrecht, the Netherlands, 2016.

14. *Role of Transcription Factors in Gastrointesinal Malignancies,* ed. G.P. Nagaraju and P.V. Bramhachari, Springer, Singapore, 2018.

TRANSCRIPTIONAL SILENCING

Transcription silencing, also known as transcription repression, is the inhibition of the synthesis of RNA coded by a DNA template. An example is the prevention of inappropriate gene expression by the polycomb-group proteins,[1] which were first identified in *Drosophila*.[2] A consideration of the literature would suggest that the term transcription silencing be used in reference of the role of heterochromatin/histones in controlling transcription.[3–7]

1. Grossniklaus, J., and Paro, R., Transcription silencing by polycomb-group proteins, *Cold Spring Harb. Pespect. Biol.* 6, a019331, 2014.

2. Bienz, M., and Müller, J., Transcriptional silencing of homeotic genes in *Drosophila*, *Bioessays* 17, 775–784, 1995.

3. Yamolinksky, M., Transcriptional silencing in bacteria, *Curr. Opin. Microbiol.* 3, 138–143, 2000.

4. Grewal, S.I., Transcriptional silencing in fission yeast, *J. Cell Physiol.* 184, 311–318, 2000.

5. Chen, L., and Widom, J., Molecular basis of transcriptional silencing in budding yeast, *Biochem. Cell Biol.* 82, 413–418, 2004.

6. Will, W.R., Navarre, W.W., and Fang, F.C., Integrated circuits: How transcriptional silencing and counter-silencing facilitate bacterial evolution, *Curr. Opin. Microbiol.* 23, 8–13, 2015.

7. Flora, P., Schowalter, S., Wong-Deyrup, S., et al., Transient transcriptional silencing alters the cell cycle to promote germline stem cell differentiation in *Drosophila*, *Dev. Biol.* 434, 84–95, 2018.

TRANSCRIPTOMICS

Transcriptomics is the study of the total messenger RNA (transcriptome) in a cell, tissue, or organism. As such, transcriptomics is the study of a relatively small amount of the total RNA in a cell.[1–6] There is current interest in single-cell transcriptomics.[7–10] RNA sequencing (RNAseq) with next-generation sequencing (NGS) is the preferred method for transcriptomics.[11,12]

1. Hu, Y.F., Kaplow, J., and He, Y., From traditional biomarkers to transcriptome analysis in drug development, *Curr. Mol. Med.* 5, 29–38, 2005.

2. Viguerie, N., Poitou, C., Cancello, R., et al., Transcriptomics applied to obesity and caloric restriction, *Biochemie* 87, 117–123, 2005.

3. Seda, O., Tremblay, J., Sedova, L., and Hamet, P., Integrating genomics and transcriptomics with geo-ethnicity and the environment for the resolution of complex cardiovascular disease, *Curr. Opin. Mol. Ther.* 7, 583–587, 2005.

4. Schnabel, R.B., Baccarell, A., Lin, H., Ellinor, P.T., and Benjamin, E.J., Next steps in cardiovascular disease genomic research—sequencing, epigenetics, and transcriptomics, *Clin. Chem.* 58, 113–126, 2012.

5. Wang, H., Zhang, Q., and Fang, X., Transcriptomics and proteomics in stem cell research, *Front. Med.* 8, 433–444, 2014.

6. Uhlén, M., Hallström, B.M., Lindskog, C., et al., Transcriptomics resources of human tissues and organs, *Mol. Syst. Biol.* 12(4), 862, 2016.

7. Spaethling, J.M., and Everwine, J.H., Single-cell transcriptomics for drug target discovery, *Curr. Opin. Pharmacol.* 13, 786–790, 2013.

8. Crosetto, N., Bienko, M., and van Oudenaarden, A., Spatially resolved transcriptomics and beyond, *Nat. Rev. Genet.* 16, 57–66, 2015.

9. Chambers, D.C., Carew, A.M., Lukowski, S.W., and Powell, J.E., Transcriptomics and single-cell RNA-sequencing, *Respirology* 24, 29–36, 2019.

10. Strell, C., Hilscher, M.M., Laxman, N., et al., Placing RNA in context and space– Methods for spatially resolved transcriptomics, *FEBS J.* 286, 1468–1481, 2019.

11. McGettigan, P.A., Transcriptomics in the RNA-seq era, *Curr. Opin. Chem. Biol.* 17, 4–11, 2013.

12. Kukurba, K.R., and Montgomery, S.B., RNA sequencing and analysis, *Cold Spring Harg. Protoc.* 2015(11), 951–969, 2015.

TRANSCYTOSIS

Transcytosis describes the movement of a particle such as peptide, drug, or protein through a cell (usually an endothelial cell and vascular wall transport) as opposed to junctional transport (paracellular pathway).[1–9] Transcytosis involves a combination of endocytotic and exocytotic pathways. Transcytosis is important in transport of immunoglobulin[10,11] and albumin[12] across various tissues.

1. Patel, H.M., Transcytosis of drug carriers carrying peptides across epithelial barriers, *Biochem. Soc. Trans.* 17, 940–942, 1989.

2. Mostov, K., The polymeric immunoglobulin receptor, *Semin. Cell Biol.* 2, 411–418, 1991.

3. Michel, C.C., Transport of macromolecules through microvascular walls, *Cardiovasc. Res.* 32, 644–653, 1996.

4. Caplan, M.J., and Rodriguez-Boulan, E., Epithelial cell polarity: Challenges and methodologies, in *Handbook of Physiology. Section 14, Cell Physiology*, ed. J.F. Hoffman and J.D. Jamieson, Oxford University Press (for the American Physiological Society), New York, Chapter 17, 1997.

5. Florence, A.T., and Hussain, N., Transcytosis of nanoparticles and dendrimer delivery systems: Evolving vistas, *Adv. Drug Deliv. Rev.* 50(Suppl 1), S69–S89, 2001.

6. Vogel, S.M., and Malik, A.B., Albumin transcytosis in mesothelium: Further evidence of a transcellular pathway in polarized cells, *Am. J. Physiol. Lung Cell Mol. Physiol.* 282, L1–L2, 2002.

7. Ghetie, V., and Ward, E.S., Transcytosis and catabolism of antibody, *Immunol. Res.* 25, 97–113, 2002.

8. Kreuter, J., Influence of the surface properties on nanoparticle-mediated transport of drugs to the brain, *J. Nanosci. Nanotechnol.* 4, 484–488, 2004.

9. Rot, A., Contribution of Duffy antigen to chemokine function, *Cytokine Growth Factor Rev.* 16, 687–694, 2005.

10. Stapleton, N.M., Einardottir, H.K., Stemerding, A.M., and Vidarsson, G., The multiple facets of FcRn in immunity, *Immunol. Rev.* 268, 253–268, 2015.

11. Armitage, C.W., O'Meara, C.P., and Beagley, K.W., Chlamydial infection enhances expression of the polymeric immunoglobulin receptor (pIgR) and transcytosis IgA, *Am. J. Reprod. Immnol.* 77(1), e12611, 2017.

12. Pyzik, M., Rath, T., Kuo, T.T., et al., Hepatic FcRn regulates albumin homeostasis and susceptibility to liver injury, *Proc. Natl. Acad. Sci.* 114, E2862–E2871, 2017.

TRANSFORMATION

Transformation is a term used to described change in a cell manifested by escape from control mechanisms generally resulting in increased growth potential, alterations in the cell surface and karyotypic abnormalities.[1] Canonical cell transformation generally occurs as result of acquisition of genetic information from a virus entering the cell.[2-4] Viral transformation of cells is a common strategy in gene therapy.[5-7] Cell transformation is the basis for most neoplasms (**oncogenic transformation, neoplasic transformation**).[8-15]

1. *Theories and Model in Cellular Transformation*, ed. L. Santi and L. Zardi, Academic Press, London, UK, 1985.
2. Enders, J.F., Cell transformation by viruses as illustrated by the response of human and hamster renal cells to Simian virus 40, *Harvey Lect.* 59, 113–153, 1965.
3. Dulbecco, R., Transformation of cells in vitro by DNA-containing viruses, *JAMA* 190, 721–726, 1964.
4. Hanafusa, H., Replication of oncogenic viruses in virus-induced tumor cells–their persistence and interaction with other viruses, *Adv. Cancer Res.* 12, 137–165, 1969.
5. Smith, A.E., Viral vectors for gene therapy, *Annu. Rev. Microbiol.* 49, 807–838, 1995.
6. McConnell, M.J., and Imperiale, M.J., Biology of adenovirus and its use as vector for ene therapy, *Human Gene Ther.* 15, 1022–1033, 2004.
7. Collesi, C., and Giacca, M., Gene transfer to promote cardiac regeneration, *Crit. Clin. Lab. Sci.* 53, 359–369, 2016.
8. Rangarajan, A., Hong, S.J., Gifford, A., and Weinberg, R.A., Species- and cell type-specific requirements for cellular transformation, *Cancer Cell* 6, 171–183, 2004.
9. Adhikary, S., and Eilers, M., Transcriptional regulation and transformation by Myc proteins, *Nat. Rev. Mol. Cell Biol.* 6, 635–645, 2005.
10. Kumar, M.S., Lu, J., Mercer, K.L., et al., Impaired microRNA processing enhances cellular transformation and tumorigenesis, *Nature Genetics* 39, 673–677, 2007.
11. Ruddon, R.W., *Cancer Biology*, Oxford University Press, New York, 2007.
12. Weinberg, R.A., *The Biology of Cancer*, Garland Science/Taylor & Francis Group, New York, 2008.
13. Zhao, L., and Vogt, P.K., Class I P13K in oncogene cellular transformation, *Oncogene* 27, 5486–5496, 2008.
14. Roy, N., and Hebrok, M., Regulation of cellular identity in cancer, *Dev. Cell* 35, 674–684, 2015.
15. Pecarino, L., *Molecular Biology of Cancer; Mechanisms, Targets, and Therapeutics*, Oxford University Press, 2016.

TRANSGENE

A transgene is a piece or segment of DNA, usually coding DNA, which is introduced into a cell or organism to modify the genome.[1-4] Derivative plants or animals are referred to as **transgenic**. Some notable applications of transgenes technology have been in plants[5-9] and mice.[10-13] **Transgenic zebrafish** have also been of interest.[14-16]

1. Gluethmann, H., and Ohashi, P.S., *Transgenesis and Targeted Mutagenesis in Immunology*, Academic Press, San Diego, 1994.
2. Dichek, D.A., Retroviral vector-mediated gene transfer into endothelial cells, *Mol. Biol. Med.* 8, 257–266, 1991.
3. Barry, M.A., and Johnston, S.A., Biological features of genetic immunization, *Vaccine* 15, 788–791, 1997.
4. Patil, S.D., Rhodes, D.G., and Burgess, D.J., DNA-based therapeutics and DNA delivery systems: A comprehensive review, *AAPS J.* 7, E61–E77, 2005.
5. Hiatt, A., *Transgenic Plants: Fundamentals and Applications,* Marcel Dekker, New York, 1993.
6. Peña, L., *Transgenic Plants: Methods and Protocols*, Humana Press, Totowa, NJ, 2005.
7. Scotti, N., and Cardi, T., Transgene-induced pleiotropic effects in transplastomic plants, *Biotechnol. Lett.* 36, 229–239, 2014.
8. Jia, S., Yuan, Q., Pei, X., et al., Rice transgene flow: Its patterns, model and risk management, *Plant Biotechnol. J.* 12, 1259–1270, 2014.
9. Doron, L., Segal, N., and Shapira, M., Transgene expression in microalgae–From tools to applications, *Front. Plant. Sci.* 7, 505, 2016.
10. Grosveld, F.G., and Kollias, G.V., *Transgenic Animals*, Academic Press, San Diego, CA, 1992.
11. Babinet, C., Morello, D., and Renard, J.P., Transgenic mice, *Genome* 31, 938–949, 1989.
12. Janne, J., Hyttinen, J.M., Peura, T., et al., Transgenic animals as bioproducers of therapeutic proteins, *Ann. Med.* 24, 273–280, 1992.
13. Wright, D.C., and Wagner, T.E., Transgenic mice: A decade of progress in technology and research, *Mutat. Res.* 307, 429–440, 1994.
14. Chen, X., Gays, D., Santoro, M.M., Transgenic zebrafish, *Methods Mol. Biol.* 1464, 107–114, 2016.
15. Chang, W.W., Chi, W.Y., Kao, T.T., et al., The transgenic zebrafish display fluorescence reflecting the expressional dynamics of dihydrofolate reductase, *Zebrafish* 14, 223–235, 2017.
16. Lissouba, A., Liao, M., Kabashi, E., and Drapeau, P., Transcriptomic analysis of zebrafish TDP-43 transgenic lines, *Front. Mol. Neurosci.* 11:463, 2018.

TRANSLATION

In biochemistry, translation is the process by which information is transferred from the mRNA to linear sequence of amino acid in a polypeptide (protein) referred as the primary structure.[1–12] The process involves the transfer of an aminoacyl-tRNA to a growing peptide chain on a RNA polynucleotide (mRNA).[13] The tRNA is directed to a specific trinucleotide sequence (**triplet base code**).[14–18] Translation follows transcription, which is the process of information transfer from DNA to RNA. **Translatomics** has been suggested to describe the process of translation.[19,20]

1. Thach, R.C., Cecere, M.A., Sundararajan, T.A., and Doty, P., The polarity of messenger translation in protein synthesis, *Proc. Natl. Acad. Sci. USA* 54, 1167–1173, 1965.
2. *Translation Mechanisms*, ed. J. Lapointe and L. Brakeir-Gingras, Landes Biosciences, Georgetown, TX/Kluwer Plenum, New York, 2003.
3. *Protein Synthesis and Translational Control: A Subject Collection from Cold Spring Harbor Perspectives in Biology*, ed. J.W.B. Hershey, N. Sonnenberg, and M.B. Matthews, Cold Spring Harbor Laboratory Press, Cold Spring Harbor, NY, 2012.
4. Liljas, A., *Structural Aspects of Protein Synthesis*, World Scientific, Hackensack, NJ, 2013.
5. *Evolution of the Protein Synthesis Machinery and Its Regulation*, ed. G. Hernández and R. Jagus, Springer Science + Business, Cham, Switzerland, 2016.
6. Phelps, C.S., and Arnstein, H.R.V., Messenger RNA and Ribosomes in Protein Synthesis, Biochemical Society, London, UK, 1982.
7. Arnstein, H.R.V., and Cox, R.A., *Protein Biosynthesis*, IRL Press, Oxford, UK, 1992.
8. Belasco, J.G., and Brawerman, G., *Control of Messenger RNA Stability*, Academic Press, San Diego, CA, 1993.
9. Ilan, J., *Translational Regulation of Gene Expression 2*, Plenum Press, New York, 1993.
10. Tymms, M.J., *In Vitro Transcription and Translation Protocols*, Humana Press, Totowa, NJ, 1995.
11. Weissman, S.M., *cDNA Preparation and Characterization*, Academic Press, San Diego, CA, 1999.
12. Schoenberg, D.R., *mRNA Processing and Metabolism: Methods and Protocols*, Humana Press, Totowa, NJ, 2004.
13. Hatfield, D.L., *Transfer RNA in Protein Synthesis*, CRC/Taylor & Francis, Boca Raton, FL, 2018.
14. Gamow, G., and Yčas, M., Statistics and correlation of protein and ribonucleic acid composition, *Proc. Natl. Acad. Sci. USA* 41, 1011–1019, 1955.
15. Lengyel, P., Speyer, J.F., and Ochoa, S., Synthetic polynucleotides and the amino acid code, *Proc. Natl. Acad. Sci. USA* 47, 1936–1942, 1961.
16. Martin, R.G., Matthaei, J.H., Jones, O.W., and Nirenberg, M.W., Ribonucleotide composition of the genetic code, *Biochem. Biophys. Res. Commun.* 6, 401–414, 1962.
17. Ochoa, S., The Chemical basis of heredity—The genetic code, *Bull. N.Y. Acad. Med.* 40, 387–411, 1964.
18. Nirenberg, M., Leder, P., Bernfield, M., et al., RNA codewords and protein synthesis, VII. On the general nature of the RNA code, *Proc. Natl. Acad. Sci. USA* 53, 1161–1168, 1965.
19. Kahlau, S., and Bock, R., Plastid transcriptomics and translatomics of tomato fruit development and chloroplast-to-chloroplast differentiation: Chromoplast gene expression largely serves the production of a single protein, *Plant Cell* 20, 856–874, 2008.
20. Zhao, J., Qin, B., Nikolay, R., Spahn, C.M.T., and Zhang, G., Translatomics: The global view of translation, *Int. J. Mol. Sci.* 20(1), E212, 2019.

TRANSLOCATION

There are several definitions for translocation in molecular and cell biology.

The movement of a ribosome along mRNA during protein synthesis: this process involved the participation of elongation factor (EF-G) and is accompanied by GTP hydrolysis.[1] Translocation also refers to the process of protein transport across the endoplasmic reticulum[2,3] and from vesicles to cytoplasmic membrane.[4] Translocation also refers to the movement of water and solutes in a plant, in particular from the roots to the shoots.[5–8] See **transcription, translocon**.

1. Belardinelli, R., Sharma, H., Peske, F., Wintermeyer, W., and Rodnina, M.W., Translocation as continuous movement through the ribosome, *RNA Biol.* 13, 1197–1203, 2016.
2. Vorhees, R.M., and Hegde, R.S., Toward a structural understanding of co-translational protein translocation, *Curr. Opin. Cell Biol.* 41, 91–99, 2016.
3. Rapaport, T.A., Li, L., and Park, E., Structural and mechanistic insights into protein translocation, *Annu. Rev. Cell Dev. Biol.* 33, 369–390, 2017.
4. Wu, J., Cheng, D., Liu, L., Lv, X., and Liu, K., TBC1D15 affects glucose uptake by regulating GLUT4 translocation, *Gene* 683, 210–215, 2019.
5. Kutchan, T.M., A role for intra- and intercellular translocation in natural products, *Curr. Opin. Plant Biol.* 8, 292–300, 2005.
6. Yang, X., Feng, Y., He, Z., and Stoffells, P.J., Molecular mechanisms of heavy metal hyperaccumulation and phytoremediation, *J. Trace Elem. Med. Biol.* 18, 339–353, 2005.
7. Thompson, M.V., Phloem: The long and the short of it, *Trends Plant Sci.* 11, 26–32, 2006.
8. Takahashi, H., Yoshimoto, N., and Saito, K., Anionic nutrient transport in plants: The molecular basis of the sulfate transporter gene family, *Genet. Eng.* (NY) 27, 67–80, 2006.

TRANSLOCON

A translocon is a multiprotein complex (composed of several ER proteins) that mediates protein transport (cotranslational protein translocation) across membranes.[1–9] A translocon interacts with single recognition particle (SRP).

1. Johnson, A.E., and van Waes, M.A., The translocon: A dynamic gateway at the ER membrane, *Annu. Rev. Cell Dev. Biol.* 15, 799–842, 1999.
2. May, T., and Soll, J., Chloroplast precursor protein translocon, *FEBS Lett.* 452, 52–56, 1999.
3. Johnson, A.E., and Haigh, N.G., The ER translocon and retrotranslocation: Is the shift into reverse manual or automatic? *Cell* 102, 709–712, 2000.
4. White, S.H., Translocons, thermodynamics, and the folding of membrane proteins, *FEBS Lett.* 555, 116–221, 2003.
5. Coombes, B.K., and Finlay, B.B., Insertion of the bacterial type III translocon: Not your average needle stick, *Trends Microbiol.* 13, 92–95, 2006.
6. Skach, W.R., The expanding role of the ER translocon in membrane protein foldng, *J. Cell Biol.* 179, 1333–1335, 2007.
7. Mattel, P.J., Faudry, E., Job, V., et al., Membrane targeting and pore formation by the type III secretion system translocon, *FEBS J.* 278, 414–426, 2011.
8. Denks, K., Vogt, A., Sachelaru, I., et al., The *Sec* translocon mediated protein transport in prokaryotes and eukaryotes, *Mol. Membr. Biol.* 31, 58–84, 2014.
9. Pfeffer, S., Dudek, J., Zimmermann, R., Förster, F., Organization of the native ribosome-tranlocon complex at the mammalian endoplasmic reticulum membrane, *Biochim. Biophys. Acta* 1860, 2122–2129, 2016.

TRANSIL

Transil is a term with several meaning. Transil does refer to a diode surge protector device.[1] Transil has also been used to describe porous silica beads which can be coated with a single phospholipid bilayers and used to study protein-lipid interactions.[2–6] Transil beads are suggested to a model for liposomes[6] and erythrocytes.[4] Transil® beads for ADMET and other studies are commercially available from Sovicell.[7]

1. Boquete, L., Ascariz, J.M.R., Cantos, J., et al., A portable wireless biometric multi-channel system, *Measurement* 45,1587–1598, 2012.
2. Schmitz, A.A., Schleiff, E., Rohrig, C., et al., Interactions of myristoylated alanine-rich kinase substrates (MARCKS)-related protein with a novel solid-supported lipid membrane system (TRANSIL), *Anal. Biochem.* 268, 343–353, 1999.
3. Loidl-Stahlhofen, A., Hartmann, T., Schottner, M., et al., Multilamellar liposomes and solid-supported lipid membranes (TRANSIL): Screening of lipid-water partitioning toward a high-throughput scale, *Pharm. Res.* 18, 1782–1788, 2001.
4. Schuhmacher, J., Kohlsdorfer, C., Bühner, K., et al., High-throughput determination of the free fraction of drugs strongly bound to plasma proteins, *J. Pharm. Sci.* 93, 816–830, 2004.
5. Longhi, R., Corbioli, S., Fontana, S., et al., Brain tissue binding of drugs: Evaluation and validation of solid supported porcine brain membrane vesicles (TRANSIL) as a novel high-throughput method, *Drug. Metab. Dispos.* 39, 312–321, 2011.
6. Golius, A., Gorb, L., Michalkova, S.A., et al., Experimental and computational study of membrane affinity for selected energetic compounds, *Chemosphere* 148, 322–327, 2016.
7. Sovicell GMBH, Leipzig, Germany, https://www.sovicell.com/index.asp.

TRANSPORTAN

Transportan is a 27-amino-acid amphipathic peptide with cell penetrating properties suggested for promoting intracellular drug delivery including gene therapy products.[1–7] Transportan 10 is a short analogue of transportan,[8,9] which is being extensively used.[10–13] Glycosamioglycans are important in the cell penetrating activity of transportan and transportan 10.[14]

1. Pooga, M., Hällbrink, M., Zorko, M., and Langel, Ü., Cell penetration by transportan, *FASEB J.* 12, 67–77, 1998.
2. Lindgren, M., Gallet, X., Soomets, U., et al., Translocation properties of novel cell penetrating transportan and petratan analogues, *Bioconjug. Chem.* 11, 619–626, 2000.
3. Pooga, M., Kut, C., Kihlmark, M., et al., Cellular translocation of proteins by transportan, *FASEB J.* 15, 1451–1453, 2001.
4. Padari, K., Säälik, P., Hansen, M., et al., Cell transduction pathways of transportans, *Bioconjug. Chem.* 16, 1399–1410, 2005.
5. Pourmousa, M., Wong-ekkabut, J., Patra, M., and Karttunen, M., Molecular dynamic studies of transportan interacting with a DPPC lipid bilayer, *J. Phys. Chem. B.* 117, 230–241, 2013.
6. Pepe, D., Carvalho, V.F., McCall, M., de Lemos, D.P., and Lopes, L.B., Transportan in nanocarriers improves skin localization and antitumor activity of paclitaxel, *Int. J. Nanomedicine* 11, 2009–2019, 2016.
7. Cosme, P.J. Ye, J., Sears, S., Wojcikiewscz, E.P., and Terentis, A.C., Label-free confocal Raman mapping of transportan in melanoma cells, *Mol. Pharm.* 15, 851–860, 2018.

8. Soomets, U., Lindgren, M., Gallet, X., et al., Deletion analogues of transportan, *Biochim. Biophys. Acta* 1467, 165–176, 2000.

9. Kilk, K., El-Andaloussi, S., Järver, P., et al., Evaluation of transportan 10 in PEI mediated plasmid delivery assay, *J. Control. Rel.* 103, 511–523, 2005.

10. Wierzbicki, L., Rybarczyk, A., Alenowicz, M., Rekowski, P., and Kmiec, Z., Protein and siRNA delivery by tranportan and transportan 10 into colorectal cancer cell lines, *Folia Histochem. Cytobiol.* 52, 270–278, 2014.

11. Xie, J., Gou, Y., Zhao, Q., et al., Antimicrobial activities and action mechanism studies of transportan 10 and its analogues against multidrug-resistant bacteria, *J. Pept. Sci.* 21, 599–607, 2015.

12. Izabela, R., Jaroslaw, R., Madgalena, A., Piotr, R., and Ivan, K., Transportan 10 improves the anticancer activity of cisplatin, *Naunyn Schmiedebergs Arch. Pharmacol.* 389, 485–497, 2016.

13. Moghal, M.M.R., Islam, M.Z., Sharmin, S., et al., Continuous detection of entry of cell-penetrating peptide transportan 10 into single vesicles, *Chem. Phys. Lipids* 212, 120–129, 2018.

14. Pae, J., Liivamägi, L., Lubenets, D., et al., Glycosaminoglycans are required for translocation of amphipathic cell-penetrating peptides across membranes, *Biochim. Biophys. Acta* 1858, 1860–1867, 2016.

TRANS-SPLICING

A process that occurs with both nucleic acids and proteins. With nucleic acids, *trans*-splicing (transsplicing) occurs as part of pre-mRNA processing where there is the transfer of an RNA segment another RNA molecule to another RNA molecule in a process, which increases mRNA diversitiy.[1–10] SL (spliced leader) *trans*-splicing[11–14] is special cases of *trans*-splicing for nucleic acids. *Trans*-splicing also occurs with proteins but is most often a technique to use intein chemistry for ligation.[15–20]

1. Bonen, L., *Trans*-splicing of pre-mRNA in plants, animals, and protists, *FASEB J.* 7, 40–46, 1993.

2. Nilsen, T.W., *Trans*-splicing: An update, *Mol. Biochem. Parasitol.* 73, 1–6, 1995.

3. Adams, M.D., Rudner, D.Z., and Rio, D.C., Biochemistry and regulation of pre-mRNA splicing, *Curr. Opin. Cell Biol.* 8, 331–339, 1996.

4. Frantz, C., Ebel, C., Paulus, F., and Imbault, P., Characterization of *trans*-splicing in Euglenoids, *Curr. Genet.* 37, 349–355, 2000.

5. Garcia-Blanco, M.A., Messenger RNA reprogramming by spliceosome-mediated RNA *trans*-splicing, *J. Clin. Invest.* 112, 474–480, 2003.

6. Mitchell, L.G., and McGarrity, G.J., Gene therapy progress and prospects: Reprogramming gene expression by *trans*-splicing, *Gene Ther.* 12, 1477–1485, 2005.

7. Yang, Y., and Walsh, C.E., Spliceosome-mediated RNA *trans*-splicing, *Mol. Ther.* 12, 1006–1012, 2005.

8. Glanz, S., and Kück, U., *Trans*-splicing of organelle introns—A detour to continuous RNAs, *Bioessays* 31, 921–934, 2009.

9. Lei, Q., Li, C., Zuo, Z., et al., Evolutionary insights into RNA *trans*-splicing in vertebrates, *Genome Biol. Evol.* 8, 562–577, 2016.

10. Müller, U.F., Design and experimental evolution of *trans*-splicing Group I intron ribozymes, *Molecules* 22, E22, 2017.

11. Agabian, N., *Trans*-splicing of nuclear premRNAs, *Cell* 61, 1157–1160, 1990.

12. Hastings, K.E., SL *trans*-splicing: Easy come or easy go? *Trends Genet.* 21, 240–247, 2005.

13. Pettitt, J., Harrison, N., Stansfield, I., Connolly, B., and Müller, B., The evolution of spiced leader *trans*-splicing in nematodes, *Biochem. Soc. Trans.* 38, 1125–1130, 2010.

14. Krchňáková, Z., Krajčovič, J., and Vesteg, M. On the possibility of an early evolutionary origin for the spliced leader *trans*-splicing, *J. Mol. Evol.* 85, 37–45, 2017.

15. Shi, J., and Muir, T.W., Development of a tandem protein *trans*-splicing system based on native and engineered split inteins, *J. Am. Chem. Soc.* 127, 6198–6206, 2005.

16. Khan, M.S., Khalid, A.M., and Malik, K.A., Intein-mediated protein *trans*-splicing and transgene containment in plastids, *Trends Biotechnol.* 23, 217–220, 2005.

17. Kwon, Y., Coleman, M.A., and Camarero, J.A., Selective immobilization of proteins onto solid supports through split-intein-mediated protein *trans*-splicing, *Angew. Chem. Int. Ed. Engl.* 45, 1726–1729, 2006.

18. Iwai, H., Zuger, S., Jin, J., and Tam, P.H., Highly efficient protein *trans*-splicing by a naturally split DnaE intein from *Nostoc punctiforms*, *FEBS Lett.* 580, 1853–1858, 2006.

19. Muralidharan, V., and Muir, T.W., Protein ligation: An enabling technology for the biophysical analysis of proteins, *Nat. Methods* 3, 429–438, 2006.

20. Mattern, J.C., Bachman, A.L., Thiel, I.V., et al., Ligation of synthetic peptides to proteins using semisynthetic protein *trans*-splicing, *Methods Mol. Biol.* 1266, 129–143, 2015.

TRANSVECTION

Transvection is literally to carry over or to carry across. In mathematics, a linear function. In biology, where gene expression is influence by *trans*-interactions between alleles depending on somatic pairing between homologous chromosome regions; it can result in partial complementation between mutant alleles.[1–5]

1. Judd, B.H., Transvection: Allelic cross talk, *Cell* 53, 841–843, 1988.

2. Rassoulzadegan, M., Magliano, M., and Cuzin, F., Transvection effects involving DNA methylation during meiosis in the mouse, *EMBO J.* 21, 440–450, 2002.

3. Duncan, I.W., Transvection effects in *Drosophila* 36, 521–556, 2002.
4. Coulhard, A.B., Nolan, N., Bell, J.B., and Hilliker, A.J., Transvection at the vestigial locus of *Drosophila melanogaster* 170, 1711–1721, 2005.
5. Fukaya, T., and Levine, M., Transvection, *Curr. Biol.* 27, R1047–R1049, 2017.

TRIBODY

The original tribody consisted of 3 Fab' fragments cross-linked via a cysteine residue in the hinge region to form a trivalent antibody.[1] Later work used scFv fragments to obtain trimeric and tetrameric products.[2] A trimer formed with scFv fragments engineered with no linker between the V_H and V_L domains. The normal linker engineered between the V_H and V_L domains is 15 residues (usually glycine and serine to promote maximum flexibility) which yields a monomer; if the linker is reduced to 10 residues, a dimer (diabody) is formed while with no linker there is a trimer or higher order polymer.[3,4] There are other methods to obtain trivalent antibody derivative. A trivalent antibody construct with two scFv fragments attached to the C-terminal ends of a Fab fragment.[5,6] Tribodies have also been obtained the self-assembly of fusion protein between the C-terminal coiled region of cartilage matrix protein and a targeting ligand.[7] This latter study showed that the targeting ligand does not have to be the paratope domain. The above works shows that there are various approaches to the preparation of a tribody and while the targeting ligands, there are other possibilities including aptamers; it is also noted that a tribody can be a homotrimer or a heterotrimer. There is clinical interest in tribodies.[8,9]

1. Schott, M.E., Frazier, K.A., and Pollock, D.K., Preparation, characterization, and in vivo distribution of synthetically cross-linked multivalent antitumor antibody fragments, *Biocong. Chem.* 4, 153–165, 1993.
2. Le Gall, E., Kipriyanov, S.M., Moldenhauer, G., and Little, M., Di-, tri- and tetrameric single chain Fv antibody fragments against human CD19: Effect of valency on cell binding, *FEBS Lett.* 453, 164–168, 1999.
3. Atwell, J.L., Breheney, K.A., Lawrence, L.J., et al., scFv multimers of th anti-neuraminidase antibody NC10: Length of the linker between V_H and V_L domains dictates precisely the transition between diabodies and triabodies, *Protein Eng.* 12, 597–604, 1999.
4. Todorovska, A., Roovers, R.C., Dolezal, O., et al., Design and application of diabodies, triabodies and tetrabodies for cancer targeting, *J. Immunol. Methods* 248, 47–66, 2001.
5. Schoonjans, R., Willems, A., Schoonooghe, S., Fiers, W., et al., Fab chains as an efficient heterodimerization scaffold for the production of recombinant bispecific and trispecific antibody derivatives, *J. Immunol.* 165, 7050–7057, 2000.
6. Willems, A., Leonen, J., Schoonooghe, S., et al., Optimizing expression and purification from cell culture of trispecific recombinant antibody derivatives, *J. Chromatog. B. Anal. Technol. Biomed. Life Sci.* 786, 161–176, 2003.
7. Kim, D., Kim, S.K., Valencia, C.A., and Liu, R., Tribody: Robust self-assembled trimeric targeting ligands with high stability and significantly improved target binding strength, *Biochemistry* 52, 7283–7294, 2013.
8. Oberg, H.H., Kellner, C., Gonnermann, D., et al., Tribody [HER2(2)xCD16] is more effective that trastuzumab in enhancing γδ T cell and natural killer cell cytotoxicity against HER2-expressing cancer cells, *Front. Immunol.* 9, 814, 2018.
9. Riccio, G., Ricardo, A.R., Passariello, M., T-cell activating tribodies as a novel approach for efficient killing of ErbB2-positive cancer cells, *J. Immunother.* 42, 1–10, 2019.

TRI REAGENTS

Tri reagent is term used to describe a solvent used to extract RNA from tissues for analysis including RNA-seq.[1] Tri reagents such as Tri-Reagent®[2,3] and TRIzol®.[4–9]

1. Marioni, J.C., Mason, C.E., Mane, S.M., Stephens, M., and Gilad, Y., RNA-seq: An assessment of technical reproducibility and comparison with gene expression arrays, *Genome Res.* 18, 1509–1517, 2008.
2. Chomczynski, P., and Sacchi, N., Single-step method of RNA isolation by acid guanidinium thiocyanate-phenol-chloroform extraction, *Anal. Biochem.* 162, 156–159, 1987.
3. Jho, E.H., Zhang, T., Domon, C., et al., Wnt/β-catenin/Tcf signaling induced the transcription of Axin2, a negative regulator of the signaling pathway, *Mol. Cell. Biol.* 22, 1172–1183, 2002.
4. Xiang, X., Qui, D., Hegele, R.D., and Tan, W.C., Comparison of different methods of total RNA extraction for viral detection in sputum, *J. Virol. Methods* 94, 129–135, 2001.
5. Barbaric, D., Dalla-Pozza, L., and Byrne, J.A., A reliable method for total RNA extraction from human bone marrow samples taken at diagnosis of acute leukaemia, *J. Clin. Pathol.* 55, 865–867, 2002.
6. Rio, D.C., Ares, M., Jr., Hannon, G.J., and Nilsen, T.W., Purificiation of RNA using TRIzol (TRI reagent), *Cold Spring Harb. Protoc.* 2010(6), pdb, prot5439, 2010.
7. Ly, W., Ma, W., Yin, X., et al., Optimization of the original TRIzol-based technique improves the extraction of circulating microRNA from serum samples, *Clin. Lab.* 61, 1953–1960, 2015.
8. Prakoso, D., Dark, M.J., Barbet, A.F., Viral enrichment methods affect the detection but not sequence variation of West Nile Virus in equine brain tissue, *Front. Vet. Sci.* 5, 318, 2018.
9. Althof, N., Trojnar, E., Böhm, T., et al., Interlaboratory validation of a method for hepatitis E virus RNA detection in meat and meat products, *Food Environ. Virol.* 11, 1–8, 2019.

TRIS-LIPIDATION

A process of linking a hydrophobic component to a peptide or protein to enhance membrane binding and drug delivery.[1-4] The hydroxyl groups of Tris are esterified with fatty acids and subsequently coupled to a peptide or protein via the amino group.

1. Whittaker, R.G., Hayes, P.J., and Bender, V., A gentle method of linking Tris to amino acids and peptides, *Pept. Res.* 6, 125–128, 1993.
2. Davey, R.A., Davey, M.W., Cullen, K.V., et al., The use of Tris-lipidation to modify drug cytotoxicity in multidrug resistant cells expressing P-glycoprotein or MRP1, *Br. J. Pharmacol.* 137, 1280–1286, 2002.
3. Walker, C., Fraser, J.M., Walton, C.E., et al., Tris lipidation – A novel drug delivery system that alters biodistribution, *J. Drug Target.* 10, 479–487, 2002.
4. Ali, M., Amon, M., Bender, V., and Manolis, N., Hydrophobic transmembrane-peptide lipid conjugation enhances membrane binding and functional activity in T-cells, *Bioconjugate Chem.* 16, 1556–1563, 2005.

TROYBODY (TROY BODY)

A troy body is a recombinant antibody which contains a V region specific for an antigen presenting cell (APC) and T-cell-specific epitopes engineered in the C domain region. The troy body is processed by the APC with the peptide contain the T-cell epitopes present an MHC II complex which the activates T-cells.[1-4] The concept can be used for other antigens.

1. Lunde, E., Rasmussen, I.B., Western, K.H., et al., "Troybodies": Recombinant antibodies that target T cell epitopes to antigen presenting cells, *Intern. Rev. Immunol.* 20, 647–673, 2001.
2. Lunde, E., Lauvrak, V., Rasmussen, I.B., et al., Troybodies and pepbodies, *Biochem. Soc. Trans.* 30, 500–506, 2002.
3. Lunde, E., Western, K.H., Rasmussen, I.B., Sandlie, I., and Bogen, B., Efficient delivery of T cell epitopes to APC by use of MHC class II-specific troybodies, *J. Immunol.* 168, 2154–2162, 2002.
4. Tunheim, G., Schjetne, K.W., Fredrikson, A.B., Sandlie, I., and Bogen, G., Human CD14 is an efficient target for recombinant immunoglobulin vaccine constructs that delivers T cell epitopes, *J. Leuk. Biol.* 77, 303–310, 2005.

TUBULIN

Tubulin is a protein which polymerizes to form microtubules as part of the cytoskeleton and critical for cell motility, cell division, and differentiation.[1-4] Tubulin is heterogeneous[5-10] and tubulin function is modulated by post-translational modification.[11,12] The combination of these various forms of tubulin in function is orchestrated by the tubulin code.[13-16] Tubulin is a focus in cancer therapy.[17-22]

1. Aher, A., and Akhmanova, A., Tipping microtubule dynamics: One protofilament at a time, *Curr. Opin. Cell. Biol.* 50, 86–93, 2018.
2. Brouhard, G.J., and Rice, L.M., Microtubule dynamics: An interplay of biochemistry and mechanics, *Nat. Rev. Mol. Cell Biol* 19, 451–463, 2018.
3. Pollard, T.D., Evolution of research on cellular motility over five decade, *Biophys. Rev.* 10, 1503–1508, 2018.
4. Zwetsloot, A.J., Tut, G., and Straube, A., Measuring microtubule dynamics, *Essays Biochem.* 62, 725–735, 2018.
5. Feit, H., Slusarek, L., and Shelanski, M.L., Heterogeneity of tubulin subunits, *Proc. Natl. Acad. Sci. USA* 68, 2028–2031, 1971.
6. Fine, R.E., Heterogeneity of tubulin, *Nat. New Biol.* 233, 283–284, 1971.
7. Murphy, D.B., Functions of tubulin isoforms, *Curr. Opin. Cell Biol.* 3, 43–51, 1991.
8. Oakley, B.R., An abundance of tubulins, *Trends Cell Biol.* 10, 537–542, 2000.
9. Dutcher, S.K., The tubulin fraternity: Alpha to eta, *Curr. Opin. Cell Biol.* 13, 49–54, 2001.
10. Tischfield, M.A., and Engle, E.C., Distinct α- and β-tubulin isotypes are required for the positioning, differentiation and survival of neurons: New support for the "multi-tubulin" hypothesis, *Biosci. Rep.* 30, 319–330, 2010.
11. Wloga, D., and Gaertig, J., Post-translational modifications of microtubules, *J. Cell Sci.* 123, 3447–3455, 2010.
12. Song, Y., and Brady, S.T., Post-translational modification of tubulin: Pathways to functional diversity of microtubules, *Trends Cell Biol.* 25, 125–136, 2015.
13. Yu, I., Garnham, C.P., and Roll-Mecak, A., Writing and reading the tubulin code, *J. Biol. Chem.* 290, 17163–17172, 2010.
14. Janke, C., The tubulin code: Molecular components, read-out mechanisms, and functions, *J. Cell. Biol.* 206, 461–472, 2014.
15. Wloga, D., Joachimiak, E., and Fabczak, H., Tubulin post-translational modification and microtubule dynamics, *Int. J. Mol. Sci.* 18(10), E2207, 2017.
16. Park, J.H., and Roll-Mecak, A., The tubulin code in neuronal polarity, *Curr. Opin. Neurobiol.* 51, 95–102, 2018.
17. Pellegrini, F., and Budman, D.R., Tubulin function, action of antitubulin drugs, and new drug development, *Cancer Invest.* 23, 264–273, 2005.
18. Nepali, K., Ojha, R., Lee, H.Y., and Liou, J.P., Early investigational tubulin inhibitors as novel cancer therapeutics, *Expert Opin. Investig. Drugs* 25, 917–936, 2016.
19. Ferrara, R., Pilotto, S., Peretti, U., et al., Tubulin inhibitors in non-small cell lung cancer: Looking back and forward, *Expert Opin. Pharmacother.* 17, 1113–1129, 2016.
20. Hardin, C., Shum, E., Singh, A.P., Perex-Soler, R., and Cheng, H., Emerging treatment using tubulin inhibitors in advanced non-small cell lung cancer, *Expert Opin. Pharmacother.* 18, 701–716, 2017.

21. Parker, A.L., Teo, W.S., McCarroll, J.A., and Kavallaris, M., An emerging role for tubulin isotypes in modulating cancer biology and chemotherapy resistance, *Int. J. Mol. Sci.* 18(7), E1434, 2017.
22. Chen, H., Lin, X., Arnst, K.E., Miller, D.D., and Li, W., Tubulin inhibitor-based antibody-drug conjugates for cancer therapy, *Molecules* 22(8), E1281, 2017.

TUMOR SUPPRESSOR GENE

A tumor suppressor gene is responsible for the encoding of products that suppress the malignant phenotype.[1–3] These gene were first identified in hybrid cells resulting from cell fusion.[4] Loss of tumor suppressor genes result in cell cycle deregulation.[5] While the canonical view of tumor suppressors genes relate to cell growth, tumor suppressor genes may have a broader role in the promotion of cellular homeostasis.[6] TP53 is one of the better-known tumor suppressor genes being responsible for p53 tumor repressor.[7–9] As with other tumor suppressors, p53 has broader functions including mitochondrial homeostasis.[10]

1. *Tumor Suppressor Genes*, ed. G. Klein, Dekker, New York, 1990.
2. *Oncogenes and Tumor Suppressor Genes in Human Malignancies*, ed. C.C. Benz and E.T. Liu, Kluwer Academic, Boston, MA, 1993.
3. *Tumor Suppressor Genes in Human Cancer*, ed. D.E. Fisher, Humana Press, Totowa, NJ, 2001.
4. Klein, G., The approaching era of the tumor suppressor genes, *Science* 238, 1539–1545, 1987.
5. Sager, R., Tumor suppressor genes: The puzzle and the promise, *Science* 246, 1406–1412, 1989.
6. Yuniati, L., Schekjen, B., van der Meer, L.T., and van Leeuwen, F.N., Tumor suppression BTG1 and BTG2: Beyond growth control, *J. Cell. Physiol.* 234, 5379–5389, 2019.
7. Levine, A.J., Tumor suppressor genes, *Bioessays* 12, 60–66, 1990.
8. Greenblatt, M.S., Bennert, W.P., Hollstein, M., and Harris, C.C., Mutations in *p53* tumor suppressor gene: Clues to cancer biology, *Cancer Res.* 54, 4855–4878, 1994.
9. Sabapathy, K., and Lane, D.P., Therapeutic targeting of p53: All mutans are equal, but some mutants are more equal than others, *Nat. Rev. Clin. Oncol.* 15, 13–30, 2018.
10. Kamp, W.M., Wang, P.Y., and Hwang, P.M., TP53 mutation, mitochondria and cancer, *Curr. Opin. Genet. Dev.* 38, 16–22, 2016.

TURBIDIMETRY

Turbidity is a measurement of the light scattered by a sample in the direct path of the electromagnetic radiation (light). However, in practice, turbidity is the decrease in the light transmitted. It represents electromagnetic radiation that is not absorbed as in spectroscopy but rather scattered. It is sometimes necessary to correct spectral measurements for turbidimetry.[1–5] Nephelometry is the measurement of light scattered by a sample. The extent to which electromagnetic radiation is scattered and measured either by turbidimetry or nephelometry depends on the size of the particle and the wavelength of the incident radiation. Turbidimetry is used in clinical chemistry,[6] platelet aggregation,[7,8] for the assay of some enzymes,[9–13] and water quality.[14–18]

1. Leach, S.J., and Scheraga, H.A., Effect of light scattering of ultraviolet difference spectra, *J. Amer. Chem. Soc.* 82, 4790–4792, 1960.
2. Schneider, A.S., Analysis of optical activity spectra of turbid biological suspensions, *Methods Enzymol.* 27, 751–767, 1973.
3. Dorman, B.P., Hearst, J.E., and Maesre, M.F., UV-absorption and circular dichroism measurements on light scattering biological specimens, fluorescent cell and related large-angle light detection techniques, *Methods Enzymol.* 27, 767–796, 1973.
4. Tracy, R.P., Andrianorivo, A., Riggs, B.L., and Mann, K.G., Comparison of monoclonal and polyclonal antibody-based immunoassays for osteocalcin: A study of sources of variation in assay results, *J. Bone Miner. Res.* 5, 451–461, 1990.
5. Barman, I., Singh, G.P., Dasari, R.R., and Field, M.S., Turbidity-corrected Raman spectroscopy for blood analyte detection, *Anal. Chem.* 81, 4233–4240, 2009.
6. Blirup-Jensen, S., Protein standardization III: Method optimization basic principles for quantitative determination of human serum proteins on automated instruments based on turbidimetry or nephelometry, *Clin. Chem. Lab. Med.* 39, 1098–1109, 2001.
7. Cruz, W.O., Platelet determination by turbidimetry, *Blood* 9, 920–926, 1954.
8. Jarvis, G.E., Platelet aggregation: Turbidimetric measurements, *Methods Mol. Biol.* 272, 65–76, 2004.
9. Rapport, M.M., Meyer, K., and Linker, A., Correlation of reductimetric and turbidimetric methods for hyaluronidase, *J. Biol. Chem.* 186, 615–623, 1950.
10. Houck, J.C., The turbidimetric determination of deoxyribonuclease activity, *Arch. Biochem. Biophys.* 82, 135–144, 1959.
11. Morsky, P., Turbidimetric determination of lysozyme with *Micrococcus lysodeikticus* cells: Reexamination of reaction conditions, *Anal. Biochem.* 128, 77–85, 1983.
12. Jenzano, J.W., and Lundblad, R.L., Effects of amines and polyamines on turbidmetric and lysoplate assays for lysozyme, *J. Clin. Microbiol.* 26, 34–37, 1988.
13. Walker, M.B., Retzinger, A.C., and Retzinger, G.S., A turbidmetric method for measuring the activity of trypsin and its inhibition, *Anal. Biochem.* 351, 114–121, 2006.

14. Rymszewicz, A., O'Sullivan, J.J., Bruen, M., et al., Measurement difference between turbidity instruments, and their implications for suspended sediment concentration and load calculations: A sensor inter-comparison study, *J. Environ. Manage.* 199, 99–108, 2017.
15. Weber, D.P., Skoutens, G., and Rahimiford, S., In-plant real-time manufacturing water content characterization, *Water Resources and Industry* 20, 37–45, 2018.
16. Wang, Y., Rajib, S.M.S.M., Collins, C., and Grieve, B., Low-cost turbidity sensor for low-power wireless monitoring of fresh water courses, *IEEE Sensors J.* 18, 4689–4696, 2018.
17. Lewis, J., Rhodes, J.J., and Bradley, C., Turbidity responses from timber harvesting, wildfire, and post-fire logging in the Battle Creek watershed, Northern California, *Environm. Manage.* 63, 416–432, 2019.
18. Mullins, D., Coburn, D., Hannon, L., et al., A novel image processing-based system for turbidity measurement in domestic and industrial wastewater, *Water Sci. Technol.* 77, 1469–1482, 2018.

TYROSINE KINASES

Tyrosine kinases are a large group of enzymes involved in intracellular signal transduction via the catalysis of the phosphorylation of tyrosine residues in target proteins.[1-5] There are a number of tyrosine kinase families[6-8] including SRC kinases,[9] FGF receptor kinases,[10] and EGF receptor kinases.[11]

1. Hardle, D.G., *Protein Phosphorylation: A Practical Approach*, Oxford University Press, Oxford, UK, 1993.
2. Woodgett, J.R., *Protein Kinases,* IRL Press at Oxford University Press, Oxford, UK, 1994.
3. *The Protein Kinase Factsbooks*, ed. D.G. Hardle and S. Hanks, Academic Press, San Diego, CA, 1995; *Protein Kinase Protocols,* ed. G. Krauss, Wiley-VCH, Weinheim, Germany, 2003.
4. *Signaling by Receptor Tyrosine Kinases: A Subject Collection from Cold Spring Harbor Perspectives in Biology,* ed. J. Schlesinger and M.A. Lemmon, Cold Spring Harbor Laboratory Press, Cold Spring Harbor, NY, 2014.
5. *Receptor Tyrosine Kinases: Structure, Function and Role in Kidney Disease,* ed. D.L. Wheeler and Y. Yarden, Humana Press, New York, 2015.
6. *Receptor Tyrosine Kinases: Family and Subfamilies,* ed. D.L. Wheeler and Y. Yarden, Springer Cham, Heidelberg, Germany, 2015.
7. *Resistance to Tyrosine Kinase Inhibitors,* ed. D. Focosi, Springer, Cham, Switzerland, 2016.
8. *Role of Tyrosine Kinases in Gastrointestinal Malignancies,* ed. G.P. Nagaraju, Springer Singapore, 2018.
9. Boggen, T.J., and Eck, M.J., Structure and regulation of Src family kinases, *Oncogene* 23, 7918–7927, 2004.
10. Farrell, B., and Breeze, A.L., Structure, activation and dysregulation of fibroblast growth factor receptor kinases: Perspectives for clinical targeting, *Biochem. Soc. Trans.* 46, 1753–1770, 2018.
11. Ushiro, H., and Cohen, S., Identification of phosphotyrosine as a product of epidermal growth factor-activated protein kinase in A-431 cell membranes, *J. Biol Chem.* 255, 8363–8365, 1980.

TYRPHOSTINS

Tyrphostins are synthetic organic compounds[1-6] which are best known as inhibitors of protein tyrosine kinases.[2,7-11] There is some interest in the therapeutic use of tyrphostins in cancer.[12-15] Tyrphostins are not specific for tyrosine kinases but may inhibit other kinases[16] as well as guanylyl cyclase.[17] It has subsequently been shown that the tyrpphostins inhibited receptor guanylyl cyclases by binding to the kinase domain of the protein (noncompetitive inhibition).[18,19]

1. Gazit, A., Yaish, P., Gilon, C., and Levitzki, A., Tryphostins I: Synthesis and biological activity of protein tyrosine kinase inhibitors, *J. Med. Chem.* 32, 2344–2352, 1989.
2. Ramdas, L., Obeyesekere, N.U., McMurray, J.S., A tryphostin-derived inhibitor of protein kinases: Isolation and characterization, *Arch. Biochem. Biophys.* 323, 237–242, 1995.
3. Kumar, N., Windisch, V., and Ammon, H.L., Photostability of some tryphostin drugs: Chemical consequences of crystallinity, *Pharm. Res.* 12, 1708–1715, 1995.
4. Ellis, A.G., Nice, E.C., Weinstrock, J., et al., High-performance liquid chromatographic analysis of the tryphostin AG1478, a specific inhibitor of the epidermal growth factor receptor tyrosine kinase, in mouse plasma. *J. Chromatogr. B Biomed. Sci. Appl.* 754, 193–199, 2001.
5. Guo, G., Arvantis, E.A., Pottorf, R.S., and Player, M.R., Solid-phase synthesis of a tryphostin ether library, *J. Comb. Chem.* 5, 408–413, 2003.
6. Ackermann, U., Tochon-Danguy, H.J., Nerrie, M., et al., Syntheis, ^{11}C labeling and biological properties of derivatives of the tryphostin AG957, *Nucl. Med. Biol.* 32, 323–328, 2005.
7. Gu, L., Zhuang, H., Safina, B., et al., Combinatorial approach to identification of tryphostin inhibitors of cytokine signaling, *Bioorg. Med. Chem.* 13, 4269–4278, 2005.
8. Levitzki, A., Gazit, A., Osherov, N., Posner, I., and Gilon, C., Inhibition of protein-tyrosine kinases by tryphostins, *Methods Enzymol.* 201, 347–361, 1991.
9. Levitzki, A., Tryphostins: Tyrosine kinase blockers as novel antiproliferative agents and dissectors of signal transduction, *FASEB J.* 6, 3275–3282, 1992.
10. Levitzki, A., and Mishani, E., Tyrphostins and other tyrosine kinase inhibitors, *Annu. Rev. Biochem.* 75, 93–109, 2006.

11. Wang, Y., Sun, H.Y., Liu, Y.G., et al., Tryphostin AG556 increases the activity of large conductance Ca^{2+}-activated K^+ channels by inhibiting epidermal growth factor receptor tyrosine kinase, *J. Cell. Mol. Med.* 21, 1826–1834, 2017.

12. Xiao, G.S., Zhang, Y.H., Wu, W., et al., Genistein and tryphostin AG556 decrease ultra-rapidly activating delayed rectified K^+ current of human aorta by inhibiting EGF receptor tyrosine kinase, *Br. J. Pharmacol.* 174, 454–467, 2017.

13. Levitzki, A., Tyrphostins—potential antiproliferative agents and novel molecular tools, *Biochem. Pharmacol.* 40, 913–918, 1990.

14. Deng, J., Grande, F., and Naemati, N., Small molecule inhibitors of Stat3 signaling pathway, *Curr. Cancer Drug Targets* 7, 91–107, 2007.

15. Yu, J.L., Xing, R., Milsom, C., and Rak, J., Modulation of the oncogene-dependent tissue factor expression by kinase suppressor of ras 1, *Thromb. Res.* 126, e6–e10, 2010.

16. Zhang, X., Lu, H., Hong, W., et al., Tyrphostin B42 attenuates trichostatin A-mediated resistance in pancreatic cancer by antagonizing IL-6/JAK2/STAT3 signaling, *Oncol. Rep.* 39, 1892–1900, 2018.

17. Daya-Makin, M., Pelech, S.L., Levitzki, A., and Hudson, A.T., Erbstatin and tyrphostins block protein-serine kinase activation and meiotic maturation of sea star, *Biochim. Biophys. Acta* 1093, 87–94, 1991.

18. Jaleel, M., Shenoy, A.R., and Visweswariah, S.S., Tyrphostins are inhibitors of guanylyl and adenyl cyclases, *Biochemistry* 43, 8247–8255, 2004.

19. Mishra, V., Goel, R., and Visweswariah, S.S., The regulatory role of the kinase-homology domain in receptor guanylyl cyclases: Nothing "pseudo" about it, *Biochem. Soc. Trans.* 46, 1729–1742, 2018.

UBIQUITIN

Ubiquitin is a small intracellular protein that functions in protein degradation by the proteasome.[1–5] This is a process of controlled proteolysis which is an integral part of normal cell function. Some functions of the ubiquitin-proteasome system included the degradation of misfolded proteins[6,7] and the production of peptides during MHC class I antigen presentation.[8–11] Ubiquitin is linked to a protein via an isopeptide bond in a process referred to as ubiquitination which is catalyzed by ubiquitin ligases.[12–14] Ubiquitin is initially "activated" by the ubiquity ligase to form a high-energy thioester bond between the enzyme and the C-terminal glycine residue of ubiquitin; the ubiquitin is then transferred to a lysine residue on the target protein forming the isopeptide peptide.[15] While the discovery of ubiquitin was based on its ability to target proteins to degradation, it is clear that there are other functions.[16–20] There is a ubiquitin family of proteins (ubiquitin-like proteins)[21–26] Some of these family members are well known such as **NEDD8**[27–30] and **SUMO** (small ubiquitin-related modifier).[31–36]

1. Ciechanover, A. The ubiquitin-proteasome proteolytic pathway, *Cell* 79, 13–21, 1994.

2. Glickman, M.H., and Ciechanover, A., The ubiquitin-proteasome proteolytic pathway: Destruction for the sake of construction, *Physiol. Rev.* 82, 373–428, 2002.

3. Varshavsky, A., The ubiquitin system, autophagy, and regulated protein degradation, *Annu. Rev. Biochem.* 86, 123–128, 2017.

4. Zuebtara-Rytter, K., and Subramani, S., The roles of ubiquitin-binding protein shuttles in the degradative fate of ubiquitinated proteins in the ubiquitin-proteasome system and autophagy, *Cells* 8, E40, 2019.

5. Hanna, J., Guerra-Moreno, A., Ang, J., and Microogullari, Y., Protein degradation and the pathological basis of disease, *Am. J. Pathol.* 189, 94–103, 2019.

6. Amm, I., Sommer, T., and Wolf, D.H., Protein quality control and elimination of protein waste: The role of the ubiquitin-proteasome system, *Biochim. Biophys. Acta* 1843, 182–196, 2014.

7. Kocaturk, N.M., and Gozuacik, D., Crosstalk between mammalian autophagy and the ubiquitin-proteasome system, *Front. Cell Dev. Biol.* 6, 128, 2018.

8. Michalek, M.T., Grant, E.P., Gramm, C., et al., A role for the ubiquitin-dependent proteolytic pathway in MHC class I-restricted antigen presentation, *Nature* 363, 552–554, 1993.

9. Sijts, A., Zaiss, D., and Kloetzel, P.M., The role of the ubiquitin-proteasome pathway in MHC class I antigen processing: Implications for vaccine design, *Curr. Mol. Med.* 1, 665–676, 2001.

10. Sijts, E.J., and Kloetzel, P.M., The role of the proteasome in the generation of MHC class I ligands and immune responses, *Cell. Mol. Life Sci.* 68, 1491–1502, 2011.

11. Inobe, T., and Matouschek, A., Paradigms of protein degradation by the proteasome, *Curr. Opin. Struct. Biol.* 24, 156–164, 2014.

12. Pavletich, N.P., Structural biology of ubiquitin-protein ligases, *Harvey Lect.* 98, 65–102, 2002–2003.

13. Robinson, P.A., and Ardley, H.C., Ubiquitin-protein ligases, *J. Cell. Sci.* 5191–5194, 2004.

14. Zheng, N., and Shabek, N., Ubiquitin ligases: Structure, function, and regulation, *Annu. Rev. Biochem.* 86, 129–157, 2017.

15. Komander, D., and Rape, M., The ubiquitin code, *Annu. Rev. Biochem.* 81, 203–229, 2012.

16. Welchman, R.L., Gordon, C., and Mayer, R.J., Ubiquitin and ubiquitin-like proteins as multifunctional signals, *Nat. Rev. Mol. Cell Biol.* 6, 599–609, 2005.

17. Chen, Z.J., Ubiquitin signaling in the NF-κB pathway, *Nat. Cell Biol.* 7, 758–765, 2005.

18. Ramanathan, H.N., and Ye, Y., Cellular strategies for making monoubiquitin signals, *Crit. Rev. Biochem. Mol. Biol.* 47, 17–28, 2012.

19. Ohtake, F., and Tsuchiya, H., The emerging complexity of ubiquitin architecture, *J. Biochem.* 161, 125–133, 2017.

20. Marsh, D.J., and Dickson, K.A., Writing histone monoubiquitination in human malignancy–The role of RING finger E3 ubiquitin ligases, *Genes (Basal)* 10, E67, 2019

21. Yet, E.T., Gong, L., and Kamitani, T., Ubiquitin-like proteins: New wines in new bottles, *Gene* 248, 1–14, 2000.
22. Schwartz, D.C., and Hochstrasser, M., A superfamily of protein tags: Ubiquitin, SUMO and related modifiers, *Trends Biochem. Sci.* 28, 321–328, 2003.
23. Catic, A., and Ploegh, H.L., Ubiquitin—Conserved protein or selfish gene? *Trends Biochem. Sci.* 30, 600–604, 2005.
24. Denison, C., Kirkpatrick, D.S., and Gygi, S.P., Proteomic insights into ubiquitin-like proteins, *Curr. Opin. Chem. Biol.* 9, 69–75, 2005.
25. van der Veen, A.G., and Ploegh, H.L., Ubiquitin-like proteins, *Annu. Rev. Biochem.* 81, 323–357, 2012.
26. Cappadocia, L., and Lima, C.D., Ubiquitin-like protein conjugation: Structure, chemistry, and mechanism, *Chem. Rev.* 118, 899–918, 2018.
27. Pan, Z.Q., Kentsis, A., Dias, D.C., Yamoah, K., and Wu, K., Nedd8 on cullin: Building an expressway to protein destruction, *Oncogene* 23, 1985–1997, 2004.
28. Xirodimas, D.P., Novel substrates and functions for the ubiquitin-like molecule NEED8, *Biochem. Soc. Trans.* 36, 802–806, 2008.
29. Mergner, J., and Scwechheimer, C., The NEED8 modification pathway in plants, *Front. Plant Sci.* 5, 103, 2014.
30. Ribet, D., and Cossart, P., Ubiquitin, SUMO, and NEDD8: Key targets of bacterial pathogens, *Trends Cell Biol.* 28, 926–940, 2018.
31. Saitoh, H., Pu, R.T., and Dasso, M. SUMO-1: Wrestling with a new ubiquitin-related modifier, *Trends Biochem. Sci.* 22, 374–376, 1997.
32. Kroetz, M.B., SUMO: A ubiquitin-like protein modifier, *Yale J. Biol. Med.* 78, 197–201, 2005.
33. Lecona, E., and Fernandez-Capetillo, O., A SUMO and ubiquitin code coordinates protein traffic and replication factories, *Bioessays* 38, 1209–1217, 2016.
34. Pichler, A., Fatouros, C., Lee, H., and Eisenhardt, N., SUMO conjugation—A mechanistic view, *Biomol. Concepts* 8, 13–36, 2017.
35. Ovaa, H., and Vetegaal, A.C.O., Probing ubiquitin and SUMO conjugation and deconjugation, *Biochem. Soc. Trans.* 46, 423–436, 2018.
36. Yang, Z., Zhang, Y., and Sun, S., Deciphering the SUMO code in the kidney, *J. Cell. Mol. Med.* 23, 711–719, 2019.

ULTRACONSERVED ELEMENTS

The canonical definition of ultraconserved elements in genomes is orthologous domains that share 100% identity over at least 200 bp in several mammalian species (e.g. mouse, rat, and human).[1-4]

1. Bejerano, G., Pheasant, M., Makunin, I., et al., Ultraconserved elements in the human genome, *Science* 304, 1321–1325, 2004.
2. Baira, E., Greschock, J., Coukos, G., and Zhang, L., Ultraconserved elements: Genomicis, function and disease, *RNA Biol.* 5, 132–134, 2008.
3. McCole, R.G., Erceg, J., Saylor, W., and Wu, C.T., Ultraconserved elements occupy specific arenas of three-dimensional mammalian genome organization, *Cell Rep.* 24, 479–488, 2018.
4. Andermann, T., Fernanes, A.M., Olsson, U., et al., Allele phasing greatly improves the phylogenetic utility of ultraconserved elements, *Syst. Biol.* 68, 32–46, 2019.

VALIDITY

External validity refers to the extent to which a specific finding from an investigation or analytical process can be generalized beyond the context of the specific investigation or analytical processes.[1] For regulatory purposes such as the manufacture of drugs and therapeutic biologicals, validity can be considered to be demonstration of the ability to reproducible repeat the process and/or assay. The validation process is the process by which an organization can demonstrate that the process is reproducible and, therefore, the process is valid. In the case of assay validation; "Method Validation: The process of demonstrating or confirming that a method is suitable for its intended purpose. Validation includes demonstrating performance characteristics such as accuracy, precision, specificity, limit of detection, limit of quantitation, linearity, range, ruggedness and robustness." Regulatory agencies such as the International Council for Harmonisation (ICH) and the Food and Drug Administration (FDA) have detailed requirements for the validation of analytical procedures[2] and manufacturing procedures.[3] In the case of manufacturing, validation is defined as "A documented program that provides a high degree of assurance that a specific process, method, or system will consistently produce a result meeting pre-determined acceptance criteria.[3] Validation is of importance in all fields of investigation including the social sciences.[4]

1. Guidelines for the Validation of Chemical Methods for the FDA FVM Program, 2nd Ed., Food and Drug Administration, Office of Foods and Veterinary Medicine, Bethesda, MD, 2015.
2. Validation of Analytical Procedures: Text and Methodology, Q2(R1), ICH, Geneva, Switzerland, 2014.
3. Good Manufacturing Practice Guide for Active Pharmaceutical Ingredients, Q7, Geneva, Switzerland, 2000.
4. Taylor, C.S., *Validity and Validation*, Oxford University Press, New York, 2013.

VARIEGATION

Variegation is literally, the state of discrete diversified coloration. In biology, this can refer to the discrete coloration patterns in leaves, or the occurrence within a tissue of sectors or clones of different phenotypes.[1–3] In genetics, it is taken to mean a chromosome position effect when particular loci are contiguous with heterochromatin. A position effect results from a different level of expression of a gene depending on location with strong expression in euchromatin and less expression in heterochromatin.[4–8] Position effect variegation has been studied extensively with the *White* gene in Drosophila where epigenetic silencing in a heterochromatin environment results in patchy eye color (red and white), a variegated effect.[8] The term variegation has been used to describe white and brown fat deposition.[9]

1. Wang, R., Zhao, J., Jia, M., et al., Balance between cytosolic and chloroplast translation affects leaf variegation, *Plant Physiol.* 176, 804–818, 2018.
2. Wang, Q.M., Cui, J., Dai, H., et al., Comparative transcriptome profiling of genes and pathways involved in leaf-patterning of *Clivia miniate* var. *variegate*, *Gene* 677, 280–288, 2018.
3. Qu, Y., Legen, J., Arndt, J., et al., Ectopic transplastomic expression of a synthetic MatK gene leads to cotyledon-specific leaf variegation, *Front. Plant. Sci.* 9, 1453, 2018.
4. Baker, W.K., Position-effect variegation, *Adv. Genet.* 14, 133–169, 1968.
5. Henikoff, S., Position-effect variegation after 60 years, *Trends Genet.* 6, 422–426, 1990.
6. Shotta, G., Ebert, A., Dorn, R., and Reuter, G., Position-effect variegation and the genetic dissection of chromatin regulation in *Drosophila*, *Semin. Cell Dev. Biol.* 14, 67–75, 2003.
7. Elgin, S.C., and Reuter, G., Position-effect variegation, heterochromatin formation, and gene silencing in *Drosophila*, *Cold SpringHarb. Perspect. Biol.* 5(8), a017780, 2013.
8. Timms, R.T., Tchasovnikarova, I.A., and Lehner, P.J., Position-effect variegation revisited: HUSHing up heterochromatin in human cells, *Bioessays* 38, 333–343, 2016.
9. Mueller, E., Understanding the variegation of fat: Novel regulators of adipocyte differentiation and fat tissue biology, *Biochim. Biophys. Acta* 1842, 352–357, 2014.

V(D)J RECOMBINATION

V(D)J recombination is the process by which three discontinuous regions, V (variable gene segment), D (diversity segment), and J (joining segment), of DNA become joined to encode the variable region of immunoglobulins.[1–3] This is the genetic process which is responsible for the diversity of immunoglobulins.[4–14]

1. Ravetch, J.V., Siebenlist, U., Korsmeyer, S., Waldmann, T., and Leder, P., Structure of the human immunoglobulin μ locus: Characterization of embryonic and rearranged J and D genes, *Cell* 27, 583–591, 1981.
2. Rocca-Serra, J., Matthes, H.W., Kaartinen, M., et al., Analysis of antibody diversity: V-D-J mRNA nucleotide sequence of four anti-GAT monoclonal antibodies. A paucigene system using alternate D-J recombinations to generate functionally similar hypervariable regions, *EMBO J.* 2, 867–872, 1983.
3. Alt, F.W., and Baltimore, D., Joining of immunoglobulin heavy chain gene segments: Implications from a chromosome with evidence of three D-J$_H$ fusions, *Proc. Natl. Acad. Sci. USA* 79, 4118–4122, 1982.
4. Alt, F.W., Oltz, E.M., Young, F., Gorman, J., Taccioli, G., and Chen, J., VDJ recombination, *Immunol. Today* 13, 306–314, 1992.
5. Jung, D., and Alt, F.W., Unraveling V(D)J recombination: Insights into gene regulation, *Cell* 116, 299–311, 2004.
6. Schatz, D.G., V(D)J recombination, *Immunol. Rev.* 200, 5–11, 2004.
7. Dudley, D.D., Chaudhuri, J., Bassing, C.H., and Alt, F.W., Mechanism and control of V(D)J recombination versus class switch recombination: Similarities and differences, *Adv. Immunol.* 86, 43–112, 2005.
8. Jung, D., Giallourakis, C., Mostoslavsky, R., and Alt, F.W., Mechanism and control of V(D)J recombination at the immunoglobulin heavy chain locus, *Annu. Rev. Immunol.* 24, 541–570, 2006.
9. Johnson, K., Chaumeil, J., and Skok, J.A., Epigenetic regulation of V(D)J recombination, *Essays Biochem.* 48, 221–243, 2010.
10. Desiderio, S., Temporal and spatial regulatory functions of the V(D)J recombinase, *Semin. Immunol.* 22, 362–369, 2010.
11. Schazt, D.G., and Swanson, P.C., V(D)J recombination: Mechanisms of initiation, *Annu. Rev. Genet.* 45, 167–202, 2011.
12. Malu, S., Malshetty, V., Francis, D., and Cortes, F., Role of non-homologous end joining in V(D)J recombination, *Immunol. Res.* 54, 233–246, 2012.
13. Proudhon, C., Hao, B., Raviram, R., Chaumeil, J., and Skok, J.A., Long-range regulation of V(D)J recombination, *Adv. Immunol.* 128, 123–182, 2015.
14. Rodgers, K.K., Riches in RAGs: Revealing the V(D)J recombinase through high-resolution structures, *Trends Biochem.* 42, 72–84, 2017.

VGF

Unfortunately VGF has two definitions that are active in the literature. One definition is a small (20 kDa) growth factor encoded by vaccinia virus[1,2] Vaccinia virus growth factor (VGF) is homologous to EGF and binds to EGF receptors.[3] There is some continuing use of the term VGF to describe the peptide growth factor encoded by vaccinia virus.[4,5] The second definition is a 712 amino acid protein encoded by the VGF gene.[6,7] VGF nerve growth factor was first found in PC12 cells and the hypothalmus[8] Expression was found to be regulated by NGF.[8,9]

The VGF nerve growth factor is processed into smaller bioactive peptides with diverse functions.[10,11]

1. Brown, J.P., Twardzik, D.R., Marquardt, H., and Todaro, D.J., Vaccinia virus encodes a polypeptide homologous to epidermal growth factor and transforming growth factor, *Nature* 313, 491–492, 1985.
2. Twardzik, D.R., Brown, J.P., Ranchalis, J.E., Todaro, G.J., and Moss, B., Vaccinia virus-infected cells release a novel polypeptide functionally related to transforming and epidermal growth factors, *Proc. Natl. Acad. Sci. USA* 82, 5300–5304, 1985.
3. Tzahar, E., Moyer, J.D., Waterman, H., et al., Pathogenic poxviruses reveal viral strategies to exploit the ErbB signaling network, *EMBO J.* 17, 5948–5963, 1998.
4. Nguyen, L.T., Yang, X.-Z., Du, X., et al., Enhancing tumor-specific intracellular delivery efficiency of cell-penetrating peptide by fusion with a peptide targeting to EGFR, *Amino Acids* 47, 997–1006, 2015.
5. Beerli, C., Yakimovich, A., Kilcher, S., et al., Vaccinia virus hijacks EGFR signalling to enhance virus spread through rapid and directed infected cell motility, *Nat. Microbiol.* 4, 216–225, 2019.
6. Salton, S.R.J., Fischber, D.J., and Don, K.-W., Structure of the gene encoding VGF, a nervous system-specific mRNA that is rapidly and selectively induced by nerve growth factor in PC12 cells, *Mol. Cell Biol.* 11, 2335–2349, 1991.
7. Hunsberger, J.G., Newton, S.S., Bennett, A.H., et al., Antidepressant actions of the exercise-regulated gene VGF, *Nat. Med.* 12, 1476–1482, 2007.
8. van den Pol, A.N, Decavei, C., Levi, A., and Peterson, B., Hypothalamic expression of a novel gene product, VGF: Immunocytochemical analysis *J. Neurosci.* 9, 4122–4137, 1989.
9. Salton, S.R., Volonté, C., and D'Ancangelo, C., Stimulation of vgf gene expression by NGF is mediated through multiple signal transduction pathways involving protein phosphorylation, *FEBS Lett.* 360, 106–110, 1995.
10. Ferri, G.L., Noli, B., Brancia, C., D'Amato, F., and Cocco, C., VGF: An inducible gene product, precursor of a diverse array of neuro-endocrine peptides and tissue-specific biomarkers, *J. Chem. Neuroanat.* 42, 249–261, 2011.
11. Lewis, J.E., Brameld, J.M., and Jethwa, P.H., Neuroendocrine role for VGF, *Front. Endocrinol.* (Lausanne) 6, 3, 2015.

VICKZ PROTEINS

VICKZ (Vg1 RBP/Vera, IMP-1,2,3, CRD-BP, KOC, ZBP1) is an acronym which was advanced to describe RNA binding proteins recognizing specific *cis*-acting elements acting on a variety of transcriptional processes involved in cell polarity and migration.[1–3] This term has seen little use in the broader literature. It is noted that zipcode binding protein-1 (ZBP-1) is included this family. Zipcode binding proteins are RNA-binding proteins which recognize a specific sequence in mRNA and assist is the localization of the mRNA to a specific subcellular compartment.[4–8]

1. Yisraeli, J.K., VICKZ proteins: A multi-talented family of regulatory RNA-binding proteins, *Biol. Chem.* 97, 87–96, 2005.
2. Oberman, F., Rand, K., Maizels, Y., Rubenstein, A.M., and Yisraeli, J.K., VICKZ proteins mediate cell migration via their RNA binding activity, *RNA* 13, 1558–1569, 2007.
3. Carmel, M.S., Kahane, N., Oberman, F., et al., A novel role for VICKZ proteins in maintaining epithelial integrity during embryogenesis, *PLoS One* 10(8), e0136408, 2015.
4. Kislauskis, E.H., Zhu, X., and Singer, R.H., Sequences responsible for intracellular localization of β-actin messenger RNA also affect cell phenotype, *J. Cell Biol.* 127, 441–451, 1994.
5. Ross, A.F, Oleynikov, Y., Kislausis, E.H., Taneja, K.L., and Singer, R.H., Characterization of a β-actin mRNA zipcode-binding protein, *Mol. Cell. Biol.* 17, 2158–2165, 1997.
6. Patel, V.L., Mitra, S., Harris, R., et al., Spatial arrangement of an RNA zipcode identifies mRNAs under post-translational control, *Genes* 26, 43–53, 2012.
7. Doyle, M., and Kiebler, M.A., A zipcode unzipped, *Genes Dev.* 26, 110–113, 2012.
8. Gallagher, C., and Ramos, A., Joining the dots—Protein-RNA interactions mediating local mRNA translation in neurons, *FEBS Lett.* 592, 2932–2947, 2018.

VIRULENCE FACTORS

Virulence can be defined as the ability of a bacterium to cause infection. In the case of language, virulence is the quality of being acrimonious or bitter. Virulence factors are those diverse materials that enable a bacteria or other pathogen such as a fungus to be infective in a host organism. This can include substances or systems which mediate bacterial adherence, cell motility, cell-to-cell communications, expression of toxins.[1] In other words, those factors which initiate and maintain an infection within a host organism.[1] Virulence factors also support the survival of the pathogen in the organism. It is necessary to an pathogen to maintain a certain density in the host organism through a process described as quorum-sensing.[2] Quorum-sensing is a cell-to-cell communication system for the determination of critical cell density for the expression of virulence factors and is a therapeutic target[3] Virulence factors are diverse including endotoxins,[4] exotoxins,[5] adhesins,[6] and the formation of biofilm.[7] Endotoxins are substances such as lipopolysaccharide (LPS) from gram-negative bacteria.[8] Exotoxins act on the cell surfaces (cytotoxins) forming pores in the host cell membrane.[9] Adhesins are bacterial surface components that mediate adherence of bacterial to eukaryotic cell surfaces by binding extracellular matrix proteins such as collagen and fibronectin. Biofilm formation is necessary for enable bacteria survival, especially on implanted devices.[10] The expression of virulence factors is regulated by virulence activated gene (*vag*).[11] Many virulence factors are two-component systems consists of a membrane-associated sensor protein and cytoplasmic transcription activation. An example if the type III secretion system.[12]

1. *Structural Biology of Bacterial Pathogens*, ed. G. Waksman, M. Caperon, and S. Hultgren, ASM Press, Washington, DC, 2005.
2. Whiteley, M., Diggle, S.P., and Greenberg, E.P., Progress in and promise of bacterial quorum sensing research, *Nature* 551, 313–320, 2017.
3. Rémy, B., Mion, S., Plener, L., et al., Interference in bacterial quorum sensing: A biopharmaceutical perspective, *Front. Pharmacol.* 9, 203, 2018.
4. Bishop, R.E., Fundamentals of endotoxin structure and function, in *Concepts in Bacterial Virulence*, ed. W. Russell and H. Herwald, pp. 1–27, Karger, Basel, Switzerland, 2005.
5. Popoff, M.R., Bacterial exotoxins, *Concepts in Bacterial Virulence*, ed. W. Russell and H. Herwald, pp. 28–54, Karger, Basel, Switzerland, 2005.
6. Talay, S.R., Gram-positive adhesins, *Concepts in Bacterial Virulence*, ed. W. Russell and H. Herwald, pp. 90–119, Karger, Basel, Switzerland, 2005.
7. Reisner, A., Høiby, N., Tolker-Neilsen, T., and Molin, S., Microbial pathogenesis and biofilm development, *Concepts in Bacterial Virulence*, ed. W. Russell and H. Herwald, pp. 114–131, Karger, Basel, Switzerland, 2005.
8. O'Donoghue, E.J., Sirisaengtaksin, N., Browning, D.F., et al., Lipopolysaccharide structure impacts the entry kinetics of bacterial outer membrane vesicles into host cells, *PLoS Pathog.* 13(11), e1006760, 2017.
9. Alonzo, F., 3rd and Torres, V.J. The bicomponent pore-forming leucocidins of *Staphylococcus aureus*, *Microbiol. Mo. Biol. Rev.* 78, 199–230, 2014.
10. Dordan, R.M., and Costerten, J.W., Biofilms: Survival mechanisms of clinically relevant microorganisms, *Clin. Microbiol. Rev.* 15, 167–193, 2002.
11. Locht, C., Lereclos, D., Rood, J.I., and Fourner, B., Regulatory systems of toxin expression, in *The Comprehensive Source Book of Bacterial Toxins*, 3rd edn., ed. J.E. Alouf and M.R. Popoff, Chapter 4, pp. 64–82, Elsevier, Academic Press, Amsterdam, the Netherlands, 2006.
12. Stebbins, C.E., Type III secretion machinery and effectors, in *Structural Biology of Bacterial Pathogenesis*, ed. G. Waksman, M. Caperon, and S. Holtgren, Chapter 9, pp. 149–177, ASM Press, Washington, DC, 2005.

VISCOSITY

Viscosity is defined as the property of a fluid indicating resistance to change in form or resistance to flow. Viscosity has also been defined as internal friction.[1] Viscid is a related concept defining a substance with glutinous or gluey characteristics. Inviscid is the quality of not being viscid while fluidity is the quality of not being viscous. The measurement of viscosity (intrinsic viscosity) is an important quantity in determining the shape of a protein.[2] In general, intrinsic viscosity is sensitive to asymmetry of a protein (or other macromolecules).[3,4] Solvent viscosity is important in protein folding[5–7] and can influence enzyme kinetics.[8–10] DNA solutions can be quite viscous[11,12] presenting problems for nucleic acid drug delivery.[13] The viscosity of DNA is an important factor purulent exudates[14] and DNAse may be a therapeutic factor in resolving abscesses.[15] There is considerable interest in the viscosity of blood as its related to cardiovascular disease.[16–19]

1. Ockendon, H., and Ockendon, J.R., *Viscous Flow*, Cambridge University Press, Cambridge, UK, 1995.
2. Kyte, J., *Structure in Protein Chemistry*, 2nd edn., pp. 578–579, Chapter 12, Physical Measurement of Structure, pp. 573–657, Garland Science/Taylor & Francis, New York, 2007.
3. Hall, C.G., and Abraham, G.N., Size, shape, and hydration of a self-associating IgG myeloma protein: Axial asymmetry as a contributing factor in serum hyperviscosity, *Arch. Biochem. Biophys.* 233, 330–337, 1984.
4. Pindros, M.A., Cole, J.L., Kaur, J., et al., Effect of aggregation on the hydrodynamic properties of bovine serum albumin, *Pharm. Res.* 34, 2250–2259, 2017.
5. Klimov, D.K., and Thirumala, D., Viscosity dependence of folding rates of proteins, *Phys. Rev. Letters* 79, 317–320, 1997.
6. Rhee, Y.M., and Pande, Y.S., Solvent viscosity dependence of protein folding dynamics, *J. Phys. Chem. B* 112, 6221–6227, 2008.
7. Hagen, S.J., Solvent viscosity and friction in protein folding dynamics, *Curr. Protein Pept. Sci.* 11, 385–395, 2010.
8. Kurz, L.C., Weitkamp, E., and Frieden, C., Adenosine deaminase: Viscosity studies and the mechanism of binding of substrate and of ground- and transition-state analogue inhibitors, *Biochemistry* 26, 3027–3032, 1987.
9. Sashi, P., and Bhuyan, A.K., Viscosity dependence of some protein and enzyme reaction rates: Seventy-five years after Kramers, *Biochemistry* 54, 4453–5561, 2015.

10. Machado, T.E.G., Gloster, T.M., and da Silva, R.G., Linear eyring plots conceal a change in the rate-limiting step in enzyme reaction, *Biochemistry* 57, 6757–6761, 2018.

11. Creeth, J.M., Gulland, J.M., and Jordan, D.O., Deoxypentose nucleic acids. Part III. Viscosity and streaming birefringence of solutions of the sodium salt of deoxypentose nucleic acid of calf thymus, *J. Chem. Soc.* 25, 1141–1145, 1947.

12. Laesecke, A., and Burger, J.L., Viscosity measurements of DNA solutions with and without condensing agents, *Biorheology* 51, 15–28, 2014.

13. Elkin, I., Weight, A.K., and Klibanov, A.M., Markedly lowering the viscosity of aqueous solutions of DNA by additives, *Int. J. Pharm.* 494, 66–72, 2015.

14. Sherry, S., and Goeller, J.P., The extent of the enzymatic degradation of desooxyribonucleic acid (DNA) in purulent exudates by streptodornase, *J. Clin. Invest.* 29, 1588–1594, 1950.

15. Ayvazian, J.H., Johnson, A.J., and Tillett, W.S., The use of parenterally administered pancreatic desoxyribonuclease as an adjunct in the treatment of pulmonary abscesses, *Am. Rev. Tuber.* 76, 1–21, 1957.

16. Somer, T., and Meiselman, H.J., Disorders of blood viscosity, *Ann. Med.* 25, 31–39, 1993.

17. Woodward, M., Rumley, A., Tunstall-Pedoe, H., and Lowe, G.D., Does sticky blood predict a sticky end? Associations of blood viscosity, haematocrit and fibrinogen with mortality in the west of Scotland, *Br. J. Haematol.* 122, 645–650, 2003.

18. Ulker, P., Alexy, T., Meiselman, H.J., and Baskurt, O.K., Estimation of infused dextran plasma concentration via measurement of plasma viscosity, *Biorheology* 43, 161–166, 2006.

19. Peters, S.A., Woodward, M., Rumley, A., Tunstall-Bedoe, H.D., and Lowe, G.D., Plasma and blood viscosity in the prediction of cardiovascular disease and mortality in the Scottish Heart Health Extended Cohort Study, *Eur. J. Prev. Cardiol.* 24, 161–167, 2017.

VITAMERS

The term vitamer refers to different chemical structural forms of a vitamin which have similar biological activity.[1–6]

1. Bender, D.A., *Nutritional Biochemistry of the Vitamins*, 2nd Edn., Cambridge University Press, Cambridge, UK, 2003.

2. Voziyan, P.A., and Hudson, B.G., Pyridoxamine. The many virtues of a Maillard reaction inhibitor, *Ann. N.Y. Acad. Sci.* 1043, 807–816, 2005.

3. Smulders, Y.M., Smith, D.E., Kok, R.M., et al., Red blood cell folate vitamer distribution in healthy subjects is determined by the methylenetetrahydrofolate reductase C677T polymorphism and by total folate status, *J. Nutri. Biochem.* 18, 693–699, 2007.

4. Clement, L., Boylan, M., Miller, V., et al., Vitamin B-6 vitamer levels in plasma and related symptoms in hemodialysis subjects taking low- and high-dose renal multivitamin supplements, *Int. J. Vitam. Nutr. Res.* 82, 130–136, 2012.

5. Justiniano, R., Williams, J.D., Perer, J., et al., The B$_6$-vitamer pyridoxal is a sensitizer of UVA-induced genotoxic stress in human primary keratinocytes and reconstructed epidermis, *Photochem. Photobiol.* 93, 990–998, 2017.

6. Loohuis, L.M., Albersen, M., de Jong, S., et al., The alkaline phosphatase (ALPL) locus is associated with B6 vitamer levels in CSF and plasma, *Genes*(Basel) 10(1), E8, 2018.

WALKER A MOTIF AND WALKER B MOTIF

The Walker A motif and Walker B motif were first described as ATP binding sequences in a number of ATP-requiring proteins consisting of a common fold in proteins for nucleotide binding.[1] It was later suggested that phosphate-binding loop (P-loop) in the Walker A domain[2–4] is an essential component in nucleotide binding proteins.[5] A cursory consideration of the literature suggests that both P-loop and Walker A domain are used to describe the conserved sequence first described by Walker and colleagues in 1982.[1] The Walker B motif has been suggested to be important in the hydrolysis of nucleotide triphosphate.[6–10]

1. Walker, J.E., Saraste, M., Runswick, M.J., and Gay, N.J., Distantly related sequences in the α- and β-subunits of ATP synthase, myosin, kinases, and other ATP-requiring enzymes and a common nucleotide binding fold, *EMBO J.* 1, 945–951, 1982.

2. Saraste, M., Sibbald, P.R., and Wittinghofer, A., The P-loop—A common motif in ATP- and GTP-binding proteins, *Trends Biochem. Sci.*15, 430–434, 1990.

3. Kinoshita, K., Sadenami, K., Kidera, A., and Go, N., Structural motif of phosphate-binding site common to various protein superfamilies: All-against-all structural comparison of protein-mononucleotide complexes, *Protein Engineer.* 12, 11–14, 1999.

4. Johnson, E.R., and McKay, D.B., Crystallographic structure of the amino terminal domain of yeast initiation factor 4A, a representative DEAD-box RNA helicase, *RNA* 5, 1526–1534, 1999.

5. Romero Romero, M.L., Yang, F., Lin, Y.R., et al., Simple yet functional phosphate-loop proteins, *Proc. Natl. Acad. Sci. USA* 115, E11943–E11950, 2018.

6. Sauna, Z.E., Müller, M., Peng, X.-H., and Ambudkar, S.V, Importance of the conserved Walker B glutamate residues, 556 and 1201, for the completion of the catalytic cycle of ATP hydrolysis by human P-glycoprotein (ABCB1), *Biochemistry* 41, 13989–14000, 2002.

7. Darbari, V.C., Lawton, E., Lu, D., et al., Molecular basis of nucleotide-dependent substrate engagement and remodeling by an AAA+ activator, *Nucleic Acids Res.* 42, 9249–9261, 2014.
8. Qiu, W., Liesa, M., Carpenter, E.P., and Shirihai, O.S., ATP binding and hydrolysis properties of ABC10 and their regulation by glutathione, *PLoS One* 10(6), e0129772, 2015.
9. Chen, L., and Duan, K., A PhoPQ-regulated ABC transporter system exports tetracycline in *Pseudomonas aeruginosa*, *Antimicrob. Agents Chemother.* 60, 3016–3024, 2016.
10. Hsu, W.L., Furuta, T., and Sakurai, M., ATP hydrolysis mechanism in a maltose transporter explored by QM/MM metadynamics simulation, *J. Phys. Chem. B* 120, 11102–11112, 2016.

WESTERN BLOTTING

Western blotting is a method for identifying proteins after electrophoretic separation by use of labeled antibody.[1–5] While the name Southern blotting, the signature blotting procedure, is based on the proper name of a distinguished scientist, the geographical connotation was established. Thus, western blotting followed the earlier development of Southern blotting (identification of a specific DNA sequence on electrophoresis by hybridization with a complementary labeled DNA) and Northern Blotting (identification of a specific RNA sequence on electrophoresis by hybridization with complementary labeled DNA). Technology for western blotting continues to develop.[6–9] As noted above, Southern blotting is derived from proper names and thus it is appropriate to capitalize. There is no need to capitalize western but there does not appear to consistent editorial consensus on this matter. See also **Southwestern blotting** and **Northwestern blot**.

1. Burnette, W.N., "Western blotting": Electrophoretic transfer of proteins from sodium dodecyl sulfate—polyacrylamide gels to unmodified nitrocellulose and radiographic detection with antibody and radioiodinated protein A, *Anal. Biochem.* 112, 195–203, 1981.
2. Burnette, W.N., Western blotting: Remembrance of things past, *Methods Mol. Biol.* 1312, 9–12, 2015.
3. Harper, D.R., Kit, M.L., and Kangrok H.O., Protein blotting: Ten years on, *J. Virol. Methods* 30, 25–39, 1990.
4. Baldo, B.A., and Tovey, E.R., *Protein Blotting: Methodology, Research, and Diagnostic Applications,* Karger, Baldo Basel, 1989.
5. Dunbar, B.S., *Protein Blotting: A Practical Approach,* IRL Press at Oxford, Oxford, UK, 1994.
6. Algenäs, C., Agaton, C., and Fagerberg, L., et al., Antibody performance in western blot applications in context-dependent, *Biotechnol. J.* 9, 435–445, 2014.
7. Gorr, T.A., and Vogel, J., Western blotting revisited: Critical perusal of unappreciated technical issues, *Proteomics Clin. Appl.* 9, 396–405, 2015.
8. Mishra, M., Tiwari, S., and Gomes, A.V., Protein purification and analysis: Next generation Western blotting techniques, *Expert Rev. Proteomics* 14, 1037–1053, 2017.
9. Bass, J.J., Wilkinson, D.F., Rankin, D., et al., An overview of technical considerations for Western blotting applications to physiological research, *Scand. J. Med. Sci. Sports* 27, 4–25, 2017.

WORMBASE

A public database for the genomics biology of *Caenorhabditis elegans* (a soil-dwelling nematode used extensively in biological research).[1–7]

1. Chen, N., Harris, T.W., Antoschechkin, I., et al., WormBase: A comprehensive data resource for *Caenorhabditis* biology and genomics, *Nucleic Acids Res.* 33, D383–D389, 2005.
2. O'Connell, K., There's no place like WormBase: An indispensable resource for *Caenorhabditis elegans* researchers, *Biol. Cell.* 97, 867–872, 2005.
3. Schwarz, E.M., Antoschechkin, I., Bastiani, C., et al., WormBase: Better software, richer content, *Nucleic Acids Res.* 34, D475–D478, 2006.
4. Harris, T.W., Baran, J., Bieri, T., et al., Wormbase 2014: New views of curated biology, *Nucleic Acids Res.* 42(database issue), D789–D793, 2014.
5. Howe, K.L., Bolt, B.J., Cain, S., et al., Wormbase 2016: Expanding to enable helminth genomic research, *Nucleic Acids Res.* 44(DI), D774–D780, 2016.
6. Lee, R.Y.N., Howe, K.L, Harris, T.W., et al., Wormbase 2017: Molting into a new stage, *Nucleic Acids Res.* 46(DI), D869–D874, 2018.
7. Grove, C., Cain, S., Chen, W.J., et al., Using Wormbase: A genome biology resource for *Caenorhhadbditis elegans* and related nematodes, *Methods Mol. Biol.* 1757, 399–470, 2018.

XENOBIOTIC

A xenobiotic is a chemical or substance that is not a normal product of an organism.[1] Benzene is an example of a xenobiotic compound.[2–4] Drugs are xenobiotic compounds but frequently discussed as separate categories of chemical compounds.[5,6] There are a variety of metabolic pathways for the metabolism/detoxification of xenobiotic compounds including drugs.[7–14] One major pathways is the formation of bioconjugates.[15–19] Xenobiotic compounds can form conjugates with proteins[20] which be immunogenic based on xenobiotic compounds acting as haptens.[21–24] There has been continuing interest in the metabolism of xenobiotics by the gut microbiota.[25–28]

1. Connell, D.W., *Bioaccumulation of Xenobiotic Compounds*, CRC Press/Taylor & Francis, Boca Raton, FL, 2018.
2. Snyder, R., Xenobiotic metabolism and the mechanism(s) of benzene toxicity, *Drug. Metab. Rev.* 36, 531–547, 2004.
3. Manini, P., De Palma, G., Andreoli, R., *et a.,* Occupational exposure to low levels of benzene: Biomarkers of exposure and nucleic acid oxidation and their modulation by polymorphic xenobiotic metabolism enzymes, *Toxicol. Lett.* 193, 229–235, 2010.
4. Renaud, H.J., Rutter, A., and Winn, L.M., Assessment of xenobiotic biotransformation including reactive oxygen species generation in the embryo using benzene as an example, *Methods Mol. Bio.* 889, 253–263, 2012.
5. Foti, R.S., and Dalvie, D.K., Cytochrome P450 and non-cytochrome P450 oxidative metabolism: Contributions of the pharmacokinetics, safety, and efficiency of xenobiotics, *Drug Metab. Dispos.* 44, 1229–1245, 2016.
6. Mackowiak, B., Hodge, J., Stern, S., and Wang, H., The roles of xenobiotic receptors: Beyond chemical composition, *Drug Metab. Dispos.* 46, 1361–1371, 2018.
7. Garattini S., Notes on xenobiotic metabolism, *Ann. N.Y. Acad. Sci.* 407, 1–25, 1983.
8. Glatt, H., Gemperlein, I., Turchi, G., et al., Search for cell culture systems with diverse xenobiotic-metabolizing activities and their use in toxicological studies, *Mol. Toxicol.* 1, 313–334, 1987–1988.
9. *Cytochromes P450: Metabolic and Toxicological Aspects*, ed. C. Ioannides, CRC Press, Boca Raton, FL, 1996.
10. *Enzyme Systems that Metabolize Drugs and Other Xenobiotics*, ed. C. Iaonnides, John Wiley & Sons, Chichester, UK, 2002.
11. *Cytochrome P450: Role in the Metabolism and Toxicity of Drugs and Other Xenobiotics*, ed. C. Iaonnides, RSC Publishing, Cambridge, UK, 2008.
12. *Biotransformation and Metabolite Elucidation of Xenobiotics*, ed. A.F. Nasser, John Wiley & Sons, Hoboken, NJ, 2010.
13. *Metabolism of Drugs and Other Xenobiotics*, ed. P. Anzenbacher and U. Zanger, *Wiley-VCH*, Hoboken, NJ, 2012.
14. *Metabolic Profiling: Disease and Xenobiotics*, ed. M. Grootveld, Royal Society of Chemistry, Cambridge, UK, 2015.
15. Paulson, G.D., Lamoureux, G.L., and Feil, V.J., Advances in methods and techniques for the identification of xenobiotic conjugates, *J. Toxicol. Clin. Toxicol.* 19, 571–608, 1982.
16. Mitchell, S.C., Xenobiotic-urea conjugates: Chemical or biological? *Xenobiotica* 44, 1055–1066, 2014.
17. Darnell, M., Breitholtz, K., Isin, E.M., Jurva, U., and Weidolf, L., Significantly different covalent binding of oxidative metabolites, acyl glucuronides, and S-acyl CoA conjugates formed from xenobiotic carboxylic acids in human liver microsomes, *Chem. Res. Toxicol.* 28, 886–896, 2015.
18. Linhart, I., Himl, M., Židková, M., et al., Metabolic profile of mephedrone: Identification of nor-mephedrone conjugates with dicarboxylic acids as a new type of xenobiotic phase II metabolites, *Toxicol. Lett.* 240, 114–121, 2016.
19. Mitchell, S.C., Xenobiotic C-sulfonate derivatives; metabolites or metabolates? *Xenobiotica* 48, 211–218, 2018.
20. Pumford, N.R., Halmes, N.C., and Hinson, J.A., Covalent binding of xenobiotics to specific proteins in the liver, *Drug. Metabolism Rev.* 29, 39–57, 1997.
21. Griem, P., Wulferink, M., Sachs, B., González, J.B., and Gleichmann, E., Allergic and autoimmune reactions to xenobiotics: How do they arise? *Immunology Today* 19, 133–141, 1998.
22. Roychowdhury, S., Vyas, P.M., and Svensson, C.K., Formation and uptake of arylhydroxylamine-haptenated proteins in human dendritic cells, *Drug Metab. Dispos.* 35, 676–681, 2007.
23. Megherbi, R., Kiorpelidou, E., Foster, B., et al., Role of protein haptenation in triggering maturation events in the dendritic cell surrogate cell line THP-1, *Toxicol. Appl. Pharmacol.* 238, 120–132, 2009.
24. Vojdani, A., Kharrazian, D., and Mukerjee, P.S., Elevated levels of antibodies against xenobiotics in a subgroup of healthy subjects, *J. Appl. Toxicol.* 35, 383–397, 2015.
25. Hänninen, O., Mucosal transformation of toxins in the gut, *Arch. Toxicol.* Suppl 8, 83–86, 1985.
26. Rowland, I.R., Factors affecting metabolic activity of the intestinal microflora, *Drug. Metab. Rev.* 19, 243–261, 1988.
27. Das, A., Srinivasan, M., Ghosh, T.S., and Mande, S.S., Xenobiotic metabolism and gut microbiomes, *PLoS One* 11(10), E0163099, 2016.
28. Koppel, N., Maini Rekdal, V., and Balskus, E.P., Chemical transformation of xenobiotics by the human gut microbiota, *Science* 356, eaag2770, 2017.

XEROGEL

A xerogel can be defined as hydrogel where water has been removed by drying under ambient conditions, while an aerogel is a hydrogel removed by supercritical drying.[1] A lyogel has been described as a hydrogel which has been lyophilized.[2] There has been interest in xerogels a drug delivery vehicle.[2–7]

1. Shimizu, T., Kanamori, K., and Nakanishi, K., Silicone-based organic-inorganic hybrid aerogels and xerogels, *Chemistry* 23, 5176–5187, 2017.
2. Guziewicz, N., Best, A., Perez-Ramirez, B., and Kaplan, D.L., Lyophilized fibroin hydrogels for sustain local delivery of therapeutic monoclonal antibodies, *Biomaterials* 32, 2642–2650, 2011.
3. Kortesuo, P., Ahola, M., Karlsson, S., et al., Sol-gel-processed sintered silica xerogel as a carrier in controlled drug delivery, *J. Biomed. Mat. Res.* 44, 162–167, 1999.
4. Xue, J.M., Tan, C.H., and Lukito, D., Biodegradable polymer-silica xerogel composite microspheres for controlled release of gentamicin, *J. Biomed. Mater. Res. B Appl. Biomater.* 78, 417–422, 2006.

5. Rigby, S.P., Fairhead, M., and van der Walle, C.F., Engineering silica particles as oral drug delivery vehicles, *Curr. Pharm. Des.* 6, 1821–1831, 2008.
6. Quintanar-Guerrero, D., Ganem-Quintanar, A., Nava-Arzaluz, M.G., and Piñon-Segundo, E., Silica hydrogels as pharmaceutical drug carriers, *Expert Opin. Drug Deliv.* 6, 485–498, 2009.
7. Iafisco, M., and Margiotta, N., Silica xerogels and hydroxyapatite nanocrystals for the local delivery of platinum-biphosphonate complexes in the treatment of bone tumors: A mini-review, *J. Inorg. Biochem.* 117, 237–247, 2012.

YEAST ARTIFICIAL CHROMOSOMES

Yeast artificial chromosomes (YACs) are yeast DNA sequences which contain large segments of foreign recombinant DNA introduced by transformation. Yeast artificial chromosomes permitted the cloning of large DNA fragments such as genes with flanking regulatory regions.[1-7] While YACs are still useful, other approaches such as bacterial artificial chromosomes,[8] mouse artificial chromosomes,[9] and human artificial chromosomes[10] are proving useful.

1. Schlessinger, D., Yeast artificial chromosomes: Tools for mapping and analysis of complex genomes, *Trends Genet.* 6, 255–258, 1990.
2. Huxley, C., and Gnirke, A., Transfer of yeast artificial chromosomes from yeast to mammalian cells, *Bioessays* 13, 545–550, 1991.
3. Anand, R., Yeast artificial chromosomes (YACs) and the analysis of complex genomes, *Trends Biotechnol.* 10, 35–40, 1992.
4. Huxley, C., Transfer of YACs to mammalian cells and transgenic mice, *Genet. Eng.* 16, 65–91, 1994.
5. Schalkwyk, L.C., Francis, F., and Lehrach, H., Techniques in mammalian genome mapping, *Curr. Opin. Biotechnol.* 6, 37–43, 1995.
6. Kouprina, N., and Larionov, V., Exploiting the yeast *Saccharomyces cerevisiae* for the study of the organization and evolution of complex genomes, *FEMS Microbiol. Rev.* 27, 629–649, 2003.
7. Sasaki, T., Matsumoto, T., Antonio, B.A., and Nagamura, Y., From mapping to sequencing, post-sequencing and beyond, *Plant Cell Physiol.* 46, 3–13, 2005.
8. Zeidler, M.G., and Saunders, T.L., Transgene recombineering in bacterial artificial chromosomes, *Methods Mol. Biol.* 1874, 43–69, 2019.
9. Uno, N., Fujimoto, T., Komoto, S., et al., A luciferase complementation assay system using transferable mouse artificial chromosomes to monitor protein-protein interactions mediated by G protein-coupled receptors, *Cytotechnology* 70, 1499–1508, 2018.
10. Dance, A., Core concept: Human artificial chromosomes offer insights, therapeutic possibilities, and challenges, *Proc. Natl. Acad. Sci. USA* 114, 9752–9754, 2017.

ZEBRAFISH

Zebrafish (*Danio rerio*) is a freshwater fish used for research in developmental biology.[1-15]

1. http://www.ncbi.nlm.nih.gov/genome?term=danio%20 rerio.
2. http://www.uoneuro.uoregon.edu/k12/ZFIN%20 Historical%20FAQs.html.
3. Stemple, D.L., and Driever, W., Zebrafish: Tools for investigating cellular differentiation, *Curr. Opin. Cell. Biol.* 8, 858–864, 1996.
4. Driever, W., Stemple, D., Schier, A., and Solnica-Krezel, L., Zebrafish: Genetic tools for studying vertebrate development, *Trends Genet.* 10, 152–159, 1994.
5. Kimmel, C.B., Genetics and early development of zebrafish, *Trends Genet.* 5, 283–288, 1989.
6. Fulwiler, C., and Gilbert, W., Zebrafish embryology and neural development, *Curr. Opin. Cell Biol.* 3, 989–991, 1991.
7. Ingham, P.W., and Kim, H.R., Hedgehog signaling and the specification of muscle cell identity in the zebrafish embryo, *Exp. Cell Res.* 306, 336–342, 2005.
8. Teh, C., Parinov, S., and Korzh, V., New ways to admire zebrafish: Progress in functional genomics research methodology, *Biotechniques* 38, 897–906, 2005.
9. Amsterdam, A., and Becker, T.S., Transgenes as screening tools to probe and manipulate the zebrafish genome, *Dev. Dyn.* 234, 255–268, 2005.
10. Hsia, N., and Zon, L.I., Transcriptional regulation of hematopoietic stem cell development in zebrafish, *Exp. Hematol.* 33, 1007–1014, 2005.
11. de Jong, J.L., and Zon, L.I., Use of the zebrafish to study primitive and definitive hematopoiesis, *Annu. Rev. Genet.* 39, 481–501, 2005.
12. Alestrom, P., Holter, J.L., Nourizadeh-Lillabadi, R., Zebrafish in functional genomics and aquatic biomedicine, *Trends Biotechnol.* 24, 15–21, 2006.
13. *Zebrafish.* ed. S.F. Perry, M. Ekkey, A.P. Ferrell, and C.J. Brauner, Academic Press/Elsevier, London, UK, 2010.
14. Harper, C., *The Laboratory Zebrafish*, CRC Press, Boca Raton, FL, 2012.
15. Bryson-Richardson, P., *Atlas of Zebrafish Development*, Academic Press/Elsevier, London, UK, 2012.

ZEOLITES

Zeolites are An aluminum silicate cage-like compounds with a negative charge which "captures" cations in the cavity.[1,2] Zeolites are used as molecular sieves for drying solvents and gases.[3,4] There has been some interest in the specific adsorption on biopolymers such as proteins on zeolites.[5-10] There are suggestions for the use of zeolites in health.[11-14]

1. Mumpton, F.A., La roca magica: Uses of natural zeolites in agriculture and industry, *Proc. Natl. Acad. Sci. USA* 96, 3463–3470, 1999.

2. Kaiser, L.G., Meersmann, T., Logan, J.W., and Pines, A., Visualization of gas flow and diffusion in porous media, *Proc. Nat. Acad. Sci. USA* 97, 2414–2418, 2000.
3. Kuznicki, S.M., Bell, V.A., Nair, S., et al., A titanosilicate molecular sieve with adjustable pores for size-selective adsorption of molecules, *Nature* 412, 720–724, 2001.
4. Yan, A.X., Li, X.W., and Ye, Y.H., Recent progress on immobilization of enzymes on molecular sieves for reactions in organic solvents, *Appl. Biochem. Biotechnol.* 101, 113–129, 2002.
5. Matsui, M., Kiyozumi, Y., Yamamoto, T., Selective adsorption of biopolymers on zeolites, *Chemistry* 7, 1555–1560, 2001.
6. Chiku, H., Matsui, M., Murakami, S., et al., Zeolites as new chromatographic carriers for proteins—Easy recovery of proteins adsorbed on zeolites by polyethylene glycol, *Anal. Biochem.* 318, 80–85, 2003.
7. Sakaguchi, K., Matsui, M., and Mizukami, F., Applications of zeolite inorganic composites in biotechnology: Current status and perspectives, *Appl. Microbiol. Biotechnol.* 67, 306–311, 2005.
8. Rahimi, M., Ng, E.P., Bakhtiarik K., et al., Zeolite nanoparticles for selective sorption of plasma proteins, *Sci. Rep.* 5, 17259, 2015.
9. Liu, G., Xu, Y., Han, Y., et al., Immobilization of lysozyme proteins on a hiercarrchial zeolitic imidazolate framework (ZIF-8), *Dalton Trans.* 46, 2114–2121, 2017.
10. Zhao, M., Zie, Y., Chen, H., and Deng, C., Efficient extraction of low-abundance peptides from digested proteins and simultaneous exclusion of large-sized proteins with novel hydrophilic magnetic zeolite imidazolate frameworks, *Talenta* 167, 392–397, 2017.
11. Pavelic, K., Hadzija, M., Bedrica, L., Natural zeolite clinoptilolite: New adjuvant in anticancer therapy, *J. Mol. Med.* 78, 708–720, 2001.
12. Zarkovic, N., Zarkovic, K., Kralj, M., et al., Anticancer and antioxidative effects of micronized zeolite clinoptilolite, *Anticancer Res.* 23, 159–1595, 2003.
13. Khodaverdi, E., Soleimani, H.A., Mohammadpour, F., and Hadizadeh, F., Synthetic zeolites as controlled-release delivery systems for anti-inflammatory drugs, *Chem. Biol. Drug Des.* 87, 849–857, 2016.
14. Yang, K., Yang, K., Chao, S., et al., A supramolecular hybrid material constructed from pillar[6]arene-based host-guest complexation and ZIF-8 for targeted drug delivery, *Chem. Commun.* (Camb) 54, 9817–9820, 2018.

ZINC FINGER MOTIFS

Zinc-finger motifs are regions in DNA- and RNA-binding proteins whose amino acids are folded into a single structural unit around a zinc atom.[1-7] In the classic zinc finger, one zinc atom is bound to two cysteines and two histidines. In between the cysteines and histidines are 12 residues which form a DNA binding fingertip. By variations in the composition of the sequences in the fingertip and the number and spacing of tandem repeats of the motif, zinc fingers can form a large number of different sequence specific binding sites. Specificity of binding to the nucleic acid is achieved by recognition of an 18 bp sequence. The binding of arsenic to zinc finger motifs is of interest for therapeutic applications.[8,9]

1. Schleif, R., DNA binding by proteins, *Science* 241, 1182–1187, 1988.
2. Struhl, K., Helix-turn-helix, zinc-finger, and leucine-zipper motifs for eukaryotic transcriptional regulatory proteins, *Trends Biochem. Sci.* 14, 137–140, 1989.
3. Bergqvist, A., Nilsson, M., Bondeson, K., and Magnusson G., Loss of DNA-binding and new transcriptional trans-activation function in polyomavirus large T-antigen with mutation of zinc finger motif, *Nucleic Acids Res.* 18, 2715–1720, 1990.
4. Summers, M.F., Zinc finger motif for single-stranded nucleic acids? Investigations by nuclear magnetic resonance, *J. Cell. Biochem.* 45, 41–48, 1991.
5. Kochoyan, M., Keutmann, H.T., and Weiss, M.A., Architectural rules of the zinc-finger motif: Comparative two-dimensional NMR studies of native and "aromatic-swap" domains define a "weakly polar switch." *Proc. Natl. Acad. Sci. USA* 88, 8455–8459, 1991.
6. Chen, Y., and Varani, G., Protein families and RNA recognition, *FEBS J.* 272, 2088–2097, 2005.
7. Lin, C.Y., and Lin, L.Y., The conserved basic residues and the charged amino acid residues at the α-helix of the zinc finger motif regulate the nuclear transport activity of triple C_2H_2 zinc finger proteins, *PLoS One* 13(1), e0191971, 2018.
8. Chen, S.J., Zhou, G.B., Zhang, X.W., et al., From an old remedy to a magic bullet: Molecular mechanisms underlying the therapeutic effects of arsenic in fighting leukemia, *Blood* 117, 6425–6437, 2011.
9. Liu, J.X., Zhou, G.B., Chen, S.J., and Chen, Z., Arsenic compounds: Revisited ancient remedies in the fight against human malignancies, *Curr. Opin. Chem. Biol.* 16, 92–98, 2012.

ZINC FINGER NUCLEASES

Zinc finger nucleases are engineered nucleases which consist of a zinc finger domain or domains fused to the nuclease domain from Fok1 restriction endonuclease. This nuclease domain is non-specific such that the sequence specificity cleavage of the zinc finger nucleases is provided from the zinc finger domain(s).[1-4] There is considerable interest in the use of zinc finger nucleases in gene editing.[5-11]

1. Kim, Y.G., Cha, J., and Chandrasegaran, S., Hybrid restriction enzymes: Zinc finger fusions to Fok I cleavage domain, *Proc. Natl. Acad. Sci. USA* 93, 1156–1160, 1996.

2. Chandrasegaran, S., and Smith, J., Chimeric restriction enzymes: What is next? *Biol. Chem.* 380, 841–848, 1999.
3. Smith, J., Bibikova, M., Whitby, F.G., and Reddy, A.R., Chandrasegaran, S., and Carroll, D., Requirements for double-strand cleavage by chimeric restriction enzymes with zinc finger DNA-recognition domains, *Nucleic Acids Res.* 28, 3361–3369, 2000.
4. Mani, M., Kandavelou, K., Dy, F.J., Durai, S., and Chardrasegaran, S., Design, engineering, and character-ization of zinc finger nucleases, *Biochem. Biophys. Res. Commun.* 335, 447–457, 2005.
5. Durai, S., Mani, M., Kandavelou, K., Wu, J., Porteus, M.H., and Chandrasegaran, S., Zinc finger nucleases: Custom-designed molecular scissors for genome engi-neering of plant and mammalian cells, *Nucl. Acid Res.* 26, 5978–5990, 2005.
6. Porteus, M.H., Mammalian gene targeting with designed zinc finger nucleases, *Mol. Ther.* 13, 438–446, 2006.
7. Urnov, F.D., Rebar, E.J., Holmes, M.C., Zhang, H.S., and Gregory, P.D., Genome editing with engineered zinc fin-ger nucleases, *Nat. Rev. Genet.* 11, 636–646, 2010.
8. Wood, A.J., Lo, T.W., Zeitler, B., et al., Targeted genome editing across species using ZFNs and TALENs, *Science* 333, 307, 2011.
9. Davies, J.P., Kumar, S., and Sastry-Dent, L., Use of zinc-finger nuclease for crop improvement, *Prog. Mol. Biol. Transl. Sci.* 149, 47–63, 2017.
10. Germini, D., Tsfasman, T., Zakharova, V.V., et al., A com-parison of techniques to evaluate the effectiveness of genome editing, *Trends Biotechnol.* 36, 147–159, 2018.
11. Rui, Y., Wilson, D.R., and Green, J.J., Non-viral deliv-ery to enable genome editing, *Trends Biotechnol.* 37, 381–293, 2019.

ZWITTERION

The term zwitterion is used to describe an electrically neutral (isoelectric) molecule with a positive change and a negative charge.[1,2] A simple example is glycine. Some ampholytes are zwitterions. Many of the Good buffers are zwitterions.[3–5] Zwitterionic ion-exchangers have potential in a variety of applications including hydrophilic interac-tion liquid chromatography (HILIC) and mixed-mode chromatography.[6,7] See also **ampholytes**.

1. Sharp, D.W.A., *Dictionary of Chemistry*, 2nd edn., Penguin Books, London, UK, 1990.
2. Ràfols, S., Subirats, X., Rubio, J., Roses, M., and Bosch, E., Lipophilicity of amphoteric and zwitterionic com-pounds: A comparative study of determination methods, *Talenta* 162, 293–299, 2017.
3. Long, R.D., Hilliard, N.P., Chhatre, S.A., et al., Com-parison of zwitterionic N-alkylaminomethanesulfonic acids to related compounds in the Good buffer series, *Beilstein J. Org. Chem.* 6, 31, 2010.

4. Koerner, M.M., Palacio, L.A., Writght, J.W., et al., Electrodynamics of lipid membrane interactions in the presence of zwitterionic buffers, *Biophys. J.* 101, 362–369, 2011.
5. Xu, X., Gevaert, B., Bracke, N., Yao, H., and Wynendaele, E., Hydrophilic interaction liquid chromatography method development and validation for the assay of HEPES zwitterionic buffer, *J. Pharm. Biomed. Anal.* 135, 227–232, 2017.
6. Kazarian, A.A., Taylor, M.R., Haddad, P.R., Nesterenko, P.N., and Pauli, B., Ion-exchange and hydrophobic inter-actions affecting selectivity for neutral and changed solutes on three structurally similar agglomerated ion-exchange and mixed-mode stationary phases, *Anal. Chim. Acta* 803, 143–153, 2013.
7. Bo, C., Wang, X., Wang, C., and Wei, Y., Preparation of hydrophilic interaction/ion-exchange mixed-mode chro-matographic stationary phase with adjustable selectiv-ity by controlling different ratios of the co-monomers, *J. Chromatog. A.* 1487, 201–210, 2017.

ZYMOGENICITY

Zymogenicity is the ratio of the activity of an active enzyme to that of the zymogen or precursor form ($A_{enzyme}/A_{zymogen}$). The term zymogenicity was first used to describe the latent state of chitin synthase in a variety of fungi and yeasts.[1] There has been some recent work on modulating the zymogenicity of tPA[2] and factor X[3] where the goal is an improved therapeutic product. The zymo-genicity of native tPA is approximately 6.7[4] which can be increased by protein engineering to greater than 100.[3] Assuming that reactivity with DFP is a reasonable assess-ment of active-site function, the zymogenicity of trypsin is on the order of 10^3 while that of chymotrypsin is on the order of 10^5. The term zymogenicity has also been used to refer to the zymogen state of other proteolytic enzymes.[6,7]

1. Gozalbo, D., Dubón, F., and Sentandreu, R., Studies on zymogenicity and solubilization of chitin synthase from *Candida albicans, Microbiol. Lett.* 26, 59–63, 1985.
2. Ivanciu, L., and Camire, R.M., Hemostatic agents of broad applicability produced by selective tuning of factor Xa zymogenicity, *Blood* 126, 94–102, 2015.
3. Tachias, K., and Madison, E.L., Converting tissue type plasminogen activator into a zymogen. Important role of Lys165, *J. Biol. Chem.* 272, 28–31, 1997.
4. Tachias, K., and Madison, E.L., Converting tissue-type plasminogen activator into a zymogen, *J. Biol. Chem.* 271, 28749–28752, 1998.
5. Neurath, H., Limited proteolysis and zymogen activa-tion, in *Proteases and Biological Control.*, ed. E. Reich, D.B. Rifkin, and E. Shaw, pp. 51–64, Cold Spring Harbor Laboratory Press, Cold Spring Harbor, NY, 1975.

6. Dall, E., and Brandstetter, H., Mechanistic and structural studies on legumain explain its zymogenicity, distinct activation pathways, and regulation, *Proc. Natl. Acad. Sci. USA* 110, 10940–10945, 2013.
7. Ponowski, A., Uson, I., Novakowska, Z., et al., Structural insights unravel the zymogenic mechanism of the virulence factor gingipain K from *Porphyromonas gingivalis*, a causative agent of gum disease from the human oral microbiome, *J. Biol. Chem.* 292, 5724–2735, 2017.

ZYMOGRAPHY

Zymography is a qualitative (usually) method for detecting enzyme activity on a matrix, usually a polyacrylamide gel or agarose gel after electrophoretic separation.[1–7] The electrophoretic separation is usually performed under native conditions.

1. Frederiks, W.M., and Mook, O.R., Metabolic mapping of proteinase activity with emphasis on in situ zymography of gelatinases: Review and protocols, *J. Histochem. Cytochem.* 52, 711–722, 2004.
2. Lombard, C., Saulnier, J., and Wallach, J., Assays of matrix metalloproteinases (MMPs) activities: A review, *Biochemie* 87, 265–272, 2005.
3. Willesman, J., Hernández, Z., Fernández, M., Contreras, L.M., and Kurz, L., Enhancement of sequential zymography technique for the detection of thermophilic lipases and proteases, *Amino Acids* 46, 1409–1413, 2014.
4. Ricci, S., D'Esposito, V., Oriente, F., Formisano, P., and Di Carlo, A., Subtrate zymography: Still worthwhile method for gelatinase anlaysis in biological samples, *Clin. Chem. Lab. Med.* 54, 1281–1290, 2016.
5. Yasumtisu, H., Ozeki, Y., and Kanaly, R.A., RAMA casein zymography: Time-saving and highly sensitive casein zymography for MMP7 and trypsin, *Electrophoresis* 37, 2959–2962, 2016.
6. Raykin, J., Snider, E., Bheri, S., Mulvihill, J., and Ethier, C.R., A modified gelatin zymography technique incorporating total protein normalization, *Anal. Biochem.* 521, 8–10, 2017.
7. Tajhya, R.B., Patel, R.S., and Beeton, C., Detection of matrix metalloproteinases by zymography, *Methods Mol. Biol.* 1579, 231–244, 2017.

ZYMOSAN

Zymosan is an insoluble polysaccharide (repeating glucose monomers joined by a β-1,3 glycosidic bond) derived from the cell wall of fungi.[1,2] More specifically, the term zymosan can be used to refer to a specific preparation which contains both protein and carbohydrate from yeast which is used in models of inflammatory disease and multi-organ dysfunction.[2] There is evidence for specific interaction with Toll receptors on macrophages.[3–7] Zymosan is used for the production of animal models of inflammation.[8–11]

1. Fitzpatrick, F.W., and DiCarlo, F.J., Zymosan, *Ann. N.Y. Acad. Sci.* 118, 233–262, 1964.
2. Ohno, N., Miura, T., Miura, N.N., Adachi, Y., and Yadomae, T., Structure and biological activities of hypochlorite oxidized zymosan, *Carb. Polymers* 44, 339–349, 2001.
3. Sigma Aldrich, https://www.sigmaaldrich.com/catalog/product/sigma/z4250?lang=en&region=US.
4. Takeuchi, O., and Akira, S., Toll-like receptors: Their physiological role and signal transduction system, *Int. Immunopharmacol.* 1, 625–635, 2001.
5. Levitz, S.M., Interactions of toll-like receptors with fungi, *Microbes Infect.* 6, 1351–1355, 2004.
6. Ikeda, Y., Adachi, Y., Ishibashi, K., Miura, N., and Ohno, N., Activation of toll-like receptor-mediated NF-kappa beta by zymosan-derived water-soluble fraction: Possible contribution of endotoxin-like substances, *Immunopharmacol. Immunotoxicol.* 27, 285–298, 2005.
7. Lamkanfi, M., Malireddi, R.K., and Kanneganti, T.D., Fungal zymosan and mannan activate the cryopyrin inflammasome, *J. Biol. Chem.* 284, 20574–20581, 2009.
8. Volman, T.J., Hendriks, T., and Goris, R.J., Zymosan-induced generalized inflammation: Experimental studies into mechanisms leading to multiple organ dysfunction syndrome, *Shock* 23, 291–297, 2005.
9. Sahan-Firat, S., Temiz-Resitoglu, M., Guden, D.S., et al., Protection by mTOR inhibition on zymosan-induced systemic inflammatory response and oxidative/nitrosative stress: Contribution of mTOR/MEK1/ERK1/2/IKKβ/IkB-α/KF-κB signalling pathway, *Inflammation* 41, 276–298, 2018.
10. Pierre, S., Zhang, D.D., Suo, J., et al., Myc binding protein 2 suppresses M2-like phenotypes in macrophages during zymosan-induced inflammation in mice, *Eur. J. Immunol.* 48, 239–249, 2018.
11. Bussmann, A.J.C., Pinho-Ribeiro, F.A., Verri, W.A.,Jr., et al., The citrus flavanone naringenin attenuates zymosan-induced mouse joint inflammation: Induction of Nrf2 expression in recruited CD45+ hematopoietic cells, *Inflammopharmacology*, 1–14, 2019.

3 List of Buffers

ACES (2-[(2-AMINO-2-OXYETHYL)AMINO]-ETHANESULFONIC ACID)

ACES is one of the several "Good" buffers.[1] As with other "Good" buffers, ACES does bind some divalent cations.[2,3]

1. Good, N.E., Winget, G.D., Winter, W., et al., Hydrogen ion buffers for biological research, *Biochemistry* 5, 467–477, 1966.
2. Pope, J.M., Stevens, P.R., Angotti, M.T., and Nakon, R., Free metal ion depletion by "Good's" buffers. II. *N*-(2-acetamido)-2-aminoethanesufonic acid (ACESH): Complexes with calcium(II), magnesium(II), manganese(II), cobalt(II), zinc(II), nickel(II), and copper(II), *Anal. Biochem.* 103, 214–221, 1980.
3. Zawisza, I., Rózga, M., Poznański, J., and Bal, W., Cu(II) complex formation by ACES buffer, *J. Inorg. Biochem.* 129, 58–61, 2013.

Some references to the use of ACES buffer:

Chappel, D.J., N-[(carbamoylmethyl)amino] ethanesulfonic acid improves phenotyping of α-1-antitrypsin by isoelectric focusing on agarose gel, *Clin. Chem.* 31, 1384–1386, 1985.
Edelstein, P.H., Improved semiselective medium for isolation of *Legionella pneumophila* from contaminated clinical and environmental specimens, *J. Clin. Microbiol.* 14, 298–303, 1981.
Flavell, R.R., von Morze, C., Blecha, J.E., et al., Application of Good's buffers to pH imaging using hyperpolarized ¹³C MRI, *Chem. Commun.*(Camb) 51, 14119–14122, 2015.
Kitamura, Y., and Itoh, T., Reaction volumes of protonic ionization for buffering agents. Prediction of pressure dependence of pH and pOH, *J. Solution Chem.* 16, 715–725, 1987.
Liu, Q., Li, X., and Sommer, S.S., pk-Matched running buffers for gel electrophoresis, *Anal. Biochem.* 270, 112–122, 1999.
Mertzman, M.B., and Foley, J.R., Effect of surfactant concentration and buffer selection on chromatographic figures of merit in chiral microemulsion electrokinetic chromatography, *Electrophoresis* 25, 3247–3256, 2004.
Roy, R.N., Roy, L.N., Fuge, M.S., et al., Buffer standards for the physiological pH of zwitterionic compound, ACES from 5°C to 55°C, *J. Solution Chem.* 38, 471–483, 2009.
Taha, M., Buffers for the physiological pH range: Acidic dissociation constants of zwitterionic compounds in various hydroorganic media, *Ann. Chim.* 95, 105–109, 2005.
Tunnicliff, G., and Smith, J.A., Competitive inhibition of gamma-aminobutyric acid receptor binding by N-hydroxyethylpiperazine-N'-2-ethanesulfonic acid and related buffers, *J. Neurochem.* 36, 1122–1126, 1981.

ACETIC ACID/SODIUM ACETATE

The acetate buffer system is widely used at pH <5.5. This includes frequent use in chromatography.[1–3] The ammonium salt (ammonium acetate) is volatile and can be removed by lyophilization.[4] It is used in the therapy for acid–base disorders and as a buffer for peritoneal dialysis. Acetate is a naturally occurring chemical and is used as a substitute for carbonate when there is a shortage of carbonate.[5] A previous work showed that acetate is a suitable substitute for bicarbonate in early dialysis studies.[6]

1. Cusumano, A., Guillarme, D., Beck, A., and Fekete, S., Practical method development for the separation of monoclonal antibodies and antibody-drug-conjugate species in hydrophobic interaction chromatography, part 2: Optimization of the phase system, *J. Pharm. Biomed. Anal.* 121, 161–173, 2016.
2. West, C., and Auroux, E., Deconvoluting the effects of buffer salt concentration in hydrophobic interaction chromatography on a zwitterionic stationary phase, *J. Chromatog. A.* 1461, 92–97, 2016.
3. Alvarez-Segura, T., Subirats, X., and Rosés, M. Retention-pH profiles of acids and bases in hydrophilic interaction liquid chromatography, *Anal. Chim. Acta* 1050, 176–184, 2019.
4. Lim, C.K., and Peters, T.J., Ammonium acetate: A general purpose buffer for clinical applications of high-performance liquid chromatography, *J. Chromatog.* 3126, 397–406, 1984.
5. Neavyn, M.J., Boyer, E.W., Bird, S.B., and Babu, K.M, Sodium acetate as a replacement for sodium bicarbonate in medical toxicology: A review, *J. Med. Toxicol.* 9, 250–254, 2013.
6. Mion, C.M., Hegstrom, R.M., Boen, S.T., and Scribner, B.H., Substitution of sodium acetate for sodium bicarbonate in the bath fluid for hemodialysis, *Trans. Am. Soc. Artif. Intern. Organs* 10, 110–115, 1964.

General references for the use of acetate buffer systems:

Ahmad, I., Anwar, Z., Iqbal, K., et al., Effect of acetate and carbonate buffers on the photolysis of riboflavin in aqueous solution: A kinetic study, *AAPS PharmSciTech.* 15, 550–559, 2014.

Barnett, G.V., Razinov, V.I., Kerwin, B.A, Hillsley, A., and Roberts, C.J., Acetate- and citrate-specific ion effects on unfolding and temperature-dependent aggregation rates of anti-Streptavidin IgG1, *J. Pharm. Sci.* 105, 1066–1073, 2016.

Cuvelier, A., Bourguignon, J., Muir, J.F., et al., Substitution of carbonate by acetate buffer for IgG coating in sandwich ELISA, *J. Immunoassay* 17, 371–382, 1996.

Frieden, C., and Alberty, R.A., The effect of pH on fumase activity in acetate buffer, *J. Biol. Chem.* 212, 859–868, 1955.

Righetti, P.G., and Gelfi, C., Capillary electrophoresis of DNA in the 20–500 bp range: Recent developments, *J. Biochem. Biophys. Methods* 41, 75–90, 1999.

Sen Gupta, K.K., Pal, B., and Begum, B.A., Reactivity of some sugars and sugar phosphates toward gold (III) in sodium acetate-acetic acid buffer medium, *Carbohydr. Res.* 330, 115–123, 2001.

Urbansky, E.T., Cooper, B.T., and Margerum, D.W., Disproportionation kinetics of hypoiodous acid as catalyzed and suppressed by acetic acid-acetate buffer, *Inorg. Chem.* 36, 1338–1344, 1997.

Watanabe, N., Shirakami, Y., Tomiyoshi, K., et al., Direct labeling of macroaggregated albumin with indium-111-chloride using acetate buffer, *J. Nucl. Med.* 38, 1590–1592, 1997.

Citations for clinical use of acetate buffers:

Maiorca, R., Cancarini, G.C., Zubani, R., et al., Differing dialysis treatment strategies and outcome, *Nephrol. Dial. Transplant.* 11(Suppl 2), 134–139, 1996.

Man, N.K., Itakura, Y., Chauveau, P., and Yamauchi, T., Acetate-free biofiltration: State of the art, *Contrib. Nephrol.* 108, 87–93, 1994.

Naka, T., and Bellomo, R., Bench-to-bedside review: Treating acid-base abnormalities in the intensive care unit – the role of renal replacement therapy, *Crit. Care* 8, 108–114, 2004; Khanna, A. and Kurtzman, N.A., Metabolic alkalosis, *J. Nephrol.* 19(Suppl 9), S86–S96, 2006.

Pfortmueller, C.A., and Fleischmann, E., Acetate-buffer crystalloid fluids: Current knowledge, a systematic review, *J. Crit. Care.* 35, 96–104, 2016.

ADA (N-(2-AMINO-2-OXOETHYL)-N-CARBOXYMETHYL GLYCINE; N-(2-ACETAMIDO) IMINODIACETIC ACID)

ADA is a "Good" buffer.[1] As with many "Good" buffers, ADA can bind divalent cations.[2,3] Its ability to bind

Cu(II) interferes with the bicinchoninic acid (BCA) assay for measuring protein concentration.

1. Good, N.E., Winget, G.D., Winter, W., et al., Hydrogen ion buffers for biological research, *Biochemistry* 5, 467–477, 1966.
2. Durham, A.C., A survey of readily available chelators for buffering calcium ion concentrations in physiological solutions, *Cell Calcium* 4, 33–46, 1983.
3. Kaushal, V., and Barnes, L.D., Effect of zwitterionic buffers on measurement of small masses of protein with bicinchoninic acid, *Anal. Biochem.* 157, 291–294, 1986.

Other general references include the following:

Bers, D.M., Hryshko, L.V., Harrison, S.M., and Dawson, D.D., Citrate decreases contraction and Ca current in cardiac muscle independent of its buffering action, *Am. J. Physiol.* 260, C900–C909, 1991.

Delaney, J.P., Kimm, G.E., and Bonsack, M.E., The influence of luminal pH on the severity of acute radiation enteritis, *Int. J. Radiat. Biol.* 61, 381–386, 1992.

Pietrzkowski, E., and Korohoda, W., Extracellular ATP and ADA-buffer enable chick embryo fibroblasts to grow in secondary culture in protein-free, hormone-free, extracellular growth factor-free media, *Folia Histochem. Cytobiol.* 26, 143–152, 1988.

Righetti, P.G., Chiari, M., and Gelfi, C., Immobilized pH gradients: Effect of salts, added carrier ampholytes and voltage gradients on protein patterns, *Electrophoresis* 9, 65–73, 1988.

Robinson, J.D., and Davis, R.L., Buffer, pH, and ionic strength effects on the (Na+, + K+)-ATPase, *Biochim. Biophys. Acta* 912, 343–347, 1987.

Roy, R.N., Gibbons, J.J., Padron, J.L., and Casebolt, R.G, Thermodynamics of the second-stage dissociation of N-(2-acetamido)iminoacetic acid in water 5°C–55°C, *Anal. Chim. Acta* 129, 247–252, 1981.

Taha, M., Buffers for the physiological pH range: Acidic dissociation constants of zwitterionic compounds in various hydroorganic media, *Ann. Chim.* 95, 105–109, 2005.

Tunnicliff, G., and Smith, J.A., Competitive inhibition of gamma-aminobutyric acid receptor binding by N-2-hydroxyethylpiperazine-N'-2-ethanesulfonic acid and related buffers, *J. Neurochem.* 36, 1122–1126, 1981.

BES (N,N-BIS(2-HYDROXYETHYL)-2-AMINOETHANESULFONIC ACID; N,N-BIS(2-HYDROXYETHYL)TAURINE)

BES is a "Good" buffer[1] not frequently used, similar to MES and HEPES. BES, as with other "Good" buffers that contain hydroxyl groups, has been shown to interfere with the CNBr-mediated ligation of phosphorylated oligonucleotide and unphosphorylated oligonucleotide.[2]

BES can also bind divalent cations such as Cu(II), which interferes with the bicinchoninic acid (BCA) assay for measurement of protein concentration.[3]

1. Good, N.E., Winget, G.D., Winter, W., et al., Hydrogen ion buffers for biological research, *Biochemistry* 5, 467–477, 1966.
2. Vogel, H., Gerlach, C., and Richert, C., Reactions of buffers in cyanogen bromide induced ligation, *Nucleos., Nucleot. Nucl.* 32, 17–27, 2013.
3. Kaushal, V., and Barnes, L.D., Effect of zwitterionic buffers on the measurement of small masses of protein with bicinchoninic acid, *Anal. Biochem.* 157, 291–294, 1986.

General reference for BES buffer:

Hosse, M., and Wilkinson, K.J., Determination of electrophoretic mobilities and hydrodynamic radii of three humic substances as a function of pH and ionic strength, *Environ. Sci. Technol.* 35, 4301–4306, 2002.
MacKerrow, S.D., Merry, J.M., and Hoeprich, P.D., Effects of buffers on testing of *Candida* species susceptibility to flucytosine, *J. Clin. Microbiol.* 25, 885–888, 1987.
Roy, R.N., Gibbons, J.J., and Baker, G.E., Acid dissociation constants and pH values for standard "bes" and "tricine" buffer solutions in 30, 40, 50 mass% dimethyl sulfoxide/water between 25°C and −25°C, *Cryobiology* 22, 589–600, 1985.
Stellwagen, N.C., Bossi, A., Gelfi, C., and Righetti, P.G., DNA and buffers: Are there any noninteracting, neutral pH buffers, *Anal. Biochem.* 287, 167–175, 2000.
Taha, M., Buffers for the physiological pH range: Acidic dissociation constants of zwitterionic compounds in various hydroorganic media, *Ann. Chim.* 95, 105–109, 2005.
Tuli, R.K., and Holtz, W., The effect of zwitterionic buffers on the feasibility of Boer goat semen, *Theriogenology* 37, 947–951, 1992.

BICINE (*N,N*-BIS-(2-HYDROXYETHYL) GLYCINE; *N,N*-BIS(2-HYDROXYETHYL) AMINO-ACETIC ACID)

Bicine is a "Good" buffer,[1] and as with other "Good" buffers, it can bind divalent cations.[2–4] Unlike some other buffers such as Tris, aqueous bicine buffer does not show a large pH change on freezing.[5] A high concentration of bovine serum albumin (40 mg/mL) mitigated the change with most buffers tested, Tris, TAPs, and phosphate buffers being an exception. A lower concentration of albumin (10 mg/mL) had less effect. It is recognized that the equilibrium effect upon freezing can be complex.[6] Other investigators have also studied the change in pH upon freezing of aqueous buffer solutions.[7] These investigators reported that the change in pH upon freezing was mitigated by the presence of glycerol (1%–5%; V/V).

1. Good, N.E., Winget, G.D., Winter, W., et al., Hydrogen ion buffers for biological research, *Biochemistry* 5, 467–477, 1966.
2. Altura, B.M., Altura, B.T., Carella, A., and Turlapaty, P.D., Ca²⁺ coupling in vascular smooth muscle: Mg²⁺ and buffer effects on contractility and membrane Ca²⁺ movements, *Can. J. Physiol. Pharmacol.* 60, 459–482, 1982.
3. Kaushal, V., and Barnes, L.D., Effect of zwitterionic buffers on measurement of small masses of protein with bicinchoninic acid, *Anal. Biochem.* 157, 291–294, 1986.
4. Seo, Y., Satoh, K., Watanabe, K., et al., Mn-bicine: A low affinity chelate for manganese ion enhanced MRI, *Magn. Reson. Med.* 65, 1005–1012, 2011.
5. Williams-Smith, D.L., Bray, R.C., Barber, M.J., et al., Changes in apparent pH on freezing aqueous buffer solutions and their relevance to biochemical electron-paramagnetic-resonance spectroscopy, *Biochem. J.* 167, 593–600, 1977.
6. Newberg, J.T., Equilibria shifts on freezing, *Fluid Ph. Equilibria* 478, 82–89, 2018.
7. Orii, Y., and Morita, M., Measurement of the pH of frozen buffer solutions by using pH indicators, *J. Biochem.* 81, 163–168, 1977.

Some general references for the use of bicine buffers:

Churchill, T.A., and Kneteman, N.M., Investigation of a primary requirement of organ preservation solutions: Supplemental buffering agents improve hepatic energy production during cold storage, *Transplantation* 65, 551–559, 1998.
Gordon-Weeks, R., Koren'kov, V.D., Steele, S.H., and Leigh, R.A., Tris is a competitive inhibitor of K+ activation of the vacuolar H+-pumping pyrophosphatase, *Plant Physiol.* 114, 901–905, 1997.
Ito, S., Takaoka, T., Mori, H., and Teruo, A., A sensitive new method for measurement of guanase with 8-azaguanine in bicine bis-hydroxy ethyl glycine buffer as substrate, *Clin. Chim. Acta* 115, 135–144, 1981.
Ito, S., Xu, Y., Keyser, A.J., and Peters, R.L., Histochemical demonstration of guanase in human liver with guanine in bicine buffer as substrate, *Histochem. J.* 16, 489–499, 1984.
Kanfer, J.N., Base exchange reactions of the phospholipids in rat brain particles, *J. Lipid Res.* 13, 468–476, 1972.
Luo, Q., Andrade, J.D., and Caldwell, K.D., Thin-layer ion-exchange chromatography of proteins, *J. Chromatog. A* 816, 97–105, 1998.
Nakon, R., Krishnamoorthy, C.R., Free-metal ion depletion by "Good's" buffers, *Science* 221, 749–750, 1983.
Rabilloud, T., Vuillard, L., Gilly, C., and Lawrence, J.J., Silver-staining of proteins in polyacrylamide gels: A general overview, *Cell. Mol. Biol.* 40, 57–75, 1994.

Roy, R.N., Gibbons, J.J, Baker, G., and Bates, R.G., Standard electromotive force of the H_2-AgCL:Ag cell in 30, 40, and 50 mass dimethyl sulfoxide/water from −20° to 25°; pK_2 and pH values for a standard "Bicine" buffer solution at subzero temperatures, *Cryobiology* 21, 672–681, 1984.

Syvertsen, C., and McKinley-McKee, J.S., Affinity labeling of liver alcohol dehydrogenase. Effects of pH and buffers on affinity labeling with iodoacetic acid and (R, S)-2-bromo-3-(5-imidazoyl)propionic acid, *Eur. J. Biochem.* 117, 165–170, 1981.

Taha, M., Buffers for the physiological pH range: Acidic dissociation constants of zwitterionic compounds in various hydroorganic media, *Ann. Chim.* 95, 105–109, 2005.

Taha, M., Thermodynamic study of the second-stage dissociation of *N,N*-bis-(2-hydroxyethyl)glycine (bicine) in water at different ionic strength and different solvent mixtures, *Ann. Chim.* 94, 971–978, 2004.

Vaidya, N.R., Gothoskar, B.P., and Banerji, A.P., Column isoelectric focusing in nature pH gradients generated by biological buffers, *Electrophoresis* 11, 156–161, 1990.

Williams, T.I., Combs, J.C., Thakur, A.P., et al., A novel Bicine running buffer system for doubled sodium dodecyl sulfate: Polyacrylamide gel electrophoresis of membrane proteins, *Electrophoresis* 27, 2984–2995, 2006.

Wiltfang, J., Arold, N., and Neuhoff, V., A new multiphasic buffer system for sodium sulfate-polyacrylamide gel electrophoresis of proteins and peptides with molecular masses 100,000–1000, and their detection with picomolar sensitivity, *Electrophoresis* 12, 352–366, 1991.

BORATE: SODIUM BORATE (SODIUM TETRABORATE/BORIC ACID; $NA_2B_4O_7$/H_3BO_3; SODIUM BORATE DECAHYDRATE IS BORAX)

Borate buffers have a long history of use in electrophoretic separations.[1–7] Borate is well known for its interaction with carbohydrates and other polyhydroxyl compounds.[7–15] The formation of a complex between carbohydrate (diols) and borate can be an important factor in electrophoresis.[16] Borate also participates in the reversible modification of arginine residues by 1,2-cyclohexanedione.[17–20]

1. Adjutantis, G., Electrophoretic separation of filter paper of the soluble liver-cell proteins of the rat using borate buffer, *Nature* 173, 539–540, 1954.

2. Consden, R., and Powell, M.N., The use of borate buffer in paper electrophoresis of serum, *J. Clin. Pathol.* 8, 150–152, 1955.

3. Cooper, D.R., Effect of borate buffer on the electrophoresis of serum, *Nature* 181, 713–714, 1958.

4. Poduslo, J.F., Glycoprotein molecular-weight estimation using sodium dodecyl sulfate-pore gradient electrophoresis: Comparison of Tris-glycine and Tris-borate-EDTA buffer systems, *Anal. Biochem.* 114, 131–139, 1981.

5. Patton, W.F., Chung-Welch, N., Lopez, M.F., et al., Tris-tricine and Tris-borate buffer systems provide better estimates of human mesothelial cell intermediate filament protein molecular weights than the standard Tris-glycine system, *Anal. Biochem.* 197, 25–33, 1991.

6. Biyani, M., and Nishigaki, K., Sequence-specific and nonspecific mobilities of single-stranded oligonucleotides observed by changing the borate buffer concentration, *Electrophoresis* 24, 628–633, 2003.

7. Zhao, Y., Yang, X., Jiang, R. et al., Chiral separation of synthetic vicinal diol compounds by capillary zone electrophoresis with borate buffer and β-cyclodextrin as buffer additives, *Anal. Sci.* 22, 747–751, 2006.

8. Zittle, C.A., Reaction of borate with substances of biological interest, *Adv. Enzymol. Relat. Sub. Biochem.* 12, 493–527, 1951.

9. Larsson, U.B., and Samuelson, O., Anion exchange separation of organic acids in borate medium: Influence of the temperature, *J. Chromatog.* 19, 404–411, 1965.

10. Lin, F.M., and Pomeranz, Y., Effect of borate on colorimetric determinations of carbohydrates by the phenol-sulfuric acid method, *Anal. Biochem.* 24, 128–131, 1968.

11. Haug, A., The influence of borate and calcium on the gel formation of a sulfated polysaccharide from *Ulva lactuca*, *Acta Chem. Scand. B.* 30, 562–566, 1976.

12. Weitzman, S., Scott, V., and Keegstra, K., Analysis of glycoproteins as borate complexes by polyacrylamide gel electrophoresis, *Anal. Biochem.* 97, 438–449, 1979.

13. Honda, S., Takahashi, M., Kakehi, K., and Ganno, S., Rapid, automated analysis of monosaccharides by high-performance anion-exchange chromatography of borate complexes with fluorometric detection using 2-cyanoacetamide, *Anal. Biochem.* 113, 130–138, 1981.

14. Rothman, R.J., and Warren, L., Analysis of IgG glycopeptides by alkaline borate gel filtration chromatography, *Biochim. Biophys. Acta* 955, 143–153, 1988.

15. Todd, P., and Elsasser, W., Nonamphometric isoelectric focusing: II. Stability of borate-glycerol pH gradients in recycling isoelectric focusing, *Electrophoresis* 11, 947–952, 1990.

16. Yamamoto, S., Nagai, E., Asada, Y., Kinoshita, M., and Suzuki, S., A rapid and highly sensitive microchip electrophoresis of mono- and mucin-type oligosaccharides labeled with 7-amino-4-methylcoumarin, *Anal. Bioanal. Chem.* 407, 1499–1503, 2015.

17. Patthy, L., and Smith, E.L., Reversible modification of arginine residues. Application to sequence studies by restriction of tryptic hydrolysis to lysine residues, *J. Biol. Chem.* 250, 557–564, 1975.

18. Patthy, L., and Smith, E.L., Identification of functional arginine residues in ribonuclease A and lysozyme, *J. Biol. Chem.* 250, 565–569, 1975.

19. Menegatti, E., Ferroni, R., Benassi, C.A., and Rocchi, R., Arginine modification in Kunitz bovine trypsin inhibitor through 1,2-cyclohexanedione, *Int. J. Pept. Protein Res.* 10, 146–152, 1977.

20. Kozik, A., Guevara, I., and Zak, Z., 1,2-Cyclohexanedione modification of arginine residues in egg-white riboflavin-binding protein, *Int. J. Biochem.* 20, 707–711, 1988.

CACODYLIC ACID (DIMETHYLARSINIC ACID)

Cacodylic acid is a buffer in the neutral pH range. It was extensively used in early biochemical studies as it had a low affinity for most divalent cations such as calcium, but it has been largely replaced because of its toxicity.[1,2]

1. Kenyon, E.M., and Hughes, M.F., A concise review of the toxicity and carcinogenicity of dimethylarsinic acid, *Toxicology* 160, 227–236, 2001.
2. Cohen, S.M., Arnold, L.L., Eldan, M., et al., Methylated arsenicals: The implications of metabolism and carcinogenicity studies in rodents to human risk management, *Crit. Rev. Toxicol.* 99–133, 2006.

General references for the use of cacodylic acid

Caswell, A.H., and Bruschwig, J.P., Identification and extraction of proteins that compose the triad junction of skeletal muscle, *J. Cell Biol.* 99, 929–939, 1984.

Chirpich, T.P., The effect of different buffers on terminal deoxynucleotidyl transferase activity, *Biochim. Biophys. Acta* 518, 535–538, 1978.

Henney, P.J., Johnson, E.L., and Cothran, E.G., A new buffer system for acid PAGE typing of equine protease inhibitor, *Anim. Genet.* 25, 363–364, 1994.

Jacobson, K.B., Murphy, J.B., and Das Sarma, B., Reaction of cacodylic acid with organic thiols, *FEBS Lett.* 22, 80–82, 1972.

Jezewska, M.J., Rajendran, S., and Bujalowski, W., Interactions of the 8-kDa domain of rat DNA polymerase beta with DNA, *Biochemistry* 40, 3295–3307, 2001.

McAlpine, J.C., Histochemical demonstration of the activation of rat acetylcholinesterase by sodium cacodylate and cacodylic acid using the thioacetic acid method, *J. R. Microsc. Soc.* 82, 95–106, 1963.

Nunes, J.F., Aguas, A.P., and Soares, J.O., Growth of fungi in cacodylate buffer, *Stain Technol.* 55, 191–192, 1980.

Parks, J.C., and Cohen, G.M., Glutaraldehyde fixatives for preserving the chick's inner ear, *Acta Otolaryngol.* 98, 72–80, 1984.

Song, A.H., and Asher, S.A., Internal intensity standards for heme protein UV resonance Raman studies: Excitation profiles of cacodylic acid and sodium selenate, *Biochemistry* 30, 1199–1205, 1991.

Travers, F., Douzou, P., Pederson, T., and Gunsalus. I.C., Ternary solvents to investigate proteins at sub-zero temperature, *Biochimie* 57, 43–48, 1975.

Young, C.W., Dessources, C., Hodas, S., and Bittar, E.S., Use of cationic disc electrophoresis near neutral pH in the evaluation of trace proteins in human plasma, *Cancer Res.* 35, 1991–1995, 1975.

CAPS (3-(CYCLOHEXYLAMINO)-1-PROPANESULFONIC ACID)

CAPS is a zwitterionic buffer similar to a "Good" buffer.[1–3] As with "Good" buffers, CAPS can bind divalent cations such as Cu(II) and interfere with the bicinchoninic acid assay for measurement of protein concentration.[4] The effect of CAPS and other zwitterionic buffers on the Lowry method for determination of protein chemistry has also been reported.[5]

1. Kanfer, J.N., Base exchange reactions of the phospholipids in rat brain particles, *J. Lipid Res.* 13, 468–476, 1972.
2. Shettawy, M.J., and Losowsky, M.S., Determination of faecel bile acids by an enzymic method, *Clin. Chim. Acta* 64, 127–133, 1975.
3. Lad, P.J., and Leffert, H.L., Rat liver alcohol dehydrogenase. I. Purification and characterization, *Anal. Biochem.* 133, 350–361, 1983.
4. Kaushal, V., and Barnes, L.D., Effect of zwitterionic buffers on measurement of small masses of protein with bicinchoninic acid, *Anal. Biochem.* 157, 291–294, 1986.
5. Himmel, H.M., and Heller, W., Studies on the interference of selected substances with two modifications of the Lowry protein determination, *J. Clin. Chem. Clin. Biochem.* 25, 909–913, 1987.

Some general references to the use of CAPS buffer:

Bienvenut, W.V., Deon, C., Sanchez, J.C., and Hochstrasser, D.F., *Anal. Biochem.* 307, 297–303, 2002.

Hautala, J.T., Wiedmer, S.K., and Riekkola, M.L., Influence of pH on formation and stability of phosphatidylcholine/phosphatidylserine coatings in fused-silica capillaries, *Electrophoresis* 26, 176–186, 2005.

Jin, Y., and Cerletti, N., Western blotting of transforming growth factor β2. Optimization of the electrophoretic transfer, *Appl. Theor. Electrophor.* 3, 85–90, 1992.

Kannamkumarath, S.S., Wuilloud, R.G., and Caruso, J.A., Studies of various elements of nutritional and toxicological interest associated with different molecular weight fractions in Brazil nuts, *J. Agric. Food Chem.* 52, 5773–5780, 2004.

Ng, L.T., Selwyn, M.J., and Choo, H.L., Effect of buffers and osmolality on anion uniport across the mitochondrial inner membrane, *Biochim. Biophys. Acta* 1143, 29–37, 1993.

Nguyen, A.L., Luong, J.H., and Masson, C., Determination of nucleotides in fish tissues using capillary electrophoresis, *Anal. Chem.* 62, 2490–2493, 1990.

Righetti, P.G., Bossi, A., and Gelfi, C., Capillary isoelectric focusing and isoelectric buffers: An evolving scenario, *J. Capillary Electrophor.* 4, 47–59, 1997.

Taha, M., Buffers for the physiological pH range: Acidic dissociation constants of zwitterionic compounds in various hydroorganic media, *Ann. Chim.* 95, 105–109, 2005.

Tu, J., Halsall, H.B., Seliskar, C.J. et al., Estimation of logP(ow) values for neutral and basic compounds by microchip microemulsion electrokinetic chromatography with indirect fluorometric detection (muMEEKC-IFD), *J. Pharm. Biomed. Anal.* 38, 1–7, 2005.

Venosa, R.A., Kotsias, B.A., and Horowicz, P., Frog striated muscle is permeable to hydroxide and buffer anions, *J. Membr. Biol.* 139, 57–74, 1994.

Zaitseva, J., Holland, I.B., and Schmitt, L., The role of CAPS buffer in expanding the crystallization space of the nucleotide-binding domain of the ABC transporter haemolysin B from *Escherichia coli*, *Acta Crystallogr. D. Biol. Crystallogr.* 60, 1076–1084, 2004.

CAPSO (3-(CYCLOHEXYLAMINO)-2-HYDROXY-1-PROPANESULFONIC ACID)

CAPSO is a zwitterionic buffer similar to a "Good" buffer. It is used infrequently.

General references to the use of CAPSO buffer:

Delaney, J.P., Kimm, G.E., and Bonsack, M.E., The influence of lumenal pH on the severity of acute radiation enteritis, *Int. J. Radiat. Biol.* 61, 381–386, 1992.

Liu, Q. Li, X., and Somer, S.S., pK-Matched running buffers for gel electrophoresis, *Anal. Biochem.* 270, 112–122, 1999.

McGregor, D.P., Forster, S., Steven, J., et al., Simultaneous detection of microorganisms in soil suspension based on PCR amplification of bacterial 16S rRNA fragments, *BioTechniques* 21, 463–466, 1996.

Okuda, M., Iwahori, K., Yamashita, I., and Yoshimura, H., Fabrication of nickel and chromium nanoparticles using the protein cage of apoferritin, *Biotechnol. Bioeng.* 84, 187–194, 2003.

Quiros, M., Parker, M.C., and Turner, N.J., Tuning lipase enantioselectivity in organic media using solid-state buffers, *J. Org. Chem.* 66, 5074–5079, 2001.

Taha, M., Buffers for the physiological pH range: Acidic dissociation constants of zwitterionic compounds in various hydroorganic media, *Ann. Chim.* 95, 105–109, 2005.

Vespalec, R., Vlckova, M., and Horakova, H., Aggregation and other intermolecular interactions of biological buffers observed by capillary electrophoresis and UV photometry, *J. Chromatog. A* 1051, 75–84, 2004.

CARBONATE/BICARBONATE(CARBONATE BUFFER) (SODIUM BICARBONATE, SODIUM CARBONATE, AMMONIUM BICARBONATE, AMMONIUM CARBONATE)

Sodium carbonate is a physiological buffer and is used in renal dialysis.[1,2] The ammonium salt is a volatile buffer that provides advantages in purification,[3,4] although there may be problems with direct analysis by mass spectrometry.[5] Ammonium bicarbonate buffers must be kept tightly sealed to maintain pH. Alkaline carbonate buffers are used for enhancing the binding of proteins to microplates.[6-13] However, alkaline treatment of antigen can decrease immunogenicity.[14]

1. McGill, R.L., and Weiner, D.E., Dialysate composition for hemodialysis: Changes and changing risk, *Semin. Dial.* 30, 112–120, 2017.

2. Lew, S.Q., Kohn, O.F., Cheng, Y.L., Kjellstand, C.M., and Ing, T.S., Three-stream bicarbonate-based hemodialysis solution delivery system revisited: With an emphasis on some aspects of acid-base principles, *Artif. Organs* 41, 509–518, 2017.

3. Miller, R.L., Guimond, S.E. Shivkumar, M., et al., Heparin isomeric oligosaccharide separation using volatile salt strong anion exchange chromatography, *Anal. Chem.* 88, 11542–11550, 2016.

4. Zlobina, M., Sedo, O., Chou, M.Y., Slepankova, L., and Lukavsky, P.J., Efficient large-scale preparation and purification of short single-stranded RNA oligonucleotides, *Biotechniques* 60, 75–83, 2016.

5. Hedges, J.B., Vahidi, S., Yue, X., and Konermann, L., Effects of ammonium bicarbonate on the electrospray mass spectra of proteins: Evidence for bubble-induced unfolding, *Anal. Chem.* 85, 6469–6476, 2013.

6. Solling, H., and Dinesen, B., The development of a rapid ELISA for IgE utilizing commercially available reagents, *Clin. Chim. Acta* 130, 71–83, 1983.

7. Ferris, N.P., Powell, H., and Donaldson, A.I., Use of precoated immunoplates and freeze-dried reagents for the diagnosis of foot-and-mouth disease and swine vesicular disease by enzyme-linked immunosorbent assay (ELISA), *J. Virol. Methods* 19, 197–206, 1988.

8. Cutler, S.J., and Wright, D.J., Comparison of immunofluorescence and enzyme linked immunosorbent assays for diagnosing Lyme disease, *J. Clin. Pathol.* 42, 869–871, 1989.

9. Oshima, M., and Atassi, M.Z., Comparison of peptide-coating conditions in solid phase assays for detection of antipeptide antibodies, *Immunol. Invest.* 18, 841–851, 1989.

10. Houen, G., and Koch, C., A non-denaturing enzyme linked immunosorbent assay with protein preadsorbed onto aluminum hydroxide, *J. Immunol. Methods* 200, 99–105, 1997.

11. Shrivastav, T.G., Basu, A., and Kariya, K.P., Substitution of carbonate buffer by water for IgG immobilization in enzyme linked immunosorbent assay, *J. Immunoassay Immunochem.* 24, 191–203, 2003.

12. Luo, Y., Zhang, B., Chen, M., et al., Sensitive and rapid quantification of C-reactive protein using quantum dot-labeled microplate immunoassay, *J. Translational Med.* 10, 24, 2012.

13. Dou, X., Zhang, H., Liu, C., et al., Fluorometric competitive immunoassay for chloropyrifos using rhodamine-modified gold nanoparticles as a label, *Microchim. Acta* 185, 41, 2018.

14. Gye, H.J., and Nichizawa, T., Treatment with carbonate buffer decreases antigenicity of nervous necrosis virus (NNV), *Aquaculture* 500, 192–196, 2019.

Some general references for the use of carbonate/bicarbonate buffers:

Asberg, P., Bjork, P., Hook, F., and Inganas, O., Hydrogels from a water-soluble zwitterionic polythiophene: Dynamics under pH change and biomolecular interactions observed using quartz crystal microbalance with dissipation monitoring, *Langmuir* 21, 7292–7298, 2005.

Bartzatt, R., Fluorescent labeling of drugs and simple organic compounds containing amine functional groups, utilizing dansyl chloride in Na_2CO_3 buffer, *J. Pharmacol. Toxicol. Methods* 45, 247–253, 2001.

Binter, A., Goodisman, J., and Dabrowiak, J.C., Formation of monofunctional cisplatinin-DNA adducts in carbonate buffer, *J. Inorg. Biochem.* 100, 1219–1224, 2006.

Cheung, S.T., and Fonda, M.L., Reaction of phenylglyoxal with arginine. The effect of buffers and pH, *Biochem. Biophys. Res. Commun.* 90, 940–947, 1979.

Chen, X.L., Sun, C.Y., Zhang, Y.Z., and Gao, P.J., Effects of different buffers on the thermostability and autolysis of a cold-adapted proteases MCP-01, *J. Protein Chem.* 21, 523–527, 2002.

Di Pasqua, A.J., Goodisman, J., Kerwood, D.J., et al., Activation of carboplatin by carbonate, *Chem. Res. Toxicol.* 18, 139–149, 2006.

Duman, M., Saber, R., and Piskin, E., A new approach for immobilization of oligonucleotides onto piezoelectric quartz crystal for preparation of a nucleic acid sensor following hybridization, *Biosens. Bioelectron.* 18, 1355–1363, 2003.

Dwight, S.J., Gaylord, B.S., Hong, J.W., and Bazan, G.C., Perturbation of fluorescence by nonspecific interactions between anionic poly(phenylenevinylene)s and proteins. Implications for biosensors, *J. Am. Chem. Soc.* 126, 16850–16859, 2004.

Horejsi, V., and Hilgert, I., Simple polyacrylamide gel electrophoresis in continuous carbonate buffer system suitable for the analysis of ascites fluids of hybridoma bearing mice, *J. Immunol. Methods* 86, 103–105, 1986.

Medda, R., Padiglia, A., Messana, T., et al., Separation of diadenosine polyphosphates by capillary electrophoresis, *Electrophoresis* 21, 2412–2416, 2000.

Nagasawa, K., and Uchiyama, H., Preparation and properties of biologically active fluorescent heparins, *Biochim. Biophys. Acta* 544, 430–440, 1978.

Ormond, D.R., and Kral, T.A., Washing methogenic cells with the liquid fraction from a Mars soil stimulant and water mixture, *J. Microbiol. Meth.* 67, 603–605, 2006.

Petersen, A., and Steckhan, E., Continuous indirect electrochemical regeneration of galactose oxidase, *Bioorg. Med. Chem.* 7, 2203–2208, 1999.

Shah, M., Meija, J., Cabovska, B., and Caruso, J.A., Determination of phosphoric acid triesters in human plasma using solid-phase microextraction and gas chromatography coupled to inductively coupled plasma mass spectrometry, *J. Chromatog. A.* 1103, 329–336, 2006.

Steinitz, M., and Tamir, S., An improved method to create nitrocellulose particles suitable for the immobilization of antigen and antibody, *J. Immunol. Methods* 187, 171–177, 1995.

Talu, G.F., and Diyamandoglu, V., Formate ion decomposition in water under UV irradiation at 253.7 nm, *Environ. Sci. Technol.* 38, 3984–3993, 2004.

Wang, Z., Gurel, O., Baatz, J.E., and Notter, R.H., Acylation of pulmonary surfactant protein-C is required for its optimal surface active interactions with phospholipids, *J. Biol. Chem.* 271, 19104–19109, 1996.

Willems, A.V., Deforce, D.L., Van Peteghem, C.H., and Van Bocxlaer, J.F., Development of a quality control method for the characterization of oligonucleotides by capillary zone electrophoresis-electrospray ionization-quadrupole time of flight-mass spectrometry, *Electrophoresis* 26, 1412–1423, 2005.

CITRIC ACID/CITRATE (2-HYDROXY-1,2,3-PROPANETRICARBOXYLIC ACID)

Citrate is a compound found in a variety of biological tissues and cells, which is involved in energy metabolism (citric acid cycle; Krebs cycle).[1] Citrate is also used as a biological buffer; citric acid has three carboxylic acid functions, which permits buffering capacity from pH 2.0 to pH 12. Citric acid also chelate divalent cations and is used as an anticoagulant for the collection of blood based on its ability to chelate calcium ions. Chelation of metal ions is responsible for the observed inhibition of many enzymes by citrate.[2–5] Citrate does have effects on some tissues that are not clearly related to the ability to chelate metals ion, in this case calcium ions.[6,7] Concentrated solutions of sodium citrate (25%w/v) promote the action of crude prothrombin.[8–10] Citrate is a polyvalent anion, and like other polyvalent anions such as phosphate and sulfate, citrate can cause a "salting-out" phenomenon.[11–15] Citrate also has an effect on partitioning in aqueous two-phase systems.[16] In what may seem to be counterintuitive considering the above statement on "salting out," citrate has proved useful in solubilization of proteins, usually, but not always, from mineralized/calcified matrices.[17–20] Citrate is useful for dissociating protein complexes in some situations by binding to specific anion-binding sites; the ability of citrate to function as a buffering at low pH is an advantage.[21] In this particular example, the dissociation is reflection of metal ion binding and is associated with the loss of biological activity.[22] There are other examples of citrate binding to anion-binding sites (anion exosites).[23–31] A special application of citrate dissociation of protein complexes is the isolation and dissociation of antigen–antibody complexes.[32–36] A more complex and poorly understood application of citrate buffers is in epitope retrieval.[37–40] Additional work has indicated that citrate is useful but not unique for epitope retrieval.[41–43] Citrate buffer has been useful in affinity chromatography.[44–47] It is also used for immunoaffinity chromatography, including chromatography on Protein A.[48–53]

1. Krebs, H.A., The citric acid cycle and the Szent-Gyorgyi cycle in pigeon breast muscle, *Biochem. J.* 34, 775–779, 1940.

2. Smith, E.G., Dipeptidases, *Methods Enzymol.* 2, 93–114, 1955.

3. McDonald, M.R., Deoxyribonucleases, *Methods Enzymol.* 2, 437–447, 1955.

4. Kornberg, A., Adenosine phosphokinase, *Methods Enzymol.* 2, 497–500, 1955.

5. Koshland, D.E., Jr., Preparation and properties of acetyl phosphatase, *Methods Enzymol.* 2, 556–556, 1955.

6. Matoba, H., and Gollnick, P.D., Influence of ionic composition, buffering agent, and pH on the histochemical demonstration of myofibrillar actomyosin ATPase, *Histochemistry* 80, 609–614, 1984.

7. Bers, D.M., Yryshko, L.V., Harrison, S.M., and Dawson, D.D., Citrate decreases contraction and Ca current in cardiac muscle independent of its buffering action, *Am. J. Physiol.* 260, C900–C909, 1991.

8. Seegers, W.H., McClaughery, R.I., and Fahey, J.L., Some properties of purified prothrombin and its activation with sodium citrate, *Blood* 5, 421–433, 1950.

9. Lanchantin, G.F., Friedman, J.A., and Hart, D.W., The conversion of human prothrombin to thrombin by sodium citrate. Analysis of the reaction mixture, *J. Biol. Chem.* 240, 3276–3282, 1965.

10. Aronson, D.L., and Mustafa, A.J., The activation of human factor X in sodium citrate: The role of factor VII, *Thromb. Haemostas.* 36, 104–114, 1976.

11. Hegardt, F.G., and Pie, A., Sodium citrate salting-out of the human blood serum proteins, *Rev. Esp. Fisiol.* 24, 161–168, 1968.

12. Carrea, G., Pasta, P., and Vecchio, G., Effect of the lyotropic series of anions on denaturation and renaturation of 20-β-hydroxysteroid dehydrogenase, *Biochim. Biophys. Acta* 784, 16–23, 1984.

13. Nakano, T., Yuasa, H., and Kanaya, Y., Suppression of agglomeration in fluidized bed coating. III. Hofmeister series in suppression of particle agglomeration, *Pharm. Res.* 16, 1616–1620, 1999.

14. Nakano, T., and Yuasa, H., Suppression of agglomeration in fluidized bed coating. IV. Effects of sodium citrate concentration on the suppression of particle agglomeration and the physical properties of HPMC film, *Int. J. Pharm.* 215, 3–12, 2001.

15. Mani, N., and Jun, H.W., Microencapsulation of a hydrophilic drug into a hydrophobic matrix using a salting-out procedure. I: Development and optimization of the process using factorial design, *J. Microencapsulation* 21, 125–135, 2004.

16. Andrews, B.A., Schmidt, A.S., and Asenjo, J.A., Correlation for the partition behavior of proteins in aqueous two-phase systems: Effect of surface hydrophobicity and charge, *Biotechnol. Bioeng.* 90, 380–390, 2005.

17. Faludi, E., and Harsanyi, V., The effect of Na_3-citrate on the solubility of cryoprecipitate (citrate effect of cryoprecipitate), *Haematologia* 14, 207–214, 1981.

18. Myllyla, R., Preparation of antibodies to chick-embryo galactosylhydroxylysyl glucosyltransferase and their use for an immunological characterization of the enzyme of collagen synthesis, *Biochim. Biophys. Acta* 658, 299–307, 1981.

19. Guy, O., Robles-Diaz, G., Adrich, Z., et al., Protein content of precipitates present in pancreatic juice of alcoholic subjects and patients with chronic calcifying pancreatitis, *Gastroenterology* 84, 102–107, 1983.

20. Collingwood, T.N., Shanmugam, M., Daniel, R.M., and Langdon, A.G., M(III)-facilitated recovery and concentration of enzymes from mesophilic and thermophilic organisms, *J. Biochem. Biophys. Meth.* 19, 281–286, 1989.

21. Kuo, T.T., Chow, T.Y., Lin, X.T., et al., Specific dissociation of phage Xp12 by sodium citrate, *J. Gen. Virol.* 10, 199–202, 1971.

22. Lark, K.G., and Adams, M.H., The stability of phage as a function of the ionic environment, *Cold Spring Harb. Symp. Quant. Biol.*, 18, 171–183, 1953.

23. Sheffery, M., and Newton, A., Reconstitution and purification of flagellar filaments from *Caulobacter crescentus*, *J. Bacteriol.* 132, 1027–1030, 1977.

24. Brooks, S.P., and Nicholls, P., Anion and ionic strength effects upon the oxidation of cytochrome c by cytochrome c oxidase, *Biochim. Biophys. Acta* 680, 33–43, 1982.

25. Berliner, L.J., Sugawara, Y., and Fenton, J.W., 2nd, Human alpha-thrombin binding to nonpolymerized fibrin-Sepharose: Evidence for an anionic binding region, *Biochemistry* 24, 7005–7009, 1985.

26. Kella, N.K., and Kinsella, J.E., Structural stability of beta-lactoglobulin in the presence of kosmotropic salts. A kinetic and thermodynamic study, *Int. J. Pept. Protein Res.* 32, 396–405, 1988.

27. Oe, H., Takahashi, N., Doi. E., and Hirose, M., Effects of anion binding on the conformations of the two domains of ovotransferrin, *J. Biochem.* 106, 858–863, 1989.

28. Polakova, K., Karpatova, M., and Russ, G., Dissociation of β-2-microglobulin is responsible for selective reduction of HLA class I antigenicity following acid treatment of cells, *Mol. Immunol.* 30, 1223–1230, 199.

29. Lecker, D.N., and Khan, A., Model for inactivation of α-amylase in the presence of salts: Theoretical and experimental studies, *Biotechnol. Prog.* 14, 621–625, 1998.

30. Rabiller-Baudry, M., and Chaufer, B., Small molecular ion adsorption on proteins and DNAs revealed by separation techniques, *J. Chromatog. B. Analyt. Technol. Biomed. Life. Sci.* 797, 331–345, 2003.

31. Raibekas, A.A., Bures, E.J., Siska, C.C., et al., Anion binding and controlled aggregation of human interleukin-1 receptor antagonist, *Biochemistry* 44, 9871–9879, 2005.

32. Woodroffe, A.J., and Wilson, C.B., An evaluation of elution techniques in the study of immune complex glomerulonephritis, *J. Immunol.* 118, 1788–1794, 1977.

33. Ehrlich, R., and Witz, I.P., The elution of antibodies from viable murine tumor cells, *J. Immunol. Methods* 26, 345–353, 1979.

34. McIntosh, R.M., Garcia, R., Rubio, L., et al., Evidence of an autologous immune complex pathogenic mechanism in acute poststreptococcal glomerulonephritis, *Kidney Int.* 14, 501–510, 1978.

35. Theofilopoulos, A.N., Eisenberg, R.A., and Dixon, F.J., Isolation of circulating immune complexes using Raji cells. Separation of antigens from immune complexes and production of antiserum, *J. Clin. Invest.* 61, 1570–1581, 1978.

36. Tomino, Y., Sakai, H., Endoh, M., et al., Cross-reactivity of eluted antibodies from renal tissues of patients with Henoch-Schonlein purpura nephritis and IgA nephropathy, *Am. J. Nephrol.* 3, 315–318, 1983.

37. Shi, S.R., Chaiwun, B., Young, L., et al., Antigen retrieval techniques utilizing citrate buffer or urea solution for immunohistochemical demonstration of androgen receptor in formalin-fixed paraffin sections, *J. Histochem. Cytochem.* 41, 1599–1604, 1993.

38. Langlois, N.E., King, G., Herriot, R., and Thompson, W.D., Non-enzymatic retrieval of antigen permits staining of follicle centre cells by the rabbit polyclonal antibody to protein gene product 9.5, *J. Pathol.* 173, 249–253, 1994.

39. Leong, A.S., Microwaves in diagnostic immunohistochemistry, *Eur. J. Morphol.* 34, 381–383, 1996.

40. Lucas, D.R., al-Abbadi, M., Teabaczka, P., et al., c-Kit expression in desmoid fibroblastosis. Comparative immunohistochemical evaluation of two commercial antibodies, *Am. J. Clin. Pathol.* 119, 339–345, 2003.

41. Imam, S.A., Young, L., Chaiwun, B., and Taylor, C.B., Comparison of two microwave based antigen-retrieval solutions in unmasking epitopes in formalin-fixed tissues for immunostaining, *Anticancer Res.* 15, 1153–1158, 1995.

42. Pileri, S.A., Roncador, G., Ceccarelli, C., et al., Antigen retrieval techniques in immunohistochemistry: Comparison of different methods, *J. Pathol.* 183, 116–123, 1997.

43. Rocken, C., and Roessner, A., An evaluation of antigen retrieval procedures for immunoelectron microscopic classification of amyloid deposits, *J. Histochem. Cytochem.* 47, 1385–1394, 1999.

44. Ishikawa, K., and Iwai, K., Affinity chromatography of cysteine-containing histone, *J. Biochem.* 77, 391–398, 1975.

45. Chadha, K.C., Grob, P.M., Mikulski, A.J., et al., Copper chelate affinity chromatography of human fibroblast and leucocyte interferons, *J. Gen. Virol.* 43, 701–706, 1979.

46. Tanaka, H., Sasaki, I., Yamashita, K., et al., Affinity chromatography of porcine pancreas deoxyribonuclease I on DNA-binding Sepharose under non-digestive conditions, using its substrate-binding site, *J. Biochem.* 88, 797–806, 1980.

47. Smith, R.L., and Griffin, C.A., Separation of plasma fibronectin from associated hemagglutinating activity by elution from gelatin-agarose at pH 5.5, *Thromb. Res.* 37, 91–101, 1985.

48. Martin, L.N., Separation of guinea pig IgG subclasses by affinity chromatography on protein A-Sepharose, *J. Immunol. Methods* 52, 205–212, 1982.

49. Compton, B.J., Lewis, M.A., Whigham, F., et al., Analytical potential of protein A for affinity chromatography of polyclonal and monoclonal antibodies, *Anal. Chem.* 61, 1314–1317, 1989.

50. Giraudi, G., and Baggiani, C., Strategy for fractionating high-affinity antibodies to steroid hormones by affinity chromatography, *Analyst* 121, 939–944, 1996.

51. Arakawa, T., Philo, J.S., Tsumoto, K., et al., Elution of antibodies from a Protein-A column by aqueous arginine solutions, *Protein Expr. Purif.* 36, 244–248, 2004.

52. Ghose, S., McNerney, T., and Hubbard, B., Protein A affinity chromatography for capture and purification of monoclonal antibody and Fc-fusion protein: Practical considerations for process development, in *Process Scale Bioseparations for the Biopharmaceutical Industry*, ed. A.A. Shukla, M.R. Etzel, and S. Gadam, CRC/Taylor & Francis Group, Boca Raton, FL, Chapter 16, pp. 462–489, 2007.

53. Makino, T., Nakamura, K., and Takahara, K., A high-performance liquid immunoaffinity chromatography method for determining transferrin-bound iron In serum, *Clin. Chim. Acta* 412, 914–919, 2011.

HEPES (4-(2-HYDROXYETHYL)-1-PIPERIZINEETHANESULFONIC ACID)

HEPES is a "Good" buffer.[1] However, reagent purity may be an issue.[2–5] There are several studies on the binding of Cu(II) by HEPES.[6,7] But one of these studies[7] showed that an impurity in HEPES was responsible for binding Cu(II).[7] The oxidation of HEPES by hydrogen peroxide[8] and Cu(II)[9] has been reported. Radical oxygen species can produce radical species from HEPES.[10] Those radical oxygen species are formed from the autooxidation of iron via the Haber-Weiss process. An Impurity in HEPES was Reported to Activate 5′-Nucleotidase.[11]

A validated method for determining the purity of HEPES products has been reported.[12] Independent of reagent purity, there may be intrinsic properties of HEPES that need to be considered. Enhanced degradation of pure magnesium metal in the presence of HEPES as compared to a bicarbonate solution has been observed.[13] An effect of HEPES on the Lowry protein assay has also been reported,[14–16] with perhaps a lesser effect on the closely related bicinchoninic acid.[16,17] HEPES buffer does not affect the assay for Cu(I) with bicinchoninic acid.[18] It is tempting to suggest that the effect of HEPES on Cu(II) in protein assays is due to impurities present in the individual HEPES preparation. HEPES is being used in the processing of tissue samples (tissue fixation) for microscopic analysis.[19,20]

1. Good, N.E., Winget, G.D., Winter, W., et al., Hydrogen ion buffers for biological research, *Biochemistry* 5, 467–477, 1966.
2. Tadolini, B., Iron autoxidation in Mops and Hepes buffers, *Free Radic. Res. Commun.* 4, 149–160, 1987.
3. Simpson, J.A., Cheeseman, K.H., Smith, S.E., and Dean, R.T., Free-radical generation by copper ions and hydrogen peroxide. Stimulation by Hepes buffer, *Biochem. J.* 254, 519–523, 1988.
4. Abas, L., and Guppy M., Acetate: A contaminant in Hepes buffer, *Anal. Biochem.* 229, 131–140, 1995.
5. Li, Y., Yang, X., Wang, D., et al., Striking effects of storage buffers on apparent half-lives of the activity *Pseudomonas aeruginosa* arylsulfatase, *Protein J.* 35, 283–298, 2016.
6. Sokolowska, M., and Bal, W., Cu(II) complexation by "non-coordinating" *N*-2-hydroxyethylpiperazine-*N'*-ethanesulfonic acid (HEPES buffer), *J. Inorg. Biochem.* 99, 1653–1660, 2005.
7. Mash, H.E., Chin, Y.-D., Siggs, L., Having, R., and Xuo, H., Complexation of copper by zwitterionic aminosulfonic (Good) buffers, *Anal. Chem.* 75, 671–677, 2003.
8. Zhao, G., and Chasteen, N.D., Oxidation of Good's buffers by hydrogen peroxide, *Anal. Biochem.* 349, 262–267, 2006.
9. Hegetschweiler, K., and Saltman, P., Interaction of Cu(II) with *N*-(2-hydroxyethyl)piperazine-*N'*-ethanesulfonic acid (HEPES), *Inorg. Chem.* 25, 107–109, 1986.
10. Grady, J.K., Chasteen, N.D., and Harris, D.C., Radicals from "Good's" buffers, *Anal. Biochem.* 173, 111–115, 1988.
11. Le Hir, M., Impurity in buffer substances mimics the effects of ATP on soluble 5'-nucleotidase, *Enzyme* 45, 194–199, 1991.
12. Xu, X., Gevaert, B., Bracke, N., et al., Hydrophilic interaction liquid chromatography method development and validation for the assay of HEPES zwitterionic buffer, *J. Pharm. Biomed. Anal.* 135, 227–233, 2017.
13. Kirkland, N.T., Waterman, J., Birbilis, N., et al., Buffer-regulated biocorrosion of pure magnesium, *J. Mater. Sci. Mater. Med.* 23, 283–291, 2012.
14. Turner, L.V., and Manchester, K.L., Interference of HEPES with the Lowry method, *Science* 170, 649, 1970.
15. Himmel, H.M., and Heller, W., Studies of the interference of selected substances with two modifications of the Lowry protein determination, *J. Clin. Chem. Clin. Biochem.* 25, 909–913, 1987.
16. Lleu, P.L., and Rebel, G., Interference of Good's buffer and other biological buffer with protein determination, *Anal. Biochem.* 192, 215–218, 1991.
17. Kaushal, V., and Barnes, L.D., Effect of zwitterionic buffers on measurement of small masses of protein with bicinchoniic acid, *Anal. Biochem.* 157, 291–294, 1986.
18. Brenner, A.J., and Harris, E.D., A quantitative test for copper using bicinchoninic acid, *Anal. Biochem.* 226, 80–84, 1995.
19. Wiedorn, K.H., Olert, J., Stacy, R.A., et al., HOPE: A new fixing technique enables preservation and extraction of high molecular weight DNA and RNA of >20 kb from paraffin-embedded tissues. Hepes-glutamic acid buffer mediated organic solvent protection effect, *Pathol. Res. Pract.* 198, 735–740, 2002.
20. Marwitz, S., Kolarova, J., Reck, M., et al., The tissue is the issue: Improved methlome analysis from paraffin-embedded tissues by application of the HOPE technique, *Lab. Invest.* 94, 927–933, 2014.

Other observations on the use HEPES buffer:

Chirpich, T.P., The effect of different buffers on terminal deoxynucleotidyl transferase activity, *Biochim. Biophys. Acta* 518, 535–538, 1978;.
Fulop, L., Szigeti, G., Magyar, J., et al., Differences in electrophysiological and contractile properties of mammalian cardiac tissues bathed in bicarbonate – and HEPES-buffered solutions, *Acta Physiol. Scand.* 178, 11–18, 2003.
Hartman, R.F., and Rose, S.D., Kinetics and mechanism of the addition of nucleophiles to alpha, beta-unsaturated thiol esters, *J. Org. Chem.* 71, 6342–6350, 2006.
Mash, H.E., Chin, Y.P., Sigg, L., et al., Complexation of copper by zwitterionic aminosulfonic, *Anal. Chem.* 75, 671-677, 2003.
Schmidt, K., Pfeiffer, S., and Mayer, B., Reaction of peroxynitrite with HEPES or MOPS results in the formation of nitric oxide donors, *Free Radic. Biol. Med.* 24, 859–862, 1998.

MES (1-MORPHOLINEETHANE-SULFONIC ACID; 2-(4-MORPHOLINO) ETHANE SULFONATE)

MES is a "Good" buffer.[1] There is a method for the evaluation of the purity of MES preparations.[2] An impurity in MES has been reported to activate a 5'-nucleotidase.[3]

MES does not appear to have an effect on the bicinchoninic acid assay for measuring protein concentration.[4] MES has been used as a buffer in hydroponic studies.[5–7] Several of these studies noted the use of an ion-exchange resin, IRC-50, as a solid-phase buffer.[5,6] Carbon quantum dots have been prepared from MES by a hydrothermal process.[8]

1. Good, N.E., Winget, G.D., Winter, W., et al., Hydrogen ion buffers for biological research, *Biochemistry* 5, 467–477, 1966.
2. Zhang, T., Hewitt, D., and Kuo, Y.H., SEC assay of polyvinylsulfonic impurities in 2(*N*-morphoolino) ethanesulfonic acid using a charged aerosol detector, *Chromatographia* 72, 142–149, 2010.
3. Le Hir, M., Impurity in buffer substances mimics the effect of ATP on soluble 5' nucleotidase, *Enzyme* 45, 194–199, 1991.
4. Kaushal, V., and Barnes, L.D., Effect of zwitterionic buffers on measurement of small masses of protein with bicinchoninic acid, *Anal. Biochem.* 157, 291–294, 1986.
5. Bugbee, B.G., and Salisbury, F.B., An evaluation of MES (2(*N*-morpholino)ethanesulfonic acid) and Amberlite 1RC-50 as pH buffers for nutrient growth studies, *J. Plant Nutr.* 8, 567–583, 1985.
6. Frick, J., and Mitchell, C.A., Stabilization of pH in solid-matrix hydroponic systems, *HortiScience* 28, 981–984, 1993.
7. Zhu, Y.G., Geng, C.N., Tong, Y.P., Smith, S.E., and Smith, F.A., Phosphorus(Pi) and arsenate uptake by two whet (*Triticum aestivum*) cultivars and their doubled haploid lines, *Ann. Bot.* 98, 631–636, 2006.
8. Samantara, A.K., Maji, S., Ghosh, A., et al., Good's buffer derived highly emissive carbon quantum dots: Excellent biocompatible anticancer drug carrier, *J. Mater. Chem.* 4, 2412–2420, 2016.

Some other studies using MES as a buffer:

Gelfi, C., Vigano, A., Curcio, M., et al., Single-strand conformation polymorphism analysis by capillary zone electrophoresis in neutral pH buffer, *Electrophoresis* 21, 785–791, 2000.
Hosse, M., and Wilkinson, K.J., Determination of electrophoretic mobilities and hydrodynamic radii of three humic substances as a function of pH and ionic strength, *Environ. Sci. Technol.* 35, 4301–4306, 2001.
Krajewska, B., and Ciurli, S., Jack bean (*Canavalia ensiformis*) urease. Probing acid-base groups of the active site by pH variation, *Plant Physiol. Biochem.* 43, 651–658, 2005.
Ozkara, S., Akgol, S., Canak, Y., and Denizli, A., A novel magnetic adsorbent for immunoglobulin-g purification in a magnetically stabilized fluidized bed, *Biotechnol. Prog.* 20, 1169–1175, 2004.
Vasseur, M., Frangne, R., and Alvarado, F., Buffer-dependent pH sensitivity of the fluorescent chloride-indicator dye SPQ, *Am. J. Physiol.* 264, C27–C31, 1993.
Walsh, M.K., Wang, X., and Weimer, B.C., Optimizing the immobilization of single-stranded DNA onto glass beads, *J. Biochem. Biophys. Methods* 47, 221–231, 2001.

MOPS (3-(*N*-MORPHOLINO) PROPANESULFONIC ACID; 4-MORPHOLINE-PROPANESULFONIC ACID)

MOPS is a "Good" buffer.[1] Incubation of peroxynitrite with MOPS buffer resulted in the formation of nitric acid donors.[2] The observation was that the incubation of peroxynitrite with endothelial cells resulted in a 12-fold increase in cGMP. Such an increase was not observed with phosphate buffer. A 20-fold increase was observed with HEPES. MOPS buffers, as well as other Good buffers such as HEPES and PIPES, interfere with the contractile response of smooth muscle.[3,4] These investigators suggested that "natural" anion buffers such as bicarbonate are critical to physiological function. MOPS (and HEPES) reacts with tetranitromethane to produce free radicals.[5] High concentrations of buffer (~1 M) of MOPS (and other buffers) may show specific interaction with proteins.[6–9]

1. Good, N.E., Winget, G.D., Winter, W., et al., Hydrogen ion buffers for biological research, *Biochemistry* 5, 467–477, 1966.
2. Schmidt, K., Pfeiffer, S., and Mayer, B., Reaction of peroxynitrite with HEPES or MOPS results in the formation of nitric oxide donors, *Free Radic. Biol. Med.* 24, 859–862, 1998.
3. Altura, B.M., Altura, B.M., Carella, A., and Altura, B.T., Adverse effects of Tris, HEPES and MOPS buffers on contractile responses of arterial and venous smooth muscle induced by prostaglandins, *Prostaglandins Med.* 5, 123–130, 1980.
4. Altura, B.M., Altura, B.T., Carella, A., and Turlapaty, P.D., Ca^{2+} coupling in vascular smooth muscle; Mg^{2+} and buffer effects on contractility and membrane Ca^{2+} movements, *Can. J. Physiol. Pharmacol.* 60, 459–482, 1982.
5. Hodges, G.R., and Ingold, K.U., Superoxide, amine buffers and tetranitromethane: A novel free radical chain reaction, *Free Radic. Res.* 33, 547–550, 2000.
6. Ishihara, H., and Welsh, M.J., Block by MOPS reveals a conformation change in the CFTR pore produced by ATP hydrolysis, *Am. J. Physiol.* 273, C1278–C1289, 1997.
7. Gupta, B.S., Taha, M., and Lee, M.J., Buffers more than buffering agents: Introducing a new class of stabilizers for the protein BSA, *Phys. Chem. Chem. Phys.* 17, 1114–1133, 2015.
8. Schmidt, J., Wei, F., Oeser, T., et al., Effect of Tris, MOPS, and phosphate buffers on the hydrolysis of polyethylene films by polyester hydrolases, *FEBS Open Biol.* 6, 919–927, 2016.
9. Zhang, J., and Hwang, T.C., Electrostatic tuning of the pre- and post-hydrolytic open states in CFTR, *J. Gen. Physiol.* 149, 355–372, 2017.

Some general references on MOPS buffer:

Corona-Izquierdo, F.P., and Membrillo-Hernandez, J., Biofilm formation in *Escherichia coli* is affected by 3-(*N*-morpholino)propane sulfonate (MOPS), *Res. Microbiol.* 153, 181–185, 2002.

Cvetkovic, A., Zomerdijk, M., Straathof, A.J., et al., Adsorption of fluorescein by protein crystals, *Biotechnol. Bioeng.* 87, 658–668, 2004.

de Carmen Candia-Plata, M., Garcia, J., Guzman, R., et al., Isolation of human serum immunoglobulins with a new salt-promoted adsorbent, *J. Chromatog. A.* 1118, 211–217, 2006.

Denizli, A., Alkan, M., Garipcan, B., et al., Novel metal-chelate affinity adsorbent for purification of immunoglobulin-G from human plasma, *J. Chromatog. B. Analyt. Technol. Biomed. Life. Sci.* 795, 93–103, 2003.

Emir, S., Say, R., Yavuz, H., and Denizli, A., A new metal chelate affinity adsorbent for cytochrome C, *Biotechnol. Prog.* 20, 223–228, 2004.

Gayán, E., Condón, S., Álvarez, I., et al., Effect of pressure-induced changes in the ionization equilibria of buffers on inactivation of *Escherichia coli* and *Staphylococcus aureus* by high hydrostatic pressures, *Appl. Environ. Microbiol.* 79, 4041–4047, 2013.

Ishihara, H., and Welsh, M.J., Block by MOPS reveals a conformation change in the CFTR pore produced by ATP hydrolysis, *Am. J. Physiol.* 273, C1278–C1289, 1997.

Janc, T., Vlachy, V., and Lukšič, M., Calorimetric studies of interaction between low molecular weight salts and bovine serum albumin in water at pH values below and above the isoionic point, *J. Mol. Liq.* 270, 74–80, 2018.

Johnson, R.A., Fulcher, L.M., Vang, K., et al., In depth, thermodynamic analysis of Ca^{2+} binding parameters, *Biochim. Biophys. Acta Proteom.* 1867, 359–366, 2019.

Mash, H.E., Chin, Y.P., Sigg, L., et al., Complexation of copper by zwitterionic aminosulfonic (good) buffers, *Anal. Chem.* 75, 671–677, 2003.

Roy, L.N., Roy, R.N., Allen, K.A., et al., Buffer standards for the physiological pH of the zwitterionic compound of 3-(*N*-morpholino)propanesulfonic acid (MOPS) from T = (278.15 to 328.15) K, *J. Chem. Thermodyn.* 47, 21–27, 2012.

Roy, R.N., Gibbons, J.J., McGinnis, T., and Woodmansee, R., Standard electromotive force of the H_2-AgCl;Ag cell in 30, 40, and 50 mass% glycerol/water from −20 to 25 degrees C: pK_2 and pH values for a standard "mops" buffer in 50 mass% glycerol/water, *Cryobiology* 22, 578–588, 1985.

Strelau, J.H., Berens, M.J., and Arnold, W.A., Minerology and buffer identity effects on RDX kinetics and intermediates during reaction with natural and synthetic magnetite, *Chemosphere* 213, 602–609, 2018.

Tadolini, B., Iron autoxidation in Mops and Hepes buffers, *Free Radic. Res. Commun.* 4, 149–160, 1987.

Tadolini, B., Iron oxidation in Mops buffer. Effect of EDTA, hydrogen peroxide and $FeCl_3$, *Free Radic. Res. Commun.* 4, 172–182, 1987.

Tadolini, B., and Sechi, A.M., Iron oxidation in Mops buffer. Effect of phosphorus containing compounds, *Free Radic. Res. Commun.* 4, 161–172, 1987.

Vrakas, D., Giaginis, C., and Tsantili-Kakoulidou, A., Different retention behavior of structurally diverse basic and neutral drugs in immobilized artificial membrane and reversed-phase high performance liquid chromatography: Comparison with octanol-water partitioning, *J. Chromatog. A.* 1116, 158–164, 2006.

PHOSPHATE

Phosphate buffers are among the most common buffers used for biological studies. It is noted that the use of phosphate solutions in early transfusion medicine lead to the discovery of the importance of calcium ions in blood coagulation.[1] Many investigators use phosphate buffer saline (PBS; generally 0.01 M sodium phosphate—0.14 M NaCl, pH 7.2). A consideration of the literature suggests that there is an incredible variation in PBS, so it is necessary to verify composition—the only common factor that this writer finds is 0.01 M (10 mM) phosphate is extensively used. The ionic strength of PBS is intended to closely resemble that of most biological fluids. Sodium phosphate buffers are the most common, but there is extensive use of potassium phosphate buffers and mixtures of sodium and potassium. Unfortunately many investigators simply refer to phosphate buffer without respect to its counter ion. Also, investigators will prepare a stock solution of sodium phosphate, usually sodium dihydrogen phosphate (sodium phosphate, monobasic) or disodium hydrogen phosphate (sodium phosphate, dibasic), and adjust the pH as required with (usually) hydrochloric acid and/or sodium hydrogen. This is not preferable and, if used, must be described in the text to permit other investigators to repeat the experiment. pH changes in phosphate buffers during freezing can be dramatic.[2–7] Phosphate binds divalent cations in solutions and can form insoluble salts; the sequestration of divalent cations can influence biological reactions by binding cations such as calcium, platinum, and iron.[8–13] Phosphate buffers have been shown to inhibit other enzymes.[14–19] There also situations where buffers such as Tris or HEPES appear to inhibit enzyme activity relative to a phosphate buffer.[20] A phosphate buffer also appeared to stabilize HEWL from fibrillation in comparison to other buffers.[21]

1. Hutchin, P., History of blood transfusion: A tercentennial look, *Surgery* 64, 685–700, 1968.
2. van den Berg, L., and Rose, D., Effect of freezing on the pH and composition of sodium and potassium phosphate solutions: The reciprocal system KH_2PO_4-Na_2PO_4-H_2O, *Arch. Biochem. Biophys.* 81, 319–329, 1959.
3. Williams-Smith, D.L., Bray, R.C., Barber, M.J, Tsopanakis, A.D., and Vincent, S.P., Changes in apparent pH on freezing aqueous buffer solutions and their relevance to biochemical electron-paramagnetic-resonance spectroscopy, *Biochem. J* 167, 593–600, 1977.

4. Murase, N., and Franks, F., Salt precipitation during the freeze-concentration of phosphate buffer solutions, *Biophys. Chem.* 34, 393–300, 1989.

5. Pikal-Cleland, K.A., and Carpenter, J.F., Lyophilization-induced protein denaturation in phosphate buffer systems: Monomeric and tetrameric beta-galactosidase, *J. Pharm. Sci.* 90, 1255–1268, 2001.

6. Gomez, G., Pikal, M., and Rodriguez-Hornedo, N., Effect of initial buffer composition on pH changes during far-from-equilibrium freezing of sodium phosphate buffer solutions, *Pharm. Res.* 18, 90–97, 2001.

7. Pikal-Cleland, K.A., Cleland, J.L., Anchorodoquy, T.J., and Carpenter, J.F., Effect of glycine on pH changes and protein stability during freeze-thawing in phosphate buffer systems, *J. Pharm. Sci.* 91, 1969–1979, 2002.

8. Staum, M.M., Incompatibility of phosphate buffer in 99^{m}Tc-sulfur colloid containing aluminum ion, *J. Nucl. Med.* 13, 386–387, 1972.

9. Frank, G.B., Antagonism by phosphate buffer of the twitch ions in isolated muscle fibers produced by calcium-free solutions, *Can. J. Physiol. Pharmacol.* 56, 523–526, 1978.

10. Hasegawa, K., Hashi, K., and Okada, R., Physicochemical stability of pharmaceutical phosphate buffer solutions. I. Complexation behavior of Ca(II) with additives in phosphate buffer solutions, *J. Parenter. Sci. Technol.* 36, 128–133, 1982.

11. Abe, K., Kogure, K., Arai, H., and Nakano, M., Ascorbate induced lipid peroxidation results in loss of receptor binding in tris, but not in phosphate, buffer. Implications for the involvement of metal ions, *Biochem. Int.* 11, 341–348, 1985.

12. Pedersen, H.B., Josephsen, J., and Keerszan, G., Phosphate buffer and salt medium concentrations affect the inactivation of T4 phage by platinum(II) complexes, *Chem. Biol. Interact.* 54, 1–8, 1985.

13. Kuzuya, M., Yamada, K., Hayashi, T., et al., Oxidation of low-density lipoprotein by copper and iron in phosphate buffer, *Biochim. Biophys. Acta* 1084, 198–201, 1991.

14. Modak, M.J., and Marcus, S.L., Purification and properties of Rauscher leukemia virus DNA polymerase and selective inhibition of mammalian viral reverse transcriptase by inorganic phosphate, *J. Biol. Chem.* 252, 11–19, 1977.

15. Doehlert, D.C., and Huber, S.C., Phosphate inhibition of spinach leaf sucrose phosphate synthase as affected by gluose-6-phosphate and glucose phosphoglucoisomerase, *Plant Physiol.* 76, 250–253, 1984.

16. Libbe, C., Wolfe, S., and Demain, A.L., Repression and inhibition of cephalosporin synthase in *Streptomyces clavuligerus* by inorganic phosphate, *Arch. Microbiol.* 140, 317–320, 1985.

17. Notomi, T., Ikeda, Y., Okadome, A., and Nagayama, A., The inhibitory effect of phosphate on the ligase reaction used for detecting *Chlamydia trachomatis*, *J. Clin. Pathol.* 51, 306–308, 1998.

18. Hartman, M.D., Figueroa, C.M., Arias, D.G., and Iglecias, A.A., Inhibition of recombinant aldolase 6-phosphate reductase from peach leaves by hexose phosphates, inorganic phosphates, and oxidants, *Plant Cell Physiol.* 58, 145–155, 2017.

19. Fukunaga, R., Loquacious PD removes phosphate inhibition of Dicer-2 processing of hairpin RNA into siRNA, *Biochem. Biophys. Res. Commun.* 498, 1022–1027, 2018.

20. Lund, P., and Wiggins, D., Inhibition of carbamoyl phosphate synthase (ammonia) by Tris and Hepes. Effect on Ka for *N*-acetylglutamate, *Biochem. J.* 243, 273–276, 1987.

21. Brudar, S., and Hribar-Lee, B., The role of buffers in wild-type HEWL amyloid fibril formation mechanism, *Biomolecules* 9, E65, 2019.

Some other studies on phosphate buffer:

Ahmad, I., Fasihullah, Z., and Vaid, F.H., Effect of phosphate buffer on photodegradation reactions of riboflavin in aqueous solution, *J. Photochem. Photobiol. B* 78, 229–234, 2005.

Buchanan, D.D., Jameson, E.E., Perlette, J., et al., Effect of buffer, electric field, and separation time on detection of aptamers-ligand complexes for affinity probe capillary electrophoresis, *Electrophoresis* 24, 1375–1382, 2003.

Gebauer, P., and Bocek, P., New aspects of buffering with multivalent weak acids in capillary zone electrophoresis: Pros and cons of the phosphate buffer, *Electrophoresis* 21, 2809–2813, 2000.

Gebauer, P., Pantuikova, P., and Bocek, P., Capillary zone electrophoresis in phosphate buffer – known or unknown?, *J. Chromatog. A* 894, 89–93, 2000.

Millsap, K.W., Reid, G., van der Mei, H.C., and Busscher, H.J., Adhesion of *Lactobacillus* species in urine and phosphate buffer to silicone rubber and glass under flow, *Biomaterials* 18, 87–91, 1997.

Taborsky, G., Oxidative modification of proteins in the presence of ferrous ion and air. Effect of ionic constituents of the reaction medium on the nature of the oxidation products, *Biochemistry* 12, 1341–1348, 1973.

Wolf, W.J., and Sly, D.A., Effects of buffer cations on chromatography of proteins on hydroxylapatite, *J. Chromatog.* 15, 247–250, 1964.

PIPES (PIPERAZINE-*N*,*N*'-BIS(2-ETHANESULFONIC ACID); 1,4-PIPERAZINEDIETHANE ACID)

PIPES is a "Good" buffer.[1] As with HEPES, PIPES has been used in tissue fixation,[2] but both buffers have been suggested to introduce artifacts.[3] PIPES has also been used for cytocemistry.[4]

PIPES has also been used in the processing of samples for electron microscopy.[5–7] PIPES, as did some other buffers, inhibited the reaction of iodoacetate with active site of liver alcohol dehydrogenase.[8] There was a lesser effect on the reaction with an affinity label (*R*,*S*-2-bromo-3-(5-imidazolyl)propionic acid. PIPES (or HEPES) was shown to promote free radical generation from H_2O_2 in the presence of Cu(II).[9,10] Data have been obtained for the binding of zinc by PIPES.[11] PIPES (also HEPES and MES) have been observed to inhibit oxidation of phenolic compounds by peroxidase.[12] PIPES (also MES and HEPES) was shown to contain an impurity that mimics ATP in the activation of 5-nucleotidase.[13] Tubulin polymerization is enhanced in the presence of PIPES buffer as compared to MES buffer.[14] Uranium(IV) was observed to be more toxic toward *Desulfovibrio desulfuricans* in the presence of PIPES than in bicarbonate.[15]

1. Good, N.E., Winget, G.D., Winter, W., et al., Hydrogen ion buffers for biological research, *Biochemistry* 5, 467–477, 1966.
2. Montanaro, J., Gruber, D., and Leisch, N., Improved ultrastructure of marine invertebrates using non-toxic buffers, *PeerJ* 4, e1860, 2016.
3. Nie, J., Mahato, S., and Zelhof, A.C., Imaging the *Drosophila* retina: Zwitterionic buffers PIPES and HEPES induce morphological artifacts in tissue fixation, *BMC Dev. Biol.* 15:10, 2015.
4. Yamamoto, K., and Ogawa, K., Effects of NaOH-PIPES buffer used in aldehyde fixative on alkaline phosphatase activity in rat hepatocytes, *Histochemistry* 77, 339–351, 1983.
5. Baur, P.S., and Stacey, T.R., The use of PIPES buffer in the fixation of mammalian and marine tissues for electron microscopy, *J. Micros.* 109, 315–327, 1977.
6. Schiff, R.I., and Gennaro, J.F., Jr., The influence of the buffer on maintenance of tissue liquid in specimens for scanning electron microscopy, *Scan. Electron Microsc.* (3), 449–458, 1979.
7. Haviernick, S., Lalague, E.D., Corvellec, M.R., et al., The use of Hanks'—pipes buffers in the preparation of human, normal leukocytes for TEM observation, *J. Microsc.* 135, 83–88, 1984.
8. Syvertsen, C., and McKinley-McKee, J.S., Affinity labeling of liver alcohol dehydrogenase. Effects of pH and buffers on affinity labelling with iodoacetic acid and (R,S-2-bromo-3-(5-imidazolyl)propionic acid, *Eur. J. Biochem.* 117, 165–170, 1981.
9. Simpson, J.A., Cheeseman, K.H., Smith, S.E., and Dean, R.T., Free-radical generation by copper ions and hydrogen peroxide. Stimulation by Hepes buffers, *Biochem. J.* 254, 519–523, 1988.
10. Prutz, W.A., The interaction between hydrogen peroxide and the DNA-Cu(I) complex: Effects of pH and buffers, *Z. Naturforsch.* 45, 1197–1206, 1990.
11. Wyrzykowski, D., Tesmar, A., Jacewicz, D., Pranczky, J., and Chmurzyński, L., Zinc(II) complexation by some biologically relevant pH buffers, *J. Mol. Recognit.* 27, 722–726, 2014.
12. Baker, C.J., Mock, N.M., Roberts, D.P., et al., Interference by Mes [2-(4-morpholino)ethanesulfonic acid] and related buffers with phenolic oxidation by peroxidase, *Free Radic. Biol. Med.* 43, 1322–1327, 2007.
13. Le Hir, M., Impurity in buffer substances mimics the effects of ATP on soluble 5′-nucleotidase, *Enzyme* 45, 194–199, 1991.
14. Waxman, P.G., del Campo, A.A., Lowe, M.C., and Hamel, E., Induction of polymerization of purified tubulin by sulfonate buffers. Marked differences between 4-morpholineethananesulfonate (Mes) and 1,4-piperazineethanesulfonate(Pipes), *Eur. J. Biochem.* 129, 129–136, 1981.
15. Sani, R.K., Peyton, B.M., and Dohnalkova, A., Toxic effects of uranium on *Desulfovibrio desulfuricans* G20, *Environ. Toxicol. Chem.* 25, 1231–1238, 2006.

Some other references to the use of PIPES buffer:

Altura, B.M., Altura, B.T., Carella, A., and Turlapty, P.D., Adverse effects of artificial buffers on contractile responses of arterial and venous smooth muscles, *Br. J. Pharmacol.* 69, 207–214, 1980.
Correla, J.J., Lipscomb, L.D., Dabrowiak, J.C., et al., Cleavage of tubulin by vandate ion, *Arch. Biochem. Biophys.* 309, 94–104, 1994.
Lee, B.H., and Nowak, T., Influence of pH on the Mn^{2+} activation of and binding to yeast enolase: A functional study, *Biochemistry* 31, 2165–2171, 1992.
Moore, S.A., Kingston, R.L., Loomes, K.M., et al., The structure of truncated recombinant human bile salt-stimulated lipase reveals bile salt-independent conformational flexibility at the active-site loop and provides insights into heparin binding, *J. Mol. Biol.* 3 12, 511–523, 2001.
Olmsted, J.B., and Borisy, G.G., Ionic and nucleotide requirements for microtubule polymerization *in vitro*, *Biochemistry* 14, 2996–3005, 1975.
Roy, R.N., Gibbons, J.J., Pardron, J.L., Buechter, K., and Faszholz, S., Sodium 1,4-piperazinedithansulfonate monohydrate ("Pipes") for measurement of pH of blood and other physiological media, *Clin. Chem.* 26, 1919–1920, 1980.
Roy, R.N., Gibbons, J.J., Padron, J.L., et al., Revised values of the paH of monosodium 1,4-piperazinediethanesulfonate ("Pipes") in water other buffers in isotonic saline at various temperatures, *Clin. Chem.* 27, 1787–1788, 1981.
Schmidt, J., Mangold, C., and Deitmer, J., Membrane responses evoked by organic buffers in identified leech neurones, *J. Exp. Biol.* 199, 327–335, 1996.
Tedokon, M., Suzuki, K., Kayamori, Y., et al., Enzymatic assay of inorganic phosphate with the use of sucrose phosphorylase and phosphoglucomutase, *Clin. Chem.* 38, 512–515, 1992.

TES (N-TRIS(HYDROXYMETHYL) METHYL-2-AMINOETHANE-SULFONIC ACID)

TES is a "Good" buffer.[1] It has been shown to complex certain divalent cations such as Cu(II) and Zn(II), but not Ca(II).[2] TES has a small effect on the bicinhoninic acid assay for protein concentration.[3] The presence of TES has been shown to induce a phase separation in a mixture of water and water-miscible organics such as acetone and acetonitrile.[4] In an early study, TES or HEPES supported the growth of several mammalian cell lines as well as bicarbonate in stoppered flasks.[5] This was not true in open cultures that required supplemental bicarbonate. Photosynthetic oxygen evolution in a blue-green alga was observed to be reduced in medium containing TES or phosphate compared to medium containing tricine.[6] Further reduction was observed with a Tris buffer. It was suggested that the effect of TES was directed toward electron transport. TES and HEPES have been shown to be useful in the use of equilibrium dialysis to study calcium binding to protein.[7]

1. Good, N.E., Winget, G.D., Winter, W., et al., Hydrogen ion buffers for biological research, *Biochemistry* 5, 467–477, 1966.
2. Nakon, R., and Krishnamoorthy, C.R., Free-metal ion depletion by "Good's" buffers, *Science* 221, 749–750, 1983.
3. Kaushal, V., and Varnes, L.D., Effect of zwitterionic buffers on measurement of small masses of protein with bicinchoninic acid, *Anal. Biochem.* 157, 291–294, 1986.
4. Taha, M., and Lee, M.J., TES buffer-induced phase separation of aqueous solutions of several water-miscible organic solvents at 298.15 K: Phase diagrams and molecular dynamic simulations, *J. Chem. Phys.* 138, 244501, 2013.
5. Itagaki, A., and Kimura, G., Tes and HEPES buffers in mammalian cell cultures and viral studies: Problem of carbon dioxide requirement, *Exp. Cell Res.* 83, 351–361, 1974.
6. Bridges, S., and Ward, B., Effect of hydrogen ion buffers on photosynthetic oxygen evolution in the blue-green alga, *Agmenellum quadruplicatum*, *Microbios* 15, 49–56, 1976.
7. Kragh-Hansen, U., and Vorum, H., Quantitative analyses of the interaction between calcium ions and human serum albumin, *Clin. Chem.* 39, 202–208, 1993.

Some additional references on the use of TES buffer:

Bhattacharyya, A., and Yanagimachi, R., Synthetic organic pH buffers can support fertilization of guinea pig eggs, but not as efficiently as bicarbonate buffer, *Gamete Res.* 19, 123–129, 1988.

Jacobs, B.R., Caulfield, J., and Boldt, J., Analysis of TEST (TES and Tris) yolk buffer effects of human sperm, *Fertil. Steril.* 63, 1064–1070, 1995.

Poole, C.A., Reilly, H.C., and Flint, M.H., The adverse effects of HEPES, TES, and BES zwitterionic buffers on the ultrastructure of cultured chick embryo epiphyseal chondrocytes, *In Vitro* 18, 755–765, 1982.

Taha, M., Buffers for the physiological pH range: Acidic dissociation constants of zwitterionic compounds in various hydroorganic media, *Ann. Chim.* 95, 105–109, 2005.

Veeck, L.L., TES and Tris (TEST)-yolk buffer systems, sperm function testing, and in vitro fertilization, *Fertil. Steril.* 58, 484–486, 1992.

TRICINE (N-[TRIS(HYDROXYMETHYL) METHYL]GLYCINE; N-[2-HYDROXY-1,1-BIS-(HYDROXYMETHYL)ETHYL] GLYCINE)

Tricine is a good buffer.[1] Tricine is also used as a chelating agent, useful for cupric ions and zinc ions.[2,3] The affinity of tricine for Cu(II) and Zn(II) permits use as a metal ion buffer.[4–6] Tricine is also used to complex technetium-99(99mTc) in cancer therapy.[7–11] Tricine interferes with the bicinchoninic acid assay for protein concentration[12] as well as the Lowry assay for protein concentration.[13,14] Tricine has been used in cell culture media[15,16] and as buffer in SDS-Gel electrophoresis.[17–19]

1. Good, N.E., Winget, G.D., Winter, W., et al., Hydrogen ion buffers for biological research, *Biochemistry* 5, 467–477, 1966.
2. Renganathan, M., and Bose, S., Inhibition of photosystem II activity by Cu++ ion. Choice of buffer and reagent is critical, *Photosynth. Res.* 23, 95–99, 1990.
3. Ramos Silva, M., Paixão, J.A., Matos, B.A., and Alte de Veiga, L., Conformational flexibility of tricine as a chelating agents in *catena*-poly-[[(tricinato)copper(II)]-μ-chloro], *Acta Chrystallogr. C* 57, 9–11, 2001.
4. Neumaier, F., Alpdogan, S., Hescheler, J., and Schneider, T., A practical guide to the preparation and use of metal ion-buffered systems for physiological research, *Acta Physiol.*(Oxf) 222, e12988, 2018.
5. Shcheglovitov, A., Vitko, I., Lazarenko, R.M., et al., Molecular and biophysical basis of glutamate and trace metal modulation of voltage-gated Ca$_v$2.3 calcium channels, *J. Gen. Physiol.* 139, 219–234, 2012.
6. Neumaier, F., Akhtar-Schäfer, I., Lüke, J.N., et al., Reciprocal modulation of Ca$_v$2.3 voltage-gated calcium channels by copper (II) ions and kainic acid, *J. Neurochem.* 147, 310–322, 2018.
7. Larsen, S.K., Soloman, H.F., Caldwell, G., and Abrams, M.J., [99mTc]tricine: A useful precursor complex for the radiolabeling of hydrazinonicotinate protein conjugates, *Bioconjugate Chem.* 6, 635–638, 1995.
8. Barrett, J.A., Crocker, A.C., Damphousee, D.J., et al., Biological evaluation of thrombus imaging agents utilizing water soluble phosphines and tricine as coligands when used to label a hydrazinonicotinamide-modified cyclic glycoprotein IIb/IIIa receptor antagonist with 99 mTc, *Bioconjug. Chem.* 8, 155–160, 1997.
9. Bangard, M., Behe, M., Guhlke, S., et al., Detection of somatostatin receptor-positive tumours using the new 99mTc-tricine-HYNIC-D-Phe1-Tyr3-octreotide: First results in patients and comparison with 111In-D-Phe1-octreotide, *Eur. J. Nucl. Med.* 27, 628–637, 2000.
10. Ananias, H.J., Yu, Z., Hoving, H.D., et al., Application of 99mTechnetium-HYNIC(tricine/TPPTS)-Aca-Bombesin (7–14) SPECT/CT in prostate cancer patients: A first-in-man study, *Nucl. Med. Biol.* 40, 933–938, 2013.

11. Shaghaghi, Z., Abedi, S.M., and Hosseinimehr, S.J., Tricine co-ligand improved the efficacy of ^{99m}Tc-HYNIC-(Ser)$_3$-J18 peptide for targeting and imaging of non-small-cell lung cancer, *Biomed. Pharmacother.* 104, 325–331, 2018.

12. Kaushal, V., and Barnes, L.D., Effect of zwitterionic buffers on measurement of small masses of protein with bicinchoninic acid, *Anal. Biochem.* 157, 291–294, 1986.

13. Bensadoun, A., and Weinstein, D., Assay of proteins in the presence of interfering materials, *Anal. Biochem.* 70, 241–250, 1976.

14. Peterson, G.L., Review of the Folin Phenol protein quantitation method of Lowry, Rosebrough, Farr and Randell, *Anal. Biochem.* 100, 201–220, 1979.

15. Garder, R.S., The use of tricine buffer in animal tissue cultures, *J. Cell Biol.* 42, 320–321, 1969.

16. Spendlove, R.S., Crosbie, R.B., Hayes, S.F., and Keeler, R.F., TRICINE-buffered tissue culture media for control of mycoplasma contaminants, *Proc. Soc. Exptl. Biol. Med.* 137, 258–263, 1971.

17. Patton, W.F., Chung-Welch, N., Lopez, M.F., et al., Tris-tricine and tris-borate buffer systems provide better estimates of human mesothelial cell intermediate filament protein molecular weights than the standard Tris-glycine system, *Anal. Biochem.* 197, 25–33, 1991.

18. Wisdom, G.B., Molecular weight determinations using polyacrylamide gel electrophoresis with tris-tricine buffers, *Methods Mol. Biol.* 73, 97–100, 1997.

19. Haider, S.R., Reid, H.J., and Sharp, B.L., Tricine-SDS-PAGE, *Methods Mol. Biol.* 1855, 151–160, 2019.

Other references of the use of tricine buffers:

Bates, R.G., Roy, R.N., and Robinson, R.A., Buffer standards of tris(hydroxymethyl)methylglycine ("tricine") for the physiological range pH 7.2–8.5, *Anal. Chem.* 45, 1663–1666, 1973.

Grande, H.J., and van der Ploeg, K.R., Tricine radicals as formed in the presence of peroxide producing enzymes, *FEBS Lett.* 95, 352–356, 1978.

Hall, M.S., and Leach, F.R., Stability of firefly luciferase in tricine buffer and in a commercial enzyme stabilizer, *J. Biolumin. Chemilumin.* 2, 41–44, 1988.

Le, Q.T., and Katunuma, N., Detection of protease inhibitors by a reverse zymography method, performed in a tris(hydroxylmethyl)aminomethane-tricine buffer system, *Anal. Biochem.* 324, 237–240, 2004.

Roy, R.N., Gibbons, J.J., and Baker, G.E., Acid dissociation constants and pH values for standard "bes" and "tricine" buffer solutions in 30, 40, and 50 mass% dimethyl sulfoxide/water between 25°C and −25°C, *Cryobiology* 22, 589–600, 1985.

Roy, R.N., Robinson, R.A., and Bates, R.G., Thermodynamics of the two dissociation steps of *N*-tris(hydroxymethyl) methylglycine ("tricine") in water from 5 to 50 degrees, *J. Amer. Chem. Soc.* 95, 8231–8235, 1973.

Silva, M.R., Paixo, J.A., Beja, A., and Alte da Veiga, L., *N*-[Tris(hydroxymethyl)methyl]glycine(tricine), *Acta Crystallogr. C.* 57, 421–422, 2001.

Su, Z.F., He, J., Rusckowski, M., and Hnatowich, D.J., In vitro cell studies of technetium-99m-labeled RGD-HYNIC peptide, a comparison of tricine and EDDA as co-ligands, *Nucl. Med. Biol.* 30, 141–149, 2003.

TRIETHANOLAMINE (TRIS(2-HYDROXYETHYL) AMINE; TEA)

TEA is used as a buffer in a variety of applications. Triethanolamine has the advantage over some other buffers is that is weakly binds divalent cations[1] permitting use in a variety of enzyme reactions.[2–7] The binding of divalent cations by TEA is somewhat enhanced in 90% DMSO. The binding of divalent cations by TEA is similar to that seen with Tris but much less than that observed with Bis-Tris. Triethanolamine has been shown to activate some enzymes.[8,9] Triethanolamine buffer has been shown to increase the adhesive strength of hydrocarbon monolayers.[10] Triethanolamine is used in mass spectrometry as a matrix and in preparing a derivative of boric acid.[11,12] Triethanolamine is used in the formulation of cosmetics.[13,14] Triethanolamine has also been evaluated as a transdermal transport agent.[15–17] Unlike Tris, TEA was not observed to catalyze an isomerization reaction.[18] There is a report on the catalysis of the cyclization of propargylic amines with carbon dioxide.[19]

1. Sigel, H., Scheller, K.H., and Prijs, B., Metal ion/buffer interactions. Stability of alkali and alkaline earth ion complexes with triethanolamine (Tea), 2-amino-2(hydroxylmethyl)-1,3-propanediol (Tris) and 2-[bis(2-hydroxyethyl)-amino-2(hydroxymethyl)-1,3-propanediol (Bistris) is aqueous and mixed solvents, *Inorg. Chim. Acta* 66, 147–155, 1982.

2. Duff, E.J., and Stuart, J.L., The use of triethanolamine in a buffer for the determination of fluoride in calcium and transition metal orthophosphates, using a fluoride-selective electrode, *Talanta* 19, 74–76, 1972.

3. Buhl, S.N., Jackson, K.Y., and Graffunder, B., Optimal reaction conditions for assaying human lactate dehydrogenase pyruvate-to-lactate at 25, 30, and 37 degrees C, *Clin. Chem.* 24, 261–266, 1978.

4. Lloyd, B., Burrin, J., Smythe, P., and Alberti, K.G., Enzymatic fluorometric continuous flow assays for blood glucose, lactate, pyruvate, alanine, glycerol, and 3-hydroxybutyrate, *Clin. Chem.* 24, 1724–1729, 1978.

5. Soga, M., Ohashi, A., Taniguchi, M., Matsui, T., and Tsuda, T., The di-peptide Trp-His activate AMP-activated protein kinase and enhances glucose uptake independently of insulin in L6 monocytes, *FEBS Open Bio.* 4, 898–904, 2014.

6. Broguiere, N., Formica, F.A., Borreto, G., and Zenobi-Wong, M., Sortase A as a cross-linking enzyme in tissue engineering, *Acta Biomater.* 77, 182–190, 2018.
7. Zhao, C., Xie, B. Zhao, R., Chen, S., and Fang, H., Intracellular amino and nonamino acids profiling of *Trichosporum cutaneum* on rich and limited nitrogen conditions for lipid production, *Biomass Bioengener.* 118, 84–92, 2018.
8. Sekiguchi, S., Hashida, Y., Yasukawa, K., and Inouye, K., Effects of amines and aminoalcohols on bovine intestine alkaline phosphatase activity, *Enzyme Microb. Technol.* 49, 171–176, 2011.
9. Li. D., Zhang, Y., Song, H., et al., Aminoalcohol-induced activation of organophosphorous hydrolase (OPH) towards diisopropylfluorophosphate (DFP), *PLoS One* 12, e11169937, 2017.
10. Ma, C.D., Wang, C., Acevedo-Vélez, C, Gellman, S.H., and Abbott, N.L., Modulation of hydrophobic interactions by proximally immobilized ions, *Nature* 517, 347–350, 2015.
11. Arita, M., Iwamori, M., Higuchi, T., and Nagai, Y., 1,1,3,3-tetramethylurea and triethanolamine as a useful matrix for fast atom bombardment mass spectrometry of gangliosides and neutral glycosphingolipids, *J. Biochem.* 93, 319–322, 1983.
12. Zeng, L.M., Wang, H.Y., and Guo, Y.L., Fast quantitative analysis of boric acid by gas chromatography-mass spectrometry coupled with a simple and selective derivatization reaction using triethanolamine, *J. Am. Soc. Mass Spectrom.* 21, 482–485, 2010.
13. Fiume, M.M., Heldreth, B., Bergfeld, W.F., et al., Safety assessment of triethanolamine and triethanolamine-containing ingredients as used in cosmetics, *Int. J. Toxicol.* 32(3 Suppl), 59S–83S, 2013.
14. Shin, K.O., and Lee, Y.M., Simultaneous analysis of mono-, di-, and tri-ethanolamine in cosmetic products using liquid chromatography coupled tandem mass spectrometry, *Arch. Pharm. Res.* 39, 66–72, 2016.
15. Fang, L., Kobayashi, Y., Numajiri, S., et al., The enhancing effect of a triethanolamine-ethanol-isopropyl myristate mixed system on the skin permeation of acidic drugs, *Biol. Pharm. Bull.* 25, 1339–1344, 2002.
16. Fang, L., Numajiri, S., Kobahashi, D., and Morimoto, D., The use of complexation with alkanolamines to facilitate skin permeation of mefenamic acid, *Int. J. Pharm.* 262, 13–22, 2003.
17. Xi, H., Cun, D., Xiang, R., et al., Intra-articular drug delivery from an optimized topical patch containing terifluomide and lornoxicam for rheumatoid arthritis treatment: Does the topical patch really enhance a local treatment, *J. Control Release* 169, 73–81, 2013.
18. Fitzgerald, J.W., The tris-catalyzed isomerization of potassium D-glucose 6-*O*-sulfate, *Can. J. Biochem.* 53, 906–910, 1975.
19. Zhao, Y., Qiu, J., Li, Z., et al., An experimental and theoretical study on the unexpected catalytic activity of triethanolamine for the carboxylative cyclization of propargylic amines with CO_2, *ChemSusChem* 10, 2001–2007, 2017.

Other references for the use of TEA:

Cao, H., and Preiss, J., Evidence for essential arginine residues at the active site of maize branching enzymes, *J. Protein Chem.* 15, 291–304, 1996.
Knaak, J.B., Leung, H.W., Stott, W.T., et al., Toxicology of mono-, di-, and triethanolamine, *Rev. Environ. Contim. Toxicol.* 149, 1–86, 1997.
Liu, Q., Li, X., and Sommer, S.S., pK-matched running buffers for gel electrophoresis, *Anal. Biochem.* 270, 112–122, 1999.
Musial, W., and Kubis, A., Effect of some anionic polymers on pH of triethanolamine aqueous solutions, *Polim. Med.* 34, 21–29, 2004.
Myohanen, T.A., Bouriotas, V., and Dean, P.D., Affinity chromatography of yeast alpha-glucosidase using ligand-mediated chromatography on immobilized phenylboronic acids, *Biochem. J.* 197, 683–688, 1981.
Sanger-van de Griend, C.E., Enantiomeric separation of glycyl dipeptides by capillary electrophoresis with cyclodextrins as chiral selectors, *Electrophoresis* 20, 3417–3424, 1999.
Shinomiya, Y., Kato, N., Imazawa, M., and Miyamoto, K., Enzyme immunoassay of the myelin basic protein, *J. Neurochem.* 39, 1291–1296, 1982.

TRIETHYLAMINE (*N,N*-DIETHYLETHANAMINE)

Triethylamine is a buffer that is better known as an ion-pair reagent for chromatography[1–13] and transdermal transport.[14–16] TEA also forms an exciplex with naphthalene in fluorescence studies.[17,18]

1. Brind, J.L., Kuo, S.W., Chervinsky, K., and Orentreich, N., A new reversed phase, paired-ion thin-layer chromatographic method for steroid sulfate separations, *Steroids* 52, 561–570, 1988.
2. Koves, E.M., Use of high-performance liquid chromatography-diode array detection in forensic toxicology, *J. Chromatog. A* 692, 103–119, 1995.
3. Cole, S.R., and Dorsey, J.G., Cyclohexylamine additives for enhanced peptide separations in reversed phase liquid chromatography, *Biomed. Chromatog.* 11, 167–171, 1997.
4. Gilar, M., and Bouvier, E.S.P., Purification of crude DNA oligonucleotides by solid-phase extraction and reversed-phase high-performance liquid chromatography, *J. Chromatog. A* 890, 167–177, 2000.
5. Loos, R., and Barcelo, D., Determination of haloacetic acids in aqueous environments by solid-phase extraction followed by ion-pair liquid chromatography-electrospray ionization mass spectrometric detection, *J. Chromatog. A.* 938, 45–55, 2001.
6. Gilar, M., Fountain, K.J., Budman, Y., et al., Ion-pair reversed phase high-performance liquid chromatography analysis of oligonucleotides: Retention prediction, *J. Chromatog. A.* 958, 167–182, 2002.

7. El-dawy, M.A., Mabrouk, M.M., and El-Barbary, F.A., Liquid chromatographic determination of fluoxetine, *J. Pharm. Biomed. Anal.* 30, 561–571, 2002.

8. Yang, X., Zhang, X., Li, A., et al., Comprehensive two-dimensional separations based on capillary high-performance liquid chromatography and microchip electrophoresis, *Electrophoresis* 24, 1451–1457, 2003.

9. Murphey, A.T., Brown-Augsburger, P., Yu, R.Z., et al., Development of an ion-pair reverse-phase liquid chromatographic/tandem mass spectrometry method for the determination of an 18-mer phosphorothioate oligonucleotide in mouse liver tissue, *Eur. J. Mass Spectrom.* 11, 209–215, 2005.

10. Gong, L., Comparing ion-pairing reagents and counter anions for ion-pair reversed-phase liquid chromatography/electrospray ionization mass spectrometry analysis of synthetic oligonucleotides, *Rapid Commun. Mass Spectrom.* 29, 2402–2410, 2015.

11. Fernández-Amado, M., Prieto-Blanco, M.C., López-Mahía, P., Muniategui-Lorenzo, S., and Prada-Rodríguez, D., Ion-pair in-tube solid phase microextraction for the simultaneous determination of phthalates and their degradation products in atmospheric particulate matter. *J. Chromatog. A.* 1520, 35–47, 2017.

12. Rahimi Kakavandi, N., Esoddin, M., Abdi, K., et al., Ion-pair switchable-hydrophilicity solvent-based homogeneous liquid-liquid microextraction for the determination of paraquat in environmental and biological samples before high-performance liquid chromatography, *J. Sep. Sci.* 40, 3703–3709, 2017.

13. Qiao, J.-Q., LIang, C., Zhu, Z.-Y., et al., Monolithic alkylsilane column: A promising separation medium for oligonucleotides by ion-pair reversed-phase liquid chromatography, *J. Chromatog. A* 1569, 168–177, 2018.

14. Xi, H., Wang, Z., Chen, Y., et al., The relationship between hydrogen-bonded ion-pair stability and transdermal penetration of lornoxicam with organic amines, *Eur. J. Pharm. Sci.* 47, 325–330, 2012.

15. Liu, N., Song, W., Song, T., and Fang, L., Design and evaluation of a novel Felbinac transdermal patch: Combining ion-pair and chemical enhancer strategy, *AAPS PharmSciTech* 17, 262–271, 2016.

16. Cui, H., Quan, P., Zhou, Z., and Fang, L., Development of a drug-in-adhesive patch combining ion pair and chemical enhancer strategy for transdermal delivery of zaltoprofen: Pharmacokinetic, pharmacodynamic and in vitro/in vivo correlation evaluation, *Drug. Deliv.* 23, 3461–3470, 2016.

17. Xie, G., Sueishi, Y., and Yamamoto, S., Analysis of the effects of protic, aprotic, and multi-component solvents on the fluorescence emission of naphthalene and its exciplex with triethylamine, *J. Fluoresc.* 15, 475–483, 2005.

18. Solis, C., Grosso, V., Faggioli, N., et al., Estimation of the solvent reorganization energy and the absolute energy of solvation of charge-transfer states from their emission spectra, *Photochem. Photobiol. Sci.* 9, 675–686, 2010.

TRIS (TRIS(HYDROXYMETHYL) AMINOMETHANE; 2-AMINO-2-(HYDROXYMETHYL)-1,3-PROPANEDIOL; THAM; TROMETHAMINE)

Tris is one of the most frequently used buffers in biochemistry and molecular biology. Tris is not without complications as it is also a nucleophile and can participate in chemical reactions. Tris has been reported to react with the thioester intermediate in intein-mediated protein cleavage.[1] Tris has been reported to react with organophosphorous compounds such as sarin.[2] Tris reacts with *p*-nitrophenyl acetate[3] and *p*-nitrophenyl phosphate.[4] It also reacts with acyl enzymes such as cinnamoylchymotrypsin and cinnamoyltrypsin.[5] Tris has been reported to reduce tetranitromethane.[6] Tris is oxidized by H_2O_2 in the presence of ferritin.[7] Tris (and HEPES) has been reported to be a competitive inhibitor of carbamoyl phosphate synthase.[8] Tris does interfere with the determination of protein by the bicinchoninic acid assay[9] and Lowry reaction.[10] Tris does strongly bind cupric ions.[11] Tris can also interfere with the biuret reaction and the Kjeldahl method.[12] The effect of Tris and other constituents of samples on protein assay can be obviated by use of the amido Schwartz reaction.[13] Tris can be used as a buffer in fermentation and cell culture. Fermentation of *Pseudomonas aeruginosa* in the presence of Tris resulted in the production of phosphatidyltris(hydroxymethyl)aminomethane.[14] Tris is used clinically a variety of applications THAM (tromethamine).[15–21] There is interest in the use of Tris in oncology to neutralize the acidity in solid tumors.[22] Attempts to use Tris buffer in a synthetic body fluid used in glass-ceramic scaffold were unsuccessful as the buffer dissolved the crystalline phase of the matrix with the formation of crystalline hydroxyapatite.[23]

1. Peroza, E.A., and Freisinger, E., Tris is a non-innocent buffer during intein-mediated protein cleavage, *Prot. Express. Purif.* 57, 217–225, 2008.

2. Stable adducts of nerve agents sarin, soman and cyclosarin with TRIS, TES and related buffer compounds-Characterization by LC-ESI-MS and NMR and implications for analytical chemistry, *J. Chromatog. B* 878, 1382–1390, 2010.

3. Jencks, W.P., and Carriuolo, J., Reactivity of nucleophilic reagents toward esters, *J. Am. Chem. Soc.* 82, 1778–1786, 1960.

4. Kirby, A.J., and Jencks, W.P., The reactivity of nucleophilic reagents toward the *p*-nitrophenyl phosphate dianion, *J. Am. Chem. Soc.* 87, 3209–3216, 1966.

5. Oliver, R.W., and Viswanatha, T., Reaction of tris(hydroxymethyl)aminomethane with cinnamoyl imidazole and cinnamoyltrypsin, *Biochim. Biophys. Acta* 156, 422–425, 1968.

6. Hodges, G.R., and Ingold, K.U., Superoxide, amine buffers and tetranitromethane: A novel free radical chain reaction, *Free Radic. Res.* 33, 547–550, 2000.

7. Zhang, B., Wilson, P.E., and Watt, G.D., Ferritin-catalyzed consumption of hydrogen peroxide by amine buffers causes the variable Fe^{2+} to O_2 stoichiometry of iron deposition in horse spleen ferritin, *J. Biol. Inorg. Chem.* 11, 1075–1086, 2006.

8. Lund, P., and Wiggins, D., Inhibition of carbamoyl phosphate synthase (ammonia) by Tris and Hepes. Effect on Ka for *N*-acetylglutamate, *Biochem. J.* 243, 273–276, 1987.

9. Kaushal, V., and Barnes, L.D., Effect of zwitterionic buffers on measurement of small masses of protein with bicinchoninic acid, *Anal. Biochem.* 157, 291–294, 1986.

10. Raj, R., and Richards, A.H., Interference by Tris buffer in the estimation of protein by the Lowry procedure, *Anal. Biochem.* 62, 240–247, 1974.

11. Hanlon, D.F., Watt, D.S., and Westhead, E.W., The interaction of divalent metal ions with Tris buffer in dilute solution, *Anal. Biochem.* 16, 225–233, 1966.

12. Robson, R.M., Goll, D.E., and Temple, M.J., Determination of proteins in "Tris" buffer by the biuret reaction, *Anal. Biochem.* 24, 339–341, 1968.

13. Sapan, C.V., and Lundblad, R.L., Review of methods for determination of total protein and peptide concentration in biological samples, *Proteomics Clin. Appl.* 9, 268–276, 2015.

14. Abbes, I., Rihouey, C., Hardouin, J., et al., *Pseudomonas aeruginosa* produces phosphatidyltris(hydroxymethyl) aminomethane and derivatives when grown in Tris-buffer medium, *Biochim. Biophys. Acta* 1861, 703–714, 2016.

15. Beich, H.L., and Schwartz, W.R., Tris buffer (THAM) – An appraisal of its physiologic effect and clinical usefulness, *New. Eng. J. Med.* 274, 782–787, 1966.

16. Elton, C.D., Gain, E.A., and Moonie, G., A clinical study on the use of T.H.A.M., for buffering A.C.D. blood prior to use in extracorporeal bypass procedures, *Can. Anaesth. Soc. J.* 10, 419–427, 1963.

17. Triana, J.R., Yanagihashi, M., and Larson, D.F., Mathematical modeling of buffer used in myocardial preservation, *Perfusion* 22, 353–362, 2007.

18. Nahas, G.G., Sutin, K.M., Fermon, C., et al., Guidelines for the treatment of acidaemia with THAM, *Drugs* 55, 191–224, 1998.

19. Holmdahl, M.H., Wiklund, L, Wetterberg, T., et al., The place of THAM in the management of acidemia in clinical practice, *Acta Anaesthesiol. Scand.* 44, 524–527, 2000.

20. Sinha, V.R., Kumar, R.V., and Singh, G., Ketorolac tromethamine formulations: An overview, *Expert Opin. Drug Deliv.* 6, 961–975, 2009.

21. Zeiler, F.A., Teitelbaum, J., Gillman, L.M., and West, M., THAM for control of ICP, *Neurocrit. Care.* 21, 332–344, 2014.

22. Ibrahim-Hashim, A., Abrahams, D., Enriquez-Navas, P.M., et al., Tris-base buffer: A promising new inhibitor for cancer progression and metasis, *Cancer. Med.* 6, 1720–1729, 2017.

23. Rohanová, D., Boccaccini, A.R., Yunos, D.M., et al., TRIS buffer in simulated body fluid distorts the assessment of glass-ceramic scaffold bioactivity, *Acta Biomater.* 7, 2623–2630, 2011.

General references for the use of Tris buffer:

AbouHaider, M.G., and Ivanov, I.G., Non-enzymatic RNA hydrolysis promoted by the combined catalytic activity of buffers and magnesium ions, *Z. Naturforsch.* 54, 542–548, 1999.

Afifi, N.N., Using difference spectrophotometry to study the influence of different ions and buffer systems on drug protein binding, *Drug Dev. Ind. Pharm.* 25, 735–743, 1999.

Ashworth, C.D., and Nelson, D.R., Antimicrobial potentiation of irrigation solutions containing tris-[hydroxymethyl] aminomethane-EDTA, *J. Am. Vet. Med. Assoc.* 197, 1513–1514, 1990.

Bernhard, S.A., Ionization constants and heats of tris(hydroxymethyl)aminomethane and phosphate buffers, *J. Biol. Chem.* 218, 961–969, 1956.

Burcham, P.C., Fontaine, F.R., Petersen, D.R., and Pyke, S.M., Reactivity of Tris(hydroxymethyl) aminomethane confounds immunodetection of acrolein-adducted proteins, *Chem. Res. Toxicol.* 16, 1196–1201, 2003.

Durst, R.A., and Staples, B.R., Tris/Tris-HCl: A standard buffer for use in physiologic pH range, *Clin. Chem.* 18, 206–208, 1972.

Kinoshita, T., Yamaguchi, A., and Tada, T., Tris(hydroxymethyl) aminomethane induced conformational change and crystal-packing contraction of porcine pancreatic elastase, *Acta Crystallograph. Sect. F. Struct. Biol. Cryst. Commun.* 62, 623–626, 2006.

Koval, D., Kasicka, V., and Zuskova, I., Investigation of the effect of ionic strength of Tris-acetate background electrolyte on electrophoretic mobilities of mono-, di-, and trivalent organic anions by capillary electrophoresis, *Electrophoresis* 26, 3221–3231, 2005.

Nakano, M., and Tauchi, H., Difference in activation by Tris(hydroxymethyl)aminomethane of Ca, Mg-ATPase activity between young and old rat skeletal muscles, *Mech. Aging. Dev.* 36, 287–294, 1986.

Niedernhofer, L.J., Riley, M., Schnez-Boutand, N., et al., Temperature dependent formation of a conjugate between tris(hydroxymethyl)aminomethane buffer and the malondialdehyde-DNA adduct pyrimidopurinone, *Chem. Res. Toxicol.* 10, 556–561, 1997.

Oliveira, L., Araujo-Viel, M.S., Juliano, L., and Prado, E.S., Substrate activation of porcine kallikrein *N*-α derivatives of arginine 4-nitroanilides, *Biochemistry* 26, 5032–5035, 1987.

Qi, Z., Li, X., Sun, D., et al., Effect of Tris on catalytic activity of MP-11, *Bioelectrochemistry* 68, 40–47, 2006.

Rapp, R.D., and Memminger, M.M., Tris (hydroxymethyl) aminomethane as an electrophoresis buffer, *Am. J. Clin. Pathol.* 31, 400–403, 1959.

Rodkey, F.L., Tris(hydroxymethyl)aminomethane as a standard for Kjeldahl nitrogen analysis, *Clin. Chem.* 10, 606–610, 1964.

Schacker, M., Foth, H., Schluter, J., and Kahl, R., Oxidation of tris to one-carbon compounds in a radical-producing model system, in microsomes, in hepatocytes and in rats, *Free Radic. Res. Commun.* 11, 339–347, 1991.

Shihabi, Z.K., Stacking of discontinuous buffers in capillary zone electrophoresis, *Electrophoresis* 21, 2872–2878, 2000.

Shiraishi, H., Kataoka, M., Morita, Y., and Umemoto, J., Interaction of hydroxyl radicals with tris (hydroxy-methyl) aminomethane and Good's buffers containing hydroxymethyl or hydroxyethyl residues produce form-aldehyde, *Free Radic. Res. Commun.* 19, 315–321, 1993.

Stambler, B.S., Grant, A.O., Broughton, A., and Strauss, H.C., Influences of buffers on dV/dtmax recovery kinetics with lidocaine in myocardium, *Am. J. Physiol.* 249, H663-H671, 1985.

Stellwagen, N.C., Bossi, A., Gelfi, C., and Righetti, P.G., DNA and buffers: Are there any noninteracting, neutral pH buffers?, *Anal. Biochem.* 287, 167–175, 2000.

Trivic, S., Leskovac, V., Zeremski, J., et al., Influence of Tris(hydroxymethyl)aminomethane on kinetic mecha-nism of yeast alcohol dehydrogenase, *J. Enzyme Inhib.* 13, 57–68, 1998.

Vasseur, M., Frangne, R., and Alvarado, F., Buffer-dependent pH sensitivity of the fluorescent chloride-indicator dye SPQ, *Am. J. Physiol.* 264, C27–C31, 1993.

Veeck, L.L., TES and Tris (TEST)-yolk buffer systems, sperm function testing, and in vitro fertilization, *Fertil. Steril.* 58, 484–486, 1992.

Visconti, M.A., and Castrucci, A.M., Tris buffer effects on melanophore aggregating responses, *Comp. Biochem. Physiol. C* 82, 501–503 1985.

Weber, R.E., Use of ionic and zwitterionic (Tris/BisTris and HEPES) buffers in studies on hemoglobin function, *J. Appl. Physiol.* 72, 1611–1615, 1992.

Williams-Smith, D.L., Bray, R.C., Barber, M.J., Tsopanakis, A.D., and Vincent, S.P., Changes in apparent pH on freezing aqueous buffer solutions and their relevance to biochemical electron-paramagnetic-resonance spectros-copy, *Biochem. J.* 167, 593–600, 1977.

4 Organic Name Reactions Useful in Biochemistry and Molecular Biology

AKABORI AMINO ACID REACTION

It was originally devised as a method for the conversion of amino acids or amino acid esters to aldehydes.[1] The Akabori reaction has been modified for use in the determination of C-terminal amino acids by performing the reaction in the presence of hydrazine and for the production of derivatives useful for mass spectrometric identification.[2–4] More recently, the Akabori reaction has been the mechanism for amino acid formation during the Maillard reaction.[5]

1. Ambach, E., and Beck, W., Metal-complexes with biologically important ligands. 35. Nickel, cobalt, palladium, and platinum complexes with Schiff-bases of α-amino acids – A contribution to the mechanism of the Akabori reaction, *Chemische Berichte-Recueil* 118, 2722–2737, 1985.
2. Bose, A.K., Ing, Y.H., Pramanik, B.N., et al., Microwave enhanced Akabori reaction for peptide analysis, *J. Am. Soc. Mass Spectrom.* 13, 839–850, 2002.
3. Pramanik, B.N., Ing, Y.H., Bose, A.K., et al., Rapid cyclopeptide analysis by microwave enhanced Akabori reaction, *Tetrahedron Lett.* 44, 2565–2568, 2003.
4. Puar, M.S., Chan, T.M., Delgarno, D., et al., Sch 486058: A novel cyclic peptide of actinomycete origin, *J. Antibiot.* 58, 151–154, 2005.
5. Nashalian, O., and Yaylayan, V.A., De novo synthesis of amino acids during the Maillard reaction: qTOR/ESI mass spectrometric evidence for the mechanism of the Akabori transformation, *J. Agric. Food Chem.* 63, 328–334, 2015.

ALDOL CONDENSATION

It is defined as the aldol condensation of one carbonyl compound with the enol/enolate form of another carbonyl compound to form a β-hydroxyaldehyde. The base-catalyzed reaction proceeds via the enolate form while the acid-catalyzed reaction proceeds via the enol form.[1–4] The basic chemistry of the aldol condensation is observed in several enzymatic reactions, including citrate synthase,[5,6] fructose-1,6-bisphosphate aldolase,[7–9] and 2-keto-4-hydroxyglutarate aldolase.[10,11] A crossed aldol refers to a condensation reaction with two different aldehydes/ketones; the second aldehyde frequently is formaldehyde as it cannot react with itself, although this is not a requirement.[12–15]

1. Evans, D.A., and McGee, L.R., Aldol diastereoselection. Zirconium enolates. Product selective, enolate structure independent condensations, *Tetrahedron Lett.* 21, 3975–3978, 1980.
2. Dalsgaard, T.K., Nielsen, J.H., and Larsen, L.B., Characterization of reaction products formed in a model reaction between pentanal and lysine-containing oligopeptides, *J. Agric. Food Chem.* 54, 6367–6373, 2006.
3. Perrin, C.L., and Chang, K.L., The complete mechanism of an aldol condensation, *J. Org. Chem.* 81, 5631–5635, 2016.
4. Abreu, I., Da Costa, N.C., van Es, A., et al., Natural occurrence of aldol condensation products in Valencia orange oil, *J. Food Sci.* 82, 2805–2815, 2017.
5. Rokita, S.E., Srere, P.A., and Walsh, C.T., 3-Fluoro-3-deoxycitrate: A probe for mechanistic study of citrate-utilizing enzymes, *Biochemistry* 21, 3765–3774, 1982.
6. van Rooyen, J.P., Mienie, L.J., Eramus, E., et al., Urinary excretion of homocitric acid and methylhomocitric acid in propionic acidemia: Minor metabolic products of the citrate synthase aldol condensation reaction, *Clin. Chim. Acta* 230, 91–99, 1994.
7. Rozova, O.N., Khmelenina, V.N., Mustakhimov, I.I., Reshetnikov, A.S., and Trotsenko, Y.A., Characterization of recombinant fructose-1,6—biphosphate aldolase from *Methylococcus capsulatus* Bath, *Biochemistry* (Moscow) 75, 892–898, 2010.
8. Du, J., Say, R.F., Lü, W., Fuchs, G., and Einsle, O., Active-site remodeling in the bifunctional fructose-1,6-biphosphate aldolase/phosphatase, *Nature* 478, 534–537, 2011.
9. Li, A., Cai, L., Chen, Z., et al., Recent advances in the synthesis of rare sugars using DHAP-dependent aldolases, *Carbohydr. Res.* 452, 108–115, 2017.
10. Lane, R.S., Hansen, B.A., and Dekker, E.E., Sulfhydryl groups in relation to the structure and catalytic activity of 2-oxo-4-hydroxyglutarate aldolase from bovine liver, *Biochim. Biophys. Acta* 481, 212– 221, 1977.
11. Grady, S.R., Wang, J.K., and Dekker, E.E., Steady-state kinetics and inhibition studies of the aldol condensation reaction catalyzed by bovine liver and *Escherichia coli* 2-keto-4-hydroxyglutarate aldolase, *Biochemistry* 20, 2497–2502, 1981.

12. Kiehlman, E., and Loo, P.W., Orientation in crossed aldol condensation of chloral with unsymmetrical aliphatic ketones, *Canad. J. Chem.* 49, 1588, 1971.

13. Findlay, J.A., Desai, D.N., and McCaulay, J.B., Thermally induced crossed aldol condensations, *Canad. J. Chem.* 59, 3303–3304, 1981.

14. Esmaelli, A.A., Tabas, M.S., Nasseri, M.A., and Kazemi, F., Solvent-free crossed aldol condensation of cyclic ketones with aromatic aldehydes assisted by microwave irradiation, *Monatshefte fur Chemie* 136, 571–576, 2005.

15. Gibson, M.Z., Nguyen, M.A., and Zingales, S.K., Design, synthesis, and evaluation of (2-(pyridinyl)methylene)-1-tetralone chalcones for anticancer and antimicrobial activity, *Med. Chem.* 14, 333–343, 2018.

AMADORI REARRANGEMENT

A reaction following the formation of the unstable reaction product between an aldehyde (reducing sugar) and a amino group (formation of a Schiff base, an aldimine) which results in a more stable ketoamine.[1–10] The Amadori rearrangement is part of the Maillard reaction which is important in food chemistry[11,12] and can result in the formation of advanced glycation end products.[13,14] The Amadori rearrangement has been used for carbohydrate conjugation.[11–17]

1. Amadori, M. *Atti. Accad. Nazl. Lincei* 2, 337, 1925.

2. Hodge, J.E., The Amadori rearrangement, *Adv. Carbohydrate Chem.* 10, 169–205, 1955.

3. Acharya, A.S., and Manning, J.M., Amadori rearrangement of glyceraldehyde-hemoglobin Schiff based adducts. A new procedure for the determination of keotamine adducts in proteins, *J. Biol. Chem.* 255, 7218–7224, 1980.

4. Acharya, A.S., and Manning, J.M., Reaction of glycoaldehyde with proteins: Latent crosslinking potential of α-hydroxyaldehydes, *Proc. Natl. Acad. Sci. USA* 80, 3590–3594, 1983.

5. Roper, H., Roper, S., and Meyer, B., Amadori- and N-nitroso-Amadori compounds and their pyrrolysis products. Chemical, analytical and biological aspects, *IARC Sci. Publ.* 57, 101–111, 1984.

6. Baynes, J.W., Watkins, N.G., Fisher, C.I., et al., The Amadori product on protein: Structure and reactions, *Prog. Clin. Biol. Res.* 304, 43–67, 1989.

7. Nacharaju, P., and Acharya, A.S., Amadori rearrangement potential of hemoglobin at its glycation sites is dependent on the three-dimensional structure of protein, *Biochemistry* 31, 12673–12679, 1992.

8. Zyzak, D.V., Richardson, J.M., Thorpe, S.R., and Baynes, J.W., Formation of reactive intermediates from Amadori compounds under physiological conditions, *Arch. Biochem. Biophys.* 316, 547–554, 1995.

9. Khalifah, R.G., Baynes, J.W., and Hudson, B.G., Amadorins: Novel post-Amadori inhibitors of advanced glycation reactions, *Biochem. Biophys. Res. Commun.* 257, 251–158, 1999.

10. Davidek, T., Clety, N., Aubin, S., and Blank, I., Degradation of the Amadori compound N-(1-deoxy-D-fructose-1-yl)glycine in aqueous model system, *J. Agric. Food Chem.* 50, 5472–5479, 2002.

11. Nguyen, H.T., van der Fels-Klerx, H.J., and van Boekel, M.A., Kinetics of N^ε-(carboxymethyl)lysine formation in aqueous model systems of sugars and casein, *Food Chem.* 192, 125–133, 2016.

12. Hemmler, D., Roullier-Gall, C., Marshal, J.W., et al., Evolution of complex Maillard chemical reactions, resolved in time, *Sci. Rep.* 7(1), 3227, 2017.

13. Salahuddin, P., Rabbani, G., and Khan, R.H., The role of advanced glycation end products in various types of neurogenerative disease: A therapeutic approach, *Cell. Mol. Biol. Lett.* 19, 407–437, 2014.

14. Ahmad, S., Khan, M.S., Akhter, F., Glycoxidation of biological macromolecules: A critical approach to halt the menace of glycation, *Glycobiology* 24, 979–990, 2014.

15. Wrodnigg, T.M., Kartusch, C., and Illaszewicz, C., The Amadori rearrangement as key reaction for the synthesis of glyconeoconjugates, *Carbohydr. Res.* 343, 2057–2066, 2008.

16. Gallas, K., Pototschnig, G., Adenitsch, F., Stütz, A.E., and Wrodnigg, T.M., The Amadori rearrangement as glycoconjugation method: Synthesis of non-natural C-glycosyl type glycoconjugates, *Beilstein J. Org. Chem.* 8, 1619–1629, 2012.

17. Hojnik, C., Müller, A., Gloe, T.E., Lindhorst, T.K., and Wrodnigg, T.M., The Amadori rearrangement for carbohydrate conjugation: Scope and limitations, *European J. Org. Chem.* 2016, 4328–4337, 2016.

BAEYER–VILLIGER REACTION

It is the oxidation of a ketone by a peroxy acid to yield an ester or a lactone.[1–5] The Baeyer–Villiger reaction is also known as the Baeyer–Villiger oxidation.[4] Early work showed that monooxygenases catalyzed the Baeyer–Villiger reaction.[6,7] Subsequent work extended these early observations.[8–11] There is considerable interest in the use of Baeyer–Villiger reaction catalyzed by monooxygenases in synthetic organic chemistry.[12–17]

1. Bayer, A., and Villiger, V., Wirkung des Caro'schen Reagents auf Ketone, *Ber. Dtsch. Chem. Ges.* 32, 3625–3633, 1899.

2. Hara, S., Baeyer-Villiger reaction of 2-oxo-A-norsteroids, *Chem. Pharm. Bull.* 12, 1531–1532, 1964.

3. Cannon, J.G., and Garst, J.E., Preparation and Baeyer-Villiger reaction of certain 2-carbalkoxycyclopropyl methyl ketones, *J. Pharm. Sci.* 64, 1059–1061, 1975.

4. Renz, M., and Meunier, B., 100 years of Baeyer-Villiger Oxidation, *Eur. J. Org. Chem.* 1999, 737–750, 1999.

5. Boronat, M., Corma. A., Renz, M., et al., A multisite molecular mechanism for Baeyer-Villiger oxidations on solid catalysts using environmentally friendly H_2O_2 as oxidant, *Chemistry* 11, 6905–6915, 2005.

6. Turfitt, G.E., The microbial degradation of steroids: Fission of the steroid molecules, *Biochem. J.* 46, 376–383, 1948.

7. Fried, J., Thomas, R.W., and Klingsberg, A., Oxidation of steroid by microorganisms. III. Side chain degradation, ring D-cleavage and dehydrogenation in ring A, *J. Amer. Chem. Soc* 75, 5764–5765, 1953.

8. Ryerson, C.C., Ballou, D.P., and Walsh, C., Mechanistic studies on cyclohexanone oxygenase, *Biochemistry* 21, 2644–2655, 1982.

9. Ougham, H.J., Taylor, D.G., and Trudgill, P.W., Camphor revisited: Involvement of a unique mono-oxygenase in metabolism of 2-oxo-Δ^3-3-4,4,4-trimethylcyclopentenylacetic acid by *Pseudomonas putida*, *J. Bacteriol.* 153, 140–152, 1983.

10. Itagaki, E., Studies on steroid monooxygenase from *Cylindrocarpon radicicola* ATCC 11011. Purification and characterization, *J. Biochem.* 99, 815–824, 1986.

11. Mihovilovic, M.D., Rudroff, E., Winninger, A., et al., Microbial Baeyer-Villiger oxidation: Stereopreference and substrate acceptance of cyclohexanone monooxygenase mutants prepared by directed evolution, *Org. Lett.* 8, 1221–1224, 2006.

12. Willetts, A., Structural studies and synthetic applications of Baeyer-Villiger monooxygenases, *Trends Biotechnol.* 15, 55–62, 1997.

13. Zambianchi, F., Pasta, P., Carrea, G., et al., Use of isolated cyclohexanone monooxygenase from recombinant *Escherichia coli* as a biocatalyst for Baeyer-Villiger and sulfide oxidations, *Biotechnol. Bioeng.* 78, 489–496, 2002.

14. Alphand, V., Carrea, G., Wohlgemuth, R., et al., Towards large-scale synthetic application of Baeyer-Villiger monooxygenase, *Trends Biotechnol.* 21, 318–323, 2003.

15. ten Brink, G.J., Arends, I.W., and Sheldon, R.A., The Baeyer-Villiger reaction: New developments toward greener procedures, *Chem. Rev.* 104, 4105–4124, 2004.

16. Torres-Paziño, D., Dudek, H.M., and Fraaije, M.W., Baeyer-Villiger monooxygenases: Recent advances and future challenges, *Curr. Opin. Chem. Biol.* 14, 138–144, 2010.

17. Bučko, M., Gemeiner, P., Schenkmayerová, A., et al., Baeyer-Villiger oxidations: Biotechnological approach, *Appl. Microbiol. Biotechnol.* 100, 6585–6599, 2016.

BECKMANN REARRANGEMENT

The canonical definition of a Beckmann rearrangement is the acid-catalyzed conversion of aldoximes and ketoximes to the corresponding amide.[1–6] There is continuing interest in the use of the Beckmann rearrangement in synthetic organic chemistry and polymer chemistry.[7–13] There is suggestion that the Beckmann rearrangement in important in biochemical reaction.[14–16]

1. Beckmann, E., Zur der Kenntwiss der Isonitroso-verbindugen, *Ber. Deutsch. Chem. Ges.* 19, 988–993, 1886.

2. Bhatt, A.H., The Beckmann Rearrangement, *Chem. Rev.* 12, 215–260, 1933.

3. Jones, B., Kinetics and mechanism of the Beckmann rearrangement, *Chem. Rev.* 35, 335–350, 1944.

4. McLaren, A.D., The Beckmann rearrangement of aliphatic ketoximes, *Science* 103, 503, 1946.

5. Lezcano-González, I., Boronat, M., and Blasco, T., Investigation on the Beckmann rearrangement reaction catalyzed by porous solids, MAS NMR and theoretical calculations, *Solid State Nucl. Magn. Reson.* 35, 120–129, 2009.

6. Darling, C.M., and Chen, C.P., Rearrangement of *N*-benzyl-2-cyano-(hydroxyimino)acetamide, *J. Pharm. Sci.* 67, 860–861, 1978.

7. De Luca, L., Giacomelli, G., and Procheddu, A., Beckmann rearrangement of oximes under very mild conditions, *J. Org. Chem.* 67, 6272–6274, 2002.

8. Furuya, Y., Ishihara, K., and Yamamoto, H., Cyanuric chloride as a mild and active Beckmann rearrangement catalyst, *J. Am. Chem. Soc.* 127, 11240–11241, 2005.

9. Torisawa, Y., Nishi, T., and Minamikawa, J., Continuing efforts on the improvement of Beckmann rearrangement of indanone oxime, *Bioorg. Med. Chem. Lett.* 17, 448–452, 2007.

10. Kiely-Collins, H.J., Sechi, I., Brennan, P.E., and McLaughlin, M.G., Mild, calcium catalyzed Beckmann rearrangement, *Chem. Commun.* 54, 654–657, 2018.

11. Gao, Y., Liu, J., Li, Z., et al., Dichloroimidazolidinedione-activated Beckmann rearrangement of ketoximes for accessing amides and lactams, *J. Org. Chem.* 83, 2040–2049, 2018.

12. Mo, X., Morgan, T.D.R., Ang, H.T., and Hall, D.G., Scope and mechanism of a true organocatalytic Beckmann rearrangement with a boronic acid/perfluoropinacol system under ambient conditions, *J. Am. Chem. Soc.* 140, 5264–5271, 2018.

13. Chapman, S., O'Malley, A.J., Parker, S.F., and Raja, R., Comprehensive vibrational spectroscopic characterization of Nylon-6 precursors for precise tracking of the Beckmann rearrangement, *Chemphyschem*, in press. doi:10.1002/cphc.201800721, 2018.

14. Gayen, A.K., and Knowles, C.O., Penetration and fate of methomyl and its oxime metabolite in insects and two spotted spider mites, *Arch. Environ. Contam. Toxicol.* 10, 55–67, 1981.

15. Mangold, B.L., and Spina, A., Rat liver aryl sulfotransferase-catalyzed sulfation and rearrangement of 9-fluorenone oxime, *Biochim. Biophys. Acta* 874, 37–43, 1986.

16. Ichino, T., Arimoto, H., and Uemura, D., Possibility of a non-amino acid pathway in the biosynthesis of marine-derived oxazoles, *Chem. Commun.* (16), 1742–1744, 2006.

BENZOIN CONDENSATION

The canonical definition is the conversion of benzaldehyde to benzoin (an aromatic α-hydroxyketone) via cyanide-mediated condensation of two benzaldehyde molecules. Other aromatic aldehydes can participate in this reaction. It has been established that the benzoin condensation can be catalyzed by benzaldehyde lyase.[1,2] This enabled the preparation of optically pure ketones for starting material for organic synthesis.[3] There has been continued interest in the study of catalysis of the benzoin condensation by benzaldehyde lyase.[4-8] The benzoin condensation is also catalyzed by benzoylformate decarboxylase[6,9,10] and other enzymes.[6] The catalysis of the benzoin condensation by antibody[11] and by a montmorillonite clay[12] has been described.

1. Demir, A.S., Pohl, M., Janzen, E., and Müller, M., Enantioselective synthesis of hydroxy ketones through cleavage and formation of acyloin linkage. Enzymatic kinetic resolultion via C-C bond cleavage, *J. Chem. Soc. Perkin Trans* 1, 633–635, 2001.
2. Dünkelmann, P., Kolter-Jung, D., Nitsche, A., et al., Development of a donor-acceptor concept for enzymatic cross-coupling reactions of aldehydes: The first asymmetric cross-benzoin dcondensation, *J. Am. Chem. Soc.* 124, 12084–12085, 2002.
3. Wildemann, H., Dünkelmann, P., Müller, M., and Schmidt, B., A short olefin metathesis-based route to enantiomerically pure arylated dihydropyrans and α,β-unsaturated δ-valero lactones, *J. Org. Chem.* 68, 799–804, 2003.
4. Chakraborty, S., Nermeria, N, Yep, A., et al., Mechanism of benzaldehyde lyase studied via thiamine diphosphate-bound intermediates and kinetic isotope effects, *Biochemistry* 47, 3800–3809, 2008.
5. Brandt, G.S., Nemeria, N., Chakraborty, S., et al., Probing the active center of benzaldehyde lyase with substitutions and the pseudosubstrate analogue benzoylphosphonic acid methyl ester, *Biochemistry* 47, 7734–7743, 2008.
6. Beigi, M., Gauchenova, E., Walter, L., et al., Regio- and stereoselective aliphatic-aromatic cross benzoin reaction: Enzyme divergent catalysis, *Chemistry* 22, 13999–14005, 2016.
7. Herández, K., Parella, T., Petrillo, G., et al., Intramolecular benzoin reaction catalyzed by benzaldehyde lyase from *Pseuomonas fluorescens* Biovar I, *Angew. Chem. Int. Ed. Engl.* 56, 5304–5307, 2017.
8. Ohs, R., Leipnitz, M., Schöpping, M., and Speiss, A.C., Simultaneous identification of reaction and inactivation kinetics of an enzyme-catalyzed carboligation, *Biotechnol. Prog.* 34, 1081–1092, 2018.
9. Iding, H., Dunnwald, T., Greiner, L., et al., Benzoylformate decarboxylase from *Pseudomonas putida* as stable catalyst for the synthesis of chiral 2-hydroxy ketones, *Chemistry* 6, 1483–1495, 2000.
10. Tural, S., Tural, B., and Demir, A.S., Heterofunctional magnetic metal-chelate-epoxy supports for the purification and covalent immobilization of benzoylformate decarbpxylase from *Pseudomonas putida* and its carboligation reactivity, *Chirality* 27, 635–642, 2015.
11. Sklute, G., Oizerowich, R., Shulman, H., and Keinan, E., Antibody-catalyzed benzoin oxidation as a mechanistic probe for nucleophilic catalysis by an active site lysine, *Chemistry* 10, 2159–2165, 2004.
12. Morales-Serna, J.A., Frontana-Uribe, B.A., Olguin, R., et al., Reaction control in heterogeneous catalysis using montmorillonite: Switching between acid-catalyzed and red-ox processes, *RSC Advances* 6, 426130–42617, 2016.

CANNIZZARO REACTION

Base-catalyzed disproportionation of an aldehyde to yield a carboxylic acid and the corresponding alcohol.[1-4] Cannazzaro observed that the addition of sodium hydroxide to benzaldehyde resulted in the formation of a solid consisting of sodium benzoate and benzyl alcohol. A crossed Cannizzaro reaction is the reaction of two different aldehydes to yield an alcohol and an acid as in the reaction of benzaldehyde and furfural (2-furaldehyde).[5] Formation of an aromatic amide and the corresponding alcohol from an aromatic aldehyde was observed with lithium amide in the presence of lanthanide chlorides.[6] A Cannizzaro-like reaction has been suggested to occur on the reaction of glyoxal and similar compounds with proteins.[7]

An internal Cannizzaro reaction was observed with a glyoxal inhibitor bound to trypsin.[8]

1. Cannizzaro, S., Ueber den der Benzoësäure entsprechenden Alkohol, *Annalen der Chemie und Pharmacie* 88, 129–130, 1853.
2. Pearl, I.A., Reactions of vanillin and its derived compounds; the Cannizzaro reaction of vanillin, *J. Org. Chem.* 12, 79–84, 1947.
3. Swain, C.G., Powell, A.L., Sheppard, A.L., and Morgan, C.R., Mechanism of the Cannizzaro reaction, *J. Amer. Chem. Soc.* 101, 3576–3583, 1979.
4. Russell, A.E., Miller, S.P., and Morken, J.P., Efficient Lewis acid catalyzed intramolecular Cannizzaro reaction, *J. Org. Chem.* 65, 8381–8383, 2000.
5. Hazlet, S.E., and Stauffer, D.A., Crossed Cannizzaro reactions, *J. Org. Chem.* 27, 2021–2024, 1962.
6. Zhang, L., Wang, S., Zhou, S., et al., Cannizzaro-type disproportionation of aromatic aldehydes to amides and alcohols by using either a stoichiometric amount or a catalytic amount of lanthanide compounds, *J. Org. Chem.* 71, 3149–3153, 2006.

7. Glomb, M.A., and Monnier, V.M., Mechanism of protein modification by glyoxal and glycoaldehyde, reactive intermediates of the Maillard reaction, *J. Biol. Chem.* 270, 10017–10026, 1995.

8. Cleary, J.A., and Malthouse, J.P.G., A new lysine derived glyoxal inhibitor of trypsin, its properties and utilization for studying the stabilization of tetrahedral adducts of trypsin, *Biochem. Biophys. Rep.* 5, 272–284, 2016.

CLAISEN CONDENSATION

The base-catalyzed condensation of two moles of an ester to give a β-keto ester or one ester with another carbonyl compound to yield a β-keto ester or lactone.[1–6] The Claisen condensation should be confused with the Claisen rearrangement (see below). The Claisen condensation is useful in the formation of carbon–carbon bonds in synthetic organic chemistry. The Claisen condensation is of great importance in the biosynthesis of fatty acids, polyketides, and hydrocarbons.[7–15] The retro-Claisen reaction is the reverse of the Claisen condensation.[16–19]

1. Claisen, L., Beiträge zur Kenntniss der Condensation Producte des Acetons, *Justus Liebeg Ann. Chem.* 180, 1–20, 1976.

2. Stuart, C.M., On the condensation-products formed by benzoic aldehyde with malonic and isosuccinic acids, *J. Chem. Soc.* 43, 403–409, 1883.

3. Claisen, L., and Lowman, O., Ueber eine neue Bildungsweise der Benzoylessigäthers, *Ber. Deutsch. Chem. Ges.* 20, 651–654, 1887.

4. Moersch, G.W., Evans, D.E., and Lewis, G.S., Steroidal γ-lactones. The Claisen condensation of 17α-acetate with 17β-acetal, *J. Med. Chem.* 10, 254–255, 1967.

5. Kamijo, S., and Dudley, G.B., Claisen-type condensation of vinylogous acyl triflates, *Org. Lett.* 8, 175–177, 2006.

6. Ishikawa, T., Kadoya, R., Arai, M., et al., Revisiting [3 + 3] route to 1,3-cyclohexanedione frameworks: Hidden aspect of thermodynamically controlled enolates, *J. Org. Chem.* 66, 8000–8009, 2001.

7. Dewar, M.J., and Dieter, K.M., Mechanism of the chain extension step in the biosynthesis of fatty acids, *Biochemistry* 27, 3302–3308, 1988.

8. Clark, J.D., O'Keefe, S.J., and Knowles, J.R., Malate synthase: Proof of a stepwise Claisen condensation using the double-isotope fractionation test, *Biochemistry* 27, 5961–5971, 1988.

9. Lee, R.E., Armour, J.W., Takayama, K., et al., Mycolic acid biosynthesis: Definition and targeting of the Claisen condensation step, *Biochim. Biophys. Acta* 1346, 275–284, 1997.

10. Olsen, J.G., Madziola, A., von Wettstein-Knowles, P., et al., Structures of β-ketoacyl-acyl carrier protein synthase I complexed with fatty acids elucidate its catalytic machinery, *Structure* 9, 233–243, 2001.

11. Heath, R.J., and Rock, C.O., The Claisen condensation in biology, *Nat. Prod. Rep.* 19, 581–596, 2002.

12. Haapalainen, A.M., Meriläinen, G., and Wierenga, R.K., The thiolase superfamily: Condensing enzymes with diverse reaction specificities, *Trends Biochem. Sci.* 31, 64–71, 2006.

13. Horsman, M.E., Hari, T.P., and Boddy, C.N., Polyketide synthetase and non-ribosomal peptide synthetase thioesterase selectivity: Logic gate or a victim of fate?, *Nat. Prod. Rep.* 33, 183–202, 2016.

14. Schäberle, T.F., Biosynthesis of α-pyrones, *Beilstein J. Org. Chem.* 12, 571–588, 2016.

15. Jensen, M.R., Goblirsch, B.R., Christenson, J.K., et al., OleA Glu117 is key to condensation of two fatty-acyl coenzyme A substrates in long-chain olefin biosynthesis, *Biochem. J.* 474, 3871–3886, 2017.

16. Grogan, G., Roberts, G.A., Bougioukou, D., Turner, N.J., and Flitsch, S.L., The desymmetrization of bicyclic β-diketones by an enzymatic retro-Claisen reaction. A new reaction of the crotonase superfamily, *J. Biol. Chem.* 276, 12565–12572, 2001.

17. Hollnagel, A., and Kroh, L.W., 3-Deoxypentosulose: An α-dicarbonyl oompound predominating in nonenzymatic browning oligosaccharides in aqueous solution, *J. Agric. Food Chem.* 50, 1659–1664, 2002.

18. Grenning, A.J., and Tunge, J.A., Deacylative allylation: Allylic alkylation via retro-Claisen activation, *J. Am. Chem. Soc.* 133, 14785–14794, 2011.

19. Hussein, M.A., Huynh, V.T., Hommelshein, R., Koenigs, R.M., and Nguyen, T.V., An efficient method for retro-Claisen-type C-C bond cleavage of diketones with tropylium catalyst, *Chem. Commun.* (Camb) 54, 12970–12973, 2018.

CLAISEN REARRANGEMENT

The rearrangement of an allyl vinyl ether or the nitrogen or sulfur analogue or allyl aryl ether to yield a γ,δ-unsaturated ketone or an *o*-allyl substituted phenol.[1–5] Chorismate mutase is an enzyme-catalyzed Claisen rearrangement.[6–8] An antibody catalyzed a Claisen rearrangement (chorismite mutase) has been described.[9–11]

1. Claisen, L., Über Umlagerung von Phenol-allyl-äthern in C-Allyl-phenole, *Ber. Dtsch. Chem. Ges.* 45, 3157–3166, 1912.

2. Rhoades, S.J., and Raulins, N.R., The Claisen and Cope Rearrangements, *Org. Reactions* 22, 1–212, 1975.

3. Ziegler, F.E., The thermal, aliphatic Claisen rearrangement, *Chem. Rev.* 1423–1452, 1988.

4. Martin Castro, A.M., Claisen rearrangement over the past nine decades, *Chem. Rev.* 104, 2939–3002, 2004.

5. Davis, C.J., Hurst, T.E., Jacob, A.M., and Moody, C.J., Microwave-mediated Claisen rearrangement followed by phenol oxidation: A simple route to naturally occurring 1,4-benzoquinones. The first synthesis of verapliquinones A and B and panicein A, *J. Org. Chem.* 70, 4414–4422, 2005.

6. Declue, M.S., Baldridge, K.K., Kast, P., and Hilvert, D., Experimental and computational investigation of the uncatalyzed rearrangement and elimination reactions of isochorismate, *J. Am. Chem. Soc.* 128, 2043–2051, 2006.

7. Guimarães, C.R., Udier-Blagović, M., Tubert-Brohman, I., and Jorgensen, W.L., Effects of Arg90 neutralization on the enzyme-catalyzed rearrangement of chorismite to prephenate, *J. Chem. Theory Comput.* 1, 617–625, 2005.

8. Wright, S.K., DeClue, M.S., Mandal, A., et al., Isotope effects on the enzymatic and nonenzymatic reactions of chorismate, *J. Am. Chem. Soc.* 127, 12957–12964, 2005.

9. Zhang, X., and Bruice, T.C., Temperature dependence of the structure of the substrate and active site of the *Thermus thermophilus* chorismate mutase E-S complex, *Biochemistry* 45, 8562–8567, 2006.

10. Hilvert, D., Carpenter, S.H., Nared, K.D., and Auditor, M.T., Catalysis of concerted reactions by antibodies: The Claisen rearrangement, *Proc. Nat. Acad. Sci. USA* 85, 4953–4955, 1988.

11. Campbell, A.P., Tarasow, T.M., Massefski, W., Wright, P.E., and Hilvert, D., Binding of a high-energy substrate conformer in antibody catalysis, *Proc. Natl. Acad. Sci. USA* 90, 8663–8667, 1993.

CURTIUS REARRANGEMENT (ALSO CURTIUS REACTION)

The formation of an isocyanate from an acyl azide.[1,2] The isocyanate can be converted to an amine. It provides a method for converting a carboxylic acid to an amine. There are a variety of studies on the application of the Curtius rearrangement.[3–14]

1. Curtius, Th., Ueber Stickstoffwasserstoftsäure (Azomid) N_3H, *Ber. Dtsch. Chem. Ges.* 23, 3023–3033, 1890.

2. Curtius, Th., Chemische Notizen, *Ber. Dtsch. Chem. Ges.* 23, 3033–3041, 1890.

3. Inouye, K., Watanabe, K., and Shin, M., Formation and degradation of urea derivatives in the azide method of peptide synthesis. Part 1. The Curtius rearrangement and urea formation, *J. Chem. Soc.* (17), 1905–1911, 1977.

4. Chorev, M., and Goodman, M., Partially modified retro-inverso peptides. Comparative Curtius rearrangements to prepare 1,1-diaminoalkane derivatives, *Int. J. Pept. Protein Res.* 21, 258–268, 1983.

5. Sasmal, S., Geyer, A., and Maier, M.E., Synthesis of cyclic peptidomimetics from aldol building blocks, *J. Org. Chem.* 67, 6260–6263, 2002.

6. Kedrowski, B.L., Synthesis of orthogonally protected (R)- and (S)-2-methylcysteine via an enzymatic desymmerization and Curtius rearrangement, *J. Org. Chem.* 68, 5403–5406, 2003.

7. Englund, E.A., Gopi, H.N., and Appella, D.H., An efficient synthesis of a probe for protein function: 2,3-diaminopropionic acid with orthogonal protecting groups, *Org. Lett.* 6, 213–215, 2004.

8. Spino, C., Tremblay, M.C., and Gobout, C., A stereo-divergent approach to amino acids, amino alcohols, or oxazolidonones of high enantiomeric purity, *Org. Lett.* 6, 2801–2804, 2004.

9. Brase, S., Gil, C., Knepper, K., and Zimmerman, V., Organic azides: An exploding diversity of a unique class of compounds, *Angew. Chem. Int. Ed. Engl.* 44, 5188–5240, 2005.

10. Lebel, H., and Leogane, O., Boc-protected amines via a mild and efficient one-pot Curitus rearrangement, *Org. Lett.* 7, 4107–4110, 2005.

11. Lebel, H., and Leogane, O., Curtius rearrangement of aromatic carboxylic acids to access protected anilines and aromatic ureas, *Org. Lett.* 8, 5717–5720, 2006.

12. Gokada, M.R., Hunter, R., Andrijevic, A., et al., Quaternized α,α′-amino acids via Curitus rearrangement of substituted malonate-imidazolidiones, *J. Org. Chem.* 82, 10650–10658, 2017.

13. Ghosh, A.K., Sarkar, A., and Brindisi, M., The Curtius rearrangement: Mechanistic insight and recent applications in natural product synthesis, *Org. Biomol. Chem.* 16, 2006–2027, 2018.

14. Ghosh, A.K., Brindisi, M., and Sarkar, A., The Curtius rearrangement: Applications in modern drug discovery and medicinal chemistry, *ChemMedChem* 13, 2351–2373, 2018.

DAKIN–WEST REACTION

Conversion of amino acids to acetamidoketones via the action of acetic anhydride in base where a carboxyl group is replaced by an acyl group in a reaction proceeding through an oxazolone intermediate.[1–5] This reaction has been used for the synthesis of enzyme inhibitors and receptor antagonists.[6–12]

1. Dakin, H.D., and West, R., Some aromatic derivatives of substituted acetylaminoacetones, *J. Biol. Chem.* 78, 757–764, 1928.

2. Cleland, G.H., and Niemann, C., Some observations on the Dakin-West reaction, *J. Am. Chem. Soc.* 71, 841–843, 1949.

3. Cornforth, J.W., and Elliott, D.F., Mechanism of the Dakin and West reaction, *Science* 112, 534–535, 1950.

4. Allinger, N.L., Wang, G.L., and Dewhurst, B.B., Kinetic and mechanical studies of the Dakin-West reactions, *J. Org. Chem.* 39, 1730–1735, 1978.

5. Dalla-Vechia, L., Santos, V.G., Godoi, M.N., et al., On the mechanism of the Dakin-West reaction, *Org. Biomol. Chem.* 10, 9013–9020, 2012.

6. Angliker, H. Wikstrom, P., Rauber, P., et al., Synthesis and properties of peptidyl derivatives of arginylfluoromethanes, *Biochem. J.* 256, 481–486, 1988.

7. Cheng, L., Goodwin, C.A., Schully, M.F., et al., Synthesis and biological activity of ketomethylene pseudopeptide analogues as thrombin inhibitors, *J. Med. Chem.* 35, 3364–3369, 1992.

8. Godfrey, A.B., Brooks, D.A., Hay, L.A., et al., Application of the Dakin-West reaction for the synthesis of oxazole-containing dual PPARα/γ agonists, *J. Org. Chem.* 68, 2623–2632, 2003.

9. Loksha, Y.M., el-Barbary, A.A., et-Barbary, M.A., et al., Synthesis of 2-(aminocarbonylmethylthio)-1*H*-imidazoles as novel Capravirine analogues, *Bioorg. Med. Chem.* 13, 4209–4220, 2005.

10. Wende, R.C, Seitz, A., Niedek, D., et al., The enantioselective Dakin-West reaction, *Angew. Chem. Int. Ed. Engl.* 55, 2719–2723, 2016.

11. Fernández, L.R., Svetaz, L., Butassi, E., et al., Synthesis and antifungal activity of bile acid-derived oxazoles, *Steroids* 108, 68–76, 2016.

12. Baumann, M., and Baxendale, I.R., Diastereoselective trifluoroacetylation of highly substituted pyrrolidines by a Dakin-West process, *J. Org. Chem.* 81, 11898–11908, 2016.

DIELS–ALDER CONDENSATION

A cycloaddition reaction between a conjugated diene (diene) and an alkene or alkyne (dienophile) resulting in the formation of alkene ring (1,4-cycloaddition).[1] This is considered one of the of the most useful reactions in synthetic organic chemistry[2–8] and has seen increasing use in biochemistry[9–11] in areas such as bioconjugate synthesis.[12] There are other cycloadditions used in chemical biology such as the azide-alkyne additions that are similar to the Diel–Alder reaction.[13] The inverse-demand Diels–Alder reaction[14,15] is used in bioorthogonal modifications.[16] The characteristics of the reaction partners are reversed in the inverse-demand Diels–Alder reactions where the "diene" is electron-poor and the "dienophile" is electron-rich. A retro-Diels–Alder is the reverse of a Diels–Alder regenerating a diene and a dienophile.[17,18]

1. Diels, O., and Alder, K., Synthesen in der Hydroaromatischen Reihe, *Justus Liebig Ann. Chem.* 460, 98–122, 1928.

2. Wasserman, A., *Diels–Alder Reactions. Organic Background and Physico-Chemical Aspects*, Elsevier, Amsterdam, the Netherlands, 1965.

3. Waller, R.L., and Recknagel, R.O., Determination of lipid conjugated dienes with tetracyanoethylene-14C: significance for study of the pathology of lipid peroxidation, *Lipids* 12, 914–921, 1977.

4. Fringuelli, F., and Taticchi, A., *The Diels–Alder Reaction. Selected Practical Methods*, John Wiley & Sons, Chichester, UK, 2002.

5. Nicolaou, K.C., Snyder, S.A., Montagnon, T., and Vassilikogiannakis, G., The Diels-Alder reaction in total synthesis, *Angew. Chem. Int. Ed. Engl.* 41, 1688–1698, 2002.

6. Boul, P.J., Reutenauer, P., and Lehn, J.M., Reversible Diels-Alder reactions for the generation of dynamic combinatorial libraries, *Org. Lett.* 7, 15–18, 2005.

7. Funel, J.A., and Abele, S., Industrial applications of the Diels-Alder reaction, *Angew. Chem. Int. Ed. Engl.* 52, 3822–3863, 2013.

8. Liu, L., Cotelle, Y., Bornhof, A.B., et al., Anion-π catalysis of Diels-Alder reactions, *Angew. Chem. Int. Ed. Engl.* 56, 13066–13069, 2017.

9. Stocking, E.M., and Williams, R.M., Chemistry and biology of biosynthetic Diels-Alder reactions, *Angew. Chem. Int. Ed.* 42, 3078–3115, 2003.

10. Gregoritza, M., and Brandl, F.P., The Diels-Alder reaction: A powerful tool for the design of drug delivery systems and biomaterials, *Eur. J. Pharm. Biopharm.* 97, 438–453, 2015.

11. Hashimoto, T., and Kuzuyama, T., Mechanistic insights into Diels-Alder reactions in natural product biosynthesis, *Curr. Opin. Chem. Biol.* 35, 117–123, 2016.

12. St. Amant, A.H., Lemen, D., Florinas, S., et al., Tuning the Diels-Alder reaction for bioconjugation to maleimide drug-linkers, *Bioconjug. Chem.* 29, 2406–2414, 2018.

13. Pickens, C.J., Johnson, S.N., Pressnall, M.M., Leon, M.A., and Berkland, C.J., Practical considerations, challenges, and limitations of bioconjugation via azide-alkyne cycloaddition, *Bioconjug. Chem.* 29, 686–701, 2018.

14. Reiner, T., and Ziglis, B.M., The inverse electron demand Diels-Alder click reaction in radiochemistry, *J. Labelled Comp. Radiopharm.* 57, 285–290, 2014.

15. Oliveira, B.L, Guo, Z., and Bernardes, G.L., Inverse electron demand Diels-Alder reactions in chemical biology, *Chem. Soc. Rev.* 46, 4895–4950, 2017.

16. Liu, D.S., Tangpeerachaikul, A., Selvaraj, R., et al., Diel-Alder cycloaddition for fluorophore targeting to specific proteins inside living cells, *J. Am. Chem. Soc.* 134, 792–795, 2012.

17. Mahajna, M., Quistad, G.B., and Casida, J.E., Retro-Diels-Alder reaction: Possible involvement in the metabolic activation of 7-oxabicylco[2.2.1]hepta-2(3),5(6)-diene-2,3-dicarboxylates and a phosphonate analog, *Chem. Res. Toxicol.* 9, 241–246, 1996.

18. Zhou, W., Zhang, H., and Chen, F., Modified lignin: Preparation and use in reversible gel via Diels-Alder reaction, *Int. J. Biol. Macromol.* 107, 790–795, 2018.

EDMAN DEGRADATION

The stepwise degradation of a peptide chain from the amino-terminal via reaction with phenylisothiocyanate.[1,2] The Edman degradation has been used for the chemical determination of the amino acid sequence of a peptide or protein.[3–14] This technology has be largely supplanted by other techniques such cDNA analysis and mass spectrometry[15,16] but is still used for the analysis of peptides and proteins.[17–22]

1. Edman, P., A method for the determination of amino acid sequence in peptides, *Arch. Biochem.* 22, 475, 1949.

2. Edman, P., Sequence determination, *Mol. Biol. Biochem. Biophys.* 9, 211–255, 1970.

3. Heinrikson, R.L., Application of automated sequence analysis to the understanding of protein structure and function, *Ann. Clin. Lab. Sci.* 8, 295–301, 1978.

4. Tsugita, A., Developments in protein microsequencing, *Adv. Biophys.* 23, 91–113, 1987.

5. Masiarz, F.R., and Malcolm, B.A., Rapid determination of endoprotease specificity using peptide mixtures and Edman degradation analysis, *Methods Enzymol.* 241, 302–310, 1994.

6. Gooley, A.A., Ou, K., Russell, J., et al., A role for Edman degradation in proteome studies, *Electrophoresis* 18, 1068–1072, 1997.

7. Wurzel, C., and Wittmann-Liebold, B., A wafer based micro reaction system for the Edman degradation of proteins and peptides, *J. Protein Chem.* 17, 561–564, 1998.

8. Walk, T.B., Sussmuth, R., Kempter, C., et al., Identification of unusual amino acids in peptides using automated sequential Edman degradation coupled to direct detection by electrospray-ionization mass spectrometry, *Biopolymers* 49, 329–340, 1999.

9. Lauer-Fields, J.L., Nagase, H., and Fields, G.B., Use of Edman degradation sequence analysis and matrix-assisted laser desorption/ionization mass spectrometry in designing substrates for matrix metalloproteinases, *J. Chromatog. A.* 890, 117–125, 2000.

10. Shively, J.E., The chemistry of protein sequence analysis, *EXS* 88, 99–117, 2000.

11. Wang, P., Arabaci, G., and Pei, D., Rapid sequencing of library-derived peptides by partial Edman degradation and mass spectrometry, *J. Comb. Chem.* 3, 251–254, 2001.

12. Brewer, M., Oost, T., Sukonpan, C., et al., Sequencing hydroxylethyleneamine-containing peptides via Edman degradation, *Org. Lett.* 4, 3469–3472, 2002.

13. Sweeney, M.C., and Pei, D., An improved method for rapid sequencing of support-bound peptides by partial Edman degradation and mass spectrometry, *J. Comb. Chem.* 5, 218–222, 2003.

14. Thakkar, A., Wavreille, A.S., and Pei, D., Traceless capping agent for peptide sequencing by partial Edman degradation and mass spectrometry, *Anal. Chem.* 78, 5935–5939, 2006.

15. Elashal, H.E., Cohen, R.D., Elashal, H.E., et al., Cyclic and lasso peptides: Sequence determination, topology analysis, and rotaxane formation, *Angew. Chem. Int. Ed. Engl.* 57, 6150–6154, 2018.

16. Hammers, C.M., Tang, H.Y., Chen, J., et al., Mass spectrometry for analysis of proteins in dermatological research, *J. Invest. Dermatol.* 138, 1236–1242, 2018.

17. Chen, W., Yin, X., and Yin, Y., Rapid and reliable peptide *de novo* sequencing facilitated by microfluidic chip-based Edmand degradation, *J. Proteome Res.* 7, 766–770, 2008.

18. Kashina, A.S., and Yates, J.R., 3rd, Analysis of arginylated peptides by subtractive Edman degradation, *Methods Mol. Biol.* 1337, 105–107, 2015.

19. Sun, W., Sun, J., Zhang, H., et al., Chemosynthesis and characterization of site-specific N-terminally PEGylated alpha-momorcharin as a potential agent, *Sci. Rep.* 8(1), 17729, 2018.

20. Hellinghausen, G., Lopez, D.A., Lee, J.T., et al., Evaluation of the Edman degradation product of vancomycin bonded to core-shell particles as a new HPLC chiral stationary phase, *Chirality* 30, 1067–1078, 2018.

21. Li, Z., Shao, S., Ren, X., et al., Construction of a sequencable protein mimetic peptide library with a true 3D diversifiable chemical space, *J. Am. Chem. Soc.* 140, 14552–14556, 2018.

22. Swaminathan, J., Boulgakov, A.A., Hernandez, E.T., et al., Highly parallel single-molecule identification of proteins in zeptomole-scale mixtures, *Nat. Biotechnol.* in press. doi: 10.1038/nbt.4278, 2019.

ESCHWEILER-CLARKE REACTION

The reductive methylation of amines with formaldehyde in the presence of formic acid.[1,2] This reaction is used to modify amines for synthetic and analytical purposes.[3–7] The reaction can be accomplished with sodium borohydride or sodium cyanoborohydride and is related to the reductively methylation/alkylation of lysine residues in proteins.[8]

1. Eschweiler, W., Ersatz von an Stickstoff gedundenen Wasserstoffatoms durch die Methylgrupe mit Hüffe von Formaldehyde, *Ber. Dtsch. Chem. Ges.* 38, 800–882, 1905.

2. Clarke, H.T., Gillespie, H.B., and Weisshaus, S.Z., The action of formaldehyde on amines and amino acids, *J. Am. Chem. Soc.* 55, 4571–4587, 1933.

3. Lindeke, B., Anderson, B., and Jenden, D.J., Specific deuteromethylation by the Escheweiler-Clarke reaction. Synthesis of differently labelled variants of trimethylamine and their use of the preparation of labelled choline and acetylcholine, *Biomed. Mass Spectrom.* 3, 257–259, 1976.

4. Boldavalli, F., Bruno, O., Mariani, E., et al., Esters of N-methyl-N-(2-hydroxyethyl or 3-hydroxypropyl)-1,3,3-trimethylbicyclo[2.2.1] heptan-2-endo-amine with hypotensive activity, *Farmaco* 42, 175–183, 1987.

5. Lee, S.S., Wu, W.N., Wilton, J.H., et al., Longiberine and O-methyllogiberine, dimeric protoberberine-benzyl tetrahydroisoqunioline alkaloids from *Thalictrum longistrylum*, *J. Nat. Prod.* 62, 1410–1414, 1999.

6. Suma, R., and Sai Prakash, P.K., Conversion of sertraline to N-methyl sertraline in embalming fluid: A forensic implication, *J. Anal. Toxicol.* 30, 395–399, 2006.

7. Ray, A., Bristow, T., Whitmore, C., and Mosely, J., On-line reaction monitoring by mass spectrometry, modern approaches for the analysis of chemical reactions, *Mass Spectrom. Rev.* 37, 565–579, 2018.

8. Lundblad, R.L., *Chemical Reagents for the Modification of Proteins*, 4th edn., CRC Press, Boca Raton, FL, 2014.

FAVORSKII REARRANGEMENT

The rearrangement of an α-ketone in the presence of an alkoxide to form a carboxylic ester; cyclic α-ketone undergo ring contraction.[1,2] Favorskii-type products have been suggested to occur in the formation oxylipins.[3,4] There is good evidence for the occurrence of the Favorskii reaction in the synthesis of enteocin, a polyketide bacteriostatic agent.[5-7]

1. March, J. *Advanced Organic Chemistry. Reactions, Mechanisms, and Structures*, 3rd edn. John Wiley & Sons, New York, 1985.
2. Zhang, L., and Koreeda, M., Stereocontrolled synthesis of kelsoene by the homo-favorskii rearrangement, *Org. Lett.* 4, 3755–3788, 2002.
3. Grechkin, A.N., Lantsova, N.V., Toporkova, Y.Y., et al., Novel allene oxide synthase product formed via Favorskii-type rearrangement: Mechanistic implications for 12-oxo-10,15-phytodienoic acid biosynthesis, *ChemBiochem* 12, 2511–2517, 2011.
4. Grechkin, A.N., Ogorodnikova, A.V., Egorova, A.M., et al., Allene oxide synthase pathway in cereal roots: Detection of novel oxylipin graminoxins, *ChemistryOpen* 7, 336–343, 2018.
5. Xiang, L., Kalaitzis, J.A., Nilsen, G., et al., Mutational analysis of the enterocin favorskii biosynthetic rearrangement, *Org. Lett.* 4, 957–960, 2002.
6. Xiang, L., Kalaitzis, J.A., and Moore, B.S., EccM, a versatile enterocin biosynthetic enzyme involved in Favorskii oxidative rearrangement, aldol condensation, and heterocycle-forming reactions, *Proc. Natl. Acad. Sci. USA* 101, 15609–15614, 2004.
7. Moore, B.S., Biosynthesis of marine natural products: Microorganisms (Part A), *Nat. Prod. Rep.* 22, 580–593, 2005.

FISCHER INDOLE SYNTHESIS

The thermal conversion of arylhydrazones in the presence of a protic acid or a Lewis acid such as zinc chloride to form an indole ring.[1-4] A solid-phase method for the Fischer indole synthesis has been developed.[5-9] This reaction has seen considerable use in synthetic organic chemistry.[10-15]

1. Fischer, E., and Jourdan, E., Uber die Hydrazine der Benztraubensäure, *Ber. Dtsch. Chem. Ges.* 16, 2241–2245, 1883.
2. Robinson, B., The Fischer indole synthesis, *Chem. Rev.* 63, 373–401, 1963.
3. Owellen, R.J., Fitzgerald, J.A., Fitzgerald, B.M., et al., The cyclization phase of the Fischer indole synthesis. The structure and significance of Pleininger's intermediate, *Tetrahedron Lett.* 18, 1741–1746, 1967.
4. Robinson, B., The Fischer indole synthesis, *Chem. Rev.* 69, 222–250, 1969.
5. Kim, R.M., Manna, M., Hutchins, S.M., et al., Dendrimer-supported combinatorial chemistry, *Proc. Natl. Acad. Sci. USA* 93, 10012–10017, 1996.
6. Brase, S., Gil, C., and Knepper, K., The recent impact of solid-phase synthesis on medicinally relevant benzoannelated nitrogen heterocycles, *Bioorg. Med. Chem.* 10, 2415–2437, 2002.
7. Rosenbaum, C., Katzka, C., Marzinzik, A., and Waldmann, H., Traceless Fischer indole synthesis on the solid phase, *Chem. Commun.* (15), 1822–1823, 2003.
8. Mun, H.S., Ham, W.H., and Jeong, J.H., Synthesis of 2,3-disubstituted indole on solid phase by the Fischer indole synthesis, *J. Comb. Chem.* 7, 130–135, 2005.
9. Patil, S.A., Patil, R., and Miller, D.D., Solid phase synthesis of biologically important indoles, *Curr. Med. Chem.* 16, 2531–2365, 2009.
10. Narayana, B., Ashalatha, B.V., Vijaya Raj, K.K., et al., Synthesis of some new biologically acivie 1,3,4-oxadiazolyl nitroindole and a modified Fischer indole synthesis of ethyl nitro indole-2-carboxylates, *Bioorg. Med. Chem.* 13, 4638–4644, 2005.
11. Schmidt, A.M., and Eilbracht, P., Tandem hydroformylation-hydrazone formation-Fischer indole synthesis: A novel approach to tryptamides, *Org. Biomol. Chem.* 3, 2333–2343, 2005.
12. Linnepe Nee Kohling, P., Schmidt, A.M., and Eilbracht, P., 2,3-Disubstituted indoles from olefins and hydrazines via tandem hydroformylation-Fischer indole synthesis and skeletal rearrangement, *Org. Biomol. Chem.* 4, 302–313, 2006.
13. Landwehr, J., George, S., Karg, E.M., et al., Design and synthesis of novel 2-amino-5-hydroxyindole derivatives that inhibit human 5-lipooxygenase, *J. Med. Chem.* 49, 4327–4332, 2006.
14. Aksenov, A.V. Smirnov, A.N., Askenov, N.A., et al., Metal-free transnnulation reaction of indoles with nitrostyrenes: A simple practical synthesis of 3-substituted 2-quinolines, *Chem. Comm.*(Cambridge) 49, 9305–9307, 2013.
15. Abdelatif, K.R., Lamie, P.F., and Omar, H.A., 3-methyl-2-phenyl-1-substituted-indole derivatives as indomethacin analogs: Design, synthesis and biological evaluation as potential anti-inflammatory and analgesic agents, *J. Enzyme Inhib. Med. Chem* 31, 318–324, 2016.

FRIEDEL–CRAFTS REACTION

The Friedel–Crafts reaction can be separated into two reactions.[1] The first, the *Friedel–Crafts alkylation* is the alkylation of an aromatic ring by an alkyl halide in the presence of a strong Lewis acid such as aluminum chloride.[2-7] The ability of an enzyme to catalyze Friedel–Crafts alkylation reactions has been demonstrated.[8] A Friedel–Crafts mechanism has been proposed for the action of histidine lyase and phenylalanine lyase.[9,10] The second Friedel–Crafts reaction, the *Friedel–Crafts acylation*, is the acylation of an aromatic ring by an acyl halide in the presence of a strong Lewis acid. Acids and acid anhydrides can replace the acyl halides.[11-15] Enzymatic catalysis of the Friedel–Crafts acylation has been reported.[16,17]

1. Olah, G.A., *Friedel–Crafts Chemistry*, John Wiley & Sons, New York, 1973.
2. Olah, G.A., Farooq, O., Farnia, S.M.F., and Olah, J.A., Friedel-Crafts chemistry. 11. Boron, aluminum, and gallium tris(trifluoromethanesulfonate)(triflate): Effective new Friedel-Crafts catalysts, *J. Am. Chem. Soc.* 110, 2560–2565, 1988.
3. Roberts, R.M., and Khalaf, A.A., *Friedel-Krafts Alkylation Chemistry: A Century of Discovery*, Marcel Dekker, New York, 1989.
4. Darbeau, R.W., Chen, Y., et al., A new look at the Friedel-Crafts alkylation reaction (1), *J. Org. Chem.* 61, 7986–7987, 1996.
5. Bandini, M., Melloni, A., and Umani-Ronchi, A., New catalytic approaches in the stereoselective Friedel-Crafts alkylation reaction, *Angew. Chem. Int. Ed. Engl.* 43, 550–556, 2004.
6. Poulsen, T.B., and Jørgensen, K.A., Catalytic asymmetric Friedel-Crafts alkylation reactions—cooper showed the way, *Chem. Rev.* 108, 2903–2915, 2008.
7. Sunke, R., Nallapati, S.B., Kumar, J.S., Shiva Kumar, K., and Pal, M., Use of AlCl$_3$ in Friedel Crafts arylation type reactions and beyond: An overview on the development of unique methodologies leading to *N*-heteroarenes, *Org. Biomol. Chem.* 15, 4042–4057, 2017.
8. Schultz, E., Braffman, N.R., Luescher, M.U., Hager, H.H., and Balskus, E.P., Biocatalytic Friedel-Crafts alkylation using a promiscuous biosynthetic enzyme, *Angew. Chem. Int. Ed. Engl.* 58, 3151–3155, 2019.
9. Rétey, J., Enzymatic catalysis by Friedel-Crafts-type reactions, *Naturwissenschaften* 83, 439–447, 1996.
10. Poppe, L., and Retéy, J., Friedel-Crafts-type mechanism the enzymatic elimination of ammonia from histidine and phenylalanine, *Angew. Chem. Int. Ed. Engl.* 44, 3668–3688, 2005.
11. White, E.H. Studer, J., Purdie, N., and Krouse, J.A., Friedel-Crafts acylation as a quality control assay for steroids, *Appl. Spectrosc.* 57, 791–796, 2003.
12. Sartori, G., and Maggi, R., Use of solid catalysts in Friedel-Crafts acylation reactions, *Chem. Rev.* 106, 1077–1104, 2006.
13. Motiwala, H.F., Verkariya, R.H., and Aubé, J., Intramolecular Friedel-Crafts acylation reaction promoted by 1,1,1,3,3,4-hexaflouro-2-propanol, *Org. Lett.* 17, 5484–5487, 2015.
14. Zhang, Y., Sun, F., Dan, W., and Fang, X., Friedel-Crafts acylation reactions of BN-substituted arenes, *J. Org. Chem.* 82, 12877–12887, 2017.
15. Li, L.H., Niu, Z.J., and Liang, Y.M., New Friedel-Crafts strategy for preparing 3-acylindoles, *Org. Biomol. Chem.* 16, 7792–7796, 2018.
16. Schmidt, N.G., Pavkov-Keler, T., Richter, N., et al., Biocatalytic Friedel-Crafts acylation and Fries reaction, *Angew. Chem. Int. Ed. Engl.* 56, 7615–7619, 2017.
17. Pavkov-Keller, T., Schmidt, N.G., Żadło-Dobrowolska, A., Kroutil, W., and Gruber, K., Structure and catalytic mechanism of a bacterial Friedel-Crafts acylase, *Chembiochem* 20, 88–95, 2019.

FRIEDLÄNDER SYNTHESIS

The base-catalyzed formation of quinoline derivatives by condensation of an *o*-aminobenzaldehyde with a ketone.[1-3] This reaction is also referred to as the Friedländer quinoline synthesis. The general utility of the reaction may be somewhat limited by the availability of *o*-aminobenzaldehyde derivatives but it has proved useful for the synthesis of a variety of organic compounds.[4-11]

1. Friedlaender, P., Ueber *o*-Aminobenzaldehyde, *Ber. Dtsch. Chem. Ges.* 15, 2572–2575, 1882.
2. Gladiali, S., Chelucci, G., Mudadu, M.S., et al., Friedlander synthesis of chiral alkyl-substituted 1,10-phenanthrolines, *J. Org. Chem.* 66, 400–405, 2001.
3. Patteux, C., Levacher, V., and Dupas, G., A novel traceless solid-phase Friedlander synthesis, *Org. Lett.* 5, 3061–3063, 2003.
4. McNaughton, B.R., and Miller, B.L., A mild and efficient one-step synthesis of quinolines, *Org. Lett.* 5, 4257–4259, 2003.
5. Maguire, M.P., Sheets, K.R., McVety, K., et al., A new series of PDGF receptor tyrosine kinase inhibitors: 3-substituted quinoline derivatives, *J. Med. Chem.* 37, 2129–2137, 1994.
6. Yasuda, N., Hsiao, Y., Jensen, M.S., et al., An efficient synthesis of an $\alpha_v\beta_3$ antagonist, *J. Org. Chem.* 69, 1959–1966, 2004.
7. Nagarajan, S., Arjun, P., Raaman, N., and Das, T.M., Regioselective facile one-pot Friedländer synthesis of sugar-based heterocyclic biomolecules, *Carbohydr. Res.* 345, 1988–1997, 2010.
8. Garrison, A.T., Abouelhassan, Y., Yang, H., et al., Microwave-enhanced Friedländer synthesis for the rapid assembly of halogenated quinolines with antibacterial and biofilm eradication activities against drug resistant and tolerant bacteria, *Medchemcomm.* 8, 720–724, 2016.
9. Chen, Y., Wei, X.R., Sun, R., et al., The fluorescent biomarkers for lipid droplets with quinoline-coumarin unit, *Org. Biomol. Chem.* 16, 7619–7625, 2018.
10. Kumar, G., Sathe, A., Krishna, V.S., Sriram, D., and Jachak, S.M., Synthesis and biological evaluation of dihydroquinoline carboxamide derivatives as anti-tubercular agents, *Eur. J. Med. Chem.* 157, 1–13, 2018.
11. Ukwitegetse, N., Saris, P.J.G., Sommer, J.R., et al., *Chemistry* 25, 1472–1475, 2019.

FRIES REARRANGEMENT

Rearrangement of a phenolic ester to yield *o*- and *p*-acyl-phenols.[1] The distribution of products between the *ortho* and *para* acyl derivates depends on reaction conditions and is a reversible process. The presence of solvent and a Lewis acid, the *para* product is preferred; with the photolytic process or at high temperature in the absence of solvent, the *ortho* derivative is preferred. The Fries rearrangement is a useful reaction in synthetic organic chemistry.[2-7] The canonical catalysis of the Fries rearrangement by Lewis acids such as $AlCl_3$ has been largely replaced by photocatalysis.[8-16] The presence of albumin in the photo-Fries reaction influences the rate and quantum yield of product.[17]

1. Fries, K., and Finck G., Über Homologue des Coumaranons und ihre Abkömmlinge, *Ber. Dtsch. Chem. Ges.* 41, 4271–4284, 1908.
2. Sen, A.B., and Bhattacharji, S., Fries' rearrangement of aliphatic esters of β-naphthol, *Curr. Sci.* 20, 132–133, 1951.
3. Kozhevnikova, E.F., Derouane, E.G., and Kozhevnikov, I.V., Heteropoly acid as a novel efficient catalyst for Fries rearrangement, *Chem. Commun.* (11), 1178–1179, 2002.
4. Girard, C., Tranchant, I., Nioré, P.A., et al., Fast, easy, and efficient method for the purification of phenolic isomers using a selective solid-phase scavenging process, *J. Comb. Chem.* 4, 640–651, 2002.
5. Seijas, J.A., Vazquez-Tato, M.P., and Carballido-Reboredo, R., Solvent-free synthesis of functionalized flavones under microwave irradiation, *J. Org. Chem.* 70, 2855–2858, 2005.
6. Yoshida, S., Uchida, K., Igawa, K., Tomooka, K., and Hosoya, T., An efficient generation method and remarkable reactivities of 3-trifyloxybenzyne, *Chem. Commun.*(Camb) 50, 15059–15062, 2014.
7. Doustkhah, E., Lin, J., Rostamnia, S. et al., Development of sulfonic-acid-functionalized mesoporous materials: Synthesis and catalytic applications, *Chemistry* 25, 1614–1635, 2019.
8. Iwasaki, S., Photochemistry of imidazolides. I. The photo-Fries-type rearrangement of *N*-substituted imidazoles, *Helv. Chim. Acta* 59, 2738–2752, 1976.
9. Castell, J.V., Gomez, M.J., MIrabet, V., et al., Photolytic degradation of benorylate: Effects of the photoproducts on cultured hepatocytes, *J. Pharm. Sci.* 76, 374–378, 1987.
10. Climent, M.J., and Miranda, M.A., Gas chromatographic-mass spectrometric study of photodegradation of carbamate pesticides, *J. Chromatog. A.* 738, 225–231, 1996.
11. Dickerson, T.J., Tremblay, M.R., Hoffman, T.Z. et al., Catalysis of the photo-Fries reaction: Antibody-mediated stabilization of high energy states, *J. Am. Chem. Soc.* 125, 15395–15401, 2003.
12. Canle Lopez, M., Fernandez, M.I., Rodriguez, S., et al., Mechanisms of direct and TiO_2-photocatalyzed degradation of phenylurea herbicides, *Chemphyschem* 6, 2064–2074, 2005.
13. Ferrini, S., Ponticelli, F., and Taddei, M., Rapid approach to 3,5-disubstituted 1,4-benzodiazepines via the photo-fries rearrangement of anilides, *J. Org. Chem.* 71, 9217–9220, 2006.
14. Martignac, M., Oliveros, E., Maurette, M.T., Claparols, C., and Benoit-Marquié, F., Mechanistic pathways of the photolysis of paracetamol in aqueous solution: An example of photo-Fries rearrangement, *Photochem. Photobiol. Sci.* 12, 527–535, 2013.
15. Iguchi, D., Erra-Balsells, R., and Bonesi, S.M., Photo-Fries rearrangement of aryl acetamides: Regioselectivity induced by the aqueous micellar green environment, *Photochem. Photobiol. Sci.* 15, 105–116, 2016.
16. Toldo, J.M., Barbatti, M., and Goncalves, P.F.B., A three-state model for the photo-Fries rearrangement, *Phys. Chem. Chem. Phys.* 19, 19103–19108, 2017.
17. Marin, M., Lhiaubet-Vallet, V., and Miranda, M.A., Site-dependent photo-Fries rearrangement within serum albumins, *J. Phys. Chem. B.* 115, 2910–2915, 2011.

GABRIEL SYNTHESIS

The conversion of an alkyl halide to alkyl amine mediated by potassium phthalimide.[1] The intermediate product of the reaction of the alkyl halide and phthalimide is hydrolyzed to the product amine by acid or by reflux in ethanolic hydrazine. There are a number of applications of the Gabriel synthesis of the preparation of biochemicals of which a few are cited herein.[2-9]

1. Gabriel, S., Ueber eine Darstellungsweise primärer Amine aus den entsprechenden Halogenverbindungen, *Ber. Dtsch. Chem. Ges.* 20, 2224–2236, 1887.
2. Mikola, H., and Hanninen, E., Introduction of aliphatic amino and hydroxy groups to keto steroids using *O*-substituted hydroxylamines, *Bioconjugate Chem.* 3, 182–186, 1992.
3. Groutas, W.C., Chong, L.S., Venkataraman, R., et al., Mechanism-based inhibitors of serine proteinases based on the Gabriel-Colman rearrangement, *Biochem. Biophys. Res. Commun.* 194, 1491–1499, 1993.
4. Konig, S., Ugi, I., and Schramm, H.J., Facile syntheses of C_2-symmetrical HIV-1 protease inhibitor, *Arch. Pharm.* 328, 699–704, 1995.
5. Zhang, X.X., and Lippard, S.J., Synthesis of PDK, a novel porphyrin-linked dicarboxylate ligand, *J. Org. Chem.* 65, 5298–5305, 2000.
6. Scozzafava, A. Saramet, I., Banciu, M.D., and Supuran, C.T., Carbonic anhydrase activity modulators: Synthesis of inhibitors and activators incorporating 2-substituted-thiazol-4-yl-methyl scaffolds, *J. Enzyme Inhib.* 16, 351–358, 2001.

7. Nicolaou, K.C., Hao, J., Reddy, M.V., et al., Chemistry and biology of diazonamide A: Second total synthesis and biological investigations, *J. Am. Chem. Soc.* 126, 12897–12906, 2004.

8. Chung, S.H., Lin, T.J., Hu, Q.Y., Tsai, C.H., and Pan, P.S., Synthesis of boron-containing primary amines, *Molecules* 18, 12346–12367, 2013.

9. Briš, A., Dud, M., and Margetić, D., Mechanochemical *N*-alkylation of imides, *Beilstein J. Org. Chem.* 13, 1745–1752, 2017.

GRIESS REACTION

The Griess reaction[1] is used for the assay of nitrites in nitric oxide research,[2–10] in biological tissues and fluids,[11–14] and in environmental testing.[15–18] The Griess reaction can be used to for the determination of nitrate but reduction to nitrite is required before analysis.[2–4,19]

1. Greiss, P., Bemerkungen zu der Abhandlung der HH Wesselsky und Benedikt "Ueber einige Azoverbindungen", *Ber. Dtsch. Chem. Ges.* 12, 426–428, 1879.

2. Tsikas, D., Analysis of nitrite and nitrate in biological fluids by assays based on the Griess reaction: Appraisal of the Griess reaction in the L-arginine/nitric oxide area of research, *J. Chromatog. B* 851, 51–70, 2007.

3. NIthipatikom, K., and Campbell, W.B., Simultaneous determination of nitrate and nitrite in biological samples by multichannel flow injection analysis, *Anal. Biochem.* 231, 383–386, 1995.

4. Greenberg, S.S., Xie, J., Spitzer, J.J., et al., Nitro containing L-arginine analogs interfere with assays for nitrate and nitrite, *Life Sci.* 57, 1949–1961, 1995.

5. Pratt, P.F., Tang, Y., Han, C., and Wang, X., Role of nitric oxide and prostaglandins in the potentiating effects of calcitonin gene-related peptide on lipopolysaccharide-induced interleukin-6 release from mouse peritoneal macrophages, *Immunology* 96, 171–175, 1999.

6. Baines, P.B., Stanford, S., Bishop-Bailey, D., et al., Nitric oxide production in meningococcal disease is directly related to disease severity, *Crit. Care. Med.* 27, 1163–1165, 1999.

7. Lee, R.H., Efron, D., Tantry, U., and Barbul, A., Nitric oxide in the healing wound: A time-course study, *J. Surg. Res.* 101, 104–108, 2001.

8. Stark, J.M., Khan, A.M., Chiappetta, C.L., et al., Immune and functional role of nitric oxide in a mouse model of respiratory syncytial virus infection, *J. Infect. Dis.* 191, 387–395, 2005.

9. Bellows, C.F., Alder, A., Wludyka, P., and Jaffe, B.M., Modulation of macrophage nitric oxide production by prostaglandin D2, *J. Surg. Res.* 132, 92–97, 2006.

10. Ghafourifar, P., Parihar, MS., Nazarewicz, R., Zenebe, W.J., and Parihar, A., Detection assays for determination of mitochondrial nitric oxides synthase activity; advantages and limitations, *Methods Enzymol.* 440, 317–334, 2008.

11. Guevara, I., Iwanejko, J., Dembińska-Kieć, A., et al., Determination of nitrite/nitrate in human biological material by the simple Griess reaction, *Clin. Chim. Acta* 274, 177–188, 1998.

12. Rabbani, G.H., Islam, S., Chowdhury, A.K., et al., Increased nitrite and nitrate concentrations in sera and urine of patients with cholera or shigellosis, *Am. J. Gastroenterol.* 96, 467–472, 2001.

13. Hufeland, M., Schünke, M., Grodzinsky, A.J., Imgenberg, J., and Kurz, B., Response of mature meniscal tissue to a single injurious compression and interleukin-1 *in vitro*, *Osteoarthritis Cartilage* 21, 209–216, 2013.

14. Georgescu, E., Oancea, A., Georgescu, F., et al., Schiff bases containing a furoxan moiety as potential nitric oxide donors in plant tissues, *PLoS One* 13(7), e0198121, 2018.

15. Feres, M.A., and Reis, B.F., A downsized flow setup based on multicommutation for the sequential photometric determination of iron(II)/iron(III) and nitrite/nitrate in surface water, *Talanta* 68, 422–428, 2005.

16. Jurado-Sánchez, B., Ballesteros, E., and Gallego, M., Automatic screening method of the preconcentration and determination of *N*-nitrosamines in water, *Talanta* 73, 498–504, 2007.

17. Daniel, W.L., Han, M.S., Lee, J.S., and Mirkin, C.A., Colorimetric nitrite and nitrate detection with gold nanoparticle probes and kinetic end points, *J. Am. Chem. Soc.* 131, 6362–6363, 2009.

18. Lee, M., Lee, Y., Soltermann, F., and von Gunten, U., Analysis of *N*-nitrosamines and other nitro(so) compounds in water by high-performance liquid chromatography with post-column UV photolysis/Griess reaction, *Water Res.* 47, 4893–4903, 2013.

19. Nithipatikom, K., Pratt, P.F., and Campbell, W.B., Nitro-L-arginine interference with the cadmium reduction of nitrate/griess reaction method of measuring nitric oxide production, *Eur. J. Clin. Chem. Biochem.* 34, 133–137, 1996.

GRIGNARD REAGENT OR GRIGNARD REACTION

The reaction of alkyl or aryl halides with magnesium in dry ether to yield derivatives,[1–6] which can be used in a variety of organic synthetic reactions.[7–15]

1. Grignard, V., Sur quelques nouvelles combinaisons organométalliques du magnesium et leur application à des syntheses d'alcools et d'hydrocarbures, *Compt. Rendu. Seances de l'Acad. des Sciences* 130, 1322–1324, 1900.

2. Maruyama, K., and Katagiri, T., Mechanism of the Grignard reaction, *J. Phys. Org. Chem.* 2, 205–213, 1988.

3. *Handbook of Grignard Reagents*, ed. G.S. Silverman and P.E. Rakita, Marcel Dekker, New York, 1996.

4. *Grignard Reagents and Transition Metal Catalysts*, ed. J. Cossy, Walter de Gruyter, Berlin, Germany, 2016.

5. Shao, Y., Liu, Z., Huang, P., and Liu, B., A unified model of Grignard reagent formation, *Phys. Chem. Chem. Phys.* 20, 11100–11108, 2018.

6. Banno, T., Hayakawa, Y., and Umeno, M., Some applications of the Grignard cross-coupling reaction in the industrial field, *J. Organometallic Chem.* 653, 288–291, 2002.

7. Agarwal, S., and Knolker, H.J., A novel pyrrole synthesis, *Org. Biomol. Chem.* 2, 3060–3062, 2004.

8. Hatano, M., Matsumara, T., and Ishihara, K., Highly alkyl-selective addition to ketones with magnesiumate complexes derived from Grignard reagents, *Org. Lett.* 7, 573–576, 2005.

9. Itami, K., Higashi, S., Mineno, M., and Yoshida, J., Iron-catalyzed cross-coupling of alkenyl sulfides with Grignard reagents, *Org. Lett.* 7, 1219–1222, 2005.

10. Wang, X.J., Zhang, L., Sun, X., et al., Addition of Grignard reagents to aryl chlorides: An efficient synthesis of aryl ketones, *Org. Lett.* 7, 5593–5595, 2005.

11. Hoffman-Emery, F., Hilpert, H., Scalone, M., and Waldmeier, F., Efficient synthesis of novel NK1 receptor antagonists: Selective 1,4-additional of Grignard reagents to 6-chloronicotinic acid derivatives, *J. Org. Chem.* 71, 2000–2008, 2006.

12. Werner, T., and Barrett, A.G., Simple method for the preparation of esters from Grigard reagents and alkyl 1-imidazolecarboxylates, *J. Org. Chem.* 71, 4302–4304, 2006.

13. Demel, P., Keller, M., and Breit, B., *o*-DPPB-directed copper-mediated and -catalyzed allylic substitution with Grignard reagents, *Chemistry* 12, 6669–6683, 2006.

14. Riva, E., Gagliardi, S., Martinelli, M., et al., Reaction of Grignard reagents with carbonyl compounds under continuous flow conditions, *Tetrahedron* 66, 3242–3247, 2010.

15. Dhakal, R.C., and Dieter, R.K., Regioselective 1,4-conjugate addition of Grignard reagents to nitrodienes in the presence of catalytic amounts of Zn(II) salts, *Org. Lett.* 16, 1362–1365, 2014.

3. Pivonka, D.E., and Empfield, J.R., Real-time *in situ* Ramen analysis of microwave-assisted organic reactions, *Appl. Spectrosc.* 58, 41–46, 2004.

4. Lai. S.M., Martin-Aranda, R., and Yeung, K.L., Knoevenagel condensation reaction in a membrane bioreactor, *Chem. Commun.* (2), 218–219, 2003.

5. Strohmeier, G.A., Haas, W., and Kappe, C.O., Synthesis of functionalized 1,3-thiazine libraries combining solid-phase synthesis and post-cleavage modification reactions, *Chemistry* 10, 2919–2926, 2004.

6. Kuster, G.J., van Berkom, L.W., Kalmoua, M., et al., Synthesis of spirohydantoins and spiro-2,5-diketopiperazines via resin-bound cyclic α,α-disubstituted α-amino esters, *J. Comb. Chem.*8, 85–94, 2006.

7. Evdokimov, N.M., Kireev, A.S., Yakovenko, A.A., et al., One-step synthesis of heterocyclic privileged medicinal scaffolds by a multicomponent reaction of malonitrile with aldehydes and thiols, *J. Org. Chem.* 72, 3443–3453, 2007.

8. Pels, K., Dickson, P., An, H., and Kodadek, T., DNA-compatible solid-phase combinatorial synthesis of β-cyanoacrylamides and related electrophiles, *ACS Comb. Sci.* 20, 61–69, 2018.

9. Sharma, A., Noki, S., Zamisa, S.J., et al., Exploiting the thiobarbituric acid scaffold for antibacterial activity, *ChemMedChem* 13, 1923–1930, 2018.

10. Klavins, M., Dipane, J., and Babre, K., Humic substances as catalysts in condensation reactions, *Chemosphere* 44, 737–742, 2001.

11. Wirz, R., Ferri, D., and Baiker, A., ATR-IR spectroscopy of pendant NH_2 groups on silica involved in the Knoevenagel condensation, *Langmuir* 22, 3698–3706, 2006.

12. Garraboui, X., Wicky, B.I., and Hilvert, D., Fast Knoevenagel condensation catalyzed by an artificial Schiff-base-forming enzyme, *J. Am. Chem. Soc.* 138, 6972–6974, 2016.

KNOEVENAGEL REACTION OR KNOEVENAGEL CONDENSATION

An amine-catalyzed reaction between active hydrogen compounds of the type $Z-CH_2-Z$, where Z can be a CHO, COOH, COOR, NO_2, SOR, or related electron withdrawing groups and an aldehyde or ketone.[1-4] The Knoevenagel reaction is useful in the development of libraries.[5-9] A variety of catalysts for the Knoevenagel reaction have been advanced.[10-12]

1. Knoevenagel, E., Condensationen zwischen Malonester und Aldhyden under den Einfluss von Amoniak und organischen Aminen, *Ber. Dtsch. Chem. Ges.* 31, 2585–2595, 1898.

2. March, J., *Advanced Organic Chemistry. Reactions, Mechanisms, and Structure*, 3rd edn., John Wiley & Sons, New York, 1985.

LEUCKART REACTION

The reductive amination of carbonyl groups by ammonium formate or formamide with heating.[1] The Leuckart reaction is used to prepare a variety of biochemicals.[2-10] The related Leuckart–Wallach reaction, which is the reductive alkylation of amines by carbonyl compounds, was developed by Wallach from the observations of Leuckart[11-15] and is a useful synthetic method.

1. Leuckart, R., Ueber eine neue Bildungsweise von Tribenzlamin, *Ber. Dtsch. Chem. Ges.* 18, 2341–2344, 1885.

2. Matsueda, G.R., and Stewart, J.M., A *p*-methylbenzhydrylamine resin for improved solid-phase synthesis of peptide amides, *Peptides* 2, 45–50, 1981.

3. Agwada, V.C., and Awachie, P.I., Intermediates in the Leuckart reaction of benzophenone with formamide, *Tetrahedron Lett.* 23, 779–780, 1982.

4. Loupy, A., Monteux, D., Petit, A., et al., Toward the rehabilitation of the Leuckart reductive amination reaction using microwave technology, *Tetrahedron Lett.* 37, 8177–8180, 1996.

5. Adger, B.M., Dyer, U.C., Lennon, I.C., et al., A novel synthesis of *tert*-leucine via a Leuckart type reaction, *Tetrahedron Lett.* 38, 2153–2154, 1997.

6. Lejon, T., and Helland, I., Effect of formamide in the Leuckart reaction, *Acta Chem. Scand.* 53, 76–78, 1999.

7. Tournier, L., and Zard, S.Z., A practical variation on the Leuckart reaction, *Tetrahedron Lett.* 46, 971–973, 2005.

8. Wang, J., Gu, J., Nguyen, M.T., Springsteen, G., and Leszczynski, J., From formamide to purine: A self-catalyzed reaction pathway provides a feasible mechanism for the entire process, *J. Phys. Chem. B* 117, 9333–9342, 2013.

9. Rani, P., Pal, D., Hegde, R.R., and Hashim, S.R., Leuckart synthesis and pharmacological assessment of novel acetamide derivatives, *Anticancer Agents Med. Chem.* 16, 898–906, 2016.

10. Skachilova, S.Ya., Zheltukhan, N.K., Seegev, V.N., and Davydova, N.K., Reductive amination of sterically hindered arylaminoketones using a modified Leuckart reaction, *Pharm. Chem. J.* 52, 545–549, 2018.

11. Wallach, O., Ueber Methylamin, *Ber. Dtsch. Chem. Ges.* 24, 3992–3993, 1891.

12. Crossley, F.S., and Moore, M.L., Studies on the Leuckart reaction, *J. Org. Chem.* 9, 529–536, 2018.

13. Kitamura, M., Lee, D., Hayashi, S., et al., Catalytic Leuckart-Wallach type reductive amination of ketones, *J. Org. Chem.* 67, 8685–8687, 2002.

14. Neochoritis, C.G., Zarganes-Tzitzikas, T., Stotani, S., Leuckart-Wallach route toward isocyanides and some applications, *ACS Comb. Sci.* 17, 493–499, 2015.

15. De, A., Ghosal, N.C., Mahato, S., et al., Scope and limitations of Leuckart-Wallach type reductive alkylation: Chemoselective synthesis of tertiary amines from aldehydes under neat conditions, *Chem. Select* 3, 4058–4066, 2018.

LOSSEN REARRANGEMENT

The formation of isocyanates on heating of *O*-acyl derivatives of hydroxamic acids or treatment by base.[1,2] The isocyanate frequently adds water *in situ* to form an amine with a chain one carbon shorter that the parent compound. The Lossen rearrangement in the presence of amines results in the formation of ureas. This reaction is important in biochemistry.[3–14]

1. Lossen, W., Ueber Benzoylderivate des Hydroxylamins, *Justus Liebig Ann. Chem.* 161, 347–362, 1872.

2. Thomas, M., J., Alsarraf, N., Araji, et al., The Lossen rearrangement from free hydroxamic acids, *Org. Biomol. Chem.* 17, 5420–5427, 2019.

3. Andersen, W., The synthesis of phenylcarbamoyl derivatives by Lossen rearrangement of dibenzohydroxamic acid, *C. R. Trav. Lab. Carlsberg.* 30, 79–103, 1956.

4. Gallop, P.M., Seifter, S., Lukin, M., and Meilman, E. Application of the Lossen rearrangement of dintirophenylhydroxamates to analysis of carboxyl groups in model compounds and gelatin, *J. Biol. Chem.* 235, 2619–2627, 1960.

5. Hoare, D.G., Olson, A., and Koshland, D.E., Jr., The reaction of hydroxamic acids with water-soluble carbodiimides. A Lossen rearrangement, *J. Am. Chem. Soc.* 90, 1638–1643, 1968.

6. Harris, R.B., and Wilson, I.B., Glutamic acid is an active site residue of angiotensin I-converting enzyme. Use of the Lossen rearrangement for identification of dicarboxylic acid residues, *J. Biol. Chem.* 258, 1357–1362, 1983.

7. Libert, R., Draye, J.P., Van Hoof, F., et al., Study of reactions induced by hydroxylamine treatment of esters for organic acids and of 3-ketoacids: Application to the study of urines from patients under valproate therapy, *Biol. Mass. Spectrom.* 20, 75–86, 1991.

8. Neumann, U., and Gutschow, M., *N*-(sulfonyloxy) phthalimides and analogues are potent inactivators of serine proteases, *J. Biol. Chem.* 269, 21561–21567, 1994.

9. Steinmetz, A.C., Demuth, H.U., and Ringe, D., Inactivation of subtilisin Carlsberg by *N*-[(*t*-butoxycarbonyl) alanylprolyl-phenylalanyl]-*O*-benzoylhydroxyl-amine: Formation of a covalent enzyme-inhibitor linkage in the form of a carbamate derivative, *Biochemistry* 33, 10535–10544, 1994.

10. Needs, P.W., Rigby, N.M., Ring, S.G., and MacDougall, A.J., Specific degradation of pectins via a carbodiimide-mediated Lossen rearrangement of methyl esterified galacturonic acid residues, *Carbohydr. Res.* 333, 47–58, 2001.

11. Hamon, E., Prié, G., Lecornué, F., and Papot, S., Cyanuric chloride: An efficient reagent for the Lossen rearrangement, *Tetrahedron Lett.* 50, 6800–6802, 2009.

12. Dobé, P., Nathel, N.F.F., Vetelino, M., et al., Carbodiimidazole-mediated Lossen rearrangement, *Org. Lett.* 11, 5622–5625, 2009.

13. Strotman, N.A., Ortiz, A., Savage, S.A., et al., Revisiting a classic transformation: A Lossen rearrangement initiated by nitriles and "pseud-catalytic" in isocyanate, *J. Org. Chem.* 82, 4044–4049, 2017.

14. Schulz-Fincke, A.C., Tikhomirov, A.S., Braune, A., et al., Design of an activity-based probe for human neutrophil elastase: Implementation of the Lossen rearrangement to induce Förster resonance energy transfers, *Biochemistry* 57, 742–752, 2018.

MAILLARD REACTION

The Maillard reaction (named after Louis-Camille Maillard)[1,2] is a reaction between a protein amino group, usually the epsilon-amino group of lysine and a reducing sugar/aldose, which can proceed to form a large number of derivative products.[3–5] The initial observation by Maillard was the formation of a yellow-brown color on heating an aqueous solution of an amine and sugar.[5] There is an initial condensation reaction to form a Schiff base which undergoes rearrangement to form an Amadori product. The Amadori product can then form a variety of products and, in the case of lysine, form crosslinks between protein chains as well as the formation of derivatives known as advanced glycation end products (AGE) or Maillard reaction products.[6] The initial reaction between amines and sugars is in essence a reaction between an aldehyde and a ketone with the initial formation of an N-substituted α-hydroxy derivative which forms a Schiff base (an imine) derivative by dehydration.[7] A Maillard-type reaction can also occur with the amino group of guanine in nucleic acid[8] generating novel taste products.[9] There is considerable interest in the Maillard reaction in food chemistry for taste. nutrition, and color.[10–15] Acrylamide is formed by a Maillard-type reaction in food in a reaction involving asparagine and a carbonyl compound.[16,17] The Maillard reaction is also involved in the tanning of animal skin.[18] In addition, the Maillard reaction In important in the action of self-tanning products.[19] AGE formed by Maillard-type reactions are also of considerable medical interest.[20–26] Finally, the reaction of sugars with proteins in the Maillard reaction is glycation as opposed to glycosylation which involves a different type of chemistry in the linking of sugars to proteins and is the result of an enzyme-catalyzed reaction. The broad interest in the Maillard reaction has resulted in the application of proteomic technology to study the various Maillard products.[27–29]

1. Nurston, H.E., *The Maillard Reaction: Chemistry, Biochemistry, and Implications*, Royal Society of Chemistry, Cambridge, UK, 2010.
2. Hellwig, M., and Henle, T., Baking, ageing, diabetes: A short history of the Maillard reaction, *Angew. Chem. Int. Ed. Engl.* 53, 10316–10329, 2014.
3. Hodge, J.E., Chemistry of the browning reactions in model systems, *J. Agric. Food Chem.* 1, 928–943, 1953.
4. Martins, S.I.F.S., Jongen, W.M.F., and van Boekel, M.A.J.S., A review of Maillard reaction in food ad implications to kinetic modeling, *Trends Food Sci. Technol.* 11, 364–373, 2001.
5. Fayle, S.E., Gerrard, J.A., and Belton, P.S., What is the Maillard reaction?, in *The Maillard Reaction*, ed. Fayle, S.E., and Gerrard, J.A., Chapter 1, pp. 1–8, Royal Society of Chemistry, Cambridge, UK, 2002.
6. Sell, D.R., Biemel, K.M., Reihl, O., Glucosepane is a major protein cross-link of the senescent human extracellular matrix. Relationship with diabetes, *J. Biol. Chem.* 280, 12310–12315, 2005.
7. Sprung, M.M., A summary of the reactions of aldehydes with amines, *Chem. Rev.* 26, 297–338, 1940.
8. Papoulis, A., al-Abed, Y., and Bucala, R., Identification of N^2-(1-carboxyethyl) guanine (CEG) as a guanine advanced glycosylation end product, *Biochemistry* 54, 648–655, 1995.
9. Suess, B., Brockhoff, A., Degenhardt, A., et al., Human taste and umami receptor responses to chemosensorica generated by Maillard-type N^2-alkyl- and N^2-arlthiomethylatkion of guanosine-5'-monophosphates *J. Agrc. Food Chem.* 62, 11429–11440, 2014.
10. *The Maillard Reaction in Foods and Nutrition*, ed. G.R. Wallen, and M.S. Feather, American Chemical Society, Washington, DC, 1987.
11. *The Maillard Reaction in Food and Medicine*, ed. J.O'Brien, H.E., Nurston, M.J.C., Crabbe and J.M. Ames, Royal Society of Chemistry, Cambridge, UK, 1998.
12. Losso, J.N., *The Maillard Reaction Reconsidered. Cooking and Eating for Health*, CRC Press, Boca Raton, FL, 2015.
13. Yin, Z., Sun, Q., Zhang, X., and Jing, H., Optimised formation of blue Maillard reaction products of xylose and glycine model systems and associated antioxidant activity, *J. Sci. Food. Agric.* 94, 1332–1339, 2014.
14. Liska, D.J., Cook, C.M., Wang, D.D., and Szpylka, J., Maillard reaction products and potatoes: Have the benefits been clearly assessed? *Food Sci. Nutr.* 4, 234–249, 2015
15. Khan, M.I., Jo, C., and Tang, M.R., Meat flavor precursors and factors influencing flavor precursors—A systemic review, *Meat Sci.* 110, 278–284, 2015.
16. Mottram, D.S., Wedzicha, B.L., and Dodsoon, A.T., Acrylamide is formed in the Maillard reaction, *Nature* 419, 448–449, 2002.
17. Stadler, R.H., Blank, I., Varga, N., et al., *Nature* 419, 2002; Zyzak, D.V., Sanders, R.A., Stajonovic, M., et al., Acrylamide formation mechanism in heated foods, *J. Agric. Food Chem.* 51, 4782–4787, 2003.
18. Painter, T.J., Lindow man, Tollund man and other peat-bog bodies: The preservative and antimicrobial action of sphagnan, a reactive glycuronoglycan with tanning and sequesting properties, *Carbohydr. Poly.* 15, 123–142, 1991.
19. Jung, K., Seifert, M., Herrling, T., and Fuchs, J., UV-generated free radicals (FR) in skin: Their prevention by sun screens and their induction by self-tanning agents, *Spectrochim. Acta A Mol. Biomol. Spectrosc.* 69, 1423–1428, 2008.
20. Smith, M.A., Taned, S., Richey, P.L., Advanced Maillard reaction end products are associated with Alzheimer disease pathology, *Proc. Natl. Acad. Sci. USA* 91, 5710–5714, 1994.
21. Njoroge, F.G., and Monnier, V.M., The chemistry of the Maillard reaction under physiological conditions: A review, *Prog. Clin. Biol. Res.* 304, 85–107, 1989.
22. Marko, D., Habermeyer, M., Keméy, M., et al., Maillard reaction products modulating the growth of human tumor cells in vitro, *Chem. Res. Toxicol.* 16, 48–55, 2003.

23. Takeguchi, M., Yamagishi, S., Iwaki, M., et al., Advanced glycation end product (age) inhibitors and their therapeutic implications in diseases, *Int. J. Clin. Pharmacol. Res.* 24, 95–1010, 2004.

24. Jing, H., and Nakamura, S., Production and use of Maillard products as oxidative stress modulators, *J. Med. Food* 8, 291–298, 2005.

25. Vistoli, G., De Maddis, D., Cipak, A., et al., Advanced glycoxidation and lipoxidation end products (AGEs and ALEs): An overview of their mechanism of formation, *Free Radic. Res.* 47 (Suppl 1), 3–27, 2013.

26. Ott, C., Jacobs, K., Haucke, E, et al., Role of advanced glycation end products in cellular signaling, *Redox. Biol.* 2, 411–429, 2014.

27. Ames, J.M., Application of semiquantiative proteomics techniques to the Maillard reaction, *Ann. N.Y. Acad. Sci.* 1043, 225–235, 2005.

28. Renzone, G., Arena, S., and Scaloni, A., Proteomic characterization of intermediate and advanced glycation end-products in commercial milk samples, *J. Proteomics* 117, 12–23, 2015.

29. Soboleva, A., Schmidt, R., Vikhnina, M., Grishina, T., and Frolov, A., Maillard proteomics: Opening new pages, *Int. J. Mol. Sci.* 18, 2677, 2017.

MALAPRADE REACTION

The Malaprade reaction[1] is the cleavage of a diol by periodate, although this term is seldom used for this extremely common reaction. However, Malprade reaction appears to be the correct terminology. Periodic acid is used for the diol cleavage in aqueous solvent, while lead tetraacetate can be used in organic solvents. The reaction also occurs when an amine group is vicinal to a hydroxyl function. It would appear that the term Malaprade reaction has been used more in description of analytical techniques for organic diols such as gluconic acid or in the assay of periodate.[2–13] The periodic acid oxidation of sugars in used the identification of glycoproteins (periodic acid-Schiff base reaction, PAS).[14]

1. Malaprade, M.L., Oxydation de quelques polyalcools par l'acide periodique, *Comp. Rend. Hebd. Séances l'Acad. Sci.* 186, 382, 1928.

2. Belcher, R., Dryhurst, G., and MacDonal, A.M., Submicro-methods for analysis of organic compounds. 22. Malaprade reaction, *J. Chem. Soc.* 3964, 1965.

3. Chen, K.P., Determination of calcium gluconate by selective oxidation with periodate, *J. Pharm. Sci.* 73, 681–683, 1984.

4. Verma, K.K., Gupta, D., Sanghi, S.K., and Jain, A., Spectrophotometric determination of periodate with amodiaquine dihydrochloride and its application to the indirect determination of some organic-compounds via the Malaprade reaction, *Analyst* 112, 1519–1522, 1987.

5. Nevado, J.J.B., and Gonzalez, P.V., Spectrophotometric determination of periodate with salicylaldehyde guanylhydrazone—indirect determination of some organic compounds using the Malaprade reaction, *Analyst* 114, 243–244, 1989.

6. Jie, N, Q., Yang, D.L., Zhang, Q.N., et al., Fluorometric determination of periodate with thiamine and its application to the determination of ethylene glycol and glycerol, *Anal. Chim. Acta* 359, 87–92, 1998.

7. Guillan-Sans, R., and Guzman-Chozas, M., The thiobarbituric acid (TBA) reaction in foods, A review, *Crit. Rev. Food Sci. Nutrition* 38, 315–330, 1998.

8. Pumera, M., Jelinek, I., Jindrich, J., et al., Determination of cyclodextrin content using periodate oxidation by capillary electrophoresis, *J. Chromatog. A* 891, 201–206, 2000.

9. Afkhami, A., and Mosaed, F., Kinetic determination of periodate based on its reaction with ferroin and its application to the indirect determination of ethylene glycol and glycerol, *Microchemical J.* 68, 35–40, 2001.

10. Afkhami, A., and Mosaed, F., Sensitive kinetic-spectrophotometric determination of trace amounts of periodate ion, *J. Anal. Chem.* 58, 588–593, 2003.

11. Mihovilovic, M.D., Spina, M., Muller, B., and Stanetty, P., Synthesis of carbo- and heterocyclic aldehydes bearing an adjacent donor group – Ozonolysis versus OsO_4/ KIO_4-oxidation, *Monatshefte für Chemie* 135, 899–909, 2004.

12. Gupta, M., Jain, A., and Verma, K.K., Optimization of experimental parameters in single-drop microextraction-gas chromatography-mass spectrometry for the determination of periodate by the Malaprade reaction, and its application to ethylene glycol, *Talanta* 71, 1039–1046, 2007.

13. Bagherian, G., Chamjangali, M.A., Goudarzi, N., and Namazi, N., Selective spectrophotometric determination of periodate based on its reaction with methylene green and its application to indirect determination of ethylene glycol and glycerol, *Spectrochim. Acta A Mol. Biomol. Spectrosc.* 76, 29–32, 2010.

14. Steinke, H., Wiersbicki, D., Speckert, M.L., et al., Periodic acid-Schiff (PAS) reaction and plastination in whole body slices. A novel technique to identify fascial tissue structures, *Ann. Anat.* 216, 29–35, 2018.

MALONIC ESTER SYNTHESIS

The synthesis of a variety of derivatives taking advantage of the reactivity (acidity) of the methylene carbon in malonic esters. The malonic ester synthesis is related to the acetoacetic ester synthesis and the Knoevenagel synthesis. The reaction is the addition to α,β-unsaturated carbonyl compounds.[1] This reaction is used to prepare compounds of biochemical and pharmaceutical interest.[2–8]

1. Smith, L.I., and Dobrovolny, F.J., The reaction between duroquinone and malonic esters, *J. Am. Chem. Soc.* 48, 1693–1709, 1928.
2. Mizuno, Y., Adachi, K., and Ikeda, K., Studies on condensed systems of aromatic nitrogenous series. XIII. Extension of malonic ester synthesis to the heterocyclic series, *Pharm. Bull.* 2, 225–234, 1954.
3. Beres, J.A., Varner, M.G., and Bria, C., Synthesis and cyclization of dialkylmalonuric esters, *J. Pharm. Sci.* 69, 451–454, 1980.
4. Kinder, D.H., Frank, S.K., and Ames, M.M., Analogues of carbamyl aspartate as inhibitors of dihydroorotase: Preparation of boronic acid transition-state analogues and a zinc chelator carbamylhomocysteine, *J. Med. Chem.* 33, 819–823, 1990.
5. Groth, T., and Meldal, M., Synthesis of aldehyde building blocks protected as acid labile *N*-boc-*N.O*-acetals: Toward combinatorial solid phase synthesis of novel peptide isosteres, *J. Comb. Chem.* 3, 34–44, 2001.
6. Hachiya, I., Ogura, K., and Shimizu, M., Novel 2-pyridine synthesis via nucleophilic addition of malonic esters to alkynyl imines, *Org. Lett.* 4, 2755–2757, 2002.
7. Strohmeier, G.A., Haas, W., and Kappe, C.O., Synthesis of functionalized 1,3-thiazine libraries combining solid-phase synthesis and post-cleavage modification methods, *Chemistry* 10, 2919–2926, 2004.
8. Coutant, E.P., Hervin, V., Gagnol, G., et al., Unnatural α-amino ethyl esters from diethylmalonate or ethyl β-bromo-α-hydroxyiminocarboxylate ester, *Beilstein J. Org. Chem.* 14, 2853–2860, 2018.

MANNICH REACTION

The canonical definition is the condensation of an amine with an carbonyl compound which can exist in an enol form, and a carbonyl compound that cannot exist as an enol.[1] The reaction frequently use formaldehyde as the carbonyl compound not existing as an enol for condensing with a secondary amine in the first phase of the reaction. There is extensive use of the Mannich reaction.[2–13] A variation described as the Petasis reaction[14] that involves the condensation of an aryl or vinyl boronic acid, an amine and certain carbonyl compounds to form complex products.[15,16]

1. Mannich, C., Eine Synthese von β-Ketonbasen, *Arch. Pharm.* 255, 261–276, 1917.
2. Britton, S.B., Caldwell, H.C., and Nobles, W.L., The use of 2-pipecoline in the Mannich reaction, *J. Am. Pharm. Assoc. Am. Pharm. Assoc.* 43, 641–643, 1954.
3. Nobles, W.L., and Thompson, B.B., Application of the Mannich reaction to sulfones. I. Reactive methylene moiety of sulfones, *J. Pharm. Sci.* 54, 576–580, 1965.
4. Thompson, B.B., The Mannich reaction. Mechanistic and technological considerations, *J. Pharm. Sci.* 57, 715–733, 1968.
5. Nobles, W.L., and Potti, N.D., Studies on the mechanism of the Mannich reaction, *J. Pharm. Sci.* 57, 1097–1103, 1968.
6. Delia, T.J., Scovill, J.P., Munslow, W.D., and Burckhalter, J.H., Synthesis of 5-substituted aminomethyluracils via the Mannich reaction, *J. Med. Chem.* 19, 344–346, 1976.
7. List, B., Pojarliev, P., Biller, W.T., and Martin, H.J., The proline-catalyzed direct asymmetric three-component Mannich reaction: Scope, optimization, and application to the highly enantioselective synthesis of 1,2-amino alcohols, *J. Am. Chem. Soc.* 124, 827–833, 2002.
8. Palomo, C., Oiarbide, M., Landa, A., et al., Design and synthesis of a novel class of sugar-peptide hybrids: *C*-linked glyco β-amino acids through a stereoselective "acetate" Mannich reaction as the key strategic element, *J. Am. Chem. Soc.* 124, 8637–8643, 2002.
9. Cordova, A., The direct catalytic asymmetric Mannich reaction, *Acc. Chem. Res.* 37, 102–112, 2004.
10. Azizi, N., Torkiyan, L., and Saidi, M.R., Highly efficient one-pot three-component Mannich reaction in water catalyzed by heteropoly acids, *Org. Lett.* 8, 2079–2082, 2006.
11. Matsuo, J., Tanaki, Y., and Ishibashi, H., Oxidative Mannich reaction of *N*-carbobenzoxy amines 1,3-dicarbonyl compounds, *Org. Lett.* 8, 4371–4374, 2006.
12. Biersack, B., Ahmed, K., Padhye, S., and Schobert, R., Recent developments concerning the application of the Mannich reaction for drug design, *Expert. Opin. Drug Discov.* 13, 39–49, 2018.
13. Martínez-Martínez, M., Rodríguez-Berna, G., Marejo, M., et al., Covalently crosslinked organophosphorous derivatives-chitosan hydrogel as a drug delivery system for oral administration of camptothecin, *Eur. J. Pharm. Biopharm.* 136, 174–183, 2019.
14. Petasis, N.A., and Boral, S., One-step three-component reaction among organoboronic acids, amines and salicylaldehydes, *Tetrahedron Lett.* 42, 530–542, 2001.
15. Candeias, N.R., Montalbano, F., Cal, P.M., and Gois, P.M., Boronic acids and esters in the Petasis-borono Mannich multicomponent reaction, *Chem. Rev.* 110, 6169–6193, 2010.
16. Ricardo, M.G., Llanes, D., Wessjohann, L.A., and Rivera, D.G., Introducing the Petasis reactions for late-stage multicomponent diversification, labeling, and stapling of peptides, *Ange. Chem. Int. Ed. Engl.* 58, 2700–2704, 2019.

MICHAEL ADDITION (MICHAEL CONDENSATION)

Formally a 1,4 addition/conjugate addition of a resonance-stabilized carbanion (the reaction of an active methylene compound such as a malonate to an α,β-unsaturated carbonyl compound or the reaction of a nucleophile with an activated α,β unsaturated system).[1] From a practical point of view in biochemistry, a Michael addition is the addition of a nucleophile to a conjugated double bond such the reaction between an acrylate and a thiolate anion.[2,3] There is extensive application of the Michael addition in biochemistry.[4–12] It should be noted that Michael addition reactions can be reversible.[13–15] One the best examples in biochemistry is the modification of cysteine residues with *N*-alkylmaleimide derivatives.[16–19] Another important example of the Michael addition in biochemistry and molecular biology is the reaction of 4-hydroxynon-2-enal and other oxidized lipids with amines (such as lysine) and sulfhydryl groups.[20–25] The reaction of oxidized lipids with lysine in protein has been referred to as protein carbonylation.[26]

1. Michael, A., Ueber die Addition von Natriumacetessig und Natriummalonsäurethern zu den Aethern ungesättigter Säuren, *J. Prakt. Chem.* 35, 349–356, 1886.
2. Nair, D.P., Podgórski, M., Chatani, S., et al., The thiol-Michael addition click reaction. A powerful and widely used tool in materials chemistry, *Chem. Mater.* 26, 724–744, 2014.
3. Saraswathy, M., Stansbury, J.W., and Nair, D.P., Thiol-functionalized nanogels as reactive plasticizers for cross-linked polymer networks, *J. Mech. Biomed. Mater.* 74, 296–303, 2017.
4. Powell, G.K., Winter, H.C., and Dekker, E.E., Michael addition of thiols with 4-methyleneglutamic acid: Preparation of adducts, their properties and presence in peanuts, *Biochem. Biophys. Res. Commun.* 105, 1361–1367, 1982.
5. Wang, M., Nishikawa, A., and Chung, F.L., Differential effects of thiols on DNA modifications via alkylation and Michael addition by α-acetoxy-*N*-nitrosopyrrolidine, *Chem. Res. Toxicol.* 5, 528–531, 1992.
6. Jang, D.P., Chang, C.W., and Uang, B.J., Highly diastereoselective Michael addition of α-hydroxy acid derivatives and enantioselective synthesis of (+)-crobarbatic acid, *Org. Lett.* 3, 983–985, 2001.
7. Naidu, B.N., Sorenson, M.E., Connolly, T.P., and Ueda, Y., Michael addition of amines and thiols to dehydroalanine amides: A remarkable rate acceleration in water, *J. Org. Chem.* 68, 10098–10102, 2003.
8. Weinstein, R., Lerner, R.A., Barbas, C.F., 3rd, and Shabat, D., Antibody-catalyzed asymmetric intramolecular Michael additional of aldehydes and ketones to yield the disfavored *cis*-product, *J. Am. Chem. Soc.* 127, 13104–13105, 2005.
9. Dai, H.X., Yao, S.P., and Wang, J., Michael addition of pyrimidine with disaccharide acrylates catalyzed in organic medium with lipase M from *Mucor javanicus*, *Biotechnol. Lett.* 28, 1503–1507, 2006.
10. Grimsrud, P.A., Xie, H., Griffin, T.J., and Berhlohr, D.A., Oxidative stress and covalent modification of protein with bioactive aldehydes, *J. Biol. Chem.* 283, 21837–21841, 2008.

11. Minko, I.G., Kozekov, I.D., Harris, T.M., et al., Chemistry and biology of DNA containing 1,*N*²-deoxyguanosine adducts of α,β-unsaturated aldehydes acrolein, crotonaldehyde, and 4-hydroxynonenal, *Chem. Res. Toxicol.* 22, 759–778, 2009.
12. Oeste, C.L., and Pérez-Sala, D., Modification of cysteine residues by cyclopentenone prostaglandins: Interplay with redox regulation of protein function, *Mass Spectrom. Rev.* 33, 110–125, 2014.
13. Johansson, M.H., Reversible Michael additions: Covalent inhibitors and prodrugs, *Mini Rev. Med. Chem.* 12, 1330–1344, 2012.
14. Freeman, B.A., O'Donnell, V.B., and Schopfer, F.J., The discovery of nitro-fatty acids as products of metabolic and inflammatory reactions and mediators of adaptive cell signaling, *Nitric Oxide* 77, 106–111, 2018.
15. Renault, K., Fredy, J.W., Renard, P.Y., and Sabot, C., Covalent modification of biomolecules through maleimide-based labeling strategies, *Bioconjug. Chem.* 29, 2497–2513, 2018.
16. Heitz, J.R., Anderson, C.D., and Anderson, B.M., Inactivation of yeast alcohol dehydrogenase by *N*-alkylmaleimides, *Arch. Biochem. Biophys.* 127, 627–636, 1968.
17. Lusty, C.J., and Fasold, H., Characterization of sulfhydryl groups of actin, *Biochemistry* 8, 2933–2939, 1969.
18. Bowes, T.J., and Gupta, R.S., Induction of mitochondrial fusion of cysteine-alklyators ethacrynic acid and *N*-ethylmaleimide, *J. Cell Physiol.* 202, 796–804, 2005.
19. Lundblad, R.L., *Chemical Reagents for Protein Modification*, 3rd edn., CRC Press, Boca Raton, FL, 2014.
20. Winter, C.K., Segall, H.J., and Haddon, W.F., Formation of cyclic adducts of deoxyguanosine with the aldehyde *trans*-4-hydroxy-2-hexenal and *trans*-4-hydroxy-2-nonenal *in vitro*, *Cancer Res.* 46, 5682–5686, 1986.
21. Sayre, L.M., Arora, P.K., Iyer, R.S., and Salomon, R.G., Pyrrole formation from 4-hydroxyonenal and primary amines, *Chem. Res. Toxicol.* 6, 19–22, 1993.
22. Hartley, D.P., Ruth, J.A., and Petersen, D.R., The hepatocellular metabolism of 4-hydroxynonenal by alcohol dehydrogenase, aldehyde dehydrogenase, and glutathione-*S*-transferase, *Arch. Biochem. Biophys.* 316, 197–205, 1995.
23. Engle, M.R., Singh, S.P., Czernik, P.J., et al., Physiological role of mGSTA4-4, a glutathione *S*-transferase metabolizing 4-hydroxynonenal: Generation and analysis of mGst4 null mouse, *Toxicol. Appl. Pharmacol.* 194, 296–308, 2004.
24. Lopachin, R.M. Gavin, T., and Barber, D.S., Type-2 alkenes mediate synaptotoxicity in neurodegenerative diseases, *Neurotoxicity* 29, 871–882, 2008.
25. Huang, H., Kozekov, I.D., Kozekova, A., et al., DNA cross-link induced by trans-4-hydroxynonenal, *Environ. Mol. Mutagen* 51, 625–634, 2010.
26. Colombo, G., Clerici, M., Garavaglia, M.E., et al., A step-by-step protocol for assaying protein carbonylation in biological samples, *J. Chromatog. B. Analyt. Technol. Biomed. Life Sci.* 1019, 178–190, 2016.

REFORMATSKY REACTION

Formation of a complex between zinc and an α-bromoester followed by condensation with an aldehyde yielding a β-hydroxyester; an α,β-unsaturated ester via dehydration following the condensation reaction.[1] The Reformatsky reaction is used in variety of synthetic reactions of interest in biochemistry.[2-14]

1. Reformatsky, E., Neue Synthese zweiatomiger einbasischer Säuren aus der Ketonen, *Ber. Dtsch. Chem. Ges.* 20, 1210–1211, 1887.
2. Tanabe, K., Studies on vitamin A and its related compounds. II. Reformatsky reaction of β-cyclocitral with methyl γ-bromosenecioate, *Pharm. Bull.* 3, 25–31, 1955.
3. Ross, N.A., and Bartsch, R.A., High-intensity ultrasound-promoted Reformatsky reactions, *J. Org. Chem.* 68, 360–366, 2003.
4. Jung, J.C., Lee, J.H., Oh., S., Synthesis and antitumor activity of 4-hydroxycoumarin derivatives, *Bioorg. Med. Chem. Lett.* 14, 5527–5531, 2004.
5. Kloetzing, R.J., Thaler, T., and Knochel, P., An improved asymmetric Reformatsky reaction mediated by (-)-N, N-dimethylaminoisoborneol, *Org. Lett.* 8, 1125–1128, 2006.
6. Moume, R. Laavielle, S., and Karoyan, P., Efficient synthesis of β₂-amino acid by homologation of α-amino acids involving the Reformatsky reaction and Mannich-type imminium electrophile, *J. Org. Chem.* 71, 3332–3334, 2006.
7. Cozzi, P.G., Reformatsky reactions meet catalysis and stereoselectivity, *Angew. Chem. Int. Ed. Engl.* 46, 2568–2571, 2007.
8. Pasunooti, K.K., Yang, R., Vedachalam, S., et al., Synthesis of 4-mercapto-L-lysine derivatives: Potential building blocks for sequential native chemical ligation, *Bioorg. Med. Chem. Lett.* 19, 6268–6271, 2009.
9. March, T.L., Johnston, M.R., Duggan, P.J., and Gardiner, J., Synthesis, structure, and biological applications of α-fluorinated β-amino acids and derivatives, *Chem. Biodivers.* 9, 2410–2441, 2012.
10. Choppin, S., Ferreiro-Medeiros, L., Barbarotto, M., and Colobert, F., Recent advances in the diastereoselective Reformatsky-type reaction, *Chem. Soc. Rev.* 42, 937–949, 2013,
11. Pellissier, H., Recent developments in the asymmetric Reformatsky-type reaction, *Beilstein J. Org. Chem.* 14, 325–344, 2018.
12. Savic, J., Dilber, S., Milenkovic, M. et al., Docking studies, synthesis and biological evaluation of β-aryl-β-hydroxy propanoic acids for anti-inflammatory activity, *Med. Chem.* 13, 186–195, 2017.
13. Lu, Z., Zhang, X., Guo, Z., et al., Total synthesis of aplysiasecosterol A, *J. Am. Chem. Soc.* 140, 9211–9218, 2018.
14. Khaniani, Y., Lipfert, M., Bhattacharyya, D., et al., A simple and convenient synthesis of unlabeled and ^{13}C-labeled 3-(3-hydroxyphenyl)-3-hydroxypropionic acid and its quantification in human urine samples, *Metabolites* 8(4), E80, 2018.

RITTTER REACTION

Acid-catalyzed nucleophilic addition of a nitrile to a carbenium ion generated from alcohol (usually tertiary, primary alcohols other than benzyl alcohol will not react) yielding an N-alkyl amide.[1,2] The Ritter reaction is used to prepare compounds of value in biochemical research.[3-16]

1. Ritter, J., and Minieri, P.P., A new reaction of nitriles. I. Amides from alkenes and mononitriles, *J. Am. Chem. Soc.* 70, 4045–4048, 1948.
2. Ritter, J., and Kalish, J., A new reaction of nitriles. II. Synthesis of t-carbinamines, *J. Am. Chem. Soc.* 70, 4048–4050, 1948.
3. Sanguigni, J.A., and Levine, R., Amides from nitriles and alcohols by the Ritter reaction, *J. Med. Chem.* 53, 573–574, 1964.
4. Radzicka, A., and Konieczny, M., Studies on the Ritter reaction. I. Synthesis of 3-/5-bartbituryl/-1propanesulfonic acids with anti-inflammatory activity, *Arch. Immunol. Ther. Exp.* 30, 421–432, 1982.
5. Van Emelen, K., De Wit, T., Hoornaert, G.J., and Compernolle, F., Diastereoselective intramolecular Ritter reaction: Generation of a cis-fused hexahydro-4aH-indeno[1,2-b] pyridine ring system with 4a,9b-diangular substituents, *Org. Lett.* 2, 3083–3086, 2000.
6. Concellon, J.M., Reigo, E., Suarez, J.R., et al., Synthesis of enantiopure imidazolines through a Ritter reaction of 2-(1-aminoalkyl)azirdines with nitriles, *Org. Lett.* 6, 4499–4501, 2004.
7. Feske, B.D., Kaluzna, I.A., and Stewart, J.D., Enantiodivergent, biocatalytic routes to both taxol side chain antipodes, *J. Org. Chem.* 70, 9654–9657, 2005.
8. Crich, D., and Patel, M., On the nitrile effect in L-rhamnopyranosylation, *Carbohydr. Res.* 341, 1467–1475, 2006.
9. Czifrák, K., Gyóllai, V., Kövér, K.E., and Somsák, L., Ritter-type reaction of C-(1-bromo-1-deoxy-D-glycopyranosyl)formamides and its application for the synthesis of oligopeptides incorporating α-amino acids, *Carbohydr. Res.* 346, 2104–2112, 2011.
10. Gandhi, S., Bisai, A., Prasad, B.A., and Singh, V.K., Studies on the reaction of aziridines with nitriles and carbonyls: Synthesis of imidazolines and oxazolidines, *J. Org. Chem.* 72, 2133–2142, 2007.
11. Valverde, E., Sureda, F.X., and Vázquez, S., Novel benzopolycyclic amines with NMDA receptor antagonist activity, *Bioorg. Med. Chem.* 22, 2678–2683, 2014.

12. Sarkar, S., Sonkar, R., Bhatia, G., and Tadigoppula, N., Synthesis of new *N*-acyl-1-amino-2-phenylethanol and *N*-acyl-10-amino-3-aryloxypropanols and evaluation of their antihyperlipidemic, LDL-oxidation and antioxidant activity, *Eur. J. Med. Chem.* 80, 135–144, 2014.

13. Chiba, M., Ishikawa, Y., Sakai, R., and Oikawa, M., Three-component, diastereoselective Prins-Ritter reaction for *cis*-fused 4-amidotetrahydropyrans toward a precursor for possible neuronal receptor ligands, *ACS Comb. Sci.* 18, 399–404, 2016.

14. Amarasekara, H., and Crich, D., Synthesis and intramolecular glycosylation of sialyl mono-esters of *o*-xylyene glycol. The importance of donor configuration and nitrogen protecting groups on cyclization yield and selectivity; isolation and characterization of *N*-sialyl acetamide indicative of participation by acetonitrile, *Carbohydr. Res.* 435, 113–120, 2016.

15. de Leon, A.C., Alonso, L., Mangadlao, J.D., Advincula, R.C., and Pentzer, E., Simultaneous reduction and functionalization of graphene oxide via Ritter reaction, *ACS Appl. Mater. Interfaces* 9, 14265–14272, 2017.

16. Bouhedja, M., Peres, B., Fhayli, W., et al., Design, synthesis and biological evaluation of novel ring-opened cromakalim analogues with relaxant effects on vascular and respiratory smooth muscle and as stimulators of elastin synthesis, *Eur. J. Med. Chem.* 144, 774–796, 2018.

SCHIFF BASE

A Schiff base is the unstable derivative which can be formed between an carbonyl (usually an aldehyde) and an amino group.[1-6] The Schiff base can be converted to a stable derivative by reduction with sodium borohydride or sodium cyanoborohydride. Schiff bases appear to be resistant to reduction with sulfhydryl-base reducing agents such as 2-mercaptoethanol or dithiothreitol and phosphines. Schiff bases are involved in a diverse group of biochemical events including protein carbonyl formation including glycation,[7-13] pyridoxal phosphate function,[14-17] drug function,[18-20] and food chemistry.[21,22] Schiff base formation is important in the Maillard reaction.[23] There is some interesting chemistry on the presence of Schiff bases in inorganic chemistry.[24-26]

1. Schiff, H., Mittheilungen aus dem Universitätslaboratorium in Pisa: Eine neue Reihe organische Basen, *Justus Liebigs Annalen Chem.* 131, 118–119, 1864.

2. Shepard, N.A., and Tickner, T.B., Researches on amines. The formation of Schiff bases from β-phenylethylamine and their reduction to alkyl derivatives of the amine, *J. Amer. Chem. Soc.* 38, 381–386, 1916.

3. McIntire, F.C., Some Schiff bases from amino acids, *J. Am. Chem. Soc.* 69, 1377–1380, 1947.

4. Puchtler, H., and Meloan, S.N., ON Schiff's bases and aldehyde-fuchsin: A review from H. Schiff to R.D. Lillie, *Histochemistry* 72, 321–332, 1981.

5. Hadjoudis, E., and Mavridis, I.M., Photochomism and thermochromism of Schiff bases in the solid state: Structural aspects, *Chem. Soc. Rev.* 33, 579–588, 2004.

6. Segura, J.L., Macheño, M.J., and Zamora, F., Covalent organic frameworks based on Schiff-base chemistry: Synthesis, properties and potential applications, *Chem. Soc. Rev.* 45, 5635–5671, 2016.

7. Feeney, R.E., Blankenhorn, G., and Dixon, H.B., Carbonyl-amine reactions in protein chemistry, *Adv. Protein. Chem.* 29, 135–203, 1975.

8. O'Donnell, J.P., The reaction of amines with carbonyls: Its significance in the nonenzymatic metabolism of xenobiotics, *Drug. Metab. Rev.* 13, 123–159, 1982.

9. Stadtman, E.R., Covalent modification reactions are marking steps in protein turnover, *Biochemistry* 29, 6232–6331, 1990.

10. Tuma, D.J., Hoffman, T., and Sorrell, M.F., The chemistry of aldehyde-protein adducts, *Alcohol Alcohol Suppl.* 1, 271–276, 1991.

11. Yim, M.B., Yim, H.S., Lee, C., et al., Protein glycation: Creation of catalytic sites for free radical generation, *Ann. N. Y. Acad. Sci.* 928, 48–53, 2001.

12. Schaur, R.J., Basic aspects of the biochemical reactivity of 4-hydroxynonenal, *Mol. Aspects Med.* 24, 149–159, 2003.

13. Kurtz, A.J., and Lloyd, R.S., $1,N^2$-deoxyguanosine adducts of acrolein, crotonaldehyde, and *trans*-4-hydroxynonenal cross-link to peptides via Schiff base linkage, *J. Biol. Chem.* 278, 5970–5975, 2003.

14. Metzler, D.E., Tautomerism in pyridoxal phosphate and in enzymatic catalysis, *Adv. Enzymol. Relat. Areas Mol. Biol.* 50, 1–40, 1979.

15. Gramatikova, S., Mouratou, B., Stetefeld, J. et al., Pyridoxal-5'-phosphate-dependent catatlytic antibodies, *J. Immunol. Methods* 269, 99–110, 2002.

16. Schackerz, K.D., Andi, B., and Cook, P.F., ^{31}P NMR spectroscopy senses the microenvironment of the 5'-phosphate group of enzyme-bound pyridoxal 5'-phosphate, *Biochim. Biophys. Acta* 1814, 1447–1458, 2011.

17. Dajnowicz, S., Parks, J.M., Hu, X., et al., Direct evidence that an extended hydrogen-bonding network influences activation of pyridoxal 5'-phosphate in aspartate aminotransferase, *J. Biol. Chem.* 292, 5970–5980, 2017.

18. Chen, H., and Rhodes, J., Schiff base forming drugs: Mechanisms of immune potentiation and therapeutic potential, *J. Mol. Med.* 74, 497–504, 1996.

19. Ganguly, A., Chakraborty, P., Banerjee, K., and Chouduri, S.K., The role of a Schiff base scaffold, *N*-(2-hydroxy acetophenone) glycinate-in overcoming multidrug resistance in cancer, *Eur. J. Pharm. Sci.* 51, 96–109, 2014.

20. Parlak, A.E., Cakmak, H., Sandal, S., et al., Evaluation of antioxidant and antiproliferative activities of 1,2-bis (*p*-amino-phenoxy) ethane derivative Schiff bases and metal complexes, *J. Biochem. Mol. Toxicol.* 33, e2247, 2019.

21. Stadler, R.H., Acrylamide formation in different foods and potential strategies for reduction, *Adv. Expt. Med. Biol.* 561, 157–169, 2005.
22. Wang, Y., and Ho, C.T., Flavour chemistry of methylglyoxal and glyoxal, *Chem. Soc. Rev.* 41, 4140–4149, 2012.
23. van Boekel, M.A., Formation of flavor compounds in the Maillard reaction, *Biotechnol. Adv.* 24, 230–233, 2006.
24. Nakoji, M., Kanayama, T., Okino, T., and Takemoto, Y., Chiral phosphine-free Pd-mediated asymmetric allylation of prochiral enolate with a chiral phase-transfer catalyst, *Org. Lett.* 2, 3329–3331, 2001.
25. Walther, D., Fugger, C. Schreer, H., et al., Reversible fixation of carbon dioxide at nickel(0) centers: A route for large organometallic rings, dimers, and tetramers, *Chemistry* 7, 5214–5221, 2001.
26. Benny, P.D., Green, J.L., Engelbrecht, H.P., Reactivity and rhenium(V) oxo Schiff base complexes with phosphine ligands: Rearrangement and reduction reactions, *Inorg. Chem.* 44, 2381–2390, 2005.

SCHMIDT REACTION/SCHMIDT REARRANGEMENT

Used to describe the reaction of carboxylic acids, aldehyde and ketones (carbonyl compounds), and alcohols/alkenes with hydrazoic acid.[1] Reaction with carboxylic acids yields amines, carbonyl compounds yield amides in a reaction involving a rearrangement, and alcohols/azides yield alkyl azides.[2–13]

1. Schmidt, K.F., Über die Einwirkung von NH auf organische Veerbindungen, *Angew. Chem.* 36, 511, 1923.
2. Rabinowitz, J.L., Chase, G.D., and Kaliner, L.F., Isotope effects of in the decarboxylation of 1-^{14}C-dicarboxylic acids studied by means of the Schmidt reaction, *Anal. Biochem.* 19, 578–583, 1967.
3. Iyengar, R., Schildknegt, K., and Aube, J., Regiocontrol in an intramolecular Schmidt reaction: Total synthesis of (+)-aspidospermidine, *Org. Lett.* 2, 1625–1627, 2000.
4. Sahasrabudhe, K., Gracias, V., Furness, K., et al., Asymmetric Schmidt reaction of hydroxyalkyl azides with ketones, *J. Am. Chem. Soc.* 125, 7914–7922, 2003.
5. Wang, W., Mei, Y., Li, H., and Wang, J., A novel pyrrolidine imide catalyzed direct formation of α,β-unsaturated ketones from unmodified ketones and aldehydes, *Org. Lett.* 7, 601–604, 2005.
6. Brase, S., Gil, C., Knepper, K., and Zimmerman, V., Organic azides: An exploding diversity of a unique class of compounds, *Angew. Chem. Int. Ed. Engl.* 44, 5188–5240, 2005.
7. Lang, S., and Murphy, J.A., Azide rearrangements in electron-deficient systems, *Chem. Soc. Rev.* 35, 146–156, 2006.
8. Zarghi, A., Zebardast, T., Hakimion, F., et al., Synthesis and biological evaluation of 1,3-diphenylprop-2-en-1-ones possessing a methanesulfonamido or an azido pharmacophore as cyclooxygenase-1/2 inhibitors, *Bioorg. Med. Chem.* 14, 7044–7050, 2006.
9. Lang, S., and Murphy, J.A., Azide rearrangements in electron-deficient systems, *Chem. Soc. Rev.* 35, 146–156, 2006.
10. Kapat, A., Kumar, P.S., and Baskaran, S., Synthesis of crispine A analogues via an intramolecular Schmidt reaction, *Beilstein J. Org. Chem.* 3, 49, 2007.
11. Katori, T., Itoh, S., Sato, M., and Yamataka, H., Reaction pathways and possible path bifurcation for the Schmidt reaction, *J. Am. Chem. Soc.* 132, 3413–3422, 2010.
12. Moreno, L.M., Quiroga, J., Abonia, R., Ramírez-Prada, J., and Isuasty, B., Synthesis of new 1,3,5-triazine-baed 2-pyrazolines as potential anticancer agents, *Molecules* 23, E1956, 2018.
13. Ding, S.L., Ji, Y., Su, Y., Li, R., and Gu, P., Schmidt reaction of ω-azido valeryl chlorides followed by intermolecular trapping of the rearrangement ions: Synthesis of assoanine and related pyrrolophenanthridine alkaloids, *J. Org. Chem.* 84, 2012–2021, 2019.

STRECKER SYNTHESIS/ STRECKER DEGRADATION

The Strecker synthesis is the synthesis of α-amino acids from aldehydes or ketones.[1] The Strecker synthesis is for the synthesis of unique amino acids.[2–4] The Strecker degradation is the formation of aldehyde from an α-amino acid by oxidation.[5] The Strecker degradation is a component of the process of advanced protein glycation including the Maillard reaction.[6–9]

1. Strecker, A., Ueber die künstliche Bildung der Milchsäure und eine neuen, dem Glycoll homologen Körper, *Justus Liebig Ann. Chem.* 75, 27–50, 1850.
2. Aiba, S., Takamatsu, N., Sasai, T., Tukunaga, Y., and Kawasaki, T., Replication of α-amino acids via Strecker synthesis with amplification and multiplication of chiral intermediate aminonitriles, *Chem. Commun.* (Camb) 52, 10834–10837, 2016.
3. Zaghari, Z., and Azizian, J., Synthesis of novel α-amidino carboxylic acids and their use as H-bond catalysts in Strecker reaction, *Comb. Chem. High Throughput Screen.* 21, 609–614, 2018.
4. Baglai, I., Leeman, M., Wurst, K., et al., The Strecker reaction coupled to Viedma ripening: A simple route to highly hindered enantiomerically pure amino acids, *Chem. Commun.* (Camb) 54, 10832–10834, 2018.
5. Strecker, A., Notiz uber eine eigenthümliche Oxydation durch Alloxan, *Justus Leibig Ann. Chem.* 123, 363–365, 1862.
6. Balance, P.E., Production of volatile compounds related to the flavor of foods from the Strecker degradation of DL-methionine, *J. Sci. Food Agric.* 12, 532–536, 1961.
7. Yaylayan, V.A., Recent advances in the chemistry of Strecker degradation and Amadori rearrangement: Implications to aroma and color formation, *Food Sci. Technol. Res.* 9, 1–6, 2007.

8. Baldensperger, T., Jost, T., Zipprich, A., and Glomb, M.A., Novel α-oxamide advanced-glycation endproducts within the N^6-carboxymethyl lysine and N^6-carboxyethyl lysine reaction cascades, *J. Agric. Food Chem.* 66, 1898–1906, 2018.

9. Scalone, G.L.L., Lamichhane, P., Cucu, T., De Kimpe, N., and De Meulenaer, B., Impact of different enzymatic hydrolysates of whey protein on the formation of pyrazines in Maillard model systems, *Food Chem.* 278, 53–544, 2019.

UGI CONDENSATION/UGI REACTION

The Ugi reaction is a four component (aldehyde, amine, isocyanide and a carboxyl group) condensation resulting in an α-aminoacyl amide.[1] There is significant use of the Ugi reaction in the development of chemical libraries for synthesis and analysis.[2–13] The Ugi reaction is also used for the synthesis of complex chemical compounds.[14–17] The enzymatic catalysis of the Ugi reaction by lipases to prepare peptide scaffolds has been described.[18,19]

1. Ugi, I., The α-addition of immonium ions and anions to isonitriles accompanied by secondary reactions, *Angewandt. Chem. Int. Ed. Engl.* 1, 1–18, 1962.

2. Liu, X.C., Clark, D.S., and Dordick, J.S., Chemoenzymatic construction of a four-component Ugi combinatorial library, *Biotechnol. Bioeng.* 69, 457–460, 2000.

3. Ugi, I., and Heck, S., The multicomponent reactions and their libraries for natural and preparative chemistry, *Comb. Chem. High Throughput Screen.* 4, 1–34, 2001.

4. Hulme, C., and Gore, V., "Multi-component reactions: Emerging chemistry in drug discovery" from 'from xylocaine to crixivan', *Curr. Med. Chem.* 10, 51–80, 2003.

5. Mironov, M.A., Ivantsova, M.N., and Mokrushin, V.S., Ugi reaction in aqueous solutions: A simple protocol for libraries production, *Mol. Divers.* 6, 193–197, 2003.

6. Liu, L., Ping Li, C., Cochran, S., and Ferro, V., Application of the four-component Ugi condensation for the preparation of glycoconjugate libraries, *Bioorg. Med. Chem. Lett.* 14, 2221–2226, 2004.

7. El Khoury, G., Rowe, L.A., and Lowe, C.R., Biomimetic affinity ligands for immunoglobulins based on the multi-component Ugi reaction, *Methods Mol. Biol.* 800, 57–74, 2012.

8. Pérez-Labrada, K., Méndez, Y., Brouard, I., and Rivera, D.G., Multicomponent ligation of steroids: Creating diversity at the linkage moiety of bis-spirostanic conjugates by Ugi reaction, *ACS Comb. Sci.* 15, 320–330, 2013.

9. Sanhueza, C.A., Cartmell, J., El-Hawiet, A., et al., Evaluation of a focused virtual library of heterobifunctional ligands for *Clostridium difficile* toxins, *Org. Biomol. Chem.* 13, 283–298, 2015.

10. Batalha, I.L., and Roque, A.C.A., New affinity tools for the enrichment of phosphorylated peptides, *J. Chromatog. B Analyt. Technol. Biomed. Life Sci.* 1031, 86–93, 2016.

11. Patil, P., Mishra, B., Sheombarsing, G., et al., A library-to-library synthesis of highly substituted α-aminomethyl tetrazoles via Ugi reaction, *ACS Comb. Sci.* 20, 70–74, 2018.

12. Moni, L., De Moliner, F., Garbarino, S., et al., Exploitation of the Ugi 5-center-4-component reaction (U-5C-4CR) for the generation of diverse libraries of polycyclic (spiro) compounds, *Front. Chem.* 6, 369, 2018.

13. Capurro, P., Moni, L., Galtini, A., Mang, C., and Basso, A., Multi-gram synthesis of enantiopure 1,5-disubstituted tetrazoles via Uga-Azide 3-component reaction, *Molecules* 23(11), E2758, 2018.

14. Bayer, T., Riemer, C., and Kessler, H., A new strategy for the synthesis of cyclopeptides containing diaminoglutaric acid, *J. Pept. Sci.* 7, 250–261, 2001.

15. Crescenzi, V., Francescangeli, A., Renier, D., and Bellini, D., New cross-linked and sulfated derivatives of partially deacylated hyaluronan: Synthesis and preliminary characterization, *Biopolymers* 64, 86–94, 2002.

16. Bu, H., Kjoniksen, A.L., Knudsen, K.D., and Nystrom, B., Rheological and structural properties of aqueous alginate during gelation via the Ugi multicomponent condensation reaction, *Biomacromolecules* 5, 1470–1479, 2004.

17. Tempest, P.A., Recent advances in heterocycle generation using the efficient Ugi multiple-component condensation reaction, *Curr. Opin. Drug Discov. Devel.* 8, 776–788, 2005.

18. Żadło-Dobrowolska, A., Kłossowski, S., Koszelewski, D., Paprocki, D., and Ostaszewski, R., Enzymatic Ugi reaction with amines and cyclic imines, *Chemistry* 22, 16684–16689, 2016.

19. Wilk, M., Brodzka, A., Koszelewski, D., et al., The influence of the isocyanoesters structure on the course of enzymatic Ugi reactions, *Bioorg. Chem.*, in press. doi:10.1016/j.bioorg.2019.02.042, 2019.

WITTIG REACTION

Synthesis of an alkene from the reaction of an aldehyde or ketone with an ylide generated from a phosphonium salt and an alkyl halide (Wittig Reagent, e.g., triphenylphosphonium).[1] It is useful way of generating double bonds during synthetic procedure. The Wittig reaction is used for synthesis of interesting biochemicals.[2–11] Triphenylarsine has been substituted for triphenylphospine.[12] The Wittig rearrangement is a separate reaction, which is the rearrangement of an ether to form an alcohol.[13–15]

1. Wittig, G., and Geissler, G., Zur Reaktionsweise des Pentaphenyl phosphors under einiger Derivate, *Justus Leibig Ann. Chem.* 582, 44–57, 1953.

2. Jorgensen, M., Iversen, E.H., and Madsen, R., A convenient route to higher sugars by two-carbon chain elongation using Wittig/dihydroxylation reactions, *J. Org. Chem.* 66, 4625–4629, 2001.

3. Magrioti, V., and Constantinou-Kokotou, V., Synthesis of (S)-α-amino oleic acid, *Lipids* 37, 223–228, 2002.

4. Rhee, J.U., and Krische, M.J., Alkynes as synthetic equivalents to stabilized Wittig reagents: intra- and inter-molecular carbonyl olefinations catalyzed by Ag(1), BF_3, and HBF_4, *Org. Lett.* 7, 2493–2495, 2005.

5. Ermolenko, L., and Sasaki, N.A., Diastereoselective synthesis of all either *l*-hexoses from L-ascorbic acid, *J. Org. Chem.* 71, 693–703, 2006.

6. Halim, R., Brimble, M.A., and Merten, J., Synthesis of the ABC tricyclic fragment of the pectenotoxins via stereocontrolled cyclization of a γ-hydroxyepoxide appended to the AB spiroacetal unit, *Org. Biomol. Chem.* 4, 1387–1399, 2006.

7. Phillips, D.J., Pillinger, K.S., Li, W., et al., Desymmerization of diols by a tandem oxidation/Wittig olefination reaction, *Chem. Commun.* 21, 2280–2282, 2006.

8. Modica, E., Compostella, F. Colombo, D., et al., Stereoselective synthesis and immunogenic activity of the *C*-analogue of sulfatide, *Org. Lett.* 8, 3255–3258, 2006.

9. Gu, Y., and Tian, S.K., Olefination reactions of phosphorus-stabilized carbon nucleophiles, *Top. Curr. Chem.* 327, 197–238, 2012.

10. Byrne, P.A., and Gilheany, D.G., The modern interpretation of the Wittig reaction mechanism, *Chem. Soc. Rev.* 42, 6670–6696, 2013.

11. Lao, Z., and Toy, P.H., Catalytic Wittig and aza-Wittig reactions, *Beilstein J. Org. Chem.* 12, 2577–2587, 2016.

12. Li, L., Stimac, J.C., and Geary, L.M., Synthesis of olefins via a Wittig reaction mediated by triphenylarsine, *Tetrahedron Lett.* 58, 1379–1381, 2017.

13. Wittig, G., and Geissler, G., Übe die kationtrope isomerization gewisser Benyläther bei Einwirkung von Phenyl-lithium, *Justus Leibig Ann. Chem.* 550, 260–268, 1942.

14. Kennedy, C.R., Guidera, J.A., and Jacobsen, E.N., Synergistic ion-binding catalysis demonstrated via an enantioselective, catalytic [2,3]-Wittig rearrangement, *ACS Cent. Sci.* 2, 416–423, 2016.

15. Rycek, L., and Hudlicky, T., Applications of the Wittig-Still rearrangement in organic synthesis, *Angew. Chem. Int. Ed. Engl.* 56, 6022–6066, 2017.

Additional information on name reactions in organic chemistry can be obtained from the below references.

Lane, T., and Plagens, A., *Named Organic Reactions*, 2nd edn., John Wiley & Sons, Chichester, UK, 2005.

Kurti, L., and Czakó, B., *Strategic Applications of Named Reactions in Organic Synthesis: Background and Detailed Mechanisms*, Elsevier, Amsterdam, the Netherlands, 2005.

Li, J.J., *Name Reactions for Homoligations. Part I*, John Wiley & Sons, Hoboken, NJ, 2009.

Li, J.J., *Name Reactions for Carboxylic Ring Formation*, John Wiley & Sons, Hoboken, NJ, 2010.

Li, J.J., *Name Reactions in Heterocyclic Chemistry* II, John Wiley & Sons, Hoboken, NJ, 2011.

Li, J.J. *Name Reactions: A Collection of Detailed Mechanisms and Synthetic Applications*, Springer, Cham, Switzerland, 2014.

5 Deamidation of Asparagine in Peptides and Proteins

The deamidation of asparagine with the associated formation of isoaspartic acid[1,2] and peptide bond cleavage[3] is one the most common causes of heterogeneity in biopharmaceutical protein products. The process of deamidation of asparagine involves the formation of a cyclic succinimide which decomposes to form aspartic acid or isoaspartic acid. Deamidation results in heterogeneity of the protein, which can result in a loss of potency.[4,5] Factors that affect deamidation of asparagine residues include the amino acid sequence around the asparagine residue, pH, buffer composition and temperature. In general, asparagine in proteins is less susceptible to deamidation than peptides.[6] Glutamine is also susceptible to deamidation.[7] Selected studies of deamidation of peptides and proteins are shown below.

REFERENCES

1. Song, Y., Schowen, R.L., Borchardt, R.T., and Topp, E.M., Effect of "pH" on the rate of asparagine deamidation in polymeric formulations: "pH"-rate profile, *J. Pharm. Sci.* 90, 141–156, 2001.
2. Reubsaet, J.L., Beijnen, J.H., Bult, A., et al., Analytical techniques used to study the degradation of proteins and peptides: Chemical instability, *J. Pharm. Biomed. Anal.* 17, 955–978, 1998.
3. Catak, S., Monard, G., Aviyente, V., and Ruiz-López, M.F., Computation study on nonenzymatic peptide bond cleavage at asparagine and aspartic acid, *J. Phys. Chem.* 112, 8752–8761, 2008.
4. Zhang, L., Martinez, T., Woodruff, B., et al., Hydrophobic interaction chromatography of soluble interleukin I receptor type II to reveal chemical degradations resulting in loss potency, *Anal. Chem.* 80, 7022–7078, 2008.
5. Nellis, D.F., Michiel, D.F., Jiang, M.S., Characterization of recombinant human IL–15 deamidation and its practical elimination through substitution of asparagine 77, *Pharm. Res.* 29, 722–738, 2012.
6. Xie, M., and Schowen, R.L., Secondary structure and protein deamidation, *J. Pharm. Sci.* 88, 8–13, 1999.
7. Bischoff, R., and Kole, H.V., Deamidation of asparagine and glutamine residues in proteins and peptides: Structural determinants and analytical methodology, *J. Chromatog. B Biomed. Appl.* 662, 261–278, 1994.

Deamidation of Asparagine and Glutamine in Peptides and Proteins

Peptide/Protein Sequence	Conditions	Rate	References
QNSLLWR (18–24 from recombinant human lymphotoxin)[a]	50 mM phosphate, pH 11 at 40°C	0.58×10^{-6} s^{-1}	1
QNSLLWR (18–24 from recombinant human lymphotoxin)[a]	50 mM phosphate, pH 11 with 4 M GuCl[b] at 40°C	17.7×10^{-6} s^{-1}	1[q] The
.....GFSLSNNSLL....(contained in 30–67 from recombinant human lymphotoxin)	50 mM phosphate, pH 11 at 40°C	0.1×10^{-6} s^{-1}	1
QNSLLWR (18–24 from recombinant human lymphotoxin)[a]	50 mM phosphate, pH 11 with 4 M GuCl[b] at 40°C	0.87×10^{6} s^{-1}	1
Ac-KQNSL-NH$_2$	50 mM phosphate, pH 11 at 40°C	8×10^{-6} s^{-1}	1
Ac-KQNSL-NH$_2$	50 mM phosphate, pH 11 with 4 M GuCl[b] at 40°C	6.6×10^{-6} s^{-1}	1
Ac-LSNNGL-NH$_2$	50 mM phosphate, pH 11 at 40°C	8.1×10^{-6} s^{-1}	1
Ac-LSNNGL-NH$_2$	50 mM phosphate, pH 11 with 4 M GuCl[b] at 40°C	9.7×10^{-6} s^{-1}	1
rhVEGF[c]	100 mM phosphate, pH 5.0/37°C	5×10^{-4} h^{-1}	2
rhVEGF[c]	100 mM phosphate, pH 8.0/37°C	4.18×10^{-3} h^{-1}	2
GQNHH	100 mM phosphate, pH 5.0/37°C	6.08×10^{-3} h^{-1}	2

(Continued)

Deamidation of Asparagine and Glutamine in Peptides and Proteins (*Continued*)

Peptide/Protein Sequence	Conditions	Rate	References
GQNHH	100 mM phosphate, pH 8.0/37°C	4.86×10^{-3} h^{-1}	2
GQNGG	100 mM sodium phosphate, pH 5.0/37°C	3.6×10^{-4} h^{-1}	3
GQNGG	100 mM sodium phosphate, pH 6.0/37°C	25.5×10^{-4} h^{-1}	3
GQNGG	100 mM sodium phosphate, pH 7.0/37°C	185.5×10^{-4} s^{-1}	3
GQNGG	100 mM sodium phosphate, pH 8.0/37°C	517.6×10^{-4} s^{-1}	3
GQNGG	100 mM sodium phosphate, pH 9.0/37°C	1211.5×10^{-4} s^{-1}	3
GQNGG	100 mM sodium phosphate, pH 10.0/37°C	2685×10^{-4} s^{-1}	3
GQNGH	100 mM sodium phosphate, pH 5.0/37°C	3.6×10^{-4} h^{-1}	3
GQNGH	100 mM sodium phosphate, pH 6.0/37°C	17.7×10^{-4} h^{-1}	3
GQNGH	100 mM sodium phosphate, pH 7.0/37°C	124.1×10^{-4} h^{-1}	3
GQNVH	100 mM sodium phosphate, pH 6.0/37°C	1.6×10^{-4} h^{-1}	3
GQNVH	100 mM sodium phosphate, pH 7.0/37°C	14.6×10^{-4} h^{-1}	3
GQNVH	100 mM sodium phosphate, pH 8.0/37°C	45.6×10^{-4} h	3
GQNHA	100 mM sodium phosphate, pH 6.0/37°C	19.6×10^{-4} h^{-1}	3
GQNHA	100 mM sodium phosphate, pH 7.0/37°C	116.9×10^{-4} h^{-1}	3
GQNHA	100 mM sodium phosphate, pH 8.0/37°C	122.1×10^{-4} h^{-1}	3
VSNGV	20 mM phosphate, pH 7.3/60°C	0.12 h$^{-1,d}$	4
VSNGV	20 mM TAPS, pH 8.0/60°C	4.1×10^{-2} h$^{-1,d}$	4
VSNGV	20 mM phosphate, pH 8.0/60°C	0.17 h$^{-1,d}$	4
VSNGV	50 mM phosphate, pH 8.0/60°C	0.26 h$^{-1,d}$	4
VSNGV	100 mM phosphate, pH 8.0/60°C	0.35 h$^{-1,d}$	4
VSNGV	20 mM CAPS, pH 10.0/60°C	0.11 h$^{-1,d}$	4
VSNGV	20 mM CAPS + 20 mM glycine, pH 10.0/60°C	0.46 h$^{-1,d}$	4
VSNGV	20 mM CAPS + 50 mM NH$_4$OH	0.63 h$^{-1,d}$	4
VSNGV	20 mM CAPS = 250 mM triethylamine	0.12 h$^{-1,d}$	4
VSNHV	20 mM phosphate, pH 7.3/60°C	2.7×10^{-2} h$^{-1,d}$	4
VSNSV	20 mM phosphate, pH 7.3/60°C	1.5×10^{-2} h$^{-1,d}$	4
VSNRV	20 mM phosphate, pH 7.3/60°C	9.1×10^{-3} h$^{-1,d}$	4
VSNLV	20 mM phosphate, pH 7.3/60°C	2.9×10^{-3} h$^{-1,d}$	4
VSNLV	20 mM CAPS, pH 10/60°C	2.1×10^{-2} h$^{-1,d}$	4
VSNAV	20 mM phosphate, pH 7.3/60°C	1.1×10^{-2} h$^{-1,d}$	4
VSNTV	20 mM phosphate, pH 7.3/60°C	2.9×10^{-3} h$^{-1,d}$	4
VSNVV	20 mM phosphate, pH 7.3/60°C	1.7×10^{-3} h$^{-1,d}$	4
VANTV	20 mM phosphate, pH 7.3/60°C	5.8×10^{-3} h$^{-1,d}$	4
VYPNGA	100 mM sodium phosphate, pH 7.4/37°C	2.1×10^{-2} h$^{-1,e}$	5
VYPNGA	100 mM sodium phosphate, pH 7.4/100°C	46.2 h$^{-1,e}$	5
VYPNLA	100 mM sodium phosphate, pH 7.4/37°C	9.9×10^{-3} h^{-1}	5
VYPNLA	100 mM sodium phosphate, pH 7.4/100°C	0.14 h^{-1}	5
VYPNPA	100 mM sodium phosphate, pH 7.4/37°C	6.5×10^{-3} h^{-1}	5
VYPNPA	100 mM sodium phosphate, pH 7.4/100°C	9.2×10^{-2} h	5
N$_{54}$ in monoclonal a antibody	100 mM Tris, pH 8.5/40°C	2.6×10^{-6} s$^{-1,f}$	6
GANAG	Phosphate, pH 7.4 ($I = 0.2$)^g/37°C	8.4×10^{-8} s^{-1}	7
GRNAG	Phosphate, pH 7.4 ($I = 0.2$)^g/37°C	4.43×10^{-7} s^{-1}	7
GDNAG	Phosphate, pH 7.4 ($I = 0.2$)^g/37°C	1.83×10^{-7} s^{-1}	7
GCNAG	Phosphate, pH 7.4 ($I = 0.2$)^g/37°C	1.17×10^{-7} s^{-1}	7
GENAG	Phosphate, pH 7.4 ($I = 0.2$)^g/37°C	1.64×10^{-7} s^{-1}	7
GGNAG	Phosphate, pH 7.4 ($I = 0.2$)^g/37°C	9.2×10^{-8} s^{-1}	7

(*Continued*)

Deamidation of Asparagine and Glutamine in Peptides and Proteins (*Continued*)

Peptide/Protein Sequence	Conditions	Rate	References
GHNAG	Phosphate, pH 7.4 ($I = 0.2$)[g]/37°C	1.77×10^{-7} s^{-1}	7
GINAG	Phosphate, pH 7.4 ($I = 0.2$)[g]/37°C	1.6×10^{-8} s^{-1}	7
GLNAG	Phosphate, pH 7.4 ($I = 0.2$)[g]/37°C	3.7×10^{-8} s^{-1}	7
GKNAG	Phosphate, pH 7.4 ($I = 0.2$)[g]/37°C	1.32×10^{-7} s^{-1}	7
GMNAG	Phosphate, pH 7.4 ($I = 0.2$)[g]/37°C	1.04×10^{-7} s^{-1}	7
GFNAG	Phosphate, pH 7.4 ($I = 0.2$)[g]/37°C	1.69×10^{-7} s^{-1}	7
GPNAG	Phosphate, pH 7.4 ($I = 0.2$)[g]/37°C	8.0×10^{-8} s^{-1}	7
GSNAG	Phosphate, pH 7.4 ($I = 0.2$)[g]/37°C	1.53×10^{-7} s^{-1}	7
GTNAG	Phosphate, pH 7.4 ($I = 0.2$)[g]/37°C	1.18×10^{-1} s^{-1}	7
GWNAG	Phosphate, pH 7.4 ($I = 0.2$)[g]/37°C	9.2×10^{-8} s^{-1}	7
GYNAG	Phosphate, pH 7.4 ($I = 0.2$)[g]/37°C	9.4×10^{-1} s^{-1}	7
GVNAG	Phosphate, pH 7.4 ($I = 0.2$)[g]/37°C	7.2×10^{-8} s^{-1}	7
GAQAG	Phosphate, pH 7.4 ($I = 0.2$)[g]/37°C	1.5×10^{-8} s^{-1}	7
GAQRG	Phosphate, pH 7.4 ($I = 0.2$)[g]/37°C	4.2×10^{-8} s^{-1}	7
GAQIG	Phosphate, pH 7.4 ($I = 0.2$)[g]/37°C	7.2×10^{-9} s^{-1}	7
GAQKG	Phosphate, pH 7.4 ($I = 0.2$)[g]/37°C	5.1×10^{-8} s^{-1}	7
GRQAG	Phosphate, pH 7.4 ($I = 0.2$)[g]/37°C	2.1×10^{-8} s^{-1}	7
GRQRG	Phosphate, pH 7.4 ($I = 0.2$)[g]/37°C	2.8×10^{-8} s^{-1}	7
GDQAG	Phosphate, pH 7.4 ($I = 0.2$)[g]/37°C	3.8×10^{-8} s^{-1}	7
GEQAG	Phosphate, pH 7.4 ($I = 0.2$)[g]/37°C	3.5×10^{-8} s^{-1}	7
GGQAG	Phosphate, pH 7.4 ($I = 0.2$)[g]/37°C	1.9×10^{-8} s^{-1}	7
GHQAG	Phosphate, pH 7.4 ($I = 0.2$)[g]/37°C	8.3×10^{-8} s^{-1}	7
GIQAG	Phosphate, pH 7.4 ($I = 0.2$)[g]/37°C	7.3×10^{-9} s^{-1}	7
GLQAG	Phosphate, pH 7.4 ($I = 0.2$)[g]/37°C	1.2×10^{-8} s^{-1}	7
GKQAG	Phosphate, pH 7.4 ($I = 0.2$)[g]/37°C	2.8×10^{-8} s^{-1}	7
GMQAG	Phosphate, pH 7.4 ($I = 0.2$)[g]/37°C	7.8×10^{-8} s^{-1}	7
GFQAG	Phosphate, pH 7.4 ($I = 0.2$)[g]/37°C	7.6×10^{-9} s^{-1}	7
GPQAG	Phosphate, pH 7.4 ($I = 0.2$)[g]/37°C	7.2×10^{-9} s^{-1}	7
GSQAG	Phosphate, pH 7.4 ($I = 0.2$)[g]/37°C	9.0×10^{-9} s^{-1}	7
GTQAG	Phosphate, pH 7.4 ($I = 0.2$)[g]/37°C	2.3×10^{-9} s^{-1}	7
GWQAG	Phosphate, pH 7.4 ($I = 0.2$)[g]/37°C	1.1×10^{-8} s^{-1}	7
GYQAG	Phosphate, pH 7.4 ($I = 0.2$)[g]/37°C	1.2×10^{-8} s^{-1}	7
GYQLG	Phosphate, pH 7.4 ($I = 0.2$)[g]/37°C	9.0×10^{-8} s^{-1}	7
GVQAG	Phosphate, pH 7.4 ($I = 0.2$)[g]/37°C	2.4×10^{-9} s^{-1}	7

[a] Recombinant human lymphotoxin was incubated under the indicated solvent conditions for 43 days at which time the protein was denatured in 8.0 M urea and subjected to tryptic hydrolysis. Peptides containing asparagine were isolated and the extent of deamination determined and used for the first-order rate constants.

[b] The incubation was performed in the presence of 4.0 M guanidine hydrochloride.

[c] rhVEGF, recombinant human vascular endothelial growth factor.

[d] Calculated for $t_{1/2}$ data $t_{1/2} = 0.693/k$.

[e] Extrapolated from date obtained at 70°C.

[f] N_{58} undergoes deamidation at a much slower rate (13% after two weeks compared to 76% for N_{54}; N_{56} is resistant to deamidation).

[g] Buffer a combination of potassium dihydrogen phosphate (potassium monobasic phosphate) and sodium monohydrogen phosphate (sodium dibasic phosphate).

References for the table on asparagine deamidation

1. Xie, M., Shabrokh, X., Kadkhodayan, M., et al., Asparagine deamidation in recombinant human lymphotoxin: Hindrance by three-dimensional structures, *J. Pharm. Sci.* 92, 869–880, 2003.
2. Goolcharran, C., Jones, A.J.S., Borchardt, R.T., Cleland, J.L., and Keck, R., Comparison of the rates of deamidation, diketopiperazine formation, and oxidation in recombinant human vascular endothelial growth factor and model peptides, *Pharm. Sci.* 2, E5, 2000.
3. Goolcharran, C., Stauffer, L.L., Cleland, J.L., and Bordchardt, R.T., The effects of a histidine residue on the C-terminal side of as asparaginyl residue on the rate of deamidation using model pentapeptides, *J. Pharm. Sci.* 89, 818–825, 2000.
4. Tyler-Cross, R., and Schirch, V., Effects of amino acid sequence, buffers, and ionic strength on the rate and mechanism of deamidation of asparagine residues in small peptides, *J. Biol. Chem.* 266, 22549–22556, 1991.
5. Geiger, T., and Clarke, S., Deamidation, isomerization, and racemization at asparaginyl and aspartyl residues in peptides, *J. Biol. Chem.* 262, 785–794, 1987.
6. Phillips, J.J., Buchanan, A., Andrews, J., et al., Rate of asparagine deamidation in a monoclonal antibody correlating with hydrogen exchange rate at adjacent downstream residues, *Anal. Chem.* 89, 2361–2368, 2017.
7. Robinson, A.B., Scotchler, J.W., and McKerrow, J.H., Rates of nonenzymatic deamidation of glutaminyl and asparaginyl residues in pentapeptides, *J. Am. Chem. Soc.* 95, 8156–8159, 1973.

General references for deamidation include the following.

Lindner H, Helliger W. Age-dependent deamidation of asparagine residues in proteins. *Exp Gerontol.* 36(9), 1551–1563, 2001. Review. PubMed PMID: 11525877.

6 Properties of Some Solvents

Properties of Some Solvents Useful in Biochemistry and Molecular Biology[a]

	Solvent	M.W	Freezing Point (°C)	Boiling Point (°C$_{760}$)	Density (°C)[b]	Viscosity (mPa s)[c]	Log P	pKa	UV Cutoff (nm)
1	H_2O	18	0	100	1.00	0.89	–	14	190
2	MeOH	32.04	−97.8	64.7	0.79	0.54	−0.77	15.3	206
3	EtOH	4607	−114	78.4	0.79	1.07	−0.31	15.9	205
4	nPrOH	60.10	−127	97.2	0.80	2.26	0.25	16.1	210
5	iPrOH	60.10	−87.9	82.3	0.79	2.04	0.05	17.1	205
6	nBuOH	74.12	−88.6	117.6	0.81	2.54	0.88	16.1	180
7	Acn	41.05	−44	81.6	0.79	0.35	−0.34		255
8	Acetone	58.08	−94.9	56.1	0.79	0.32	−0.24		265
9	HOAc	60.05	16.7	118	1.05	1.06	−0.17	4.76	255
10	EtOAc	88.10	−83.8	77.1	0.90	0.42	0.73		265
11	EG	60.07	−13	197.6	1.1	16.9	1.93[1]		
12	HCOOH	46.03	8.4	100.8	1.2	1.6	−0.54		
13	TFA	144.2	−15.4	72.4	1.5	0.93	−0.25	0.3	
14	DMSO	78.13	18.5	189	1.1	2.47	−1.35	35.1	286
15	Formamide[2]	45.05	2.5	211	1.1	3.34	−1.51		275
16	DMF	73.09	−60.3	152.8	0.94	0.80	−1.01		263
17	$CHCl_3$	119.38	−63.4	61.2	1.48	5.63	1.27		245
18	CCl_4	153.83	−23	76.8	1.59	2.03	2.83		233
19	$CHCl_2$	84.93	−95	40	1.33	0.44	1.25		233
20	Dioxane	88.11	11.8	101.2	1.03	1.18	−0.27		215
21	THF	72.16	−108.5	65	0.89	0.53	0.46		212
22	DMAc	87.12	−20	163	0.94	0.92	−0.77		268
23	n-heptane	100.2	−90.5	98.4	0.68	0.42	4.66		200
24	n-hexane	86.18	−95.4	68.7	0.66	0.33	3.90		200
25	Toluene	92.14	−94.9	110.6	0.86	0.56	2.73		284

Abbreviations: DMF, dimethyl formamide; DMSO, dimethyl sulfoxide; EG, ethylene glycol (Ethane, 1,2-diol); TFA, trifluoroacetic acid; DMAc, N,N-dimethylacetamide

[1] T value of −1.36 has also been reported for the log P for ethylene glycol.

[2] For additional discussion of the use of formamide as a solvent for capillary zone electrophoresis, see Porras, S.P., and Kenndler, E., Formamide as solvent for capillary zone electrophoresis, *Electrophoresis* 25, 2946–2958, 2004.

[a] This information has been obtained from a variety of sources. For general reference, the following references are recommended.

1. Pubchem https://pubchem.ncbi.nih.gov.
2. Weast, Robert C., Melvin J. Astle, and William H. Beyer. *CRC Handbook of Chemistry and Physics*, CRC Press/Taylor & Francis Group, Boca Raton, FL, 1988.
3. *The Merck Index: An Encyclopedia of Chemicals, Drugs, and Biologicals*, ed. M.J. O'Neil, Royal Society of Chemistry, Cambridge, UK, 2013 (and previous editions published by Merck and Company, Whitehouse Station, NJ).
4. Shugar, G.J., and Dean, J.A., *The Chemists Ready Reference Handbook*, McGraw-Hill, New York, 1990.
5. Lide, D.R., *Basic Laboratory and Industrial Chemicals*, CRC Press, Boca Raton, FL, 1993.
6. Bruno, T.J., and Svaronos, P.D.N., *Handbook of Basic Tables for Chemical Analysis*, CRC Press, Boca Raton, FL, 1989.
7. Ramis-Ramos, G., García-Álvarez_Coque, M.C., Solvent selection in liquid chromatography, in *Liquid Chromatography Fundamental and Instructions*, ed. S. Fanali, P.R. Haddad, C.R. Poole, P. Schoenmakers, and D. Lloyd, Chapter 10, pp. 225–249, Elsevier, Amsterdam, the Netherlands, 2013.
8. Seaver, C., and Sadek, P., Solvent selectoin. Part I. UV absorption characteristics, *LCGC* 12, 742, 1994.

[b] Normalized to water = 1.00 g/cm^3 (1 cm^3 = 1 mL)

[c] miilepascals second (mPa s); millepascals second = centipoise

Change in pH on Addition of Solvent to Several Buffers Systems

Buffer	$_w^w$pH	$_w^s$pH						
		20% ACN	40% ACN	60% ACN	20% MeOH	40% MeOH	60% MeOH	80% MeOH
0.01 M acetate	3.50	3.83	4.16	4.48	3.75	4.09	4.48	4.90
	4.00	4.45	4.90	5.36	4.30	4.71	5.17	5.68
	5.00	5.46	5.91	6.37	5.30	5.72	6.19	6.70
0.05 M acetate	3.50	3.95	4.39	4.84	3.79	4.19	4.65	5.14
	4.00	4.46	4.91	5.37	4.30	4.71	5.17	5.68
	5.00	5.46	5.91	6.37	5.30	5.71	6.18	6.68
0.01 M citrate	4.00	4.31	4.62	4.94	4.31	4.75	5.24	5.78
	6.00	6.40	6.79	7.19	6.38	6.89	7.49	8.13
	7.50	7.90	8.30	8.69	7.87	8.38	8.96	9.59
0.05 M citrate	4.00	4.32	4.64	4.96	4.32	4.76	5.26	5.81
	6.00	6.38	6.75	7.13	6.37	6.87	7.44	8.07
	7.50	7.88	8.25	8.63	7.86	8.36	8.92	9.54
0.01 M phosphate	3.50	3.77	4.04	4.30	3.82	4.27	4.77	5.32
	6.50	6.88	7.20	7.55	6.90	7.45	8.08	8.76
	8.00	8.35	8.70	9.05	8.38	8.91	9.51	10.16
0.05 M phosphate	3.50	3.84	4.18	4.53	3.88	4.39	4.99	5.63
	6.50	6.84	7.18	7.53	6.90	7.44	8.06	8.74
	8.00	8.34	8.68	9.03	8.39	8.92	9.52	10.18
0.01 M NH$_4$	8.00	7.88	7.76	7.64	7.86	7.73	7.59	7.45
	10.00	9.88	9.76	9.64	9.87	9.73	9.60	9.47
0.05 M NH$_4$	8.00	7.88	7.76	7.64	7.86	7.73	7.59	7.45
	10.00	9.94	9.76	9.64	9.86	9.73	9.59	9.46

Source: Data are taken from Subirats, X., Rosés, M., and Bosch, E., On the effects of organic solvent composition on the pH of buffer HPLC mobile phases and the pK_a of analytes: A review, *Sep. Purif. Rev.*, 36, 231–255, 2007.

Effect of Acetonitrile or Methanol on the p*Ka* of Some Organic Acids

Buffer	Water	pKa					
		20% Acn	40% Acn	60% Acn	20% MeOH[e]	40% MeOH[e]	60% MeOH[e]
Formic acid[a,b]	3.72	3.96(3.99)[c]	4.40(4.54)	4.87(5.33)	–	–	–
Acetic acid[d]	4.74	(5.17)	(5.76)	(6.62)	5.05	5.43	5.66
Citrate (k$_1$)[d]	3.16	(3.49)	(3.90)	(4.45)	3.44	3.84	4.30
Citrate (k$_2$)[d]	4.79	(5.14)	(5.60)	(6.28)	6.40	7.39	7.96
Boric acid[a]	9.23	9.85(9.88)	10.43(10.57)	11.00(11.45)			
Carbonic acid	10.35	10.82(10.85)	11.31(11.45)	11.62(12.08)			
H$_3$PO$_4$	2.21	(2.62)	(3.11)	(3.75)	2.63	3.09	3.68
H$_2$PO$_4^-$	7.23	(7.60)	(8.08)	(8.73)	7.55	8.04	8.75
Tris	8.08	7.94(7.97)	7.85(7.99)	7.72(8.18)			
NH$_4$	9.29	(9.21)	(9.19)	(9.34)	9.11	8.97	8.82

[a] Subirats, X., Bosch, E., and Rosés, M., Retention of ionizable compounds on high-performance liquid chromatography XVII pH variation in mobile phases containing formic acids, piperazine, tris, boric acid and carbonate as buffering systems and acetonitrile as organic modified, *J.Chromatog. A* 1216, 2491–2498, 2009.

(Continued)

Effect of Acetonitrile or Methanol on the p*Ka* of Some Organic Acids (*Continued*)

[b] The p*Ka* values for neutral acids increases with addition of organic solvent with a sharp increase in pH above 60–70% solvent, while cationic acids (e.g. Tris, ammonia) shows a decrease in p*Ka* to about 80% solvent with a sharp increase in p*Ka* at higher concentrations (Cox, B.G., Acids, bases, and salts in mixed-aqueous solvents, *Org. Process Res. Dev.* 19, 1800–1808, 2015).

[c] Numbers in parentheses are value obtained with a solvent-containing reference buffer ($_s^s$p*Ka*); value without parentheses use the aqueous reference buffer ($_w^s$p*Ka*). This is IUPAC nomenclature, where the subscript indicates the media of the sample (s being solvent) while the subscript indicate the media for the reference solvent (w being water) (*IUPAC Compendium of Analytical Nomenclature. Definitive Rules 1997*, Blackwell, Oxford, England, 1998).

[d] Subirats, X., Bosch, E., and Rosés, M., Retention of ionizable compounds on high-performance liquid chromatography XV. Estimation of the pH variation of aqueous buffers with the change of the acetonitrile fraction of the mobile phase, *J. Chromatog. A* 1059, 33–42, 2004.

[e] Subirats, X., Bosch, E., and Rosés, M., Retention of ionizable compounds on high-performance liquid chromatography XVII. Estimation of the pH variation of aqueous buffers with the change in methanol fraction of the mobile phase, *J. Chromatog. A* 1138, 203–214, 2007.

Effect of Organic Solvents on the p*Ka* of Various Acids

Compound	$_w^w$p*Ka*	$_w^s$p*Ka*							
		MeOH[a]	EtOH	EG	PG	Me$_2$SO	DMF	Dioxane	THF
GlyGly (p*Ka*1)	3.15	3.47	3.46	3.43	3.44	3.55	3.46	3.63	3.51
HOAc	4.59	4.90	4.95	4.82	4.86	4.96	4.95	5.28	5.29
Benzoic acid[b]	3.98	4.53	–	–	–	4.51	4.52	4.59	4.95
Imidazole	7.13	6.88	6.88	7.02	6.92	6.72	6.58	6.79	–
HEPES (p*Ka*1)	2.94	2.84	2.88	3.10	2.96	2.87	2.86	2.94	2.88
HEPES (p*Ka*2)	7.54	7.46	7.47	7.66	7.52	7.46	7.38	7.51	7.45
MES	6.14	6.07	6.04	6.30	6.18	6.04	5.97	6.08	–
Tris	8.23	8.16	8.12	8.31	8.24	8.14	8.04	8.20	–
TAPS	8.46	8.45	8.43	8.54	8.48	8.37	8.32	8.52	8.43
Boric acid	9.29	9.42	9.90	8.18[c]	7.98[c]	10.50	10.23	10.12	–
KH$_2$PO$_4$	6.91	7.39	7.40	7.24	7.25	7.64	7.44	7.49	–

Source: Data are taken from Grace, S., and Dunaway-Mariano, D., Examination of the solvent perturbation technique as a method to identify enzyme catalytic groups, *Biochemistry*, 22, 4238–4247, 1983.

Abbreviations: HOAc, acetic acid; HEPES, *N*-(2-hydroxyethyl)-piperazine-*N'*–2-ethanesulfonic acid; MES, 2-(*N*-morpholino)-ethanesulfonic acid; Tris, tris(hydroxymethyl)aminomethane; TAPS, 3-[[tris(hydroxymethyl)methyl]amino]propanesulfonic acid; MeOH, methanol; EtOH, ethanol; EG, ethylene glycol; PG, propylene glycol; Me$_2$SO, dimethyl sulfoxide; DMF, dimethylformamide; THF, tetrahydrofuran.

[a] Solvent at 25%(V/V by preparation).

[b] A more detailed study on the effect of organic solvents (Rubino, J.T., and Berryhill, W.S., Effects of solvent polarity on the acid dissociation-constants of benzoic acid, *J.Pharm. Sci.* 75, 182–186, 1986).

[c] The effect of ethylene glycol and propylene glycol on boric acid reflect the complexation of polyhydroxy compounds with boric acids resulting a decrease in pH. A similar effect has been observed with monosaccharides (Shubhada, S., and Sundaram, P.V., The role of pH change caused by the addition of water-miscible organic solvents in the destabilization of an enzyme, *Enzyme Microb. Technol.* 17, 330–335, 1994).

Polarity of Solvents Used in Chromatography[a]

	Solvent	Solvent Polarity (P')[b]	Solvent Polarity (P')[b,c]	Solvent Polarity (P')[d]	Eluuotropic Solvent Strength (E°)[e] Al_2O_3	Solvent Polarity[f] (E_T^N)	Solvation Ability (A)[g]	Dielectric Constant (E_r)[h]
1	H_2O	10.2	1.00			1.00	2.00	80.1
2	MeOH	5.1	0.5		0.95	0.762	1.25	33
3	EtOH	4.3	0.4	4.4		0.654	1.11	25.3
4	nPrOH	3.9	0.4	4.1		0.617	1.08	20.8
5	iPrOH	3.9	0.4	3.9	0.82	0.546		20.2
6	nBuOH	3.9	0.4	4.1		0.586		17.8
7	Acn	5.8	0.6	5.6	0.79	0.460	1.22	36.6
8	Acetone					0.355	1.06	21.0
9	HOAc	6.0	0.6	6.1		0.228	1.06	6.2
10	EtOAc	4.4	0.4	4.2	0.58	0.221	0.79	6.1
11	EG	6.9	0.7			0.790	1.62	41.4
12	HCOOH				6.1	0.728		51.1
13	TFA						1.72	8.4
14	DMSO	7.2	0.7		7.3	0.444		47.2
15	Formamide	9.6	0.9			0.775	1.65	111
16	DMF	6.4	0.6	6.3		0.386	1.23	38.3
17	$CHCl_3$	4.1	0.4	4.3	0.40	0.259	1.15	4.7
18	CCl_4	1.6	0.2	1.6	0.18	0.052	0.43	2.2
19	$CHCl_2$	3.1.	0.3	4.3	0.42	0.309	1.13	8.9
20	Dioxane	4.8		5.3	0.63	0.164	0.86	2.2
21	THF	4.0		4.3		0.207	0.84	7.5
22	DMAc	6.5		6.5				38.9
23	n-heptane							1.9
24	n-hexane	0.1		−0.14				1.9
25	Toluene	2.4		2.7				2.4

Abbreviations: DMF, dimethyl formamide; DMSO, dimethyl sulfoxide; EG, ethylene glycol (Ethane, 1,2-diol); TFA, trifluoroacetic acid; DMAc, N,N-dimethylacetamide

[a] This information has been obtained from a variety of sources. For general reference, the following references are recommended.

1. Pubchem, https://pubchem.ncbi.nih.gov.
2. *CRC Handbook of Chemistry and Physics*, CRC Press/Taylor & Francis Group, Boca Raton, FL.
3. O'Neil, M.J. et al., *The Merck Index: An Encyclopedia of Chemicals, Drugs, and Biologicals*, ed. Royal Society of Chemistry, Cambridge, UK, 2013. (and previous editions published by Merck and Company, Whitehouse Station, NJ.)
4. Shugar, G.J., and Dean, J.A., *The Chemists Ready Reference Handbook*, McGraw-Hill, New York, 1990.
5. Lide, D.R., *Basic Laboratory and Industrial Chemicals*, CRC Press, Boca Raton, FL, 1993.
6. Bruno, T.J., and Svaronos, P.D.N., *Handbook of Basic Tables for Chemical Analysis*, CRC Press, Boca Raton, FL, 1989.
7. Ramis-Ramos, G., García-Álvarez_Coque, M.C., Solvent selection in liquid chromatography, in *Liquid Chromatography Fundamental and Instructions*, ed. S. Fanali, P.R. Haddad, C.R. Poole, P. Schoenmakers, and D. Lloyd, Chapter 10, pp. 225–249, Elsevier, Amsterdam, Netherlands, 2013.
8. Seaver, C., and Sadek, P., Solvent selectoin. Part I. UV absorption characteristics, *LCGC* 12, 742, 1994.
9. Welch, J., Brkovic, T., Schafer, W., and Gong, X., Performance to burn? Re-evaluating the choice of acetonitrile as the platform solvent for analytical HPLC, *Green Chem.* 11, 1232–1238, 2009.

(*Continued*)

Polarity of Solvents Used in Chromatography (*Continued*)

[b] Solvent polarity (P′) as defined by L.R. Snyder (Snyder, L.R., Classification of the solvent properties of common liquids, *J. Chromatog. Sci.* 16, 223–234, 1978). P′ is a global estimation of solvent strength (polarity) including acidity, basicity, and dipolar characteristics.

[c] Normalized to water = 1; not taken to more significant figures than original data.

[d] Solvent polarity (P′) slightly. (Modified Rutan, S.C., Carr, P.W., Cheung, W.J., *et al.*, *J. Chromatog. A.*, 463, 21–37, 1989.)

[e] Eluotropic is a measure of the adsorption interaction of a solvent with a specific stationary phase. In this example, the stationary phase is a normal phase thin layer (planar) chromatography. (From Gocan, S., Eluotropic series of solvents for TLC, in *Encyclopedia of Chromatography*, 3rd edn., ed. J.Cazes, pp. 730–735, CRC Press/Taylor & Francis Group, Boca Raton, FL, 2010.)

[f] E_T^N is $E_T^{(30)}$ normalized to water = 1. $E_T(30)$ is an empirical scale of solvent polarity. (From Reichardt, C., *Pure Appl. Chem.*, 76, 19093–1919, 2004.) Data shown are taken. (From Reichardt, C., *Chem. Rev.* 94, 2319–2358, 1994.) $Et_T^{(30)}$ is the molar electronic transition energy of pyridinium N-phenolate betaine dye; E_T^N is obtained from the normalization of $E_T(30)$ use water as the most polar solvent and tetramethylsilane as the most nonpolar solvent. Units of $E_T(30)$ are kcal mol^{-1} while E_T^N is dimensionless.

[g] A measure of solvation—a combination of anion-solvating ability and cation-solvating ability considered a measure of solvent polarity. (Form Reichardt, C., and Welton, T., *Solvents and Solvent Effects in Organic Chemistry*, 4th edn., Wiley-VCH, Weinheim, NJ, 2011.)

[h] Also referred to as permittivity; shown here is the relative permittivity, which is the ratio of actual permittivity to permittivity in a vacuum.

Polarity of Solvents Used in Chromatography (Continued)

7 Partial Volumes

Partial Molal Volumes for Some Biochemicals[a]

Substance	A[b]	B[c]	cm³ m⁻¹ C[c]	cm³ m⁻¹ D[c]	E[c]	F[b,d]
α-Aminobutyric Acid	75.5		75.5	76.5		
ε-Aminocaproic Acid				104.9		
Urea		44.23		44.3	44.23	
Thioacetamide		66.42			66.42	44.2
Thiourea					54.79	
Dextrose		112.04			112.04	
D-Fructose						110.2
D-Glucose						110.3
D-Ribose		95.21			95.21	95.8
Sucrose		211.32			211.32	
Succinic acid		82.67			82.67	
Norleucine			107.93			
Norvaline			91.7			
Formic acid				34.7		
Foramide				38		
Acetic acid				50.7		
Acetamide	55.6			55	55.6	
Propionic acid				67.9		
Butyric acid				84.3		
Glycine				43.5		
Glycinamide				60.3		
Leucinamide				123.8		
Pyridine				76.7		
1,4-Dioxane					80.94	

[a] Values at 298.15 K (25°C)
[b] Partial molar volume
[c] Partial molal volume
[d] This study contains partial molal volume data for a large number of chemicals including detergents.

REFERENCES

A. Singh, S.K., and Kishore, N., Volumetric properties of amino acids and hen-egg white lysozyme in aqueous Triton X-100 at 298.15 K, *J. Solution Chem.* 33, 1411–1427, 2004.

B. Milero, F.J., and Huang, F., The partial molal volumes and compressibilities of nonelectrolytes and amino acids in 0.725 M NaCl, *Aquat. Geochem.* 22, 1–16, 2016.

C. Mishra, A.K., and Abluwalla, J.C., Apparent molal volumes of amino acids, N-acetylamino acids, and peptides in aqueous solution, *J. Phys. Chem,* 88, 86–92, 1984.

D. Edsall, J.T., Apparent molal volume, heat capacity, compressibility and surface tension of dipolar ions in solutions, in *Proteins, Amino Acids and Peptides as Ions and Dipolar Ions,* ed. J.T., Edsall and E.J. Cohn, Chapter 7, pp. 155–176, Reinhold Publishing, New York, 1943.

E. Lo Surdo, A., Chin, C., and Millero, F.J., The apparent molal volumes and adiabatic compressibility of some organic solutes in water at 25°C, *J. Chem. Eng. Data* 23, 197–201, 1978.

F. Durchschlag, H., and Zipper, P., Calculation of the partial volume of organic compounds and polymers, *Prog. Colloid Polymer Sci.* 94, 20–39, 1994.

Partial Molar Volumes of Some Nucleic Acid Bases, Nucleosides, and Related Biochemicals[a]

	A	B	B[e]	B[f]	C	C[g]	C[h]	D[i]
Acetyl-CoA	545.3[c]							
Acetyl-CoA	500.9[d]							
FMN(Na)								281.5
NAD(free acid)[b]								409.4
NAD(Na)[b]								394.3
Cytosine		73.6	74.14	72.61		74.3	75.8	
Cytidine		154.19	155.37	155.7		156.7	157.4	
Uracil		72.29	71.74	71.58		72.9	73.3	
Uridine		152.32	153.39	153.25		153.6	154	
Thymine		88.75	86.37	87.07		88.6	87.4	
Thymidine		168.03	168.74	169.19		168.3	168.6	
Adenine		90.49	86.41					
Adenosine		171.43	171.08	171.49		170.6	172.3	
AMP(Na)					189.1	203		
ATP(2Na)					238.9	257.7	271.3	

[a] A values at 298.15 K (25°C) unless otherwise indicated
[b] 20°C
[c] Free acid
[d] Sodium salt
[e] 1 molal glucose
[f] 1 molal sucrose
[g] 1 molal NaCl
[h] 1 molal CaCl$_2$
[i] This study contains calculated and experimental partial molal volume data for a large number of chemicals.

REFERENCES

A. Durchschlag, H., and Zipper, P., Calculation of partial specific volumes and other volumetric properties of small molecules and polymers. *J. Appl. Cryst.* 30, 803–807, 1997.

B. Kishore, N., Bhat, R., and Ahluwalia, J.C., Thermodynamics of some nucleic acid bases and nucleosides in water, and their transfer to aqueous glucose solutions at 298.15 K, *Biophys. Chem.* 33, 227–236, 1989.

C. Kishore, N., and Ahluwalia, J.C., Partial molar heat capacities and volumes of transfer of nucleic acid bases, nucleosides and nucleotides from water to aqueous solutions of sodium and calcium chloride at 25°C, *J. Solution Chem.* 19, 51–64, 1990.

D. Durchschlag, H., and Zipper, P., Calculation of the partial volume of organic compounds and polymers, *Prog. Colloid Polymer Sci.* 94, 20–39, 1994.

Partial Molar/Molal Volumes of Amino Acids[a]

	A^b	B^b	$C^{b,c}$	$C^{b,d}$	D^b	E^e	F^b	G^e	H^e
					cm³ m⁻¹				
Ala	60.45	60.4	63.9	60.5	60.43	60.43	60.43	60.42	60.6
Arg	123.7		123.6	127.3		127.34		123.86	
Asn	77.18		76.8	77.3				95.63	78
Asp	71.79		69	73.8		73.83		74.8	58.9
(Cys)2	148								
Cys	73.62		74.3	73.4		73.44			
Gln	94.36		93.5	93.6				93.61	
Glu	89.36		82.9	85.9		85.88		89.85	
Gly	43.25	43.12	48.8	43.2	43.14	43.19	43.14	43.19	43.5
His	99.14	98.81	94.9	98.9		98.79		98.3	99.3
Ile	105.45		105.5	105.7				195.8	
Leu	107.57		104.6	107.8	107.72		107.72	107.83	
Lys	108.71		115.5	108.5	125.9		125.9	124.76	108.5
Met	105.3		106.9	104.8		105.35		105.57	
Phe	121.92		111.8	121.5		121.48		122.2	121.3
Pro	82.65		84.7	82.5		82.83		82.63	81
Ser	60.62	60.32	66.5	60.6				60.62	60.8
Thr	76.84	76.84	81.9	76.9				76.83	
Trp	144		123.9	143.4		143.91		143.8	144.1
Tyr	123		113.1	124.3				124.4	
Val	90.79		90.6	90.8	90.39	90.78		90.65	
Hypro									84.4
NorLeu								107.93	
NorVal								91.7	

[a] Values obtained at 298.15 K (25°C)

[b] Partial molar volume

[c] Calculated using the Kirkwood–Buff equation and a three-dimensional reference interaction site model (3D-RISM) integral equation theory for molecular liquids

[d] Experimental value

[e] Partial molal volume.

REFERENCES

A. Jolicoeur, C., Riedl, B., Desrochers, D., et al., Solvation of amino acid residues in water and urea-water mixtures: Volumes and heat capacities of 20 amino acid in water and 8 M urea at 25°C, *J. Solution Chem.* 15, 109–128, 1986.

B. Shen, J.-L., Li, Z.-F., Wang, B.-H., and Zhang, Y.-M., Partial molar volumes of some amino acids and a peptide in water, DMSO, NaCl, and DMSO/NaCl aqueous solutions, *J. Chem. Thermodyn.* 32, 805–819, 2000.

C. Harano, Y., Imai, T., Kovalenko, A., Kimoshito, M., and Hirata, F., Theoretical study for partial molar volume of amino acids and polypeptides by three-dimensional reference interaction model, *J. Chem. Phys.* 114, 9506–9511, 2001.

D. Singh, S.K., and Kishore, N., Volumetric properties of amino acids and hen-egg white lysozyme in aqueous Triton X-100 at 298.15 K, *J. Solution Chem.* 33, 1411–1427, 2004.

E. Milero, F.J., and Huang, F., The partial molal volumes and compressibilities of nonelectrolytes and amino acids in 0.725 M NaCl, *Aquat. Geochem.* 22, 1–16, 2016.

F. Singh, S.K., Kundu, A., and Kishore, N., Interaction of some amino acids and glycine peptides with aqueous sodium dodecyl sulfate and cetylmethylammoniumbromideat T = 298.15 K: A volumetric approach, *J. Chem. Thermodynam.* 36, 7–16, 2004.

G. Mishra, A.K., and Abluwalla, J.C., Apparent molal volumes of amino acids, N-acetylamino acids, and peptides in aqueous solution, *J. Phys. Chem,* 88, 86–92, 1984.

H. Cohn, E.J., McMeekin, T.L., Edsall, J.T., and Blanchard, M.H., Studies in the physical chemistry of amino acids, peptides and related substances. I. The apparent molal volume and electrostriction of the solvent, *J. Am. Chem. Soc.* 56, 784–794, 1934.

Partial Volumes of Amino Acids and Amino Acid Residues

AA	A[a]	B[b,c]	C[b]	D[e,f]	E[e]	F[g]	G[h]
	$\times 10^{-3}$ nm^3	cm^{-3}mL^{-1}					
Ala	87.2	17.75	17.20	13.0–15.34	12.7	0.17	0.74
Arg	181.3		80.48	13.0–26.05		0.676	0.70
Asn	117.4	35.43	33.93			0.344	0.62
Asp	114.6		28.54	13.0–21.09		0.304	0.60
Cys	106.7		105[d]	13.0–21.10			0.61
Cys/2			30.37			0.299	
Gln	142.4		51.11			0.50	0.67
Glu	141.4		46.11	13.0–23.24		0.467	0.66
Gly				8.68–13.1	13.5	0.0	0.64
His	152.4	58.0	55.89	10.8–29.40	10.8	0.555	0.67
Ile	168.9	65.32	62.20			0.636	
Leu	168.9	65.43	64.32	13.0–23.39		0.636	
Lys	174.3		65.45		18.3	0.647	0.82
Met	163.1	63.18	62.01	13.0–22.33		0.613	0.75
Phe	187.9		78.67	13.3–27.44	13.7	0.774	0.77
Pro	122.4		39.40	9.54–14.27	13.8	0.373	0.76
Ser	91.0		17.37	12.9–17.2	12.9	0.172	0.63
Thr	117.4		33.61			0.334	0.70
Trp	228.5		100.71	15.1–29.15	15.1	1.0	0.74
Tyr	192.1		80			0.796	0.71
Val	141.4		47.54	13.1–22.33		0.476	

[a] These values are a consensus of amino acid residue volumes from six sets of data (see reference A).

[b] Partial molar amino acid residue volume.

[c] Obtained from the analysis of the tripeptide, gly-X-gly (Hedwig, G.R., Partial molar volumes of amino acid sidechains of proteins in aqueous solution: Some comments on their estimates using partial molar volumes of amino acids and small peptides, *Biopolymers* 32, 537–540, 1992).

[d] Calculated data (see also reference A).

[e] Value for electrorestriction. Electrorestriction, in this context, is the observed decrease in volume due to interaction of the dipolar amino acid with solvent (Greenstein, J.P., Wyman, J., Jr., and Cohn, E.J., Studies of multivalent amino acids and peptides. III. The dielectric constants and electrorestriction of the solvent in solutions of tetrapoles, *J. Am. Chem. Soc.* 57, 637–642, 1935; Linderstrøm-Lang, K., and Jacobsen, C.F., The contraction accompanying break-down of proteins, *Enzymologia* 10, 97–126, 1941).

[f] Three methods were used to calculate the value for electroconstriction, and the range of values is shown.

[g] Residue volume; it is assumed that this is amino acid residue specific volume.

[h] Specific volume of the residue obtained by dividing molal volume by molecular weight.

REFERENCES

A. Perkins, S.J., Protein volumes and hydration effects. The calculation of partial specific volumes, neutron scattering matchpoints and 280-nm absorption coefficients for proteins and glycoproteins from amino acid sequences, *Eur. J. Biochem.* 157, 169–180, 1986.

B. Hedwig, G.R., Partial molar heat capacities volumes and compressibilities of aqueous solutions of some peptides that model the side chains of proteins, *Pure Appl. Chem.* 66, 387–397, 1994.

C. Jolicoeur, C., Riedl, B., Desrochers, D., et al., Solvation of amino acid residues in water and urea-water mixtures: Volumes and heat capacities of amino acids in water and in 8 M urea at 25°C, *J. Solution Chem.* 15, 109–128, 1986.

D. Millero, E.J., Lo Surdo, A., and Shin, C., The apparent molal volumes and adiabatic compressibilities of aqueous amino acids at 25°C, *J. Phys. Chem.* 82, 784–792, 1976.

E. Cohn, E.J., McMeekin, T.L., Edsall, J.T., and Blanchard, M.H., Studies in the physical chemistry of amino acids, peptides and related substances. I. The apparent molal volume and the electrostriction of the solvent, *J. Am. Chem. Soc.* 56, 784–794, 1934.

F. Goodarza, H., Katanforoush, A., Torabi, N., and Najafabadi, H.S., Solvent accessibility, residue charge and residue volume, the three ingredients of a robust amino acid substitution matrix, *J. Theoret. Biol.* 245, 715–725, 2007.

G. Cohn, E.J., and Edsall, J.T., Density and apparent specific volume of proteins, in *Proteins, Amino Acids and Peptides as Ion and Dipolar Ions*, ed. E.J. Cohn and J.T. Edsall, Chapter 16, pp. 370–381, Reinhold Publishing, New York, 1943.

Effect of Solvent on Partial Molar Volume[a]

Amino Acid	Water[a]	0.10 M DMSO[a]	2.0 M NaCl[a]	0.75 M NaCl[b]	8.0 M Urea[c]
		cm^{-3}m^{-1}			
Gly	43.12	43.12	46.02	42.68	47.33
Ala	60.4	60.3	62.9	60.4	64.2
Ser	60.32	60.68	63.73		64.97
Thr	76.84	76.81	79.64		81.1
L-His	98.81	98.68	101.84		103.52

[a] Shen, J.-L., et al., *J. Chem. Thermodyn.*, 32, 805–819, 2000.

[b] Millero, F.J., and Huang, F., *Aquatic Geochem.*, 22, 1–16, 2016.

[c] Jolilcoeur, C., et al., *J. Solution Chem.*, 15, 109–128, 1986.

8 A List of Log P Values, Water Solubility, and Molecular Weight for Some Selected Chemicals

Compound	M.W.	Log P[a]	Water Solubility(g/L)[b]
Acetamide	59.07	−1.26	2.25×10^3
Acetic acid	60.05	−0.17	10×10^3
Acetic anhydride	102.09	−0.58	1.2×10^2
Acetoacetic acid	102.1	−0.98	1×10^3
Acetoin	88.11	−0.36	1×10^3
Acetone	58.08	−0.24	1×10^3
Acetophenone	120.15	1.58	6.13
N-Acetylcysteinamide	162.21	−0.29	5.8
N-Acetylcysteine		−0.64	
N-Acetylmethionine		−0.49	
Acetylsalicylic acid	180.16	1.19	4.6
Acridine	179.22	3.40	0.03
Acrolein	56.06	−0.01	2.13×10^2
Acrylamide	71.08	−0.67	6.4×10^2
Adenine	135.13	−0.09	1.0
Adenosine	267.25	−1.05	8.2
Alanine	89.09	−2.96	1.7×10^2
Aldosterone		1.08	
9-Aminoacridine	194.23	2.74	0.02
4-Aminobenzoic acid (p-aminobenzoic acid; PABA)	151.17	1.03	9.89
4-Aminobutyric acid (γ-aminobutyric acid; GABA)	103.12	−3.17	1.3×10^3
6-Aminohexanoic acid (ε-aminocaproic acid)	131.18	−2.95	5.05×10^2
Aminopyrine [4-(dimethylamino)-1,5-dimethyl-2-phenylpyrazol-3-one]	231.4	0.5	23.8
Ammonium picrate	246.14	−1.40	1.6×10^2
Aniline		0.9	
Anisole		2.11	
ANS (1-amino-2-naphthalenesulfonic acid)	222.25	−0.97	2.23
Anthracene		4.45	
Arabinose	150.13	−3.02	10^3
Arginine	174.20	−4.20	1.82×10^2
Ascorbic acid	176.13	−1.64	1×10^3
Asparagine	132.12	−3.82	29.4
Aspartic acid	133.10	−3.89	5.0
Aspirin (Acetylsalicylicacid; 2-acetoxybenzoic acid)	180.16	1.23	7
Barbital (5,5-diethylbarbituric acid)	184.20	0.65	7
Barbituric acid	128.1	−1.47	
Benzamide	121.14	0.64	13.5
Benzamidine	120.16	0.65	27.9

(Continued)

Compound	M.W.	Log P[a]	Water Solubility(g/L)[b]
Benzene	78.11	2.13	0.002
Benzoic acid	122.12	1.87	3.4
Betaine	117.15	−4.93	6.11×10^2
Biuret (imidodicarbonicacid)	103.08		1.5
Bromoacetic acid	138.95	0.41	93
2-Bromopropionic acid	152.98	0.92	29.9
Bufexamac[2-(4-butoxyphenyl)-*N*-hydroxyacetamide]	223.3	0.77	1.1
2,3-Butanediol	90.12	−0.36	7.6×10^2
2,3-Butanedione	86.09	−1.34	2×10^2
Butyl urea	116.16	0.41	46.3
3-Butyl hydroxy urea	132.16	0.32	23.5
Cacodylic acid	138.00	0.36	2×10^3
Carbon tetrachloride	153.82	2.83	0.8
Cholesterol	386.67	8.74	0.9
Chloroacetamide	93.51	−0.53	90
Chloroacetic anhydride	170.98	−0.07	68
Chloroacetyl chloride	112.94	−0.22	1.6×10^2
Chloroform	119.38	1.97	8
6-Chloroindole	151.60	3.25	0.1
p-Chloromercuribenzoic acid	357.16	1.48	0.3
Chlorosuccinic acid	152.54	−0.57	1.8×10^2
Cholic acid	405.58	2.02	0.2
Citric acid	192.13	−1.72	5.92×10^2
Congo red	696.68	2.63	1.2×10^2
Corticosterone		1.94	
Cortisone		2.88	
Creatine	132.14	−3.72	13.3
Creatinine	113.12	−1.76	80
Crotonaldehyde (2-butenal)	70.09	0.60	1.8×10^2
Cyanoacetic acid	85.06	−0.76	7.7×10^2
Cyanogen	52.04	0.07	1.2×10^2
Cyanuric acid	129.08	0.61	2
Cyclohexanone		0.81	
Cysteine	121.16	−2.49	1.1×10^2
Cystine	240.30	−5.08	0.2
Cytidine	243.22	−2.51	1.8×10^2
Cytosine	111.10	−1.73	8
Deoxycholic acid	392.58	3.50	0.04
Deoxycorticosterone		2.88	
Dexamethasone		2.01	
Diazomethane	42.04	2.00	2
Dichloromethane		1.2	
Diclofenac acid (2-[2-(2,6-dichloroanalino)phenyl]acetic acid)	295.14	4.5	0.002
Diclofenac acid (2-[2-(2,6-dichloroanalino)phenyl]acetate, sodium salt)	318.13	0.7	
Dicumarol	336.30	2.07	0.1
Diethyl ether (ethyl ether; ether)	74.1	0.9	
Diethylsuberate	230.31	3.35	0.7
Diethylsulfone	122.19	−0.59	1.4×10^2
N,N-Diethyl urea	116.2	0.1	4
Dihydroxyacetone	88.11	−0.49	16.2

(Continued)

Compound	M.W.	Log P[a]	Water Solubility(g/L)[b]
Diisopropyl fluorophosphate (DFP)	184.15	1.17	15.4
Diketene	84.08	−0.39	5.3×10^2
Dimethylformamide		−1.04	
Dimethylguanidine	87.13	−0.95	1.6
Dimethylsulfoxide	78.13	−1.35	1×10^3
Dimethylphthalate		1.56	
1,4-Dinitrobenzene		1.47	
2,4-Dinitrophenol		1.55	
EDTA	292.25	−3.86	1
EDTA, tetrasodium salt	360.17	−13.17	5.0×10^2
Ethanol (ethyl alcohol)	46.07	−0.31	1×10^3
N-Hydroxy-1-ethylurea	104.11	−0.10	7
N-Ethylnicotinamide	150.18	0.31	41.2
Estradiol		2.69	
N-Ethylthiourea	104.17	−0.21	24
Ethylurea	88.11	−0.74	26.4
Ethylene glycol	2.07	−1.36	1×10^3
Ethylene oxide	44.05	−0.30	1×10^3
Flufenamic acid (2[3-(trifluoromethyl)anilino]benzoic acid)	281.23	5.25	0.009
Fluorescein	333.32	3.35	0.05
Fluoroacetone	76.07	−0.39	286
Flurbiprofen [2-(3-fluoro-4-phenylphenyl)propionic acid]	244.26	4.16	0.008
Folic acid	441.41	−2.00	0.002
Formaldehyde	30.03	0.35	400
Formic acid	48.03	−0.54	1×10^3
Galactose	180.16	−2.43	683
Glucose	180.16	−3.00	$\geq 1 \times 10^3$
Glutamic acid	147.10	−3.69	8.6
Glutamine	146.15	−3.64	41
Glycerol	92.10	−1.76	1×10^3
Glycine	75.10	−3.21	2.5×10^2
Glyoxal	58.04	−1.66	1×10^3
Glyoxylic acid	74.04	−1.40	1×10^3
Guanidine	59.07	−1.63	1.8
Guanine	151.13	−0.91	2.1
Guanosine	283.25	−1.90	0.7
Hexanal	100.16	1.78	6
Hydroxyproline	131.13	−3.17	395
Hydroxyurea (N-hydroxyurea)	76.06	−1.80	200
N-Hydroxy-1-ethylurea	104.11	−0.10	7
Indole	117.15	2.14	4
Inositol	180.16	−2.08	143
Iodoacetamide	184.96	−0.19	76
Isoleucine	131.18	−1.70	34
Isopropanol	60.10	0.05	1×10^3
Ketoprofen [2-(3-benzoylphenyl)propanoic acid]	254.28	3.12	0.02
Lactic acid	90.08	−0.72	1×10^3
Lactose	342.30	−5.43	195
Leucine	131.18	−1.52	22
Linoleic acid	280.45	7.05	0.00004

(Continued)

Compound	M.W.	Log P[a]	Water Solubility(g/L)[b]
Lysine	146.19	−3.05	1×10^3
Maleic anhydride	98.06	1.62	5
Maltose	342.30	−5.43	780
Mannitol	182.17	−3.10	216
Mefenamic acid (2-[2(2,3-dimethylphenyl)amino]benzoic acid)	241.29	5.12	0.020
Mercaptoacetic acid	92.12	0.09	1×10^3
2-Mercaptobenzoic acid	154.19	2.39	0.7
Methane	16.04	1.09	0.002
Methanol	32.04	−0.77	1×10^3
Methionine	149.21	−1.87	57
Methotrexate	454.45	−1.85	2.6
Methylene blue	319.86	5.85	44
N-Methyl glycine	89.09	−2.78	300
5-Methylindole	131.18	2.68	0.5
Methyl isocyanate	57.05	0.79	29
Methylmalonic acid	118.09	−0.83	680
Methyl methacrylate	86.09	0.80	49
Methylmethane sulfonate	110.13	−0.66	1×10^3
Methyl thiocyanate	73.12	0.73	32
N-Methyl thiourea	119.21	−0.69	240
Methyl urea	74.08	−1.40	100
Naphthalene	128.17	3.29	0.031
Naproxen	230.26	3.18	0.016
Nicotinic acid	123.11	0.36	18
Ornithine	132.16	−4.22	1×10^3
Orotic acid	156.10	−0.83	2
Oxalic acid	90.06	−2.22	
Oxindole	133.15	1.16	9
Palmitic acid	256.43	7.17	0.0008
Paraldehyde	132.16	0.67	112
Pentobarbital	226.28	2.10	0.7
Phenol	94.11	1.46	83
Phenylalanine	165.19	−1.52	22
Phosgene	98.02	−0.71	475
Proline	115.13	−2.54	131
Prostaglandin E2	352.48	2.82	0.006
Propylamine	59.11	0.48	1×10^3
Propylene oxide	58.08	0.03	595
Pyridine	79.10	0.65	1×10^3
Pyridoxal	203.63	−3.32	500
Pyridoxal-5-phosphate	247.15	0.37	20
Pyridoxine	169.18	−0.77	282
Pyruvic acid	88.06	−1.24	1×10^3
Ribose	150.13	−2.32	
Salicylic acid	138.12	2.26	2.24
Sarin	140.10	0.72	1×10^3
Serine	105.09	−3.07	425
Sorbic acid	112.13	1.33	2
Sorbitol	182.17	−2.20	3×10^3
Stearic acid	284.49	8.23	0.03

(*Continued*)

Compound	M.W.	Log P[a]	Water Solubility(g/L)[b]
Succinic anhydride	100.07	0.81	24
Succinimide	99.09	−0.85	196
Sucrose	342.30	−3.70	2.12×10^3
Testosterone	288.43	3.32	0.03
Tetrahydrofuran	72.11	0.46	1×10^3
Threonine	119.12	−2.94	97
Toluene	92.14	2.73	0.5
2,4,6-Trinitrobenzene	257.12	0.23	21
Tryptophan	204.23	−1.06	12
Urea	60.06	−2.11	545
Valine	117.15	−2.26	60

Source: Adapted from Howard, P.H., and Meylan, W.M. ed. *Handbook of Physical Properties of Organic Chemicals*, CRC Press, Boca Raton, FL, 1997 and other numerous other sources including PubChem.

[a] Log P = log concentration in oil/concentration in water, a partition coefficient, K = oil/water; see above Howard and Meylan and following for discussion of log P.

[b] Solubility values taken from various literature sources and in some cases are approximations. Data is assumed at 20°C–25°C. Some values are estimates. A value of 1×10^3 g/L means approximately 1 gm solute in 1 mL H_2O or, in the case of a liquid, the liquid is miscible with H_2O.

REFERENCES

Abrahams, M.H., Du, C.M., and Platts, J.A., Lipophilicity of the nitrophenols, *J.Org. Chem.* 65, 7114–7718, 2000.

Avdeef, A., Physicochemical profiling (solubility, permeability and charge state), *Curr. Top. Med. Chem.* 1, 277–351, 2001.

Chuman, H., Mori, A., and Tanaka, H., Prediction of the 1-octanol/H_2O partition coefficient, Log P, by *Ab Initio* calculations: Hydrogen-bonding effect of organic solutes on Log P, *Analyt. Sci.* 18, 1015–1020, 2002.

Halling, P.J., Thermodynamic predictions for biocatalysis in nonconventional media: Theory, tests, and recommendations for experimental design and analysis, *Enzyme Microb. Technol.* 16, 178–206, 1994.

Hansch, C., and Leo, A., *Exploring QSAR. Fundamentals and Applications in Chemistry and Biology*, American Chemical Society, Washington, DC, 1995.

Lipinski, C.A., Lombardo, F., Dominy, B.W., and Feeney, P.J., Experimental and computational approaches to estimate solubility and permeability in drug discovery and development settings, *Adv. Drug. Deliv. Rev.* 46, 3–26, 2001.

Uttamsingh, V., Keller, D.A., and Anders, M.W., Acylase I-catalyzed deacetylation of *N*-acetyl-L-cysteine and *S*-Alkyl-*N*-acetyl-L-cysteines, *Chem. Res. Toxicol.* 11, 800–809, 1998.

Valko, K., Du, C.M., Bevan, C., Reynolds, D.P., and Abraham, M.H., Rapid method for the estimation of octanol/water partition coefficient (Log P_{oct}) from gradient RP-HPLC retention and a hydrogen bond acidity term ($\Sigma\alpha_2^H$), *Curr. Medicin. Chem.* 8, 1137–1146, 2001.

Yalkowsky, S.H., and He, Y., *Handbook of Aqueous Solubility Data*, CRC Press, Boca Raton, FL, 2003.

Index